THE OXFORD HANDBOOK OF

CLINICAL
GEROPSYCHOLOGY

THE OXFORD HANDBOOK OF

CLINICAL GEROPSYCHOLOGY

Edited by

NANCY A. PACHANA

and

KEN LAIDLAW

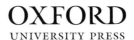

OXFORD
UNIVERSITY PRESS

OXFORD
UNIVERSITY PRESS

Great Clarendon Street, Oxford, OX2 6DP,
United Kingdom

Oxford University Press is a department of the University of Oxford.
It furthers the University's objective of excellence in research, scholarship,
and education by publishing worldwide. Oxford is a registered trade mark of
Oxford University Press in the UK and in certain other countries

Published in the United States of America by Oxford University Press
198 Madison Avenue, New York, NY 10016, United States of America

British Library Cataloguing in Publication Data
Data available

Library of Congress Control Number: 2014943850

ISBN 978–0–19–966317–0

Printed and bound by
CPI Group (UK) Ltd, Croydon, CR0 4YY

FOREWORD

CLINICAL geropsychology has been growing as a field for several decades and a book like this *Oxford Handbook of Clinical Geropsychology* summarizes where the field is at now but also calls attention to its growth from being the preoccupation of a few dedicated psychologists in the 1960s and 1970s to a worldwide and globalized science and profession in the twenty-first century. In fact, one of my first responses to looking at the book was that there are many more authors in this volume than there were geropsychologists early in my career.

There are two broad perspectives in mental health and ageing. One is to see older adults as a special population that needs certain types of specialty services. While true in some ways, this view tends to lead to a focus on older adults with dementia and with physical frailty and reinforces the perception of older adults as 'others'. The other perspective is to emphasize the roots of clinical geropsychology in lifespan developmental psychology. The lifespan perspective puts older adults into developmental perspective, reminds us that we are all ageing, and focuses attention on normative and successful ageing as well as highlighting the needs of those growing old less successfully as being due to causes other than ageing itself. The chapters of this volume pay attention to the lifespan perspective, the importance of longitudinal studies and longitudinal thinking about ageing, and the need to consider trajectories of cognitive change in addition to simple one-time snapshots of cognitive functioning.

The understanding of the developmental psychopathology of late-life has advanced a great deal within clinical geropsychology. This book calls attention to and explains a wide variety of psychopathology in later life including the neurocognitive disorders (formerly known as the dementias), depression, anxiety, substance abuse, psychosis, personality disorder, and insomnia. There is also considerable attention paid to the interconnection of these psychopathologies with physical illnesses and the interconnection of psychological factors and pain. This coverage will please, but likely not surprise, specialists in geropsychology. This level of nuanced understanding is, however, in my experience considerably beyond the general thinking of the nonspecialist physical health, mental health, and social service professionals who often serve older adults. They have moved from thinking of all older adults who act strangely as having dementia, as was the case in the 1980s, to recognizing that depression is also an issue. But for far too many, the understanding of mental health problems in later life stops there. Hopefully, this book and those who read it can continue the work of educating nonspecialist colleagues and the general public about the full range of potential psychological disorders affecting older adults seeking help, and the interactions of those psychological disorders with physical health maladies.

The range of interventions covered here is similarly broad with attention to cognitive-behavioural therapy, interpersonal therapy, acceptance and commitment therapy, cognitive analytic therapy, reminiscence-based approaches, and family therapy. Several of these chapters focus on the use of therapy in helping older adults address some of the specific challenges of later life: (1) physical illness and functional disability including end-of-life issues, (2) grief, and (3) care-giving. The attention to the effects of physical exercise and to healthy life styles as factors in improving mental health and possibly reducing risk of cognitive decline is an important reminder that not all helpful interventions are psychological or psychopharmacological.

The coordination of psychotherapy and medication is covered as are the issues in taking psychological assessment and treatment into particular social contexts such as primary medical care, long-term care, and into the courts with capacity assessments. All work with older adults involves the need to work with other professionals, and so having the knowledge base, attitudes, and skills to work well in interprofessional teams is of critical importance. Geropsychologists also need to be prepared to work with a variety of older adults with a full range of individual diversity, including older gays and lesbians.

The range of nations represented among the contributors is inspiring proof of the extent to which clinical geropsychology has grown and spread around the world. It is especially gratifying to see signs of the spread going beyond the western world of Europe, North America, Australia, and New Zealand and into other nations such as China.

The attention to normative and positive ageing is heartening. This focus is of critical importance for clinical geropsychologists who can lose track of the fact that our patients, clients, and residents are a selected group from the wider population of older people in the world. Focusing on those who are not doing well and are in need of help is the main reason for there being a field of clinical geropsychology, but we cannot allow this focus to lead us to view ageing itself as always having negative consequences and so to reinforce societal ageism in ourselves and others.

Finally, technology perhaps gives us a glimpse into the future of the post-retirement life style and also into the future of psychological intervention. It provides an important reminder to those of us earlier born geropsychologists who are gradually moving into the digital age that the world and the way we communicate and heal are changing. It is likely to come more naturally to later born geropsychologists, and they can be prepared to work effectively with the future cohorts of older adults in need of psychological assessment and treatment.

Bob G. Knight, PhD
Director, Tingstad Older Adult Counseling Center
The Merle H. Bensinger Professor of Gerontology
Professor of Psychology and Medicine
University of Southern California
Los Angeles, CA 90089-0191
USA

Contents

PART III SOURCES OF PSYCHOLOGICAL DISTRESS

PART IV INTERVENTIONS

PART V NEW HORIZONS

LIST OF CONTRIBUTORS

Professor Kristine J. Ajrouch, Survey Research Center, Institute for Social Research, University of Michigan, USA

Professor Kaarin J. Anstey, Centre for Research on Ageing, Health & Wellbeing, The Australian National University, Australia

Professor Toni C. Antonucci, Survey Research Center, Institute for Social Research, University of Michigan, USA

Ms Maria E. A. Armento, Menninger Department of Psychiatry & Behavioral Sciences, Baylor College of Medicine, USA

Associate Professor Deborah K. Attix, Department of Psychiatry and Behavioral Sciences, Duke University, USA

Associate Professor Duncan R. Babbage, Auckland University of Technology, Centre for eHealth and Centre for Person Centred Research, New Zealand

Dr Alex Bahar-Fuchs, Centre for Research on Ageing, Health & Wellbeing, The Australian National University, Australia

Dr MaryBeth Bailar-Heath, Clinical Neuropsychologist, USA

Mr Christopher Barmann, Alliant International University California, School of Professional Psychology, USA

Dr Liora Bar-Tur, Collman College of Management Academic Studies, Rishon LeZion, Israel

Associate Professor Kristen L. Barry, University of Michigan, Department of Psychiatry, USA

Dr John R. Beard, Department of Ageing and Life Course, World Health Organization, Switzerland

Dr Sunil S. Bhar, Faculty of Life and Social Sciences, Swinburne University of Technology, Australia

Professor Frederic C. Blow, University of Michigan, Department of Psychiatry, USA

Assistant Professor Simone Brockman, Department of Psychiatry and Clinical Neurosciences, Fremantle Hospital, University of Western Australia, Australia

Professor Gerard J. Byrne, School of Medicine, The University of Queensland, Australia

Ms Jennifer Ceglowski, Department of Psychiatry, University of California, San Diego, USA

Professor Gordon J. Chelune, Center for Alzheimer's Care, Imaging and Research University of Utah, USA

Dr Kysa M. Christie, Spinal Cord Injury Center, VA Boston Healthcare System, USA

Professor Yeates Conwell, University of Rochester Medical College, USA

Assistant Adjunct Professor Colin Depp, Department of Psychiatry, University of California, San Diego, USA

Ms Elizabeth A. DiNapoli, Department of Psychology, University of Alabama, USA

Ms Laura Vergel de Dios, Department of Psychiatry, University of California, San Diego, USA

Associate Professor Kevin Duff, Center for Alzheimer's Care, Imaging and Research, University of Utah, USA

Professor Barry A. Edelstein, University of West Virginia, USA

Professor Dr Paul M. G. Emmelkamp, Universiteit van Amsterdam, the Netherlands

Professor Rocío Fernández-Ballesteros, Catedrática Emérita Universidad Autónoma de Madrid, España

Professor Dolores Gallagher-Thompson, Department of Psychiatry and Behavioral Sciences, Stanford University School of Medicine, USA

Mr Alistair Gaskell, Older People's Mental Health Services, Cambridgeshire and Peterborough Foundation Trust, UK

Dr Lindsay A. Gerolimatos, West Virginia University, USA

Dr David Gillanders, School of Health in Social Science, University of Edinburgh, UK

Mr Xianmin Gong, Developmental Psychology Institute, Beijing Normal University, Beijing, People's Republic of China

Mr Jeffrey J. Gregg, West Virginia University, USA

Dr Michelle Hamill, Deputy Head of Clinical Psychology for Older Adults, Newham Mental Health Care of Older People, UK

Assistant Professor Dustin B. Hammers, Center for Alzheimer's Care, Imaging and Research, University of Utah, USA

Dr Gregory A. Hinrichsen, Albert Einstein College of Medicine, USA

Associate Professor Kathryn Hyer, Florida Policy Exchange Center on Aging, University of South Florida, USA

Dr Marie-Geneviève Iselin, Zucker Hillside Hospital, USA

Dr M. Lindsey Jacobs, University of Alabama, Center for Mental Health and Aging and Department of Psychology, USA

Professor Ian A. James, Consultant Clinical Psychologist, Newcastle Challenging Behaviour Service, Newcastle General Hospital, UK

Dr. Michele J. Karel, Psychogeriatrics Coordinator, Mental Health Services, Office of Patient Care Services, Veterans Health Administration, Washington DC, USA

Dr Julia E. Kasl-Godley, VA Hospice and Palliative Care Center, VA Palo Alto Health Care System, USA

Dr Eva-Marie Kessler, Heidelberg University, Network Aging Research (NAR) and Institute of Psychology, Germany

Professor Douglas C. Kimmel, City College, City University of New York, USA

Professor Paul Kingston, Staffordshire University, UK

Professor Bob G. Knight, School of Gerontology, University of Southern California, USA

Associate Professor Candace Konnert, Department of Psychology, University of Calgary, Canada

Professor Andreas Kruse, Heidelberg University, Institute of Psychology, Germany

Professor Ken Laidlaw, Department of Clinical Psychology, Norwich Medical School, University of East Anglia, Norwich, UK

Professor Yunhwan Lee, Department of Preventive Medicine and Public Health and Institute on Aging, Ajou University School of Medicine, Republic of Korea

Professor Eric Lenze, Washington University School of Medicine, USA

Professor Kenneth L. Lichstein, Department of Psychology, University of Alabama, USA

Professor Rebecca G. Logsdon, School of Nursing, University of Washington, USA

Professor Andrés Losada Baltar, Universidad Rey Juan Carlos Campus de Alcorcón, Spain

Professor Jeffrey M. Lyness, Professor of Psychiatry and Senior Associate Dean for Academic Affairs, University of Rochester School of Medicine and Dentistry, USA

Professor Susan M. McCurry, School of Nursing, University of Washington, USA

Assistant Professor Ellen L. McGough, Department of Rehabilitation Medicine, University of Washington, USA

Dr Ruth Malkinson, International Centre for the Study of Loss Bereavement and Resilience, Haifa University, Israel

Dr María Oliva Márquez, Universidad Autónoma de Madrid, Spain

Dr María Márquez-González, Universidad Autónoma de Madrid, Spain

Professor Mike Martin, Department of Gerontology and Gerontopsychology and University Research Priority Program (URPP) "Dynamics of Healthy Aging", University of Zurich, Switzerland

Dr Katharina Meyerbröker, Academic Medical Centre, Department of Psychiatry, Universiteit van Amsterdam, the Netherlands

Beyon Miloyan, School of Psychology, The University of Queensland, Australia

Professor Victor Molinari, School of Aging Studies, College of Behavioral and Community Sciences, University of South Florida, USA

Dr Philip E. Mosley, Neuropsychiatry Fellow, Asia-Pacific Centre for Neuromodulation, University of Queensland, UQ Centre for Clinical Research, Australia

Dr Jennifer Moye, Staff Psychologist, VA Boston Healthcare System, USA and Associate Professor, Harvard Medical School, USA

Associate Professor Karen Pallesgaard Munk, Centre for Research on Health and Humanities, Department of Philosophy, University of Aarhus, Denmark

Dr Nageen Mustafa, Staffordshire University, UK

Professor Galit Nimrod, Department of Communication Studies and Center for Multidisciplinary Research in Aging, Ben-Gurion University of the Negev, Israel

Dr Alisa A. O'Riley, University of Rochester Medical College, USA

Professor Nancy A. Pachana, School of Psychology, The University of Queensland, Australia

Professor Constança Paúl, CINTESIS, Institute of Biomedical Sciences Abel Salazar, University of Porto, Portugal

Ms Sojung Park, University of Michigan, USA

Ms Ana Petrovic-Poljak, Department of Psychology, University of Calgary, Canada

Professor Dr Martin Pinquart, Department of Psychology, Philipps University, Marburg, Germany

Professor Sara Honn Qualls, University of Colorado at Colorado Springs, USA

Dr Rosa Romero-Moreno, Department of Psychology, Universidad Rey Juan Carlos, Madrid, Spain

Dr Megan E. Ruiter Petrov, University of Alabama at Birmingham, USA

Dr Phillip D. Ruppert, Postdoctoral Fellow in Neuropsychology, Department of Psychiatry and Behavioral Sciences, Division of Medical Psychology, Duke University Medical Center, USA

Professor Joel Sadavoy, University of Toronto, Canada

Assistant Professor Marta Santacreu, Department of Psychobiology and Health, Universidad Autónoma de Madrid, Spain

Dr Kerry Sargent-Cox, Centre for Research on Ageing, Health & Wellbeing, The Australian National University, Australia

Dr Vera Schumacher, Department of Gerontology and Gerontopsychology, University of Zurich, Switzerland

Professor Forrest R. Scogin, Department of Psychology, University of Alabama, USA

Assistant Professor Colette M. Smart, Department of Psychology, University of Victoria, Canada

Associate Professor A. Lynn Snow, University of Alabama, Center for Mental Health and Aging and Department of Psychology, USA

Associate Professor Silvia Sörensen, University of Rochester Medical Center, School of Medicine and Dentistry, Rochester, New York, USA

Professor Melinda A. Stanley, Menninger Department of Psychiatry & Behavioral Sciences, Baylor College of Medicine, USA

Professor Sergio E. Starkstein, Department of Psychiatry and Clinical Neurosciences, Fremantle Hospital, University of Western Australia, Australia

Associate Professor Ann M. Steffen, Department of Psychology University of Missouri-St. Louis, USA

Dr Nardi Steverink, Department of Sociology, ICS University of Groningen, the Netherlands

Associate Professor Jill A. Stoddard, Alliant International University California, School of Professional Psychology, USA

Professor Linda Teri, Department of Psychosocial and Community Health, Director, Northwest Research Group on Aging, University of Washington, USA

Professor Larry W. Thompson, Department of Psychiatry and Behavioral Sciences, Stanford University School of Medicine, USA

Professor Linda A. Travis, College of Psychology and Behavioral Sciences, Argosy University, USA

Professor Holly A. Tuokko, Department of Psychology, University of Victoria, Canada

Ms Marian Tzuang, Stanford Geriatric Education Centre, Stanford University School of Medicine, USA

Dr Kimberly Van Orden, University of Rochester Medical College, USA

Dr Gregory S. Vander Wal, The University of Alabama, USA

Ms Elizabeth Vongxaiburana, School of Aging Studies, University of South Florida, USA

Professor Dr Hans-Werner Wahl, Heidelberg University, Institute of Psychology, Germany

Dr Dahua Wang, Developmental Psychology Institute, Beijing Normal University, Beijing, People's Republic of China

Dr Julie L. Wetherell, VA San Diego Healthcare System and University of California, San Diego, Department of Psychiatry, USA

Antonette M. Zeiss, Department of Veterans Affairs, USA

Dr Jacqueline Zöllig, Department of Gerontology and Gerontopsychology and International Normal Aging and Plasticity Imaging Center, University of Zurich, Switzerland

PART I

CLINICAL GEROPSYCHOLOGY: AN INTRODUCTION

CHAPTER 1

....

CLINICAL GEROPSYCHOLOGY

A Lifespan Perspective

....

EVA-MARIE KESSLER, ANDREAS KRUSE,
AND HANS-WERNER WAHL

Introduction

....

CLINICAL geropsychology is a subdiscipline in psychology that covers a broad spectrum of topics at the intersection of clinical psychology, lifespan developmental psychology, and neuropsychology. In this chapter, it is our aim to describe and discuss key concepts, issues, and challenges of clinical geropsychology. Within the broader field of the psychology of ageing, clinical geropsychology has a major focus on pathological ageing, as indicated by mental health problems, dysfunction, and disorder in old age. At the same time, clinical geropsychology considers older individuals' resources, plasticity, and potential for normal and successful ageing. In this chapter, we argue that it is important to integrate these two perspectives in order to understand and to deal with the enormous complexity of mental health/mental illness in old age. Specifically, our approach to maladaptive behaviour and psychopathology in old age is guided by a lifespan perspective.

The chapter is organized as follows: (1) We start with a definition and conceptualization of mental health/mental illness in old age as emerging from lifespan developmental theory and research; (2) thereafter, we offer four central propositions that guide clinical geropsychology in both research and practice; (3) we then propose a taxonomy of clinical phenomena that combine to create the subject matter of clinical geropsychology; (4) after this, we describe three types of intervention strategy currently offered by clinical geropsychology; (5) we then briefly discuss how negative subjective representations of ageing and structural age barriers have restrained members of the current cohort of older people from sufficiently profiting from intervention; and (6) we close with practical implications and a summary.

Mental Health in Old Age: A Lifespan Perspective

Paradigms of lifespan theory

According to lifespan developmental psychology (Baltes, Lindenberger, and Staudinger 2006; Lerner 1984; Settersten 2003), individual development is a lifelong and dynamic process driven by biological (e.g. basic cognitive capacity, physical health), psychological (e.g. coping strategies, knowledge, self-efficacy), and sociocultural (e.g. healthcare provisions, social relations, financial resources, social status) factors. Additional tenets of lifespan developmental psychology include the concepts of multidimensionality and multidirectionality. Multidimensionality means that human development always covers a range of psychological domains, which may follow different developmental paths (e.g. cognitive, social, and emotional development). Multidirectionality implies that development is a dynamic and simultaneous balancing of gains (resources) and losses (deficits). In addition, a lifespan view assumes that all life periods are characterized by unique developmental experiences that can only be fully understood when the inter-relations with previous life periods are taken into consideration. This implies that each life period possesses specific characteristics needed for and significantly contributing to a complete life cycle (Erikson 1980). Another fundamental premise is that people are, to a large extent, agents of their own development (Brandtstädter 2007; Lerner and Busch-Rossnagel 1981). Taken together, human development is the result of a complex product of factors incorporating biology, culture, and, last but not least, the actions and reactions of the developing individual her—or himself while negotiating developmental challenges over the lifespan.

In such a view, ageing is an integral part of development that comes with growth and decline, as does every other life period. At the same time, some defining characteristics of the final phase of life deserve reflection. First, biological resources and capacities show a strong normative decline over the adult lifespan—and certainly after adulthood. Increasing levels of multimorbidity, sensory impairment, and functional limitations lead to a growing gap between biological potential and individual-cultural goals. Theories of normal and successful ageing assume that people continuously adapt to such changing biological requirements by allocating their resources primarily to maintenance and recovery, rather than to growth (as in childhood and early adulthood) (Staudinger, Marsiske, and Baltes 1995). Second, old age is characterized as a life period where one is challenged to finally complete the life cycle in a meaningful manner and to unfold its potential in the nearness of death (Erikson 1980). Third, the life period of old age has, by definition, the most cumulative 'learning history', which in the domain of personality development may come with normative advantages (gains in personality adjustment, e.g. a large repertoire of coping styles and compensatory strategies) and disadvantages (e.g. flattening of the personality-growth trajectory, e.g. stable or even declining levels of openness to experience and self-insight) (see Staudinger and Kessler 2009, for further reading).

Defining Mental Health in Old Age

It is in light of such reasoning that we conceptualize mental health in old age as a result of the multiplicative transaction among biological, psychological, and sociocultural factors across the whole lifespan (Fiske, Wetherell, and Gatz 2009; Gatz, Kasl-Godley, and Karel 1996; Whitbourne and Meeks 2011). In other words, mental health is not the result of chronological age, per se (cf. Busse and Maddox 1985). According to prominent definitions of mental health, such as the World Health Organization (WHO) definition, mental health is usually defined as a state, without explicitly including development and ageing. From a lifespan perspective, we define an older individual's mental health as a *unique configuration* of risk factors and protective factors having accumulated over the whole life course that is potentially reflected in various degrees of adaptive behaviour. Consequently, a lifespan perspective situates risk and protective factors of mental health *developmentally* (Fiske et al. 2009; Whitbourne and Meeks 2011).

A lifespan approach also proposes that people across the whole lifespan actively and purposefully select and create developmental contexts. Specifically, individuals define, prioritize, adjust, and possibly give up developmental aims and respective goal criteria, thereby contributing to their own mental health. This proposition of an 'intentional' character of mental health certainly has to be seen in conjunction with the increasingly unfinished biological and cultural architecture of human ontogenesis (Baltes, Lindenberger, and Staudinger 2006). With age, plasticity—as indexed by an individual's change potential— decreases; furthermore, the genetic material, associated genetic mechanisms, and genetic expressions, become less effective. In other words, mental health is increasingly challenged by the 'age-unfriendliness' of the biological system. Furthermore, old age and particularly advanced old age are the culturally least defined life periods, as compared to all other periods. There is a significant lag between the current potential of old age and the existing societal opportunity structures serving to unfold such potential (Riley, Kahn, and Foner 1994). As a consequence, many decisions of individuals operate in kind of a 'cultural vacuum'. Therefore, contexts such as social networks, the healthcare system, new media technology, and living environments are crucial elements of mental health in old age. In other words, *mental health dysfunction* in old age is a characteristic attributed to a specific *constellation* of biological, psychological, and sociocultural factors that operate as primarily stressful, rather than as protective. This approach reflects a contextual (rather than a trait-oriented) understanding of resilience in old age, as defined in lifespan developmental psychology (Staudinger et al. 1995). Accordingly, resilience conveys the idea that individuals can regain normal levels of functioning after developmental setbacks, as well as the idea that they can avoid negative outcomes, despite the presence of significant risk factors of the environment—both without *and* with the help of external interventions.

Mental Illness in Old Age

Given the lack of sociocultural resources, biological losses, nearness to death, and potential accumulation of disadvantages (see above), avoiding mental health distress and achieving well-being is a challenge for ageing individuals. Mental illness occurs if the individual's bio-logical, psychological, and sociocultural deficits outweigh that individual's resources, result-ing in clinically significant problems that interfere with daily functioning and quality of life in old age. Mental health problems normally go along with subjective complaints, as well as behaviour that deviates from social norms (Zarit 2009). We refer to *mental health disorders* as a pattern of symptoms meeting established criteria for psychiatric diagnoses, as provided by the *Diagnostic and Statistical Manual of Mental Disorders* (*DSM-IV-TR; DSM-5*) and the *International Classification of Diseases* (*ICD-10*).

POSITIVE MENTAL HEALTH IN OLD AGE

In clinical psychology, *positive mental health* is conceptualized to be more than just the absence of mental disorders. Positive mental health in old age results from individu-als' biological, psychological, and sociocultural resources outweighing respective deficits. Within a lifespan framework, this is usually the case when individuals' primary allocation of resources is successfully directed to maintenance and recovery in old age, and even to further well-being and growth (Staudinger et al. 1995). One central facet of positive men-tal health is subjective well-being (SWB), as indicated by life satisfaction and high lev-els of positive and low levels of negative affect (e.g. Diener and Suh 1997). Going beyond hedonic well-being, autonomy, environmental mastery, personal growth, positive rela-tions with others, purpose in life, and self-acceptance are regarded as central dimensions of positive mental health in adulthood and old age, according to Ryff's (1989) prominent and lifespan-oriented framework of *psychological well-being*.

Historically, much of the research in positive mental health in adulthood originated from now classic psychosocial models of human development, drawing from humanistic and psychodynamic research traditions. According to these models, development is regu-larly conceptualized as a lifelong task, reaching its endpoint only in advanced age; positive mental health is achieved as the end of an ideal trajectory. Erikson (1980) described lifelong personality development as a series of eight characteristic, age-related, psychosocial crises. Successful solution of psychosocial crises in late adulthood is regarded as a prerequisite of positive mental health and requires an integration of two conflicting forces: ego integrity vs despair. Achievement of ego integrity is perceived as the final aim of lifelong development, including the ability to perceive continuity and meaning in life, to accept one's own life as lived, including finitude, definitiveness, failure, and omissions.

Following Tornstam's theory of gero-transcendence (Tornstam 1989, 1996), the endpoint of personality development implies giving up a materialistic, rational perspective in favour of a more cosmic and transcendent perspective. In this view, development in very old age is ideally characterized by changes on three levels. On a cosmic level, people achieve a closer integration of past, present, and future; intense feelings of connectedness to following gen-erations; decreased fear of death; enhanced receptiveness to the allegedly meaningless; and a general acceptance of the mystic dimension of life. On the level of the self, people discover new aspects of their identity and have a higher ability to integrate success and failure experi-ences. On the level of social relationships, changes particularly include increases in selectiv-ity, i.e. focusing more on emotionally meaningful relationships, deeper understanding of the difference between self and role, increased consciousness of relativity of material values, and more profound judgments.

According to the analytical psychology approach of Jung (1976), individuation is a life-long psychological task. In younger ages, establishing a distinct identity implies accentuating individual attributes against the collective. In later life, people become increasingly aware of unconscious and conscious feelings, rejoin collective experiences, and reunite with humankind. At this time, personality is less defined by the conscious 'I', but more and more by a whole 'self', including unconscious, repressed, suppressed, and disowned thoughts and feelings. Within this framework, positive mental health in old age is conceptualized as self-realization that requires integration of the shadow, i.e. not yet fully developed personal attributes, orientations, and abilities beyond societal norms and demands (i.e. the persona).

Overall, models of psychosocial development have extensively described indicators of positive mental health—including ways of achieving and failing—thereby complementing the complex picture of mental health in old age beyond mental health dysfunction.

ADDITIONAL CORE PROPOSITIONS OF CLINICAL GEROPSYCHOLOGY

Ageing research over the last years has refuted one-sided deficit-oriented models of ageing. Pervasive theoretical and empirical arguments for *heterogeneity, aetiological complexity, plasticity*, and *historical embeddedness* of mental health in old age have been provided.

Heterogeneity

A frequently met, stereotypical conception is that ageing is accompanied by senility, depression, tiredness in life, and negative feelings. Clinical geropsychology challenges this assumption by pointing to the enormous heterogeneity of mental health and well-being in old age. In old age, heterogeneity is reflected in the co-existence of both highly vulnerable/mentally ill and highly resilient/healthy older individuals. For example, people over the age of 60 have the highest rates of suicide in almost two-thirds of countries worldwide (WHO 2007). Men over the age of 75 are the group most at risk, being twice as likely to commit suicide as men aged 25 to 34. Moreover, among 90- to 100-year-olds, dementia has a prevalence of about 50% (Helmchen et al. 1999). At the same time, epidemiological research has consistently shown that older people have lower prevalence rates of depression and anxiety that fulfil the criteria of a mental health diagnosis than do young and middle-aged adults (e.g. Blazer, George, and Hughes 1991; Kessler et al. 2003). Furthermore, there is cross-sectional and longitudinal evidence that levels of negative affect do *not* increase in the normal population of older and very old people, while life satisfaction and high-arousal positive affect (e.g. excitement) are stable and show only a small decline in very old age (see Charles and Carstensen 2010; Kessler and Staudinger 2010, for an overview).

Together, these examples illustrate older people's enormous inter-individual variability in mental health resources in old age. Simultaneously, a large proportion of older adults seem to be able to maintain subjective well-being in the face of an increasing amount of losses. Various attempts have been undertaken to understand the underlying mechanisms behind this 'well-being paradox of old age'. It has been suggested that people, as they age, become increasingly better at adjusting to losses and negative events—for example, by selecting environments that meet one's needs, optimizing skills, and compensating for losses by practical means (as addressed in the *Model of Selective Optimization with Compensation*, Baltes and Baltes 1990); disengaging from blocked goals, re-scaling personal expectations to the given, or letting go of self-images that do not fit the actual self any more (as addressed by the *Dual-Process Model of Assimilative and Accommodative Coping*, Brandtstädter and Rothermund 2002); or by avoiding attention to and memory of negative information (as addressed by *Socioemotional Selectivity Theory*, Charles and Carstensen 2010).

Aetiological complexity

According to lay theories of development and ageing, mental health dysfunction in old age is the inevitable result of limitations and losses 'naturally' occurring in old age. Given the multiplicative relationship among biological, psychological, and sociocultural factors, clinical geropsychology conceptualizes mental health and mental health problems as *probable* rather than determined, and, as such, never fully predictable (Gottlieb 1970). Moreover, different aetiological pathways can result in similar clinical syndromes and presentations. As a simplified example, patients may develop depressive symptoms, following an accumulation of various stressful life events that started in childhood (with or without meeting the criteria of a manifest mental health disorder)—or within the context of a physical or neurological illness in old age, together with a lack of social support. This observation corresponds to the paradigm of *equifinality* in lifespan theory (Kruglanski 1996).

For heuristic reasons and in line with central assumptions of developmental psychopathology (Sameroff, Lewis, and Miller 2000), we distinguish three pathways to psychopathology in old age (see Figure 1.1). Frequently, mental health problems start in the first half of life and then persist into old age. In the case of *long-term overt pathways*, mental health problems manifest in clinically relevant disorders during childhood, adolescence, or adulthood (typically labelled as mental health disorder 'with early onset'). In contrast, in the case of *long-term hidden pathways*, individuals perform at the level of normal development during the first half of life, but simultaneously hold significant vulnerabilities that are only manifested in old age under the condition of age normativity (e.g. basic cognitive decline, retirement), idiosyncratic stressors (e.g. death of a child, lethal disease), and/or a lack of sociocultural support. Finally, other individuals may develop a mental health disorder 'with late onset' despite high levels of resources/protective factors and low levels of deficits/risks in the first half of life (*short-term pathway*). These individuals typically fail to maintain and regain adequate levels of mental health in the face of age-related risk factors and losses because of a lack of coping mechanisms, or as a result of pathological ageing of the brain (see below). By distinguishing between these three pathways, our framework qualifies the classical diathesis-stress-model considering a lifespan approach to human development. In line with this reasoning, Gatz and colleagues (1996) have proposed a 'lifespan developmental diathesis-stress model' as a framework for late-life depression.

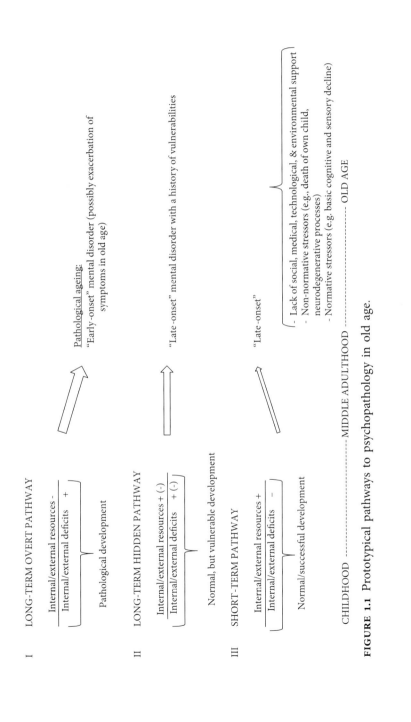

FIGURE 1.1 Prototypical pathways to psychopathology in old age.

In clinical practice, it is a challenging task to uncover the different aetiological pathways behind similar clinical presentations. In the case of depression, for example, clinical ger-opsychological research has identified indicators that help to discern different developmental trajectories and causes. Specifically, depression presents differently among patients with neurological syndromes (Fiske et al. 2009, for an overview). Depression following stroke is less likely to include dysphoria and is more strongly characterized by vegetative symptoms than are other forms of late-life depression. Depression associated with Parkinson's disease (PD) is a milder form of depression and is associated with dysphoria and anhedonia less frequently than is depression in older adults without neurological illness. Depression linked with vascular dementia, compared to depression linked with Alzheimer's disease (AD), is characterized by more vegetative symptoms, such as fatigue, muscular weakness, and weight loss.

The greater spectrum of aetiological pathways leading to mental illnesses also seems to be the central reason behind many clinicians' observation that there are differences in presentation between older and younger adults suffering from depression. Indeed, older adults are often reported to be less likely to report cognitive-affective symptoms of depression, including dysphoria and worthlessness/guilt, than are younger adults (Gallo, Anthony, and Muthén 1994). Subjective complaints of poor memory and concentration are also common among depressed older adults. Slower cognitive processing speed and decreases in executive function are frequent findings from objective testing (Butters et al. 2004). Indeed, physical factors, functional impairment, disease chronicity, and most probably cohort membership and ageing self-stereotypes (see below), lead to differences in clinical presentations. In each case, we should be critical about statements that older people would 'express depression in a different manner', especially by expressing somatic symptoms. From a lifespan psychological perspective, it seems to be more appropriate to argue that there is a greater *uniqueness* of symptom presentation in older people with depression and other mental disorders, with some symptom clusters being highly age-related. This is the case in the 'depression executive dysfunction syndrome of late life' (formerly 'vascular depression'), which encompasses dysfunction that may not be exclusively caused by vascular disease (Alexopoulos et al. 2005). In our view, the well-documented finding that sub-syndromal depression symptoms increase in old age also has to be interpreted against the background of increasing heterogeneity and aetiological complexity (including somatic and contextual pathways to depression) rather than as an indicator of less severe forms of depression. Interestingly, the positive age trends in subsyndromal forms of depression have been shown to be based on loss of interest, poor ability to concentrate, and anhedonia rather than on negative affective states (i.e. tearfulness, a wish to die, negative emotions) (Prince et al. 1999). In line with this interpretation, it has been shown that one characteristic of subthreshold depression is comorbidity with somatic illness and physical disability, and that a substantial group of older people with subthreshold depression require treatment (Geiselmann, Linden, and Helmchen 2001).

Plasticity and resilience

It is commonly assumed that as people age, they become increasingly rigid and less able to learn. Ageing research has challenged this common assumption and its resulting therapeutic nihilism. While brain plasticity decreases with age, there is growing substantial evidence that old age is still indexed by a large (yet limited) amount of biological, cognitive, motivational, and emotional plasticity and reserve capacity—even in older people with mental disorders. Three examples should illustrate older individuals' potential for change and growth, even under the condition of mental distress. As a first example, in a recent meta-analysis of fifty-seven controlled intervention studies, Pinquart, Duberstein, and Lyness (2007) assessed the effects of psychotherapy and other behavioural interventions on depressive symptoms in clinically depressed older patients. On average, self-rated depression improved by d = 0.84 standard deviation units. Effect sizes were medium for psychodynamic therapy, psychoeducation, physical exercise, and supportive interventions. Effect sizes were large for cognitive-behavioural therapy (CBT) and reminiscence, demonstrating that these forms of intervention are the most effective forms of depression treatment.

Our second example illustrates that psychological interventions can lead to positive changes, even in the case of beginning organic mental disorders. In a series of experimental studies, Belleville et al. (2011) investigated the efficacy of training that is focused on teaching episodic-memory strategies in samples of persons with mild cognitive impairment (MCI). Specifically, participants were trained using interactive imagery, the method of loci, face-name associations, hierarchical organization, and semantic organization techniques (six weekly sessions, approximately 120 minutes each). Compared to normal older participants who did not receive the intervention, the brains of those patients with MCI who received the episodic-memory training remained able to recruit new neural circuits to perform the demanding memory tasks. In line with earlier research, positive effects of the training were also found in measures of subjective memory and well-being.

Plasticity also refers to possibilities of *prevention* in old age. Our third example illustrates that plasticity exists—to a limited degree—even in the early onset of neurodegenerative disorders. Recent findings have shown that stimulating activities, either mentally or socially oriented, may protect against dementia. For example, Wang and colleagues (2002) used data from the 1987–1996 Kungsholmen Project—a longitudinal population-based study carried out in Sweden—to examine whether engagement in different activities in the preceding 6.4 years leading up to dementia diagnosis was related to a decreased incidence of dementia. After adjustment for major control variables, frequent engagement in mental and social activities was inversely related to dementia incidence. This result also illustrates that resilience is not only a 'naturally-occurring' phenomenon, but that resilience can be supported and enhanced by individual life styles, as well as by 'age-friendly' social environments.

Cohort flow and historical embeddedness

Lifespan developmental psychology not only points to pronounced inter-individual differences within age groups, but also to the role of historical embeddedness of ageing processes and resulting differences between birth cohorts. Findings from the *Seattle Longitudinal Study* show that large proportions of cross-sectional age differences in mental abilities do not—as traditionally hypothesized—reflect age-correlated declines and deficits, but rather, cohort-specific levels, resulting from differences in education, health, and lifelong opportunities for development (Schaie 1996, 2005). In addition, living conditions and functional status, particularly in the 'third age', have continuously improved over recent decades. Due to modern cultural and societal efforts—not least, advances in medicine and industrial technology—biological-physiological losses of individual development are largely compensated for in this period of life (Baltes 1999). Because of, on average, better health, higher education, increased familiarity with education and learning contexts, and more financial resources, future cohorts of older people can be expected to be able to lead an independent and self-responsible life, maintain reciprocity in social relationships, and take responsibility for development of other people (as well as of society) for longer.

Seemingly paradoxically, there is also substantial evidence that more recent cohorts have higher risks of developing depression as compared to previous cohorts. For example, in their analysis of data from the National Comorbidity Survey Replication (NCS-R), based on a representative sample of 9282 participants, Kessler et al. (2005) estimated the lifetime risk for *DSM-IV* disorders at age 75 from age-of-onset reports in four successive cohorts (1970 or later, 1955–1969, 1940–1954, and earlier than 1940). Significant inter-cohort differences were found for most diagnoses, with more recent cohorts having consistently higher odds ratios of onset. Similar trends were reported in other studies, with samples from the US (Yang 2007) and China (Lee et al. 2007). Possible explanations include that because of an expansion of health definitions, more recent cohorts may be more likely to perceive and report health-related problems (Clarke et al. 2003). Additional interpretations may refer to altered lifetime experiences of the more recent cohorts. For example, war and poverty experience may have strengthened the resilience resources of earlier cohorts, while increased stress related to work may have increased the vulnerability of mental health development in later life in more recent cohorts.

In conclusion, the aforementioned studies on (partially conflicting) cohort trends illustrate the complex interplay between structural changes and individual lives. As a consequence, clinical geropsychology must be sensitive not only to possible age effects and cohort effects, but also to cohort-specific ageing processes and age-specific cohort differences.

A Taxonomy of Clinical Phenomena Addressed by Clinical Geropsychology

In the following, we propose a taxonomy of clinical phenomena that are addressed by clinical geropsychology. Accordingly, three phenomena combine to create a unique characterization of the subject matter of clinical geropsychology: (1) dysfunctional psychological reactions to normal ageing (as well as to life events occurring in high frequency in old age)—as exemplified in an older patient with complicated grief disorder after the death of his/her spouse; (2) mental health problems in the course of pathological ageing of the brain—as exemplified in an older patient with PD; and (3) mental health problems as a result of pathological developmental processes that started earlier in life and persisted into old age—as exemplified in an older patient with a long history of recurrent depressive episodes and comorbid dependent personality disorder.

Dysfunctional psychological reactions to normal ageing

As described above, the relatively high level of mental health and well-being in old age is well documented in a large body of empirical research. However, acute and chronic exposure to normative age-related losses or common events in old age can massively interfere with daily functioning and well-being. The loss of a romantic partner, retirement, or chronic illness are three examples of events that are considered to be common stressors that increase distress for older adults and set limits to resilience in a significant proportion of older people. Older adults who are widowed are at high risk of developing depression and/or anxiety disorders, according to a systematic review (Onrust and Cuijpers 2006). The percentage of people who reported symptoms meeting the criteria for major depressive disorder (MDD) a year following the death of the spouse was estimated at 16%, compared to the 4–8% observed in same-aged, non-bereaving samples (Clayton and Darvish 1979; Zisook and Shuchter 1991). In the case of retirement, men who retire early may experience an elevated risk of depression, even though retirement is not associated with depression in the older population in general (Butterworth et al. 2006). Furthermore, chronic illness predicts changes in depressive symptoms in late life, with functional impairment probably accounting for most of the association between chronic illness and depression. Notably, dysfunctional reactions to ageing-related losses often do not fulfil the criteria of any particular non-organic mental disorder (such as depression, anxiety, or post-traumatic stress disorder). These reactions can be rather subsyndromal (see above) or show a specific pattern of symptoms, as in the case of the 'post-fall anxiety syndrome' or the syndrome of complicated grief disorder.

Mental health problems in the course of pathological ageing of the brain

A second focus of clinical geropsychology is pathological processes in the ageing brain that are—directly or indirectly—associated with mental health problems. Even though these pathological processes are not part of normal ageing, they are highly correlated with chronological age—and in that sense, typical 'late-life diseases'. The most prominent example of late-life disease is AD, which is characterized by loss of neurons and synapses in the cerebral cortex and certain subcortical regions. Typical psychological symptoms of AD are short-term and long-term memory loss, confusion, irritability and aggression, mood swings, and problems with language. This disease typically does not become manifest until age 70, with the exception of the 5–10% of people suffering from 'early-onset' AD (i.e. diagnosed before the age of 65). After age 70, however, incidence increases markedly (Helmchen et al. 1999).

Furthermore, clinical geropsychology addresses the psychological correlates and consequences of other age-related neurodegenerative conditions, such as PD, as well as those of cerebrovascular events, such as stroke (going along with a broad range of cognitive, affective, motivational, and behavioural dysfunctions) (Cockburn 2008; Hobson 2008). Within the ICD-10, these mental health problems are classified as 'organic mental disorders'. They account for the largest proportion of mental disorders in old age (i.e. if insomnia is not considered a primary disease, but rather a comorbid condition to depression and anxiety).

For example, in the Berlin Aging Study, a representative German sample of people aged 70 to more than 100 years, the prevalence of dementia, depression, and anxiety were 17%, 9%, and 5%, respectively (insomnia: 19%) (Helmchen et al. 1999).

Chronic pathological processes persisting from earlier life periods

Clinical geropsychology is not only concerned with the psychological problems associated with normal and pathological ageing. Rather, clinical geropsychology is also focused on mental health dysfunction starting in the first half of life and persisting or recurring in old age ('long-term hidden pathway to psychopathology', see above). It is routine for clinicians to see older patients for whom mental health problems have been a long-standing or recurrent matter across their life courses. Within the *ICD-10* and *DSM-5*, these mental health disorders are characterized as chronic or recurrent mental health disorders.

Indeed, distinguishing between individuals who first experienced mental illness earlier in life and those whose first encounter with mental illness occurs in old age is an important heuristic in clinical practice and is supported by empirical research. This is well illustrated in the example of depression in old age. There is consensus that the distinction between 'late-onset' depression (arising in adults 60–70 years and older) and 'early-onset' depression portends differences in aetiology and prognosis. Those with early-onset depression are more likely than those with late-onset depression to have a family history of depression (e.g. Heun et al. 2001), and are also more likely to have a higher prevalence of personality disorder or elevated scores on neuroticism (e.g. Brodaty et al. 2001). Those with late-onset manifestation of depression often show a history of cerebrovascular disease. Typically, these patients show psychomotor retardation, anhedonia, and concomitant executive-functioning deficits (Fiske et al. 2009). Neurological findings, including white-matter hyperintensities or leukoencephalopathy, are reported as common among late-onset but not among patients with early-onset depression (Krishnan 2002).

LIMITATIONS OF THE OFFERED TAXONOMY

Although we see heuristic value in using the taxonomy described above, it is also important to highlight its limitations. We do this not as an academic exercise, but rather in order to further elaborate on the complexity of mental health in old age. As a first limitation, pathological and normal ageing processes cannot always be classified as distinct processes. For example, recent studies suggest that AD is a continuum, starting with subjective cognitive impairment (SCI; no supporting objective evidence from neuropsychological testing or evidence of functional decline), moving to MCI, and culminating in full-blown dementia. It is still unclear whether cognitive deficits observed in people with AD and other forms of dementia are exaggerated or accelerated versions of normal ageing on this continuum. According to a recent study (Walters 2010), differences in neuropsychological test performance between adults diagnosed with dementia of the Alzheimer's type and comparably aged nondemented adults are quantitative, rather than qualitative. Postmortem studies have found only quantitative differences in neurofibrillary tangles and amyloid plaques in the brains of people previously diagnosed with AD and those without dementia (Caselli et al. 2006). As another example, it is sometimes difficult in clinical practice to distinguish between normal grief, pathological grief, and depression, after the death of a spouse (e.g. Whitbourne and Meeks 2011), even on the basis of the clearly defined criteria of bereavement-related disorder (see above). For example, 'conversations' with the deceased on a weekly basis can either be a sign of common grief or of psychopathology.

As a second limitation of our taxonomy, late-onset mental health problems often cannot clearly be separated from vulnerabilities and dysfunctional dispositions in the first half of life. In line with the assumption of lifespan diathesis-stress models of depression (Fiske et al. 2009), a recent study showed that certain types of childhood trauma continue to constitute risk factors for depression in old age, possibly moderated by alterations in the serotonin gene-linked promoter region (5-HTTLPR) (Ritchie et al. 2009). Notably, childhood trauma outweighed more proximal causes, such as widowhood, recent life events, or vascular and neurologic disorder. As another example, brain chemistry changes in patients with inherited forms of AD can be detected up to twenty years before the expected age of symptomatic onset (Bateman et al. 2011), pointing to longstanding biological dispositions over the lifespan.

Finally, psychological dysfunction as a direct effect of pathological ageing of the brain cannot be clearly distinguished from its indirect psychological effects, such as changes in social networks, financial resources, living environment, etc. For example, depression symptoms in the course of PD are regarded as an interaction between several vulnerabilities, including genetic factors, cognitive diathesis, age-associated neurobiological changes, and stressful events in late life (Fiske et al. 2009). For pragmatic reasons and in order to avoid under-diagnosing depression in PD, an inclusive diagnostic approach has been recommended in which all symptoms are 'counted' toward a diagnosis of major depression, even if they overlap with PD symptoms (Marsh et al. 2006).

INTERVENTION STRATEGIES IN CLINICAL GEROPSYCHOLOGY

A taxonomy of intervention strategies

Clinical geropsychology currently utilizes a wide variety of strategies, frequently implemented in cooperation with other disciplines, such as geriatric medicine, rehabilitation science, the health sciences, and occupational therapy. Intervention strategies offered by clinical geropsychology serve different functions, the most important of which are: (1) enrichment of normal late-life development to facilitate optimal ageing; (2) therapy and rehabilitation after the occurrence of mental health problems; and (3) prevention in order to counteract possible and avoidable loss and support positive development in the longer run of late-life development. An important distinction exists between *genuine* psychological interventions—i.e. interventions that are strictly based on psychological theory and principles at the treatment scheme and outcome level (e.g. psychotherapy based on cognitive-behavioural principles may reduce negative affect)—and interventions with major impact on psychological outcomes, which are not based on solely psychological theories and principles (e.g. a physical activity training programme may improve cognitive functioning and well-being). There are also genuine psychological interventions, which show positive impact on non-psychological outcomes (e.g. a psychological intervention aimed to enhance self-efficacy may change health-related behaviour or the course and outcome of a somatic disease).

One can distinguish between psychosocial intervention strategies, training-oriented intervention and person-environment-related interventions. In the following, we address some of the most prominent and widely used examples for these three types of intervention strategies. Note that these examples differ in the degree to which they have been supported by empirical evidence so far.

First, clinical geropsychology most typically uses a full set of *psychosocial intervention strategies*. The classic treatment under this label is the full bandwidth of psychotherapeutic approaches with the two dominant models of CBT (Laidlaw et al. 2003) and psychodynamic therapy (Davenhill 2008). In addition, classic approaches, such as interpersonal therapy (Markowitz and Weissmann 2004), and couples therapy (Snyder, Castellani, and Whisman 2006) have also gained in importance, the latter not the least in the area of dealing with a family member with dementia. In some places, recent developments in mindfulness-based psychotherapeutic approaches were conducted with older people (Smith, Graham, and Senthinathan 2007). The psychosocial interventions mentioned above were not primarily developed to match specific problems of older people, but they were sometimes more or less adapted and modified for old age. At the same time, there are psychosocial interventions that have been developed with the aim to psychosocially support older adults in crisis situations such as widowhood, relocation to a long-term–care institution, or after the diagnosis of dementia (Kurz et al. 2012). These interventions were sometimes used as a prevention strategy (Steverink, Lindenberg, and Slaets 2005). In addition, intervention approaches with the aim of initiating successful coping with chronic diseases that typically occur in old age—such as diabetes, stroke, or sensory impairment—have gained prominence in the recent two decades (e.g. Mohlman 2009). Such approaches, operating under the heading of disease management or self-management programmes, are frequently implemented in a group format under the supervision of a clinical psychologist (Jonker et al. 2009; Wahl et al. 2006). In our view, there is only one treatment approach that was specifically developed for old age: life review therapy/reminiscence therapy (e.g. Pinquart and Forstmeier 2012; Serrano et al. 2004). During reminiscence therapy, the older patient reconstructs his/her biography by examining both positive and negative experiences. The overall purpose is to provide perspective and acceptance of one's life, get control of positive life experiences, and to solve conflicting themes in the past. Unfortunately, we have to realize that there are a lack of gero-psychological interventions that both allow existential experience and help older adults to successfully cope with death, dying, and finitude.

A second type of intervention strategy that is typically used by clinical geropsychology is *training-oriented interventions*. Behaviour modification programmes have been applied to change a wide range of behaviours of older adults such as to increase independent self-care or social behaviour in nursing homes residents (Baltes, Neumann, and Zank 1994) or to reduce noncognitive symptoms, such as aggressive behaviours, in those with dementia (Burgio 1996). Cognitive interventions rely on extensive exercise in cognitive operations such as inductive reasoning or episodic memory. Their aim is to enhance everyday cognitive functioning as well as everyday competence (Willis et al. 2006). Such training is also applied in older adults with major impairment (Sitzer, Twamley, and Jeste 2006). Notably, the existing cognitive training interventions have been shown to promote specific cognitive skills (typically mnemonic strategies) rather than fluid intelligence per se. By contrast, physical activity interventions using aerobic exercise and muscle strength training—being rooted in the health and exercise sciences—proved to have positive effects on the cognitive (particularly executive control), social, and well-being domain; this demonstrated strong health and preventive effect on the cardiovascular system at large, as well as the reduction of falls (Netz et al. 2005). There is also evidence that such programmes come with improvement at the brain level, including brain tissue and synaptic density (Kramer, Erickson, and Colcombe 2006). Finally, contributions by clinical geropsychologists to neuro-rehabilitation programmes for older people primarily include the provision of cognitive remediation programmes, e.g. cognitive linguistic therapies with language deficits after left-hemisphere stroke, interventions for functional communication deficits with traumatic brain injury, goal-management training, training in formal problem-solving, and self-monitoring strategies for persons with deficits in executive functioning (see Crossley 2008, for an overview).

As a third type of intervention strategy, a range of *person-environment—related interventions* have been found to be of importance for the older client. This category encompasses interventions targeting the social as well as the physical, spatial, and technological environment (Wahl, Iwarsson, and Oswald 2012). The fundamental assumption behind this approach is that older adults, particularly those with physical and mental health problems, are highly sensible for contextual factors, when it comes to developmental outcomes such as autonomy or well-being (Wahl and Gitlin 2007). A key intervention at the social environment level aims to reduce burden in family care-givers, particularly those serving older adults with dementia-related disorders (Sörensen, Pinquart, and Duberstein 2002). Additionally, programmes have been developed to improve the professional expertise of care-givers in institutional settings and home healthcare, based on psychological principles such as social learning theory. As has been shown, respective interventions also come with positive effects, such as increased independent self-care behaviours in older adults involved in care interactions (Baltes et al. 1994). At the level of the physical-spatial environment, substantial linkages between environmental barriers and hazards in the home and disability-related outcomes have been confirmed (Wahl et al. 2009). Interventions targeting the physical-spatial environment may serve to support the effect and sustainability of psychotherapeutic interventions by improving the natural settings, in which older adults exert their day-to-day life. This also applies to the increasing role of new technology in the areas of smart mobility, robotics, and information and communication technology (Rogers and Fisk 2010; Wahl et al. 2012). For example, the internet has become a major medium for health education and diverse training purposes including psychosocial consultation and the science of robotics, innovations that will possibly shape care in old age dramatically in the not-too-distant future (e.g. by providing assistance with daily tasks, or with behavioural shaping via machine-based voice control).

BARRIERS TO TREATMENT OF OLDER ADULTS: THE ROLE OF AGE ATTITUDES AND AGE STEREOTYPES

Studies of attitudes toward older people among health professionals in the US, UK, and Germany found that they are more positive and more complex than had been assumed (Knight et al. 2006). Despite these encouraging findings, it seems fair to argue that across age and professional groups, stereotypical thinking still infiltrates the area of mental health in old age, both at the level of individuals and healthcare organizations and institutions. Experimental work has shown that the patient's age has a major influence on treatment decisions by physicians and nurses. In one vignette study (Barnow et al. 2004), the question of whether patients who expressed the wish to die should receive treatment was answered with 'yes' by both physicians and nurses significantly less frequently when the real age of the old patient was known; whereas when a lower patient age (–20 years) was given, they more often saw the need for psychotherapy or other medical interventions. At the structural level, the still suboptimal provision of health services for older people as well a widespread lack of specific training opportunities for psychotherapists are only two examples that may in part reflect that negative stereotypical thinking about mental health in old age still exists.

One reason for the inconsistent pattern of results reported above may be that explicit beliefs and attitudes towards older people tend to operate independently of implicit beliefs (Levy 2003). Although age attitudes tend to be negative on both the implicit and explicit levels, they tend to be more negative on the implicit level. Although both positive and negative age stereotypes coexist, negative age stereotypes outnumber positive age stereotypes, have a greater accessibility, and are persistent and rigid (Levy 2009). Clinicians must be aware that these stereotypes operate in many older patients themselves and can go along with their perception that mental health problems are a result of factors that they cannot change. When individuals reach old age, the ageing stereotypes, internalized in childhood, and then reinforced for decades, become self-stereotypes (Levy 2009).

PRACTICAL IMPLICATIONS

As we have argued, a lifespan approach to psychopathology in old age is vital to both diagnostic and treatment considerations. A defining feature of mental dysfunction and disorder in old age is deviance from normative behaviour including its developmental history. This emphasizes the importance of understanding normal ageing as well as cohort flow and cultural contexts when working with older adults with mental disorders.

Furthermore, adequate assessment in geropsychological practice encompasses the use of multiple data sources from a variety of disciplines, including the whole bandwidth of biological, psychological, and social-environmental factors. In order to gain a full appreciation of the driving forces of ageing, clinicians should assess both deficits *and* resources. Most importantly, a thorough assessment of the wide range of risk and protective factors clearly goes beyond a person's present deficits. Furthermore, the understanding of psychopathology that first emerges in later adulthood must consider a different set of influential factors as compared to psychopathology that has either intermittently or chronically been present for much of an individual's adult life. A lifespan-informed approach to mental health in old age also considers the possibility that mental health dysfunction is not the endpoint of an individual's development, but can rather be a precursor for a variety of pathological pathways, as well as releasing a cascade of developmental growth. In the face of heterogeneity and aetiological complexity, neither consensus on intervention aims nor means-end relationships can be taken for granted. Treatment considerations in geropsychological practice should be strictly grounded in individual assessment—not only of symptoms and problems, but also of individual goals and aspirations. Development and implementation of intervention measures must proceed from a comprehensive understanding of individual life-long goals, goal pursuit, and goal adjustment. In addition to individual diagnostic results, clinicians should have state-of-the-art knowledge of the range of life-long plasticity in various mental health disorders, including organic as well as non-organic mental health disorders. This is a key prerequisite to focus the treatment schema on either maintenance of psychological function (or even further growth), or at least on the attenuation and delay of symptom presentation. One central challenge in clinical practice is to combine existing measures from the already large 'tool box' of clinical geropsychology (e.g. combining training programmes from the health and exercise sciences with psychotherapeutic interventions) and to implement them in a wide array of intervention settings (laboratory environments, nursing homes and day care centres, rehabilitation units, the family setting, and the community at large). Last, but not least, clinicians should reflect on their patients' self-perceptions of ageing as well as of their own subjective representations and potential stereotypes of old age.

Summary

In this chapter, we argued that mental health dysfunction is best conceptualized as a complex product of biological, cognitive, emotional, and motivational deficits and resources that have accumulated over the whole life course. Mental health disorders are transient 'endpoints' of the highly multifaceted lifespan trajectories. As a consequence, clinical geropsychology must confront the task of limited generalizability—not only of aetiological hypotheses—but also of intervention methods and aims. This reasoning underscores the idea that no single discipline's efforts to study mental health in old age are likely to be adequate. Rather, the study of mental health in old age, with all its facets, is a fundamentally multidisciplinary enterprise. Its aim is to promote individuals, as they age, in realizing their full psychological potential. The realization of this aim must also include changing social norms and structures so that they allow for minimizing risks and maximizing possibilities for loss management, maintenance, and growth (see Caplan 1964).

Key References and Sources for Further Reading

Baltes, P. B., Lindenberger, U., and Staudinger, U. M. (2006). 'Life-span Theory in Developmental Psychology'. In W. Damon and R. M. Lerner (eds), *Handbook of Child Psychology: Vol. 1. Theoretical Models of Human Development* (6th edn, pp. 569–664). New York: Wiley.

Fiske, A., Wetherell, J. L., and Gatz, M. (2009). 'Depression in Older Adults'. *Annual Review of Clinical Psychology* 5(1): 363–389. doi:10.1146/annurev.clinpsy.032408.153621.

Kessler, E.-M. and Staudinger, U. M. (2010). 'Emotional Resilience and Beyond: A Synthesis of Findings from Lifespan Psychology and Psychopathology'. In P. S. Frey and C. L. Keyes (eds), *New Frontiers of Resilient Aging* (pp. 258–282). Cambridge: Cambridge University Press.

Knight, B. G., Kaskie, B., Shurgot, G. R., and Dave, J. (2006). 'Improving the Mental Health of Older Adults'. In J. E. Birren and K. W. Schaie (eds), *Handbook of Psychology and Aging* (6th edn, pp. 408–425). New York: Academic Press.

Staudinger, U. M. and Kessler, E.-M. (2009). 'Adjustment and Personality Growth: Two Trajectories of Positive Personality Development across Adulthood'. In M. C. Smith and T. J. Reio (eds), *The Handbook on Adult Development and Learning* (pp. 241–268). Mahwah, NJ: Lawrence Erlbaum Associates.

Zarit, S. H. (2009). 'A Good Old Age: Theories of Mental Health and Aging'. In V. Bengtson, M. Silverstein, N. Putney, and D. Gans (eds), *Handbook of Theories of Aging* (pp. 675–692). New York: Springer.

References

Alexopoulos, G. S., Katz, I. R., Bruce, M. L., Heo, M., Have, T. T., Raue, P., et al. (2005). 'Remission in Depressed Geriatric Primary Care Patients: A Report from the PROSPECT Study'. *American Journal of Psychiatry* 162(4): 718–724. doi:10.1176/appi.ajp.162.4.718.

Baltes, P. B. and Baltes, M. M. (1990). 'Psychological Perspectives on Successful Aging: The Model of Selective Optimization with Compensation'. In P. B. Baltes and M. M. Baltes (eds), *Successful Aging: Perspectives from the Behavioral Sciences* (pp. 1–34). Cambridge: Cambridge University Press.

Baltes, M. M., Neumann, E.-M., and Zank, S. (1994). Maintenance and rehabilitation of independence in old age: An intervention program for staff. *Psychology and Aging*, 9: 179–188. doi: 10.1037/0882-7974.9.2.179.

Baltes, P. B. (1999). 'Altern und Alter als unvollendete Architektur der Humanontogenese'. [Aging and age as incomplete architecture of human ontogenesis]. *Zeitschrift für Gerontologie und Geriatrie* 32: 433–448.

Baltes, P. B., Lindenberger, U., and Staudinger, U. M. (2006). 'Life-span Theory in Developmental Psychology'. In W. Damon and R. M. Lerner (eds), *Handbook of Child Psychology: Vol. 1. Theoretical Models of Human Development* (6th edn, pp. 569–664). New York: Wiley.

Barnow, S., Linden, M., Lucht, M., and Freyberger, H.-J. (2004). 'Influence of Age of Patients Who Wish to Die on Treatment Decisions by Physicians and Nurses'. *American Journal of Geriatric Psychiatry* 12(3): 258–264.

Bateman, R., Aisen, P., De Strooper, B., Fox, N., Lemere, C., Ringman, J., et al. (2011). 'Autosomal-dominant Alzheimer's Disease: A Review and Proposal for the Prevention of Alzheimer's Disease'. *Alzheimer's Research and Therapy* 3(1): 1. doi:10.1186/alzrt59.

Belleville, S., Clément, F., Mellah, S., Gilbert, B., Fontaine, F., and Gauthier, S. (2011). 'Training-related Brain Plasticity in Subjects at Risk of Developing Alzheimer's Disease'. *Brain* 134(6): 1623–1634. doi:10.1093/brain/awr037.

Blazer, D. G., George, L. K., and Hughes, D. (1991). 'Generalised Anxiety Disorder'. In L. N. Robins and D. A. Regier (eds), *Psychiatric Disorders in America: The Epidemiological Catchment Area Study* (pp. 180–203). New York: The Free Press.

Brandtstädter, J. and Rothermund, K. (2002). 'The Life-course Dynamics of Goal Pursuit and Goal Adjustment: A Two-process Framework'. *Developmental Review* 22(1): 117–150. doi:http://dx.doi.org/10.1006/drev.2001.0539.

Brandtstädter, J. (2007). 'Causality, Intentionality, and the Causation of Intentions: The Problematic Boundary'. In M. Ash and T. Sturm (eds), *Psychology's Territories: Historical and Contemporary Perspectives from Different Disciplines* (pp. 51–66). Mahwah, NJ: Erlbaum.

Brodaty, H., Luscombe, G., Parker, G., Wilhelm, K., Hickie, I., Austin, M.-P., et al. (2001). 'Early and Late Onset Depression in Old Age: Different Aetiologies, Same Phenomenology'. *Journal of Affective Disorders* 66(2–3): 225–236. doi:http://dx.doi.org/10.1016/S0165-0327(00)00317-7.

Burgio, L. (1996). 'Interventions for the Behavioral Complications of Alzheimer's Disease: Behavioral Approaches'. *International Psychogeriatrics* 8(S1): 45–52. doi:10.1017/S1041610296003079.

Busse, E. W. and Maddox, G. L. (eds) (1985). *The Duke Longitudinal Studies of Normal Aging: 1955–1980: Overview of History, Design, and Findings.* New York: Springer.

Butters, M. A., Whyte, E. M., Nebes, R. D., Begley, A. E., Dew, M. A., Mulsant, B. H., et al. (2004). 'The Nature and Determinants of Neuropsychological Functioning in Late-life Depression'. *Archives of General Psychiatry* 61(6): 587–595. doi:10.1001/archpsyc.61.6.587.

Butterworth, P., Gill, S. C., Rodgers, B., Anstey, K. J., Villamil, E., and Melzer, D. (2006). 'Retirement and mental health: Analysis of the Australian national survey of mental health and well-being'. *Social Science and Medicine* 62(5): 1179–1191. doi:http://dx.doi.org/10.1016/j.socscimed.2005.07.013.

Caplan, G. (1964). '*Principles of Preventive Psychiatry*'. New York: Basic Books.

Caselli, R. J., Beach, T. G., Yaari, R., and Reiman, E. M. (2006). 'Alzheimer's Disease a Century Later'. *The Journal of Clinical Psychiatry* 67: 1784–1800.

Charles, S. T. and Carstensen, L. L. (2010). 'Social and Emotional Aging'. *Annual Review of Psychology* 61: 383–409. doi:10.1146/annurev.psych.093008.100448.

Clarke, A. E., Mamo, L., Fishman, J. R., Shim, J. K., and Fosket, J. R. (2003). 'Biomedicalization: Technoscientific Transformations of Health, Illness, and U.S. Biomedicine'. *American Sociological Review* 68(2): 161–194. doi:10.2307/1519765.

Clayton, P. J. and Darvish, H. S. (1979). 'Course of Depressive Symptoms Following Stress of Bereavement'. In J. E. Barrett, R. M. Rose, and G. L. Klerman (eds), *Stress and Mental Disorder* (pp. 121–136). New York: Raven Press.

Cockburn, J. (2008). 'Stroke'. In R. Woods and L. Clare (eds), *Handbook of the Clinical Psychology of Ageing* (2nd edn, pp. 201–217). Chichester: Wiley. doi: 10.1002/9780470773185.ch13.

Crossley, M. (2008). 'Neuropsychological Rehabilitation in Later Life: Special Considerations, Contributions and Future Directions'. In B. Woods and L. Clare (eds), *Handbook of the Clinical Psychology of Ageing*. Chichester: Wiley. doi: 10.1002/9780470773185.ch30.

Davenhill, R. (2008). 'Psychoanalysis in Old Age'. In R. Woods and L. Clare (eds), *Handbook of the Clinical Psychology of Ageing* (2nd edn, pp. 201–217). Chichester: Wiley. doi: 10.1002/9780470773185.ch13.

Diener, E. and Suh, M. E. (1997). 'Subjective Well-being and Age: An International Analysis'. In K. W. Schaie and M. P. Lawton (eds), *Annual Review of Gerontology and Geriatrics* (vol. 17, pp. 304–324). New York: Springer.

Erikson, E. H. (1980). *Identity and the Life Cycle* (2nd edn). New York: Norton.

Fiske, A., Wetherell, J. L., and Gatz, M. (2009). 'Depression in Older Adults'. *Annual Review of Clinical Psychology* 5(1): 363–389. doi:10.1146/annurev.clinpsy.032408.153621.

Gallo, J. J., Anthony, J. C., and Muthen, B. O. (1994). 'Age Differences in the Symptoms of Depression: A Latent Trait Analysis'. *Journal of Gerontology* 49(6): P251–P264. doi:10.1093/geronj/49.6.P251.

Gatz, M., Kasl-Godley, J. E., and Karel, M. J. (1996). 'Aging and Mental Disorders'. In J. E. Birren and K. W. Schaie (eds), *Handbook of the Psychology of Aging* (4th edn, pp. 367–382). San Diego, CA: Academic Press.

Geiselmann, B., Linden, M., and Helmchen, H. (2001). 'Psychiatrists' Diagnoses of Subthreshold Depression in Old Age: Frequency and Correlates'. *Psychological Medicine* 31(1): 51–63.

Gottlieb, G. (1970). 'Conceptions of Prenatal Behavior'. In L. R. Aronson, E. Tobach, D. S. Lehrman, and J. S. Rosenblatt (eds), *Development and Evolution of Behavior: Essays in Memory of T.C. Schneirla* (pp. 11–137). San Francisco, CA: Freeman.

Helmchen, H., Baltes, M. M., Geiselmann, B., Kanowski, S., Linden, M., Reischies, F. M., et al. (1999). 'Psychiatric Illness in Old Age'. In P. B. Baltes and K. U. Mayer (eds), *The Berlin Aging Study: Aging from 70 to 100* (pp. 167–196). Cambridge: Cambridge University Press.

Heun, R., Papassotiropoulos, A., Jessen, F., Maier, W., and Breitner, J. C. S. (2001). 'A Family Study of Alzheimer Disease and Early- and Late-onset Depression in Elderly Patients'. *Archives of General Psychiatry* 58(2): 190–196. doi:10.1001/archpsyc.58.2.190.

Hobson, P. (2008). 'Parkinson's disease'. In B. Woods and L. Clare (eds), *Handbook of the Clinical Psychology of Ageing* (pp. 187–199). Chichester: Wiley. doi: 10.1002/9780470773185.ch12.

Jonker, A. A. G. C., Comijs, H. C., Knipscheer, K. C. P. M., and Deeg, D. J. H. (2009). 'Promotion of Self-management in Vulnerable Older People: A Narrative Literature Review of Outcomes of the Chronic Disease Self-Management Program (CDSMP)'. *European Journal of Ageing* 6(4): 303–314. doi:10.1007/s10433-009-0131-y.

Jung, C. G. (1976). 'Die Lebenswende' [Turning in life]. In M. Niehus-Jung, L. Hurwitz-Eisner, F. Riklin, L. Jung-Merker, and E. Rüf (eds), C. J. Jung, *Gesammelte Werke* [Collected works], *Band 8: Die Dynamik des Unbewussten* [Dynamic of the unconcious] (2nd edn, pp. 425–442). Olten: Walter.

Kessler, R. C., Barker, P. R., Colpe, L. J., Epstein, J. F., Gfroerer, J. C., Hiripi, E., et al. (2003). 'Screening for Serious Mental Illness in the General Population'. *Archives of General Psychiatry* 60(2): 184–189. doi:10.1001/archpsyc.60.2.184.

Kessler, R. C., Berglund, P., Demler, O., Jin, R., Merikangas, K. R., and Walters, E. E. (2005). 'Lifetime Prevalence and Age-of-onset Distributions of DSM-IV Disorders in the National Comorbidity Survey Replication'. *Archives of General Psychiatry* 62(6): 593–602. doi:10.1001/archpsyc.62.6.593.

Kessler, E.-M. and Staudinger, U. M. (2010). 'Emotional Resilience and Beyond: A Synthesis of Findings from Lifespan Psychology and Psychopathology'. In P. S. Frey and C. L. Keyes (eds), *New Frontiers of Resilient Aging* (pp. 258–282). Cambridge: Cambridge University Press.

Knight, B. G., Kaskie, B., Shurgot, G. R., and Dave, J. (2006). 'Improving the Mental Health of Older Adults'. In J. E. Birren and K. W. Schaie (eds), *The Handbook of the Psychology of Aging* (6th edn, pp. 407–424). San Diego: Academic Press.

Kramer, A. F., Erickson, K. I., and Colcombe, S. J. (2006). 'Exercise, Cognition, and the Aging Brain'. *Journal of Applied Physiology* 101(4): 1237–1242. doi:10.1152/japplphysiol.00500.2006.

Krishnan, K. R. R. (2002). 'Biological Risk Factors in Late Life Depression'. *Biological Psychiatry* 52(3): 185–192. doi:10.1016/S0006-3223(02)01349-5.

Kruglanski, A. W. (1996). 'Goals as Knowledge Structures'. In P. M. Gollwitzer and J. A. Bargh (eds), *The Psychology of Action: Linking Cognition and Motivation to Behavior* (pp. 599–618). New York: Guilford Press.

Kurz, A., Thöne-Otto, A., Cramer, B., Egert, S., Frölich, L., Gertz, H.-J., et al. (2012). 'CORDIAL: Cognitive Rehabilitation and Cognitive-behavioral Treatment for Early Dementia in Alzheimer Disease: A Multicenter, Randomized, Controlled Trial'. *Alzheimer Disease and Associated Disorders* 26(3): 246–253. doi:10.1097/WAD.0b013e318231e46e.

Laidlaw, K., Thompson, L. W., Siskin-Dick, L., and Gallagher-Thompson, D. (2003) *Cognitive Behavioural Therapy with Older People*. Chichester: Wiley.

Lee, S., Tsang, A., Zhang, M.-Y., Huang, Y.-Q., He, Y.-L., Liu, Z.-R., et al. (2007). 'Lifetime Prevalence and Inter-cohort Variation in DSM-IV Disorders in Metropolitan China'. *Psychological Medicine* 37(1): 61–71. doi:10.1017/S0033291706008993.

Lerner, R. M. and Busch-Rossnagel, N. (eds) (1981). *Individuals as Producers of their Development: A Life Span Perspective*. New York: Academic Press.

Lerner, R. M. (1984). *On the Nature of Human Plasticity*. New York: Cambridge University Press.

Levy, B. R. (2003). 'Mind Matters: Cognitive and Physical Effects of Aging Self-stereotypes'. *The Journals of Gerontology Series B: Psychological Sciences and Social Sciences* 58(4): 203–211. doi:10.1093/geronb/58.4.P203.

Levy, B. R. (2009). 'Stereotype Embodiment: A Psychosocial Approach to Aging'. *Current Directions in Psychological Science* 18(6): 332–336. doi:10.1111/j.1467-8721.2009.01662.x.

Markowitz, J. C. and Weissman, M. M. (2004). 'Interpersonal Psychotherapy: Principles and Applications'. *World Psychiatry* 3: 136–139.

Marsh, L., McDonald, W. M., Cummings, J., and Ravina, B. (2006). 'Provisional Diagnostic Criteria for Depression in Parkinson's Disease: Report of an NINDS/NIMH Work Group'. *Movement Disorders* 21(2): 148–158. doi:10.1002/mds.20723.

Mohlman, J. (2009). 'Cognitive Self-consciousness—a Predictor of Increased Anxiety Following First-time Diagnosis of Age-related Hearing Loss'. *Ageing and Mental Health* 13(2): 246–254.

Netz, Y., Wu, M.-J., Becker, B. J., and Tenenbaum, G. (2005). 'Physical Activity and Psychological Well-being in Advanced Age: A Meta-analysis of Intervention Studies'. *Psychology and Aging* 20(2): 272–284. doi:10.1037/0882-7974.20.2.272.

Onrust, S. A. and Cuijpers, P. (2006). 'Mood and Anxiety Disorders in Widowhood: A Systematic Review'. *Aging & Mental Health* 10: 327–334. doi:10.1080/13607860600638529.

Pinquart, M., Duberstein, P. R., and Lyness, J. M. (2007). 'Effects of Psychotherapy and Other Behavioral Interventions on Clinically Depressed Older Adults: A Meta-analysis'. *Aging & Mental Health* 11(6): 645–657. doi:10.1080/13607860701529635.

Pinquart, M. and Forstmeier, S. (2012). 'Effects of Reminiscence Interventions on Psychosocial Outcomes: A Meta-analysis'. *Aging & Mental Health* 16(5): 541–558. doi:10.1080/13607863.2011.651434.

Prince, M., Beekman, A., Deeg, D., Fuhrer, R., Kivela, S., Lawlor, B., et al. (1999). 'Depression symptoms in late life assessed using the EURO-D scale - Effect of age, gender and marital status in 14 European centres'. *British Journal of Psychiatry*, 174, 339–345.

Riley, M. W., Kahn, R. L., and Foner, A. (eds) (1994). *Age and Structural Lag: Society's Failure to Provide Meaningful Opportunities in Work, Family, and Leisure*. Oxford: Wiley.

Ritchie, K., Jaussent, I., Stewart, R., Dupuy, A.-M., Courtet, P., Ancelin, M.-L., et al. (2009). 'Association of Adverse Childhood Environment and 5-HTTLPR Genotype with Late-life Depression'. *The Journal of Clinical Psychiatry* 70(9): 1281–1288. doi:10.4088/JCP.08m04510.

Rogers, W. A. and Fisk, A. D. (2010). 'Toward a Psychological Science of Advanced Technology Design for Older Adults'. *Journal of Gerontology: Psychological Sciences* 65B: 645–653. doi:10.1093/geronb/gbq065.

Ryff, C. D. (1989). 'Happiness is Everything, or Is It? Explorations on the Meaning of Psychological Well-being'. *Journal of Personality and Social Psychology* 57(6): 1069–1081. doi:10.1037/0022-3514.57.6.1069.

Sameroff A.J., Lewis M., and Miller S. M. (eds) (2000). *Handbook of Developmental Psychopathology* (2nd edn). New York: Springer.

Schaie, K. W. (1996). *Intellectual Development in Adulthood. The Seattle Longitudinal Study*. Cambridge: Cambridge University Press.

Schaie, K. W. (2005). 'What can we Learn from Longitudinal Studies of Adult Intellectual Development?' *Research in Human Development* 2(3): 133–158. doi:10.1207/s15427617rhd0203_4.

Serrano, J. P., Latorre, J. M., Gatz, M., and Montanes, J. (2004). 'Life Review Therapy Using Autobiographical Retrieval Practice for Older Adults with Depressive Symptomatology'. *Psychology and Aging* 19(2): 272–277. doi: 10.1037/0882-7974.19.2.272.

Settersten, R.A., Jr (ed.) (2003). *Invitation to the Life Course: Toward a New Understanding of Later Life*. Amityville, NY: Baywood.

Sitzer, D. I., Twamley, E. W., and Jeste, D. V. (2006). 'Cognitive Training in Alzheimer's Disease: A Meta-analysis of the Literature'. *Acta Psychiatrica Scandinavica* 114(2): 75–90. doi:10.1111/j.1600-0447.2006.00789.x.

Smith, A., Graham, L., and Senthinathan, S. (2007). 'Mindfulness-based Cognitive Therapy for Recurring Depression in Older People: A Qualitative Study'. *Aging & Mental Health* 11(3): 346–357. doi:10.1080/13607860601086256.

Snyder, D. K., Castellani, A. M., and Whisman, M. A. (2006). 'Current Status and Future Directions in Couple Therapy'. *Annual Review of Psychology* 57(1): 317–344. doi:10.1146/annurev.psych.56.091103.070154.

Sörensen, S., Pinquart, M., and Duberstein, P. (2002). 'How Effective are Interventions with Caregivers? An Updated Meta-analysis'. *The Gerontologist* 42(3): 356–372. doi:10.1093/geront/42.3.356.

Staudinger, U. M., Marsiske, M., and Baltes, P. B. (1995). 'Resilience and Reserve Capacity in Later Adulthood: Potentials and Limits of Development across the Life Span'. In D. Cicchetti and D. Cohen (eds), *Developmental Psychopathology: Vol. 2. Risk, Disorder and Adaptation* (pp. 801–847). New York: Wiley.

Staudinger, U. M. and Kessler, E.-M. (2009). 'Adjustment and Personality Growth: Two Trajectories of Positive Personality Development across Adulthood'. In M. C. Smith and T. J. Reio (eds), *The Handbook on Adult Development and Learning* (pp. 241–268). Mahwah, NJ: Lawrence Erlbaum Associates.

Steverink, N., Lindenberg, S., and Slaets, J. (2005). 'How to Understand and Improve Older People's Self-management of Wellbeing'. *European Journal of Ageing* 2(4): 235–244. doi:10.1007/s10433-005-0012-y.

Tornstam, L. (1989). 'Gero-transcendence: A Meta-theoretical Re-formulation of the Disengagement Theory'. *Aging* 1: 55–63.

Tornstam, L. (1996). 'Caring for the Elderly: Introducing the Theory of Gero-transcendence as a Supplementary Frame of Reference for Caring for the Elderly'. *Scandinavian Journal of Caring Sciences* 10: 144–150.

Wahl, H.-W., Kämmerer, A., Holz, F., Miller, D., Becker, S., Kaspar, R., and Himmelsbach, I. (2006). 'Psychosocial Intervention for Age-related Macular Degeneration: A Pilot Project'. *Journal of Visual Impairment and Blindness*, 100: 533–544.

Wahl, H.-W. and Gitlin, L. N. (2007). 'Environmental Gerontology'. In J. E. Birren (ed.), *Encyclopedia of Gerontology: Age, Aging, and the Aged* (2nd edn, pp. 494–501). Oxford: Elsevier.

Wahl, H.-W., Fänge, A., Oswald, F., Gitlin, L. N., and Iwarsson, S. (2009). 'The Home Environment and Disability-related Outcomes in Aging Individuals: What Is the Empirical Evidence?' *The Gerontologist* 49(3): 355–367. doi:10.1093/geront/gnp056.

Wahl, H.-W., Iwarsson, S., and Oswald, F. (2012). 'Aging Well and the Environment: Toward an Integrative Model and Research Agenda for the Future'. *The Gerontologist* 52(3): 306–316. http://gerontologist.oxfordjournals.org/content/52/3/306. doi:10.1093/geront/gnr154.

Walters, G. D. (2010). 'Dementia: Continuum or Distinct Entity?' *Psychology and Aging* 25(3): 534–544. doi:10.1037/a0018167.

Wang, H.-X., Karp, A., Winblad, B., and Fratiglioni, L. (2002). 'Late-life Engagement in Social and Leisure Activities is Associated with a Decreased Risk of Dementia: A Longitudinal Study from the Kungsholmen Project'. *American Journal of Epidemiology* 155(12): 1081–1087. doi:10.1093/aje/155.12.1081.

Whitbourne, S. K. and Meeks, S. (2011). 'Psychopathology, Bereavement, and Aging'. In K. W. Schaie and S. L. Willis (eds), *Handbook of the Psychology of Aging* (7th edn, pp. 311–323). San Diego, CA: Academic Press.

WHO (2007). 'Suicide prevention (SUPRE)'. http://www.who.int/mental_health/prevention/suicide/suicideprevent/en/index.html. Retrieved 3 January 2008.

Willis, S. L., Tennstedt, S. L., Marsiske, M., Ball, K., Elias, J., Koepke, K. M., et al. (2006). 'Long-term Effects of Cognitive Training on Everyday Functional Outcomes in Older Adults'. *Journal of the American Medical Association* 296(23): 2805–2814. doi:10.1001/jama.296.23.2805.

Yang, Y. (2007). 'Is Old Age Depressing? Growth Trajectories and Cohort Variations in Late-life Depression'. *Journal of Health and Social Behavior* 48(1): 16–32. doi:10.1177/002214650704800102.

Zarit, S. H. (2009). 'A Good Old Age: Theories of Mental Health and Aging'. In V. Bengtson, M. Silverstein, N. Putney, and D. Gans (eds), *Handbook of Theories of Aging* (pp. 675–692). New York: Springer.

Zisook, S. and Shuchter, S. R. (1991). 'Early Psychological Reaction to the Stress of Widowhood'. *Psychiatry: Journal for the Study of Interpersonal Processes* 54: 320–333.

CHAPTER 2

....

THE DEMOGRAPHY
AND EPIDEMIOLOGY
OF POPULATION AGEING

....

JOHN R. BEARD

INTRODUCTION

....

POPULATION ageing may be the most predictable of all the major changes that society will experience in the first half of the twenty-first century. Its impact is also likely to be among the most far-reaching.

The shift to older populations is a global phenomenon. While it started in wealthy regions such as Europe and North America, it is now low- and middle-income countries that are experiencing the greatest change. By 2050, 80% of older people will live in these settings, and countries like Chile, China, and the Islamic Republic of Iran will have a greater proportion of older people than the US (United Nations Department of Social and Economic Affairs (UNDESA) 2010).

These demographic changes are occurring alongside other major global trends such as urbanization, globalization, an epidemiological transition to non-communicable disease and technological change (Beard et al. 2012). These trends are interrelated, and understanding the relationships between them is important if we are to develop innovative and successful models of ageing that are appropriate for the twenty-first century.

At the individual level, chronological age is a poor measure of the many physical, mental, and social changes that have been associated with increasing age. These are neither smooth nor well defined, and one of the hallmarks of ageing is increased inter-individual variability (Lazarus and Harridge 2010).

Older populations are therefore typified by marked heterogeneity. They will include fit and energetic 'old' people wishing to continue to participate in social and occupational activities at levels little different from younger populations. For this subpopulation, a key challenge will be overcoming ageism, discrimination that prevents their ongoing social contribution.

But older populations will also include less healthy individuals requiring significant health and social care. Others will live in isolation or struggle financially. In poorer countries, few will have access to even the most basic healthcare and many will need to continue to work until their last days. An event like a stroke may be catastrophic, not just for their own well-being, but for the economic security of their whole family.

Yet, addressing the needs of older people in less developed countries need not be unaffordable. For example, a number of low-income countries have recently introduced small, universal, tax-funded pensions to provide some financial security for these older populations. Recent analysis suggests this may add less than 1% to GDP in most settings (UNDESA 2007). However, these small pensions can be quickly diverted to healthcare costs unless older people also have access to affordable and appropriate care.

Population ageing will therefore present societies with many challenges: strains on social security systems, increased demand for acute and primary healthcare, demand for a larger and more appropriately trained health workforce and increased need for long-term and other social care (Sikken et al. 2008). But older people also make significant contributions to their families and communities, as well as in the formal workforce. Older populations therefore represent a significant human resource on which society can draw (Oxley 2009).

The challenge for countries rich and poor is to maximize these benefits of demographic change, while effectively managing the risks (United Nations Population Fund and HelpAge International 2012). This will require a better understanding of the causes of population ageing, the health challenges faced by older people around the world and the many social changes that are taking place alongside this global transition.

Population Ageing and Socioeconomic Development

Population ageing can be considered a consequence of socioeconomic development. While each country experiences this in a unique way, common patterns emerge. Initially, improving living conditions and increasing access to healthcare result in falling infant and maternal mortality. As families become aware that their children are more likely to survive, and as women gain more access to contraception, fertility falls. But the lag between falling mortality and falling fertility creates a population spike that quickly moves through to traditional working age. When combined with the fall in the proportion of younger people needing to be supported, these workforce changes can have major impacts on economic growth (UNDESA 2007). For example, up to one-third of East Asia's economic gains between 1965 and 1990 may have been the result of these demographic shifts alone (Bloom, Canning, and Fink 2010).

But the population bulge eventually moves into older age. Over the past twenty years, this has been accompanied by increasing longevity, particularly in the developed world, which further increases the proportion of older people in the population (Christensen et al. 2009). Combined, these changes dramatically shift population structures from a dominance of younger ages to one where all age groups are more equally represented. With continued low fertility and improved survival at all ages, these trends are likely to continue. Figure 2.1 illustrates the example of Brazil to highlight how significant these structural changes can be in a rapidly developing country.

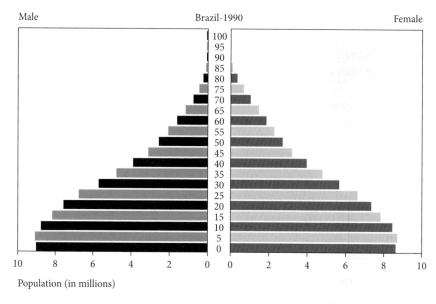

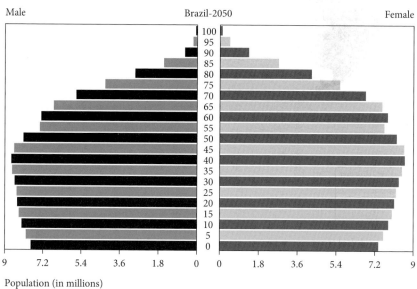

FIGURE 2.1 Changing population age structure for Brazil 1990–2050.

Reproduced from United States Census Bureau, International Database.

THE GLOBAL DEMOGRAPHY OF AGEING

Population ageing is a global phenomenon, and not one that is limited to Europe and North America (see Figure 2.2). Indeed, it is middle-income countries and emerging economies that will experience some of the most dramatic demographic change in the next thirty years.

Percentage of the total population aged 60 years and over, 2012

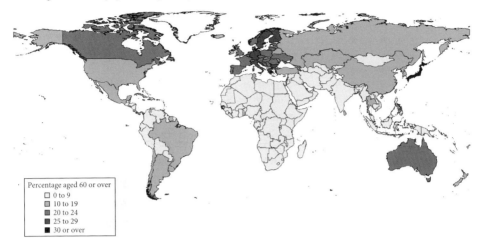

Percentage of the total population aged 60 years and over, 2050

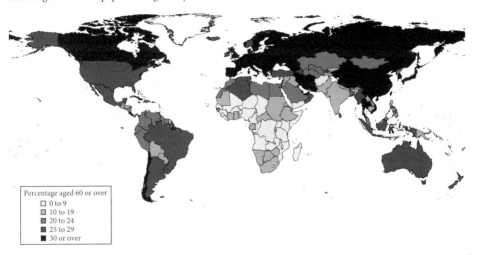

FIGURE 2.2 Global ageing trends: percentage of the total population aged 60 years and over 2012.

Similar trends are also occurring for the oldest age groups. The global population over the age of 80 years will increase from fourteen million in the mid-twentieth century to around four hundred million in 2050. One hundred million of these older people will be living in a single country: China.

The pace of demographic change has also increased. For example, it took France over a hundred years for the proportion of those aged 65 or older to increase from 7% to 14%. For countries like China, Thailand, and South Korea, the same demographic shift will take just over twenty years (Figure 2.3). This gives them less time to put in place the appropriate infrastructure and policies to meet the needs of this older population. However, the pace of ageing is generally matched by the pace of economic development in these countries, so while the task is urgent, it is still achievable.

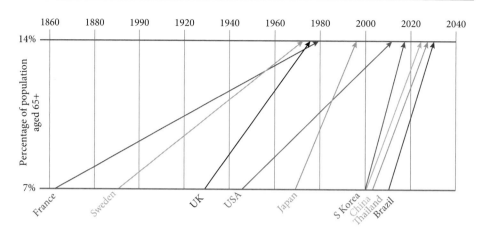

FIGURE 2.3 The speed of population ageing: time required or expected for population aged 65 or older to increase from 7% to 14%.

Reproduced from United States Census Bureau, International Database.

Changing social patterns

Population ageing interacts with many other social trends to influence physical and mental well-being in older age. For example, until the twenty-first century, most of the world's population lived in rural areas (United Nations Population Fund (UNFPA) 2007) and older people tended to live as part of extended families comprising relatively large proportions of younger people. These structures allowed even frail older people to continue to make a family contribution (e.g. through child care or food preparation), and older people could, in turn, expect younger family members to assist them if they became unable to fully look after themselves.

But population ageing is changing the relative proportion of older people within families, and changing the balance of this reciprocal relationship between young and old. At the same time, family structures are changing. Older people are becoming much more likely to live alone. For example, in 1960, 87% of older people in Japan lived with their children. By 2005, this had fallen to 47% (National Institute of Population and Social Security Research 2012). In some European countries, nearly 50% of women aged 65 or older now live by themselves (Central Statistics Office 2007).

These patterns are reinforced by broader social trends. Rapid urbanization is often accompanied by internal migration of younger people from rural areas seeking work. The older family members who are left behind in their rural homes may have to survive without the extended family support they might have otherwise expected. On the other hand, these older members of the family may accompany their younger relatives to the city and then need to adjust to an urban environment that may not provide the same social support they might have anticipated in their rural community of origin. The younger migrants themselves will age, often at a distance from other family members. Combined, these shifts mean that by 2050, almost a quarter of urban populations in less developed countries will be over the age of 60, while, in developed countries, 80% of older people already live in urban areas (UNFPA 2007).

But globalization is also resulting in increased external migration of younger family members to other countries, further exacerbating these impacts. While population ageing itself will also influence migration patterns as countries may seek external additions to their workforce to overcome shortages, only very high rates of migration impact significantly on a country's rate of population ageing (UNDESA 2007).

THE EPIDEMIOLOGY OF POPULATION AGEING

Life expectancy at birth reflects both survival at younger ages and how long survivors tend to live. Table 2.1 shows life expectancy at birth for different regions of the World Health Organization (WHO) and highlights the twenty-year gap between high-income and low-income countries. This is heavily influenced by the higher risk of dying at an early age (generally from communicable disease) in poorer countries, but greater longevity in the rich world is also a factor.

A better perspective on how long people are living can be gained by examining the number of additional years that someone who has already attained the age of 60 might expect to live. Variation in 'Life expectancy at age 60' is significantly less than for life expectancy at birth. For example, a 60-year-old woman in sub-Saharan Africa can expect to live for another fourteen years, while a 60-year-old woman in a high-income country can expect to live twenty-five years (Table 2.1). But life expectancy at 60 is increasing twice as fast in high-income countries compared to low- and middle-income countries in general, and eight times as fast as in sub-Saharan Africa.

Is there a limit to the age humans can hope to reach? The evidence on this is mixed. While it seems intuitive that there must be an upper age limit beyond which individual humans cannot survive, data on the countries with the highest average life expectancies between 1840 and 2007 show a steady increase (Figure 2.4). While the country with the highest average life expectancy has varied over time, there is little evidence that, at least at a national level, a limit is being approached. This is likely to reflect a greater proportion of the population reaching a maximum possible individual age.

Table 2.1 Life expectancy at birth and at age 60 by WHO Region 2009

WHO Region	Life expectancy at birth (years) male/female	Life expectancy at 60 years (years) male/female
World	66/71	18/21
Africa	52/56	14/16
Americas	73/79	21/24
Eastern Mediterranean	64/67	16/18
Europe	71/79	19/23
South East Asia	64/67	15/18
Western Pacific	72/77	19/22

Source: WHO (2011). *World Health Statistics.* Geneva: WHO

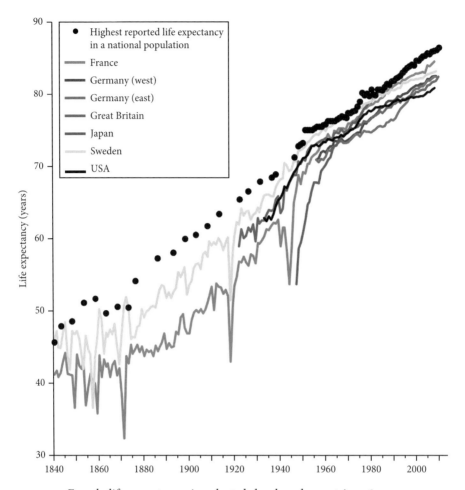

FIGURE 2.4 Female life expectancy in selected developed countries, 1840–2009.

Causes of mortality in older age

The demographic transition to older populations is being accompanied by an epidemiological transition to a predominance of chronic, rather than communicable, disease. This is true for both developed and less developed countries.

One way of characterizing the importance of different diseases is to look at the deaths they cause and to calculate the number of years each person might have lived if, instead, they had been able to survive to the highest observed life expectancies globally. Theoretically, this ideal is reachable with current technology and resources since it is already being achieved in at least one country. Death at any age younger than this ideal can be considered premature, and this can be quantified as 'Years Of Life Lost' depending on how many years earlier than the ideal it occurred.

Figure 2.5 shows the fifteen greatest causes of Years of Life Lost for every 100 000 people aged 60 and over by different country income group. Regardless of the level of economic development, the three biggest causes of premature death are non-communicable

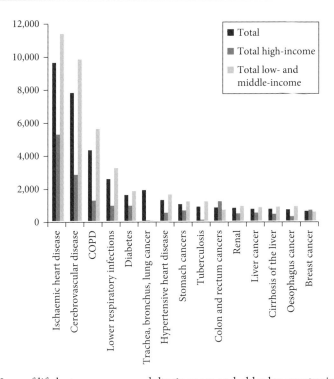

FIGURE 2.5 Years of life lost per 100,000 adults 60 years and older by country income group.
Reproduced from Good Health Adds Life to Years: Global Brief for World Health Day 2012 p. 14 © World Health Organization, 2012.

diseases: ischaemic heart disease, cerebrovascular disease (stroke), and chronic obstructive pulmonary disease (COPD).

However, comparison of the relative impact of each of these conditions in different economic settings shows that, perhaps surprisingly, the burden of premature mortality from non-communicable diseases in older people is much higher in low- and middle-income countries than for high-income countries. More than three times as many years of life are lost from stroke among the same number of older people living in a low-income country as in a high-income country. In low-income countries, more than twice as many years of life are lost to heart disease and four times as many years of life are lost to chronic obstructive pulmonary disease.

Disability in later life

While it is important to reduce mortality in later life, it is also vital that any extra years are healthy ones. Unfortunately, despite very clear evidence that people are living longer, we do not yet know whether they are living longer and healthier lives, or if these added years are associated with extended periods of illness and disability.

This is a crucial issue for society since, if people are living for longer periods of ill health, this will result in increased pressure on health and social systems at the same time as the proportion of people of traditional working age is falling. On the other hand, if people are

Table 2.2 Prevalence in adults over age 60 of moderate and severe disability (in millions), by leading health condition associated with disability, and by country income group

	High-income countries	Low- and middle-income countries
Visual impairment	15.0	94.2
Hearing loss	18.5	43.9
Osteoarthritis	8.1	19.4
Ischaemic heart disease	2.2	11.9
Dementia	6.2	7.0
Chronic obstructive pulmonary disease	4.8	8.0
Cerebrovascular disease	2.2	4.9
Depression	0.5	4.8
Rheumatoid arthritis	1.7	3.7

Source: Reproduced from WHO (2012). *Good Health Adds Life to Years: Global Brief for World Health Day 2012,* Geneva: WHO, p. 17, Table 4 © World Health Organization 2012

experiencing more years of healthy life, this will require less support from health and social systems and create opportunities for more extended periods of social participation that may at least partly balance any increased costs. Understanding which of these scenarios is occurring is therefore fundamental if we are to plan effectively for the future.

The evidence on this crucial question is conflicting. While research in the US suggests that ageing has been associated with less severe disability in older age, an assessment of patterns of milder disability in OECD countries found that it had decreased in some countries, increased in others, and in others remained the same (Lafortune and Balestat 2007; Manton, Gu, and Lamb 2006).

We do know, however, the main causes of disability in older age. In low- and middle-income countries, visual disturbances are by far the biggest problem. In high-income countries, the biggest burden of disability is from dementia. Other common impairments in both settings are hearing loss and osteoarthritis. Table 2.2 shows the absolute number of older people around the world who are affected by these and other conditions.

In low-income countries, the most common causes of visual impairment are refractive errors and cataracts. It is startling to think that millions of people around the world are still limited in their daily activities by lack of access to such simple refractive lenses. Similarly, surgery for cataracts is simple and relatively cheap. Yet twenty million people around the world are blinded due to lack of access to this cheap procedure.

Common mental disorders in older age

There is ongoing debate about the prevalence of mental disorders in older age. While evidence remains sparse on some common conditions such as anxiety disorders, there is now a considerable body of evidence on depression in older age (Byrne and Pachana 2010). Since this stage of life is often associated with an increase in stressful life events such as the loss of a spouse or partner and change of social role, it might be anticipated to precipitate a greater prevalence of common disorders. Yet estimates of major depression in older people living in the community range from less than 1% to about 5% (Hybels and Blazer 2003). These low prevalences do not appear to be the result of misattribution of depressive symptoms to physical disorders. Furthermore, some studies suggest that sense of well-being can increase in older age, particularly in developed countries. Combined, these results point to psychological changes in older age that increase resilience and reduce vulnerability to life stressors.

Prevalence of depression does appear to rise among those with significant loss of function (13.5%) and in hospitalized older people (11.5%) (Hybels and Blazer 2003). It may be even higher among nursing home residents, with one recent study finding a prevalence of clinically significant depression of 21.2%, with a twelve-month incidence rate of 14.9% and a persistence rate of 44.8% (Barca et al. 2010). These findings may relate in part to an association of depression with cognitive decline and dementia, although there is increasing evidence that this is a two-way relationship (Byrne and Pachana 2010).

The global challenge of dementia

One way of measuring the severity, as well as the incidence and duration of disability in older populations is to assess 'Years Lost to Disability' per 100 000 older adults. Using this measure, the greatest burden from disability in high-income countries, and the second greatest in low- and middle-income countries, is dementia (WHO and Alzheimer's Disease International 2012).

Globally, it is estimated that 35.6 million suffered from dementia in 2010 and this is projected to nearly double every twenty years, to 65.7 million in 2030 and 115.4 million in 2050. Nearly 7.7 million new cases of dementia are diagnosed each year, and this will increase dramatically as populations age (Figure 2.6).

In 2010, the total worldwide costs of dementia were estimated at US$604 billion. Alzheimer's International has estimated that if dementia care were a country, it would be the world's eighteenth largest economy, ranking between Turkey and Indonesia. If it were a company, it would be the world's largest by annual revenue exceeding Wal-Mart (US$414 billion) and Exxon Mobil (US$311 billion) (Wimo and Prince 2010).

In low-income and lower to middle-income countries care is usually provided unpaid by the family. However, as the proportion of younger family members falls, and as more women pursue careers, it is likely that fewer family members will be available to provide this care in the coming decades.

Disease risk factors

Despite the importance of non-communicable disease in older age and the well-known preventable risk factors for these conditions, current approaches to their control in

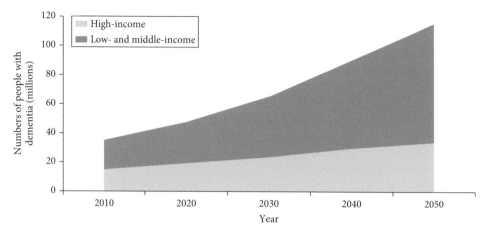

FIGURE 2.6 Growth in numbers of persons with dementia in high-income and low-and middle-income countries.

Reproduced from World Health Organization & Alzheimer's Disease International 2012 Dementia: A Public Health Priority Geneva, World Health Organization, p. 19, figure 2.3 © World Health Organization, 2012.

developing countries do not appear to be succeeding (Table 2.3). For example, the WHO Study on Global Aging and Adult Health (SAGE) suggests that while the prevalence of high blood pressure in people over 50 in Ghana and South Africa is around 55% and 75%, respectively, only 4% and 8%, respectively, are receiving effective treatment (WHO 2012).

SUMMARY

This brief review of the epidemiology of population ageing highlights the importance of chronic disease for older people, and the marked inequity between the experience of ageing in the rich and poor worlds. It also emphasizes the heterogeneity of the ageing experience, even for individuals living in the same setting.

The overwhelming burden of disease in older age relates to non-communicable diseases. Much of this burden is preventable, either through reduction in risk behaviours or treatment of metabolic risk factors. In high-income settings, addressing these risks and treating their consequences appears to be increasing the proportion of people living to older ages. However, in low-income settings, the burden of these diseases is up to four times as high, and little infrastructure is in place to meet this challenge.

What is not captured by these crude data is the importance for older people of mental health and well-being. This is explored in other chapters in this Handbook. However, as with the measures this chapter has focused on, mental health and well-being are inextricably linked with the many social changes that are accompanying population ageing. Changing family dynamics, changing intergenerational relations and changing aspirations among older people will all need to be considered if we are to develop effective strategies to support active and healthy ageing in the twenty-first century.

Table 2.3 Prevalence of risk factors by age and gender among aged 50 and older across six countries

Risk factor	China		Ghana		India		Mexico		Russian Federation		South Africa	
	Male	Female	Male	Female	Male	Female	Male	Female	Male	Female	Male	Female
Current daily smoker	50.9	3.0	11.3	3.7	62.9	30.2	18.8	8.5	39.5	4.9	22.9	16.6
Heavy drinker	15.2	0.8	4.1	1.2	1.2	0.1	14.9	0.6	20.3	3.4	6.0	2.5
Insufficient nutrition	33.6	33.7	69.6	67.3	87.9	93.5	74.6	86.0	78.9	77.2	63.2	70.4
Obese	3.4	7.8	6.3	13.6	1.3	3.0	21.7	34.5	28.0	41.7	38.2	50.6
High risk waist–hip ratio	45.9	68.8	67.0	89.5	73.8	83.9	91.9	78.2	68.7	57.5	56.0	70.4
Hypertension	49.3	51.4	50.2	54.7	24.4	26.8	48.7	51.4	52.2	53.7	66.6	69.4
Low physical activity	26.8	30.6	22.0	29.0	23.4	26.1	33.2	44.9	21.9	23.4	56.8	63.0

KEY REFERENCES AND SOURCES FOR FURTHER READING

Crimmins, E. M. and Beltrín-Sínchez, H. (2011). 'Mortality and Morbidity Trends: Is There Compression of Morbidity?' *The Journals of Gerontology, Series B: Psychological Sciences and Social Sciences* 66B(1): 75–86.

Ellis, G., Whitehead, M. A., Robinson, D., O'Neill, D., and Langhorne, P. (2011). 'Comprehensive Geriatric Assessment for Older Adults Admitted to Hospital: Meta-Analysis of Randomised Controlled Trials'. *British Medical Journal* 34: d6553.

He, W., Muenchrath, M. N., and Kowal, P. (2012). *Shades of Gray: A Cross-Country Study of Health and Well-Being of the Older Populations in SAGE Countries 2007–2010*. Washington, DC: US Government Printing Office.

Michel, J. P., Newton, J. L., and Kirkwood, T. B. (2008). 'Medical Challenges of Improving the Quality of a Longer Life'. *Journal of the American Medical Association* 299(6): 688–690.

REFERENCES

Barca, M. L., Engedal, K., Laks, J., and Selbaek, G. (2010). 'A 12 Months Follow-up Study of Depression among Nursing-home Patients in Norway'. *Journal of Affective Disorders*, 120(1–3): 141–148.

Beard, J. R., Biggs, S., Bloom, D. E., Fried, L. P., Hogan, P., et al. (2012). *Global Population Ageing: Peril or Promise?* Geneva: World Economic Forum.

Bloom, D. E., Canning, D., and Fink, G. (2010). 'Implications of Population Aging for Economic Growth'. *Oxford Review of Economic Policy* 26(4): 583–612.

Byrne, G. J. and Pachana, N. A. (2010). 'Anxiety and Depression in the Elderly: Do We Know Any More?' *Current Opinion in Psychiatry* 23(6): 504–509.

Central Statistics Office (2007). *Ageing in Ireland*. Dublin: Government of Ireland.

Christensen, K., Doblhammer, G., Rau, R., and Vaupel, J. W. (2009). 'Ageing Populations: The Challenges Ahead'. *Lancet* 374(9696): 1196–1208.

Hybels, C. F. and Blazer, D. G. (2003). 'Epidemiology of Late-life Mental Disorders'. *Clinics in Geriatric Medicine* 19(4): 663–696.

Lafortune, G. and Balestat, G. (2007). *Trends in Severe Disability Among Elderly People: Assessing the Evidence in 12 OECD Countries and the Fututre Implications*. Paris: OECD Publishing.

Lazarus, N. R. and Harridge, S. D. (2010). 'Exercise, Physiological Function, and the Selection of Participants for Aging Research'. *Journals of Gerontology, Series A: Biological Sciences and Medical Sciences* 65(8): 854–857.

Manton, K. G., Gu, X., and Lamb, V. L. (2006). 'Change in Chronic Disability from 1982 to 2004/2005 as Measured by Long-term Changes in Function and Health in the U.S. Elderly Population'. *Proceedings of the National Academy of Sciences* 103(48): 18374–18379.

National Institute of Population and Social Security Research (2012). *Population Statistics of Japan 2008*. Tokyo: Japan National Institute of Population and Social Security Research.

Oxley, H. (2009). *Policies for Healthy Ageing: an Overview*. Paris, OECD.

Sikken, B. J., Davis, N., Hayashi, C., and Olkkonen, H. (2008). *The Future of Pensions and Healthcare in a Rapidly Ageing World*. Geneva, World Economic Forum.

United Nations Department of Social and Economic Affairs (2007). *World Economic and Social Survey 2007: Development in an Ageing World*. New York: UNDESA.

United Nations Department of Social and Economic Affairs (2010). *World Population Prospects: The 2008 Revision Population Database*. New York: United Nations Population Division.

United Nations Population Fund (2007). *State of World Population 2007: Unleashing the Potential of Urban Growth*. New York: UNPF.

United Nations Population Fund and HelpAge International (2012). *Ageing in the Twenty-first Century: A Celebration and a Challenge*. New York: UNPF and HelpAge International.

World Health Organization (2012). *Good Health Adds Life to Years: Global Brief for World Health Day 2012*. Geneva: WHO.

World Health Organization and Alzheimer's Disease International (2012). *Dementia: A Public Health Priority*. Geneva: WHO.

Wimo, A. and Prince, M. (2010). *World Alzheimer Report*. London: Alzheimer's Disease International.

CHAPTER 3

LONGITUDINAL STUDIES AND CLINICAL GEROPSYCHOLOGY

KAARIN J. ANSTEY, ALEX BAHAR-FUCHS, AND KERRY SARGENT-COX

OVERVIEW OF LONGITUDINAL RESEARCH

IMPORTANT research questions in developmental and psychiatric research revolve around change across time. How do cognitive, emotional, and social processes develop across the lifespan? What is the trajectory of physical and health changes in late life? Is personality stable across adulthood? Can we identify patterns of change in symptoms and behaviours that may predict mental health or identify those at risk? To answer such questions repeated measurements are needed to allow us to describe developmental trends and distinguish normal from non-normal trajectories. Longitudinal studies (also called panel studies and prospective studies) involve following a sample or samples of participants over time and assessing them on two or more occasions. They are usually designed to enable observations of individual or household characteristics over time. Longitudinal studies are differentiated from cross-sectional studies, in which a sample is measured once.

There are two main objectives of this chapter. First, to provide an overview of the longitudinal design, its advantages and disadvantages, and the types of design and analysis that longitudinal data affords. The second objective is to examine how longitudinal data are used to inform clinical geropsychology, outline the strengths and limitations of longitudinal research designs within this field, and highlight issues and challenges that are yet to be addressed in geropsychology. This second objective will be illustrated by examining three central topics in geropsychology: cognitive disorders, depression, and anxiety.

Advantages and Limitations
of Longitudinal Studies

Inferences about ageing and mental disorders are often made from cross-sectional studies with wide age ranges. However, in such studies, any age differences are confounded by possible cohort effects (Hofer and Sliwinski 2001). Cohort effects relate to the broader societal conditions that influence each birth cohort. An example of the confounding of ageing with cohort effects may be seen if one compares prevalence of depression in 20-year-olds and 80-year-olds in the same year, and inferred differences in prevalence are due to ageing. Without following a sample from age 20 to age 80, it is not possible to estimate the true effect of ageing on depression prevalence as the comparison of different ages includes cohort effects plus ageing effects. Within a longitudinal study it is possible to study how individuals change over time, or ageing effects. Cross-sectional studies are limited in the extent to which they provide evidence of causal or temporal relationships because they measure all variables simultaneously. In a longitudinal study, the temporal ordering of events is observed and this enables falsification of some hypotheses. However, causality cannot be established in a longitudinal study because there is no manipulation of independent variables, and the environment in which the study occurs cannot be controlled except through statistical methods.

In the study of mental disorders, a key advantage of longitudinal designs is the capacity to follow individuals as they move in and out of diagnoses. Longitudinal studies allow the estimation of the incidence of disorders, and the long-term evaluation of impact of environmental and social factors on the risk of mental disorders. They also allow for the evaluation of changes in treatment patterns, access to services, and the impact of general, broader socio-economic conditions on long-term mental health.

From a methodological perspective, a key strength of longitudinal studies is that they enable the variance in independent variables to be classified as either within person or between person (Curran and Bauer 2011). Within-person variance refers to intra-individual change. Between-person variance refers to individual differences from one person to another. Longitudinal studies also allow for analysis of between-person differences in intra-individual change, i.e. how people differ in the degree to which they change over time.

However, longitudinal studies are not without their limitations. These include selection bias in the initial sample (which may also occur in cross-sectional studies); incomplete data within occasions of measurement; and loss to follow-up due to illness, death, or refusal (Allen, Frier, and Strachan 2004). This latter problem is called sample attrition, and in samples of older adults results in a strong healthy survivor effect whereby the sample becomes increasingly less representative and healthier than the population, over time. For example, research has shown that participants with cognitive impairment are more likely to discontinue their participation in longitudinal studies (Anstey and Luszcz 2002) and to have missing cognitive test data on the occasions on which they are assessed within a study. Longitudinal studies are also expensive to conduct and maintain, and require long-term commitment on the part of researchers and funding bodies.

Longitudinal research requires sensitivity to issues of measurement and research design. For example, in longitudinal studies of older adults, it is possible that the apparent decline in prevalence of anxiety among older persons reflects in part a reduced sensitivity of assessment measures to detecting geriatric anxiety. More recently, scales have been developed that were designed to measure symptoms of anxiety specifically in older adults—for example, the Geriatric Anxiety Inventory (GAI; Pachana et al. 2007), and the Geriatric Anxiety Scale (Yochim et al. 2011). Longitudinal studies may vary in their design characteristics, such as the interval between assessments, whether new cohorts are introduced at various time points (cohort sequential), and whether they include measurement bursts. Measurement bursts are intense phases of assessment (e.g. eight assessments within two weeks) that provide data on change in a characteristic that may be particularly influenced by events occurring on a small time scale, such as life stressors (Rast, MacDonald, and Hofer 2012; Sliwinski, Almeida et al. 2009). A challenge that is of particular importance in neurocognitive research is the improvement sometimes seen in performance on cognitive measures over repeated testing, a phenomenon known as 'practice effects'. Practice effects on cognitive tests may lead to an underestimation of cognitive decline depending on the type of test and how susceptible it is to practice (Collie et al. 2003).

Analysis of longitudinal datasets requires knowledge of various longitudinal methods for modelling longitudinal change, time until events, and time until death. It also requires careful consideration of missing data so that sample attrition and resulting sample bias are accounted for when interpreting the results of research. Statistical techniques for analysing longitudinal data are well described elsewhere (Singer and Willett 2003) and are available in statistical packages such as IBM SPSS, SAS, and STATA, which provide modules for analysing longitudinal data. Data analysis approaches vary according to whether they focus on estimating mean level change at the population level, or describe trajectories of subgroups. Longitudinal analyses allow for modelling of time-varying covariates and estimates of inter-individual variation in intra-individual rates of change.

WHAT CAN LONGITUDINAL STUDIES CONTRIBUTE TOWARDS CLINICAL GEROPSYCHOLOGY?

Clinical geropsychology may be informed by longitudinal studies as they observe individuals, their symptoms, and whether they meet diagnostic criteria for a psychiatric disorder over time (Anstey and Hofer 2004). Long-term follow-up of cohorts has been used to delineate new psychiatric syndromes in ageing, such as apathy (Withall et al. 2011). Longitudinal research is used to evaluate current diagnostic criteria and has been used to inform the development of the definition of depression in *DSM-5* (Mojtabai 2011). Longitudinal research allows for the natural history of disorders to be described, and risk and protective factors to be identified. Risk and protective factors may be demographic, biological, psychosocial, or cultural. For example, in a longitudinal study it is possible to identify whether particular groups defined by their geographical location, education level, gender, or cultural background have higher incidence of mental disorders. It is possible to evaluate whether the onset of particular medical conditions or different genotypes predispose individuals to developing a psychiatric disorder concurrently or later in life. Within a longitudinal study, retrospective life-history data may also be obtained which can then be linked to risk of disorders. For example, self-report of child abuse may be a risk factor for depression in adulthood (Korkeila et al. 2010).

Another important strength of longitudinal studies that observe individuals over extended periods of time is the information they provide on normative developmental change; this assists in identifying abnormal development or the development of a disorder. Within a large cohort, individual differences in change can be estimated, and large variations from typical or normative change identified statistically (Evans 2006). This is particularly relevant in cognitive ageing because cognitive decline in the population may be non-pathological or it may be pathological and predictive of impending dementia.

In the field of geropsychology, there are specific health, social transition, and biological factors that feature prominently in longitudinal research. In particular, older adults are more likely to experience spousal bereavement and transition into widowhood (d'Epinay, Cavalli, and Guillet 2009) than younger adults. This may affect their psychological and social well-being (Ott et al. 2007). Physical changes occurring in ageing that lead to functional impairment and changes in the ageing brain, also increase the risk of developing mental disorders. In particular, vascular disease increases the risk of stroke, dementia, and depression in late life (Alexopoulos et al. 1997). Hence, geropsychology research requires a multidisciplinary approach to study design and the inclusion of measures of physical health and disability, and, wherever possible, biological markers and measures of brain structure and function.

The availability of longitudinal data allows researchers to test hypotheses about the temporal ordering of events and disorders, and the temporal relationships between the onset of eventual comorbid disorders. Within a longitudinal study it is possible to estimate effect sizes of specific risk factors for mental disorders. It is also possible to answer questions about how risk factors are moderated by other risk factors (e.g. does bereavement create greater risk for depression among those with pre-existing cardiovascular disease?). Long-term follow-up of cohorts also provides opportunities to examine the impact of treatments such as psychotropic medication on mental and physical health.

Finally, longitudinal studies with a representative sample of a nation's population enable the estimate of incidence of disorders; that is, the rate at which new cases of a disorder occur each year. This information is essential for planning of health services and for evaluation of prevention policies.

USE OF LONGITUDINAL DESIGNS TO INFORM GEROPSYCHOLOGY: COGNITIVE DISORDERS, DEPRESSION, AND ANXIETY

The most common mental disorders in late life include neurocognitive, depressive, and anxiety disorders. The following sections demonstrate the importance of longitudinal research for geropsychology in these three key areas.

Cognitive disorders

Neurocognitive disorders in late life include mild cognitive impairment and dementia. The most frequent cause of dementia is Alzheimer's disease (AD), followed by cerebrovascular disease. Longitudinal research is particularly important for understanding cognitive decline and cognitive impairment because cognitive decline tends to occur gradually, and it is often difficult to distinguish pathological from non-pathological cognitive decline in the early stages of neurocognitive disease. Longitudinal research allows for the clinical characterization of the prodromal period of disorders. For example, with AD there may be changes in personality and weight loss several years prior to diagnosis (Knopman et al. 2007; Roman et al. 1993). Longitudinal research has also led to the characterization of the cascade of changes that occur in the development of AD, typically commencing with the deposition of beta amyloid, followed by tau mediated neuronal injury, changes in brain structure, cognition and function (Jack, Knopman et al. 2013).

Normal cognitive changes in ageing

Rather than being a stable characteristic, cognitive abilities follow a developmental trajectory. Verbal or crystallized abilities often improve during adulthood, and decline often reflects the presence of neurological disease or injury. In comparison, more 'fluid' cognitive abilities and processes, such as information processing speed, reasoning, and working memory, tend to peak in early adulthood (usually in the late twenties) and thereafter show gradual decline until about the mid-sixties, when a more rapid decline takes place (Horn 1982; Salthouse 2004). Memory abilities also differ in their trajectories over the life course. Episodic memory is most vulnerable to ageing and specifically linked to early hippocampal atrophy that occurs in AD (Ehreke et al. 2011; Mormino et al. 2009).

Much of the focus of longitudinal research in the field of cognitive ageing is on identifying the difference between normal and pathological decline. This is increasingly being informed by the inclusion of biomarkers of disease pathology such as beta amyloid deposition associated with AD, which can be detected on positron emission tomography (Luck et al. 2011). Cognitive decline develops gradually over several years before reaching the required threshold for classification as 'impairment', particularly in cases where individuals have high premorbid levels of ability. Hence, without longitudinal follow-up it is not possible to identify rates of decline that are abnormal when absolute performance may be in the normal range. A third form of decline observed in longitudinal studies is the 'terminal drop', an acceleration in loss of cognitive abilities occurring in the few years prior to death (MacDonald, Hultsch, and Dixon 2011).

Prevalence and incidence

Original definitions of mild cognitive impairment (Petersen et al. 2001) have been revised to improve their accuracy in defining a preclinical dementia syndrome (Ritchie and Tuokko 2010; Winblad et al. 2004). Prevalence and incidence of cognitive disorders and dementia are generally obtained from longitudinal studies that use standard research diagnostic criteria such as the *DSM-IV* or NINCDS-ADRDA criteria (Roman et al. 1993). Prevalence rates of mild cognitive disorders in community samples of older adults are notably variable (Tuokko and McDowell 2006) and have ranged from 3 to 36% (Anstey et al. 2008; Busse et al. 2003; Luck et al. 2010b). Likewise, there is wide variation in the reported conversion rates from mild cognitive disorders to dementia, ranging from 1 to 36% per year (Tuokko and McDowell 2006). Reasons proposed for this variability include variation in sampling frame, diagnostic criteria, underlying neuropathology, and sample age (Kumar et al. 2005). In a review of nineteen longitudinal studies published between 1991 and 2001, it was concluded that the major source of variability in the conversion rate is the study setting with the memory clinic attendees having higher conversion rates compared to epidemiological samples (Bruscoli and Lovestone 2004).

Prevalence and incidence rates for dementia also vary among studies. Approximately 6.6% of adults aged 65 and older suffer from dementia (Jorm, Dear, and Burgess 2005). Rates are thought to double approximately every five years starting at 0.7% between 60 and 64, increasing to 10.5% between 80 and 84, and 38.6% between 90 and 94 (see Figure 3.1).

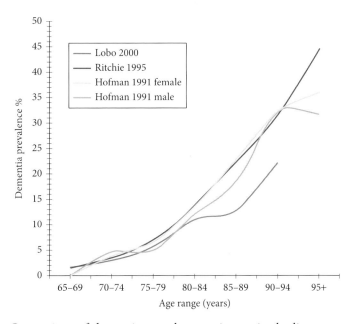

FIGURE 3.1 Comparison of dementia prevalence estimates in the literature.

Data from Hofman, A., W. A. Rocca, et al., The prevalence of dementia in Europe: a collaborative study of 1980–1990 findings, *International Journal of Epidemiology* 20, pp. 736–748, 1991, Oxford University Press. Ritchie, K. and D. Kildea, Is senile dementia "age-related" or "ageing-related"?—evidence from meta-analysis of dementia prevalence in the oldest old, *Lancet* 346(8980), pp. 931–934, 1995, Elsevier. Lobo, A., L. J. Launer, et al., Prevalence of dementia and major subtypes in Europe: A collaborative study of population-based cohorts. Neurologic Diseases in the Elderly Research Group, *Neurology*, 54(11 Suppl 5), pp. S4–9, 2000, American Academy of Neurology.

Risk and protective factors of cognitive decline

One of the most significant contributions of longitudinal studies has been their capacity to shed light on risk and protective factors for AD, vascular dementia and non-pathological cognitive decline. Interestingly, while some factors occurring in mid-life increase the risk of late-onset dementia, the same factors may not be risk factors if they occur in late life. Again, longitudinal studies have been able to demonstrate these complex relationships and provide a life course perspective on how risk factors vary at different ages (Whalley, Dick, and McNeill 2006). The risk of developing dementia increases with age and in some studies has been higher for women than men. (AccessEconomics 2009; Anstey et al. 2010; Jorm et al. 2005; Lobo et al. 2000; Ritchie and Kildea 1995). Risk factors for cognitive decline may be socio-demographic, medical, life-style-related, genetic, or related to the physical environment.

After age, a low level of education is arguably the most significant socio-demographic risk factor for dementia, as has been demonstrated in a systematic review of sixteen cohort studies and six case control studies (Caamano-Isorna et al. 2006).

In the medical field, neurological conditions such as traumatic brain injury and stroke increase the risk of dementia (Launer et al. 1999; Plassman et al. 2000; Schofield, Tang et al. 1997). More recently, cardiovascular risk factors have been recognized as risk factors for dementia, both directly and indirectly via their influence on cerebrovascular disease. These risk factors include diabetes, hypertension, high cholesterol, excess body fat, and smoking.

In a systematic review of eight longitudinal studies, diabetes was identified as a risk factor for AD and dementia (Lu, Lin, and Kuo 2009; Williams et al. 2010). A systematic review of prospective studies on the association between body mass index (BMI) and risk of AD and vascular dementia found that BMI in mid-life was associated with dementia risk but not BMI in late-life (Luck et al. 2010). Specifically, low, overweight and obese BMI in mid-life increased the risk of dementia in late life.

Longitudinal research has also shown that total serum cholesterol level is a risk factor for AD (Anstey, Lipnicki, and Low 2008). However, studies vary in how the exposure variable is measured and whether they use self-report of serum measures of high cholesterol (Williams et al. 2010).

Life style factors have also been shown by longitudinal research to be important determinants of dementia risk. There is consistent evidence from meta-analyses and individual longitudinal studies that physical activity reduces the risk of AD (Hamer and Chida 2009; Scarmeas et al. 2009; Williams et al. 2010) and this has led to clinical recommendations of physical activity as a secondary prevention strategy for AD (Savica and Petersen 2011). Longitudinal studies have also shown that smoking increases the risk of dementia (Anstey et al. 2007a). At present, there is insufficient information to establish whether former smokers have an increased risk of dementia, or whether there is a critical length of time required after smoking cessation before risk is reduced. Longitudinal research on ex-smokers is needed to inform this issue. Alcohol consumption has been evaluated as a risk factor for dementia in a meta-analysis of fifteen longitudinal studies including 14 646 participants (Anstey, Mack, and Cherbuin 2009). This review showed that alcohol abstainers had an increased risk of AD compared to light to moderate drinkers. The only dietary factor reliably linked to the risk of AD is fish consumption. This was found to be protective against cognitive decline and AD in three longitudinal studies (Barberger-Gateau et al. 2007; Huang et al. 2005; Williams et al. 2010). Two large cohort studies have reported a reduced risk of AD in older adults who engage in cognitively stimulating activities (Akbaraly et al. 2009; Wilson et al. 2007).

Longitudinal studies have shown that a measure of social engagement comprised of marital status, social network size, level of social activities, and living arrangements is associated with risk of dementia with low levels of social engagement increasing risk (Bassuk, Glass, and Berkman 1999; Fratiglioni et al. 2000; Helmer et al. 1999; Saczynski et al. 2006).

Prevention and treatment

Future longitudinal research in geropsychology is likely to focus on evaluation of preventive strategies for cognitive decline. Researchers are increasingly focusing on long-term multi-domain interventions, rather than single-domain interventions (Gillette-Guyonnet et al. 2009). Currently, cognition-focused interventions to prevent dementia and cognitive decline tend to focus on the training of memory and other cognitive abilities. Despite some promising results showing the benefits of cognitive training for reducing cognitive decline (Willis et al. 2006), to date there has been insufficient research on the effects of cognitive training for the prevention of neurocognitive disorders to determine their efficacy. Secondary prevention of dementia, targeting individuals with mild cognitive disorders, also includes the treatment of modifiable life-style and cardiovascular risk factors (Luck et al. 2010a).

Depression

Trajectory of depression in late-life

Longitudinal studies allow the examination of the onset, trajectories, and natural history, of depression across the lifespan. While lifespan longitudinal studies of this nature are rare, the contribution that this type of research has made to the understanding of depression in late-life is examined here.

Within a lifespan perspective, late-life depression is recognized as the first onset of depression appearing after the age of 60 (Blazer 2003). Prevalence of major depressive disorders in community-dwelling adults over 65 in most large epidemiological studies across the globe is quite low at 1–5% (Fiske, Wetherell, and Gatz et al. 2009). Including subthreshold depressive symptoms dramatically increases prevalence rates to approximately 12–15%, and these rates may increase over time in adults over 65 years old (Beekman et al. 2001). Furthermore, a gender gap in prevalence rates of depression remains apparent in older adults, with females showing higher rates (see Figure 3.2 showing percentage of males and females with high depressive symptoms scores from the PATH through Life Study in the 60–64 year cohort over four years). Interestingly, this gender gap may widen in late-life over time. Heikkinen and Kauppinen (2004) found that at the age of 85 the prevalence figure for women increased by a significant 8.1% (from 36.6% to 44.7%) from the age of 75 years, whereas for males the prevalence rate had only increased 2.3% (27.4% to 29.7%).

There is great variability in the reported incidence rates of depression in late-life. This may be due to methodological differences, particularly those related to the length of time over which the incidence rates are calculated. For example, over three years Beekman and colleagues (2001) found the incidence rate of depression in adults over 65 years to be 9.7%. In contrast, Luijendijk and colleagues (2008) found the incidence rate for community-dwelling

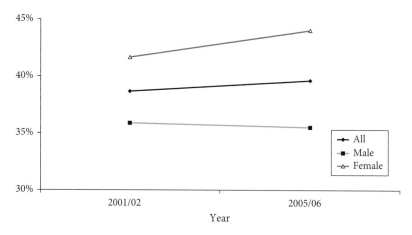

FIGURE 3.2 Percentage of PATH Through Life Respondents aged 60 to 64 with high depressive symptoms over four years.

adults (aged 56+) over eight years was low at 7/1000 person years for depressive syndromes, and the recurrence rate was 27.5/1000 person years using *DSM-IV*-defined categories.

The majority of studies indicate very poor outcomes of late-life depression in terms of recurrence and persistence levels, with older adults showing greater risk of recurrence compared to younger cohorts (Mueller et al. 2004). It is estimated that one in three older adults with depression develops a chronic course of their symptoms (Licht-Strunk et al. 2007). Beekman and colleagues (Beekman et al. 2001) found that 50.4% of the community-based sample who were depressed at baseline remained classified as depressed three years later. Of particular interest is that older adults who have higher baseline-level depression are less likely to change depressive symptoms over time—indicating a strong persistence of symptoms at this chronic level (Hong, Hasche, and Bowland 2009).

Longitudinal research designs are of particular benefit when used to answer questions of the natural history of conditions and their persistence. For example, using fourteen measurement periods over six years, Beekman and colleagues (Beekman et al. 2002) identified four patterns of persistence and remission in older adults: (1) 23% were classified as in remission (defined as decline in symptoms and remaining non-depressed); (2) 12% were in remission with recurrence (recurrence of symptoms after decrease); (3) 32% showed a chronic/intermittent course (defined as greater than 1 remission followed by recurrence of symptoms); and (4) 32% suffered a chronic course (where they were classified as depressed for 80% or more of the observations).

Incidence and prevalence

Understanding prevalence and incidence rates of depression in older populations are confounded by potential differences in rates for community-dwelling vs institutionalized adults. Many epidemiological studies exclude institutionalized adults, resulting in less accurate figures. It is argued that nursing home patients are more likely to have chronic depression with high persistent rates (Barca et al. 2010). Anstey and colleagues (2007b) found a vast difference in prevalence of depression (CESD> = 16) with residential care older adults showing over twice the prevalence (32%) of those living in the community (14.4%). These high figures for institutionalized adults are reflected in a study conducted by Barca et al. (2010), who found a depression prevalence rate of 21.2%, and a high incidence rate over twelve months of 14.4%. Barca and colleagues showed that the risk of incidence increased for those who had been in the nursing home for shorter periods of time, suggesting that the move to the nursing home, with its associated changes in dependence and autonomy, may lead to depression during a period of adaptation.

Risk and protective factors for late-life depression

Recent longitudinal studies have highlighted differences in risk factors and aetiology of late-life-onset depression compared to that of early-onset. For example, early onset of depression is more strongly associated with a genetic component (i.e. family history) than is late-life onset. In contrast, Heikkinen and Kauppinen (2004) revealed very old adults were more likely to become depressed when negative health and life changes occurred. That is, a higher risk of depression was found if individuals also reported loneliness, poor self-rated health, decline in visual acuity, and perceived negative changes in life over a ten-year period. Similarly, Beekman and colleagues (2001) showed that risk for persistence of depressive symptoms over a three-year period in adults over 55 years was largely based on the presence of chronic physical illness and the psychological construct of external locus of control.

In the few longitudinal studies that have looked at protective factors for late-life depression, psychological and social resources are emerging as important. Over time, self-efficacy, and a strong sense of personal control have been found to be protective of late-life depression in older adults (Yang 2006), while neuroticism and low mastery has been found to be strongly associated with recurrence and persistence of depression in older adults (Kendler et al. 2006; Steunenberg et al. 2010). Spousal or significant other relationships appear to be protective for depression over time in older adults (Takkinen et al. 2004). In a similar vein, social activity participation is espoused as protective of well-being in late-life. In a recent longitudinal study older adults who had higher levels of participation, which included a wide range of activities such as volunteering, social outings, talking on the phone, and exercising, had lower initial depressive symptoms, and were less likely to have an increase in symptoms over a six-year period, than those who had low participation (Hong et al. 2009). Perceptions of having 'enough' social activities were also protective against depression across time. The authors note that those older adults in the low participation category also had very poor health status, further exacerbating the barriers to engaging in activities as well as being a high correlate of depression itself.

Comorbidity

Cross-sectional studies have consistently shown a high association between depression and dementia. However, this relationship is not as straightforward when examined using longitudinal methodology. Greater degree of dementia (as reflected in higher scores on the Clinical Dementia Rating Scale) at baseline is not predictive of worsening depression over time (Barca, Selbaek et al. 2009). However, good cognitive functioning is associated with a significant decrease in depressive symptoms over eight years (Anstey et al. 2007b). Exploring the temporal nature of depressive symptoms and cognitive functioning, Bielak et al. (2011) showed that depressive symptoms predicted subsequent change in perceptual speed rather than vice versa (i.e. perceptual speed did not predict change in depressive symptoms). These findings indicate that depression may drive cognitive changes in late-life. There are a number of potential explanations for this effect: depression may elicit clinical symptoms of cognitive decline; depression may be an early prodromal indicator of cognitive decline; and depression may deplete cognitive resources, thereby increasing the risk of cognitive decline. While these hypotheses remain speculative, longitudinal research such as that of Bielak and colleagues provides substantive steps towards piecing together the puzzle.

While poor health is related to depression in older adults in cross-sectional research, the relationship is less clear longitudinally. For example, depression appears to be more robustly associated with physical functioning over time than with general poor health. In Anstey and colleagues' (2007b) longitudinal study of risk factors for depression in community and residential care samples, rate of change in depression scores was dependent on having physical and functional difficulties and worsening self-rated health, but was not related to medical conditions. Furthermore, transition from no functional difficulties to more than one was found to significantly increase depression scores. Functional limitations have been shown to be the strongest predictor of a chronic course of depression in late-life, signifying a high impact and level of disability between these two factors (Beekman et al. 2002).

Treatment

A recent 2009 meta-regression analysis (Cuijpers et al. 2009) showed that psychological therapies, including CBT were found to be as effective in older as younger adults. However, there was great heterogeneity among the studies included in the analysis, and the number of studies that directly compared younger and older cohorts was very rare. RCT placebo trials suggest that the efficacy of anti-depressants for treatment in late-life depression is reduced in adults over 65 years of age compared to those between 55 and 64 years (Tedeschini et al. 2011). It is not clear why this poor outcome for pharmacological treatments in older adults exists, though the link found between vascular burden and late-onset depression, along with poorer treatment outcomes found in those with vascular depression (Sheline et al. 2010), may provide answers in future research.

In another systematic review, the effectiveness of physical activity for reducing depressive symptoms in older adults was investigated (Blake et al. 2009). Again, there was great heterogeneity among studies, particularly relating to the type of physical activity (including tai chi, Qigong, gardening, and resistance /weight training), intensity and duration of the activities, and the follow-up periods. Nevertheless, the results were positive; indicating that engaging in some type of physical activity is beneficial for reducing depression symptoms and maintaining positive well-being over time.

ANXIETY

Anxiety disorders in older adults are understudied relative to mood and cognitive disorders. However, anxiety disorders are common and are associated with significant burden and disability. Most of what is known about the prevalence, risk factors, comorbidities, and treatment of anxiety in older adults is based on data from cross-sectional studies or short follow-up studies. As is the case with cognition and depression, however, certain questions regarding anxiety in older age can only be adequately answered through longitudinal designs.

Prevalence and incidence

Estimates of the prevalence of anxiety disorders in older adults show considerable variation, with studies reporting prevalence rates ranging from 4% to 14%. For example, data from the National Comorbidity Survey Replication (NCS-R) suggests that the twelve-months prevalence of any anxiety disorder in older persons is 7% (Gum, King-Kallimanis, and Kohn 2009), whereas using the same dataset Byers et al. (2010) reported this prevalence to be 12%. It is not the purpose of this chapter to provide an exhaustive review of the epidemiological evidence base regarding anxiety in older adults, but the interested reader is referred to a recent comprehensive review (Wolitzky-Taylor, Castriotta et al. 2010). Briefly, the variability in these estimates is likely to reflect mostly methodological differences in epidemiological studies with respect to such things as the age cut-off used to define older people, measures of anxiety used, diagnostic criteria applied, and which specific anxiety disorders are included.

Despite some inconsistency among researchers as to the prevalence of anxiety in older adults, there is a relative consensus that anxiety disorders are more prevalent in younger than in older adults, with estimates of anxiety disorders in younger adults ranging from 7.3% to 35.1% (see Wolitzky-Taylor et al. 2010, for a recent review).

Within the older adult population, cross-sectional studies generally report a decline in the prevalence of anxiety disorders with advancing age (Goncalves, Pachana, and Byrne 2011; Mackenzie et al. 2011). Some support for this hypothesis comes from the Longitudinal Aging Study Amsterdam (LASA), which showed that 31% of individuals who had an anxiety disorder at baseline (n = 112) were at complete remission at the six-year follow-up (Schuurmans et al. 2005). Importantly, 23% continued to meet diagnostic criteria by the six-year follow-up and a further 47% continued to display subclinical levels of anxiety. Taken together with the estimated incidence of anxiety disorders in older age (see below), these data seem to support the results from cross-sectional studies suggesting that the prevalence of anxiety disorders generally declines with age.

Recent reports from the National Epidemiological Survey of Alcohol and Related Conditions (NESARC, n = 8012, age > 60) provided some much-needed data on the incidence of mood, anxiety, and alcohol-related disorders in persons aged 55 and over. Using *DSM-IV* criteria, the one- and three-year incidence rates were found to be 0.4% and 0.8% for panic disorder, 0.1% and 0.6% for social phobia, 0.2% and 1.3% for specific phobia, and 0.7% and 1.6% for generalized anxiety disorder (Chou et al. 2011; Grant et al. 2008). When all anxiety disorders are considered together, these data suggest a 1.4% incidence over one year, or 4.3% over three years for any anxiety disorder.

Using data from LASA, Vink and colleagues (2009) reported a 5.6% incidence of clinically relevant anxiety symptoms in isolation (based on a cut-off of equal to or greater than 7 on the HADS-A), or 11.6% when combined with depression, over a nine-year period (n = 1,712) (Vink et al. 2009). This figure can be translated into a 1.3% incidence of clinically relevant symptoms of anxiety (either alone or in combination with depression), which interestingly closely echoes the findings by Chou et al. (2011) noted above.

Risk factors

Risk factors in relation to anxiety in older adults have been mostly studied in the context of cross-sectional study designs. However, insight into those factors that are associated with change in anxiety symptoms over time can only be gained using longitudinal approaches.

Examining three-year follow-up data, de Beurs and colleagues (2000) found that changes in anxiety over time were best predicted by female sex and neuroticism. Hearing and eyesight problems and distress due to life events were associated with becoming anxious, but not with persistence of anxiety. Over six years, however, neuroticism was found to be the single strongest predictor of persistent anxiety (Schuurmans et al. 2005). Examining the nine-year follow-up data, Vink and colleagues found death or illness of a partner/relative to be predictive of the onset of clinically significant anxiety symptoms, whereas loneliness and being a victim of crime predicted the development of combined anxiety and depression symptoms (Vink et al. 2009). Of note, in a model combining all predictors, the development of anxiety symptoms alone (i.e. without concomitant depression) was best predicted by greater anxiety symptoms at baseline, a finding which was also reported by Schoevers and colleagues using data from the Amsterdam Study of the Elderly (AMSTEL; Schoevers et al. 2005). Interestingly, in the study by de Beurs and colleagues (2000), although both vulnerability factors (e.g. demographic or personality characteristics) and stress factors (i.e. stressful life events between the two measurement time points) were found independently to predict change in anxiety over time, no interaction was found between vulnerability and stress-related factors.

Using three-year incidence data from the NESARC study, Chou et al. (2011) found that persons older than 80 years of age, and persons with a high income were at a higher risk of developing a first incident of panic disorder over three years than persons aged 60–69, or those on a low income. Furthermore, like de Beurs et al., these authors found that older women were more likely than older men to develop generalized anxiety disorder. Having a diagnosis of post-traumatic stress disorder (PTSD) at baseline increased the risk of incident panic disorder, specific phobia, and generalized anxiety disorder. Finally, meeting criteria for narcissistic personality disorder at baseline was related to an increased risk of developing generalized anxiety disorder over the three years. Importantly, unlike the study by de Beurs et al., Chou and colleagues found no evidence of an increase in the chance of newly diagnosed anxiety disorders over three years as a function of stressful life events or health-related factors during the study period. An important limitation of the study by Chou and colleagues is the unavailability of analysis of attrition data. Therefore, it is not possible to ascertain that the participants who dropped out of the study were not different in important ways from those who remained in the study.

Comorbidity

Anxiety often co-occurs with other psychological and medical conditions, and while such associations have been mostly detected and explored in the context of cross-sectional studies, longitudinal studies are necessary to characterize the nature and direction of such relationships.

Mood disorders, particularly depression, appear to be the most commonly reported comorbidity (Gonçalves et al. 2011). It is less clear, however, whether one disorder typically precedes the other or plays a role in its development. Others have indeed proposed a dimensional model in which depression and anxiety are part of the same continuum of psychopathology (Schoevers et al. 2003). Wetherell, Gatz, and Pedersen (2001) explored these issues in a longitudinal design over six years in middle-aged and older adults. Using structural equation modelling and confirmatory factor analysis, they found that although anxiety and depression were highly correlated, a model in which both appeared separately fitted the data better than a model which included a single mental health factor, or a model that included a positive and negative affect factor. Further, these authors found that anxiety was more stable than depression, and that over a period of six years, anxiety consistently led to depression, but depression did not consistently lead to anxiety (Wetherell et al. 2001). Wetherell and colleagues interpreted their findings to suggest that anxiety was more likely to be associated with a pervasive personality trait such as neuroticism, whereas depression tended to fluctuate more.

Support for a temporal sequencing of depression and anxiety in older persons comes from the AMSTEL study (n = 4,051). Schoevers et al. (2005) found that among those who met criteria for generalized anxiety disorder (GAD) at baseline (n = 25), 48% were in full remission by the three-year follow-up. However, for those 52% who were not in remission, the outcome was not favourable: 12% had persistent anxiety, 24% developed depression, and a further 16% developed comorbid depression and GAD. Conversely, only 2% of those who had depression at baseline met criteria for GAD at the three-year follow-up, with a further 13.6% developing comorbid anxiety and depression. Out of the 258 persons with psychopathology at baseline, 34 (13%) had comorbid anxiety and depression. Remission in this group was lowest, with only 27% in full remission at the three-year follow-up. Progression from GAD to comorbid anxiety/depression was associated with the presence of a comorbid medical illness.

Treatment

Studies have shown that in younger adults (aged less than 55 years) anxiety disorders show a chronic but variable course with intermittent periods of waxing and waning of symptoms when left untreated. In older adults, evidence suggests that pharmacological and non-pharmacological interventions alike are more effective than no treatment in improving symptoms (Gonçalves and Byrne 2011). In a two-year longitudinal study of community-dwelling adults in Quebec, Canada, Preville et al. (2011) reported that less than half (46.9%) of the older adults with a diagnosis of either depression or anxiety (n = 279) were treated with anti-depressants for an average of 400 days during the two years of the study. Conversely, 59% of individuals with a 'mental health' disorder used benzodiazepines (BZs) for a period of 338 days on average during the study period. Interestingly, those participants who during the follow-up evaluation were either in partial or full remission from a mental disorder (either depression or anxiety) were no different than those with persistent mental health issues in terms of the duration of anti-depressant or BZs use. The authors also found that over 10% of participants without a diagnosis of a mental health condition at either baseline or follow-up were nevertheless taking anti-depressants. This longitudinal study raised questions regarding the effectiveness and prescription practices of psychotropic medication for mental health issues among older community-dwellers.

Summary

Longitudinal research provides an essential resource for the understanding of psychiatric and neurocognitive disorders, how they differ from normative life-course development, predisposing factors, prognosis, and the efficacy and side effects of treatments. Longitudinal studies continue to be the only method available for linking risk factors occurring in early life, or adulthood, with late-life cognitive decline, depression, and anxiety. As more findings from these studies are published and as cohorts age, the body of evidence about the impact of health, environment, and life style on late-life mental disorders will increase.

Within a lifespan perspective, late-life onset of disorders such as depression and anxiety are less well understood than are early-onset depression and anxiety. A sample of the longitudinal work that has been done in this area has been presented in this chapter. Clinicians may refer to longitudinal research, as well as conduct their own time-dependent research, to learn of the validity of diagnostic criteria, expected prognosis of disorders and factors that may modify outcomes. The existing longitudinal datasets allow for questions to be answered that would otherwise be beyond the capacity of any cross-sectional or case study. This rich resource within the research community will continue to grow in significance with the inclusion of biomarkers, neuroimaging, life-history data, and linkage of datasets to health services registries.

Key References and Sources for Further Reading

Anstey, K. J. and Hofer, S. M. (2004). 'Longitudinal Designs, Methods and Analysis in Psychiatric Research'. *Australian and New Zealand Journal of Psychiatry* 38(3): 93–104.

Anstey, K. J., von Sanden, C., Sargent-Cox, K. and Luszcz, M. A. (2007b). 'Prevalence and Risk Factors for Depression in a Longitudinal, Population-based Study Including Individuals in the Community and Residential Care'. *American Journal of Geriatric Psychiatry* 15: 497–505.

Newsom, J. T., Jones, R. N., and Hofer, S. M. (eds) (2012). *Longitudinal Data Analysis: A Practical Guide for Researchers in Aging, Health and Social Sciences*. New York: Routledge.

Singer, J. D. and Willett, J. B. (2003). *Applied Longitudinal Data Analysis: Modeling Change and Event Occurrence*. Oxford: Oxford University Press.

Sutin, A. R., Terracciano, A., Milaneschi, Y., An, Y., Ferrucci, L. and Zonderman, A B. (2013). 'The Trajectory of Depressive Symptoms across the Adult Life Span'. *JAMA Psychiatry* 70(8): 803–811. doi:10.1001/jamapsychiatry.2013.193.

References

AccessEconomics (2009). *Keeping Dementia Front of Mind: Incidence and Prevalence 2009–2050*. Canberra, Alzheimer's Australia.

Akbaraly, T. N., Portet, F., Fustinoni, S., Dartigues, J.-F., Artero, S., Rouaud, O., et al. (2009). 'Leisure Activities and the Risk of Dementia in the Elderly: Results from the Three-City Study'. *Neurology* 73(11): 854–861.

Alexopoulos, G. S., B. S. Meyers, Kelber, S. T., and Prigerson, H. G. (1997). '"Vascular Depression" Hypothesis'. *Archives of General Psychiatry* 54(10): 915–922.

Allen, K. V., Frier, B. M., and Strachan, M. W. (2004). 'The Relationship between Type 2 Diabetes and Cognitive Dysfunction: Longitudinal Studies and their Methodological Limitations'. *European Journal of Pharmacology* 490(1–3): 169–175.

Anstey, K. J. and Luszcz, M. A.(2002). 'Mortality Risk Varies according to Gender and Change in Depressive Status in Very Old Adults'. *Psychosomatic Medicine* 64(6): 880–888.

Anstey, K. J. and Hofer, S. M. (2004). 'Longitudinal Designs, Methods and Analysis in Psychiatric Research'. *Australian and New Zealand Journal of Psychiatry* 38(3): 93–104.

Anstey, K. J., von Sanden, C., Salim, A., and O'Kearney, R. (2007a). 'Smoking as a Risk Factor for Dementia and Cognitive Decline: A Meta-analysis of Prospective Studies'. *American Journal of Epidemiology* 166(4): 367–378.

Anstey, K. J., von Sanden, C., Sargent-Cox, K., and Luszcz, M. A. (2007b). 'Prevalence and Risk Factors for Depression in a Longitudinal, Population-based Study Including Individuals in the Community and Residential Care'. *American Journal of Geriatric Psychiatry* 15: 497–505.

Anstey, K. J., Cherbuin, N., Christensen, H., Burns, R., Reglade-Meslin, C., Salim, A., et al. (2008). 'Follow-up of Mild Cognitive Impairment and Related Disorders over Four Years in Adults in their Sixties: The PATH Through Life Study'. *Dementia and Geriatric Cognitive Disorders* 26(3): 226–233.

Anstey, K. J., Lipnicki, D. M., and Low, L. F. (2008). 'Cholesterol as a Risk Factor for Dementia and Cognitive Decline: A Systematic Review of Prospective Studies with Meta-analysis'. *American Journal of Geriatric Psychiatry* 16(5): 343–354.

Anstey, K. J., Mack, H. A., and Cherbuin, N. (2009). 'Alcohol Consumption as a Risk Factor for Dementia and Cognitive Decline: Meta-analysis of Prospective Studies'. *American Journal of Geriatric Psychiatry* 17(7): 542–555.

Anstey, K. J., Burns, R. A., Birrell, C. L., Steel, D., Kiely, K. M., and Luszcz, M. A. (2010). 'Estimates of Probable Dementia Prevalence from Population-based Surveys Compared with Dementia Prevalence Estimates Based on Meta-analyses'. *BMC Neurology* 10: 62–73.

Barberger-Gateau, P., Raffaitin, C. Letenneur, L., Berr, C., Tsourio, C., Dartigues, J. F., et al. (2007). 'Dietary Patterns and Risk of Dementia—The Three-city Cohort Study'. *Neurology* 69(20): 1921–1930.

Barca, M. L., Selbaek, G., Laks, J., and Engedal, K. (2009). 'Factors Associated with Depression in Norwegian Nursing Homes'. *International Journal of Geriatric Psychiatry* 24: 417–425.

Barca, M. L., Engedal, K., Laks, J., and Selbaek, G. (2010). 'A 12 Months Follow-up Study of Depression among Nursing-home Patients in Norway'. *Journal of Affective Disorders* 120: 141–148.

Bassuk, S. S., Glass, T. A., and Berkman, L. F. (1999). 'Social Disengagement and Incident Cognitive Decline in Community-dwelling Elderly Persons'. *Annals of Internal Medicine* 131(3): 165–173.

Beekman, A., Deeg, D., Geerlings, S. W., Schoevers, R. A., Smit, J. H., and van Tilbur, W. (2001). 'Emergence and Persistence of Late Life Depression: A 3 Year Follow-up of the Longitudinal Aging Study Amsterdam'. *Journal of Affective Disorders* 65: 131–138.

Beekman, A., Geerlings, S. W., Deeg, D. J., Smit, J. H., Schoevers, R. S., de Beurs, E., et al. (2002). 'The Natural History of Late-life Depression: A 6-year Prospective Study in the Community'. *Archives of General Psychiatry* 59: 605–611.

de Beurs, E., Beekman, A., Deeg, D. J., Van Dyck, R., and van Tilburg, W. (2000). 'Predictors of Change in Anxiety Symptoms of Older Persons: Results from the Longitudinal Aging Study Amsterdam'. *Psychological Medicine* 30(03): 515–527.

Bielak, A. A. M., Gerstorf, D., Kiely, K. M., Anstey, K. J., and Luszcz, M. (2011). 'Depressive Symptoms Predict Decline in Perceptual Speed in Older Adults'. *Psychology and Aging* 6(3): 576–583. doi: 10.1037/a0023313.

Blake, H., Mo, P., Malik, S., and Thomas, S. (2009). 'How Effective are Physical Activity Interventions for Alleviating Depressive Symptoms in Older People? A Systematic Review'. *Clinical Rehabilitation* 23: 873–888.

Blazer, D. (2003). 'Depression in Late Life: Review and Commentary'. *Journal of Gerontology: Medical Sciences* 58A: 249–265.

Bruscoli, M. and Lovestone, S. (2004). 'Is MCI Really Just Early Dementia? A Systematic Review of Conversion Studies'. *International Psychogeriatrics* 16(2): 129–140.

Busse, A., Bischkopf, J., Riedel-Heller, S. G., and Angermeyer, M. C. (2003). 'Mild Cognitive Impairment: Prevalence and Incidence according to Different Diagnostic Criteria. Results of the Leipzig Longitudinal Study of the Aged (LEILA75+)'. *British Journal of Psychiatry* 182: 449–454.

Byers, A. L., Yaffe, K., Covinsky, K. E., Friedman, M. B., and Bruce, M. L. (2010). 'High Occurrence of Mood and Anxiety Disorders among Older Adults: The National Comorbidity Survey Replication'. *Archives of General Psychiatry* 67(5): 489–496.

Caamano-Isorna, F., Corral, M., Montes-Martínez, A., and Takkouche, B. (2006). 'Education and Dementia: A Meta-analytic Study'. *Neuroepidemiology* 26(4): 226–232.

Chou, K.-L., Mackenzie, C. S., Liang, K., and Sareen, J. (2011). 'Three-Year Incidence and Predictors of First-Onset of DSM-IV Mood, Anxiety, and Substance Use Disorders in Older Adults: Results From Wave 2 of the National Epidemiologic Survey on Alcohol and Related Conditions'. *Journal of Clinical Psychiatry* 72(2): 144–155.

Collie, A., Maruff, P., Darby, D. G., and McStephen, M. (2003). 'The Effects of Practice on Cognitive Test Performance of Neurologically Normal Individuals Assessed at Brief Test-retest Intervals'. *The Journal of the International Neuropsychological Society* 9: 419–428.

Cuijpers, P., van Straten, A., Smit, F., and Andersson, G. (2009). 'Is Psychotherapy for Depression Equally Effective in Younger and Older Adults? A Meta-regression Analysis'. *International Psychogeriatrics* 21: 16–24.

Curran, P. J. and Bauer, D. J. (2011). 'The Disaggregation of Within-person and Between-person Effects in Longitudinal Models of Change'. *Annual Review of Psychology* 62: 583–619.

Ehreke, L., Luck, T., Luppa M, König, H. H., Villringer, A., Riedel-Heller, S. G., et al. (2011). 'Clock Drawing Test—Screening Utility for Mild Cognitive Impairment according to Different Scoring Systems: Results of the Leipzig Longitudinal Study of the Aged (LEILA 75+)'. *International Psychogeriatrics* 23(10): 1592–1601.

d'Epinay, C. J., Cavalli, S., and Guillet, L. A. (2009). 'Bereavement in Very Old Age: Impact on Health and Relationships of the Loss of a Spouse, a Child, a Sibling, or a Close Friend'. *Omega* 60(4): 301–325.

Evans, A. C. (2006). 'The NIH MRI Study of Normal Brain Development'. *NeuroImage* 30(1): 184–202.

Fiske, A., Wetherell, J. L., and Gatz, M. (2009). 'Depression in Older Adults'. *Annual Review of Clinical Psychology* 5: 363–389.

Fratiglioni, L., Wang, H. X., Ericsson, K., Maytan, M., and Winblad, B. (2000). 'Influence of Social Network on Occurrence of Dementia: A Community-based Longitudinal Study'. *Lancet* 355(9212): 1315–1319.

Gillette-Guyonnet, S., Andrieu, S., Dantoine, T., Dartiques, J. F., Touchon, J., Vellas, B. et al. (2009). 'Commentary on "A Roadmap for the Prevention of Dementia II. Leon Thal Symposium 2008": The Multidomain Alzheimer Preventive Trial (MAPT): A New Approach to the Prevention of Alzheimer's Disease'. *Alzheimer's and Dementia* 5(2): 114–121.

Gonçalves, D. C. and Byrne, G. J. (2011). 'Interventions for Generalized Anxiety Disorder in Older Adults: Systematic Review and Meta-Analysis'. *Journal of Anxiety Disorders* 26(1): 1–11.

Gonçalves, D. C., Pachana, N. A., and Byrne, G. J. (2011). 'Prevalence and Correlates of Generalized Anxiety Disorder among Older Adults in the Australian National Survey of Mental Health and Well-Being'. *Journal of Affective Disorders* 132(1–2): 223–230.

Grant, B. F., Goldstein, R. B., Chou, S. P., Huang, B., Stinson, F. S., Dawson, D. A., et al. (2008). 'Sociodemographic and Psychopathologic Predictors of First Incidence of DSM-IV Substance Use, Mood and Anxiety Disorders: Results from the Wave 2 National Epidemiologic Survey on Alcohol and Related Conditions'. *Molecular Psychiatry* 14(11): 1051–1066.

Gum, A. M., King-Kallimanis, B., and Kohn, R. (2009). 'Prevalence of Mood, Anxiety, and Substance-abuse Disorders for Older Americans in the National Comorbidity Survey-replication'. *American Journal of Geriatric Psychiatry* 17(9): 769.

Hamer, M. and Chida, Y. (2009). 'Physical Activity and Risk of Neurodegenerative Disease: A Systematic Review of Prospective Evidence'. *Psychological Medicine* 39(1): 3–11.

Heikkinen, R.-L. and Kauppinen, M. (2004). 'Depressive Symptoms in Late Life: A 10-Year Follow-up'. *Archives of Gerontology and Geriatrics* 38: 239–250.

Helmer, C., Damon, D., Letenneur, L., Fabrigoule, C., Barberger-Gateau, P., Lafont, S., et al. (1999). 'Marital Status and risk of Alzheimer's Disease: A French Population-based Cohort Study'. *Neurology* 53(9): 1953–1958.

Hofer, S. M. and Sliwinski, M. J. (2001). 'Understanding Ageing: An Evaluation of Research Designs for Assessing the Interdependence of Ageing-related Changes'. *Gerontology* 47(6): 341–352.

Hofman, A., Rocca, W. A., Brayne, C., Breteler, M. M., Clarke, M., Cooper, B., et al. (1991). 'The Prevalence of Dementia in Europe: A Collaborative Study of 1980–1990 Findings'. *International Journal of Epidemiology* 20: 736–748.

Hong, S.-I., Hasche, L., and Bowland, S. (2009). 'Structural Relationships between Social Activities and Longitudinal Trajectories of Depression among Older Adults'. *The Gerontologist* 49: 1–11.

Horn, J. L. (1982). 'The Aging of Human Abilities'. In B. B. Wolman (ed), *Handbook of Developmental Psychology* (pp. 847–869). Englewood Cliffs, NJ: Prentice Hall.

Huang, T. L., Zandi, P. P., Tucker, K. L., Fitzpatrick, A. L., Kuller, L. H., Fried, L. P., et al. (2005). 'Benefits of Fatty Fish on Dementia Risk Are Stronger for Those without APOE epsilon4'. *Neurology* 65(9): 1409–1414.

Jack, C. R., Jr, Knopman, D., Jagust, W. J., Petersen, R. C., Weiner, M. W., Aisen, P. S., et al. (2013). 'Tracking Pathophysiological Processes in Alzheimer's Disease: An Updated Hypothetical Model of Dynamic Biomarkers'. *The Lancet Neurology* 12: 207–216.

Jorm, A. F., Dear, K. B., and Burgess, N. M. (2005). 'Projections of Future Numbers of Dementia Cases in Australia with and without Prevention'. *The Australian and New Zealand Journal of Psychiatry* 39(11–12): 959–963.

Kendler, K. S., Gatz, M., Gardner, C. O., and Pedersen, N. L. (2006). 'Personality and Major Depression: A Swedish Longitudinal, Population-based Twin Study'. *Archives of General Psychiatry* 63: 1113–1120.

Knopman, D. S., Edland, S. D., Cha, R. H., Petersen, R. C., and Rocca, W. A. (2007). 'Incident Dementia in Women is Preceded by Weight Loss by at least a Decade'. *Neurology* 69(8): 739–746.

Korkeila, J., Vahtera, J. Nabi, H., Kivimäki, M., Korkeila, K., Sumanen, M., et al. (2010). 'Childhood Adversities, Adulthood Life Events and Depression'. *Journal of Affective Disorders* 127(1–3): 130–138.

Kumar, R., Dear, K. B., Christensen, H., Ilschner, S., Jorm, A. F., Meslin, C., et al. (2005). 'Prevalence of Mild Cognitive Impairment in 60- to 64-year-old Community-dwelling Individuals: The Personality and Total Health through Life 60+ Study'. *Dementia and Geriatric Cognitive Disorders* 19(2–3): 67–74.

Launer, L. J., Andersen, K. Dewey, M. E., Letenneur, L., Ott, A., Amaducci, L. A., et al. (1999). 'Rates and Risk Factors for Dementia and Alzheimer's Disease: Results from EURODEM Pooled Analyses. EURODEM Incidence Research Group and Work Groups. European Studies of Dementia'. *Neurology* 52(1): 78–84.

Licht-Strunk, E., van der Windt, D. A. W. M., van Marwijk, H. W., de Haan, M., Beekman, A. T. (2007). 'The Prognosis of Depression in Older Patients in General Practice and the Community. A Systematic Review'. *Family Practice* 24: 168–180.

Lobo, A., Launer, L. J., Fratiglioni, L., Andersen, K., Di Carlo, A., Breteler, M. M., et al. (2000). 'Prevalence of Dementia and Major Subtypes in Europe: A Collaborative Study of Population-based Cohorts. Neurologic Diseases in the Elderly Research Group'. *Neurology* 54(11 Suppl. 5): S4–9.

Lu, F.-P., Lin, K.-P., and Kuo, H.-K. (2009). 'Diabetes and the Risk of Multi-System Aging Phenotypes: A Systematic Review and Meta-Analysis'. *PLoS One* 4(1): e4144. doi:10.1371/journal.pone.0004144.

Luck, T., Luppa, M., Briel, S., Matschinger, H., König, H. H., Bleich, S., et al. (2010a). 'Mild Cognitive Impairment: Incidence and Risk Factors: Results of the Leipzig Longitudinal Study of the Aged'. *Journal of the American Geriatrics Society* 58(10): 1903–1910.

Luck, T., Luppa, M., Briel, S., and Riedel-Heller, S. G. (2010b). 'Incidence of Mild Cognitive Impairment: A Systematic Review'. *Dementia and Geriatric Cognitive Disorders* 29(2): 164–175.

Luck, T., Luppa, M., Angermeyer, M. C., Villringer, A., König, H. H., and Riedel-Heller, S. G. (2011). 'Impact of Impairment in Instrumental Activities of Daily Living and Mild Cognitive Impairment on Time to Incident Dementia: Results of the Leipzig Longitudinal Study of the Aged'. *Psychological Medicine* 41(5): 1087–1097.

Luijendijk, H., van den Berg, J. F., Dekker, M. J., van Tuijl, H. R., Otte, W., Smit, F., et al. (2008). 'Incidence and Recurrence of Late-life Depression'. *Archives of General Psychiatry* 65: 1394–1401.

MacDonald, S. W. S., Hultsch, D. F., and Dixon, R. A. (2011). 'Aging and the Shape of Cognitive Change before Death: Terminal Decline or Terminal Drop?' *The Journals of Gerontology: Series B Psychological Science Social Science* 66B: 292–301.

Mackenzie, C. S., Reynolds, K., Chou, K. L., Pagura, J., and Sareen, J. (2011). 'Prevalence and Correlates of Generalized Anxiety Disorder in a National Sample of Older Adults'. *American Journal of Geriatric Psychiatry* 19(4): 305–315.

Mojtabai, R. (2011). 'Bereavement-related Depressive Episodes: Characteristics, 3-year Course, and Implications for the DSM-5'. *Archives of General Psychiatry* 68(9): 920–928.

Mormino, E. C., Kluth, J. T., Madison, C. M., Rabinovici, G. D., Baker, S. L., Miller, B. L., et al. (2009). 'Episodic Memory Loss is Related to Hippocampal-mediated Beta-amyloid Deposition in Elderly Subjects'. *Brain* 132(Pt 5): 1310–1323.

Mueller, T. I., Kohn, R., Leventhal, N., Leon, A. C., Solomon, D., Coryell, W., et al. (2004). 'The Course of Depression in Elderly Patients'. *American Journal of Geriatric Psychiatry* 12: 22–29.

Ott, C. H., Lueger, R. J., Kelber, S. T., and Prigerson, H. G. (2007). 'Spousal Bereavement in Older Adults: Common, Resilient, and Chronic Grief with Defining Characteristics'. *The Journal of Nervous and Mental Disease* 195(4): 332–341.

Pachana, N. A., Byrne, G. J., Siddle, H., Koloski, N, Harley, E, and Arnold, E. (2007). 'Development and Validation of the Geriatric Anxiety Inventory'. *International Psychogeriatrics* 19(1): 103–114.

Petersen, R. C., Doody, R., Kurz, A., Mohs, R. C., Morris, J. C., Rabins, P. V., et al. (2001). 'Current Concepts in Mild Cognitive Impairment'. *Archives of Neurology* 58(12): 1985–1992.

Plassman, B. L., Havlik, R. J., Steffens, D. C., Helms, M. J., Newman, T. N., and Drosdick, D., et al. (2000). 'Documented Head Injury in Early Adulthood and Risk of Alzheimer's Disease and Other Dementias'. *Neurology* 55(8): 1158–1166.

Preville, M., Vasiliadis, H.-M., Bossé, C., Dionne, P. A., Voyer, P., and Brassard, J. (2011). 'Pattern of Psychotropic Drug Use among Older Adults Having a Depression or an Anxiety Disorder: Results from the Longitudinal ESA Study'. *Canadian Journal of Psychiatry-Revue Canadienne De Psychiatrie* 56(6): 348–357.

Rast, P., MacDonald, S. W. S., and Hofer, S. M. (2012). 'Intensive Measurement Designs for Research on Aging'. *Geropsych: The Journal of Gerontopsychology and Geriatric Psychiatry* 25: 45–55.

Ritchie, K. and Kildea, D. (1995). 'Is Senile Dementia "Age-related" or "Ageing-related"?—Evidence from Meta-analysis of Dementia Prevalence in the Oldest Old'. *Lancet* 346(8980): 931–934.

Ritchie, L. J. and Tuokko, H. (2010). 'Patterns of Cognitive Decline, Conversion Rates, and Predictive Validity for 3 Models of MCI'. *American Journal of Alzheimer's Disease and Other Dementias* 25(7): 592–603.

Roman, G. C., Tatemichi, T. K., Erkinjuntti, T., Cummings, J. L., Masdeu, J. C., Garcia, J. H., et al. (1993). 'Vascular Dementia: Diagnostic Criteria for Research Studies. Report of the NINDS-AIREN International Workshop'. *Neurology* 43(2): 250–260.

Saczynski, J. S., Pfeifer, L. A., Masaki, K., Korf, E. S., Laurin, D., White, L., et al. (2006). 'The Effect of Social Engagement on Incident Dementia: The Honolulu-Asia Aging Study'. *American Journal of Epidemiology* 163(5): 433–440.

Salthouse, T. A. (2004). 'What and When of Cognitive Aging'. *Current Directions in Psychological Science* 13(4): 140–144.

Savica, R. and Petersen, R. C. (2011). 'Prevention of Dementia'. *The Psychiatric Clinics of North America* 34(1): 127–145.

Scarmeas, N., Luchsinger, J. A., Schupf, N., Brickman, A. M., Cosentino, S., Tang, M. X., et al. (2009). 'Physical Activity, Diet, and Risk of Alzheimer Disease'. *Journal of the American Medical Association* 302(6): 627–637.

Schoevers, R., Beekman, A., Deeg, D. J., Jonker, C., and van Tilburg, W. (2003). 'Comorbidity and Risk-patterns of Depression, Generalised Anxiety Disorder and Mixed Anxiety-depression in Later Life: Results from the AMSTEL Study'. *International Journal of Geriatric Psychiatry* 18(11): 994–1001.

Schoevers, R. A., Deeg, D., van Tilburg, W., and Beekman, A. T. (2005). 'Depression and Generalized Anxiety Disorder: Co-occurrence and Longitudinal Patterns in Elderly Patients'. *American Journal of Geriatric Psychiatry* 13(1): 31–39.

Schofield, P. W., Tang, M., Marder, K., Bell, K., Dooneief, G., Chun, M. et al. (1997). 'Alzheimer's Disease after Remote Head Injury: An Incidence Study'. *Journal of Neurology, Neurosurgery & Psychiatry* 62(2): 119–124.

Schuurmans, J., Comijs, H., Beekman, A. T., de Beurs, E., Deeg, D. J., Emmelkamp, P. M., et al. (2005). 'The Outcome of Anxiety Disorders in Older People at 6-year Follow-up: Results from the Longitudinal Aging Study Amsterdam'. *Acta Psychiatrica Scandinavica* 111(6): 420–428.

Sheline, Y. I., Pieper, C. F., Barch, D. M., Welsh-Boehmer, K., McKinstry, R. C., MacFall, J. R., et al. (2010). 'Support for the Vascular Depression Hypothesis in Late-life Depression: Results of a 2-ste, Prospective, Antidepressant Treatment Trial'. *Archives of General Psychiatry* 67(3): 277–285.

Singer, J. D. and Willett, J. B. (2003). *Applied Longitudinal Data Analysis: Modeling Change and Event Occurrence*. Oxford: Oxford University Press.

Sliwinski, M. J., Almeida, D. M., Smyth, J., and Stawski, R. S. (2009). 'Intraindividual Change and Variability in Daily Stress Processes: Findings from Two Measurement-burst Diary Studies'. *Psychology and Aging* 24: 828–840.

Steunenberg, B., Beekman, A., Deeg, D. J., and Kerkhof, A. J. (2010). 'Personality Predicts Recurrence of Late-life Depression'. *Journal of Affective Disorders* 123: 164–172.

Takkinen, S., Gold, C. H., Pedersen, N. L., Malmberg, B., Nilsson, S., and Rovine, M. (2004). 'Gender Differences in Depression: A Study of Older Unlike-sex Twins'. *Aging & Mental Health* 8: 187–195.

Tedeschini, E., Levkovitz, Y., Lovieno, N., Ameral, V. E., Craig, N. J., and Papakostas, G. L. (2011). 'Efficacy of Antidepressants for Late-life Depression: A Meta-analysis and Meta-regression of Placebo-controlled Randomized Trials'. *The Journal of Clinical Psychiatry* 72: 1660–1668.

Tuokko, H. A. and McDowell, I. (2006). 'An Overview of Mild Cognitive Impairment'. In H. A. Tuokko and D. F. Hultsch (eds), *Mild Cognitive Impairment: International Perspectives* (pp. 3–28). New York: Taylor and Francis.

Vink, D., Aartsen, M. J., Comijs, H. C., Heymans, M. W., Penninx, B. W., Stek, M. L., et al. (2009). 'Onset of Anxiety and Depression in the Aging Population: Comparison of Risk Factors in a 9-Year Prospective Study'. *American Journal of Geriatric Psychiatry* 17(8): 642–652.

Wetherell, J. L., Gatz, M., and Pedersen, N. L. (2001). 'A Longitudinal Analysis of Anxiety and Depressive Symptoms'. *Psychology and Aging* 16(2): 187–195.

Whalley, L. J., Dick, F. D., and McNeill, G. (2006). 'A Life-course Approach to the Aetiology of Late-onset Dementias'. *Lancet Neurology* 5(1): 87–96.

Williams, J. W., Plassman, B. L., Burke, J., Holsinger, T., and Benjamin, S. (2010). 'Preventing Alzheimer's Disease and Cognitive Decline'. Evidence Report/Technology Assessment 193. Report No.: 10-E005. Rockville, MD: Agency for Healthcare Research and Quality (US).

Willis, S. L., Tennstedt, S. L., Marsiske, M., Ball, K., Elias, J., Koepke, K. M., et al. (2006). 'Long-term Effects of Cognitive Training on Everyday Functional Outcomes in Older Adults'. *Journal of the American Medical Association* 296(23): 2805–2814.

Wilson, R. S., Scherr, P. A., Schneider, J. A., Tang, Y., and Bennett, D. A. (2007). 'Relation of Cognitive Activity to Risk of Developing Alzheimer Disease'. *Neurology* 69(20): 1911–1920.

Winblad, B., Palmer, K., Kivipelto, M., Jelic, V., Fratiglioni, L., Wahlund, L. O., et al. (2004). 'Mild Cognitive Impairment—Beyond Controversies, towards a Consensus: Report of the International Working Group on Mild Cognitive Impairment'. *Journal of Internal Medicine* 256(3): 240–246.

Withall, A., Brodaty, H., Attendorf, A., and Sachdev, P. (2011). 'A Longitudinal Study Examining the Independence of Apathy and Depression after Stroke: The Sydney Stroke Study'. *International Psychogeriatrics* 23(2): 264–273.

Wolitzky-Taylor, K. B., Castriotta, N., Lenze, E. J., Stanley, M. A., and Craske, M. G. (2010). 'Anxiety Disorders in Older Adults: A Comprehensive Review'. *Depression and Anxiety* 27(2): 190–211.

Yang, Y. (2006). 'How Does Functional Disability Affect Depressive Symptoms in Late Life? The Role of Perceived Social Support and Psychological Resources'. *Journal of Health and Social Behavior* 47: 355–372.

Yochim, B. P., Mueller, A. E., June, A., and Segal, D. L. (2011). 'Psychometric Properties of the Geriatric Anxiety Scale: Comparison to the Beck Anxiety Inventory and Geriatric Anxiety Inventory'. *Clinical Gerontologist* 34(1): 21–33.

CHAPTER 4

META-ANALYSES IN CLINICAL GEROPSYCHOLOGY

MARTIN PINQUART AND SILVIA SÖRENSEN

INTRODUCTION

CLINICIANS and other practitioners need skills for obtaining and (critically) evaluating up-to-date information from scientific sources. Evidence-based practice (EBP) has become the norm for effective clinical practice. It includes the use of best scientific evidence integrated with clinical experience and patient values and preferences in the practice of professional patient care (Sackett et al. 2000). EBP is founded on a hierarchy of scientific evidence with (1) *meta-analysis* of randomized controlled trials (RCTs) being considered the highest level of research evidence, followed by (2) evidence from at least one RCT, (3) evidence from at least one controlled study without randomization, (4) evidence from at least one other type of quasi-experimental study, (5) evidence from nonexperimental descriptive studies, such as comparative studies, correlation studies, and case control studies, and (6) opinions and/or clinical experience of respected authorities as the lowest level of evidence (Shakelle et al. 1999).

In the present chapter, we briefly summarize the meta-analytic approach and discuss advantages and disadvantages of meta-analysis. Subsequently, we summarize the results of recent meta-analyses in clinical geropsychology focusing on studies of the effects of behavioural and psychotherapeutic interventions with older adults that have been published in the last decade.

THE META-ANALYTIC APPROACH

Meta-analysis is a research review method that combines the evidence of multiple primary studies by employing *statistical methods*, thus enhancing the objectivity and validity of findings (Glass 1976). It presupposes a clear definition of the research question, the systematic search of the available literature, and a precise definition of eligibility criteria for individual studies. Three kinds of inclusion criteria have to be fulfilled: first, there are content-specific criteria, for example regarding the age range studied. Second, included studies should meet predefined criteria of quality, such as the use of a well-described study population, sampling procedure, valid measures, and appropriate statistical tests, as well as sufficient numbers of completers (80% and higher), adequate study design (e.g. RCT in intervention research), measures, and lack of serious flaws (e.g. control for confounding variables; Valentine 2009). Third, the studies included in the analysis must provide sufficient statistical information for computing effect sizes. When the direction of the effect is provided without exact effect size, the effect sizes can be estimated with statistical procedures (e.g. Bushman and Wang 1995). Although these estimations may differ somewhat from the exact effect size, the inclusion of these estimations leads to lower bias than excluding this study or setting its effect size to zero.

The statistical procedures of meta-analyses encompass five steps (Borenstein et al. 2009; Lipsey and Wilson 2001, Figure 4.1):

- *Step 1.* Because available studies often use different assessments (e.g. different depression scales), the effect sizes of these studies must be made comparable, using three standardized measures:
  (a) standardized mean differences (e.g. difference between post-test scores of the intervention group and the control group, divided by the pooled standard deviation);

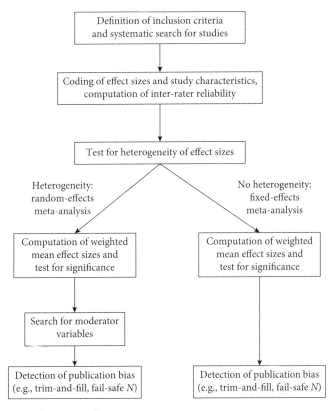

FIGURE 4.1 Steps of meta-analyses.

(b) odds ratios, which is the ratio of the odds of an event occurring in one group (e.g. remission) to the odds of it occurring in another group; or

(c) correlation coefficients (when analysing the size of association between two variables).

Inter-rater reliability of the effect sizes and other coded characteristics of the studies should be reported in meta-analyses. The effect sizes can be adjusted for sources of bias, such as the overestimation of effect sizes in small samples.

- *Step 2*. The heterogeneity of effect sizes is tested; that is, whether they vary between studies beyond random measurement error.
- *Step 3*. The weighted overall effect size is computed across all studies that fulfil the inclusion criteria. A significant advantage of the meta-analysis method is that larger, more reliable studies receive a larger weight. Subsequently, it is tested whether the weighted mean effect size differs statistically significant from zero. Because meta-analyses pool the results of studies, they have more test power than individual studies for identifying small or even very small effects. Two statistical estimations can be used. *Fixed effects models* assume that the studies included in the meta-analysis estimate the same underlying 'true' effect that is 'fixed', and that the observed differences across studies are due to random error. *Random effects models* are preferred when there is significant between-study variability of the effect sizes. In random effects models it is assumed that the studies included in the meta-analysis are only a random sample of a theoretical universe of all possible studies on a given research question, and that these studies vary in the size of their effects. The random effects model and the fixed effects model yield similar results if the variability of effect sizes between studies is low.
- *Step 4*. If the effect sizes are heterogeneous, careful investigation of the potential causes must be accomplished. The general approach is to test whether the effect sizes of the individual studies vary by study characteristics, such as the number of sessions of the intervention or participant age (moderator analysis). This analysis is important for identifying optimal characteristics of an intervention (e.g. regarding number of sessions needed for highest effects) or defining a group of persons who will benefit most from it.
- *Step 5*. Several procedures have been suggested for dealing with the fact that it is usually impossible to collect all available studies and that studies with non-significant effects may be less likely to be published (the 'file-drawer problem,' Rosenthal 1979). The fail-safe number estimates the number of unidentified studies with null results that would be needed to reduce the average effect size to a point of non-significance (Rosenthal 1979). Duval and Tweedie (2000) developed a method of imputing missing studies, based on the assumption that in funnel plots the effect sizes of individual studies should be equally distributed on both sides of the mean effect size. However, the results of the so-called trim-and-fill procedure have to be interpreted with caution because publication bias is difficult to detect in the case of small numbers of studies, and criteria other than the missing of studies could lead to an asymmetrical distribution of effect sizes (Borenstein et al. 2009). Nonetheless, these analyses provide important information about the robustness of the statistical effects.

Special software for meta-analysis is available, such as Comprehensive Meta-analysis (CMA), MetAnalysis, MetaWin, MIX, RevMan, and WEasyMA, with CMA and MIX scoring highest on usability and having the most complete set of analytical features (Bax et al. 2007). Most meta-analytical procedures can also be computed with macros developed for general statistical packages, such as SPSS and SAS (Lipsey and Wilson 2001) as well as STATA (Bradburn et al. 2003).

Useful formal guides for writing meta-analyses and interpreting the quality of reporting of meta-analyses have been published, such as the guidelines for meta-analyses evaluating diagnostic tests (Irwig et al. 1994), the QUOROM (Quality of Reporting of Meta-analyses) guidelines for meta-analyses of controlled trials (Moher et al. 1999), the MOOSE guidelines (Meta-analysis of Observational Studies in Epidemiology; Stroup et al. 2000), the American Psychological Association Meta-Analysis Reporting Standards (MARS) (APA Publications and Communications Board Working Group on Journal Article Reporting Standards 2008), and the PRISMA Statement (Preferred Reporting Items for Systematic Reviews and Meta-Analyses) (Moher et al. 2009). These guidelines refer to the report of all relevant aspects of the meta-analysis. However, the quality of a meta-analysis also strongly depends upon content-related criteria, namely measures used for getting access to all relevant studies (e.g. search in all relevant electronic databases, attempts often made to obtain missing data from authors of primary studies), application of adequate inclusion criteria (e.g. use of randomized controlled studies in intervention research), high inter-rater reliability, use of adequate statistical procedures (e.g. computation of random effects in the case of heterogeneous effect sizes), assessment of possible publication bias, and correct interpretation of the results.

In addition, the Cochrane Collaboration, an international network of more than 28,000 researchers from over 100 countries prepares systematic reviews and meta-analyses according to a standardized protocol (Higgins and Green 2011). These reviews are published online in the *Cochrane Library*. As Cochrane reviews include only studies of the highest quality, the final number of included studies is often very low and the analyses have low statistical power. Therefore, many researchers prefer to include relevant lower-quality studies and to test whether effect sizes vary by study quality. If there is not such variation, these more inclusive meta-analyses tend to yield more robust estimations of effect sizes.

In sum, meta-analyses provide a compact overview over a field of research and they can guide practitioners in the selection of evidence-based interventions. Their main advantages are:

(a) the inclusion of large numbers of studies on a particular topic (while qualitative reviews often restrict the number of included studies for reasons of clarity and comprehensibility);
(b) quantification of mean effect sizes;
(c) statistical testing of the significance and homogeneity of the effect sizes across available studies;
(d) identification of small effects that would be overlooked in studies with small sample sizes and in qualitative reviews that report only the number of studies with statistically significant results;
(e) use of standardized criteria for interpreting the effect sizes (e.g. Cohen 1992);
(f) testing whether the results may be affected by a publication bias; and
(g) testing for moderating effects of study characteristics.

Meta-analyses are less error-prone than qualitative reviews, due to the use of standardized statistical procedures. For example, Bushman and Wells (2001) report that qualitative reviewers are influenced by the titles of studies (i.e. whether they refer to statistically significant effects). In contrast, reviewers with some experience in meta-analysis judged studies on the basis of the effect sizes in the results sections, irrespective of the study's title.

Nonetheless, some limitations of meta-analyses exist. First, meta-analyses cannot integrate the results from qualitative studies. If quantitative and qualitative research is available on a topic, it may be useful to combine the meta-analysis of quantitative results with a systematic qualitative review of the qualitative results. Second, a minimum number of empirical studies is needed for computing a meta-analysis to be worthwhile. Although meta-analytics can be performed, in principle, for only two studies, these results are unlikely to be robust when additional studies become available. Third, available studies have to show sufficient similarity (e.g. regarding the kind of intervention and assessed outcome variables). The critique that meta-analyses mix apples and oranges holds true if the included studies do not share many similarities. Nonetheless, meta-analyses can test whether subgroups of studies find identical effects and whether apples and oranges can therefore be combined into a category of 'fruits'. Fourth, the results of meta-analyses depend upon the quality of the available studies. For example, if randomized controlled intervention studies are lacking, the conclusions drawn from meta-analysis about a particular kind of intervention will be limited. Finally, meta-analyses tend to be more cost-intensive than narrative reviews as they often include larger numbers of studies and because most meta-analyses use special commercial software (Bax et al. 2007).

META-ANALYSES IN THE FIELD OF CLINICAL GEROPSYCHOLOGY

Meta-analyses on correlational studies in geropsychology

In principle, meta-analyses can be applied in all fields of clinical geropsychology as long as there is sufficient quantitative research. We highlight four areas of focus and cite some representative studies for each.

Epidemiological data on mental health problems in old age

Based on 69 studies, a meta-analysis by Mitchell et al. (2010) reported an average prevalence of late-life depression in geriatric patients and nursing home residents of 29.2%. Possibly attributable to limited power, prevalence did not differ between inpatients, outpatients, and residents of nursing homes.

Risk factors for mental health problems in older adults

A meta-analysis of twenty studies by Cole and Dendukuri (2003) identified disability, new medical illness, poor health status, prior depression, poor self-perceived health, and bereavement as risk factors for depression in old age. Meta-analysing twenty-five studies, Kraaij,

Arensman, and Spinhoven (2002) found that almost all negative life events appeared to have a small but significant correlation with geriatric depression (e.g. death of a significant other $r = .10$; severe illness of significant others $r = .10$). The total number of negative life events ($r = .15$) and the total number of daily hassles ($r = .41$) appeared to have the strongest relationship with depression. Finally, Tenev, Robinson, and Jorge (2010), using six studies, showed that a severe stressor (stroke) had a stronger effect on the risk for depression if the patient showed elevated vulnerability as indicated by a family history of depression. More concretely, family history of depression increased the average risk for post-stroke depression by 46%.

Accuracy of diagnostic instruments

In a meta-analysis of eleven studies, Heo, Murphy, and Meyers (2007) showed that the Hamilton Depression Rating Scale and the Montgomery-Asberg Depression Rating Scale yield very similar results, with aggregated correlations between the two measures ranging from $r = .80$ to $.88$. Sensitivity refers to the ability of an instrument to detect a specified disease whereas specificity refers to the ability of an instrument to correctly identify disease-free individuals. Mitchell et al. (2010) compared the diagnostic validity of different versions of the Geriatric Depression Scale (GDS) across sixty-nine studies. The GDS30, GDS15, and the GDS4/5 did not differ significantly with regard to sensitivity (81.9%–92.5%) and specificity (73.8%–77.7%), thus indicating that fewer items did not impair the ability of the instrument to detect clinical depression in old age. Compared to self-ratings in the prediction of depression, subjective memory complaints showed low sensitivity in predicting dementia (18.5%–43.0%) although the specificity of these scales was high (85.8%–86.9%; Mitchell et al. 2010).

The course of diseases

Han et al. (2000) reported that across thirty-seven studies, older adults with Alzheimer's disease show an average decline of the Mini Mental State Examination (MMSE) scores of 3.3 scale points per years. However, the decline was stronger in the case of higher MMSE scores at pre-test, thus indicating non-linear change.

META-ANALYSES IN THE FIELD OF PREVENTION AND INTERVENTION

We will summarize the meta-analyses on available behavioural and psychotherapeutic interventions that have been published in the last decade (see Table 4.1). The meta-analyses were identified with a literature search in the electronic databases Medline, PsycINFO, and the Cochrane Library. If not otherwise stated, we report effect sizes of interventions that control for non-specific change in the control condition. The magnitude of the effect size (d) represents group differences in standard deviation units. Effect sizes of $d = .20$ to $.49$ are interpreted as small; $d = .50$ to $.79$ indicates medium-sized effects, and $d \geq .80$ indicates large effect sizes, as suggested by Cohen (1992).

Table 4.1 Summary of recent meta-analyses in the field of behavioural/psychotherapeutic interventions (ordered by topic and year of publication)

Authors	Target problem	Intervention	Number and kind of studies included[1]	Age	Mean controlled standardized effect size
Treatment or prevention of depression					
Pincuart and Sörensen (2001)	depressive symptoms	psychosocial and psychotherapeutic interventions	122 CT	55+	d = .43 (self-rated depression)
					d = 1.03 (clinician–rated depression)
Bohlmeijer et al. (2003)	depression	reminiscence	15 RCT, 5 NCT, REM	65+	d = .84 (self-rated depression)
Pinquart et al. (2007)	depression	behavioural interventions, psychotherapy	50 RCT, 7 NCT	60+	d = .87 (self-rated depression)
					d = .93 (clinician–rated depression)
Wilson (2009)	depression	psychotherapy	9 RCT	55+	d = 1.77 (CBT, no-treatment control, HDRS)
					d = .77 (CBT, active control, HDRS)
					d = .32 (CBT, active control, GDS)
Kang-Yi and Gellis (2010)	depression	community-based health interventions for homebound older adults with heart disease	10 RCT	64+	d = .10
Dai et al. (2011)	depression in Chinese inpatients	psychotherapy	12 RCT	60+	d = .80
Forsman et al. (2011)	depression	prevention	15 RCT, 4 NCT	60+	d = .17
Pinquart and Forstmeier (2012)	depression	reminiscence	69 RCT, 47 NCT	60+	d = .53 (total)
					d = 1.09 (depressed patients)
Treatment of anxiety					
Nordhus and Pallesen (2003)	anxiety	behavioural interventions	15 UCT/CT	55+	d = .55
Pinquart and Duberstein (2007)	anxiety disorders	behavioural interventions	12 RCT, 1 NCT, 6 UCT	60+	d = .80

Study	Condition	Intervention	Studies	Age	Effect size
Hendricks et al. (2008)	anxiety disorders	cognitive-behavioural therapy	7 RCT	60+	*d* = **.44** (compared to WLC); *d* = **.55** (compared to active control condition)
Thorp et al. (2009)	anxiety symptoms or anxiety disorders	cognitive-behavioural therapy, relaxation	14 CT, 5 UCT	63+	*d* = **.90** (relaxation training); *d* = .00–.33 (CBT without/with relaxation training)
Jung et al. (2010)	fear of falling	education, exercise, encouragement…	3 RCT, 3 NCT	75+	*d* = **.21**

Treatment of symptoms of dementia

Study	Condition	Intervention	Studies	Age	Effect size
Woods et al. (2005)	cognitive symptoms	reminiscence	4 RCT	60+	*d* = .27 (post-test); *d* = **.50** (follow-up)
Woods (2008)	memory problems	cognitive training	9 RCT	66+	*d* = -.06–**52**
Sizer et al. (2006)	cognitive symptoms	cognitive training	14 RCT, 3 NCT	66+	*d* = **.47**
Kong et al. (2008)	agitation in dementia	behavioural interventions	14 RT	Not specified	*d* = **1.07** (sensory interventions)
Zetteler (2008)	challenging behaviour	simulated presence therapy	4 CT	64+	*d* = **.70**

Treatment of insomnia

Study	Condition	Intervention	Studies	Age	Effect size
Irwin et al. (2006)[1]	insomnia	behavioural (CBT, relaxation)	8 RCT	55+	*d* = -.19 (sleep time) to *d* = **.73** (wakenings after sleep onset)
Montgomery and Dennis (2009)	insomnia	cognitive-behavioural treatment	6 RCT	59+	Only nonstandardized effect sizes

Interventions with care-givers of older adults

Study	Condition	Intervention	Studies	Age	Effect size
Acton and Kang (2001)	burden of dementia care-givers	care-giver interventions (support, education, respite,...)	17 CT, 7 UCT	not specified	*d* = -.08
Yin et al. (2002)	burden of mixed care-givers	care-giver interventions (support, education, respite,...)	11 RCT, 15 NCT	not specified	*d* = **.41**

(continued)

Table 1 Continued

Authors	Target problem	Intervention	Number and kind of studies included[1]	Age	Mean controlled standardized effect size
Sörensen et al. (2002)	psychological outcomes of mixed care-givers	care-giver interventions	78 CT	M = 62.3	$d = .41$ (knowledge) $d = .37$ (pos. well-being) $d = .20$ (symptoms of care recipient) $d = .15$ (burden) $d = .14$ (care-giver depression) $d = .15$ (benefits)
Brodaty et al. (2003)	psychological outcomes of dementia care-giving	care-giver interventions	21 RCT, 10 NRT	55+	$d = .51$ (knowledge) $d = .31$ (distress) $d = .09$ (burden) $d = .68$ (patient mood)
Pinquart and Sörensen (2006)	psychological outcomes of dementia care-giving	care-giver interventions	127 CT	M = 63	$d = .12$ (burden) $d = .24$ (depression) $d = .31$ (positive well-being) $d = .46$ (knowledge) $d = .17$ (symptoms of care recipient) $OR = .77$ (risk for institutionalization)
Lee et al. (2007)	mental health of stroke care-givers	care-giver interventions	4 RCT	M = 61.1	$d = .28$
Northouse et al. (2010)	mental health of cancer care-givers	care-giver interventions	29 RCT	M = 55	$d = .25$ (self-efficacy) $d = .22$ (burden) $d = .20–.47$ (coping) $d = .16–.29$ (psychol. distress) $d = .17$ (benefits) $d = -.06$ to .06 (depression)
Chien et al. (2011)	psychosoc. outcomes of dementia care-givers	support groups	20 RCT, 10 NCT	44+	$d = .44$ (psych. well-being) $d = .40$ (depression) $d = .40$ (social outcomes) $d = .23$ (burden)

Vernooij-Dassen et al. (2011)	mental health of dementia care-givers	cognitive reframing interventions	11 RCT	M = 59	*d* = **.66** (depression) *d* = **.64** (self-efficacy) *d* = **.24** (stress) *d* = **.21** (anxiety) *d* = .21 (memory /behav. problems of care recipient) *d* = .14 (burden)

Bereavement interventions

Currier et al. (2008)	psychological distress after bereavement	bereavement interventions	61 CT	M = 40.4	*d* = **.16** (randomized studies) *d* = **.51** (non-randomized studies)
Wittouck et al. (2011)	complicated grief after bereavement	bereavement interventions	14 RCT	M = 41	*d* = **.53** (therapy) *d* = .00 (prevention)

Improvement of broad indicators of positive well-being

Pinquart and Sörensen (2001)	positive well-being	psychosocial and psychotherapeutic interventions	122 CT	55+	*d* = **.45**
Chin (2007)	positive well-being	reminiscence	12 RCT, 3 NCT		*d* = **1.09** (happiness) *d* = **.55** (self-esteem) *d* = .22 (life-satisfaction)
Bohlmeijer et al. (2007)	positive well-being	reminiscence	13 RCT, 2 NCT	60+	*d* = **.54**
Pinquart and Forstmeier (2012)[1]	positive well-being, ego-integrity	reminiscence	69 RCT, 47 NCT	60+	*d* = **.63** (ego-integrity) *d* = **.36** (pos. well-being)

Notes. [1] If the meta-analysis also reports results for younger adults, we included only the results of older adults. CBT = cognitive-behavioural therapy; CT = controlled trial; *d* = effect size (in standard deviation units; positive scores indicate improvement); GDS = Geriatric Depression Scale; HDRS = Hamilton Depression Rating Scale; NCT = non-randomized controlled trial; OR = odds ratio (scores < 1 indicate that the intervention reduced the odds of a defined event); RCT = randomized controlled trial; RT = randomized trial; UCT = uncontrolled trials; WLC = wait-list control condition. Significant improvements are printed in bold.

Among the ageing population, depression and anxiety are the most prevalent mental health problems (Iliffe and Manthorpe 2002). Thus, larger numbers of intervention studies and meta-analyses have dealt with behavioural treatments of depressive symptoms and anxiety in old age.

Depression

In the first large meta-analysis on psychological interventions in old age, Pinquart and Sörensen (2001) analysed the effects of controlled psychosocial and psychotherapeutic interventions on self-rated depression (ninety-one interventions) and clinician-rated depression of older adults (thirty-one interventions). The studies included both individuals with and without a clinical depression diagnosis. Psychotherapeutic interventions showed moderate improvements of self-rated depression ($d = .64$) while non-therapeutic interventions (such as self-help groups) had only small effects ($d = .28$). In addition, large improvements of clinician-rated depression were observed in therapeutic interventions ($d = 1.07$) as compared to moderate improvements in non-therapeutic interventions ($d = .63$).

In a meta-analysis of fifty-seven controlled studies of behavioural and psychotherapeutic interventions with depressed older adults, Pinquart, Duberstein, and Lyness (2007) found that self-rated depression improved by $d = .84$ and clinician-rated depression improved by $d = .93$. Significant improvements of self-rated ($d = .49$) and clinician-rated depression ($d = 1.01$) were also found at follow-up (about thirty-one weeks after the end of the intervention). Effect sizes at post-test were large for cognitive and behavioural therapy (CBT; $d = 1.06$) and reminiscence ($d = 1.00$); and medium for psychodynamic therapy ($d = .76$), psychoeducation ($d = .70$), physical exercise ($d = .73$), and supportive interventions ($d = .57$). Effects did not vary between group format and one-to-one format, or by number of sessions. However, effect sizes were smaller for individuals with medical comorbidities or cognitive impairments.

Another meta-analysis by these authors showed that improvements of clinician-rated depression were significantly higher in psychotherapeutic interventions ($d = 1.09$) than in pharmacological interventions ($d = .69$) while both kinds of interventions had similar effects on self-rated depressive symptoms ($d = .83$ versus $d = .62$; Pinquart, Duberstein, and Lyness 2006). However, the relatively smaller effect of pharmacological intervention on clinician-rated depression was due to the fact that these studies used an active placebo control condition while many psychotherapeutic studies did not. This reduced the size of relative improvement of pharmacotherapeutic interventions compared to the control condition. In fact, studies with a pharmacotherapeutic and a psychotherapeutic arm showed similar effects for both kinds of intervention.

Two meta-analyses focused on effects of *reminiscence* and *life-review* on depression. Bohlmeijer, Smit, and Cuijpers (2003) found a mean effect of $d = .84$. Larger improvements were observed in the case of high depressive symptoms at pre-test ($d = 1.23$) than in other studies ($d = .37$). In this meta-analysis the effect sizes were disattenuated, thus the mean effect size indicates the strength of reminiscence interventions if measures were perfectly reliable.

In an updated meta-analysis by Pinquart and Forstmeier (2012),[1] participants of reminiscence interventions showed, on average, moderate improvements of depressive symptoms

(d = .53). However, large effects were found for individuals with elevated levels of depressive symptoms or diagnosed depressive disorders at pre-test (d = 1.09) and among those who received life-review *therapy* in particular (d = 1.28). In life-review therapy, the structured (re)evaluation of one's life is often accompanied by techniques that have been developed in other therapeutic frameworks, such as cognitive therapy, problem-solving therapy, or narrative therapy.

Wilson, Mottram, and Vassilas (2009) analysed the effect of *CBT* and *psychodynamic therapy* approaches on geriatric depression. Based on five trials, CBT was more effective than wait-list controls in studies that used the Hamilton Rating Scale for Depression (d = 1.78). CBT was also superior to active control conditions when using the Hamilton Depression Rating Scale (d = .77), but equivalent when using the Geriatric Depression Scale (d = .32). No significant differences were found when comparing effects of CBT and psychodynamic therapy.

Two meta-analyses focused on the treatment of depressive symptoms for older adults with chronic medical illness. Dai, Li, and Cuijpers (2011) found large effects of psychotherapy on Chinese older adults with clinical depression and chronic physical illness (d = .80). However, a meta-analysis on heterogeneous (non-therapeutic) behavioural interventions for homebound older adults with heart disease (e.g. meditation, Tai Chi, telehealth) found no significant effect on depression symptoms (d = .11; Kang-Yi and Gellis 2010).

Finally, Forsman, Schierenbeck, and Wahlbeck (2011) summarized the results on the *prevention* of depression in old age. Overall, prevention programmes had a very small but statistically significant effect on depression symptoms (d = .17). In comparison with no-intervention controls, only social activities (e.g. volunteering) were effective in preventing depression symptoms (d = .41), but this result was only based on two studies. No significant preventive effects were found for physical exercise, skill training, reminiscence, and multicomponent interventions.

In sum, these meta-analyses show large immediate effects of CBT and reminiscence on older adults with clinical depression with and without physical comorbidity. Effects of psychotherapy on depression in old age are comparable to those of pharmacotherapy. Non-therapeutic interventions and prevention programmes tend to have small to very small effects on depression symptoms, which is, in part, based on the fact that these interventions are most often offered to older adults with low levels of depression at pre-test.

Anxiety

Available meta-analyses on the treatment of anxiety in old age have had to rely on a smaller database than meta-analyses on geriatric depression. This has often led to the inclusion of uncontrolled studies. Two available meta-analyses included a broad range of treatment programmes while three others focused on specific kinds of treatments or non-psychotherapeutic interventions.

Nordhus and Pallesen (2003) analysed the effects of (uncontrolled and controlled) behavioural intervention studies for the treatment of anxiety in old age. A combined effect size of d = .55 was reported. When controlling for nonspecific change in the control group, a meta-analysis by Pinquart and Duberstein (2007) found anxiety symptoms in the intervention condition to improve by d = .80. These relative improvements were significantly larger if clinician ratings were used ($d = 1.15$) than when self-ratings of the older adults were used ($d = .53$). Improvements of anxiety were maintained at follow-up (with a mean interval of thirty-seven weeks). The *relative* improvement of anxiety symptoms in behavioural interventions (after controlling for nonspecific change of anxiety symptoms in the control condition) was similar to that observed in pharmacological intervention studies ($d = .83$). However, relative improvements are difficult to compare because pharmacological studies use pill placebos as a control condition, whereas behavioural interventions primarily use wait-list control conditions. In fact, the level of *absolute* improvement of anxiety symptoms of pharmacological interventions ($d = 1.76$) was significantly larger than absolute improvements of these symptoms in behavioural interventions ($d = .81$).

Hendricks et al. (2008) included only CBT studies that had both a no-treatment control condition and an active control condition (attention placebo). Anxiety symptoms were reduced in comparison to the wait-list control condition ($d = .44$) and to the active control condition ($d = .51$).

A meta-analysis by Thorp et al. (2009) compared CBT and relaxation in the treatment of anxiety in old age. Unfortunately, most of their analyses focused on effect sizes that did not control for nonspecific change in the control condition. Large uncontrolled effect sizes were observed for CBT alone ($d = 1.18$), as well as for relaxation training alone ($d = .91$), and CBT plus relaxation ($d = .86$), and these effect sizes did not differ significantly from each other. When controlling for nonspecific change in the active control condition, only relaxation training alone showed a significant effect on anxiety symptoms ($d = .90$). The fact that improvements of anxiety in CBT trials were not significantly larger than in an active control condition should be interpreted with caution because only three controlled studies were available for CBT alone and for CBT plus relaxation training.

Finally, a meta-analysis on interventions targeted at fear of falling found small mean effects ($d = .21$; Jung, Lee, and Lee 2009). These interventions used exercise, education, encouragement, socializing, and hip protectors rather than cognitive-behavioural strategies or relaxation.

In sum, these meta-analyses show that behavioural interventions cause moderate to large improvements of anxiety symptoms but that these effects are lower than those of pharmacological interventions. CBT and relaxation tend to show similar effects but more comparative research is needed. In addition, non-therapeutic interventions, such as encouragement, have small effects at best.

Dementia

Dementia is the most common neurological disorder in old age (Hirtz et al. 2007); it is associated with cognitive impairment as well as behavioural symptoms, such as agitation and challenging behaviour (e.g. hitting, wandering, or constant repetition of sentences). Most behavioural interventions have focused on cognitive impairment.

Sitzer, Twamley, and Jeste (2006) analysed the effects of seventeen controlled trials on cognitive training with patients with Alzheimer's disease. They found average improvements of cognitive performance of $d = .47$ standard deviation units. Mean effect sizes at post-test were larger for restorative ($d = .54$) strategies that train lost cognitive abilities than for compensatory strategies aimed at building new compensatory skills ($d = .36$). At the follow-up of 4.5 months, a mean effect size of $d = .30$ was found. Unfortunately, these authors did not report whether the improvements were statistically significant.

Clare and Woods (2008) analysed the effects of nine randomized controlled trials of memory training on dementia patients' cognitive performance. No significant overall improvements of test performance and patient-reported memory problems were found, but low numbers of studies per outcome variable precluded the identification of significant improvements. Informant report on participant memory performance improved significantly ($d = .52$) but this effect was based on only two studies.

Based on four randomized controlled trials, Woods et al. (2005) found no statistically significant positive effects of reminiscence on cognitive performance at post-test ($d = .27$), although a significant moderate improvement was observed at six-weeks follow-up ($d = .50$).

Scientific evidence about behavioural treatments of agitation and challenging behaviour is even more limited. A meta-analysis by Kong, Evans, and Guevara (2008) reported that sensory interventions (aromatherapy, thermal bath, and calming music and hand massage) had a large statistical effect on agitation ($d = 1.07$), while effects of social contact, activities, environmental modification, care-giver training, combined interventions, and behavioural therapy interventions were not significant. However, these results should be interpreted with caution because only three or fewer effects sizes were available per analysis. Zetteler (2008) analysed the effect of simulated presence therapy on nursing home residents with dementia. The intervention consists of playing an audio or videotape that has been personalized by the care-giver and describes positive experiences from the client's life and shared memories involving family and friends. A moderate average effect on challenging behaviour was reported ($d = .70$).

In sum, the scientific evidence for effects of behavioural interventions with patients with dementia is still very limited. Nonetheless, the meta-analyses indicate that it is promising to conduct more research on that field.

Sleep problems

Nearly half of older adults report difficulty initiating and maintaining sleep, more than in any other age group (Roepke and Ancoli-Israel 2010). Briefly, sleep hygiene teaches persons about the impact of life-style habits on sleep; stimulus control aims to help individuals renew the association of bed and bedtime stimuli with sleep rather than sleep disruption; sleep restriction limits the time spent in bed at night and obviates sleep during the day; and cognitive therapy breaks dysfunctional beliefs and attitudes about sleep that lead to emotional distress and further sleep problems. Irwin, Cole, and Nicassio (2006) analysed the effects of randomized trials on behavioural interventions for insomnia. Both middle-aged adults and persons older than 55 years of age showed similar robust improvements in sleep quality ($d = .60$), sleep latency ($d = .51$), and wakening after sleep onset ($d = .73$). No significant effect was found on the total time of sleep. Intervention effects on sleep efficiency and total sleep time were smaller for older than for middle-aged adults, while no age differences were found for other outcomes.

In another meta-analysis of six RCTs on CBT with older adults with sleep problems, Montgomery and Dennis (2009) found a significant effect only on sleep efficiency at the three-month follow-up, but no other sleep measures. Lack of effects may have been attributable to low statistical power, as several analyses were computed for subsets of the six studies.

Care-giving

Most support for frail and chronically ill older adults is provided by family members, and spouses and adult children in particular. Care-giving activities often produce strain on care-givers themselves, referred to as 'care-giver burden', and they are often associated with compromised psychological health. While two meta-analyses focused on interventions with care-givers in general, others restricted their focus to dementia care-givers or care-givers of older adults with a chronic physical illness.

Based on twenty-six intervention studies, Yin, Zhou, and Bashford (2002) found improvement of burden of care-givers of family members with dementia or physical illness ($d = .41$). In the same year, a meta-analysis by Sörensen, Pinquart, and Duberstein (2002) found smaller effects on the levels of burden of these care-givers ($d = .15$). The primary difference between these two meta-analyses was in the number of studies included. Yin et al. (2002) did not include some available intervention studies with very small effects. Sörensen et al. (2002) included seventy-five studies and also found significant improvements of depression ($d = .14$), positive well-being ($d = .37$), and perceived abilities/knowledge of the care-givers ($d = .41$), as well as of symptoms of the care recipient ($d = .20$) across all care-giver interventions. Interventions with dementia care-givers had, on average, lower effects than interventions with care-givers of older adults with physical illness or mixed care-givers.

Four meta-analyses focused exclusively on interventions for dementia care-givers. Acton and Kang (2001) found, on average, no effect on care-giver burden. When comparing different forms of intervention, only multicomponent interventions significantly reduced care-giver burden ($d = .46$). However, this meta-analysis probably underestimated intervention effects because it included seven uncontrolled studies and thus could not control for possible increases in care-giver burden among participants not receiving an intervention.

Brodaty et al. (2003) included thirty studies on controlled interventions with informal care-givers for family members with dementia. These interventions improved knowledge about the disease and available sources of support ($d = .51$), psychological distress ($d = .31$), and patient mood ($d = .68$). Effects on care-giver burden did not reach statistical significance ($d = .09$).

Pinquart and Sörensen (2006) integrated the results of 127 controlled intervention studies with dementia care-givers. Interventions had, on average, statistically significant but small effects on burden ($d = .12$), depression ($d = .24$), positive well-being ($d = .31$), ability/knowledge ($d = .46$), and symptoms of care recipient ($d = .17$). Effects on burden ($d = .14$), depression ($d = .17$), and ability/knowledge ($d = .42$) were maintained at follow-up at an average of eleven months. Psychoeducational interventions that require active participation of care-givers had the broadest effects ($d = .15$ to $d = .55$). Effects of other interventions were domain specific. For example, CBT had the strongest effect on care-giver depression ($d = .70$) and an additional small effect on burden ($d = .36$). Counselling and case management ameliorated only care-giver burden ($d = .50$), and respite care was associated with a reduction of care-giver burden ($d = .26$) and depression ($d = .12$) as well as an increase in positive well-being of the care-giver (d = .27). Only multicomponent interventions reduced the risk for institutionalization (OR = .65).

Recently, Vernooij-Dassen et al. (2011) summarized effects of cognitive reframing interventions (e.g. CBT, problem-solving training) with dementia care-givers. Positive effects were found on psychological morbidity, specifically anxiety (d = .21), depression (d = .66), and psychological distress in general (d = .23). No significant effects were found for coping, care-giver burden, reactions to their relatives' behaviours, or institutionaliza-tion of the care recipient. However, the statistical test power for identifying effects was low because each of the eleven studies that were included provided data for only a subset of outcome variables.

Another recent meta-analysis of group-based interventions for care-givers of patients with dementia (mutual support groups or psychoeducational groups) found positive effect on care-givers' psychological well-being (d = .44), depression (d = .40), burden (d = .23), and social outcomes (d = .40; Chien et al. 2011). However, this effect was driven by (psycho-) educational interventions. Peer support groups had no significant effects on the outcome variables.

Finally, two meta-analyses focused on care-givers of older adults with chronic physical illness. Lee, Soeken, and Picot (2007) found a small effect of care-giving interventions on mental health outcomes of stroke care-givers (d = .28). A meta-analysis of interventions for care-givers of patients with cancer by Northouse et al. (2010) reported statistically signifi-cant but small improvements of self-efficacy beliefs (d = .25), care-giver burden (d = .22), coping (d = .20–.47), and general measures of psychological distress (d = .16–.29). No sig-nificant improvements of depression symptoms were found.

In sum, these meta-analyses show that care-giver interventions have, on average, small positive effects on a wide range of outcome variables. The interventions are most suc-cessful for increasing care-giver knowledge. In addition, effects of most interventions are domain-specific. In clinical practice, interventions need to be carefully selected with regard to the needs of the care-givers and the desired outcomes.

Bereavement

Bereaved individuals are at increased risk for mental and physical disorders. Both preven-tion and treatment of symptoms of psychological distress are indicated. Unfortunately, available meta-analyses are primarily focused on age-heterogeneous samples.

Two meta-analyses summarized the effects of interventions for bereaved individuals. Currier, Neimeyer, and Berman (2008) analysed the effect of controlled bereavement inter-ventions. There were small intervention effects at post-test but none at follow-up, on average thirty-six weeks after the end of the intervention.

Recently, Wittouck et al. (2011) analysed the effects of RCTs for prevention and treatment of complicated grief. Prevention trials with bereaved individuals who did not show elevated grief symptoms had neither significant effects at post-test nor follow-up. In contrast, treat-ment studies with individuals with elevated grief symptoms at pre-test showed significant improvements of grief symptoms at post-test (d = .53) and follow-up (d = 1.38). It remains unclear whether the results of these two meta-analyses can be generalized to older adults as the mean age of the participants of both meta-analyses was about 40 years. Nonetheless, the available studies indicate that bereavement interventions are most effective for individuals with elevated levels of psychological distress.

Improvement of positive well-being

Many interventions with older adults have focused on the improvement of positive well-being (e.g. happiness, life-satisfaction) rather than on the reduction of mental health problems. Pinquart and Sörensen (2001) found, on average, moderate improvements of positive well-being in psychotherapeutic interventions ($d = .51$) and small improvements in non-psychotherapeutic interventions ($d = .39$). Above-average improvements were found in control-enhancing interventions with institutionalized older adults ($d = 1.03$), CBT ($d = .78$), and relaxation training ($d = .72$). Small effects were observed in supportive interventions ($d = .37$), and psychoeducational interventions ($d = .37$) and no significant effects were found for the promotion of the general level of activity.

Bohlmeijer et al. (2007) found that reminiscence interventions led to moderate improvements of positive psychological well-being ($d = .54$). The structured life review was more effective ($d = 1.04$) than less structured simple reminiscence ($d = .40$). Another meta-analysis compared effects of reminiscence on different aspects of positive well-being. Improvements of positive affect ($d = 1.09$) but not of self-esteem or life-satisfaction were found to be statistically significant (Chin 2007). More recently, Pinquart and Forstmeier (2012)[1] found that reminiscence interventions showed moderate improvements of older adults' ego-integrity ($d = .63$) and small improvements of positive well-being at post-test ($d = .36$). The latter was found for positive affect ($d = .41$), life-satisfaction ($d = .22$), and self-esteem ($d = .20$). In addition, life-review therapy had stronger effects on positive well-being ($d = 1.02$) than non-therapeutic life-review ($d = .38$) and simple reminiscence ($d = .24$).

ARE THE RESULTS OF SOME AVAILABLE META-ANALYSES BIASED?

Problems with the design and execution of individual intervention studies raise questions about the validity of their findings. Thus, it is important to test whether the results of studies vary by methodological quality, such as randomized assignment to intervention and control group, blinding of the raters, lack of selective attrition, and provision of sufficient data for computing the exact effect size. For most of the meta-analyses reviewed here, the size of intervention effects did not vary by study quality (reminiscence: Bohlmeijer et al. 2003; Pinquart and Forstmeier 2012; anxiety treatments: Pinquart and Duberstein 2007; care-giver interventions: Brodaty et al. 2003; Chien et al. 2011). Three meta-analyses found smaller effect sizes among studies with higher quality (bereavement interventions: Currier et al. 2008; treatment of geriatric depression: Pinquart et al. 2007; care-giver interventions: Pinquart and Sörensen 2006) and one found weaker effects in studies with lower methodological quality for behavioural and psychotherapeutic interventions (Pinquart and Sörensen 2001). Thus, sources of bias are likely to vary in magnitude and direction (Higgins and

Green 2011), and some quality problems cause random error when larger numbers of studies are pooled (e.g. random differences between baseline characteristics of the intervention and control group).

A second important question is whether the studies included in meta-analyses are a biased collection of studies with large effect sizes because studies with non-significant effects are less likely to be published (Rosenthal 1979). Unfortunately, this question has not been addressed in most meta-analyses in clinical geropsychology. Pinquart and Forstmeier (2012) found some evidence for a file-drawer problem with regard to two out of nine outcomes of reminiscence interventions, and one effect size was no longer significant after applying the trim-and-fill procedure that corrects for this source of bias (Duval and Tweedie 2000). However, effects of reminiscence on two other variables *increased* after applying the trim-and-fill algorithm, thus indicating that factors other than the file-drawer problem may lead to asymmetrical distributions of effect sizes. In fact, consistent with Bohlmeijer et al.'s (2003) observations, Pinquart and Forstmeier (2012) found that the direct comparison of effects of published and unpublished studies suggests similar effects in both groups.

Implications for Practice

Meta-analyses are useful tools for practitioners and policy makers for selecting evidence-based diagnostic instruments and interventions. The meta-analyses reviewed here show that behavioural and psychotherapeutic interventions have moderate to large effects on depression symptoms, anxiety symptoms, and sleep problems. There are rather small effects on dementia patients' cognitive performance and distress among individuals coping with care-giving and bereavement. Nonetheless, small or very small improvements in a statistical sense can be practically meaningful if they have low costs per participant or if they reduce costs, as is, for example, the case with a delay of institutionalization of care recipients.

More convincing results are observed when testing whether behavioural and psychotherapeutic treatments have an *overall* effect on psychological and psychosomatic symptoms than when comparing different treatment *modalities*. Given the fact that the average number of included studies was twenty-nine (with a range from 3 to 127), the statistical power of several of the meta-analyses reviewed here was limited. This was the case particularly with regard to subgroup analysis. Thus, our review of existing meta-analyses highlights the need for further research on behavioural interventions with patients with dementia and interventions with bereaved older adults.

Summary

The growth of empirical studies in the field of clinical gerontology is reflected in a growing number of meta-analyses that summarize available research. This raises the question whether these meta-analyses come to similar conclusions or whether their results are as heterogeneous as the results of individual trials. Comparisons of the results of different meta-analyses on the same topic (e.g. reminiscence, treatment of depression, care-giver interventions) suggest that their results are quite robust. Nonetheless, robustness of results presupposes that larger numbers of effect sizes are included in the meta-analysis. The results of meta-analyses on very small numbers of studies may or may not be replicated in future meta-analyses (e.g. effects of social activity on the prevention of depression; Forsman et al. 2011). Including a larger number of studies increases the chance of finding statistically significant and situationally robust results, provided the meta-analysis does not include a highly selective sample of studies (e.g. Yin et al. 2002). Thus, if a meta-analysis is based on a small number of studies (e.g. ten or fewer), researchers and practitioners should regularly check whether updated meta-analyses become available. A regular update of meta-analyses is accomplished through the Cochrane Library.

Notes

1. Because twelve of the included 128 studies of that meta-analysis focused on adults younger than 60 years, we will only summarize the results of the remaining studies.

Key References and Sources for Further Reading

Lipsey, M. W. and Wilson, D. B. (2001). *Practical Meta-Analysis*. Thousand Oaks, CA: Sage.

Moher, D., Cook, D. J., Eastwood, S., Olkin, I., Rennie, D., and Stroup, D. F. (1999). 'Improving the Quality of Reports of Meta-analyses of Randomized Controlled Trials: The QUOROM Statement. *Lancet* 354: 1896–900.

References

Acton, G. J. and Kang, J. (2001). 'Interventions to Reduce the Burden of Caregiving for an Adult with Dementia: A Meta-analysis'. *Research in Nursing and Health* 24: 349–60.

APA Publications and Communications Board Working Group on Journal Article Reporting Standards (2008). 'Reporting Standards for Research in Psychology. Why Do We Need Them? What Might They Be?' *American Psychologist* 63: 839–851.

Bax, L., Yu, L. M., Ikeda, N., and Moons, K. G. (2007). 'A Systematic Comparison of Software Dedicated to Meta-analysis of Causal Studies'. *BMC Medical Research Methodology* 7: 40.

Bohlmeijer, E., Smit, F., and Cuijpers, P. (2003). 'Effects of Reminiscence and Life Review on Late-Life Depression: A Meta-analysis'. *International Journal of Geriatric Psychiatry* 18: 1088–1094.

Bohlmeijer, E., Roemer, M., Cuijpers, P., and Smit, F. (2007). 'The Effects of Reminiscence on Psychological Well-being in Older Adults: A Meta-analysis'. *Aging & Mental Health* 11: 291–300.

Borenstein, M., Hedges, L. V., Higgins, J. P. T., and Rothstein, H. R. (2009). *Introduction to Meta-Analysis*. Chichester: Wiley.

Bradburn, M. J., Deeks, J. J., and Altman, D. G. (2003). 'Metan—an Alternative Metaanalysis Command' (Metan 1.81). *Stata Technical Bulletin* 44(sbe24): 4–15.

Brodaty, H., Green, A., and Koschera, A. (2003). 'Meta-analysis of Psychosocial Interventions for People with Dementia'. *Journal of the American Geriatrics Society* 51: 657–664.

Bushman, B. J. and Wang, M. C. (1995). 'A Procedure of Combining Sample Correlation Coefficients and Vote Counts to Obtain an Estimate and a Confidence Interval for the Population Correlation Coefficient'. *Psychological Bulletin* 117: 530–546.

Bushman, B. J. and Wells, G. L. (2001). 'Narrative Impressions of Literature: The Availability Bias and the Corrective Properties of Meta-analytic Approaches'. *Personality and Social Psychology Bulletin* 27: 1123–1130.

Chien, L.-Y., Chu, H., Guo, J. L., Liao, Y. M., Chang, L. I., Chen, C. H., et al. (2011). 'Caregiver Support Groups in Patients with Dementia: A Meta-analysis'. *International Journal of Geriatric Psychiatry* 26: 1089–1098.

Chin, A. M. (2007). 'Clinical Effects of Reminiscence Therapy in Older Adults: A Meta-analysis of Controlled Trials'. *Hong Kong Journal of Occupational Therapy* 17: 10–22.

Clare, L. and Woods, B. (2008). 'Cognitive Rehabilitation and Cognitive Training for Early-stage Alzheimer's Disease and Vascular Dementia'. *Cochrane Library* 4: CD003260.

Cohen, J. (1992). 'A Power Primer'. *Psychological Bulletin* 112: 155–159.

Cole, M. G. and Dendukuri, N. (2003). 'Risk Factors for Depression among Elderly Community Subjects: A Systematic Review and Meta-analysis'. *American Journal of Psychiatry* 160: 1147–1156.

Currier, J.M., Neimeyer, R.A., and Berman, J. S. (2008). 'The Effectiveness of Psychotherapeutic Interventions for Bereaved Persons: A Comprehensive Quantitative Review'. *Psychological Bulletin* 134: 648–661.

Dai, B., Li, J., and Cuijpers, P. (2011). 'Psychological Treatment of Depressive Symptoms in Chinese Elderly Inpatients with Significant Medical Comorbidity: A Meta-analysis'. *BMC Psychiatry* 11: 92–100.

Duval, S. J. and Tweedie, R. L. (2000). 'Trim and Fill: A Simple Funnel Plot-based Method of Testing and Adjusting for Publication Bias in Meta-analysis'. *Biometrics* 56: 455–463.

Forsman, A. K., Schierenbeck, I., and Wahlbeck, K. (2011). 'Psychosocial Interventions for the Prevention of Depression in Older Adults: Systematic Review and Meta-analysis'. *Journal of Aging and Health* 23: 387–416.

Glass, G. V. (1976). 'Primary, Secondary and Meta-analysis of Research'. *Educational Researcher* 5: 3–8.

Han, L, Cole, M., Bellavance, F., McCusker, J., and Primeau, F. (2000). 'Tracking cognitive decline in Alzheimer's disease using the Mini-Mental State Examination: A Meta-analysis'. *International Psychogeriatrics* 12: 231–247.

Hendriks, G. J., Oude Voshaar, R. C., Keijsers, G. P. J., Hoogduin, C. A. L., and van Balkom, A. J. (2008). 'Cognitive-behavioural Therapy for Late-life Anxiety Disorders: A Systematic Review and Meta-analysis'. *Acta Psychiatrica Scandinavica* 117: 403–411.

Heo, M., Murphy, C. F., and Meyers, B. S. (2007). 'Relationship between the Hamilton Depression Rating Scale and the Montgomery-Asberg Depression Rating Scale in Depressed Elderly: A Meta-analysis'. *American Journal of Geriatric Psychiatry* 15: 899–905.

Higgins, J. P. T. and Green, S. (2011) (eds). *Cochrane Handbook for Systematic Reviews of Interventions* Version 5.1.0 [updated March 2011]. The Cochrane Collaboration, Available from http://www.cochrane-handbook.org.

Hirtz, D., Thurman, D. J., Gwinn-Hardy, K., Mohamed, M., Chaudhuri, A. R., and Zalutsky, R. (2007). 'How Common are the "Common" Neurologic Disorders?'. *Neurology* 68: 326–337.

Iliffe, S. and Manthorpe, J. (2002). 'Depression, Anxiety and Psychoses in Later Life'. *Reviews in Clinical Geropsychology* 12: 327–341.

Irwig, L., Tosteson, A. N., Gatsonis, C., Lau, J., Colditz, G., and Chalmers, T. C., et al. (1994). 'Guidelines for Meta-analyses Evaluating Diagnostic Tests'. *Annals of Internal Medicine* 120: 667–676.

Irwin, M. R., Cole, J. C., and Nicassio, P. M. (2006). 'Comparative Meta-analysis of Behavioral Interventions for Insomnia and their Efficacy in Middle-aged Adults and in Older Adults 55+ Years of Age'. *Health Psychology* 25: 3–14.

Jung, D., Lee, J., and Lee, S.-M. (2009). 'A Meta-analysis of Fear of Falling Treatment Programs for the Elderly'. *Western Journal of Nursing Research* 31: 6–16.

Kang-Yi, C. D. and Gellis, Z. D. (2010). 'A Systematic Review of Community-based Health Interventions on Depression for Older Adults with Heart Disease'. *Aging & Mental Health* 14: 1–19.

Kong, E.-H., Evans, L. K., and Guevara, J. P. (2008). 'Nonpharmacological Intervention for Agitation in Dementia: A Systematic Review and Meta-analysis'. *Aging & Mental Health* 13: 512–520.

Kraaij, V., Arensman, E., and Spinhoven, P. (2002). 'Negative Life Events and Depression in Elderly Persons: A Meta-analysis'. *Journals of Gerontology: Psychological and Social Sciences* 57B: P87–94.

Lee, H. J., Soeken, K., and Picot, S. J. (2007). 'A Meta-analysis of Interventions for Informal Stroke Caregivers'. *Western Journal of Nursing Research* 29: 344–356.

Lipsey, M. W. and Wilson, D. B. (2001). *Practical Meta-analysis*. Thousand Oaks, CA: Sage.

Mitchell, A. J., Bird, V., Rizzo, M., and Meader, N. (2010). 'Which Version of the Geriatric Depression Scale is Most Useful in Medical Settings and Nursing Homes? Diagnostic Validity Meta-analysis'. *American Journal of Geriatric Psychiatry* 18: 1066–1077.

Moher, D., Cook, D. J., Eastwood, S., Olkin, I., Rennie, D., and Stroup, D. F. (1999). 'Improving the Quality of Reports of Meta-analyses of Randomized Controlled Trials: The QUOROM Statement'. *Lancet* 354: 1896–1900.

Moher, D., Liberati, A., Tetzlaff, J., and Altman, D. G. (2009). 'Preferred Reporting Items for Systematic Reviews and Meta-analyses: The PRISMA Statement'. *Plos Medicine* 6: e1000097.

Montgomery, P. and Dennis, J. A. (2009). 'Cognitive Behavioural Interventions for Sleep Problems in Adults Aged 60+'. *Cochrane Library* 1: CD003161.

Nordhus, I. H. and Pallesen, S. (2003). 'Psychological Treatment of Late-life Anxiety: An Empirical Review'. *Journal of Consulting and Clinical Psychology* 71: 643–651.

Northouse, L. L., Katapodi, M. C., Song, L., Zhang, L., and Mood, D. W. (2010), 'Interventions with Family Caregivers of Cancer Patients: Meta-analysis of Randomized Trials'. *Cancer Journal for Clinicians* 60: 317–339.

Pinquart, M. and Sörensen, S. (2001). 'How Effective are Psychotherapeutic and Other Psychosocial Interventions with Older Adults? A Meta-analysis'. *Journal of Mental Health and Aging* 7: 207–243.

Pinquart, M. and Sörensen, S. (2006). 'Gender Differences in Caregiver Stressors, Social Resources, and Health: An Updated Meta-analysis'. *Journals of Gerontology Series B: Psychological Sciences and Social Sciences* 61(1): 33–45.

Pinquart, M., Duberstein, P., and Lyness, J. M. (2006). 'Treatments for Later Life Depressive Conditions: A Meta-analytic Comparison of Pharmacotherapy and Psychotherapy'. *American Journal of Psychiatry* 163: 1493–1501.

Pinquart, M. and Duberstein, P. R. (2007). 'Treatment of Anxiety Disorders in Older Adults: A Meta-analytic Comparison of Behavioral and Pharmacological Interventions'. *American Journal of Geriatric Psychiatry* 15: 639–651.

Pinquart, M., Duberstein, P.R., and Lyness, J. M. (2007). 'Effects of Psychotherapy and Other Behavioral Interventions on Clinically Depressed Older Adults: A Meta-analysis'. *Aging & Mental Health* 11: 645–657.

Pinquart, M. and Forstmeier, S. (2012). 'Effects of Reminiscence Interventions on Psychosocial Outcomes: A Meta-analysis'. *Aging & Mental Health* 16: 541–558.

Roepke, K. and Ancoli-Israel, S. (2010). 'Sleep Disorders in the Elderly'. *Indian Journal of Medical Research* 131: 302–310.

Rosenthal, R. (1979). 'The "File Drawer Problem" and Tolerance for Null Results'. *Psychological Bulletin* 85: 638–641.

Sackett, D. L., Straus, S. E., Richardson, W. S., Rosenberg, W., and Haynes, R. B. (2000). *Evidence-based Medicine: How to Practice and Teach EBM* (Vol. 2). London: Churchill Livingstone.

Shakelle, P. G., Woolf, S. H., Eccles, M., and Grimshaw, J. (1999). 'Developing Guidelines'. *British Medical Journal* 318: 593–596.

Sitzer, D. I., Twamley, E. W., and Jeste, D. V. (2006). 'Cognitive Training in Alzheimer's Disease: A Meta-analysis of the Literature'. *Acta Psychiatrica Scandinavia* 114: 75–90.

Sörensen, S., Pinquart, M., and Duberstein, P. (2002). 'How Effective are Interventions with Caregivers? An Updated Meta-analysis'. *Gerontologist* 42: 356–372.

Stroup, D. F., Berlin, J. A., Morton, S. C., Olkin, I., Williamson, G. D., and Rennie, D. (2000). 'Metaanalysis of Observational Studies in Epidemiology: A Proposal for Reporting'. *Journal of the American Medical Association* 283: 2008–2012.

Tenev, V. T., Robinson, R. G., and Jorge, R. E. (2010). 'Is Family History of Depression a Risk Factor for Poststroke Depression? Meta-analysis'. *American Journal of Geriatric Psychology* 17: 276–280.

Thorp, S. R., Ayers, C. R., Nuevo, R., Stoddard, J. A., and Sorrell, J. T. (2009). 'Meta-analysis Comparing Different Behavioral Treatments for Late-life Anxiety'. *American Journal of Geriatric Psychiatry* 7: 105–115.

Valentine, J. C. (2009). 'Judging the Quality of Primary Research'. In H. Cooper, L. V. Hedges, and J. C. Valentine (eds), *Handbook of Research Synthesis and Meta-analysis* (2nd edn, pp. 129–146). New York: Sage.

Vernooij-Dassen, M., Draskovic, I., McCleery, J., and Downs, M. (2011). 'Cognitive Reframing for Carers of People with Dementia'. *Cochrane Database of Systematic Reviews* 11: CD005318.

Wilson, K., Mottram, P. G., and Vassilas, C. (2009). 'Psychotherapeutic Treatments for Older Depressed People'. *Cochrane Database of Systematic Reviews* 1: CD004853.

Wittouck, C., Van Autreve, S., De Jaegere, E., Portzky, G., and van Heeringen, K. (2011). 'The Prevention and Treatment of Complicated Grief: A Meta-analysis'. *Clinical Psychology Review* 31: 69–78.

Woods, B., Spector, A., Jones, C., Orrell, M., and Davies, S. (2005). 'Reminiscence Therapy for Dementia'. *Cochrane Database of Systematic Reviews* 2: CD001120.

Yin, T., Zhou, Q., and Bashford, C. (2002). 'Burden on Family Members Caring for Frail Elderly: A Meta-analysis of Interventions'. *Nursing Research* 51: 199–208.

Zetteler, J. (2008). 'Effectiveness of Simulated Presence Therapy for Individuals with Dementia: A Systematic Review and Meta-analysis'. *Aging & Mental Health* 12: 779–85.

CHAPTER 5

SUCCESSFUL DEVELOPMENT
AND AGEING

Theory and Intervention

NARDI STEVERINK

INTRODUCTION

HEALTH and well-being, along with the question how to maintain them for as long as possible into old age, continue to intrigue scientists, policy makers, clinical professionals, as well as older adults themselves. The trend of population ageing encourages a search for workable insights and interventions to support and serve increasing numbers of older adults. In the last decades phrases like 'healthy ageing', 'ageing well', 'active ageing', and 'successful ageing' have become guiding themes in both the scientific field of gerontology and in policy development concerning the ageing population (e.g. WHO 2002). Although there is still little consensus about the criteria of 'success' (Depp and Jeste 2006), a clear development in the field is that the common deficit approach to ageing has been modified and the challenge has become how to understand the mechanisms by which ageing individuals are able to remain healthy and happy for as long as possible. Today, it is generally accepted that ageing successfully is not just a matter of having the right genes or having the right material resources; it is also a matter of how individuals actively regulate their life and their behaviours such that health and well-being are optimized. Knowing more about these self-regulatory aspects of successful ageing will enhance the design of interventions and public health policies.

Two general trends underline the importance of knowing more about active self-regulation in the process of ageing well. First, the still increasing numbers of older people and the related threat of an overloaded healthcare and welfare system make it increasingly important that older adults themselves are optimally able to stay healthy and happy for as long as possible. Second, increasing life expectancy, with more remaining years of life after retirement but few social structures and socially defined roles (Freund, Nikitin, and Ritter 2009; Riley and Riley 1994; Walker 1999), urges older people to find their way in the life stage that has been called the 'third age'. Because increasingly more people reach this 'third age', more and more people need adequate self-regulatory skills if they want to (keep) feeling well and living a meaningful life into old age. But how can successful development and ageing be understood, and effectively become the focus of interventions and public health policy?

In the remainder of this chapter, first the question will be addressed of how successful development and ageing are being approached in research and in the development of interventions. Next, a selection of existing approaches to successful development and ageing will be reviewed. One of these approaches, the Self-management of Well-being Theory (SMW), will be elaborated in more detail, because this theory has been shown to be useful as a basis for concrete and effective interventions aimed at the improvement of self-regulation and well-being in older adults. A short description of these interventions will be given. Finally, some suggestions for the future will be discussed.

SUCCESSFUL AGEING: A LIFESPAN DEVELOPMENTAL PERSPECTIVE

Many of the perspectives on ageing that have emerged in the last decades nuanced the dominant biological deficit approach to ageing by recognizing the importance of the multidimensionality of the ageing process (i.e. ageing is not just a biological process, but occurs also at social and psychological domains of functioning). Moreover, interest in the multidirectionality of the ageing process grew (i.e. ageing is characterized by gains and losses, many of which occur at individually different points and rates during the lifespan). The recognition of these two important insights resulted, first, in much more attention being paid to the psychological and social phenomena of ageing, and, second, in new ideas about the differences between 'usual' and 'successful' ageing (Rowe and Kahn 1987). Both had specific implications for theorizing about ageing, but also for the design of interventions aimed at supporting older adults in ageing well.

With regard to the increased attention to the social and psychological domains of ageing, it became much clearer that ageing is not just a biological process. Rather, it covers also the social and psychological domains of life (Rowe and Kahn 1987). Moreover, these domains interact with each other. For example, robust evidence is found that a diversity of social factors influence morbidity (Cohen 2004; House, Landis, and Umberson 1988; Seeman 1996) and even mortality (Holt-Lunstad, Smith, and Layton 2010). The same holds for mental health outcomes (Steverink et al. 2011). Additionally, interacting ageing-related changes and losses across several domains may result in self-reinforcing spirals of change and challenge. For example, loss of mobility may negatively affect people's social life, which, in turn, may negatively affect one's mood, which may then undermine the energy to take care of one's physical health and condition. The latter may subsequently lead to a further decline in social activities, and may lead to loneliness, and so on. Thus, an initial (small) loss in one domain may affect resources in other, perhaps multiple, domains. When there is a declining reserve capacity to compensate fully for certain resource losses, this process may be accelerated and lead to declines in well-being. The complex interplay of different life domains and interacting influences most likely holds for the entire lifespan, but seems to be accelerated in later life (Hawkley and Cacioppo 2007).

However, in addition to possibly negative spirals, positive spirals also seem to occur in ageing. Important work in the field of positive ageing has been done by Carol Ryff, who has criticized the neglect of the possibilities for continued growth and development in old age (Ryff 1989). The field of positive psychology also identified a wide variety of human strengths that potentially increase during old age, such as serenity, wisdom, feeling more relaxed, developing new social relationships (e.g. with grandchildren), and having a broader capacity for the analysis of intellectual and social problems (e.g. Fernández-Ballesteros 2003). Additionally, recent studies showed the positive influence of happiness and subjective well-being on health and longevity (Veenhoven 2008). Although still relatively few studies exist on this matter, the findings consistently show that high levels of subjective well-being significantly lower the risk of mortality and disability, when controlling for other risk factors (e.g. Collins, Goldman, and Rodriquez 2008; Ostir et al. 2000). Therefore, the complex interplay of gains and losses in different domains of functioning deserves specific attention in ageing individuals. Successful ageing thus not only implies the management of these interacting challenges and cumulative losses, but also the prevention or postponement of them in different domains of functioning, as well as the development and maintenance of strengths.

The second main insight—multidirectionality in the ageing process—points to the fact that there is a substantial heterogeneity within age groups, and that there are many individual differences in the ageing process, for multiple domains of functioning. This insight has also led to the differentiation between 'usual' and 'successful' ageing (Rowe and Kahn 1987). 'Usual' ageing refers to how most people age: to typical physical, cognitive, and social processes. The other concept, 'successful ageing', refers to relatively high levels of physical, cognitive, and social functioning, as is visible in individuals who do better than the general population. The latter perspective is appealing because it challenges older adults themselves, as well as clinical professionals and researchers, to address the optimal potential and possibilities for continued growth and resilience at later life stages, instead of focusing on decline and increasing losses. As such, the perspective of successful ageing is a helpful construct, too, for designing interventions and policy. However, the phrase 'successful' has often been criticized, because it would imply a value judgment, and it would imply that people who do not achieve or keep objective high levels of functioning could not age 'successfully'. Therefore, it might be more acceptable to speak of 'ageing well', and emphasize that the ultimate criterion of 'ageing well' must be the subjective experience of well-being and quality of life, not some objective indicators of high functioning (cf. George 2006). Ultimately, the key criterion of 'success' in successful ageing can only be the subjective perception of well-being, because older adults who experience declines in physical and cognitive functioning, and who suffer from disability or who lack social engagement, still can rate their well-being as high. Conversely, older adults who show objectively high levels of physical, cognitive, and social functioning still may not feel happy. So, the key criterion of 'success' ultimately can only be the subjective experience of well-being, not the mere sum of objective indicators of high functioning (see also Huber et al. 2011). Nevertheless, there may be specific objective antecedents and determinants that lead to the subjective experience of elevated well-being in most people. Therefore, the challenge is to discover these universal determinants, in order to address them in interventions and policy.

But what are the antecedents and determinants of high levels of subjective well-being for most people at later ages? Several external and internal circumstances have been identified. For example, health, social integration and social support, and socio-economic status have been found to be important external determinants of high levels of subjective well-being (for a review see George 2006). Additionally, psychosocial characteristics—as internal circumstances—play a role, such as the individual's belief that he or she is in control, and is able to manage his or her own life. Moreover, often these psychosocial factors are found to have both direct effects on subjective well-being, as well as indirect effects via mediating the effects of objective circumstances on subjective well-being. So, ageing with high levels of subjective well-being—and thus, ageing successfully—is more likely when certain external circumstances are present, together with certain psychosocial characteristics and skills. In other words, successful ageing is about both achieving and maintaining the right external resources and the right internal resources (psychosocial characteristics).

Because of the specific issues of multidimensionality and multidirectionality of the ageing process, it may be especially important that older adults have a diverse repertoire of self-regulatory capacities to manage life proactively and break possible downward spirals. This repertoire should include abilities to reinforce one's strengths, thereby consolidating important resources for ageing successfully. So the question is how, by what self-regulatory capacities and behavioural strategies, people are able to age successfully. This is the question of *how* (to age well). Moreover, we need to know what it means to be 'well'; this is the question of *what*. Only when we *understand* (i.e. by a theory that provides explicit *explanations*) *how* people age well, and *what* it means to be 'well', are we able to design interventions. As Bengtson et al. (1999) have stated it: 'If you don't understand the problem, how can you fix it?' (7).

Several models and theories exist that try to answer the questions of *what* and *how*. In the following section we will briefly discuss some of the main models and theories, and see to what extent they are concrete and explicit about 'how' and 'what', and thus useful as a basis for the design of interventions.

Existing Models and Theories about Successful Development and Ageing

Several important theoretical approaches to successful ageing exist. Here we will discuss four important models and theories, the first being Carol Ryff's model of Psychological Well-being (Ryff, 1989; Ryff and Keyes 1995), which is especially concrete about the 'what' question, i.e. what it means to be 'well'. The second and third models are especially concrete about the 'how' question, i.e. about the behavioural processes that lead to ageing well. These are the Selection, Optimization and Compensation (SOC) model (Baltes and Baltes 1990) and the Motivational Theory of Life-span Development (Heckhausen, Wrosch, and Schulz 2010; Schulz and Heckhausen 1996). The fourth theory, finally, is a theory that is concrete and explicit about both the 'how' *and* 'what' questions: the Self-management of Well-being theory (SMW; Steverink, Lindenberg, and Slaets 2005). The latter will be elaborated on in somewhat more detail.

Carol Ryff's model of Psychological Well-being

The model of Psychological Well-Being of Carol Ryff (Ryff 1989; Ryff and Keyes 1995) is a general model of psychological well-being, which examines perceived thriving in the face of existential challenges over the lifespan. The model basically describes six dimensions of well-being: self-acceptance, positive relationships, autonomy, environmental mastery, purpose in life, and personal growth. These dimensions are based on the integration of insights from lifespan developmental theories, clinical theories of personal growth, and mental health approaches (Ryff 1989; Ryff and Keyes 1995). The core assumption of this model is that well-being is not so much an outcome or end state, but rather a process of fulfilling or actualizing one's potentials. Living and ageing well, according to this model, imply that people fulfil their potential, which will be visible in high levels on all six dimensions. As such, the six dimensions of psychological well-being can be seen as criteria of 'success'. Ryff and colleagues have also developed a scale for measuring the six dimensions (Ryff and Keyes 1995).

The Selection, Optimization and Compensation (SOC) model

The SOC model (Baltes and Baltes 1990; Freund and Baltes 2007) is a general model of successful ageing, which describes behavioural processes of adaptation throughout the lifespan. Due to the changing balance between gains and losses, including decreasing reserve capacity, selection, optimization, and compensation are assumed to be important processes if people desire to age with 'success'. Selection refers to the selection of and commitment to a specific goal or set of goals. Facing physical, social, and cultural constraints, it includes concentration on a limited set of alternatives. Optimization refers to the acquisition, application, and investment of resources such that desired outcomes are attained in selected domains.

Compensation refers to processes aimed at maintaining functioning in the face of impending or actual losses by substituting available resources as alternative means. The three processes of selection, optimization, and compensation are presumed to work in orchestration, and to lead to the experience of mastery and adaptability across the lifespan and into old age. Regarding the definition of 'success' in successful ageing, the authors of the SOC model state that criteria for success are necessarily relative to social and cultural values. Therefore, they conclude that success can only be defined at a very abstract level, and they conceptualize successful ageing as a process encompassing the simultaneous maximization of gains and minimization of losses (Freund and Baltes 2007).

The Motivational Theory of Life-span Development (MTLSD)

The MTLSD (Heckhausen et al. 2010) is a recent integration of earlier theories on successful development and ageing by the same authors (Heckhausen and Schulz 1995; Schulz and Heckhausen 1996). The new theory focuses on the major challenges faced by individuals throughout the life course and on the motivational and self-regulatory processes that people use to meet these challenges. As in the SOC model, it is assumed that the individual needs to master two fundamental regulatory challenges: selectivity of resource investment, and compensation of failure and loss. When people succeed in this, a sense of control is maintained. The processes by which these challenges are mastered are, according to the Motivational Theory of Life-span Development, processes of primary and secondary control. Primary control processes are conceptualized as being directed at bringing the environment into line with one's wishes, whereas secondary control processes are defined as changing the self to bring oneself into line with environmental forces (Rothbaum, Weisz, and Snyder 1982). Heckhausen et al. (2010) conceptualize the secondary control processes explicitly as auxiliary motivational processes that support short-term or long-term primary control striving, not as alternatives or even processes opposed to primary control. Somewhat different than the SOC model, the process of optimization is placed at a meta-level, referring to a higher-level universal motivational process of maximizing control. With this latter aspect, the MTLSD is a more explicit motivational theory than the SOC model. Regarding the definition of 'success', the authors are clear that the criteria that differentiate adaptive from maladaptive outcomes of development should be specified. For them, the key criterion for adaptive development is the extent to which the individual realizes control of his or her environment (i.e. primary control) across different domains of life (e.g. work, family, health, leisure) as well as across the lifespan (Heckhausen et al. 2010, p.35).

The Self-management of Well-being theory (SMW)

The SMW theory (Steverink et al. 2005) is basically an extension of the SPF-Successful Ageing theory (Steverink and Lindenberg 2006; Steverink, Lindenberg, and Ormel 1998), which in turn is based on the general theory of Social Production Functions (SPF theory; Lindenberg 1996; Ormel 2002; Ormel et al. 1999). In the following section the SMW theory will be described in more detail, because this theory is especially concrete and explicit about both the criteria of 'success' and about the behavioural mechanisms leading to 'success'. This makes this theory especially useful as a basis for the design of interventions. In the following, first, the basic premises of the theory of SPF will be briefly described, after which the subsequent elaborations that resulted in the integrated SMW theory will be described.

THE SMW THEORY

The origin: SPF theory

Social Production Function theory, in its basic form, is a general theory of well-being, applicable to individuals of all ages. SPF theory integrates two core premises: one about human basic needs and related goals and resources, and one about basic behavioural and motivational processes. The first core premise of SPF theory describes a hierarchy of universal human needs, instrumental goals, and resources. 'Needs' refer to specific basic physical and social needs that must at least be minimally fulfilled for an individual to experience a sense

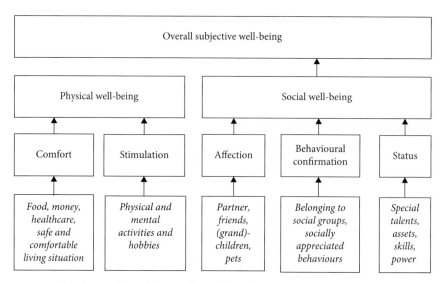

FIGURE 5.1 The hierarchy of basic physical and social needs (upper three layers) as specified by the theory of SPF, and examples of resources in the lowest (fourth) layer.

Reproduced from *Social Indicators Research*, 46(1), pp. 61–90, Subjective Well-Being and Social Production Functions, Johan Ormel, (c) 1999, Springer Science and Business Media. With kind permission from Springer Science and Business Media.

of well-being (see also Deci and Ryan 2000). The social needs—if fulfilled—provide social well-being, while the physical needs—if fulfilled—provide physical well-being. Together, social and physical well-being contribute to overall well-being. So, the better an individual's needs are fulfilled, the higher the individual's overall subjective well-being will be. In SPF theory, needs are by definition inherent, universal, and relevant to people of all ages. Moreover, they are conceptually distinguished from goals and resources. The needs are the top three layers in the hierarchy, and goals and resources—lower in the hierarchy—refer to the means and instruments by which the needs can be fulfilled. Figure 5.1 shows the hierarchy of basic needs, goals and resources as specified by the theory of SPF.

For example, a close relationship is a resource (lower in the hierarchy) to fulfil the need for affection (higher in the hierarchy). When, however, a close relationship has not yet been achieved, it can also be a goal. Goals and resources are thus two sides of the same coin. In addition to two basic physical needs (comfort and stimulation), SPF theory identifies three basic social needs (affection, behavioural confirmation and status).

Comfort refers to physical comfort, i.e. the satisfaction of basic physical needs such as food, drink, rest, warmth, the absence of pain, fatigue, etc. Stimulation refers to the pleasant range of activation (physically and mentally), i.e. the absence of boredom and the right amount of exposure to novelty, challenges, and interesting events. Affection is the feeling that you are liked, loved, trusted and accepted, understood, empathized with, know that your feelings are reciprocated, feel that others are willing to help without expecting something in return, feel that your well-being is intertwined with others, and feel that others like to be either emotionally or physically close to you (e.g. to hug). Affection thus refers to the love you get for being who you are, regardless of your assets (status) or actions (behavioural confirmation). Behavioural confirmation is the feeling of doing the 'right' thing in the eyes of 'relevant' others and yourself; it includes doing good things, doing things well, being a good person, being useful, contributing to a common goal, and being part of a functional group. Behavioural confirmation thus results primarily from what you do, rather than what kind of person you are (affection), or what you have or can do (status). The final and third social need, status, is the feeling that you are being treated with respect and are being taken seriously, are independent or autonomous, achieve more than others, have influence, realize yourself, and are known for your achievements, skills, or assets.

The physical needs are intuitively appealing and generally recognized as present and important, but the social needs have also received considerable support. For example, evolutionary theory has shown that human beings are not only biologically hardwired to connect to others in close relations, but also aspire to be confirmed by their group, and to strive for status within the group (for reviews, see Baumeister and Leary 1995; Buss and Kenrick 1998; Reis, Collins, and Berscheid 2000). Additionally, there are empirical studies that support the idea of the five basic needs as proposed by SPF theory (Nieboer et al. 2005; van Bruggen 2001).

The second core premise of SPF theory describes basic behavioural and motivational processes, and states that human beings are basically motivated to improve their situation. This means, concretely, that there is a basic motivation to improve levels of physical and social need fulfilment. This premise largely overlaps with the notion of 'optimization' in the motivational theory of Heckhausen et al. (2010). Note that, although a basic motivation for improvement is assumed, this does not mean that individuals are always successful in this striving. Human cognitive functioning is subject to the effects of goal-framing, which makes them vulnerable to one-sidedness in their goal striving, and thus to failures (see Lindenberg 2013).

Because of the basic motivation for improvement, people will also try to substitute or compensate for the increasing difficulty of fulfilment of one need by an increased effort to fulfil other needs. For example, when the need for status becomes more difficult to fulfil, people will try to maintain overall social need fulfilment by concentrating more on fulfilling the other two social needs (i.e. behavioural confirmation and affection). As Nieboer and Lindenberg (2002) have shown empirically, people with difficulty achieving high status do, indeed, use their resources for the fulfilment of the needs for affection and behavioural confirmation more than people with accomplished high status do.

The processes of substitution and compensation also show how the physical and social needs of SPF theory overlap with, for example, Maslow's hierarchy of needs (Maslow 1970). Yet, the theoretical approach is basically different (for a detailed discussion see Lindenberg 1996) because of the possibility of substitution and compensation in the fulfilment of different needs. In SPF theory, contrary to Maslow's hierarchy of needs, individuals need a certain minimum fulfilment of both physical and social needs, but beyond this minimum, they can substitute one need fulfilment by that of another need. Thus, individuals may be willing to sacrifice physical need fulfilment for an improvement in social need fulfilment. For example, adolescents are often willing to undergo physically painful initiation rites in order to be accepted by their group, and adults are often willing to sacrifice sleep and rest for working on their career.

From the two core premises of SPF theory (i.e. basic needs, and basic strivings, including maintaining need fulfilment by substitution and compensation) it becomes possible to analyse (1) what happens with need fulfilment in the process of ageing; (2) what would be criteria of 'success' in ageing healthily and well; and (3) by what behavioural processes would 'success' be possible and likely. This we have elaborated in the SMW theory. In the following sections this theory will be explained in more detail.

The SPF theory applied to ageing well

In applying the SPF theory to the question of how to understand the process of ageing successfully, the two core premises of the theory are in need of some specification. First, does the basic premise of the importance of the five basic human needs for subjective well-being still hold when, due to increasing losses in resources, the fulfilment of these needs will become more difficult? Second, does the basic primary motivation as presumed in SPF theory—namely, improvement of need fulfilment—still hold when losses in resources increase in the process of ageing and people can only try to maintain their resources as much as possible, or even to manage losses as much as possible? The SMW theory, based on SPF theory, addresses both questions (Steverink et al. 2005).

Patterned change in resources and need fulfilments

The first basic tenet of the SMW theory is that, although universal human needs basically remain the same across the entire lifespan, the relative ease with which they can be fulfilled changes because the opportunities and resources that are available for fulfilling them change and decline. Important resources include physical resources (such as energy, health, mobility, etc.) and social resources and opportunities. For instance, fulfilment of the need for status often depends on having a paid job, or being recognized for having specific assets or skills, such as being a top athlete or famous singer. At advanced ages, it often becomes relatively more difficult to fulfil the need for status, not only because of retirement, but also because of age-related physical declines that may undermine specific skills. To a lesser degree, the same holds for fulfilment of the needs for behavioural confirmation and stimulation. The fulfilment of both the needs for behavioural confirmation and stimulation requires physical and social resources that may show age-related declines. Still, by and large, opportunities to fulfil both behavioural confirmation and stimulation decline more slowly with ageing than those for fulfilling the need for status. For example, the need for behavioural confirmation can be fulfilled through voluntary work, or by helping others. Fulfilment of the needs for affection and comfort, finally, seems relatively easy to maintain, because these two depend much less on performance and physical strengths than the other needs so that, even when physical and social resources decline considerably, a person may still be able to fulfil the needs for affection and comfort to a certain extent.

So an ageing-specific process regarding need fulfilment must be considered, framed as the 'patterned change' hypothesis (Steverink et al. 1998). This process refers to the fact that the availability of resources for the fulfilment of basic needs changes over the lifespan, with, in general, resources for status need fulfilment declining first and fastest, and with resources for the fulfilment of affection and comfort declining last and slowest. This 'patterned change' hypothesis has been empirically supported: older adults indeed seem to lose their resources for needs fulfilment over time in a specific order: first their resources for status, then for behavioural confirmation and stimulation, and last (if at all) their resources for affection and comfort (Steverink 2001). The patterned change hypothesis also implies a specific process of substitution and compensation regarding the need fulfilments, due to the lifespan patterned changes in resources (Steverink and Lindenberg 2006; Steverink et al. 1998). This means that loss of status need fulfilment will (at least partially) be compensated by increased efforts to satisfy the needs for behavioural confirmation and affection, and loss of need fulfilment for behavioural confirmation will (at least partially) be compensated by increased effort to fulfil the need for affection. In the same vein, loss of need fulfilment for stimulation will be compensated by increased effort to fulfil the need for comfort.

The core self-management abilities

As mentioned previously, the core tenet of the Self-management of Well-being theory is that ageing individuals are basically motivated to improve levels of physical and social need fulfilment, but in the process of ageing it must be taken into account that this motivation increasingly will manifest itself as *maintaining* levels of need fulfilment, and *managing failures and losses* in need fulfilment. But the question is: how do people achieve, maintain, and manage resources such that need fulfilment—and thus overall well-being—remains to be optimized?

In the SMW theory (Steverink et al. 2005), we identified six core self-management abilities that we consider to be key abilities for managing resources in such a way that need fulfilment is achieved and maintained, and that losses are managed optimally. These six abilities together make up overall self-management ability as the orchestrated use of various active self-management abilities. According to the theory of SMW, the achievement and maintenance of well-being over the lifespan depends on whether people have adequate resources for fulfilling their basic physical and social needs, and, more importantly, whether they have the skills or abilities to manage these resources such that these resources are indeed achieved and maintained, and eventually compensated or restored during the lifespan. Thus, overall self-management ability is defined as a generative capacity (consisting of several sub-abilities) to take care of one's own important resources, i.e. resources that help to fulfil the five basic needs that thus contribute to well-being.

What abilities have been specified? This can be made clear most easily by an example. Let us take friendship, as a resource for fulfilment of the need for affection, to explicate the six sub-abilities and illustrate the explicit link between the abilities and concrete need fulfilment. Prerequisites in achieving and maintaining friendship are the ability to take initiatives in making friends and the ability to be self-efficacious with regard to one's own behaviour in making friends and being a friend. The maintenance of a friendship furthermore requires the ability to invest in the friendship, which, in turn, is helped by the ability to have a positive frame of mind with regard to this friendship in the future. Moreover, there is a self-management ability that helps to create synergetic effects and thus optimize the outcome of friendship for well-being: the ability to achieve and maintain multifunctionality in a friendship. A multifunctional friend is a person who can satisfy one's need for affection, but at the same time supports the fulfilment of other important needs such as the need for stimulation, for example by jointly participating in interesting activities. The underlying assumption is that the synergetic effects created by mutually reinforcing activities yield more overall well-being than unifunctional activities (Nieboer and Lindenberg 2002). Finally, there is a self-management ability that reduces the negative effects of loss on well-being: the ability to take care of variety with regard to friendship. Ensuring variety simply means not putting all of one's eggs in one basket, i.e. to have a variety of friends. If something happens to one friendship, there are others to buffer the negative effect.

Although these six abilities can be specified theoretically as distinct abilities, in reality they will relate to each other and mutually reinforce each other. For instance, self-efficacy reinforces the taking of initiatives, and a positive frame of mind reinforces investment behaviour, and vice versa. Moreover, the theoretical derivation of these six abilities does not imply that other abilities may not also be important for ageing successfully. But from the resources- and basic needs-based approach presented here, these six abilities emerge as interacting key abilities. In the literature, most of these abilities have commonly been analysed and investigated separately (see Steverink et al. 2005, for a review). Here, we integrate them into a larger framework of SMW because it is likely that they are jointly important for sustainable well-being, especially when they are directed at fulfilling the five basic needs (Steverink and Lindenberg 2008). So, although each of the six sub-abilities is considered important in itself, it is the combined and orchestrated use of all six which makes people better self-managers in the process of achieving and maintaining higher levels of resources for the fulfilment of well-being needs in the process of ageing (Steverink and Lindenberg 2008). The confirmatory factor-analyses that were executed in the development studies of a scale measuring this orchestrated concept of self-management ability showed that, indeed, overall self-management ability could be measured reliably as a composite concept of interrelated abilities (Schuurmans et al. 2005; see also Cramm et al. 2012).

Criteria of 'success' in the SMW theory

With its explicit notions about basic human needs and core self-management abilities, the SMW theory is very explicit about what ageing successfully means and, moreover, what the key criterion of 'success' should be. Individuals are most likely to age successfully if they are able to maintain—by using the core self-management abilities—important resources for the fulfilment of the five basic needs; need fulfilment will lead to the experience of overall subjective well-being. 'Success', thus, is the experience of subjective well-being that results from the fulfilment of the five basic physical and social needs: comfort, stimulation, affection, behavioural confirmation, and status. For the measurement of these five need fulfilments—together being conceptualized as overall subjective well-being—a scale has been developed (Nieboer et al 2005).

This criterion also implies that the most important external circumstances that contribute to overall well-being are clear and concrete: important external circumstances are those that deliver resources for the fulfilment of the needs for comfort, stimulation, affection, behavioural confirmation, and status. It is this specificity of needs and resources that makes the SMW theory most explicit about the criteria of 'success' and, together with the concreteness of the core self-management abilities, especially suitable as a basis for the design of interventions.

IMPLICATIONS FOR PRACTICE

Effective interventions aimed at supporting older adults in ageing successfully become ever more important with the still increasing numbers of older adults in the population. Effective interventions in the realm of successful ageing must be interventions that fit the characteristic processes that are typical at the later stages of life. As argued above, these processes are characterized by multidimensionality and multidirectionality. This means that interventions are needed that cover these multiple dimensions, as well as the diversity and heterogeneity of the ageing process. So far, most evidence-based interventions in the realm of supporting older adults in managing ageing-related challenges are unidimensional. Moreover, they are often focused only on the physical domain. For example, many effective self-management interventions exist that address specific health-related problems, such as chronic diseases (Lawn and Schoo, 2010).

In the psychosocial domain, evidence-based interventions also exist, but they are much fewer in number. These are basically also unidimensional: for example, interventions for managing depression (e.g. Serrano et al. 2004) or loneliness (e.g. Routasalo et al. 2008). Yet, as argued in the previous section, ageing individuals often face multiple challenges (physical, social, and psychological) simultaneously, which could be better managed simultaneously. For example, mobility loss may lead to isolation, which may lead to loneliness or depression, which then may further affect mobility loss, etc. So, ageing-related changes and losses often accumulate and interact, creating downward spirals of decreasing resources. Moreover, often people's self-regulatory capacity itself is decreasing with such accumulating losses. Ironically, people need their self-regulatory capacity most just when losses loom larger than gains, including the loss of self-management ability itself. Therefore, self-management interventions aiming at successful ageing should not just focus on one specific physical health problem, or one specific mental health problem, but cover all core aspects of well-being, including maintaining or regaining self-management ability itself. In other words, integrative and proactive interventions are needed, focusing on several important dimensions of well-being at the same time, and on effective self-management abilities that have reactive and proactive functions at the same time. So far, such integrative and proactive interventions—addressing not only health, but also social and psychological well-being—are relatively scarce (cf. Pinquart and Sörensen 2001). Moreover, relatively few interventions are designed explicitly to focus on the achievement and maintenance of overall well-being in later life, by teaching preventive and (pro)active self-regulatory skills for ageing successfully. What seems to be especially needed are effective self-management interventions that provide older adults with a general repertoire of cognitive and behavioural abilities for dealing with different and interacting ageing-related challenges, and at the same time, reinforce their strengths for achieving their well-being.

The first thing that is needed for the design of effective integrative interventions is adequate theory (Bengtson et al. 1999; Hendricks, Applebaum, and Kunkel 2010; Putney and Bengtson 2008). This is no different for larger programmes than for individualized interventions. The SMW theory, as presented in the previous section, is such an integrative theory. This theory can be, and has been, used for the design of integrative and proactive interventions. The interventions based on the SMW theory aim to improve self-management abilities as well as overall well-being by focusing on multiple domains of well-being, including both physical and psychosocial domains. Additionally, they include proactive strategies.

The interventions based on the SMW theory run under the names of GRIP & GLEAM (in Dutch: GRIP & GLANS). The GRIP & GLEAM (G&G) courses are intended for older people who have lost—or are at risk of losing—resources in several domains of functioning, which may lead to a diminished capacity for managing new losses or changes. The interventions thus deal with the issue of the multiple challenges that we discussed earlier. Moreover, the G&G approach is based on an explicitly positive concept, in the sense that they focus on what individuals are still able to do and not only on abilities they have lost. Additionally, the self-management abilities taught are not only intended as a response to loss but also as a tool to be used before loss has occurred. The G&G approach is therefore also strongly proactive and preventive in nature.

The G&G interventions are driven by the application of the theory of the SMW, as explicated above (Steverink et al. 2005). This theory postulates that if people lose resources, they are not only at risk of losing well-being, but also of losing self-management capacity. Therefore, self-management abilities need to be strengthened together with important resources for physical and social well-being. If people have good self-management abilities—that is, skills enabling them adequately to handle their physical and social resources—it may be expected to lead to physical and social well-being, and subsequently to overall psychological well-being. The SMW theory defines five core domains of well-being and six core self-management skills. Both the dimensions of well-being and the self-management abilities are explicitly linked, as shown in Figure 5.2.

This matrix of abilities and domains of well-being basically states that each of the six abilities needs to be applied to each of the five dimensions of well-being in order to yield overall well-being (see Steverink et al. 2005 for more details). As such, the matrix basically constitutes the 'blueprint' for the design of the G&G interventions and thus also for the concrete ingredients of the interventions. In order to be able also to evaluate the effectiveness of G&G interventions, the 'blueprint' has been used as the basis for the development of a measurement instrument to measure the level of self-management ability, the Self-management Ability Scale (SMAS-30; Schuurmans et al. 2005). This scale, and also a shorter version of it (Cramm et al. 2012), measures the six self-management abilities as separate abilities, and also provides an overall index of overall self-management ability. The scale is being applied

Dimensions of well-being → Self-management abilities ↓	Comfort	Stimulation	Affection	Behavioural confirmation	Status
Self-efficacy beliefs					
Positive frame of mind					
Taking the initiative					
Investment behaviour					
Multifunctionality of resources					
Variety in resources					

FIGURE 5.2 The matrix of the six Self-management Abilities and the five Dimensions of Well-being as specified by the Self-management of Well-being theory.

Reproduced from *European Journal of Ageing*, 2(4), pp. 235–244, How to understand and improve older people's self-management of wellbeing, Nardi Steverink, Siegwart Lindenberg, and Joris P. J. Slaets © 2005, Springer Science and Business Media. With kind permission from Springer Science and Business Media.

widely in intervention research (e.g. Alma et al. 2011; Frieswijk et al. 2006; Kremers et al. 2006; Martina, Stevens, and Westerhof 2012; Schuurmans 2004). Additionally, the scales have been used in other research projects and surveys (e.g. Cramm et al. 2013; Schuurmans et al. 2004; Steverink and Lindenberg 2008).

The G&G courses have been evaluated in randomized controlled trials and have proven to be effective regarding the improvement of self-management ability and well-being in different groups of older people. Schuurmans (2004) evaluated the G&G home visits course in frail older community-dwelling people. Kremers et al. (2006) evaluated the G&G group course in lonely older women. Frieswijk et al. (2006) evaluated the G&G self-help method in slightly frail community-dwelling older people. In all three studies positive effects were found on both self-management ability and subjective well-being. These effects were still present after four to six months.

Two specific strengths of the G&G approach need to be mentioned explicitly. First, the G&G approach not only addresses the improvement of concrete self-management abilities (i.e. behaviours and strategies), but explicitly also what the self-management abilities should be directed at (i.e. the important domains of well-being). Self-management abilities can only be 'efficient' when they are directed at core dimensions of well-being—both the physical and psychosocial dimensions. Therefore, both the abilities and the dimensions of well-being are being addressed in orchestration. A second specific strength of the G&G approach is that, although the basic approach is integrative and general, at the same time it allows every individual older adult to apply it to his or her unique personal situation and preferences. Thus, the general character of the universal needs makes it possible to apply the interventions to a wide range of different people in a personalized way. For example, all five needs are universal, but perhaps not all needs require intervention: one can choose which need fulfilment to work on. Then, when, for example, selecting to work on the need for affection, people can chose their personal way of how to go about fulfilling this need: one older adult can choose to improve her contact with a specific grandchild; another can choose to buy a dog. It is this latter aspect that makes the interventions particularly well-tailored to clinical application.

Summary

The trend of population ageing makes it crucial to search for workable insights and interventions to support and serve increasing numbers of older adults in their ability to age successfully. Both the growth in numbers of older people and the related threat of an overloaded healthcare and welfare system, together with ever-increasing life expectancy, make it increasingly important that older adults themselves become good self-managers in their own ageing process. This is all the more urgent because life expectancy is increasing without an adequate increase in socially defined roles for older adults. This urgency is also in line with the expressed desire of many older people: they wish to remain in control of their own lives and of their own well-being for as long as possible. Supportive interventions for self-management ability and well-being thus seem a valuable tool to maintain the health and welfare of older people. Yet, the question remains as to how successful development and ageing can best be understood and approached in interventions and policy.

In the last decades, the biological deficit approach to ageing has become less dominant through an increasing recognition that successful ageing is a phenomenon that covers multiple domains, ranging from societal and social to physical and psychological domains. Moreover, the finding that 'usual' ageing can be distinguished from 'successful' ageing has inspired many to look at possible strengths and resilience in ageing rather than just deficits, leading to the search for adequate theories about the behavioural and social pathways to successful ageing that could guide the development of interventions and policy.

Four important models and theories on successful development and ageing that take the new perspectives on ageing into account are Ryff's model of Psychological Well-being (PWB), the model of Selection, Optimization and Compensation (SOC), the Motivational Theory of Life-span Development, and the theory of Self-management of Well-being (SMW theory). Three of the four models partly overlap in their behavioural and motivational aspects, because they all consider optimization to be the most general basic motivational drive, and selection and compensation as strategies to cope with changes and losses or failures. With regard to interventions, however, it is also essential to be as concrete as possible about what the 'success' in 'successful ageing' might mean. Ryff's model is explicit about the criteria of 'success', but does not specify behavioural aspects. Only the SMW theory is explicit on both the behavioural and motivational aspects *and* the criteria of 'success', because it specifies the goals at which the adaptive and proactive behavioural processes should be directed in order to arrive at 'success'. Concretely, these goals are directly related to the five basic needs, as proposed by the theory of SMW. In other words, the SMW theory not only specifies behavioural processes, but also specifies what people should select and optimize, and what they should find compensation for if they aim to age successfully. In addition, the SMW theory is explicit about the core self-management abilities, which, in turn, have to be related to the fulfilment of basic needs. It is this concreteness of goals (related to basic needs) and self-management abilities that makes the SMW theory most explicit about the criteria of 'success' and thereby especially suitable as a basis for the design of interventions.

Indeed, concrete interventions have been developed on the basis of the SMW theory: the GRIP & GLEAM (G&G) interventions (in Dutch: GRIP & GLANS). The G&G interventions are theory-driven and they are innovative because they cover the whole spectrum of well-being rather than just one specific aspect, as most other interventions do. Moreover, they are basically positive and proactive, focusing on what people still have and are willing to do and develop, rather than on losses and problems. Broad self-management interventions such as the G&G interventions are also important for prevention. Ageing healthily and happily often requires that people begin to learn at younger ages how to manage their resources adequately. Therefore, the G&G interventions—addressing the broad spectrum of self-management ability in orchestration with core aspects of well-being—are not only a tool in reactive management (i.e. addressing losses that have already occurred), they are also a tool in positive (i.e. building on one's strengths) and proactive management (i.e. building resources before losses occur). Finally, the G&G interventions are evidence-based, and research is in progress on the implementation of the interventions in Dutch health- and social-care organizations, and on their cost-effectiveness (Kuiper et al. 2012). Many indications exist that psychosocial interventions can save medical costs. Thus, interventions such as the G&G

interventions may be an important complementary tool in health and social care for older adults.

FUTURE OUTLOOK

The field of psychosocial interventions that support older adults in ageing successfully is growing. Such clinical approaches, like the G&G interventions, usually take an individual-centred focus. This has been shown to be beneficial to many older people. However, the insight is growing that individuals are inherently social beings (Cacioppo and Patrick 2008), and their ability to self-manage depends largely on their social connections and social networks. Consequently, it becomes increasingly clear that in the end interventions might be more effective when not just the individual older adult but also his or her social network are taken into account in the intervention process. So far, approaches to incorporate social networks into programmes of self-management are mostly found in the field of chronic disease self-management (e.g. Vassilev et al. 2011). However, ageing-related self-management, if it is to be successful, may in the end be a matter of how the individual together with others in the informal social network is co-producing successful outcomes, just as they might do to increase livability in neighbourhoods (see Frieling, Lindenberg, and Stokman 2012). So future developments of interventions may benefit from new insights on the role of others and the wider social network in adequate self-management during the process of ageing. Paying more attention to the build-up of self-management ability and well-being, both in older and in younger people, together with attention to the social environment of individuals, may lead to higher levels of successful ageing in both individual older adults and their social networks and groups, and so for society as a whole.

KEY REFERENCES AND SOURCES FOR FURTHER READING

Holt-Lunstad, J., Smith, T. B., and Layton, J. B. (2010). 'Social Relationships and Mortality Risk: A Meta-analytic Review'. *PLoS Medicine* 7: 1–20.

Huber, M., Knottnerus, J. A., Green, L., Van der Horst, H., Jadad, A. R., et al. (2011). 'How Should We Define Health?' *British Medical Journal* 343: d4163. doi:10.1136/bmj.d4163.

Rowe, J. W. and Kahn, R. L. (1987). 'Human Aging: Usual and Successful'. *Science* 237: 143–49.

Steverink, N. and Lindenberg, S. (2006). 'Which Social Needs are Important for Subjective Wellbeing? What Happens to them with Aging?' *Psychology and Aging* 21: 281–90.

Steverink, N., Lindenberg, S., and Slaets, J. P. J. (2005). 'How to Understand and Improve Older People's Self-management of Wellbeing'. *European Journal of Ageing* 2: 235–44.

REFERENCES

Alma, M. A., Van der Mei, S. F., Feitsma, W. N., Groothoff, J. W., Van Tilburg, T. G., et al. (2011). 'Loneliness and Self-management Abilities in the Visually Impaired Elderly'. *Journal of Aging and Health* 23(5): 843–861. doi:10.1177/0898264311399758.

Baltes, P. B. and Baltes, M. M. (1990). 'Psychological Perspectives on successful Aging: The Model of Selective Optimization with Compensation'. In P. B. Baltes and M. M. Baltes (eds), *Successful Aging: Perspectives from the Behavioral Sciences* (pp. 1–34). Cambridge: Cambridge University Press.

Baumeister, R. F. and Leary, M. R. (1995). 'The Need to Belong: Desire for Interpersonal Attachments as a Fundamental Human Motivation'. *Psychological Bulletin* 117: 497–529.

Bengtson, V. L., Rice, C. J., and Johnson, M. L. (1999). 'Are Theories of Aging Important? Models and Explanations in Gerontology at the Turn of the Century'. In V. L. Bengtson and K. W. Schaie (eds), *Handbook of Theories of Aging* (pp. 3–20). New York: Springer.

van Bruggen, A. (2001). *Individual Production of Social Well-being: An Exploratory Study*. Dissertation. Groningen: Groningen University. http://dissertations.ub.rug.nl/faculties/gmw/2001/a.c.van.bruggen/.

Buss, D. M. and Kenrick, D. T. (1998). 'Evolutionary Social Psychology'. In D. T. Gilbert, S. T. Fiske, and G. Lindzey (eds), *The Handbook of Social Psychology* (4th edn; pp. 982–1026). New York: McGraw-Hill.

Cacioppo, J. T. and Patrick, W. (2008). *Loneliness: Human Nature and the Need for Social Connectedness*. New York: W.W. Norton & Company.

Cohen, S. (2004). 'Social Relationships and Health'. *American Psychologist* 59: 676–684.

Collins, A. L., Goldman, N., and Rodriguez, G. (2008). 'Is Positive Well-being Protective of Mobility Limitations among Older Adults?' *Journal of Gerontology: Psychological Sciences* 63: P321–P327.

Cramm, J. M., Strating, M. M. H., de Vreede, P. L., Steverink, N., and Nieboer, A. P. (2012). 'Validation of the Self-management Ability Scale (SMAS) and Development and Validation of a Shorter Scale (SMAS-S) among Older Patients Shortly after Hospitalization'. *Health and Quality of Life Outcomes* 10(9). http://www.hqlo.com/content/10/1/9.

Cramm, J. M., Hartgerink, J. M., Steyerberg, E. W., Bakker, T. J., Mackenbach, J. P., et al. (2013). 'Understanding Older Patients' Self-management Abilities: Functional Loss, Self-management, and Well-being'. *Quality of Life Research* 22: 85–92. doi:10.1007/s11136-012-0131-9.

Deci, E. L., and Ryan, R. M. (2000). 'The "What" and "Why" of Goal Pursuits: Human Needs and the Self-determination of Behavior'. *Psychological Inquiry* 11: 227–268.

Depp C. A. and Jeste, D. V. (2006). 'Definitions and Predictors of Successful Aging: A Comprehensive Review of Later Quantitative Studies'. *American Journal of Geriatric Psychiatry* 14: 6–20.

Fernández-Ballesteros, R. (2003). 'Light and Dark in the Psychology of Human Strengths: The Example of Psychogerontology'. In L. G. Aspinwall and U. M. Staudinger (eds), *A Psychology of Human Strengths: Fundamental Questions and Future Directions for a Positive Psychology* (pp. 131–47). Washington, DC: American Psychological Association.

Freund, A. M. and Baltes, P. B. (2007). 'Toward a Theory of Successful Aging: Selection, Optimization, and Compensation'. In: R. Fernández-Ballesteros (ed.), *Geropsychology: European Perspectives for an Aging World* (pp. 239–254). Göttingen: Hogrefe.

Freund, A. M., Nikitin, J., and Ritter, J. O. (2009). 'Psychological Consequences of Longevity: The Increasing Importance of Self-regulation in Old Age'. *Human Development* 52: 1–37. doi:10.1159/000189213.

Frieling, M., Lindenberg, S., and Stokman, F. N. (2012). 'Collaborative Communities through Coproduction: Two Case Studies'. *American Review of Public Administration*. doi:10.1177/0275074012456897.

Frieswijk, N., Steverink, N., Buunk, B. P., and Slaets, J. P. J. (2006). 'The Effectiveness of a Bibliotherapy in Increasing the Self-management Ability of Slightly to Moderately

Frail Older People'. *Patient Education and Counseling* 61: 219–227. doi:10.1016/j. pec.2005.03.011.

George, L. K. (2006). 'Perceived Quality of Life'. In R. H. Binstock and L. K. George (eds), *Handbook of Aging and the Social Sciences* (6th edn; pp. 320–436). San Diego, CA: Academic Press.

Hawkley, L. C. and Cacioppo, J. T. (2007). 'Aging and Loneliness: Downhill Quickly?' *Current Directions in Psychological Science* 16: 187–191.

Heckhausen, J. and Schulz, R. (1995). 'A Life-span Theory of Control'. *Psychological Review* 102: 284–304.

Heckhausen, J., Wrosch, C., and Schulz, R. (2010). 'A Motivational Theory of Life-span Development'. *Psychological Review* 117: 32–60. doi:10.1037/a0017668.

Hendricks, J., Applebaum, R., and Kunkel, S. (2010). 'A World Apart? Bridging the Gap between Theory and Applied Social Gerontology'. *Gerontologist* 50: 284–293. doi:10.1093/geront/gnp167.

Holt-Lunstad, J., Smith, T. B., and Layton, J. B. (2010). 'Social Relationships and Mortality Risk: A Meta-analytic Review'. *PLoS Medicine* 7: 1–20.

House, J. S., Landis, K. R., and Umberson, D. (1988). 'Social Relationships and Health'. *Science* 241: 540–545.

Huber, M., Knottnerus, J. A., Green, L., van der Horst, H., Jadad, A. R., et al. (2011). 'How Should We Define Health?' *British Medical Journal* 343: d4163. doi: 10.1136/bmj.d4163.

Kremers, I. P., Steverink, N., Albersnagel, F. A., and Slaets, J. P. J. (2006). 'Improved Self-management Ability and Well-being in Older Women after a Short Group Intervention'. *Aging & Mental Health* 10: 476–484.

Kuiper, D., Sanderman, R., Reijneveld, S. A., and Steverink, N. (2012). 'Implementation of the GRIP and GLEAM Interventions for Older Adults: Preliminary Results of a Process Evaluation'. Paper presented at the 11th National Conference of the Dutch Gerontological Society: Ede, The Netherlands. http://www.nardisteverink.nl/index.php?content=publications.

Lawn, S. and Schoo, A. M. (2010). 'Supporting Self-management of Chronic Health Conditions: Common Approaches'. *Patient Education and Counseling* 80: 205–211.

Lindenberg, S. (1996). 'Continuities in the Theory of Social Production Functions'. In S. M. Lindenberg and H. B. G. Ganzeboom (eds), *Verklarende sociologie: opstellen voor Reinhard Wippler* [Explanatory Sociology: Essays in Honor of Reinhard Wippler] (pp. 169–184). Amsterdam: Thesis Publishers.

Lindenberg, S. (2013). 'Social Rationality, Self-regulation and Well-being: The Regulatory Significance of Needs, Goals, and the Self'. In R. Wittek, T. A. B. Snijders, and V. Nee (eds), *Handbook of Rational Choice Social Research* (pp. 72–112). Stanford: Stanford University Press.

Martina, C. M. S., Stevens, N. L., and Westerhof, G. J. (2012). 'Promotion of Self-management in Friendship'. *Aging & Mental Health* 16(2): 245–253.

Maslow, A. H. (1970). *Motivation and Personality* (2nd edn). New York: Harper & Row.

Nieboer, A. P. and Lindenberg, S. (2002). 'Substitution, Buffers and Subjective Wellbeing: A Hierarchical Approach'. In E. Gullone and R. A. Cummins (eds), *The Universality of Subjective Wellbeing Indicators* (pp. 175–189). Dordrecht: Kluwer Academic.

Nieboer, A. P., Lindenberg, S., Boomsma, A., and van Bruggen, A. C. (2005). 'Dimensions of Wellbeing and their Measurement: The SPF-IL Scale'. *Social Indicators Research* 73: 313–53.

Ormel, J., Lindenberg, S., Steverink, N., and Verbrugge, L. M. (1999). 'Subjective Wellbeing and Social Production Functions'. *Social Indicators Research* 46: 61–90.

Ormel, J. (2002). 'Social Production Function (SPF) Theory as an Heuristic for Understanding Developmental Trajectories and Outcomes'. In L. Pulkkinen and A. Caspi (eds), *Paths to*

Successful Development: Personality in the Life Course (pp. 353–379). New York: Cambridge University Press.

Ostir, G. V., Markides, K. S., Black, S. A., and Goodwin, J. S. (2000). 'Emotional Well-being Predicts Subsequent Functional Independence and Survival'. *Journal of the American Geriatrics Society* 48: 473–478.

Pinquart, M. and Sörensen, S. (2001). 'How Effective are Psychotherapeutic and Other Psychosocial Interventions with Older Adults? A Meta-analysis'. *Journal of Mental Health and Aging* 7: 207–243.

Putney, N. M. and Bengtson, V. L. (2008). 'Theories of Aging'. In D. Carr, R. Crosnoe, M. E. Hughes, and A. Pienta (eds), *Encyclopedia of the Life Course and Human Development* (pp. 413–423). Farmington Hills, MI: Gale Group.

Reis, H. T., Collins, W. A., and Berscheid, E. (2000). 'The Relationship Context of Human Behavior and Development'. *Psychological Bulletin* 126: 844–872.

Riley, M. W. and Riley, J. W. (1994). 'Structural Lag: Past and Future'. In M. W. Riley, R. L. Kahn, and A. Foner (eds), *Age and Structural Lag: Society's Failure in Work, Family and Leisure* (pp. 15–36). New York: Wiley.

Rothbaum, F., Weisz, J. R., and Snyder, S. S. (1982). 'Changing the World and Changing the Self: A Two Process Model of Perceived Control'. *Journal of Personality and Social Psychology* 42: 5–37.

Routasalo, P. E., Tilvis, R. S., Kautiainen, H., and Pitkala, K. H. (2008). 'Effects of Psychosocial Group Rehabilitation on Social Functioning, Loneliness and Well-being of Lonely, Older People: Randomized Controlled Trial'. *Journal of Advanced Nursing* 65: 297–305.

Rowe, J. W. and Kahn, R. L. (1987). 'Human Aging: Usual and Successful'. *Science* 237: 143–149.

Ryff, C. D. (1989). 'Beyond Ponce de Leon and Life Satisfaction: New Directions in Quest of Successful Ageing'. *International Journal of Behavioral Development* 12: 35–55.

Ryff, C. D. and Keyes, C. L. M. (1995). 'The Structure of Psychological Well-being Revisited'. *Journal of Personality and Social Psychology* 69(4): 719–727.

Schulz, R. and Heckhausen, J. (1996). 'A Life-span Model of Successful Aging'. *American Psychologist* 51: 702–714.

Schuurmans, H. (2004). *Promoting Well-being in Frail Elderly People: Theory and Intervention.* Dissertation. Groningen: Groningen University. http://dissertations.ub.rug.nl/faculties/medicine/2004/j.e.h.m.schuurmans/.

Schuurmans, H., Steverink, N., Lindenberg, S., Frieswijk, N., and Slaets, J. P. J. (2004). 'Old or Frail: What Tells us More?' *Journal of Gerontology: Medical Sciences* 59: M962–M965.

Schuurmans, H., Steverink, N., Frieswijk, N., Buunk, B. P., Slaets, J. P. J., et al. (2005). 'How to Measure Self-management Abilities in Older People by Self-report. The Development of the SMAS-30'. *Quality of Life Research* 14: 2215–2228.

Seeman, T. E. (1996). 'Social Ties and Health: The Benefits of Social Integration'. *Annals of Epidemiology* 6: 442–451.

Serrano, J. P., Latorre, J. M., Gatz, M., and Montanes, J. (2004). 'Life Review Therapy Using Autobiographical Retrieval Practice for Older Adults with Depressive Symptomatology'. *Psychology and Aging* 19: 272–277.

Steverink, N., Lindenberg, S., and Ormel, J. (1998). 'Towards Understanding Successful Ageing: Patterned Change in Resources and Goals'. *Ageing and Society* 18: 441–467.

Steverink, N. (2001). 'When and Why Frail Elderly People Give Up Independent Living: The Netherlands as an Example'. *Ageing and Society* 21: 45–69.

Steverink, N., Lindenberg, S., and Slaets, J. P. J. (2005). 'How to Understand and Improve Older People's Self-management of Wellbeing'. *European Journal of Ageing* 2: 235–244.

Steverink, N. and Lindenberg, S. (2006). 'Which Social Needs are Important for Subjective Wellbeing? What Happens to them with Aging?' *Psychology and Aging* 21: 281–290.

Steverink, N. and Lindenberg, S. (2008). 'Do Good Self-managers Have Less Physical and Social Resource Deficits and More Well-being in Later Life?' *European Journal of Ageing* 5: 181–190.

Steverink, N., Veenstra, R., Oldehinkel, A. J., Gans, R. O. B., and Rosmalen, J. G. M. (2011). 'Is Social Stress in the First Half of Life Detrimental to Later Physical and Mental Health in both Men and Women?' *European Journal of Ageing* 8: 21–30.

Vassilev, I., Rogers, A., Sanders, C., Kennedy, A., Blickem, C., et al. (2011). 'Social Networks, Social Capital and Chronic Illness Self-management: A Realist View'. *Chronic Illness* 7: 60–86.

Veenhoven, R. (2008). 'Healthy Happiness: Effects of Happiness on Physical Health and the Consequences for Preventive Health Care'. *Journal of Happiness Studies* 9: 449–469.

Walker, A. (1999). 'Public Policy and Theories of Aging: Constructing and Reconstructing Old Age'. In V. L. Bengtson and K.W. Schaie (eds), *Handbook of Theories of Aging* (pp. 361–378). New York: Springer.

World Health Organization (2002). *Active Ageing: A Policy Framework*. Geneva: WHO.

CHAPTER 6

SOCIAL CAPITAL AND GENDER

Critical Influences on Living Arrangements and Care-giving in Old Age

TONI C. ANTONUCCI, KRISTINE J. AJROUCH, AND SOJUNG PARK

INTRODUCTION

SHIFTING population demographics make it clear that the age structure of most countries is changing radically. People are living longer, although for the most part people are also healthier. Nevertheless, it is clear that we live in a time of constrained resources during which vulnerable populations, such as older adults, are often at increased risk. In this chapter, we consider the resources of older people, specifically social capital and gender, as they relate to two, almost universal, concerns of ageing: the living environment and care-giving.

We begin by outlining the perspectives that form the theoretical grounding of the chapter. We consider social capital by focusing on social relations, specifically the individual's convoy of social relations. Much of the social capital an individual builds over the years is based on the social relationships that people develop. These can create assets or vulnerabilities that vary by gender depending on the nature of these long-time, often life-time, social relations. We also outline the usefulness of considering social capital as a phenomenon especially relevant to gender and the ageing experience by focusing on the intersectionality framework. As people age they develop unique ways to cope with the challenges they face, and these strategies are shaped by whether one is a man or woman.

We use these theoretical perspectives to examine living arrangements and care-giving. We consider the different types of living arrangements, the increasing tendency to wish to age in place but also to acknowledge that where that 'place' is is likely to vary depending on the resources or social capital of the ageing individual. Similarly, we consider care-giving, its provision and receipt, as a common challenge of ageing. We examine the influence of social capital and gender on how the care-giving situation is experienced. We believe this unique approach to considering two common challenges of ageing, i.e. an optimal living environment and the availability of care-giving when needed, through the lenses of social capital and gender provides important insights concerning how to maintain or achieve a healthy older population.

THEORETICAL PERSPECTIVES: SOCIAL CAPITAL AND THE CONVOY MODEL

Social capital 'is created when the relations among persons change in ways that facilitate action' (Coleman 1990: 304). In fact, relationships, as social capital, are considered a resource. In this chapter we consider relationships as a resource via the concept of the convoy model. Convoys represent an assembly of family and friends who surround the individual and are available as resources in times of need. As such, convoys of social relations may be thought of as a resource, a form of social capital. The convoy model of social relations offers a framework within which to consider links between gender, age, and the availability of social capital. Convoys are thought to be dynamic and lifelong, changing in some ways, but remaining stable in others, across time and situations (Antonucci 1985; Kahn and Antonucci 1980).

As outlined in Figure 6.1 and for the purposes of this chapter, we focus primarily on the links between personal characteristics (which include, age, gender, race, ethnicity, and socio-economic status) and the multiple dimensions of social relations. The convoy model of social relations acknowledges and identifies the multidimensionality inherent in relationships. In particular, dimensions of structure, type, and quality are elaborated. Each dimension represents a specific resource type. The structure of relationships includes network size, composition, contact frequency, and geographic proximity. Network structure signifies whether or not resources are available in the first place. This is important because if there are no people identified as network members, there is no possibility for a relationship or for support to be received from that relationship. The size of a network identifies the number of people available in an individual's convoy. Some are large and others small, though most people have five to seven people to whom they feel close. Composition refers to the nature of the individual's relationship with their network members, i.e. family or friends, neighbours. Contact frequency simply identifies how often network members are in touch with each other, whether by phone, email, Skype or in person, and geographic proximity represents how close, geographically, network members are to each other.

Of critical importance is the type of support network members exchange. The most common types of support are instrumental, emotional, and informational. Instrumental support refers to the exchange of tangible goods such as money, while emotional support refers to less tangible support such as love and affection. And, finally, informational support refers to the exchange of knowledge or facts. Support can be provided or received. This dimension represents the types of resources available from and exchanged within a relationship. Quality of support draws attention to the experiences of both positive and negative elements of relationships, illustrating psychological resources available through relationships. Research now clearly indicates that support can be of a primarily positive quality as well as a primarily negative quality. In addition, recent research has made clear that some networks include both

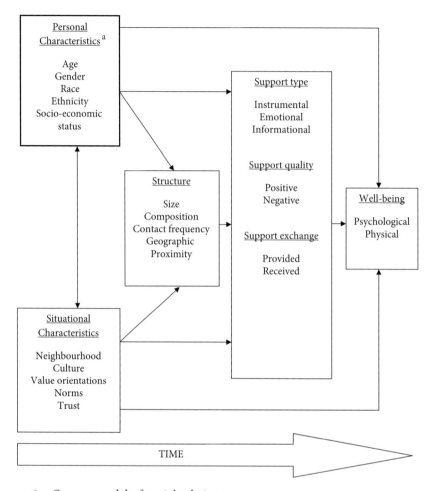

FIGURE 6.1 Convoy model of social relations.

[a] The personal characteristics box is in bold to signify intersectionality, i.e. each aspect of personal characteristics informs each of the other aspects.

positive and negative quality relationships, and can even include both positive and negative quality within the same relationship. Thus, the convoy model identifies the complexity of social relations as a resource, providing key insights into the nature of social capital.

The convoy model has been used to guide understanding of how network characteristics may differ according to life stage as well as by socio-economic status (SES) differentially for men and women (Ajrouch, Blandon, and Antonucci 2005). Findings point to the importance of recognizing gendered statuses over the life course. For instance, including the category of 'homemakers' as an occupation suggests that this category of women may differentially benefit from the SES level of their husband during the life course. Using women's own level of education or occupation may underestimate their socio-economic status (see Grundy and Holt 2001). Furthermore, findings elaborated the gendered characteristics of convoys over the life course (Moen 2001). Network structure did not vary much among men at different ages; nevertheless, life-stage effects emerged particularly among women in late-life, with those aged 75+ differing most in network structure from their middle-aged counterparts. When one considers that these findings are especially relevant for women aged 75+ years, it may be the case that their children have moved away and/or are busy with their own family obligations, leaving less time to devote to their parents. This is particularly important because at this stage of life, there is often a need for greater resources, but less likelihood of acquiring new access to these resources. Research findings suggest that the structure of personal networks in later life stages do not provide the same levels of potential capital for women as they do for women in mid-life. Such resource changes are less likely among men. It appears that various social resources available to women are especially sensitive to different measures of SES and that life stage represents an important means by which to understand social resources available to women and men (Ajrouch et al. 2005). In sum, the convoy model provides a flexible framework to ascertain both continuity and change in men's and women's social ties at various life stages.

Convoys also call attention to situational factors such as cultural context (Ajrouch and Antonucci 2014). Social capital exists within a broader context, conditioned by larger social forces including culture. Culture signifies value orientations, which in turn shape the nature of relationships, and hence the ways in which they serve as a resource. Cultural approaches to the study of social relations often introduce specific values and norms. The accumulating literature identifies several value dimensions to elaborate cultural variations in the structure and quality of social relationships. Some of those most widely accepted include: individualism/collectivism, relatedness/separateness, traditional/secular, and self-expression/survival (Hofstede 1980; Inglehart and Welzel 2005; Markus and Kitayama 1991; Triandis et al. 1988). For example, cultures that are individualistic/separate and value self-expression are said to: focus on maintaining relationships that are seen as beneficial for personal goals; include parents' investments in children that are more psychological than economic; have people who feel obligated to family but perceive this obligation as voluntary; have people who feel at ease interacting with strangers; and consider people to be separate, non-overlapping entities. Individualism is also associated with more direct goal-oriented conversation styles (Kagitcibasi 1996; Oyserman, Coon, and Kemmelmeier 2002). On the other hand, cultures ascribing to collectivism, relatedness, and/or survival tend to believe that group membership is unchangeable and that in-group exchanges are based on principles of equality and generosity (Oyserman et al. 2002; Takahashi et al. 2002). They tend to have extended families in which: young people provide direct financial help to older family members; there is greater preference for sons; fertility rates are higher; and there is an old-age-security value of children. These cultures are more likely to have social interactions with in-group members, engage in indirect communication styles, and be more concerned with a partner's feelings. As a result, cultural orientations shape the ways in which relationships serve as potential resources to older adults. Convoys of social relations, therefore, are likely to develop and function differently depending on cultural orientations and are likely to have different implications for living arrangements and care-giving.

The ways in which culture shapes social capital by gender are less clear. For instance, it appears that, regardless of cultural orientation, men and women hold similar cultural norms concerning close ties, trust norms, and obligation (Felmlee and Muraco 2009). However, while women tend to be more relationally oriented than men in western societies (e.g. Barer 1994; Cornwell 2011; Davidson 2004), men and women have been characterized as equally relational in non-western cultures (e.g. Joseph 1993; Xu and Norstrand 2012). Social networks may, nevertheless, differ for men and women in how they serve as resources in non-western cultures. For instance, recent research on convoys of social relations in Lebanon shows the importance of income levels in predicting the structure and quality of social networks for men and women in later life (Antonucci, Ajrouch and Abdulrahim 2010). Findings indicate that among the highest income groups, unique age patterns were evident for women; those 60 and older reported 75% of their networks live in Lebanon compared to over 90% for those in middle and younger age groups. Age differences in relationship closeness with siblings were most pronounced among younger men (18–39), who reported higher closeness ratings on average than middle-aged or older men. Low-income older women reported lowest relationship closeness with spouse. These patterns suggest that both older men and women may be more vulnerable in terms of the capital available through their social relationships than their younger counterparts, though such vulnerabilities for older women are especially sensitive to socio-economic position.

The ways in which gender shapes access to social capital must be understood as contingent on larger cultural forces, dynamic and changing over the life course (Calasanti 2010). Convoys form and are maintained in response to such conditions but they also provide opportunities for the development of various pathways (e.g. social support, immune system function) that ultimately influence health. While pathways between social relations and health receive a fair amount of attention, an area in need of further elaboration is the intersection of gender and age and their influence on convoy characteristics. An examination of the influence of pathways between gender and social relations on living arrangements and care-giving in later life will offer a more theoretically developed understanding of life-course social capital.

GENDER, AGEING, AND INTERSECTIONALITY

Gender structures the entire life course, impinging on relationships that range from the interpersonal to the institutional. Social capital varies by gender and usually accumulates over time. Hence, the presence of resources in middle and old age derives from the nature and type of relations with others developed across the life course. The social construction of gender has been widely addressed in the literature, with identified insights for better understanding the ageing process. Gender refers to ideals of masculinity and femininity, each of which provide distinguishing characteristics believed appropriate and core to being a man or a woman (Phillips, Ajrouch, and Hillcoat-Nalletamby 2010). Gender constitutes a critical social force in the experience of ageing, and is considered a pervasive marker of inequality. Though gender issues may vary depending on the social, cultural, and political context in which people grow older, research suggests that areas where older men and older women differ include life expectancy, health, social relations, and socio-economic resources. For instance, women live longer than men, but they also report a higher prevalence of chronic illness and disability (Barer 1994; Verbrugge 1985). However, the meanings associated with health status and symptoms in later life are often gendered (Alex 2010; Andermann 2010; Solimeo 2008). Women tend to emphasize more intimate relational activities such as understanding others and connectedness; men, on the other hand, focus on relational aspects that emphasize taking responsibility for close others' well-being and maintaining a position of authority. Moreover, roles, expectations, and social network characteristics vary depending on whether one is a man or woman (Ajrouch et al 2005; Moen 2001). Finally, men accumulate financial resources over the life course that often exceed those earned by women (Hartmann and English 2009). Some argue that with age, differences that distinguished men and women earlier in life tend to disappear, and therefore inequalities based on gender diminish (Neugarten and Guttmann 1958). For instance, gender gaps in depressive symptoms documented during earlier parts of the life course diminish in old age so that men and women's experiences of depressive symptoms do not vary greatly from one another (Akiyama and Antonucci 2002). Nevertheless, men and women often differ with regard to earlier life-course opportunities and encounters, which then shape situations later in life. Gender may be key to understanding the development of, use of, and access to social capital, especially in the form of living arrangements and care-giving.

The development of the intersectionality paradigm emerged as an interdisciplinary project that builds from notions that identities, such as gender, are social constructions, made meaningful within specific contexts through social relationships. We incorporate this perspective into the convoy model of social relations. In Figure 6.1, the personal characteristics box is in bold to signify intersectionality, i.e. each aspect of personal characteristics informs each of the other aspects. The intersectionality perspective moves beyond the notion that advantages or disadvantages associated with gender simply accumulate additively. Instead, intersectionality advocates understanding how gender operates in tandem with other factors such as race, ethnicity, and SES, each influencing the other (Dill and Zambrana 2009; Mullings and Schulz 2006; Shields 2008; Stoller and Gibson 2000), thus having multiplicative rather than simple additive effects. For example, the meaning of manhood and womanhood may vary by racial or ethnic group, and vice versa the meaning of being Black, Asian, Latino, Native American, or Arab may depend on whether one is a man or woman. The strength of the intersectionality framework lies in the attention it draws to focusing on multiple identities (e.g. gender, race, ethnicity) and multiple dimensions of social organization (e.g. power dynamics) simultaneously (Dill and Zambrana 2009). We propose to apply this framework with the added variable of age. In other words, we advance that the experience of old age varies depending on gender, race, ethnicity, and SES, and that, simultaneously, manhood and womanhood are shaped by age. As is now widely understood, men and women are perceived to be old at different ages (Toothman and Barrett 2011). Moreover, the ways in which men and women experience social capital may vary. Social capital among men is often understood to be part of the public sphere, the result of accomplishments at work or in the community, but among women it is often part of the private sphere, the result of investments in family and friends (Hyyppa 2010). This chapter considers the latest research in the areas of gender, age, and social capital to highlight strengths as well as challenges in using intersectionality and the convoy model of social relations as theoretical frameworks to clarify developments in the field. We specifically address two areas in which gender and social capital may be of particular importance in later life: living arrangements and care-giving. We then consider implications for practice and future directions.

LIVING ENVIRONMENTS

Living environments represent those sites where people spend much of their time over the life course (Wahl 2003). Options for where to live clearly differ depending on accumulated social capital and gender. Recent developments indicate that decisions concerning where to age and whether to age in place may be an issue for older adults living in the community, as well as for those who choose planned living environments. Research on community-dwelling older adults tends to focus on physical and mental health as part of the process of ageing at home, or on examining the risks and protective factors influencing relocation to a long-term care facility. Alternatively, research on planned living environments of older adults, including assisted living facilities (ALF), continuous care retirement communities (CCRCs), and others, tend to examine broader quality-of-life issues. One aspect of living environments needing attention includes the experience of social relations, and how those experiences vary by gender and race.

Older people's living environments intersect with the way gender, race, and social capital shape their life. After all, the term 'living environments' does not only refer to the location or physical features of living, but also represents a key context for the ageing process. Living environments create a primary social space in which older adults are physically and socially embedded both in everyday life as well as over the life course. The intersectionality perspective suggests that older adults' multidimensional social relations vary by larger social forces including gender, race, ethnicity, and SES. As both a location for and process of ageing in place, living environments represent an important social context, serving a variety of functions and meanings for older adults (Wahl 2003). We review the extent to which empirical research on ageing in place in varied living environments, including community living and planned living environments, has focused on gender, race, and social relations.

Community living

The limited amount of research focusing on social capital and gender in the community living context suggests important variations for men and women (Arber and Ginn 1995; Qu and Weston 2003). It has been argued that women may grow more powerful and autonomous in old age, possibly assuming new roles and duties as they get older, while women's dual roles as care-givers and receivers, especially amongst women with disabilities, has been underestimated (Arber and Ginn 1995). Based on this perspective, Boneham and Sixsmith's (2006) research investigated the processes through which social capital is differently created and maintained by men and women. The findings from this study contradict the perception that older women in the community are passive dependent beings and simply recipients of care from family, friends, and neighbours. Instead, the findings propose that older women collect social capital created and maintained through bonding ties and assume a major role in their families' health and in their communities.

Another important line of research has examined how social relations affect older adults' admission to long-term care facilities. Research has shown that people who successfully age in place in the community tend to possess greater social capital in the form of larger social networks. Family and friends, sufficient social support resources, and extensive family networks decrease the likelihood of nursing home placement and hence increase the probability of successfully ageing in place (Cutchin 2003; Gaugler et al. 2007; Lawler 2001; McCann et al. 2005; Tang and Lee 2011). Gender discrepancies arise, however. In a longitudinal study, Freedman et al. (1994) found that for men, entry to a nursing home was associated with the lack of a spouse but not with network size. For women, the composition of the network was not important, but size of the network predicted admission to a nursing home. Compared to women with more contact with relatives, the risk of entry to a nursing home for women with no contacts was almost three times higher. Other research has examined the effect of care-giver gender of the older adult care-giver on nursing home admission. Jette, Tennstedt, and Crawford (1995) found that the probability of entering a nursing home was over twice as great for older adults whose primary care-giver was male compared with those whose primary care-giver was female. Such findings indicate that network composition is an aspect of social relations that not only varies by gender, but also significantly influences the likelihood of moving from the community to a nursing home. In general, however, research in this field has tended to ignore gender. Little research has examined how the dynamic between social relations and gender is associated with nursing home placement among community-dwelling older adults.

In addition to relations with family and friends, the social capital perspective permits a broader examination of older adults' social relations with their community. Research has established that retaining connections to the community is a major factor predicting the possibility of ageing in place (Sabia 2008). Community involvement through neighbourly socialization, religious participation, volunteering, and organized group involvement strengthens connectedness to the community, as well as an individual's sense of and use of community (Stephens 2008), especially among the oldest-old (ages 75+) (Cornwell, Laumann, and Schumm 2008).

Research on social participation has also shown that women of older ages are more active than similarly aged men in terms of volunteer work, group membership, and attendance at social events (Davidson, Daly, and Arber 2003; Wilson 1995). Other research has indicated that older men and women differently experience changes in the community in terms of sentiments of 'belonging to' or 'investment in' a place. Older women were found to serve as 'neighbourhood keepers' in the sense of being more attentive to changes in local areas. They expressed greater concern for community deterioration than did older men (Phillipson et al. 1999). Other research has examined neighbourhood perceptions of women (aged from 75 to 93) residing in areas of varying socio-economic conditions. Based on features related to social capital such as networks, norms, and trust (Putnam 1995), Walker and Hiller (2007) found that social capital was fundamental to women's satisfaction with their surroundings and their continuance of relatively independent lives. This study also demonstrated that women did not view themselves as passive recipients of support or inactive social network members, but rather considered themselves to be engaged in active reciprocal relationships with family, friends, and neighbours. This seemed to be considerably less true of men.

As social capital is shaped by the broader cultural context, the ways in which an individual's social convoy is manifested in their community is likely to vary by culture. Increasingly, research has examined diverse ethnic/race groups within and across countries to consider how older adults' community participation varies by gender. Kim and Harris (2012) investigated the impacts of social capital on health status among older Korean immigrants (aged 60 years and older), one of the fastest growing segments in the older US population. Consistent with other research on social capital and health, they found positive effects of social engagement on health among Korean Americans in the US. Interestingly, a clearly diverging pattern in community participation by gender was also evident. Men reported a significantly higher level of participation (ranging from

74–86%) in the community in all the aspects examined in their study including political participation in the community, and sharing information with their community, organizations, and government, as well as with others. For women, however, only half reported being involved in the community. This gendered pattern seems to mirror the findings of the study on Korean older adults in Korea (cf. Lee et al. 2008). Traditional cultural values regarding gender-specific social roles may be retained in older Korean Americans partly because their social interactions tend to be restricted to local Korean ethnic community settings (Wong, Yoo, and Stewart 2005). Importantly, what these findings suggest is the possibility that in addition to the cultural influence on the lower level of participation among Korean women, due to other contextual factors such as lack of opportunity for social activities outside of the ethnic enclave, Korean American older women may be at a particularly disadvantaged position in social participation (Park, Jang, Lee, Haley, and Chiriboga 2012: 199).

Neighbourhood is another form of social capital that can influence living arrangements. However, the accumulating research suggests that the effect of neighbourhood on social relations may be moderated by gender and race. For older adults, due to increasing impairments and declining health, neighbourhood level conditions may be more influential particularly in the formation of social relationships. Schieman (2005) showed that in disadvantaged neighbourhoods, black women were found to both provide more and receive more social support if the neighbourhood had higher levels of residential stability. In contrast, white women were found to receive less and white men give less social support only under conditions of low residential stability. More recently, neighbourhood research has begun to examine the contingent effects of race and gender on the social relations of community-dwelling older adults and how it affects their health and well-being. One study examined how a neighbourhood social environment is associated with the social support and mental health of older adults (Brown et al. 2009). This study focused on older Hispanic immigrants (aged 70 to 100) in Florida who were thought to be at particularly high risk for poorer mental health because of social isolation, low socio-economic status, and the neighbourhood's disadvantageous environment. Findings indicate that neighbourhood environment was significantly related to perceived social support and that perceived social support was significantly related to reduced psychosocial distress. Brown et al. (2009) also found that the neighbourhood environment is indirectly related to psychosocial distress.

In countries with a weak welfare state, heavy reliance on families surfaces as key to social security for older adults. In such situations, neighbourhoods are comprised of close and significant others, often including family members. For instance, the emergence of quasi-co-residence is emerging in the Lebanese context, where older adults, especially older women, are increasingly living alone, but often their child lives next door, or at least in the same apartment building (Ajrouch et al. 2013). Such arrangements facilitate transfers between generations (e.g. economic and/or instrumental support), as well as enable close relational ties that become activated in times of need (Yount and Sibai 2009). A focus on quasi-co-residence permits more detailed insight into the ways in which social capital arises for men and women and influences well-being in weak-welfare-state nations.

There is considerable theoretical basis for suggesting the effects of macrosocial factors including gender and race on social relationships. Nevertheless, in general, there is still little empirical research on how gender and race together intersect and influence social capital as experienced in the lives of older people in the context of community living (Boneham and Sixsmith 2006; Schieman 2005; Sixsmith, Boneham, and Goldring 2001).

Planned living environments

Social relations in planned living environments are likely to differ from those of community-living older adults since residential care environments both provide and restrict social opportunities (Eckert et al. 2009). Relatively less attention to date has been directed towards social relations within newer types of living environments such as ALF and CCRCs (Gaugler and Kane 2007). ALFs are meant to provide housing options for older adults with functional limitations that make living independently difficult, yet where the level of help needed does not necessarily require nursing care. CCRCs, on the other hand, offer housing arrangement options that range from independent living to skilled nursing home care. The novelty of the CCRC housing situation is that older persons may remain in the same living community, but have the option for advanced levels of care depending on needs that change over time. Evidence is accumulating to indicate a differential shaping of social relations resulting from varying physical environments in nursing homes and urban/rural regions (Wahl and Lang 2004). Jungers (2010) examined the meaning and process of the experiences of older adults (aged 75 years and older) who shifted from private homes to ALFs. While varying degrees of loneliness were observed among residents, a sense of relatedness or connectedness to family, new and established friendships, and the staff were all identified as having a significant role in their well-being. Multiple research efforts in ALFs have indicated that residents possess varying social opportunities. Some retain active community connections (Yamasaki and Sharf 2011), while others depend exclusively on visitors, workers, and other residents in the ALF for social interaction (Ball et al. 2005). Although family support is indeed important, some residents have none, and most family members are unavailable on a daily basis (Ball et al. 2005). Research on relationships among residents suggests that resident–resident relationships influence life satisfaction (Park 2009), subjective well-being (Street and Burge 2012), and quality of life (Ball et al. 2005; Street et al. 2007). These findings suggest that the social capital of social relations accumulates over a lifetime and can be acquired at any point in life.

Limited research has examined gender-based differences in social networks among older adults residing in planned living environments. Such research is increasingly drawn from social convoy theory and examination of the dynamic nature of social relations in planned living environments in terms of gender. Research involving married couples in ALFs indicates that they remain a minority. Spouses often focus on their relationship with one another, to the exclusion of others (Kemp et al. 2012). Kemp (2008) discussed a potential variation of social relations by gender among resident relations within ALFs since women tend to maintain larger and more varied networks than do men (Antonnuci 1990). Men tend to be in the minority in later life and therefore may have fewer opportunities for same-sex friendships, especially in ALFs. Kemp et al. (2012) have recently reported that men indeed had fewer same-sex and more opposite-sex relationship opportunities compared to women.

Kemp and colleagues (2012) examined patterns of social relations across three ALFs and identified influencing factors at multiple levels including personal characteristics, the physical and social environment of the facility, and policies affecting the community. They examined dynamic patterns of social relationships ranging from stranger to friend from which they derived two major types of relationship including 'neighbouring' (supportive and pleasant) and 'anti-neighbouring' (bullying and name calling). Neighbouring was the most common way of relating in ALFs. Helping and providing support was found across relationship types. One interesting finding is that the formation of social relations varies by race, ethnicity, and culture. This suggests that relationships are not universally supportive and 'anti-neighbouring' behaviours may have a potential negative impact on certain subgroups of individuals.

Another study examined the social support networks of older adults living in CCRCs (Van Dussen and Morgan 2009). Drawing on the social convoy model, this research considered changes in older adults' social support networks. They noted shifts in relationships over time as well as different patterns of relationships by marital status and age in conjunction with gender. The findings indicate the convergences between CCRC residents and their peers outside senior housing. Unmarried respondents showed a different distribution of supporters, with a much heavier reliance on less close network members (friends/other category) while the oldest group was likely to have smaller support networks. Furthermore, the support networks of unmarried women extended more to friends and extended kinships, such as nieces and grandchildren, compared to married couples and men.

Research on planned living is at a fairly early stage in its development. Several gaps in this field are found as compared to the research on community living. Most conspicuous is a lack of attention to race. While research on community living has begun to examine the association between race and social relations, little empirical evidence is available in the emerging research on planned living. Another limitation involves the scope of research. Research on community living has examined a range of physical and psychosocial well-being including long-term care admission, but research on planned living environments mainly focuses on the nature and change of social relations with little attention paid to how relationships serve as a form of social capital that influences well-being or mental health within the facility. Research focusing on older adults living in the community examines a broader level of social participation to consider links between social relations as social capital and its effect on overall well-being. Comparatively, the focus of research on planned living environments tends to narrowly consider social relations and how they might vary by gender within the housing environment.

Given the increasing trend toward ageing in place both in the community and in planned living environments, the current gaps found in the two living environments literature suggest fruitful future directions for research on planned living. The intersectionality perspective can be a promising guide for future research endeavours. For example, future research should systematically examine to what extent the formation of social relations varies by different living environments. Also of interest is the effect of social relations on the physical and psychosocial well-being of older adults as shaped by race and gender over time. It would be very informative to gain a better understanding of the dynamic process of ageing in place for men and women, and ways in which social capital arises in those spaces as well as the ways in which social capital predicts the likelihood of various living arrangements in different types of living space such as within physical living quarters, the neighbourhood, and the larger community.

CARE-GIVING EXPERIENCES

Next to the living environment of older people, one of the most important experiences of ageing is care-giving—both providing care to others and receiving care from others. Care-giving can be of the formal or informal type, that is, provided by paid professionals or by unpaid family and friends. Research most often focuses on informal care-giving since this constitutes the majority of care and can vary considerably depending on the resources available to the individual. In addition, most care-giving is provided by women—mothers, wives, daughters, and daughters-in-law—making it not only a resource but also a gender issue as well. Thus, informal care-giving is related to an individual's convoy of social relations, and is often particularly influenced by whether the recipient (and provider) is male or female. In fact, care-giving can be viewed as a benefit of earned social capital that is the result of long-term and ongoing social relations.

Viewing care-giving as a form of social capital based on longitudinal as well as current social relations makes the characteristics of social networks especially important. Fortunately, considerable information is now available about adult social networks both in the US and in other parts of the world. We turn next to a description of social networks across the lifespan and across cultures. We also consider how these characteristics are likely to influence the availability of informal care-giving.

Informal care-giving is often exchanged between close family members. These relationships are part of the individual's convoy and have usually developed over long periods of time, representing a lifespan phenomenon. Almost everyone spends their lives as part of a convoy of social relations. Relations exist from birth to death, often with the same people. A case in point is the parent–child relationship that begins from the child's infancy through the parent's old age. The accumulated experiences, positive and negative, become either an underlying resource, in the form of social capital or deficit, i.e. the lack thereof. Antonucci (1985) has suggested that people maintain an informal Support Bank that monitors the support provided and the support received. Those providing a great deal of support feel they have an accumulation of social capital upon which to draw while those receiving such support are likely to feel more comfortable receiving that support if they have provided support in the past. A classic example is the adult child's expectation to provide care to parents in late life in return for the care those parents provided when the child was young. Research examining the notion of reciprocity in social relations suggests that while there are cultural differences in expectations (Akiyama, Antonucci, and Campbell 1997), there is an overwhelming desire for exchanges to be reciprocal. Interestingly, when they are not concurrently reciprocal people feel better about receiving support in the present if they have provided it in the past, i.e. if they feel they acquired the social capital in the past upon which they might rely in the present or future.

The availability of social relations and the social capital upon which to draw informal care-giving as needed is especially important because we now recognize that poor social relations can lead to depression and illness and that effects in the opposite direction are also possible, i.e. the networks of sick people are often restricted to close family members (Webster, Fuller-Iglesias, and Antonucci 2012). Lonely people have been shown to be more susceptible to colds and infection (Cohen and Williamson 1991). Increasingly, researchers are recognizing the multilevel influences of social relations. We are now aware of the fact that social relations can have an impact from cell to society and every level in between. Thus, convoys of social relations can have far-reaching influences on the health and well-being of individuals and societies.

As noted above, most informal care-giving is based on social relations. These social relations develop over time and reflect the individual's change and development over time, e.g. as the child develops from an infant to an adolescent and then an adult, and as relationships develop over time, beginning with the infant–mother dyad, evolving over time as the infant develops into adulthood and as the young mother matures from young adulthood through old age. The interactions of both intra-individual change and inter-individual exchanges form the critical bases of both their convoys, which in turn influence what their care-giving relationship is likely to be. This includes whether there is an expectation of care-giving from both parties and what the type and quality of that care-giving will be. Much data suggests that these expectations are influenced by the accumulation of social capital and by the quality of the relationship. We turn next to a consideration of what we know about convoy membership in several cultures.

Several research efforts have compared the social networks of men and women in different cultures. Antonucci, Akiyama and Takahashi (2004) compared convoy composition across the lifespan in representative samples from Japan and the US. Their findings indicate that in both the US and Japan adults aged 21 to 39 name their mothers first and spouse second. In the US the next most frequently mentioned person is a child, whereas in Japan the third most frequently mentioned person is a father. Among 30- to 59-year-olds the convoy composition is the same in both countries for the closest convoy members: spouse, child, and then mother. Fathers are no longer mentioned by respondents in either country. In the next two decades, i.e. among those in their 60s and 70s, the closest two people nominated are spouse and children in both countries, with siblings also nominated in the US. Mothers are no longer mentioned. Among those in their 80s to 90s, spouse and children continue to be mentioned and grandchildren are mentioned for the first time. Siblings are no longer mentioned but friends are, not among the very closest convoy members, but still among relationships respondents consider close. These data point to both the general continuity of close relationships, as mentioned earlier, and specifically highlight which individuals are likely to be available to provide care. Indeed, in a recent paper by Ryan and colleagues (2012) which examined potential care-givers across multiple cohorts in the US, the prevalence of married older adults and adult children is clearly declining, suggesting that the usual sources of care-giving, i.e. spouse and children, are likely to be unavailable for future generations of older individuals. In a related line of research, Sherman (in press; Sherman and Boss 2007) has documented the increasing prevalence of remarried spousal care-givers with adult step-children among Alzheimer's disease care-givers. Her findings indicate that this frequently creates a difficult situation of isolation and negativity for spousal care-givers, often threatening their mental health.

Another recent study examined convoys of social relations among older people in four countries: France, Germany, Japan, and the US (Antonucci et al. 2002). They examined both network structure and resource deficits. Measures of network structure included network size, while resource deficits were defined as widowhood and illness. Interestingly, results are fairly similar across cultures. Younger individuals, i.e. those 70 to 79 years old tended to report larger networks than 80- to 90-year-olds. This difference was significant in France, Germany, and the US. In addition, there was a significant effect of resource deficit in both France and Germany with people who were widowed, ill, or both, reporting fewer people in their convoy of social relations.

These findings emphasize the importance of social relations to the care-giving experience. Although both sets of findings are cross-sectional, they do suggest that lifetime social relations or convoys represent a critical link to meeting the care-giving needs of the older population. Given women's central role in the care-giving relationship, gender differences in social relations are also critical. Among the findings reported above on network structure, interestingly, there were no effects of gender. Other research suggests that this lack of gender difference in network structure is because both men and women report more women than men in their networks (Antonucci and Akiyama 1987). In fact, a recent study replicated this finding twenty-five years later (Antonucci 2008), again indicating that both men and women report more women in their networks.

On the other hand, research focusing on gender differences in care-giving suggests that the situation is complicated but that women are at risk. Pinquart and Sörensen (2006), in their recent meta-analysis of gender differences in care-giver stressors, social relations, and health, noted that while some differences were small, women's mental health was clearly affected. Women generally reported higher levels of burden and depression and lower levels of subjective well-being and health. Informal female care-givers provided more informal care, did more in terms of actual care-giving tasks and provided care for more hours and for individuals who had more behavioural problems than did men. Recent research placing the care-giving literature within a feminist perspective highlights the unpaid but fundamental contribution women are making to their families and society. Unfortunately, this contribution has gone largely unrecognized at the societal level, even though it is often provided at great personal cost (Chappell and Funk 2011).

IMPLICATIONS FOR PRACTICE

The clearest and most evident implication for clinical practice from a consideration of the influence of social capital and gender in the lives of older people is that women are especially vulnerable as they age. They are less likely to have the amount of social capital and social resources that men do. They are also more likely to be in at-risk living environments and to be providing care, especially to a spouse. Attention should be paid to protecting these vulnerable older members of the community in recognition of the fact that such protection will permit them to maintain optimal living circumstances longer and to provide care to their loved ones for longer. Such protection will lead to a healthier quality of life for all concerned.

This review also suggests the need to be mindful of the intersectionality of gender, age, race, and culture. The literature reviewed points to the paucity of studies that consider the intersectionality framework as it relates to social capital. Yet empirical findings suggest that such a framework may yield important insights into links between gender, age, and social capital. In particular, such a framework helps to uncover a more nuanced understanding of vulnerabilities in later life. It is also clear that in the US, as well as in other western and non-western settings, socio-economic status affects experiences that older women have with access to social capital in more pronounced ways than it does for men. Applying an intersectionality lens asks us to consider the ways in which culture and socio-economic status shape gendered experiences, and, moreover, how whether one is a man or woman shapes the ageing experience with regard to social capital. By attending to the ways in which gender, age, ethnicity, and SES mutually constitute one another and together influence social capital access, practitioners may address vulnerabilities more effectively. In other words, gender alone does not explain the situations of older men and women. The socio-economic position of men and women, as well as their ethnic background are also key. Attention to these intersections will enhance the ability of clinical geropsychology practitioners to better serve the mental health needs of and foster well-being among older adults.

Summary

In this chapter we have focused on the influence of social capital and gender on living arrangements and care-giving in old age. We began by considering social relations with a frame of social capital across the lifespan and over the life course as the basis for a convoy of social relations that is influenced by both individual and societal circumstances. We note that these relations are a source of social capital that both helps individuals meet their own needs and encourages them to provide assistance to others. A focus on older people led to a more detailed consideration of the influence of social capital and gender on both living environments and care-giving.

Multiple types of living environments were considered, from independent community dwellings to planned living environments While each of these housing arrangements is different, as we noted above, successfully adapting to these environments, especially while confronting the challenges of ageing—be they physical or mental, acute or chronic—is very much influenced by the availability of social capital in the form of convoys of social relations. Although the structure and composition of social convoys tend to be similar for men and women, the nature of the support exchanges and the availability of social capital do tend to differ by gender. We note the importance of considering the intersectionality both of age and gender, as well as other factors such as race, culture, and SES.

We also considered care-giving as a special issue of an ageing society. We note that it is well documented that women provide the preponderance of care and are often made more vulnerable because of it. While men do sometimes provide care, they tend to do so far less often, for fewer hours, and in less demanding or taxing situations. In addition, men are most often cared for by their wives, while women are cared for by their spouse, if they have one, and their, mostly female, children.

This chapter has highlighted both the stable and changing aspects of ageing specifically with regard to social capital and gender. Patterns of social capital acquisition and gender differences in ageing continue but there are new aspects of these experiences. Changing demographics mean people are living longer, and experiencing as well as experimenting, either through choice or necessity, with different living arrangements. People ageing in place have the highest likelihood of benefiting from accumulated social capital, but may also be threatened by inhospitable architecture or geography. Similarly, with age often comes the need for care. Traditional care-giving draws on social capital accumulated with spouse and children over a lifetime. However, fewer people are entering old age married and people of all ages are having fewer children, thus reducing the availability of these sources of care-giving. Future research should recognize the intersectionality of race, gender, and age while focusing on new ways to benefit from a lifetime of accumulated social capital.

KEY REFERENCES AND SOURCES FOR FURTHER READING

Akiyama, H. and Antonucci, T. C. (2002). 'Gender Differences in Depressive Symptoms: Insights from a Life Span Perspective on Life Stages and Social Networks'. In J. A. Levy and B. A. Pescosolido (eds), *Social Networks and Health*: Vol. 8 (pp. 343–358). London: Elsevier Science.

Stoller, E. P. and Gibson, R. C. (2000). *Worlds of Difference: Inequality in the Aging Experience* (3rd edn). Thousand Oaks, CA: Pine Forge Press.

REFERENCES

Ajrouch, K. J., Blandon, A., and Antonucci, T. C. (2005). 'Social Networks among Men and Women: The Effects of Age and Socioeconomic Status'. *Journal of Gerontology: Social Sciences* 60: 311–317.

Ajrouch, K. J., Yount, K., Sibai, A. M., and Roman, P. (2013) 'A Gendered Perspective on Well-being in Later Life: Algeria, Lebanon, and Palestine'. In S. McDaniel and Z. Zimmer (eds), *Global Ageing in the 21st Century: Challenges, Opportunities and Implications* (pp. 49–78). Farnham: Ashgate.

Ajrouch, K. J. and Antonucci T. C. (2014). 'Using Convoys of Social Relations to Understand Culture and Forgiveness from an Arab American Perspective'. In S. Nasser-McMillan, K. J. Ajrouch, and J. Hakim-Larson (eds), *Biopsychosocial Perspectives on Arab Americans: Culture, Development, and Health* (pp. 127–146). New York: Springer.

Akiyama, H., Antonucci, T. C., and Campbell, R. (1997). 'Exchange and Reciprocity among Two Generations of Japanese and American Women'. In J. Sokolovsky (ed.), *Cultural Context of Aging: Worldwide Perspectives* (2nd edn, pp. 127–138). Westfort, CT: Greenwood Press.

Akiyama, H. and Antonucci, T. C. (2002). 'Gender Differences in Depressive Symptoms: Insights from a Life Span Perspective on Life Stages and Social Networks'. In J. A. Levy and B. A. Pescosolido (eds), *Social Networks and Health: Vol. 8* (pp. 343–358), London: Elsevier Science.

Alex, L. (2010). 'Resilience among Very Old Men and Women'. *Journal of Research in Nursing* 15(5): 419–431.

Andermann, L. (2010). 'Culture and the Social Construction of Gender: Mapping the Intersection with Mental Health'. *International Review of Psychiatry* 22(5): 501–512.

Antonucci, T. C. (1985). 'Personal Characteristics, Social Support, and Social Behavior'. In E. Shanas and R. H. Binstock (eds), *Handbook of Aging and the Social Sciences* (pp. 94–128). New York: Academic Press.

Antonucci, T. C. and Akiyama, H. (1987). 'An Examination of Sex Differences in Social Support among Older Men and Women'. *Sex Roles* 17(11/12): 737–749.

Antonucci, T. C. (1990). 'Social Supports and Social Relationships'. In R. H. Binstock and L. K. George (eds), *The Handbook of Aging and the Social Sciences* (3rd edn, pp. 205–226). San Diego, CA: Academic Press.

Antonucci, T. C., Lansford, J. E., Akiyama, H., Smith, J., Baltes, M. M., Takahashi, K., Fuhrer, R., and Dartigues, J.-F. (2002). 'Differences between Men and Women in Social Relations, Resource Deficits, and Depressive Symptomatology during Later Life in Four Nations'. *Journal of Social Issues* 58: 767–783.

Antonucci, T. C., Akiyama, H., and Takahashi, K. (2004). 'Attachment and Close Relationships across the Life Span'. *Attachment and Human Development* 6: 353–370.

Antonucci, T. C. (2008). 'Convoy Model of Social Relations: Replication and Extension'. Paper presented at the 37th annual meeting of the Canadian Association of Gerontology, London, Ontario.

Antonucci, T. C., Ajrouch, K. J., and Abdulrahim, S. (2010). 'A Descriptive Analysis of Social Relations'. Paper presented at Linking Research to Policy in the Middle East Region: Family Ties and Aging Workshop, American University of Beirut, Lebanon.

Arber, S. and Ginn, J. (1995). 'The Mirage of Gender Equality: Occupational Success in the Labour Market and within Marriage'. *The British Journal of Sociology* 46(1): 21–43.

Ball, M. M., Perkins, M. M., Whittington, F. J., Hollingsworth, C., King, S. V., and Combs, B. L. (2005). *Communities of Care: Assisted Living for African American Elders*. Baltimore, MD: Johns Hopkins University Press.

Barer, B. M. (1994). 'Men and Women Aging Differently'. *International Journal of Aging and Human Development* 38(1): 29–40.

Boneham, M. A. and Sixsmith, J. A. (2006). 'The Voices of Older Women in a Disadvantaged Community: Issues of Health and Social Capital'. *Social Science and Medicine* 62: 269–279.

Brown, S. C., Mason, C. A., Spokane, A. R., Cruza-Guet, M. C., Lopez, B., and Szapocznik, J. (2009). 'The Relationship of Neighborhood Climate to Perceived Social Support and Mental Health in Older Hispanic Immigrants in Miami, Florida'. *Journal of Aging and Health* 21: 431–459.

Calasanti, T. (2010). 'Gender Relations and Applied Research on Aging'. *The Gerontologist* 50(6): 720–734.

Chappell, N. L. and Funk, L. M. (2011). 'Social Support, Caregiving and Aging'. *Canadian Journal on Aging* 30(3): 355–370.

Cohen, S. and Williamson, G. M. (1991). 'Stress and Infectious Disease in Humans'. *Psychological Bulletin* 109(1): 5–24. doi:10.1037/0033-2909.109.1.5.

Coleman, J. S. (1990). *Foundations of Social Theory*. Cambridge, MA: Harvard University Press.

Cornwell, B., Laumann, E. O., and Schumm, L. P. (2008). 'The Social Connectedness of Older Adults: A National Profile'. *American Sociological Review* 73(2): 185–203.

Cornwell, B. (2011). 'Independence through Social Networks: Bridging Potential among Older Women and Men'. *Journal of Gerontology: Social Sciences* 66(6): 782–794.

Cutchin M. P.(2003). 'The Process of Mediated Aging-in-place: A Theoretically and Empirically Based Model'. *Social Science and Medicine* 57: 1077–1090.

Davidson, K., Daly, T., and Arber, A. (2003). 'Older Men, Social Integration, and Organisational Activities'. *Social Policy and Society* 2(2): 81–89.

Davidson, K. (2004). '"Why Can't a Man Be More Like a Woman?": Marital status and Social Networking of Older Men'. *Journal of Men's Studies* 13(1): 25–43.

Dill, B. T. and Zambrana, R. E. (eds) (2009). *Emerging Intersections: Race, Class and Gender in Theory, Policy, and Practice*. New Brunswick, NJ: Rutgers University Press.

Eckert, J. K., Carder, P. C., Morgan, L. A., Frankowski, A. C., and Roth, E. G. (2009). *Inside Assisted Living: The Search for Home*. Baltimore, MD: Johns Hopkins University Press.

Felmlee, D. and Muraco, A. (2009). 'Gender and Friendship Norms among Older Adults'. *Research on Aging* 31(3): 318–344.

Freedman, V. A., Berkman, L. F., Rapp, S. R., and Ostfeld, A. M. (1994). 'Family Networks: Predictors of Nursing Home Entry'. *American Journal of Public Health* 84(5): 843–845.

Gaugler, J., Duval, S., Anderson, K., and Kane, R. (2007). 'Predicting Nursing Home Admission in the U.S.: A Meta-analysis'. *BMC Geriatrics* 7: 13, http://www.biomedcentral.com/1471-2318/7/13.

Gaugler, J. E. and Kane, R. L. (2007). 'Families and Assisted Living'. *The Gerontologist*, 47(suppl. 1): 83–99.

Grundy, E. and Holt, G. (2001). 'The Socioeconomic Status of Older Adults: How Should We Measure it in Studies of Health Inequalities'. *Journal of Epidemiology and Community Health* 55: 895–904.

Hartmann, H. and English, A. (2009). 'Older Women's Retirement Security: A Primer'. *Journal of Women, Politics & Policy* 30(2–3): 109–140.

Hofstede, G. (1980). *Culture's Consequences: International Differences in Work-related Values*. Beverly Hills, CA, and London.

Hyyppa, M. T. (2010). *Healthy Ties: Social Capital, Population Health and Survival*. New York: Springer.

Inglehart, R. and Welzel, C. (2005). *Modernization, Cultural Change and Democracy: The Human Development Sequence*. New York: Cambridge University Press.

Jette, A. M., Tennstedt, S., and Crawford, S. (1995). 'How Does Formal and Informal Community Care Affect Nursing Home Use?' *Journal of Gerontology: Social Sciences* 50B(1): S4–S12.

Joseph, S. (1993). 'Connectivity and Patriarchy among Urban Working Class Families in Lebanon'. *Ethos* 21(4): 452–484.

Jungers, C. M. (2010). 'Leaving Home: An Examination of Late-life Relocation among Older Adults'. *Journal of Counseling & Development* 88(4): 416–423.

Kagitcibasi, C. (1996). *Family and Human Development across Cultures*. Mahwah, NJ: Erlbaum.

Kahn, R. L. and Antonucci, T. C. (1980). 'Convoys over the Life Course: Attachment, Roles, and Social Support'. In P. B. Baltes and O. G. Brim (eds), *Life-span Development and Behavior* (pp. 254–283). New York: Academic Press.

Kemp, C. L. (2008). 'Negotiating Transitions in Later Life: Married Couples in Assisted Living'. *Journal of Applied Gerontology* 27: 231–251.

Kemp, C. L., Ball, M. M., Hollingsworth, C., and Perkins, M. M. (2012). 'Strangers and Friends: Residents' Social Careers in Assisted Living'. *Journals of Gerontology Series B: Psychological Sciences and Social Sciences* 67(4): 491–502.

Kim, B.J. and Harris, L. M. (2012). 'Social Capital and Self-rated Health among Korean Immigrants'. *Journal of Applied Gerontology* 20(10): 1–18. doi:10.1177/0733464812448528.

Lawler, E. J. (2001). 'An Affect Theory of Social Exchange'. *American Journal of Sociology* 107: 321–352.

Lee, H. Y., Jang, S. N., Lee, S., Cho, S. I., and Park, E. O. (2008). 'The Relationship between Social Participation and Self-rated Health by Sexed Age: A Cross-sectional Survey'. *International Journal of Nursing Studies* 45: 1042–1054. doi:10.1016/j.ijnurstu.2007.05.007.

McCann, J. J., Liesi, E. H., Yan, L., Wolinsky, F. D., Gilley, D. W., Aggarwal, N. T., Miller, J. M., and Evans, D. A. (2005). 'The Effect of Adult Day Care Services on Time to Nursing Home Placement in Older Adults with Alzheimer's Disease'. *The Gerontologist* 45(6): 754–763.

Markus, H. R. and Kitayama, S. (1991). 'Culture and the Self: Implications for Cognition, Emotion, and Motivation'. *Psychological Review* 98(2): 224–253.

Moen, P. (2001). 'The Gendered Life Course'. In L. K. George and R. H. Binstock (eds), *Handbook of Aging and the Social Sciences* (5th edn, pp. 179–196). San Diego, CA: Academic Press.

Mullings, L. and Schulz, A. J. (2006). 'Intersectionality and Health: An introduction'. In A. J. Schulz and L. Mullings (eds), *Gender, Race, Class, & Health: Intersectional Approaches* (pp. 3–17). San Francisco, CA: Jossey-Bass.

Neugarten, B. L. and Guttmann, D. L. (1958). 'Age-sex and Personality in Middle Age: A Thematic Apperception Study'. *Psychological Monographs, General and Applied* 72(17): 1–33. doi:10.1037/h0093797.

Oyserman, D., Coon, H. M., and Kemmelmeier, M. (2002). 'Rethinking Individualism and Collectivism: Evaluation of Theoretical Assumptions and Meta-analyses'. *Psychological Bulletin* 128(1): 3–72.

Park, N. S. (2009). 'The Relationship of Social Engagement to Psychological Well-being of Older Adults in Assisted Living Facilities'. *Journal of Applied Gerontology* 28(4): 461–481.

Park, N. S., Jang, Y., Lee, B. S., Haley,W. E., Chiriboga, D. A. (2012). 'The Mediating Role of Loneliness in the Relation between Social Engagement and Depressive Symptoms among Older Korean Americans'. *Journal of Gerontology, Series B: Psychological Sciences and Social Sciences* 68(2): 193–201. doi:10.1093/geronb/gbs062.

Phillips, J., Ajrouch, K., Hillcoat-Nalletamby, S. (2010). *Key Concepts in Social Gerontology*. Thousand Oaks, CA: Sage.

Phillipson, C., Bernard, M., Phillips, J., and Ogg, J. (1999). 'Older People in Three Urban Areas: Household Composition, Kinship And Social Networks'. In S. McRae (ed.), *Changing Britain* (pp. 229–247). Oxford: Oxford University Press.

Pinquart, M. and Sörensen, S. (2006). 'Gender Differences in Caregiver Stressors, Social Resources, and Health: An Updated Meta-analysis'. *Journals of Gerontology Series B: Psychological Sciences and Social Sciences* 61(1): 33–45.

Putnam, R. D. (1995). 'Bowling Alone: America's Declining Social Capital'. *Journal of Democracy* 6: 65–78.

Qu, L. and Weston, R. (2003). 'Ageing, Living Arrangements and Subjective Wellbeing. Australian Institute of Family Studies'. *Family Matters* 66: 26–33.

Ryan, L. H., Smith, J., Antonucci, T. C., and Jackson, J. S. (2012). 'Cohort Differences in the Availability of Informal Caregivers: Are the Boomers at Risk?' *The Gerontologist* 52: 177–188. doi:10.1093/geront/GNR142.

Sabia, J. J. (2008). 'There's No Place like Home: A Hazard Model Analysis of Aging in Place among Older Homeowners in the PSID'. *Research on Aging* 30: 3–35.

Schieman, S. (2005). 'Residential Stability and the Social Impact of Neighborhood Disadvantage: A Study of Gender-and-race-Contingent Effects'. *Social Forces* 83: 1031–1064.

Sherman, C. W. and Boss, P. (2007). 'Spousal Dementia Caregiving in Context of Late-life Remarriage'. *Dementia* 6: 245–269.

Sherman, C. W. (2012). 'Remarriage as Context for Dementia Caregiving: Implications of Qualitative Reports of Positive Support and Negative Interactions for Caregiver Well-being'. *Research on Human Development* 9(2): 165–182.

Shields, S. A. (2008). 'Gender: An Intersectionality Perspective'. *Sex Roles* 59(5–6): 301–311.

Sixsmith, J., Boneham, M., and Goldring, J. (2001). *Final Report: The Relationship between Social Capital, Health and Gender: A Case Study of a Deprived Community*. London: Health Development Agency.

Solimeo, S. (2008). 'Sex and Gender in Older Adults' Experience of Parkinson's Disease'. *Journal of Gerontology: Social Sciences* 63(1): S42–S48.

Stephens, C. (2008). 'Social Capital in its Place: Using Social Theory to Understand Social Capital and Inequalities in Health'. *Social Science and Medicine* 66(5): 1174–1184.

Stoller, E. P. and Gibson, R. C. (2000). *Worlds of Difference: Inequality in the Aging Experience* (3rd edn). Thousand Oaks, CA: Pine Forge Press.

Street, D., Burge, S., Quadagno, J., and Barrett, A. (2007). 'The Salience of Social Relationships for Resident Well-being in Assisted Living'. *Journals of Gerontology Series B: Psychological Sciences and Social Sciences* 62(2): S129–S134.

Street, D. and Burge, S. W. (2012). 'Residential Context, Social Relationships, and Subjective Well-being in Assisted Living'. *Research on Aging* 34(3): 365–394.

Takahashi, K., Ohara, N., Antonucci, T. C., and Akiyama, H. (2002). 'Commonalities and Differences in Close Relationships among the American and the Japanese: A Comparison by the Individualism/Collectivism Concept'. *International Journal of Behavioral Development* 26: 453–465.

Tang, F. and Lee, Y. (2011). 'Social Support Networks and Expectations for Aging in Place and Moving'. *Research on Aging* 33(4): 444–464.

Toothman, E. L. and Barrett, A. E. (2011). 'Mapping Midlife: An Examination of Social Factors Shaping Conceptions of the Timing of Middle Age'. *Advances in Life Course Research* 16: 99–111.

Triandis, H. C., Bontempo, R., Villareal, M. J., Asai, M., and Lucca, N. (1988). 'Individualism and Collectivism: Cross-cultural Perspectives on Self-ingroup Relationships'. *Journal of Personality and Social Psychology* 54(2): 323–338.

Van Dussen, D. J. and Morgan, L. A. (2009). 'Gender and Informal Caregiving in CCRCs: Primary Caregivers or Support Networks?' *Journal of Women & Aging* 21(4): 251–265.

Verbrugge, L. M. (1985). 'Gender and Health: An Update on Hypotheses and Evidence'. *Journal of Health and Social Behavior* 26(3): 156–182.

Wahl, H. W. (2003). 'Research on Living Arrangements in Old Age for What?' In K. W. Schaie, H. W. Wahl, H. Mollenkopf, and F. Oswald (eds), *Aging Independently*. New York: Springer.

Wahl, H. W. and Lang, F. R. (2004). 'Aging in Context across the Adult Life Course: Integrating Physical and Social Environmental Research'. In H. W. Wahl, R. J. Scheidt, P. G. Windley, and K. W. Schaie (eds), *Annual Review of Gerontology and Geriatrics* (pp.1–33): New York: Springer.

Walker, R. B. and Hiller, J. E. (2007). 'Places and Health: A Qualitative Study to Explore How Older Women Living Alone Perceive the Social and Physical Dimensions of their Neighbourhoods'. *Social Science & Medicine* 65(6): 1154–1165.

Webster, N. J., Fuller-Iglesias, H. R., and Antonucci, T. C. (2012). 'Health Influences on Social Network Change: The Contextualizing Role of Socio-Economic Status'. Paper presented at the 107th annual meeting of the American Sociological Association, Denver, CO.

Wilson, G. (1995). ' "I'm the Eyes and She's the Arms": Changes in Gender Roles in Advanced Old Age'. In S. Arber and J. Ginn (eds), *Connecting Gender and Ageing: A Sociological Approach*. Buckingham: Open University Press.

Wong, S. T., Yoo, G. J., and Stewart, A. L. (2005). 'Examining the Types of Social Support and the Actual Sources of Support in Older Chinese and Korean Immigrants'. *International Journal of Aging & Human Development* 61: 105–121.

Xu, Q. and Norstrand, J. A. (2012). 'Gendered Social Capital and Health Outcomes among Older Adults in China'. *Aging in China: Implications to Social Policy of a Changing Economic State, International Perspectives on Aging* 2: 147–168.

Yamasaki, J. and Sharf, B. F. (2011). 'Opting out while Fitting in: How Residents Make Sense of Assisted Living and Cope with Community Life'. *Journal of Aging Studies* 25(1): 13–21.

Yount, K. M. and Sibai, A. M. (2009). 'Demography of Ageing in Arab Countries'. In P. Uhlenberg (ed), *International Handbook of Population Ageing* (pp. 227–315). Dordrecht: Springer.

CHAPTER 7

COGNITIVE DEVELOPMENT IN AGEING

JACQUELINE ZÖLLIG, MIKE MARTIN, AND VERA SCHUMACHER

INTRODUCTION

COGNITIVE development in ageing is a multidimensional and multidirectional phenomenon characterized by age-related changes in the plasticity of different dimensions of cognitive functions. Gains, stability, and losses can be observed across abilities and across people as they age. Although with the closeness to death losses are predominant, several cognitive abilities on average show stability and even increases well into extreme old age. Importantly, the individually differing uses of the ability to learn, and cognitive as well as neural plasticity can explain the heterogeneity of cognitive ageing. In fact, behavioural and neurophysiological research on the plasticity of cognitive abilities has demonstrated that there is a high learning potential up until extreme old age. Based on different approaches to cognitive ageing, different training methods have been introduced over the past years focusing on cognitive processes, primary mental abilities, higher-order cognitive constructs, and global cognition involving multiple cognitive domains. The study of the normal and the maximal course of changes in different cognitive abilities, their interrelations, and their relations to environmental factors demonstrates the possibilities to improve cognitive functioning and to extend the phase of autonomous living for several years. A more recent and promising concept is the integration of the existing approaches within a functional approach to cognitive development. Within this approach, specific elementary cognitive abilities are conceptualized as being actively and simultaneously recruited by individuals to stabilize a high level of everyday functioning in variable environments. Even when reduced elementary abilities are observed, function stabilization may still be possible through multiple compensatory processes and activities. Due to its applicability to resource orchestration at all levels of functioning it has implications for the understanding of everyday cognitive performances and clinical practice.

THEORETICAL OVERVIEW

There is a long tradition of examining elementary cognitive abilities and their development across the lifespan. One strand of this research is the lifelong development of intelligence as a general ability to reason and adapt to varying environmental conditions. This general ability can be divided into fluid and crystallized intelligence, the first referring to the ability to master new and unfamiliar tasks, the latter to succeed in tasks requiring experiential and culture-specific knowledge. Another strand is the focus on the characteristics of information-processing resources, speed of processing, and inhibitory functioning. While many longitudinal studies have examined intelligence development, most studies examining age effects in information processing are experimental. Both strands typically use a normative approach assuming that cognitive abilities are rather stable characteristics of individuals, and that an exact measurement of the 'building blocks' of more complex, higher-order performances allows us to make reliable predictions about everyday performance in terms of academic or professional success. In terms of interventions, the approach suggests improving elementary skills should transfer to other, non-trained skills and should improve higher-order abilities requiring the use of elementary abilities.

More recently, with the advancement of experimental and neuroimaging methods, the plasticity of cognitive abilities has become the focus of cognitive ageing research (e.g. Kramer et al. 2004; Raz 2000). It distinguishes plasticity of brain structure and plasticity of brain function and relates brain plasticity to behavioural plasticity and development across the lifespan. The approach of examining equally successful performances of younger and older adults and to determine the differences in contributing processes turns the classical cognitive ageing research on its head. There the dependent variable typically is success vs failure in a particular performance measure. In terms of interventions, exploiting the plasticity of the brain should optimize the developmental trajectory of elementary skills, and measures aiming at structural plasticity (e.g. intensive practice of single elementary processes such as finger tapping) will differ from measures aiming at functional plasticity (e.g. variable use of multiple elementary processes to solve complex cognitive tasks). In addition, interventions may focus on how the same level of performance can be achieved through adapting the processes contributing to the performance.

The next step in cognitive ageing research will be the integration of the existing approaches within a functional approach of cognitive development. This assumes that multiple elementary processes are dynamically recruited to allow optimal performance across various tasks. Thus this approach requires a precise analysis of the complexity of task requirements in tasks of high individual relevance, and a theoretical model of how multiple cognitive skills have to be orchestrated to perform the task successfully, as well as how task performance may be stabilized when either environmental conditions or cognitive skills change.

GENERAL COGNITIVE ABILITIES

The study of the lifespan development of cognitive abilities originated in the examination of age differences in a single general intelligence factor 'g' (Spearman 1904). The first studies aimed to find the age of maximum performance and the beginning of age-related decline. Although the findings suggested maximum intelligence at the age of 13–16 years (Terman 1916; Yerkes 1921), Wechsler (1939) also found substantial differences in the eleven intelligence tests he used. A more detailed analysis revealed that tests measuring the processing of new information such as inductive reasoning showed different age trends compared to tests measuring experience—and culture-dependent performances such as verbal knowledge. Since then, the literature distinguishes between measures of fluid and of crystallized intelligence, the latter referring to the experience-dependent tests. Eventually, Schaie (1996) in his Seattle Longitudinal Study (SLS; the longest active study on the lifespan development of intelligence) examined five independent primary intelligence factors of inductive reasoning, spatial orientation, number skills, verbal abilities, and word fluency.

The data from the SLS display a large degree of variability in the development of intellectual abilities. First, mean trajectories differ between the five abilities. Although maximum values are achieved between 32 and 67 years of age, i.e. much later than suggested by the first studies on the topic, maximum performance in verbal abilities is achieved much later than maximum performance in word fluency or inductive reasoning (see Figure 7.1). Second, there are inter-individual differences in the trajectories. Third, at

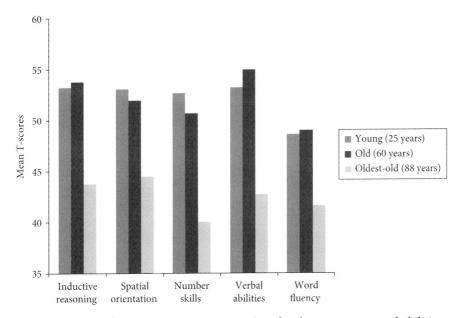

FIGURE 7.1 Estimated age effects from 28-year data for the primary mental abilities.

Data from Schaie, K. W., 1996, Intellectual Development in Adulthood: The Seattle Longitudinal Study, p. 120, figure 5.4 Cambridge University Press.

any age, the SLS observed individuals with longitudinal declines, stability, and improvement. Thus, intelligence does not necessarily, automatically, or generally decline with age. Instead, stable and improving individuals suggest that there must be activities and environmental conditions supporting these activities that can positively influence performance in all ages.

Assuming that standard intelligence tests with their rather formal or abstract tests may be less relevant or practised in older age, measures of everyday intellectual functioning have also been examined. Measures of practical intelligence focus on everyday problem-solving such as interpreting bus schedules, maps, medication labels, or vending machines. Existing data support that practical intelligence on average remains stable until very old age. However, the tasks used are cognitively so simple that only individuals with cognitive impairments will produce any errors, but unimpaired individuals will all be at the ceiling of possible test performance. Measures of wisdom focus on expertise in dealing with difficult conflict situations. Individuals would score highest when they have more factual knowledge about the circumstances of such conflicts, have more strategies to deal with the consequences of decisions, and are integrating a lifespan and a contextual perspective in their judgment (Staudinger and Baltes 1996). The available data on wisdom development suggest that there is no significant age effect between 20 and 89 years and that wisdom is a stable ability well into old age.

INFORMATION-PROCESSING RESOURCES

Another approach to study cognitive development is to focus on elementary information-processing resources (see Table 7.1). Assuming that a detailed task analysis will allow determination of which resources are required to solve the task, the approach allows predictions of performance in complex higher-order performances by combining the knowledge of individual abilities in each of the processing resources. A limitation of these resources results in a deficit in encoding information into memory and then for retrieving information from memory. Since older people tend to demonstrate restricted processing resources, they are more likely to have problems in carrying out resource

Table 7.1 Table of memory components

Retrospective memory		Prospective memory
Long-term storage	Short-term storage	Task
Long-term memory	Short-term memory	Time based
Declarative memory	Working memory	Event based
Procedural memory	Central executive	
Episodic memory	Phonological loop	
Semantic memory	Visuospatial sketchpad	
Source memory	Episodic buffer	
Autobiographical memory		

demanding operations such as updating a word, in encoding and retrieving information in a systematic way, and in dual tasking (Craik 1986). To find out more about the relations between age, information-processing resources and memory, many studies have been conducted analysing age effects on memory in all its variants. One major distinction in memory research is between retrospective memory and prospective memory. Retrospective memory refers to the encoding and later retrieving of information and prospective memory to the self-initiated execution of an earlier-formed intention (Baddeley, Eysenck, and Anderson 2009).

Retrospective memory may be further divided into long-term and short-term storage. Within long-term memory one can distinguish declarative (storing consciously retrievable facts) and procedural memory (storing learning experiences that are not accessible to conscious report). Declarative memory furthermore can be divided into episodic and semantic memory. Episodic memory refers to the ability to remember events one took part in. It is typically tested through recall tests of word lists, sentences, stories, or pictures. An important aspect of episodic memory is source memory, i.e. the memory for the context in which information was encoded. Source memory performance is lower in older adults, and this explains why older adults may have a good sense that they have seen a particular face, but are more likely to have difficulties remembering in which context. Episodic memory performance is typically lower in older vs younger adults, and age differences are typically larger compared to semantic memory. In addition, age differences increase with increasing processing demands at the retrieval of the prior learned information. Thus, free recall tests show large age differences whereas recognition tests of the same material often show small or no age differences. These findings can be explained by the observation that although young and old individuals profit from retrieval cues, older adults use them less frequently when not specifically instructed. Thus, in recognition tests in which the items displayed earlier serve as cues, there are only small age differences.

A particular type of episodic memory is autobiographical memory that contains memory of events that sometimes occurred decades earlier. Most individuals perceive their autobiographical memory to be intact because memories from the past often appear to be very clear and detailed compared to more recently experienced events. Furthermore, with increasing age, older people tend to retrieve emotionally positive autobiographical memories (positivity effect). One reason is that there is a tendency to retrieve mood-congruent memories, and compared to depressed individuals normal individuals are more often in a positive mood. Another reason is that memory retrieval may serve to regulate emotions so that one retrieves more positive memories to overcome a sad mood. To the degree that depressed individuals are impaired in their ability to regulate their emotions they are also less likely to retrieve positive emotions to overcome their depressed mood. One way to measure autobiographical memory is to ask for personal memories of the past and then to date them relative to well-established factual events such as one's wedding. Age-comparative studies show that memories produced by older adults take longer to retrieve, are less specific, and are more positively evaluated (Rubin 2000). Some aspects of autobiographical memory seem to be age-invariant. In all age groups memory is less accurate and detailed the longer ago an event occurred, and all age groups report most events in the age range between ten and thirty years ('reminiscence bump'). This is either because there are more major events in this period of the lifespan or many of the events in this phase are emotionally highly salient and are particularly well encoded.

The second aspect of declarative memory is semantic memory. This is the ability to remember factual knowledge. General knowledge, one of the tests of this ability and part of the Wechsler intelligence test battery, typically shows an age-related increase well into old age. However, word-finding problems and problems recalling the names of people are more frequent in old age. This may have to do with the fact that general knowledge can be verbally expressed in synonymous ways, whereas very specific knowledge without the option to use synonymous descriptions shows larger age differences.

Non-declarative learning and memory is called procedural memory. It refers to the acquisition of cognitive and motor skills such as bicycling, driving a car, counting, or spelling. These skills can become automatized and do not require remembering the context in which the skill was acquired. Therefore one defines these skills as implicit memory processes, and there are typically no or small age differences (cf. Park and Schwarz 2000).

As opposed to long-term memory, short-term memory (STM) and working memory (WM) are limited in duration and capacity. However the distinction between STM and WM is not that simple. There are contradictory opinions as to whether STM is part of WM, or if they are independent; sometimes the terms 'short-term memory' and 'working memory' are even used interchangeably (Baddeley 2012). Yet more recent research (Cowan 2008) tends to see STM and WM as closely related. Short-term memory, sometimes called primary memory (more restricted than short-term memory), refers to the short term, relatively passive storage of presented information. Since the capacity of short-term memory is limited, only a small number of items can be held temporarily accessible. While age differences in short-term memory are typically small, they are larger in working memory. Although working memory is capacity-limited, unlike short-term memory it is based on active processes of simultaneously storing and operating upon the stored information (Bopp and Verhaeghen 2005). This is particularly relevant for everyday functioning, because working memory skills are central to numerous higher-order cognitive skills.

One of the most prominent working memory models is the one developed by Baddeley and Hitch (1974). Originally it consisted of three components—the central executive, the visuospatial sketchpad system, and the phonological loop system—and was later on complemented with the episodic buffer. Thereby, the central executive works as planner organizing the utilization and the combination of the other so-called slave systems. While age has nearly no influence on the phonological loop system (the system which temporarily stores verbal information and consists of a phonological store and an articulatory rehearsal process) and only moderate influence on the visuospatial sketchpad system (system which is in charge of the temporary maintenance and manipulation of visuospatial information), it is clearly associated with performance reduction in tasks involving the central executive. These age-associated deficits can be seen when people have to keep a string of information in mind and consistently update and complement this string. One way to measure this capacity is with the reading span task developed by Daneman and Carpenter (1980). In this task participants are requested to read a certain number of sentences aloud (two to six sentences) and to remember the last word of each sentence. Afterwards, the last word of each sentence has to be recalled in the same order the sentences had been presented before. Normally, older people not only recall fewer words, but also commit more intrusion errors compared to younger adults (lack of inhibition) (Van Den Noort et al. 2008). The same results are found when older people perform memory updating tasks such as remembering the smallest item of a given list (De Beni and Palladino 2004). Another approach to measure the effect of ageing on executive control processes is with tasks involving the online modulation of attentional and response processes such as dual tasks (Cohen, Botvinick, and Carter 2000). The idea behind dual tasks is the simultaneous performance of two or more abilities of either the same or different modalities which leads to limitation or conflicts in cognitive resource allocation (Hiscock 1986). In fact, when older adults are instructed to recall a word list while they are walking on a narrow track, they demonstrate greater dual task cost in both domains (Lindenberger, Mariske, and Baltes 2000). If people with extremely low information-processing resources such as patients with Alzheimer's disease have to perform a dual task this can lead to complete prioritization of one or the other task. Concerning the example with thinking and walking on a narrow track, such patients tend either to enumerate fewer or non-words or slow down, stumble, or fall ('stops walking when talking'). Hence the results indicate that adult age differences in executive control processes are adjusted through the extent to which the mental representations of multiple task sets need to be activated (Baltes, Freund, and Li 2005).

The previously discussed memory components are closely related to people, words, or events that are associated with the past as opposed to prospective memory, which is linked to future events such as taking medicine before going to bed. Prospective memory problems are the most frequently reported memory mistakes of everyday life (Kliegel and Martin 2003). Older people, especially, may find these memory problems can cause serious health threats, for example when medications are not taken or are taken repeatedly (commission error; Scullin, Bugg, and McDaniel 2012). Such memory failures become even more obvious in the case of polypharmacy when for example the intake of five or more chronically administered medications has to be managed (Murray and Kroenke 2001).

Although there is no consistent agreement about the effect age has on prospective memory, most researchers point out that prospective memory performance decreases in old age. According to Park et al. (1997) older people tend to make more errors in time-based than event-based tasks. This means that they have more problems remembering and initiating an action which is linked to a point in time (e.g. medicine has to be taken at eight o'clock) rather than to an event (e.g. medicine has to be taken before going to bed). However this lower performance in time-based tasks could also be due to fundamental age deficits in time monitoring rather than to prospective memory. Interestingly, these age associated deficits in prospective memory are only found in laboratory settings and not in real-life situations. In prospective memory tasks of everyday life older people even tend to outperform younger people (Phillips, Henri, and Martin 2008). This effect even occurs when the difficulty level of the laboratory task and everyday task is comparable and when in both cases it is possible to combine the prospective action with automated, highly regular activities such as having dinner. Thus, this difference is most likely due to the effects of familiarity with the sequence of relevant cuing events; whereas in a laboratory and unfamiliar situation, participants would have to monitor the environment continuously to detect the relevant cues, in familiar environments older individuals profit from reducing attentional effort at times of low probabilities for a cuing event (Zöllig et al. 2012).

Speed of Processing

The processing-speed theory of Salthouse (1996: 403) states that 'a major factor contributing to age-related differences in memory and other aspects of cognitive functioning is a reduction with increasing age in the speed with which many cognitive operations can be executed'. This theory has its roots in the observation of mental slowing in old age and is based on two mechanisms, namely the limited time and simultaneity mechanisms. The idea behind the limited time mechanism is that if a sequence of operations has to be executed, the time to perform later operations is restricted when a large proportion of the available time is occupied by earlier operations. For example, when asking for directions to the railway station, one has to process the given information quickly enough to keep up with the further instructions to find the right destination. The simultaneity mechanism is based on the assumption that the product of an earlier operation is forgotten by the time the later operation is completed. For example, when translating a sentence, one might forget the translation of the first word when too much time is needed until reaching the last word of the sentence. Therefore, age differences in working memory tasks such as operation span or digit span backward can be explained, on the one hand, by a slowed processing of the first operations, which takes too much time to do later operations or, on the other hand, through a forgetting of the results of earlier operations when needing them at a later point in time. The age-related slowing of information-processing speed when tested with instruments such as the digit symbol substitution test from the Wechsler Intelligent Scale-Revised (Wechsler 1981) is well documented. What is more, Salthouse (1996) found a median correlation of $r = .45$ between age and measures of speed across a very wide range of behavioural measures.

Inhibitory Functioning

According to the inhibitory framework, a successful cognitive performance requires the ability to inhibit access to temporarily irrelevant information. Older adults tend to demonstrate a decrease in their ability to disregard irrelevant information and to suppress overlearned behaviour when it is not appropriate in a given situation (Lustig, Hasher, and Zacks 2007). Hasher and Zacks (1988) differentiate between three functions of inhibition namely controlling access to attention's function (access function), deleting irrelevant information from attention and working memory (deletion function), and suppressing or restraining strong but inappropriate responses (restraint function). Deficits in the access function lead to an interference of the processing of target stimuli by either disrupting or facilitating performance, depending on the relation between interference factor and the targets. Common instruments to measure access function are tests such as the digit symbol substitution test (e.g. Wechsler 1981). By contrast, the deletion function helps to correctly delete information when it is not needed. That means that sometimes it is useful to forget information in the service of better memory for relevant information (May et al. 1999). This function is especially important for working memory tasks or memory updating tasks described earlier. The restraint function means the ability to suppress behaviour which is inappropriate in a given situation. This function is often measured with Go/No-go or Stop signal tasks requiring participants to perform an action given certain cue stimuli and to inhibit that action seeing other stimuli. Although older adults on average demonstrate a decrease in inhibitory function, additional factors such as individual differences and circadian cycle should be taken into account when looking at test performance of the earlier mentioned tasks.

PLASTICITY

Lifespan theory (Baltes 1990) maintains that development is modifiable or plastic at all phases of development; however, there are constraints and limits on developmental plasticity and these constraints and limits vary by period of development. A major goal of lifespan developmental research has been to examine the range and limits of plasticity at various phases of the lifespan (for an overview see Willis, Schaie, and Martin 2009). Cognitive plasticity has been defined as an individual's capacity to acquire cognitive skills (Mercado 2008). Recently, there is increasing interest both in the conceptual relation between cognitive plasticity and neural plasticity and also in experimental studies that examine cortical changes occurring concurrently with the behavioural training or intervention efforts (Nyberg et al. 2003). In the study of cognitive ageing within neuropsychology, there has been considerable interest in the capability of the individual to continue to function at an adequate cognitive level when there have been neural deficits or pathology. Stern (2002) proposes the concept of cognitive reserve to the study of this phenomenon. *Passive reserve* is defined in terms of the amount of neuropathology that can be sustained before reaching a threshold for clinical expression. *Active cognitive reserve*, by contrast, is based on the premise that the brain may actively attempt to cope with and compensate for deficits by using alternative pre-existing cognitive processes or by enlisting compensatory resources (Stern 2007). Rather than positing that brains of individuals with high levels of cognitive reserve are anatomically different from those for individuals' with less reserve, the cognitive reserve hypothesis proposes that high-functioning individuals process tasks in a more efficient manner, allowing maintenance of cognitive performance levels longer in the face of pathological changes in the brain. So far, only indirect measures of cognitive reserve exist. They either assess potential precursors of reserve such as cognitive engagement (Nucci, Mapelli, and Mondini, 2012) or are based on comparisons between individuals of similar pathology, but different levels of education (Liao et al. 2005). Ideally, to determine cognitive reserve on an individual basis, one would have to measure performance and brain pathology repeatedly to establish which degree of pathology can be tolerated without performance declines.

Neural plasticity

Both brain structure and brain function have been studied in relation to cognitive plasticity in old age (Kramer et al. 2004). While the concept of neural plasticity, i.e. the potential for changes in neural structures, has been closely related to the concept of cognitive or behavioural plasticity, i.e. the potential for behavioural changes in cognitive performance, the exact relation between the two concepts has not been fully explicated. It has been assumed that neural plasticity contributes to or underlies cognitive-behavioural plasticity; however, Stern's concept of cognitive reserve, i.e. the potential for maintaining or stabilizing cognitive performance levels when pathological changes occur in the brain, would suggest that cognitive reserve can exist even when neural plasticity has been compromised. Neural plasticity refers to the capacity of neural circuits to change in response to fluctuations in neural or glial activity (Kempermann, Gast, and Gage 2002) and is associated with changes in synaptic connections between neurons, addition of new neurons (neurogenesis), increased myelinization of axons, or change in the size or shape of a neuron. With regard to brain function, PET and fMRI research has resulted in at least two tentative general findings. First, older adults show lower levels of activation in a wide variety of tasks and brain regions. While one explanation of reduced activation holds that ageing is associated with loss of neural resources, another explanation is that neural resources are available, but not adequately recruited. Instruction in strategy use, for example, has been shown to reduce under-recruitment (Logan et al. 2002). Second, older adults exhibit nonselective recruitment of brain regions (Kramer et al. 2004). Older adults, compared to young adults, show recruitment of different brain regions in addition to those activated in younger adults. This observation of bilateral activation has led to the Hemispheric Asymmetry Reduction in Older Adults (HAROLD) model of neurocognitive ageing (Hayes and Cabeza 2008). The model suggests and finds in functional neuroimaging studies that brain activity in the prefrontal cortex tends to be less lateralized in older than younger adults when performing episodic-memory, working-memory, perception, and inhibitory-control tasks. The finding has been replicated across PET and fMRI studies and suggests clearly that it is a general age effect, not a specific task effect.

Neural plasticity: availability, reconfigurability, customizability

To integrate the existing conceptual approaches of plasticity and reserve and to explain the empirical findings, Mercado (2008) has recently argued that three key processes impact cortical modules and thus indirectly neural and cognitive plasticity and reserve: availability, reconfigurability, and customizability. *Availability* refers to the number and diversity of cortical modules that are available for differentiating stimulus representations. Larger brain regions provide room for more complex circuitry, more dendritic expansion, more synapses, thicker myelin, more neurons, and larger neurons—all of which increase functional capacity. *Reconfigurability* refers to the brain's ability to flexibly develop new configurations of cortical modules, and to switch rapidly between them as a function of task demands. This refers to the flexibility in using the same modules for different cognitive tasks and even within tasks as one progresses in learning increasingly better ways to perform the task. There are clear indications that to stabilize cognitive performance, as people age they tend to recruit different neural circuits than they did as younger adults (HAROLD; Cabeza 2002), and that it might actually be adaptive to use different neural circuits across task trials to perform well in the same cognitive task. *Customizability* refers to the brain's capacity dynamically to adjust the selectivity of cortical modules based on experience. That is, the degree to which repeated experience in turn shapes the structure of the brain to perform well-learned tasks more efficiently or more accurately. It is an empirically open question if customizability changes with age or exposure to particular types or durations of experiences. A major question regarding neural plasticity is the issue of how experience or cognitive stimulations impact(s) the brain and enhances brain functioning. Kramer et al. (2004) have suggested two alternative hypotheses regarding the relationship between cognitive stimulation including training and plasticity in neural structure and function. On the one hand, enhanced neuronal structure and brain function may occur as a result of additional environmental stimulation and play a protective function against neuronal degradation (Fillit et al. 2002). Alternatively, enhanced neuronal networks fostered through cognitive experiences may delay cognitive decline even in the face of morphological and functional deterioration in the ageing brain.

Cognitive plasticity has been examined at multiple behavioural levels (see Willis et al. 2009). Cognitive training research has focused on cognitive processes (e.g. processing speed, inhibition), primary mental abilities (e.g. inductive reasoning, spatial orientation, episodic memory), higher-order cognitive constructs (fluid intelligence, executive functioning), and global cognition involving multiple cognitive domains. In addition, the impact of noncognitive interventions (exercise, nutrition) on cognition have been examined. Key behavioural indicators of intellectual capacity include: the capacity to learn a cognitive skill, the rate at which the skill is learned, and the highest performance (asymptote) reached.

The contexts in which behavioural cognitive plasticity have been most commonly studied have been the behavioural training studies that target those fluid- and process-based abilities that exhibit relatively early age-related decline. Overall, training-induced improvements in elementary cognitive functions have been repeatedly demonstrated (for an overview see Martin et al. 2011). While there is increasing evidence that cognitive plasticity is possible during all developmental periods, constraints and limits on plasticity at each level become more evident with increasing age. At the neural level, there are constraints due to degradation of the neural structure (brain atrophy, number of neurons, synaptic density). Likewise, there are constraints at the functional level in the brain. Flexibility in reconfiguration of cortical networks or in customization of cortical modules is reduced with advancing age. At the behavioural level, there appear to be constraints in terms of the asymptotic level of performance attainable with increasing age. Although cognitive interventions result in significant behavioural improvement, the highest level attained is lower for older adults compared to young adults. Likewise, efficiency of new skill acquisition appears to be compromised with age under conditions of 'testing the limits'. For example, increasing the speed at which older adults must perform, or requiring the engagement in dual tasks compromises the performance of older adults to a greater extent than those younger in the lifespan.

FUNCTIONAL INTEGRATIVE APPROACH

Functional integrative approaches to development have a long tradition within cognitive psychology (e.g. Hultsch and Hertzog 1988). They aim to explain how individuals through the variation in the recruitment of multiple elementary cognitive subprocesses manage to adapt to varying environmental conditions and contingencies. In essence, the focus is on which changes, i.e. in process recruitment or maximum process availability, are needed to stabilize everyday functioning. Applied to cognitive performance, Hultsch and Hertzog (1988) point out three central implications of this approach: (1) a focus on the active individual orchestrating multiple cognitive subprocesses such as memory retrieval and mnemonic strategies to achieve a stable performance in the higher-order process of intentional behaviour; (2) a focus on the dynamic, temporal nature of mental and behavioural activity; and (3) the need to examine cognitive operations as they occur under actual living conditions (e.g. Verhaeghen, Martin, and Sedek 2012). Thus, the functional approach suggests that the plasticity within each elementary process is a requirement to stabilize higher-order functions, and a larger range of plasticity in more elementary processes should make it easier to maintain higher-order functioning longer and in more variable environmental conditions.

A functional integrative approach assumes that individuals, as they age and experience changes in cognitive capabilities, may be able to stabilize individually relevant outcomes such as autonomous living or quality of life in everyday life through processes of orchestrating the goal-directed recruitment and sequencing of cognitive (and noncognitive) subprocesses. The approach assumes that successfully ageing individuals actively manage their everyday environments, their everyday activities, their everyday goal-setting and motivation, their relevant cognitive and noncognitive resources to lead idiosyncratically meaningful lives. Thus, elementary cognitive processes are conceptualized as part of this orchestration process and the research question changes from a change-focused 'how much can a single ability be improved through training?' to a stabilization-focused 'which abilities and orchestrating mechanisms allow a particular individual to keep leading a productive or meaningful life?' If one assumes, that the same individual may from one situation to another be able to recruit high vs low levels of a particular cognitive skill to achieve the same outcome, then trying to predict everyday performance from a single measurement of a single cognitive skill will necessarily lead to small amounts of detectable transfer and small effect sizes. That is, the functional orchestration approach in essence argues that the best cognitive performance is when individuals manage to produce it in varying environments. Thus, cognitive performance is a process and can only be understood when its longitudinal dynamics are examined.

As a basis for the examination of cognitive adaptation processes, an orchestration model is helpful as an analogy. In this analogy, the individual is the orchestrator deciding what piece to play for a particular audience, how to select the instruments or resources, and how to sequence the resource recruitment. The active individual also decides how to improve particular resources through making use of their plasticity through training. Alternatively, when resources are not improvable, the individual may improve resource–environment fit through selecting other music pieces or audiences, i.e. environments. If successful in the orchestrating process, each orchestra at different points in time will objectively sound different, but could at each point in time produce the optimal fit between environments, the orchestrator's goals, available resources, and resource plasticity. To improve and test improvement, longitudinal approaches are needed to demonstrate the adaptability of the orchestration to changes in any or multiple elements of the orchestration. Practically speaking, a cognitive intervention based on the functional orchestration approach is an individualized intervention based on evidence for the effects of the tools recommended to support individuals' orchestration (Eschen, Zehnder, and Martin 2013).

Such an intervention has two major components: assessment and intervention recommendations. The assessment serves to determine a person's general participation motives, self-assessments of current cognitive functions, important environmental demands and goals that may be affected by reported or expected cognitive problems, and major internal or external factors influencing cognitive health. Based on these data, individually important cognitive abilities and factors influencing these cognitive abilities are assessed with objective measures. Participants then receive feedback on the assessment results and recommendations for suitable interventions and their successful implementation. Thus, the individualized intervention targets resources, environmental demands, goals, their fit, their subjective evaluations and change expectations, as well as knowledge about effective interventions and their adequate implementation relevant for persons' satisfaction with their cognitive health. By giving recommendations and leaving implementation of these recommendations to the participants, it assigns the participants an active role in managing their cognitive health. Consequently, such an intervention differs from other gerontological interventions that try to modify cognitive health, such as memory clinics or cognitive training, by its multifactorial nature, by taking into account both objective and subjective measures of relevant variables, its level of individualization, by making the participants the agents of change, and by considering the participants' satisfaction with their cognitive health as the main outcome variable.

Implications for Practice

Different approaches to cognitive ageing have been presented. From a practical perspective, they differ substantially in their implications. Changes in cognitive performance typically become clinically relevant when the performance level in a particular cognitive resource decreases enough that it affects an individual's ability to function independently in everyday life, and, most often, leads to a substantial decrease in quality of life. Based on the cognitive resource approach, one would recommend focused training of the affected cognitive ability to increase performance and, as a consequence, improve quality of life and independence. In fact, different studies have reliably demonstrated that ability-specific training leads to an increase in the trained ability over a time period of up to seven years (Baltes and Willis 1982). However, since these trainings are highly task-specific, hardly any transfer to non-trained abilities can be observed. As a consequence, with multiple deficits one would have to practise all affected abilities independently, resulting in the need for extensive amounts of training that are often not practical. In addition, from a prevention perspective, individuals can hardly be motivated to practise multiple abilities separately and extensively when everyday functioning is not affected and there is no transfer.

A more economical way might be to focus on higher-order metacognitive abilities such as multi-tasking, working memory, executive functions, or strategy use. As these are conceptualized as superordinate abilities directing the recruitment of elementary cognitive subprocesses, one may assume that their improvement should more likely generalize to non-trained tasks. In fact, it has been reliably shown that multi-tasking trainings increase performance in the practised tasks, but can also lead to the acquisition of generalizable task-coordination and task-management skills (Kramer, Larish, and Strayer 1995). From a prevention perspective, these training approaches are more promising because of the higher likelihood of transfer. However, to improve such metacognitive skills, relatively large amounts of practice are needed to demonstrate improvements, and it would still be necessary to prioritize and select the most relevant ones.

The functional orchestration model has quite different implications. It conceptualizes all cognitive abilities and all noncognitive abilities and resources from a functional point of view. That is, it assumes that individuals actively, sequentially, and simultaneously recruit different combinations of cognitive and noncognitive abilities to achieve functional outcomes such as autonomy or quality of life. This approach can explain why increasing elementary or, more generally, single abilities does not necessarily transfer to effects in everyday life. It does so only to the degree that the increase is of functional value for an individual. If there is a major decline in one or more abilities that affect quality of life, then the increase in performance in this or these particular abilities is, in fact, functional, i.e. this improves quality of life. However, once quality of life or autonomy is stabilized, many combinations of recruiting cognitive abilities can be functional to maintain or stabilize quality of life. This implies that functional activities in everyday life, by definition, are associated with the simultaneous and sequential activation of several cognitive abilities and, thus, provide for multiple ability orchestration training. This explains findings of higher environmental complexity being related to better cognitive outcomes (Schooler 1999). From a practical perspective this approach implies that identifying one or more subjectively relevant functional outcomes is key to trigger this type of training. Providing individuals with opportunities to engage their orchestration activity through the variation of environmental demands, e.g. performing non-routine activities, exposition to new environments and individuals, creating the need for support, should suffice to trigger individual activities to adapt to these environmental variations. Eventually, more orchestration should lead to better adaptivity to varying environments and stable or even higher levels in basic information-processing resources. Practically, the approach can be used to develop individualized cognitive interventions making use of the evidence from training studies (see Figure 7.2).

From a prevention perspective, the orchestration approach has an additional advantage. The approach can be used at all ages and all levels of functioning, in impaired as well as healthy ageing individuals. Consider that many individuals are motivated to stabilize, rather than improve, cognitive functioning well into old age, and are motivated to perform activities promising such an outcome. Then, based on the model, this can be achieved by reducing environmental demands in impaired individuals, and by increasing environmental demands in healthy individuals—which level would be optimal is still an empirical question. This can be obtained either by adaptive process-based training or by functional training integrating different theoretical approaches. Adaptive process-based training is characterized, on the one hand, by individually adjusted levels of task difficulty (adapted throughout the training progress) and, on the other hand, by task complexity preventing the generation of strategies. In contrast, functional training has the advantage of training abilities important for everyday life, thus leading to stronger and broader training effects. Furthermore, by integrating and orchestrating multiple resources the training remains highly demanding and many different abilities are trained simultaneously.

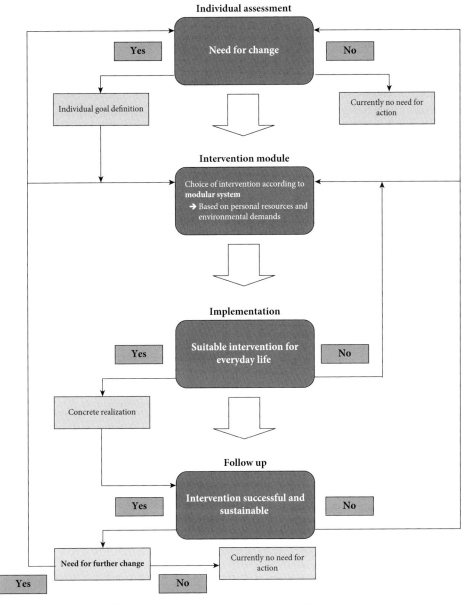

FIGURE 7.2 Course of individualized intervention approach.

SUMMARY

Cognitive ability changes in old age are characterized by their multidimensionality, multidirectionality, and plasticity. There are substantial individual differences in the developmental patterns of cognitive abilities, and cognitive abilities are differentially relevant for everyday performance. Approaches focusing on specific cognitive impairments in elementary cognitive resources and their negative effects on quality of life and independence have led to the development of effective rehabilitative training interventions with typically little transfer to non-trained abilities. Approaches focusing on higher-order metacognitive skills are the basis for effective training interventions with some transfer to non-trained abilities and tasks. Different from both approaches assuming that increasing specific abilities should positively affect everyday performance, the functional orchestration approach to cognitive ageing assumes that multiple cognitive and noncognitive resources are actively orchestrated to maintain everyday functioning and quality of life. This approach focusing on stabilization of functioning in old age emphasizes the equivalence and compensatory potential of cognitive and noncognitive resources. It suggests an individualized intervention approach integrating the importance of individual goal functions, multiple resource orchestration, and environmental variation and adaptation to stabilize functioning, and can be applied at both normal and clinical levels of performance.

KEY REFERENCES AND SOURCES FOR FURTHER READING

Kliegel, M., Mcdaniel, M. A., and Einstein, G. O. (2008). *Prospective Memory: Cognitive, Neuroscience, Developmental, and Applied Perspectives*. Mahwah, NJ: Erlbaum.

Martin, M., Schneider, R., Eicher, S., and Moor, C. (2012). 'The Functional Quality of Life (fQOL) Model: A New Basis for Quality of Life-enhancing Interventions in Old Age'. *Journal of Gerontopsychology and Geriatric Psychiatry* 25: 33–40.

Naveh-Benjamin, M., Moscovitch, M., and Loediger, H. L. (2001). *Perspectives on Human Memory and Cognitive Aging: Essays in Honour of Fergus Craik*. New York: Psychology Press.

Park, D. C. and Schwarz, N. (2000). *Cognitive Aging: A Primer*. Philadelphia, PA: Psychology Press.

Schaie, K. W. (2005). *Developmental Influences on Adult Intelligence: The Seattle Longitudinal Study*. New York: Oxford University Press.

Willis, S. L., Tennstedt, S. L., Marsiske, M., Ball, K., Elias, J., Koepke, K. M., et al. (2006). 'Long-term Effects of Cognitive Training on Everyday Functional Outcomes in Older Adults'. *The Journal of the American Medical Association* 296: 2805–2814.

Willis, S. L., Schaie, K. W., and Martin, M. (2009). 'Cognitive Plasticity'. In: V. Bengtson, M. Silverstein, N. Putney, and D. Gans (eds), *Handbook of Theories of Aging*. New York: Springer, pp. 295–322.

REFERENCES

Baddeley, A. D. and Hitch, G. J. (1974). 'Working Memory'. In: G. A. Bower (ed.) *Recent Advances in Learning and Motivation* (pp. 47–90). New York: Academic Press.

Baddeley, A. D., Eysenck, M. W., and Anderson, M. C. (2009). *Memory*. Hove: Psychology Press.

Baddeley, A. (2012). 'Working Memory: Theories, Models, and Controversies'. *Annual Review of Psychology* 63: 1–29.

Baltes, P. B. and Willis, S. L. (1982). 'Plasticity and Enhancement of Intellectual Functioning in Old Age: Penn State's Adult Development and Enrichment Project (ADEPT)'. In F. I. M. Craik and S. E. Trehub (eds), *Aging and Cognitive Processes* (pp. 353 389). New York: Plenum Press.

Baltes, P. B. (1990). 'Life-span Developmental Psychology: Basic Theoretical Principles'. *Psychologische Rundschau* 41(1): 1–24.

Baltes, P. B., Freund, A. M., and Li, S.-C. (2005). 'The Psychological Science of Human Aging' In M. Johnson, V. L. Bengston, P. G. Coleman, and T. B. L. Kirkwood (eds), *The Cambridge Handbook of Age and Ageing* (pp. 47–71). Cambridge: Cambridge University Press.

Bopp, K. L. and Verhaeghen, P. (2005). 'Aging and Verbal Memory Span: A Meta-analysis'. *The Journals of Gerontology Series B: Psychological Sciences and Social Science* 60: 223–233.

Cabeza, R. (2002). 'Hemispheric Asymmetry Reduction in Older Adults: The HAROLD Model'. *Psychology and Aging* 17: 85–100.

Cohen, J. D., Botvinick, M., and Carter, C. S. (2000). 'Anterior Cingulate and Prefrontal Cortex: Who's in Control?' *Nature Neuroscience* 3: 421–423.

Cowan, N. (2008). 'What are the Differences between Long-term, Short-term, and Working Memory?' *Progress in Brain Research* 169: 323–338.

Craik, F. I. M. (1986). 'A functional account of age differences in memory'. In F. Klix and H. Hagendorf (eds), *Human Memory and Cognitive Capabilities: Mechanisms and Performances* (pp. 409–422). Amsterdam: Elsevier Science.

Daneman, M. and Carpenter, P. A. (1980). 'Individual Differences in Working Memory and Reading'. *Journal of Verbal Learning and Verbal Behavior* 19: 450–466.

De Beni, R. and Palladino, P. (2004). 'Decline in Working Memory Updating through Ageing: Intrusion Error Analyses'. *Memory* 12: 75–89.

Eschen, A., Zehnder, F., and Martin, M. (2013). 'Cognitive Health Counseling 40+: A New Individualized Cognitive Intervention'. *Zeitschrift für Gesundheitspsychologie* 21: 24–33.

Fillit, H. M., Butler, R. N., O'connell, A. W., Albert, M. S., Birren, J. E., Cotman, C. W., et al. (2002). 'Achieving and Maintaining Cognitive Vitality with Aging'. *Mayo Clinic Proceedings* 77: 681–696.

Hasher, L. and Zacks, R. T. (1988). 'Working Memory, Comprehension, and Aging: A Review and New View'. In G. H. Bower (ed.), *The Psychology of Learning and Motivation: Advances in Research and Theory* (pp. 193–225). New York: Academic Press.

Hayes, S. M. and Cabeza, R. (2008). 'Imaging Aging: Present and Future'. In S. M. Hofe and D. F. Alwin (eds), *Handbook of Cognitive Aging: Interdisciplinary Perspectives* (pp. 308–326). Los Angeles: Sage.

Hiscock, M. (1986). 'Lateral eye movements and dual-task performance'. In H. J. Hannay (ed.), *Experimental Techniques in Human Neuropsychology* (pp. 264–308). New York: Oxford University Press.

Hultsch, R. A. and Hertzog, C. (1988). 'Adult Memory and Metamemory Development'. In F. E. Weinert and M. Perlmutter (eds), *Memory Development*. Hillsdale, NJ: Erlbaum.

Kempermann, G., Gast, D., and Gage, F. H. (2002). 'Neuroplasticity in Old Age: Sustained Fivefold Induction of Hippocampal Neurogenesis by Long-term Environmental Enrichment'. *Annals of Neurology* 52: 135–143.

Kliegel, M. and Martin, M. (2003). 'Prospective Memory Research: Why Is It Relevant?' *International Journal of Psychology* 38: 193–194.

Kramer, A. F., Larish, J. F., and Strayer, D. L. (1995). 'Training for Attentional Control in Dual-task Settings—A Comparison of Young and Old Adults'. *Journal of Experimental Psychology-Applied* 1: 50–76.

Kramer, A. F., Bherer, L., Colcombe, S. J., Dong, W., and Greenough, W. T. (2004). 'Environmental Influences on Cognitive and Brain Plasticity during Aging'. *Journals of Gerontology Series B: Biological Sciences and Medical Science* 59: M940–57.

Liao, Y. C., Liu, R. S., Teng, E. L., Lee, Y. C., Wang, P. N., Lin, K. N., et al. (2005). 'Cognitive Reserve: a SPECT Study of 132 Alzheimer's Disease Patients with an Education Range of 0–19 Years'. *Dementia and Geriatric Cognitive Disorders* 20: 8–14.

Lindenberger, U., Marsiske, M., and Baltes, P. B. (2000). 'Memorizing while Walking: Increase in Dual-task Costs from Young Adulthood to Old Age'. *Psychology and Aging* 15: 417–436.

Logan, J. M., Sanders, A. L., Snyder, A. Z., Morris, J. C., and Buckner, R. L. (2002). 'Under-recruitment and Nonselective Recruitment: Dissociable Neural Mechanisms Associated with Aging'. *Neuron* 33: 827–840.

Lustig, C., Hasher, L., and Zacks, R. (2007). 'Inhibitory Deficit Theory: Recent Developments in a "New View"'. In D. S. Gorfein and C. M. Macleod (eds), *The Place of Inhibition in Cognition* (pp. 145–162). Washington, DC: American Psychological Association.

Martin, M., Clare, L., Altgassen, A. M., Cameron, M. H., and Zehnder, F. (2011). 'Cognition-based Interventions for Healthy Older People and People with Mild Cognitive Impairment'. *Cochrane Database of Systematic Reviews* 1: CD006220.

May, C. P., Zacks, R. T., Hasher, L., and Multhaup, K. S. (1999). 'Inhibition in the Processing of Garden-path Sentences'. *Psychology and Aging* 14: 304–313.

Mercado, E. (2008). 'Neural and Cognitive Plasticity: From Maps to Minds'. *Psychological Bulletin* 134: 109–137.

Murray, M. D. and Kroenke, K. (2001). 'Polypharmacy and Medication Adherence: Small Steps on a Long Road'. *Journal of General Internal Medicine* 16: 137–139.

Nucci, M., Mapelli, D., and Mondini, S. (2012). 'Cognitive Reserve Index Questionnaire (CRIq): A New Instrument for Measuring Cognitive Reserve'. *Aging: Clinical and Experimental Research* 24(3): 218–226.

Nyberg, L., Sandblom, J., Jones, S., Neely, A. S., Petersson, K. M., Ingvar, M., et al. (2003). 'Neural Correlates of Training-related Memory Improvement in Adulthood and Aging'. *Proceedings of the National Academy of Sciences* 100: 13728–13733.

Park, D. C., Hertzog, C., Kidder, D. P., Morrell, R. W., and Mayhorn, C. B. (1997). 'Effect of Age on Event-based and Time-based Prospective Memory'. *Psychology and Aging* 12: 314–327.

Park, D. C. and Schwarz, N. (2000). *Cognitive Aging: A Primer*. Philadelphia, PA: Psychology Press.

Phillips, L. H., Henry, J. D., and Martin, M. (2008). 'Adult Aging and Prospective Memory: The Importance of Ecological Validity'. In M. Kliegel, M. A. McDaniel and G. O. Einstein (eds), *Prospective Memory: Cognitive, Neuroscience, Developmental, and Applied Perspectives* (pp. 161–186). Mahwah, NJ: Erlbaum.

Raz, N. (2000). 'Aging of the Brain and its Impact on Cognitive Performance: Integration of Structural and Functional Findings'. In F. I. M. Craik and T. A. Salthouse (eds), *The Handbook of Aging and Cognition* (pp. 1–90). Mahwah, NJ: Erlbaum.

Rubin, D. C. (2000). 'Autobiographical Memory and Aging'. In D. Park and N. Schwarz (eds), *Cognitive Aging: A Primer*. Philadelphia, PA: Psychology Press.

Salthouse, T. A. (1996). 'The Processing-speed Theory of Adult Age Differences in Cognition'. *Psychological Review* 103: 403–428.

Schaie, K. W. (1996). *Intellectual Development in Adulthood: The Seattle Longitudinal Study*. Cambridge: Cambridge University Press.

Schooler, C. (1999). 'The Workplace Environment: Measurement, Psychological Effects, and Basic Issues'. In S. L. Friedman and D. T. Wachs (eds), *Measuring Environment across the Life Span* (pp. 229–246). Washington, DC: American Psychological Association.

Scullin, M. K., Bugg, J. M., and McDaniel, M. A. (2012). 'Whoops, I Did it Again: Commission Errors in Prospective Memory'. *Psychology and Aging* 27: 46–53.

Spearman, C. (1904). ' "General intelligence," Objectively Determined and Measured'. *American Journal of Psychology* 15: 201–293.

Staudinger, U. M. and Baltes, P. B. (1996). 'The Psychology of Wisdom'. *Psychologische Rundschau* 47: 57–77.

Stern, Y. (2002). 'What is Cognitive Reserve? Theory and Research Application of the Reserve Concept'. *International Neuropsychological Society* 8: 448–460.

Stern, Y. (2007). *Cognitive Reserve Theory and Applications*. New York: Taylor and Francis.

Terman, L. M. (1916). *The Uses of Intelligence Tests*. Boston: Houghton Mifflin.

Van Den Noort, M., Bosch, P., Haverkort, M., and Hugdahl, K. (2008). 'A Standard Computerized Version of the Reading Span Test in Different Languages'. *European Journal of Psychological Assessment* 24: 35–42.

Verhaeghen, P., Martin, M., and Sedek, G. (2012). 'Reconnecting Cognition in the Lab and Cognition in Real Life: The Role of Compensatory Social and Motivational Factors in Explaining How Cognition Ages in the Wild'. *Aging Neuropsychology and Cognition* 19: 1–12.

Wechsler, D. (1939). *The Measurement of Adult Intelligence*. Baltimore: Williams and Wilkins.

Wechsler, D. (1981). *Manual for the Wechsler Adult Intelligence Scale-Revised*. New York: Psychological Corporation.

Willis, S. L., Schaie, K. W., and Martin, M. (2009). 'Cognitive plasticity'. In V. Bengtson, M. Silverstein, N. Putney and D. Gans (eds), *Handbook of Theories of Aging* (pp. 295–322). New York: Springer.

Yerkes, R. M. (1921). 'Psychological Examining in the United States Army'. *Memoirs of the National Academy of Sciences* 15: 1–890.

Zöllig, J., Mattli, F., Sutter, C., Aurelio, A., and Martin, M. (2012). 'Plasticity of Prospective Memory through a Familiarization Intervention in Old Adults'. *Neuropsychology, Development, and Cognition: Section B, Aging, Neuropsychology and Cognition* 19: 168–194.

CHAPTER 8

TRANSITIONS IN LATER LIFE

KAREN PALLESGAARD MUNK

INTRODUCTION

How does the 'empty nest' feel when the children whom for years you have given your time, love, concern, and money leave home and manage their own lives independently of you? What is it like to leave the labour market and become part of the anonymous group of retirees who are not heard and are even considered to be a burden to society? What is it like to have a spouse with Alzheimer's disease or another kind of long-term terminal disease? What is it like to become a widow? What is it like to become ill and disabled and dependent on other people's assistance with the most intimate processes of your body? What is it like to give up your home and move to an institution where unfamiliar people decide the rules of your daily life? What is it like to follow the decline of your physical looks, and your functional competence, and see death coming? In other words, what is it like to become old? These questions express the typical modern ideas of transitions in later life. In geropsychology they are traditionally called 'exit-life events', indicating to an individual that the life course is coming to an end.

These perspectives, however, give a rather one-dimensional picture of later life only as a period of loss, and of human beings as passive subjects of a biological fate. Another reason why these perspectives are too limited is that they represent a view that separates old age and transitions from other parts of life and treats the old individual as a person living in a historical vacuum. The way personal life trajectories have been shaped as one ages is in many respects crucial to health and quality of life in later life. What matters here is access to social and material resources throughout life and hence the opportunities of a given society (National Institute of Public Health 2007).

Furthermore, if the one-dimensional view of later life as a period of decline is true, older adults should be depressed and unsatisfied with their lives. They are not. Research on life satisfaction in different age groups shows that older adults in general are as satisfied with their lives as younger people (Mehlsen 2011).[1] In addition, it may come as a surprise to learn that people in later life do not experience more depressive episodes than younger people (Munk 2007a, 2007b). There is a fundamental truth, however, to the presence of more loss in old age than in any other part of life because of the fact that we all die some day (Munk 1999; Cole 1992 Katz 2009). In that respect, old age is also 'an age of resignation' because of the individual's confrontation with the biological facts of life, not only in relation to oneself, but also in relation to significant others and contemporaries. This fact seems to cause more depressive *symptoms* among older people than among younger people and is a challenge to mental health (Munk 1999; Munk 2007a). How older adults cope with these 'hard facts of life' is a complicated story, which will be described and discussed later in this chapter. Due to approaching death, ageing is also, according to Katz (2009: 20)

> a great equalizer precisely because it submits all forms of life and matter to common prin-
> ciples of truth and provides us with the communal opportunities to share our lives through
> time, narrative, memory, generation, and heritage. These are the realities that bolster genu-
> ine anti-ageism and counteract the illusory appeal of being 'forever young'. In his essay on
> 'The End of Temporality' Frederic Jameson asserts that the end of temporality is a 'situation of
> postmodernity'.

The conclusion is, however, that the idea of ageing as a universal process that is the same for everyone does not hold true. Transitions in later life are, on the contrary, highly contingent on history, society, culture, and the individual life course, and consequently subject to changes and variations—however, they are still connected with the biological body and its reality (Hareven 1982; Katz 2009; Thorsen 2005). The ageing process is therefore subject to the dynamic and discursive processes of society, its structures and spirits, but also extremely influenced by the material living conditions of the individual. The broad terms 'premodern', 'modern', and 'late modern' seem to grasp many of the significant changes to how ageing has been looked upon, handled, and lived for the last two hundred years.

Scientifically, the subject of the life course and its transitions is a crossroads for diverse human disciplines: history, sociology, culture studies, and psychology (Baltes, Reese and Lipsitt 1980; Elder 1985a; Hareven 1982; Katz 2009; Thorsen 2005). This is because the life course is part of an ongoing continuum of historical change linked to the individual's biography through collective behaviour (Bronfenbrenner 1979; Hareven 1982). Apart from being a biological reality and the last part of life, ageing is also a socially constructed phenomenon mediating the cultural production of ideas, because human beings are at the same time 'constructors' and subjects of a biological destiny.

The idea of constructivism can be seen as an overarching 'umbrella' of all kinds of theories about the lifespan. As to psychology, Harré and Van Langenhove (1999) point out that there are many versions of social constructivism in the discipline. They all share, however, an anti-nativist position, meaning that they do not support the idea of a universal social reality, and they also have in common the following principles, which are especially important to bear in mind when we are up against 'naturalized' ideas of old age, decline, and passivity (directly after Harré and Van Langenhove 1999: 2):

1. What people do, publicly and privately, is intentional, that is, directed to something beyond itself, and normatively constrained, that is, subject to such assessments as correct/incorrect, proper/improper, and so on.
2. What people are, to themselves and to others, is a product of a lifetime of interpersonal interactions superimposed over a very general ethological endowment.

This chapter is divided into two parts. The first and main part will analyse the life course and transitions in later life. This is done from a theoretical perspective referring to the importance of the cultural and social context and its different concepts of time, the constitution of transitions from a system's approach, and the ideas of normativity associated with transitions. The last part will focus more specifically on the current late-modern period and will finally deal with actual knowledge about how losses, and especially death as the final transition in life, are coped with.

FUNDAMENTAL PRINCIPLE: INDIVIDUAL TRAJECTORIES IN COLLECTIVE HUMAN SYSTEMS—CONTEXT AND TIME

The analytical unit of psychology is the individual and his or her formation and changes throughout life. However, given the special conditions of the human species as learning and construction-dependent, two dimensions are important. The first is *horizontal*, consisting of other humans and the *context* they form in transactions with each other. The second is *vertical*, covering *time* and *change* as the other crucial dimension.

The context and the individual

In order to stress the importance of context the late American developmental psychologist Bronfenbrenner (1979) compared the human condition with Russian dolls nested inside one another. This does not mean that people are completely determined by their surroundings, but that the context influences and becomes integrated in the person in many respects. Another way of expressing it is that you can find 'big society' in every person's life. However, the relationship is 'transactional', which means that the individual also influences society—represented by parents, the school system, the labour market, and so on. It is in the transactional meeting that the more or less negotiated constructs between the parts will have consequences for the person and for society (Featherman, Smith, and Peterson 1993; Sameroff and Chandler 1975). Throughout this chapter it will be demonstrated how important this principle is to understanding transitions in life, individual development, personal and social identity, and the living conditions of the individual. According to Bronfenbrenner (1979), development can be 'defined as the person's evolving conception of the ecological environment, and his relation to it, as well as the person's growing capacity to discover, sustain, or alter its properties' (9). The 'capacity to discover, sustain, or alter its properties' covers the whole life course. 'Ecological environment' here refers to the relational context in which people live and participate. The Danish psychologist Ole Dreier (1999) calls the life course 'the trajectory of individual participation in concrete social practices', because every role or position is an expression of a diversity of practices related to a given society. Like the person, the ecological context is plastic and thus subject to (re-)construction through transaction. The crossroads of individual lives and the lives of social institutions such as the school system, universities, workplaces, family, day care, hospitals, nursing homes, etc. imply that in biography we are not only dealing with individual lifetime, but also with time related to changes in society and culture with implications for the individual.

The concepts of time related to the dynamics of society and the individual life course

Studies of ageing and development are by definition based on the idea of change and that means *time*. The time dimension is associated with any culture and individual; nobody can escape it. Briefly, it can be stated that the life course of every individual is a movement from birth to death in a structure in motion: the changing society. Even if a culture is premodern or without institutional complexity and isolated, it is changing given the biological foundation of life: its members are maturing, growing old and dying, new ones are born, and so on. Due to the influence of the changing context ageing research has to operate with different levels of time, which can be traced through personal lives and their transitions (Baltes et al. 1980; Schaie 1988, 2000). The more complex and fast changing a society is, the more important those different concepts of time are when it comes to understanding the individual, the life course, and its composition of transitions. The concepts of time in ageing research are:

- *Age*: number of years after birth of the individual
- *Cohort*: time of the birth of a peer generation
- *Period*: current historical time and the changes connected with it
- *Personal:* the individual biography of roles and transitions.

Age

The historically new idea that numerical age is a fundamental characteristic of a human being has become pervasive. The inhabitants of the modern society and the users of its institutions are segregated by numerical age, which in many respects now sets the norms for the formation of the life course and its transitions: our age decides when we can go to day care and school, leave school, get an education, enter and leave the labour market, be punished, have legal sexual relationships, vote, drive a car, and so on. Age has become the structuring factor per se in modern society contrary to premodern times (Gillis 1991; Neugarten 1996; Petersen 2006). The institutional age segregation and the historically new preoccupation with age have contributed to a homogeneous picture of groups of people of the same age that does not hold true—neither according to levels of functioning nor to personality. It seems as if older adults in particular have been subject to this idea of a homogeneous group (Kirk 1995).

Cohort

The lifespan cannot be understood as a simple course of biological stages separated by numerical age running from birth to death, because the life cycle of human beings is deeply influenced on many levels by the concrete and historically changing context in which people live (Thorsen 2005). That is why the concept of cohorts is so important to understand in order to prevent the typical confusion of *age* and *cohort*. Every generation is established under certain cultural and institutional conditions that influence the individual life course until old age and death. Dominant examples are the educational systems and material living conditions during childhood (Elder 1985). The concept of cohorts is meaningful as a tool that can tell us about the difference between the generations based on their different conditions of life with regard to the collective distribution of resources, i.e. access to education and to the labour market, but also about the differences in behavioural norms influencing the rules of transitions given by the former generation.

From public arguments between the generations one is able to study aspects of the cohort effect. The Norwegian geropsychologist Kirsten Thorsen says that every generation has a 'symbolic dialect of its own' (2005: 69). Generational debates about behavioural norms and the distribution of material privileges can be quite harsh and bitter. According to the Swedish historian David Gaunt (1983), this was also seen in premodern times. Currently the generations are giving each other nicknames, such as the 'grasshopper' generation (the 1968 generation who is said to 'eat everything' and leave nothing to its successors) vs the 'surfer' or 'me-me' generations (the superficial young who are not interested in their surroundings, only in themselves). There seems to be a distinctive pattern in these debates: the young are without historical understanding, and yet older adults have forgotten what it is like to be young.

But a cohort is, of course, not a homogeneous group. This means that even if a population can be divided into cohorts with some common cultural characteristics, exposure to historical events and ongoing changes of society will have various consequences within any cohort. This is, for example, shown in the famous cohort study 'Children of the Great Depression. Social Change in Life Experience' by Glen Elder Jr (1999 [1974]). Experiences of change will differ according to gender, class, ethnicity, etc., and will sometimes deeply influence the life trajectory of the individual and have consequences for old age (Elder 1985; Hareven 1982).

Period

The concept of current time is called *period*. This means that generational impacts in the first ten to twenty years of life are not the only cultural influences on a given population. The currently changing society—also in a global perspective—has consequences for the whole population, regardless of numerical age. A good example from the present is the computerization of society. In the near future the public administration of Denmark will only communicate with its citizens through the internet. This means that older adults in Denmark are compelled to take computer courses, even if they have finished their professional lives. This new condition of life is common to the entire society and typical for the historically new 'internet period'.

Personal time

This refers to the individual lifetime embedded in *age, cohort,* and *period*. How were the roles and transitions distributed in a particular life? Did they follow the normative schedule of the given culture and social group? Or were there any non-normative transitions in the life trajectory—by choice or by fate? In relation to personal time, non-normative transitions refer to 'wrong' timing, that is, when they come too early or too late, or transitions one should avoid no matter what, for example becoming a criminal. Non-normativity can also refer to a life course with too few transitions due to illness or a handicap that prevents the person from participating in social life. The early death of the mother is another example of how 'fate' can change a life course, giving the child a new role as a 'motherless child'.

> ### Box 8.1 Implications for practice
>
> It is important not to generalize about older adults of the same numerical age. In many respects they are very different due to different backgrounds and different personalities. Older adults are carrying with them different trajectories of life and various narratives of the past that could be interesting for younger staff to explore, thus strengthening and uncovering the hidden identities of the older inhabitants.

The transitional pattern of a person's life course tells a lot about the person; he or she *is* the biography so to speak. According to Baltes et al. (1980), the accumulation of non-normative events has increasing impact on the life of the individual over the life course as an expression of 'personal time' (Box 8.1).

TRANSITION AS A THEORETICAL CONCEPT AND THE LIFE COURSE AS A CHAIN OF TRANSITIONS

The concept of transition is connected with different kinds of theories and disciplines, but seems to be a key concept related to the idea of social position, time, change, and development in the disciplines of psychology and sociology. According to the *Macmillan English Dictionary* (2007: 1593), a transition in everyday speech means: 'The process of changing from one situation, form or state to another.' The word comes from the Latin word 'transitio', which means 'change'. When the concept is related to psychology and sociology, we are usually not dealing with situational fluctuations or psychological states, but long-term changes related to structures in the crossroads of personal lives and societies called *roles* or *social positions*. The concept of transition has primarily been related to role theory and systems theory. A transition is a shift in role or position in a social system; and as a human being living among other human beings, a person is always a role possessor related to other role possessors. In other words, one cannot understand the concept of transition without understanding the concept of role, because it is the roles that constitute the transitions. A transition is discrete and by definition limited in time, but can, however, have long-term consequences. Transitions, furthermore, constitute the trajectories of the life course, which can be defined as chains of transitions that give the trajectories form and meaning (Elder 1985a). According to George (1993), transitions and trajectories are key concepts in life course research.

The concept of roles and social systems

The concept of *role* refers to the theatre and manuscripts and thus to the idea that behaviour is also decided by others and embedded in cultural schemes (Bronfenbrenner 1979; Mead 1934). Through the years there has been a development in role theory (George 1993). Bronfenbrenner (1979) is an example of a psychologist who has integrated the theory with a theory of lifespan development, which he has called the 'ecology of human development'. This means that he combines individual development with role theory and systems theory, including all layers of a modern society and its complex structure of relationships; in total, this is the 'ecology'. In the theory a role is defined as 'a set of behaviours and expectations associated with a position in society, such as of that of mother, baby, teacher, friend, and so on' (Bronfenbrenner 1979: 25). According to Bronfenbrenner's theory of development, it is the roles—and hence the transitions—of a society that are the most important forces in development. Development cannot take place without the experience of role performance, which is necessary in order to become a participating member of society. This is the core of socialization, providing individuals with the skills needed to master transitions and perform new roles.

Roles cannot be understood outside the context in which they are created; they are constituted of networks of relationships. The quality of the relationships between the role inhabitants is crucial for successful development (and for quality of life) (Bronfenbrenner 1979). Roles are also connected to the kinds of practices that constitute and enable a given society to survive. It can, however, be more or less clear how a role should be addressed, particularly in later life. The role of a mother or of a school child holds core elements. A 'mother' has given birth to or adopted a child and is—in most cultures—meant to look after it, at least at a certain stage of development, and a 'school child' has to go to school in order to be educated. It is less clear, however, what the content of the typical roles of old age is: a 'retiree' and a 'nursing home inhabitant'. These positions are primarily negatively defined by the *absence* of the activity of work and self-care. They are associated with the modern welfare state and the historically new ideas of protecting older adults through retirement systems and professionalization of care, and new kinds of structures of work life (Giddens 1991). That is probably also why some lifespan researchers use the rather non-theoretically founded notion of 'well-structured' and 'well-defined' *tasks* in the first part of life contrary to more 'ill-defined' and 'ill-structured' tasks in the latter part of life (Featherman, Smith, and Peterson 1993) (Box 8.2).

Normativity, deviance, and change of roles

The concept of role is useful in many ways, for example for understanding:

- the dynamics of social life and its regularities;
- the relationship between the social structure of society and the individual;
- the expectations and the behaviour of individual persons;
- the practices of the individual;
- questions of identity, which cannot be separated from the roles of society.

Box 8.2 Implications for practice

A challenge in later life is the absence of contents of roles and meaning of life. For nursing home staff, this means that it should be obligatory to integrate its inhabitants in the daily life of the institution. For that reason it is important to be familiar with the role biography of the inhabitants.

Box 8.3 Implications for practice

Be aware that an older adult's 'role biography' and the way the person managed his or her roles in the past could be a good basis for dialogue about the person's life story.

Every culture offers a normative behavioural framework to its inhabitants through socialisation to rules and standards for proper role behaviour. This makes daily life easier because it protects people from the demands of reflecting and making conscious choices all the time, and it gives life a certain amount of predictability (George 1993). The whole system is, to some extent, tuned to certain expectations and behaviours.

Not only are the types of roles and role behaviour crucial to normativity, but also to the 'timetable' for proper role entry and exit. When does 'entry' and 'exit' occur in the course of life? And what is the duration of each role before the person leaves it or before the active part of the role stops? Hareven (1982) points out that timing is influenced by social changes in several areas, such as demographic changes in mortality, fertility, and marriage patterns; economic changes in the opportunity structure determine the relationship to the labour force; and governmental changes decide when individuals enter and leave societal institutions such as school, and when different age groups enter and leave the labour force.

Some roles persist throughout life, primarily family roles based on biology, so to speak. The roles of mother and father persist throughout life, but normally the content of these roles changes dramatically as the child becomes an adult. This example also shows the dualistic nature of many types of roles; they are mutually dependent. This is especially evident from the configuration of the family, which changes when a member of the family goes through a transition. The developments and transitions of one member also make the other members go through a transition, as their roles will be changed too. A divorce has consequences for the life courses of the whole family. Timing is also important and can have lifelong consequences; for example, becoming a parent early in life enhances the person's chances of becoming a great-grandparent.

The order and amount of roles are other important normative aspects of the life course. According to Thorsen (2005), the individual trajectories cover the patterns or branches of and relations between the roles a person has through life—at work, in the family, during education, and in other parts of society. Many branches of roles in a person's life trajectory mean more transactions and possibilities for development and a richer life, according to Bronfenbrenner (1979). Experience also facilitates role performance (Bronfenbrenner 1979; George 1993) (see Box 8.3).

The dark side of normativity is of course deviance, exclusion, and sanctions, which are handled very differently in different cultures. Part of the inevitable destiny of being allocated roles in society is social sanction if one fails to meet the expectations of role behaviour. Being a criminal is a common example of a role connected with social sanctions and feelings of shame urging the person to hide this part of life in order to avoid sanctions (Goffman 1990 [1963]; Munk 2012; Nussbaum 2004; Pfuhl and Henry 1993) (Box 8.4).

Rules about right behaviour do not only entail role behaviour, but also how one enters and leaves a role, and at what point during the life course. Hence, what is deviant today can be a norm tomorrow. For example, the norms of sexuality and marriage have changed

---

Box 8.4 Implications for practice

The biography of an older adult can encompass more or less 'shameful' deviances. Only expect the normative aspects of a life story to be unveiled when a person tells his or her story of life.

Box 8.5 Implications for practice

It is important to recognize that the clinical staff and the inhabitants of a nursing home belong to different generations and, to some extent, probably have different values and ideas about normativity. What one generation finds shameful can be difficult for another generation to understand.

---

radically in Europe through the twentieth century with modernity (Gaunt 1983b). Fifty years ago it was very shameful to become a mother without being married or engaged to be married. Similarly, the child was identified as a child of an unmarried woman and therefore 'illegitimate'. Both parts made a 'wrong' entry into their new roles. In Denmark it was noted in the parish records if a mother was unmarried and the child had no formal father (the Danish State Archives: Church Books of the Parish of Vestervig). This followed the persons throughout life and became a crucial part of their identity (Munk 1999). In the 1970s, however, it—almost 'overnight'—became so common that nobody noticed any more; thus, this particular deviance disappeared, probably because of women's liberation. Hence, a very direct way of studying changes in a society is to study the changes of roles and their normative rules. This is also a typical result in relation to different cohorts, as mentioned earlier (Box 8.5).

LIFE AS A JOURNEY

In the social and cultural sciences life trajectories are often compared to a journey: the 'journey of life' (Cole 1992), which refers to movement, newness, and discovery. One has to move forward, unsure about what is waiting around the next corner—even if the journey has been carefully planned. But contrary to a journey after which most people return to their well-known home, the journey of life does not involve a return, but in some respects always a path into something new and unknown: new conditions—sooner or later and in one way or another. Even if role theorists claim that the schemata of role behaviour in a society prepare the life path of its inhabitants in order to tell them how to behave and when, one will be astonished about *how it really is*. No matter how normative a life seems to be, and how much the order of transitions can be planned and normatively lived, life is always new in the sense that one has never tried the next step oneself. What one has observed and known of from a distance is one thing, but being in the middle of it, in person, is another. What is it like to become a mother, a grandmother, a father, etc.? We can be pretty sure that for several reasons these very well-known transitions will have lots of surprises in store for us: for

---

Box 8.6 Implications for practice

The analogy of a journey should remind us that it might be less 'natural' for an older adult to be old than we might think. Clinical staff have almost never experienced the bodily changes their clients have been through: from a young person with a youthful appearance to bodily decline in appearance and function. This fact could easily make the staff 'naturalize' the old-age condition and forget that in the minds of the older adults it may feel like only 'yesterday' that they were young and agile.

---

example, does and should a grandparent in 2012 behave in the same way as the grandparent that person knew from his or her own childhood? It should be seriously doubted. In addition, even if we have known older people our entire life, we do not really know what it means to be there ourselves in body and mind. The analogy between a journey and life trajectories seems to be quite suitable (Box 8.6).

Modern Longevity, Freedom from Role Obligations, and Transitional Changes

The life patterns of older adults are changing rapidly in modern society. In late modernity late-life trajectories are changing in several ways, mirroring changes in society: new gender patterns, family structures, and working roles. In particular, the new family patterns reflect the demographic changes. The modern family is *vertical*, so to speak, with three or four or perhaps even five generations and few members in each generation; this is contrary to the premodern family which had fewer generations and many members in each (Jeune 2002), because grandparents and great-grandparents most often died before the birth of their grandchildren and great-grandchildren. Today grandparents and their parents continue to live longer. Furthermore, still more families in Denmark, for example, have only one parent, not because the other parent has died, but—most often—because the mother chooses to stay single (Statistics Denmark 2012).

According to Giddens (1991) and Rydström (2000), the historic transition of society from 'premodern' to 'modern' radically changed the conditions of life for the individual. The most distinctive change is a reorganization of time and space (disembedding), setting the individual free from his or her ecological niche and tradition, and moving time from local practices into a universal matter. Giddens (1991) claims that the postmodern detachment from tradition has had a considerable impact on the self as 'a reflexively organised endeavour' (5), where the self continuously reconstructs his or her life narrative, and subjects are able to choose between different life-styles. It is no longer so obvious who a person is. A person's identity has become detached from his or her origin. Experience has become still more mediated, and in daily life, negotiating a multiplicity of options, self-reflexivity has become an outstanding trait in late modernity.

This also has consequences for older adults; however, the modern prospect of life seems to be very diverse for elderly people around the world. In general, longevity and good health after 60 seems to be an expanding pattern. It seems crucial how many resources one has accumulated before old age. This means that the poor, including the poor in later life, do not have the same opportunities to make free life-style choices as the more well-off (Giddens 1991). To many people, at least in the more wealthy parts of the world such as Scandinavia, life after 60 has become a stage of freedom with good pension savings and freedom from social obligations such as meeting at work every day and looking after small children. Good health, money, and social freedom offer new opportunities to live out one's dreams—even for people who have not been too well-off in the course of life. On the other hand, in many parts of the world old age is not synonymous with good fortune. The implications of the demographics of an ageing world are globally very different; Asia and Southern Europe, for example, have an increasing amount of poor ageing adults, and these states lack the sufficient infrastructure to cope with the health and economic consequences of this.

But the new family patterns are not only created by the younger generations, to which an increasing divorce rate for couples over 60 testifies. In ten years the number of 'senior divorces', i.e. divorces after thirty to forty-five years of marriage, has doubled in Denmark (Statistics Denmark 2010). Serial monogamy no longer stops with the onset of old age. Serial monogamy has become a prevailing marriage pattern in late modernity, meaning that people go through more marriages and divorces, but only have one spouse at the time. The more optimistic prospects of a longer life probably make people more intolerant of unfruitful marriages. Some retired couples find it challenging to spend more time together than before. Some discover that they have little in common, making a divorce the only solution.

The large number of transitions or displacements in and across generations is no longer primarily caused by death, but by changing norms. In the future we will also see working careers in later life due to demographic necessity. This may also entail that exit events or exit transitions from the labour market when workers are in their 60s become rare or blurred because of an increasing amount of 'bridge arrangements' between work life, and retirement with part-time engagement in both positions (Rasmussen 2006).

Postmodern end of temporality and emancipation from localities

According to Katz (2009), the typical modern notion of old age as a distinct stage in life is now disappearing. Modern longevity creates a new era of ageing, which Katz (2009) calls the 'new ageing cultures' characterized by new ways of growing old, which remind us of Giddens' modern complex of life-styles options. This entails new kinds of relationships to one's ageing body and mind as well as social freedom, because the life course is no longer based on a prescribed timetable of beginnings and endings of life roles, but rather a combination of overlapping beginnings and endings and life transitions of all kinds, especially in later life. These new ageing cultures will also be integrated with new kinds of identities among older adults and will probably also mean a change in the way we talk about 'seniors'. It is obvious that the cultural ideals of 'staying young forever' are invading the new ageing cultures. The new seniors have become life-style specialists in the neo-liberalistic dream of 'the end of state-supported dependency' with a totally new profile of old age that we normally

> ### Box 8.7 Implications for practice
>
> Due to a life period with increasing wealth in some parts of the west, not least in Northern Europe and America, 'the end of temporality generation' could be a challenge to the clinic, because this generation is used to an expanding life perspective and has little experience with resignation and renunciation.

associate with being young: activity, consumerism, risk-taking—it is certainly very far from a 'the end is near' attitude, stretching middle age into timelessness (Katz 2009). The ageing body can, to some extent, be manipulated to look younger with updated clothes, plastic surgery, and hair dye, and even become younger by slowing down the ageing process with no smoking, physical exercise, and a healthy diet.

Somehow one could say that the late modern endeavour to stay young (and free) is fundamentally an attempt to loosen the ties not only to time, but also to specific locations. As 'snowbirds', older adults can travel to milder climates, as daily life with work and family obligations no longer restrain them. This means that the blurring of traditional life-course boundaries is typical of the late modern ageing process. It is, however, important to remember that it requires a certain amount of economic resources to be able to create the illusion of escaping from history, which excludes poor older adults from this late-modern endeavour.

This overview of how historically and culturally embedded a life course is has shown that it is difficult to point out typical transitions in later life—or at least we have seen that the early modern way of characterizing them exclusively as exit events does not hold true. We seem to be moving away from defined stages to ongoing processes in life development. However, perpetual vigour and geographical freedom notwithstanding, biology catches up with all humans sooner or later. Whatever people do to postpone death, they know that it is coming and have very different attitudes to and ways of coping with this fact (Box 8.7).

THE SAD 'FAREWELL'

It is a common idea in psychology that human beings by nature wish to control and influence the most important aspects of their lives (Heckhausen and Schulz 1995). No matter how much cultural artefacts have changed our life conditions and life course, we have not been able to change our deadly fate and the shorter or longer periods of weakness that precede it. That is probably the reason why the coping perspective has prevailed for years in gerontology (Munk 1999). In early modern gerontology old age is considered to be a stressful period of life, including the unavoidable 'exit events' mentioned at the beginning of this chapter. The late modern endeavour to enjoy later life due to better health and economy has, of course, contributed to high levels of life satisfaction in this part of life. Munk (1999) has shown that successful older adults of the generation born before the First World War experienced another process beneath the surface of life satisfaction, successful ageing, etc.—a process of resignation due to adaptation to the final transitions, i.e. the inevitable loss of loved ones and one's own death. It seems to be a double-layered process, where older adults living an active, outgoing life at the same time seem to prepare for all the endings in a slow and silent process of resignation. This means that the traditional discussion in gerontology about the dichotomies of 'activity' vs 'disengagement' appears to be too simplistic (Tornstam 1992). I here distinguish between two types of resignation:[2] *adaptive resignation* and *active resignation*. Adaptive resignation is understood as a slow and widely hidden process of recognition that the conditions of life are changing in irreversible ways. This is what you find when you ask older adults about their future, and it is not connected with depression (Munk 1999). Very slowly their expectations to life change with the help of all kinds of indications telling them that time is running out. Active resignation, on the other hand, is a process related to more abrupt loss, where the person acknowledges the loss in a realistic manner and after a period of grief is able to go on with life (Petersen 1985).

It is unclear, however, when people fully understand that they are not immortal. Logically, of course, the adaptive process of resignation should be stimulated by the accumulation of birthdays, telling us that we cannot possibly be alive when we reach twice the number of our age. One can study how people 'read' or perceive the signs of time passing: people your own age or even younger die, your children become adults and middle aged, recent photographs of you are very different from the ones taken when you were younger, and so on. Of course, as mentioned earlier, a lot of things can be done to slow down the process; a healthy diet, exercise, plastic surgery, hair dye, etc. can help a person win some time. One could imagine that the current endeavour to stop temporality makes it more difficult for some people to confront the facts of death. It is quite possible that late-modern narcissistic attitudes will make it more difficult to grow old than before, when life was determined by God or by fate and certainly not by individualistic endeavours.

Older adults also prepare themselves through so-called 'death rehearsals': How do you want your death to be? What do you want to leave behind? And who is going to inherit? The social and physical circumstances can be of such a kind that a person actually longs to die. For young and healthy persons this feeling can be difficult to understand. The living conditions can, so to speak, 'help' older adults in their adaption process, making them think that life is no longer 'worth' it. The mind might help to create good narratives that make the 'inevitable' more acceptable. It was surprising how older adults in Munk's study (1999) talked about their restricted sense of future without depression or tears, but with some sadness (p. 452): 'I have no future.' (p. 401) 'And of course, when you reach the age of 80…or more. Then you cannot go on living. You have to understand that.' (p. 402) 'I only hope to live as long as to experience the 250th anniversary of the family farm.' (p. 398) (Munk 1999) (Box 8.8).

Box 8.8 Implications for practice

In clinical practice it is important to create an 'unforgettable' present for older adults with no sense of a future. In general, the present is important, but for people with a shrinking future it may become difficult to 'catch' or create happy and meaningful hours in the present.

Box 8.9 Implications for practice

It is important for clinical staff to be able to detect if the inhabitants have no consoling narratives about loss. It should be an important endeavour to help them formulate narratives that reduce their feelings of guilt, if that is the problem, and focus on positive aspects in one way or another.

Box 8.10 Implications for practice

If older adults develop clinical depression due to a breakdown in life, it is important to avoid treating this only medically. Pills cannot replace practical help, talk, and understanding.

The active resignation process is mediated by a specific narrative, which could be called the 'narrative of consolation' (Munk 1999). The grief associated with the loss of loved ones is somehow unbearable, and we try to comfort ourselves with reformulated positive perspectives on the incident. The narrative of active resignation or consolation has to be threefold if it is going to meet this objective. First, the person is engaged in an explanation of the cause of the incident. The most important thing is that the person in question is not responsible for what happened and consequently has no feelings of guilt. The explanation of an older spouse just widowed or older people experiencing the loss of other relatives could be, 'He died because he was old,' (p. 283) or 'Only God knows how long you shall live,' (p. 339) or 'That is how nature is: You die someday' (p. 303) (Munk 1999). The second part of the narrative is a paradox: an explanation of why this awful thing is a good thing. 'How fortunate that he died. Had he lived on, his life would have been awful. Death freed him from that' (p. 267). The third and last part of the narrative is about the remaining positive aspects of life: why life is still worth living. 'I have good health,' 'I have enough money in the bank,' or 'I have nice children.' (p. 293; 342). It seems important that the grieving person is able to formulate the whole narrative in order to regain a certain quality of life. But, of course, many processes of active resignation in the last part of life also contribute to the adaptive process towards the end (pp. 317–318) (Box 8.9).

The last part of life, however, is not always a smooth process of resignation. Research on depression late in life shows that especially older adults who have suffered many losses and a deteriorating health are in danger of suffering from depression (Munk 2007a), because these circumstances make it more difficult for them to reconstruct a satisfying life and a consoling narrative about the positive aspects of loss (Box 8.10).

SUMMARY

Transitions in later life are a combination of personally, biologically, and socially initiated life-stage transitions rooted in the previous life course, but no rules can be given for the course of later life. A person's own death and the loss of loved ones, however, are unavoidable and create a paradox in connection with the new, late-modern prospect of successful ageing and the endeavour to end temporality.

Notes

1. The concept of life satisfaction in later life is, however, more complex than that of younger life (Mehlsen 2011).
2. This differentiation is developed by the Danish psychologist, Emeritus Professor Eggert Petersen, Aarhus University (Petersen 1985).

Key References and Sources for Further Reading

Goldberg, E. (2005). *The Wisdom Paradox. How your Mind Grows Stronger as your Brain Grows Older*. London: Free Print.

Hockey, J. and James, A. (2003). *Social Identities across the Life Course*. New York: Palgrave Macmillan.

Katz, S. (1996). *Disciplining Old Age. The Formation of Gerontological Knowledge*. Charlottesville and London: University Press of Virginia.

Larsen, L. (ed.) (2011). *Geropsychology. The Psychology of the Ageing Person*. Aarhus: Aarhus University Press.

Thompson, N. (1998). 'The Ontology of Ageing.' *British Journal of Social Work* 28: 695–707.

References

Baltes, P. B., Reese, H. W., and Lipsitt, L. P. (1980). 'Life-Span Developmental Psychology'. *Annual Review of Psychology* 31: 65–110.

Bronfenbrenner, U. (1979). *The Ecology of Human Development. Experiments by Nature and Design*. Cambridge, MA: Harvard University Press.

Cole, T. (1992). *The Journey of Life: A Cultural History of Aging in America*. Cambridge: Cambridge University Press.

Danish State Archives: Church Books of the Parish of Vestervig, http://www.sa.dk/ao/.

Dreier, O. (1999). 'Personal Trajectories of Participation across Contexts of Social Practice'. *Outlines. Critical Practice Studies* 1: 5–32.

Elder, G. H., Jr (1985). *Life Course Dynamics. Trajectories and Transitions, 1968–1980*. Ithaca and London: Cornell University Press.

Elder, G. H. (1999). *Children of the Great Depression. Social Change in Life Experience*. (25th anniversary edn). Boulder: Westview Press. [First published in 1974.]

Featherman, D. L., Smith, J., and Peterson, J. G. (1993). 'Succesful Aging in a Post-retired Society'. In P. B. Baltes and M. M. Baltes (eds), *Succesful Aging: Perspectives from the Behavioural Sciences* (pp. 50–93). Cambridge: Cambridge University Press.

Gaunt, D. (1983). *Familjeliv i Norden* [Family Life in The Nordic Countries]. Malmö: Gidlunds.

George, L. (1993). 'Sociological Perspectives on Life Transitions'. *Annual Review of Sociology* 19: 353–373.

Giddens, A. (1991). *The Consequences of Modernity*. Stanford, CA: Stanford University Press.

Gillis, J. R. (1985). *For Better, For Worse: Marriages 1600 to the Present*. Oxford: Oxford University Press.

Gillis, J. R. (1991). 'Barn, ung, voksen, unge-gamle og gamle-gamle'. *HUG*, 60: 35–41.

Goffman, E. (1990). *Stigma. Notes on the Management of Spoiled Identity*. London: Penguin. [First published 1963.]

Hareven, T. K. (1982). 'The Life Course and Aging in Historical Perspective'. In T. K. Hareven and K. J. Adams (eds), *Aging and Life Course Transitions: An Interdisciplinary Perspective* (pp. 1–26). New York, Guilford Press.

Harré, R. and Van Langenhove, L. (1999). *Positioning Theory: Moral Contexts of Intentional Action*. Malden: Blackwell.

Heckhausen, S. M. and Schulz, R. (1995). 'A Life-span Theory of Control'. *Psychological Review* 102: 284–304.

Jeune, B. (2002). *Længe leve!? Om udforskningen af det lange liv*. [Longevity!? About exploration of longevity]. København: Fremad.

Katz, S. (2009). *Cultural Aging. Life Course, Lifestyle, and Senior Worlds*. Ontario and New York: University of Toronto Press.

Kirk, H. (1995). *Da alderen blev en diagnose(—konstruktionen af kategorien 'alderdom' i 1800-tallets lægelitteratur—en medicinsk-idehistorisk analyse*. [When Age became a Diagnosis—on the Construction of 'Old Age' in the Medical Literature of the Nineteenth Century—a Medical Historical Analysis]. Cophenhagen: Gyldendal.

Macmillan Education (2007). *MacMillan English Dictionary for Advanced Learners*. London: Macmillan.

Mead, G. H. (1934). *Mind Self and Society from the Standpoint of a Social Behaviorist*, ed. Charles W. Morris. Chicago: University of Chicago.

Mehlsen, M. (2011). 'Life Satisfaction in Old Age'. In L. Larsen (ed), *Geropsychology. The Psychology of the Ageing Person*. Aarhus: Aarhus University Press.

Munk, K. (1999). *Belastninger i alderdommen* [Strain in Old Age]. Sundhed, Menneske og Kulturs Skriftserie: Aarhus Universitet.

Munk, K. (2007a). 'Late-life Depression. Also a Field for Psychotherapists!' Part One. *Nordic Psychology* 59(1): 7–26.

Munk, K. (2007b). 'Late-life Depression. Also a Field for Psychotherapists!' Part Two. *Nordic Psychology* 59(1): 27–44.

Munk, K. P. (2012). *Coping. Manual til kvalitativ mikroanalyse*. [Coping. Manual for Qualitative Micro Analysis]. Aarhus: Aarhus Universitetsforlag.

National Institute of Public Health (2007). *Report on Public Health*. Odense: University of Southern Denmark.

Neugarten, B. L. (1996). The Meanings of Age: selected papers of Bernice L. Neugarten. Chicago: The University of Chicago Press

Nussbaum, M. (2004). *Hiding from Humanity: Disgust, Shame, and the Law*. Princeton: Princeton University Press.

Petersen, E. (1985). *Træk af resignationens psykologi samt en model af det danske samfund under krisen ud fra livskvalitetskriterier* [Aspects of the Psychology of Resignation and a model of the Danish Society during the Crisis built on Criteria of Quality of Life]. Psykologisk Skriftserie 10(7): Aarhus: Aarhus University.

Petersen, J.-H. (2006). *Det Aldrende Samfund 2030* [The Ageing Society 2030]. Danish Agency for Science, Technology and Innovation.

Pfuhl, E. H. and Henry, S. (1993). *The Deviance Process*. New York: Aldine de Gruyter.

Rasmussen, V. J. (2006). 'Seniorpolitik og ældres arbejdsressourcer' [Senior Policy and the Resources of the Elderly]. In J.-H. Petersen (ed), *Det Aldrende Samfund 2030* [The Ageing Society 2030]. Cophenhagen: Danish Agency for Science, Technology and Innovation.

Rydström, J. (2000). ' "Sodomitical Sins are Threefold": Typologies of Bestiality, Masturbation, and Homosexuality in Sweden, 1880–1950'. *Journal of the History of Sexuality* 9(3): 240–276.

Sameroff, A. J. and Chandler, M. J. (1975). 'Reproductive Risk and the Continuum of Caretaking Causality'. In F. D. Horowitz (ed), *Review of Child Development Research* (Vol. 4, pp. 187–244). Chicago: University of Chicago Press.

Schaie, K. W. (1988). 'The Impact of Research Methodology on Theory Building in the Developmental Sciences'. In J. E. Birren and V. L. Bengtson (eds), *Emergent Theories of Aging*. New York: Springer.

Schaie, K. W. (2000). 'The Impact of Longitudinal Studies on Understanding Development from Young Adulthood to Old Age'. *International Journal of Behavioral Development* 24(3): 257–266.

Statistics Denmark. 2010. http://www.dst.dk/en

Thorsen, K. (2005). 'Et livsløbsperspektiv på aldring [Ageing from a Life Course Perspective]. *Nordisk Psykologi* 57(1): 64–85.

Tornstam, L. (1992). *Åldrandets Socialpsykologi* [The Social Psychology of Ageing]. Stockholm: Raben and Sjögren.

PART II

ASSESSMENT AND FORMULATION

···

CHAPTER 9

INTERVIEWING OLDER ADULTS

···

LINDSAY A. GEROLIMATOS, JEFFREY J. GREGG, AND BARRY A. EDELSTEIN

INTRODUCTION

THE clinical interview is frequently the first, and often the only, assessment method used by health and mental health professionals when assessing older adults (Edelstein, Martin, and Gerolimatos 2012). It can serve multiple functions, including screening potential clients, examining mental status, formulating the presenting problem, and establishing a diagnosis. In addition, the interview is important for establishing rapport and a working alliance. Interviews with older adults can be a challenge for any detective worth his or her salt. First, older adults can be considerably more recalcitrant than typical young adults. For example, older adults are more likely to refuse participation in surveys (e.g. DeMaio 1980; Herzog and Rodgers 1988) and respond 'don't know' (Colsher and Wallace 1989) to questions. The complexities of age-related cognitive and physiological changes, coupled with chronic diseases, polypharmacy, and medication adverse effects and interactions collectively militate against attempts by the clinician to assemble clues in a meaningful fashion.

This chapter will familiarize readers with age-related interviewing issues associated with various types of interviews, age-related biological, medical, and physiological factors, ethnicity and culture, interview settings, and interview content (e.g. mental disorders, suicide, sleep, substance abuse, elder abuse). Other important issues (e.g. trust, language use, interview format) will also be addressed. The discussion of the foregoing issues will be accompanied by recommendations for how one might make accommodations for these issues. Finally, suggestions for additional reading will be provided. Our goal is to enable readers to have a greater appreciation for the complexities of interviewing older adults and strategies that we and others have found useful in addressing these complexities. Interested readers are referred to specific chapters in this Handbook for more information regarding specific disorders or clinical issues such as depression and suicide.

Types of Clinical Interview

Clinical interviews with older adults range from casual, free-flowing conversations to carefully scripted diagnostic interviews that include a series of branching questions and prompts. Despite the obvious differences, each interview format (i.e. structured, semi-structured, unstructured) has strengths and weaknesses based on the primary goal. Common goals of the clinical interview include characterizing the presenting problem(s) and contextual factors, arriving at a diagnosis, and planning treatment, among others. The interviewer can opt for more or less structure, or use multiple interview approaches, based on the purpose of the interview.

Structured and semi-structured interviews

Structured and semi-structured interviews offer strong reliability and diagnostic validity. Several diagnostic interviews have been validated for use with older adults, including the Structured Clinical Interview for *DSM-IV* Axis I Disorders (SCID; First et al. 1996), the Diagnostic Interview Schedule IV (DIS; Robins et al. 1999), the Anxiety Disorders Interview Schedule-IV (ADIS; Brown, DiNardo, and Barlow 1994), and the Mini International Neuropsychiatric Inventory (MINI; Lecrubier et al. 1997). Several of these have been translated and validated cross-culturally. For example, the SCID and the MINI are available in over fifteen languages.

These interviews range in their level of structure. For instance, the DIS is highly structured, whereas the SCID allows for more flexibility. In general, greater structure in clinical interviews leads to greater validity and reliability. Though the semi-structured nature of interviews like the SCID allows for greater flexibility, there are downsides. On each occasion where one skips questions or probes for more information, opportunities for error are produced that may influence reliability and validity. Nevertheless, studies have demonstrated that many structured and semi-structured clinical interviews demonstrate high levels of inter-rater reliability, interviewer experience notwithstanding (e.g. Ventura et al. 1998).

With regard to structured and semi-structured interviews with older adults, one principal concern is fatigue. Many structured and semi-structured interviews are time-consuming, especially if all sections of the interview are administered. One can reduce fatigue attributable to time by administering modules specific to the presenting complaint. In addition, some of the semi-structured interviews are briefer than others (e.g. the MINI). Overall, structured interviews have been shown to be superior to self-report instruments in assessing the presence and severity of disorders and in monitoring change in symptoms over time (Dennis, Bodding, and Funnell 2007).

Unstructured interviews

The principal advantage of unstructured interviews is their flexible and permissive nature. Unstructured interviews permit the rephrasing of questions that are unclear to interviewees and allow the interviewer to pursue areas related to the presenting problem as they unfold (Edelstein et al. 2003). Despite the benefits of unstructured interviews, their lack of structure results in poor psychometric properties. However, unstructured interviews can be used to build rapport with older adult clients, acquire information to use in case conceptualizations, and supplement background information for the strategic selection of additional assessment instruments (Koerner, Hood, and Antony 2011).

Issues Related to Interviewing Older Adults

Numerous factors can influence the process and outcome of the interview. These include, but are not limited to, age-related sensory, cognitive, health, biological, ethnic, and cultural issues.

Age-related sensory changes

Of the sensory systems, age-related changes in the visual and auditory systems are most likely to influence the process and outcome of the interview. These two sensory systems are affected by normative changes, physical disease processes, and medications. Age-related hearing loss (presbycusis) typically occurs gradually, with approximately 33% of adults in the world over the age of 65 having disabling hearing loss (World Health Organization (WHO) 2013). The prevalence of disabling hearing loss is greatest in South Asia, Asia Pacific, and sub-Saharan Africa (WHO 2013). Sounds experienced by individuals with presbycusis are less clear and of lower volume. That, coupled with the age-related hearing loss for higher-pitched sounds, can lead to difficulty understanding speech, particularly high-pitched speech (e.g. women's speech). The sounds of 's' and 'th' are difficult to discriminate, and conversations pose hearing challenges in the presence of background noises (National Institute on Deafness and Other Communicative Disorders (NIDCD) 2010). One common cause of impaired hearing is tinnitus (the perception of sounds in one or both ears in the absence of an auditory stimulus), which can cause difficulty hearing the interviewer.

Hearing loss can have psychological and psychosocial consequences that are potentially relevant to the interview process and presenting problems. Older adults with impaired hearing are less likely to hear questions and orally presented instructions. Hearing-impaired older adults are less likely to participate in leisure activities and tend to experience more depressive symptoms (Horowitz 2003). Hearing impairment can also affect the outcome of cognitive assessment in the interview (e.g. attention, memory).

The following recommendations have been offered by various sources (e.g. NIDCD 2010; Reuben et al. 2011; Saxon, Etten, and Perkins 2010; Storandt 1994) to facilitate hearing and accommodate the individual with hearing loss. One should be aware that a hearing impairment can be embarrassing or stigmatizing for older adults, and they may deny or attempt to conceal the impairment. When interviewing older adults, one's face should be well lighted, and one should face the interviewee throughout the interview. If individuals are capable of reading lips, the interviewer should be careful not to exaggerate words or cover their mouth. One should speak distinctly and at a normal rate, and pause briefly between phrases or ideas. It is advisable to speak slightly more loudly than usual but not to shout, as shouting could distort speech. Background noise, which can mask speech, should be decreased. If the individual has a hearing aid or personal amplifier, encourage its use. Finally, the principal interview questions can be provided in written form for individuals who are capable of reading.

Visual impairment is a serious health problem for older adults, with the most common causes of visual impairment being macular degeneration, cataracts, glaucoma, and diabetic retinopathy (Prevent Blindness America 2008). The prevalence of visual impairment and blindness, and their causes, varies across countries. Age-related macular degeneration is the major cause of low vision and blindness among older adults in the Netherlands, followed by glaucoma, cataract, and diabetic eye disease (World Blind Union 2011). In Bulgaria, Armenia, and Turkmenistan, cataracts are the major cause of low vision and blindness (World Blind Union 2011). In the US, cataracts are the most common visual condition across all racial and ethnic groups, affecting 68.3% of adults aged 80 and older (National Eye Institute 2011). In addition to these disorders, age-related changes in the cornea, iris, pupil, lens, vitreous humour, and retina all contribute to diminished vision.

Visual impairment is associated with a variety of physical, medical, psychosocial, and psychological problems that are relevant to the assessment interview, including falls and injuries (Ivers et al. 2000), depression and social isolation (Horowitz 2003; Jones et al. 2009), anxiety (de Beurs et al. 2000), chronic health conditions (Crews, Jones, and Kim 2006), impairment in daily functioning (US Census Bureau 2010), and mortality (Lee et al. 2002).

The implications of visual impairment for the clinical interview are considerable. Cataracts result in the dulling of colours and substantial increases in glare caused by brightly lit objects and surfaces. Cataracts, presbyopia, diminished accommodation, retinopathy, and macular degeneration can each increase the difficulty of reading text, slow or impair cognitive processing (Glass 2007), and reduce speed on time-limited assessment tasks.

Several steps can be taken to minimize the effects of visual impairment. When presenting visual stimuli to older adults, particularly those with cataracts, it is best to avoid the use of materials printed on glossy surfaces (Storandt 1994). One should strike a balance between the glare of light and the need for sufficient illumination (Edelstein, Martin, and Koven 2003). For older adults with presbyopia, printed material should be presented in a large point size, preferably 14-point (Vanderplas and Vanderplas 1981). Older adults should not face a brightly lit window. Older adults who use reading glasses should be encouraged to use them, as some older adults often forget to use them or initially refuse to do so. Interviewers can keep a supply of inexpensive reading glasses and magnifiers to use as needed.

Cognitive changes

Age-related changes in cognitive functioning represent a unique challenge for the interviewer, due in part to inter-individual differences in cognitive deficits (Salthouse 2010), and in part to the interviewer's reliance upon the client's cognitive abilities for the extraction of relevant information. Age-related cognitive deficits occur in working and episodic memory, reasoning, spatial visualization, inhibitory processes, and processing speed (Park and Schwarz 2000; Salthouse 2010).

Deficits in memory and processing speed are likely the most apparent age-related deficits. The interviewer should encourage the interviewee to bring relevant information to the interview (e.g. a list of prescription medications, their sleep diary). When possible, an informed second party (e.g. care-giver, relative, or friend) can be encouraged to participate if the memory of the client is significantly impaired. Questions should be brief to reduce working memory and cognitive processing load, and concrete to reduce the level of reasoning required. Double-barrelled questions that touch upon more than one issue should be avoided. When long delays are encountered following queries, the interviewer can ask if the client would like the question repeated, or whether the client understood the question. Finally, providing anchors in time (e.g. mealtime, specific incident) when asking about the onset or duration of symptoms can help (Gould, Edelstein, and Ciliberti 2010).

Cognitive deficits may not be apparent in the daily activities of older adults, particularly when they are performing familiar tasks in familiar situations (Park and Schwarz 2000). In addition, older adults may report no cognitive deficits but experience difficulties in the activities of daily living. Thus, one could encounter discrepancies between self-reported difficulties regarding cognitive functioning and what is observed in the interview. Consequently, one should be cautious in generalizing from interview-based indices of cognitive functioning to the performance of everyday activities of the older adult.

Ethnicity and culture

Psychological symptoms may present differently for older adults across ethnic groups. Somatization, for example, is especially common among individuals from Asian and African cultures (Kirmayer and Young 1998). Descriptions of symptoms may also differ, such as using 'nerves' or 'nervios' to describe anxiety instead of 'anxious' or 'worried' (Kirmayer 2001). Some disorders are unique to specific cultures. For example, Japanese clients may exhibit a disorder resembling social phobia, but anxiety results from upsetting others rather than embarrassing the self (Kirmayer 2001). Another potential issue when working with ethnic-minority older adults includes difference in language or dialect between the interviewer and client. Racism and acculturative stress may contribute to psychological distress (Conner et al. 2010), and clinicians should assess for these stressors when interviewing ethnic-minority older adults.

Ethnic-minority older adults tend to attach stigma to mental illness. For example, older Koreans may believe that mental health problems bring shame to the family and indicate personal weakness (Jang, Chriboga, and Okazaki 2009). Across numerous countries, research has shown that stigma regarding mental health remains a significant barrier to mental health treatment for ethnic minorities, regardless of age (see Saxena et al. 2007). Therefore clinicians must be mindful of older adults' reluctance to discuss mental health problems. That ethnic-minority older adults may not readily discuss mental health problems could also be because they may be less knowledgeable about mental illness and may not regard their symptoms as part of a psychological syndrome (Choi and Gonzalez 2005; Conner et al. 2010).

Professionals need to increase their knowledge about various cultures (American Psychological Association (APA) 2003), and assess for culturally relevant content areas. Clinicians must be careful not to stereotype members of an ethnic group, as there is much variability within groups. The interviewer must be aware of any assumptions about the interviewee. For example, lack of eye contact may be interpreted as rude, but may be a culturally appropriate behaviour. If the client is unfamiliar with mental health practice, the interviewer should explain the interview process at the outset (Choi and Gonzalez 2005). Professionals must be mindful of the limitations of assessment methods for ethnic-minority older adults. For older adults who are wary of the clinical process, clinicians could elicit the support of family members to ease the interview process (Choi and Gonzalez 2005). Family members may also be elicited to help with translation. However, older adults may be less candid about their problems with a family member present. Additionally, the family member may alter or edit the interviewer's questions or client's responses. If one cannot refer the older client to a professional who speaks the language, paid translators, who sign confidentiality agreements, are informed on the nature of assessments, and are instructed to translate speech exactly, may be optimal.

Medical and biological considerations

Health problems and medications

Ageing is accompanied by a progressive accumulation of risk factors for disabling chronic diseases (e.g. hypertension, heart disease, arthritis, diabetes, cancer; Nolte and McKee 2008). The prevalence of chronic diseases varies across countries of the world, with the highest incidence of chronic diseases in high-income countries. However, within these countries, low-income individuals carry the highest chronic disease burden (Busse et al. 2010).

The prevalence of chronic diseases also varies by race and ethnicity. For example, non-Hispanic white older adults report lower levels of hypertension and diabetes than non-Hispanic black older adults (Federal Interagency Forum on Aging Related Statistics 2010). Health problems complicate the assessment interview in many ways. Symptoms of physical disease (e.g. pancreatic cancer, hyperthyroidism) mimic the symptoms of psychiatric disorders (e.g. depression, anxiety). Medications taken to control diseases can have side-effects that appear as psychiatric symptoms. Finally, psychiatric disorders may be comorbid with physical disorders (e.g. anxiety disorders and chronic obstructive pulmonary disease, Parkinson's disease and depression, diabetes and depression; Edelstein et al. 2012). In light of the foregoing, access to a thorough medical history is important for determining the possible causes of presenting psychological symptoms.

Pain

Approximately 25–50% of community-dwelling older adults (Gagliese 2009) and 27–83% of those in institutional settings (Malmstrom and Tait 2010) experience persistent pain that impairs functioning. Older adults have a higher threshold for pain than younger adults but are less tolerant of persistent pain (Malmstrom and Tait 2010). Unfortunately, older adults are at considerable risk of not being adequately treated for pain (Gagliese 2009). Thus, screening for pain is important when assessing older adults, particularly for older adults who cannot reliably report pain. A variety of measures are discussed by Malmstrom and Tait (2010).

Circadian rhythms

Biological clocks or circadian rhythms regulate a wide range of processes (e.g. hormone secretions, sleep/wake cycles). There is evidence that cognitive processes are influenced by circadian rhythms through a twenty-four-hour cycle, such that peaks in cognitive performance are associated with peak periods of physiological arousal (Schmidt et al. 2007). Older adults tend to experience their peak cognitive performance in the morning (Yoon, May, and Hasher 1999). Thus, one will likely see differences in cognitive functioning across different times of the day. It may not always be possible to assess older adults during times of peak cognitive performance. Interviewers are encouraged to record the time of the interview so that interpretations of the interview outcome can be informed by knowledge of the client's position on his or her performance cycle. One circadian-related issue is fatigue. Older adults may get tired more quickly than younger adults, particularly during a time of day that they are not performing at their peak level. The interviewer should consider breaking the interview into shorter intervals with opportunities for client respite. The combination of fatigue and diminished age-related inhibitory control can quickly diminish attention and motivation.

SETTING OF THE INTERVIEW

Clinical interviews with older adults occur in various settings (e.g. primary care, outpatient mental health centres, long-term care, or inpatient institutions; Segal, June, and Marty 2010). Each of these settings places unique demands on the interviewer and interviewee. Older adults are most likely to seek help for mental health problems from their primary care physician (Karlin, Duffy, and Gleaves 2008). Referrals to mental health professionals in primary care settings are often made by physicians, and the older adult may be reluctant to discuss mental health issues (Segal et al. 2010). One can explain that one's intention is to provide comprehensive care, which can ease the older client into discussing psychological issues. Individuals in primary healthcare settings are likely to have comorbid health problems and this information will be available in the client's medical chart. The interviews tend to be brief (Segal et al. 2010), necessitating prioritization of questions. The clinician has less opportunity for behavioural observations and may be less likely to gain collateral information.

Older adults are least likely to seek help in outpatient mental health centres (Karlin et al. 2008). In an outpatient setting, more time is afforded to rapport building and comprehensive assessment. The interviewer may not have access to the older client's medical records and may need to obtain a release from the client to request records. If the client refuses, the clinician must rely on self-report, recognizing that there may be inaccuracies.

Finally, older adults may be interviewed in residential settings, such as long-term care facilities. A primary limitation in these settings is the lack of privacy. Many residents have roommates, and there may be few other available rooms in the facility. The clinician contends with frequent interruptions from staff and other residents. Interviewers should make arrangements to conduct interviews in quiet, private locations, and attempt to schedule interviews around activities. Because privacy may not be guaranteed, interviewers should address its impact on confidentiality (Segal et al. 2010; Zarit and Zarit 2007). Older adults in residential settings are likely to have complicated medical histories and take numerous medications (Dwyer et al. 2010). Lastly, older adults in these facilities often present with cognitive problems that may interfere with the interview. Clinicians can interview collateral sources, such as facility staff and family members, to gain supplemental information. Measures such as the Cornell Scale for Depression in Dementia (Alexopoulos et al. 1988) and the Rating for Anxiety in Dementia (RAID) scale (Shankar et al. 1999) include interviews with proxies.

Other issues related to interviews

Rapport building

As with all clients, rapport building requires warmth, appropriate eye contact, genuineness, attentive listening, and professionalism. Interviewers must avoid speaking in a condescending or belittling manner. Older adults tend to be less familiar with mental health evaluations than younger age groups and may be anxious about the interview. At the start of the interview, an explanation of the process, with ample opportunity for questions, can lessen uncertainty associated with the evaluation (Mohlman et al. 2011).

At times, the older client may be resistant to answering questions or may conceal details. This tendency may be related to stigma associated with mental health disorders among older adults or perceived threats to independence (Koven, Shreve-Neiger, and Edelstein 2007). To circumvent these problems, clinicians should communicate warmly and non-judgmentally and acknowledge difficulty discussing sensitive topics. Koven and colleagues recommend using a 'plus minus approach', in which the interviewer alternates between more and less threatening questions. Though these are general rules for rapport building, one must take care to tailor one's approach to be consistent with the culture of the client and setting.

Trust

Client trust of the interviewer is often ignored in the assessment literature, yet resides at the heart of a client's willingness to disclose important and sensitive information in the interview (Edelstein and Semenchuk 1996). It is a critical element of the helping relationship (Cormier and Cormier 1991). When interviewing older adults, we are asking them temporarily to suspend the reciprocity we expect in social exchanges and to engage in risk-taking behaviour. That is, by disclosing information, the older adult hopes the clinician will not respond negatively and that, in the long run, something positive will result (e.g. resolution of presenting problems). Alberts and Edelstein (1992) examined therapist trust among adult clients and revealed several behaviours that suggested whether a therapist could be trusted (e.g. behaviours suggesting positive regard or interest in the client, being directive and structuring therapy sessions). Attention to trustworthy behaviours (see Edelstein and

Semenchuk for a complete list) may help the interviewer quickly gain the client's trust in the interview or avoid a breach in trust.

Language of the interview

The interview should be conducted at a comprehension level that is suitable for the client, with a sixth-grade reading level typically being appropriate. Jargon, idioms, and slang terms should be avoided. Interviewers should offer several descriptors of psychological symptoms. For example, older adults may not 'worry' or feel 'anxious', but may be more likely to note 'concern' or 'nervousness' (Stanley and Novy 2000). When administering a structured interview, rephrase questions as appropriate to ensure the client understands the items (Mohlman et al. 2011).

Length and format of the interview

Interviews with older adults often take more time than with younger adults, given older adults' slower processing speeds and longer histories. Lengthier interviews may cause client fatigue. It may be necessary to divide the interview into several sessions and prioritize the order of questions (i.e. begin with the most important questions; Mohlman et al. 2011). Older adults have a propensity to tell stories (Zarit and Zarit 2007). To limit the number of stories, the clinician can delineate the goals of the interview beforehand, acknowledge time constraints, and discuss the importance of remaining on-task throughout the interview. Interviewers may feel uncomfortable interrupting and redirecting the client, but doing so politely often does not hinder the interview process (Mohlman et al. 2011). This goal may also be accomplished gracefully with humour. Asking direct and specific questions can also curtail digressions.

Questions can be yes/no, Likert-type, or open-ended formats. Older adults tend to have difficulty with Likert-type scales (Mohlman et al. 2011). Some older adults may forget the question or the format of the response scale. Repeating the question as needed is appropriate. To ease the burden of remembering the response choices, clinicians can provide the response scales on cards (Mohlman et al. 2011). The clinician should check periodically that the older adult client understands the response scale. Finally, the clinician should allow adequate time for answers. Long response latencies suggest the clinician may need to repeat the question.

Disinhibition

Older adults with dementia or executive dysfunction may display inappropriate behaviours (e.g. sexual or aggressive behaviours) or verbalizations during the interview. The behaviours may relate to frustration associated with the interview, communicative difficulties, or pain (Talerico, Evans, and Strumpf 2002). Ascertaining the function of the behaviour and altering the contingencies (e.g. managing the pain) may decrease the behaviour, though some clients simply cannot control their behaviours. When inappropriate behaviours occur, the clinician can firmly and directly tell the client that the specific behaviour is inappropriate. The clinician should explain and model appropriate behaviours (Koven et al. 2007). Periodically, the clinician may have to redirect the client back to the question. If the behaviours prevent the continuation of the interview, behavioural observations or interviews with family or staff can provide information.

CONTENT AREAS FOR ASSESSMENT

Older adults may have unique experiences or symptom presentations that are important to address in the interview. Though it is impossible to discuss all relevant content areas in this chapter, we will highlight some common clinical disorders and problem areas with an eye to age-related factors that inform the interview. These areas include psychological disorders (depression, anxiety, personality disorders), suicide, substance abuse, sleep, and elder abuse.

Psychological disorders

Depression

Though less prevalent in older adulthood than in younger adulthood, late-life depression is associated with increased social and functional impairment, decreased cognitive functioning, and increased risk of all-cause mortality (Blazer 2003). Even subsyndromal symptoms of depression are linked to similar negative health outcome (Lavretsky, Kurbanyan, and Kumar 2004); thus, including questions related to depression in interviews with older adults is important. Late-life depression differs from depression in other age groups in several ways. Older adults are less likely to endorse symptoms of depressed affect, guilt, and suicidal ideation, and more likely to report hopelessness, helplessness, psychomotor retardation, and somatic symptoms compared to younger age groups (Fiske, Wetherell, and Gatz 2009). Somatic symptoms of depression are often difficult to disentangle from symptoms of other medical conditions associated with ageing. Evidence suggests that changes in appetite and sexual drive are not related to depression in late life, whereas other somatic symptoms, such as sleep disturbances and chronic pain, are (Nguyen and Zonderman 2006).

It may be necessary to use fewer psychopathology-laden terms (e.g. 'depressed'). Asking older clients informal questions like 'How are your spirits today?' can open a dialogue regarding recent life events and symptoms of depression (Gallo and Rabins 1999). Interviewers should be aware of age-related medical conditions that are associated with depressive syndromes. For example, individuals with cerebrovascular disease are at increased risk of developing vascular depression. Vascular depression is characterized by increased language difficulties and more vegetative symptoms (e.g. apathy) compared to other forms of depression (Alexopoulos 2004). Depressive symptoms also may be due to side-effects of prescription medications or the interaction between two or more medications. Interviewers should inquire about somatic symptoms and other non-dysphoric symptoms of depression (e.g. 'Have you had any unusual aches or pains lately?' or 'Have you been keeping up with your favourite hobbies recently?'). Endorsement of these symptoms may indicate a depressive syndrome, though somatic symptoms should be interpreted with caution (Edelstein, Drozdick, and Ciliberti 2010).

Anxiety

Anxiety disorders are the most commonly diagnosed psychiatric disorders among older adults (Kessler et al. 2005). Generalized anxiety disorder and phobic disorders are the most common, with lower prevalence rates of social anxiety disorder and panic disorder (Bryant, Jackson, and Ames 2008). As with late-life depression, symptoms of anxiety and worry are common among older adults and even subsyndromal levels are related to functional and social impairment, sleep difficulties, and poorer quality of life (Gould and Edelstein 2010; Wetherell, Le Roux, and Gatz 2003). Thus, assessing for anxiety in clinical interviews is important with older adult clients.

There are several key concepts related to interviewing older adults about anxiety-related topics. Older clients tend to prefer colloquial terms for anxiety and worry such as 'fret' or 'concern' compared to psychological terms (Stanley and Novy 2000). They are also more likely to emphasize physical symptoms (e.g. shortness of breath, chest pain, gastrointestinal distress) compared to cognitive or behavioural symptoms (e.g. worry, fear, avoidance; Lenze et al. 2005). The propensity for older adults to endorse physical symptoms of anxiety makes the detection of anxiety disorders challenging, given that these symptoms may overlap with medical conditions and anxiety-related side-effects of medications. Yet, it is critical that interviewers assess for physical symptoms of anxiety and attempt to rule out underlying medical causes.

One of the greatest differences in anxiety disorders across age groups is the content of anxiety or worry symptoms. Compared to younger age groups, older adults tend to worry less about work-related problems and more about family, health, and finances (Hunt, Wisocki, and Yanko 2003). Older adults often experience anxiety in different social situations than younger adults, such as forgetting information and using technology in front of others (Ciliberti et al. 2011). Physiological changes such as declines in vision, hearing, memory, and continence may affect specific anxiety or worry symptoms in social anxiety disorder or generalized anxiety disorder. Interviewers are encouraged to make adjustments to questions related to worry and anxiety content when assessing older adults.

Personality disorders

The prevalence of personality disorders declines in later life. However, roughly 10% of older adults meet criteria for at least one personality disorder (Zweig 2008). Though many older adults that were diagnosed with a personality disorder in young adulthood no longer meet diagnostic criteria for a personality disorder, negative consequences associated with these disorders (e.g. interpersonal problems) appear to persist into older adulthood (Balsis et al. 2007).

There are at least two possible reasons for the decline in personality disorders in late life, both of which are pertinent to clinical interviewing. First, many of the diagnostic criteria for personality disorders in the *DSM-IV-TR* contained age bias (Balsis et al. 2007). For example, one criterion of antisocial personality disorder involves aggression, as evidenced by the presence of repeated physical altercations. This feature may not be applicable to frail older adults, who may express aggression in non-physical ways (e.g. yelling, cursing; Edelstein and Segal 2011). Thus, even if older adults do not meet criteria for a personality disorder, it may still be important to assess for personality disorder symptomatology (i.e. interpersonal problems, emotional lability, maladaptive behavioural traits). Second, symptoms of personality disorder may be disregarded in older adults due to negative stereotypes of ageing (e.g. that older adults are inflexible, stingy, cantankerous, depressed, or needy). Depression, anxiety, and personality disorders are not part of normal ageing, and interviewers of older adults should take care not to fall victim to these biases. Conversely, interviewers must consider and attempt to rule out the presence of physiological or neurological syndromes that may account for overlapping symptoms.

Suicide

The World Health Organization reports that suicide rates worldwide have increased by 60% in the last forty-five years (WHO 2011). The global mortality rate is estimated to be 16 per 100,000 deaths. Older adults, particularly older men, are disproportionally affected by suicide compared to other groups. In the US, older adults accounted for 16% of all deaths by suicide in 2008, but comprised only 12.7% of the population (McIntosh 2011). Suicidal behaviour in older adults has greater lethality compared to younger adults (Chan, Draper, and Banerjee 2007). Many older adults had visited their physician within one month of committing suicide, and the majority had visited a physician in the prior year (Luoma, Martin, and Pearson 2002). Comprehensive screening for suicidal ideation or intent in clinical interviews is one route for preventing death by suicide.

The conceptual model of suicide risk presented by Bryan and Rudd (2006) may be useful for the clinical interview. According to their model, suicide risk is an amalgamation of baseline risk factors (i.e. demographic, historical factors) and acute risk factors (i.e. short-term, exacerbating factors). For older adults with high baseline risk, a difficult life transition (e.g. widowhood) could be enough to induce suicidal ideation or intent. Conwell (2004) identified several risk and protective factors specific to suicide in late life. Baseline risk factors in older adults include white race, male gender, older age (80+), marital status (with single, divorced, or widowed at higher risk), prior suicide attempts, a history of psychopathology, and recent suicide plans or attempts. Acute risk factors in later life include social isolation, recent bereavement, family discord, financial stressors, access to lethal means, hopelessness, perceived burdensomeness, and the presence of a suicide plan or method. Risk factors for special populations of older adults (e.g. institutionalized) may differ from those listed above. For example, nursing home residents at facilities with lower levels of patient autonomy have a higher risk of suicide than residents in facilities allowing greater patient autonomy (Reiss and Tishler 2008). In addition to risk factors, protective factors (e.g. religious beliefs, concerns about family, etc.) should be considered.

Given the high degree of lethality of suicidal behaviour in older adults, it is especially beneficial for clinicians to have standardized procedures for evaluating suicide risk in older adults. The Suicidal Older Adult Protocol (SOAP), a semi-structured clinical interview, is one assessment instrument designed for this purpose (Fremouw et al. 2009). Interviewers should also assess for protective factors. The Reasons for Living—Older Adults Scale (RFL-OA) is a sixty-nine-item, copyright-free measure that assesses for protective factors particular to older individuals, including family and friends, religious beliefs, and moral objections to suicide, to name a few (Edelstein et al. 2009).

Substance abuse

With the ageing of the baby boomer generation, the prevalence of substance abuse disorders among older adults is increasing (Gfroerer et al. 2003). Older adults are more likely to present with alcohol use disorders than illicit drug use disorders (Lin et al. 2011). Misuse of prescription medications is most common among older adults (Schonfeld et al. 2010) as older adults are likely to be taking several medications (Dwyer et al. 2010). Substance abuse tends to begin in young adulthood and remit over the life course, though late-onset substance abuse does occur (Sattar, Petty, and Burke 2003). Substance abuse is generally associated with male gender, younger age, being divorced or separated, recent major life events, and poor social support (King et al. 1994; Lin et al. 2011). Substance abuse can be a means by which older adults cope with psychological distress, such as depression (Rodriguez et al. 2010).

Assessment of substance abuse is complicated by the presence of comorbid medical problems, medication use (King et al. 1994; Lin et al. 2011), and psychiatric disorders (King et al. 1994; Sorocco and Ferrell 2006), which may mask or resemble symptoms of substance abuse. Cognitive impairment associated with prolonged substance abuse, especially chronic alcohol use, can hinder the clinical interview and diagnostic process. Diagnostic criteria for substance abuse may not be well suited to older adults. For example, older adults may engage in fewer activities (e.g. they may be retired, frail), which can make it difficult to determine whether substance use causes significant interference in daily life (Sorocco and Ferrall 2006). Older adults may be especially unlikely to admit to problems of substance use or may not understand what constitutes substance use problems.

When assessing for substance abuse, a respectful, non-judgmental attitude should be adopted to help the older client feel more comfortable discussing substance use (Sattar et al. 2003). Language used in the interview is important. Older adults seldom admit to using 'street drugs', but may be more likely to give an affirmative response if referred to as 'recreational drugs' (Mohlman et al. 2011). Considerations of medical and psychological disorders are important in making a differential diagnosis. Few screeners of substance abuse have been validated with older adults, though several exist for alcohol abuse. Interested readers are referred to Barry and Blow (2010) for a discussion of screening measures.

Sleep

Considering sleep in the assessment interview cannot be overemphasized. Older adults report sleeping approximately the same amount of time as young adults (Stepnowsky and Ancoli-Israel 2008), but the architecture of sleep changes with age, with a reduction in non-REM sleep, a longer latency to sleep onset, and an increase in the number of awakenings. The latter results in fragmented and lighter sleep and lower sleep efficiency (Beck and Ralls 2011). Some older adults experience Delayed Sleep Phase Syndrome, in which the individual falls asleep at progressively later times. In contrast, other older adults may experience Advanced Sleep Phase Syndrome, which involves earlier sleep onset and earlier wakening. These phase shifts can be influenced by factors such as decreased exposure to light, decreased physical activity, and irregular meal times (Ancoli-Israel and Ayalon 2006). Insomnia complaints also increase with age, with substantially more women than men reporting difficulties falling asleep, maintaining sleep, or awakening early (Lichstein et al. 2006). These age-related sleep changes can contribute to poorer quality and quantity of sleep, which can result in impaired cognitive functioning. Poor sleep is also associated with a variety of psychiatric symptoms and disorders (e.g. anxiety disorders, mood disorders). Consequently, it is important to question the older adult about his or her sleep and, if necessary, employ a brief self-report measure of sleep quality (e.g. Pittsburgh Sleep Quality Index; Buysse et al. 1991).

Elder abuse

Elder abuse is intentional actions that cause harm to a vulnerable older adult by a trusted person and includes physical, sexual, or emotional abuse, financial exploitation, abandonment, neglect, and self-neglect (National Research Council 2003). The rate at which professionals report elder abuse to authorities is less than actual incidents (Cooper, Selwood, and Livingston 2009). This trend may be explained by professionals' lack of awareness of signs of abuse, poor methods for assessing abuse, or lack of knowledge of reporting procedures. Victims may not report abuse because of shame and embarrassment or the desire to protect the abuser, especially if the abuser is a family member. Elder abuse is associated with higher rates of psychological disorders (Acierno et al. 2003), underscoring the importance of assessing for elder abuse.

Victims of elder abuse are more likely to be female (Laumann, Leitsch, and Waite 2008), have less social support, and display greater cognitive and functional impairment (Fulmer et al. 2005). Older adults living with non-spouse family or friends are more likely to be abused than those living in institutionalized settings or with a spouse (Vida, Monks, and Des Rosiers 2002). Offenders of elder abuse are more likely to be acquaintances and male (Krienert, Walsh, and Turner 2009). These characteristics are important to consider when interviewing older adults about elder abuse.

Given the sensitive nature of elder abuse, clinicians must maintain a warm, non-judgmental demeanour during the interview. It can be helpful to give definitions and descriptive examples of different types of abuse to elicit accurate answers (Acierno et al. 2003). It is prudent to ask care-givers or staff members to leave the room during questioning (Mohlman et al. 2011). Affirmative responses of elder abuse necessitate additional assessment. Follow-up assessment should include behavioural observations, interviews with others, as well as the use of screening instruments, such as the Hwalek-Sengstock Elder Abuse Screening Test (Hwalek and Sengstock 1986) and the Indicators of Abuse Screen (Reis and Nahmiash 1998).

Reporting elder abuse is mandatory in some jurisdictions, yet some professionals do not report abuse out of fear of damaging the therapeutic alliance or decreasing the client's quality of life (Rodriguez et al. 2006). However, research indicates these fears are unsupported. Consequently, when elder abuse is detected, clinicians should refer to reporting guidelines and act accordingly.

SUMMARY

Assessment of older adults requires the interviewer to act as a detective: to consider various explanations for behaviours or symptoms, and systematically deduce the underlying cause. To do so, the clinician must address numerous factors that influence the interview process and conclusions drawn from information gathered in the interview.

Numerous interviewing tools, including structured, semi-structured, or unstructured interviews, can be used with older adults. Often, it is appropriate to modify the interview. Age-related changes in the visual and auditory systems may require changes to the testing environment, such as completing the interview in a well-lit and quiet location. Cognitive changes, including slowed processing speed and impaired memory, suggest that the interviewer change the interview format or collect collateral information. The setting of the interview (e.g. nursing home, outpatient mental health clinic) will place unique demands on the interviewer and interviewee. Finally, the interviewer should be aware that older adults have peaks and troughs in cognitive performance across the day, and note the time at which interviews are conducted.

The interviewer must gather as much information as possible, which can assist in selecting interview questions and interpreting information. When working with ethnic-minority older adults, knowledge of culture-specific presenting symptoms is important. It is essential to attain an accurate medical history and a list of current medications for the older adult client, which ought to factor into case conceptualizations.

As always, it is important to build rapport with older adult clients, as they may be less familiar with the interview process than other age groups. Establishing trust is crucial, as it will help the older adult to feel more comfortable providing answers regarding potentially sensitive information. Professionalism, warmth, and politeness will likely put the older adult client at ease.

There are a number of content areas for which the clinician can assess. Though this chapter discusses only a few psychological disorders and behaviours relevant to older adults, the overall message is that older adults often have unique symptom presentations and experiences that should be addressed in the interview. The clinician should thoroughly read relevant material before interviewing an older adult to gain an understanding of issues specific to older adults.

Interviewing older adults can be complicated. An understanding of issues related to the interview process, with appropriate modifications, can help the clinician gather accurate information. Knowledge of older adult development, ethnic and cultural issues, mental and physical health problems, and age-related behaviours will enhance the quality of the interview with an older adult client.

KEY REFERENCES AND SOURCES FOR FURTHER READING

Mohlman, J., Sirota, K. G., Papp, L. A., Staples, A. M., King, A., and Gorenstein, E. E. (2011). 'Clinical Interviewing with Older Adults'. *Cognitive and Behavioral Practice* 19(1): 89–100. doi:10.1016/j.cbpra.2010.10.001.

Segal, D. L., June, A., and Marty, M. A. (2010). 'Basic Issues in Interviewing and the Interview Process'. In D. L. Segal and M. Hersen (eds), *Diagnostic Interviewing* (4th edn). New York: Springer.

Zarit, S. H. and Zarit, J. M. (2007). *Mental Disorders in Older Adults: Fundamentals of Assessment and Treatment* (2nd edn). New York: Guilford Press.

REFERENCES

Acierno, R., Resnick, H., Kilpatrick, D., and Stark-Riemer, W. (2003). 'Assessing Elder Victimization: Demonstration of a Methodology'. *Social Psychiatry and Psychiatric Epidemiology* 38: 644–653.

Alberts, G. and Edelstein, B. (1992). *Identifying and Measuring Therapist Behavior Associated with Client-perceived Trustworthiness*. Paper presented at meeting of the Association for Advancement of Behavior Therapy, Boston, MA.

Alexopoulos, G. S. (2004). 'Late-life Mood Disorders'. In J. Sadavoy, L. F. Jarvik, G. T. Grossberg, and B. B. Meyers (eds), *Comprehensive Textbook of Geriatric Psychiatry* (pp. 609–653). New York: W. W. Norton and Co.

Alexopoulos, G. S., Abrams, R. C., Young, R. C., and Shamoian, C. A. (1988). 'Cornell Scale for Depression in Dementia'. *Biological Psychiatry* 23: 271–284.

American Psychological Association (2003). 'Guidelines on Multicultural Education, Training, Research, Practice, and Organizational Change for Psychologists'. *American Psychologist* 58: 377–402.

Ancoli-Israel, S. and Ayalon, L. (2006). 'Diagnosis and Treatment of Sleep Disorders in Older Adults'. *American Journal of Geriatric Psychiatry* 14(2): 95–10. doi: 10.1097/01. JGP.0000196627.12010.d1.

Balsis, S., Gleason, M. E., Woods, C. M., and Oltmanns, T. F. (2007). 'An Item Response Theory Analysis of DSM-IV Personality Disorder Criteria across Younger and Older Age Groups'. *Psychology and Aging* 22: 171–185.

Barry, K. L. and Blow, F. C. (2010). 'Screening, Assessing, and Intervening for Alcohol and Medication Misuse in Older Adults'. In P. Lichtenberg (ed), *Handbook of Assessment in Clinical Gerontology* (pp. 307–330). London: Academic Press.

Beck, A. A. and Ralls, F. M. (2011). 'Sleep Disorders in Aging'. In M. L. Albert and J. E. Knoefel (eds), *Clinical Neurology of Aging* (3rd edn, pp. 545–556). New York: Oxford University Press.

de Beurs, E., Beekman, A. T. F., Deeg, D. J. H., Van Dyck, R., and van Tillburg, W. (2000). 'Predictors of Change in Anxiety Symptoms of Older Persons: Results from the Longitudinal Aging Study Amsterdam'. *Psychological Medicine* 30: 515–527.

Blazer, D. G. (2003). 'Depression in Late Life: Review and Commentary'. *Journal of Gerontology A: Biological Sciences and Medical Sciences* 58: 249–265.

Brown, T., DiNardo, P., and Barlow, D. (1994). *Anxiety Disorders Inteview Schedule Adult Version (ADIS-IV): Client Interview Schedule*. New York: Oxford University Press.

Bryan, C. J. and Rudd, M. D. (2006). 'Advances in the Assessment of Suicide Risk'. *Journal of Clinical Psychology: In Session* 62: 185–200.

Bryant, C., Jackson, H., and Ames, D. (2008). 'The Prevalence of Anxiety in Older Adults: Methodological Issues and a Review of the Literature'. *Journal of Affective Disorders* 109(3): 233–250. doi:10.1016/j.jad.2007.11.008.

Busse, R. Blümel, M., Scheller-Kreinsen, D., and Zentner, A. (2010). '*Tackling Chronic Disease in Europe: Strategies, Interventions and Challenges*'. Albany, NY: World Health Organization.

Buysse D. J., Reynolds, C. F., Monk, T. H., Hoch, C. C., Yeager, A. L., and Kupfer, D. J. (1991). 'Quantification of Subjective Sleep Quality in Healthy Elderly Men and Women Using the Pittsburgh Sleep Quality Index (PSQI)'. *Sleep* 14: 331–338.

Chan, J., Draper, B., and Banerjee, S. (2007). 'Deliberate Self-harm in Older Adults: A Review of the Literature from 1995 to 2004'. *International Journal of Geriatric Psychiatry* 22(8): 720–732.

Choi, N. G. and Gonzalez, J. M. (2005). 'Barriers and Contributors to Minority Older Adults' Access to Mental Health Treatment'. *Journal of Gerontological Social Work* 44(3): 115–135.

Ciliberti, C., Gould, C., Smith, M., Chorney, D., and Edelstein, B. (2011). 'A Preliminary Investigation of Developmentally Sensitive Items for the Assessment of Social Anxiety in Late Life'. *Journal of Anxiety Disorders* 25: 686–689.

Colsher, P. and Wallace, R. B. (1989). 'Data Quality and Age: Health and Psychobehavioral Correlates of Item Nonresponse and Inconsistent Responses'. *Journal of Gerontology: Psychological Sciences* 44: 45–52.

Conner, K. O., Lee, B., Mayers, V., Robinson, D., Reynolds, C. F., III, Albert, S., et al. (2010). 'Attitudes and Beliefs about Mental Health among African American Older Adults Suffering from Depression'. *Journal of Aging Studies* 24: 266–277.

Conwell, Y. (2004). 'Suicide'. In S. Roose and H. Sackeim (eds), *Late Life Depression* (pp. 95–106). Oxford: Oxford University Press.

Cooper, C., Selwood, A., and Livingston, G. (2009). 'Knowledge, Detection, and Reporting of Abuse of Health and Social Care Professionals: A Systematic Review'. *American Journal of Geriatric Psychiatry* 17: 826–838.

Cormier, S. and Cormier, W. (1991). *Interviewing Strategies for Helpers* (2nd edn). Pacific Grove, CA: Brooks-Cole.

Crews, J. E., Jones, G. C., and Kim, J. H. (2006). 'Double Jeopardy: The Effects of Comorbid Conditions among Older People with Vision Loss'. *Journal of Visual Impairment and Blindness* 100: 824–848.

DeMaio, T. (1980). 'Refusals: Who, Where and Why'. *Public Opinion Quarterly* 44: 223–233.

Dennis, R. E., Boddington, S. J., and Funnell, N. J. (2007). 'Self-report Measures of Anxiety: Are they Suitable for Older Adults?' *Aging & Mental Health* 11: 668–677.

Dwyer, L. L. Han, B., Woodwell, D. A., and Rechtsteiner, E. A. (2010). 'Polypharmacy in Nursing Home Residents in the United States: Results of the 2004 National Nursing Home Survey'. *American Journal of Geriatric Pharmacotherapy* 8: 63–72.

Edelstein, B. and Semenchuk, E. (1996). 'Interviewing Older Adults'. In L. Carstensen, B. Edelstein, and L. Dornbrand (eds), *The Practical Handbook of Clinical Gerontology*. Beverly Hills, CA: Sage.

Edelstein, B. A., Koven, L., Spira, A., and Shreve-Neiger, A. (2003). 'Older Adults'. In M. Hersen and S. Turner (eds), *Diagnostic Interviewing* (3rd edn, pp. 433–455). New York: Kluwer/Plenum.

Edelstein, B., Martin, R., and Koven, L. (2003). 'Psychological Assessment in Geriatric Settings'. In J. R. Graham and J. A. Naglieri (eds), *Comprehensive Handbook of Psychology: Vol. 10: Assessment Psychology* (pp. 389–414). New York: Wiley.

Edelstein, B. A., Heisel, M. J., McKee, D. R., Martin, R. R., Koven, L. P., Duberstein, P. R., et al. (2009). 'Development and Psychometric Evaluation of the Reasons for Living—Older Adults Scale: A Suicide Risk Assessment Inventory'. *The Gerontologist* 49(6): 736–745.

Edelstein, B. A., Drozdick, L. W., and Ciliberti, C. M. (2010). 'Assessment of Depression and Bereavement in Older Adults'. In P. A. Lichtenberg (ed.), *Handbook of Assessment in Clinical Gerontology* (pp. 3–44). New York: Wiley.

Edelstein, B. A. and Segal, D. L. (2011). 'Assessment of Emotional and Personality Disorders'. In K. W. Schaie and S. L. Willis (eds), *Handbook of the Psychology of Aging* (pp. 325–337). London: Elsevier.

Edelstein, B. A., Martin, R. R., and Gerolimatos, L. A. (2012). 'Assessment in Geriatric Settings'. In J. R. Graham and N. A. Naglieri (eds), *Handbook of Psychology: Vol. 10: Assessment Psychology* (2nd edn, pp. 425–448). New York: Wiley.

Federal Interagency Forum on Aging Related Statistics (2010). 'Older Americans 2010: Key Indicators of Well Being'. http://www.agingstats.gov/agingstatsdotnet/main_site/default. aspx.

First, M. B., Spitzer, R. L., Gibbon, M., and Williams, J. B. W. (1996). '*Structured Clinical Interview for DSM-IV Axis I Disorders: Non-patient Edition (SCID-NP, v. 2.0)*'. New York: New York State Psychiatric Institute.

Fiske, A., Wetherell, J. L., and Gatz, M. (2009). 'Depression in Older Adults'. *Annual Review of Clinical Psychology* 5: 363–389.

Fremouw, W., McCoy, K., Tyner, E. A., and Musick, R. (2009). 'Suicidal Older Adult Protocol—SOAP'. In J. A. Allen, E. Wolf, and L. VandeCreek (eds), *Innovations in Clinical Practice: A 21st Century Sourcebook* (pp. 203–212). Sarasota, FL: Professional Resource Press/Professional Resource Exchange.

Fulmer, T., Paveza, G., VandeWeerd, C., Fairchild, S., Guadagno, L., Botlon-Blatt, M., et al. (2005). 'Dyadic Vulnerability and Risk Profiling for Elder Neglect'. *The Gerontologist* 45: 525–534.

Gagliese, L. (2009). 'Pain and Aging: The Emergence of a New Subfield of Pain Research'. *The Journal of Pain* 10: 343–353.

Gallo, J. J. and Rabins, P. V. (1999). 'Depression without Sadness: Alternative Presentations of Depression in Late Life'. *American Family Physician* 60: 820–826.

Gfroerer, J., Penne, M., Pemberton, M., and Folsom, R. (2003). 'Substance Abuse Treatment Need among Older Adults in 2020: The Impact of the Aging Baby-boom Cohort'. *Drug and Alcohol Dependence* 69: 127–135.

Glass, J. M. (2007). 'Visual Function and Cognitive Aging: Differential Role of Contrast Sensitivity in Verbal versus Spatial Tasks'. *Psychology and Aging* 22(2): 233–238.

Gould, C. E. and Edelstein, B. A. (2010). 'Worry, Emotion Control, and Anxiety Control in Older and Younger Adults'. *Journal of Anxiety Disorders* 24: 759–766.

Gould, C., Edelstein, B., and Ciliberti, C. (2010). 'Older Adults'. In D. Segal and M. Hersen (eds), *Diagnostic Interviewing* (4th edn, pp. 467–494). New York: Springer.

Herzog, A. R. and Rodgers, W. L. (1988). 'Age and Response Rates to Interview Sample Surveys'. *Journal of Gerontology: Social Sciences* 43: S200–S205.

Horowitz, A. (2003). 'Depression and Vision and Hearing Impairments in Later Life'. *Generations* 27: 32–38.

Hunt, S., Wisocki, P., and Yanko, J. (2003). 'Worry and Use of Coping Strategies among Older and Younger Adults'. *Anxiety Disorders* 17: 547–560.

Hwalek, M. and Sengstock, M. (1986). 'Assessing the Probability of Abuse of the Elderly: Toward Development of a Clinical Screening Instrument'. *Journal of Applied Gerontology* 5: 153–173.

Ivers, R. Q., Norton, R., Cumming, R. G., Butler, M., and Campbell, A. J. (2000). 'Visual Impairment and Risk of Hip Fracture'. *American Journal of Epidemiology* 152: 633–639.

Jang, Y., Chiriboga, D.A., and Okazaki, S. (2009). 'Attitudes toward Mental Health Services: Age-group Differences in Korean American Adults'. *Aging & Mental Health* 13: 127–134.

Jones, G. G., Rovner, B. W., Crews, J. E., and Danielson, M. L. (2009). 'Effects of Depressive Symptoms on Health Behavior Practices among Older Adults with Vision Loss'. *Rehabilitation Psychology* 54: 164–172.

Karlin, B. E., Duffy, M., and Gleaves, D. H. (2008). 'Patterns and Predictors of Mental Health Service Use and Mental Illness among Older and Younger Adults in the United States'. *Psychological Services* 5: 275–294.

Kessler, R. C., Chiu, W. T., Demler, O., Merikangas, K. R., and Walters, E. E. (2005). 'Prevalence, Severity, and Comorbidity of 12-month DSM-IV Disorders in the National Comorbidity Survey Replication'. *Archives of General Psychiatry* 62: 617–627.

King, C. J., Van Hasselt, V. B., Segal, D. L., and Hersen, M. (1994). 'Diagnosis and Assessment of Substance Abuse in Older Adults: Current Strategies and Issues'. *Addictive Behaviors* 19: 41–55.

Kirmayer, L. J. and Young, A. (1998). 'Culture and Somatization: Clinical, Epidemiological, and Ethnographic Perspectives'. *Psychosomatic Medicine* 60: 420–430.

Kirmayer, L. J. (2001). 'Cultural Variations in the Clinical Presentation of Depression and Anxiety: Implications for Diagnosis and Treatment'. *Journal of Clinical Psychiatry* 62: 22–28.

Koerner, N., Hood, H. K., and Antony, M. M. (2011). 'Interviewing and Case Formulation'. In D. H. Barlow (ed.), *The Oxford Handbook of Clinical Psychology* (pp. 225–253). New York: Oxford University Press.

Koven, L. P., Shreve-Neiger, A., and Edelstein, B. A. (2007). 'Older Adults'. In M. Hersen and J. C. Thomas (eds), *Handbook of Clinical Interviewing with Adults* (pp. 392–406). Thousand Oaks, CA: Sage.

Krienert, J. L., Walsh, J. A., and Turner, M. (2009). 'Elderly in America: A Descriptive Study of Elder Abuse Examining National Incident-based Reporting System (NIBRS) Data, 2000–2005'. *Journal of Elder Abuse and Neglect* 21: 325–345.

Laumann, E. O., Leitsch, S. A., and Waite, L. J. (2008). 'Elder Mistreatment in the United States: Prevalence Estimates from a Nationally Representative Study'. *Journals of Gerontology: Series B: Psychological Sciences and Social Sciences* 63B: S248–S254.

Lavretsky, H., Kurbanyan, K., and Kumar, A. (2004). 'The Significance of Subsyndromal Depression in Geriatrics'. *Current Psychiatry Reports* 6: 25–31.

Lecrubier Y., Sheehan D., Weiller E., Amorim, P., Bonora, I., Sheehan, K. H., et al. (1997). 'The MINI International Neuropsychiatric Interview (M.I.N.I.) A Short Diagnostic Structured Interview: Reliability and Validity according to the CIDI'. *European Psychiatry* 12: 224–231.

Lee, D. J., Gomez-Marin, O., Lam, B. L., and Zheng, D. D. (2002). 'Visual Acuity Impairment and Mortality in US Adults'. *Archives of Ophthalmology* 120: 1544–1550.

Lenze, E. J., Karp, J. F., Mulsant, B. H., Blank, S., Shear, M. K., Houck, P. R., et al. (2005). 'Somatic Symptoms in Late-life Anxiety: Treatment Issues'. *Journal of Geriatric Psychiatry and Neurology* 18: 89–96.

Lichstein, K. L., Stone, K. C., Nau, S. D., McCrae, C. S., and Payne, K. L. (2006). 'Insomnia in the Elderly'. *Sleep Medicine Clinics* 1: 221–229.

Lin, J. C., Karno, M. P., Grella, C. E., Warda, U., Liao, D. H., Hu, P., et al. (2011). 'Alcohol, Tobacco, and Nonmedical Drug Use Disorders in US Adults Aged 65 Years and Older: Data from the 2001–2002 National Epidemiologic Survey of Alcohol and Related Conditions'. *American Journal of Geriatric Psychiatry* 19: 292–299.

Luoma, J. B., Martin, C. E., and Pearson, J. L. (2002). 'Contact with Mental Health and Primary Care Providers before Suicide: A Review of the Evidence'. *American Journal of Psychiatry* 159(6): 909–916.

McIntosh, J. L. (2011). '*U.S.A. Suicide 2008: Official Final Data*. Washington, DC: American Association of Suicidology'. (24 October). http://www.suicidology.org.

Malmstrom, T. K. and Tait, R. C. (2010). 'Pain Assessment and Management in Older Adults'. In P. Lichtenberg (ed.), *Handbook of Assessment in Clinical Gerontology* (pp. 647–678). New York: Elsevier.

Mohlman, J., Sirota, K. G., Papp, L. A., Staples, A. M., King, A., and Gorenstein, E. E. (2011). 'Clinical Interviewing with Older Adults'. *Cognitive and Behavioral Practice* 19(1): 89–100. doi:10.1016/j.cbpra.2010.10.001.

National Eye Institute (2011). 'Prevalence of Blindness Data'. http://www.nei.nih.gov/eyedata/pbd_tables.asp.

National Institute on Deafness and Other Communicative Disorders (2010). 'Presbycusis'. http://www.nidcd.nih.gov/health/hearing/pages/presbycusis.aspx.

National Research Council (2003). *Elder Mistreatment: Abuse, Neglect, and Exploitation in an Aging America*, R. J. Bonnie and R. B. Wallace (eds). Panel to review risk and prevalence of elder abuse and neglect, Committee on National Statistics and Committee on Law and Justice, Division of Behavioral and Social Sciences and Education. Washington, DC: National Academics Press.

Nguyen, H. T. and Zonderman, A. B. (2006). 'Relationships between Age and Aspects of Depression: Consistency and Reliability across Two Longitudinal Studies'. *Psychology and Aging* 21: 119–126.

Nolte, E. and McKee, M. (2008). '*Caring for People with Chronic Conditions: A Health System Perspective*'. Maidenhead: Open University Press.

Park, D. and Schwarz, N. (2000). *Cognitive Aging: A Primer*. Philadelphia: Psychology Press.

Prevent Blindness America, National Eye Institute (2008). *The Vision Problems in the U.S.: Prevalence of Adult Vision Impairment and Age-Related Eye Disease in America*. Bethesda, MD: National Institutes of Health.

Reis, M. and Nahmiash, D. (1998). 'Validation of the Indicators of Abuse (IOA) Screen'. *The Gerontologist* 38(4): 471–480.

Reiss, N. S. and Tishler, C. L. (2008). 'Suicidality in Nursing Home Residents: Part I. Prevalence, Risk Factors, Methods, Assessment, and Management'. *Professional Psychology: Research and Practice* 39(3): 264–270.

Reuben, D. R., Herr, K. A., Pacala, J. T., Pollock, B. G., Potter, J. F., and Semla, T. P. (2011). *Geriatrics at your Fingertips: 2011* (13th edn). New York: American Geriatrics Society.

Robins, L. N., Cotler, L. B., Bucholz, K. K., Compton, W. M., North, C., and Rourke, K. (1999). *The Diagnostic Interview Schedule for DMS-IV (DIS-IV)*. St. Louis, MO: Washington University School of Medicine.

Rodriguez, M. A., Wallace, S. P., Woolf, N. H., and Mangione, C. M. (2006). 'Mandatory Reporting of Elder Abuse: Between a Rock and a Hard Place'. *Annals of Family Medicine* 4: 403–409.

Rodriguez, C. A., Schonfeld, L., King-Kallimanis, B., and Gum, A. M. (2010). 'Depressive Symptoms and Alcohol Abuse/Misuse in Older Adults: Results from the Florida BRITE Project'. *Best Practices in Mental Health* 6: 90–102.

Salthouse, T. A. (2010). *Major Issues in Cognitive Aging*. New York: Oxford University Press.

Sattar, S. P., Petty, F., and Burke, W. J. (2003). 'Diagnosis and Treatment of Alcohol Dependence in Older Alcoholics'. *Clinical Geriatric Medicine* 19: 743–761.

Saxena, S., Thornicroft, G., Knapp, M., and Whiteford, H. (2007). 'Resources for Mental Health: Scarcity, Inequity, and Inefficiency'. *The Lancet* 370: 878–889.

Saxon, S. V., Etten, M. J., and Perkins, E. A. (2010). *Physical Change and Aging: A Guide for the Helping Professions* (5th edn). New York: Springer.

Schmidt, C., Fabienne, C., Cajochen, C., and Peigneux, P. (2007). 'A Time to Think: Circadian Rhythms in Human Cognition'. *Cognitive Neuropsychology* 24: 755–789.

Schonfeld, L., King-Kallimanis, B. L., Duchene, D. M., Etheridge, R. L., Herrera, R. L., Barry, K. L., et al. (2010). 'Screening and Brief Intervention for Substance Misuse among Older Adults: The Florida BRITE Project'. *American Journal of Public Health* 100(1): 108–114.

Segal, D. L., June, A., and Marty, M. A. (2010). 'Basic Issues in Interviewing and the Interview Process'. In D. L. Segal and M. Hersen (eds), *Diagnostic Interviewing* (4th edn, pp. 1–21). New York: Springer.

Shankar, K. K., Walker, M., Frost, D., and Orrell, M. W. (1999). 'The Development of a Valid and Reliable Scale for Rating Anxiety in Dementia (RAID)'. *Aging & Mental Health* 3: 39–49.

Sorocco, K. H. and Ferrall, S. W. (2006). 'Alcohol Use among Older Adults'. *The Journal of General Psychology* 133: 453–467.

Stanley, M. A. and Novy, D. M. (2000). 'Cognitive-behavior Therapy for Generalized Anxiety in Late Life: An Evaluative Review'. *Journal of Anxiety Disorders* 14: 191–207.

Stepnowsky, C. J. and Ancoli-Israel, S. (2008). 'Sleep and its Disorders in Seniors'. *Sleep Medicine Clinics* 3(2): 281–293. doi:10.1016/j.jsmc.2008.01.011.

Storandt, M. (1994). 'General Principles of Assessment of Older Adults'. In M. Storandt and G. R. VandenBos (eds), *Neuropsychological Assessment of Dementia and Depression in Older Adults: A Clinician's Guide* (pp. 7–32). Washington, DC: American Psychological Association.

Talerico, K., Evans, L., and Strumpf, N. (2002). 'Mental Health Correlates of Aggression in Nursing Home Residents with Dementia'. *The Gerontologist* 42: 169–177.

US Census Bureau (2010). 'Disability Characteristics: 2010 American Community Survey 1-year Estimates (American FactFinder Table S1810)'. http://factfinder2.census.gov/faces/tableservices/jsf/pages/productview.xhtml?pid=ACS_10_1YR_S1810andprodType=table.

Vanderplas, J. H. and Vanderplas, J. M. (1981). 'Effects of Legibility on Verbal Test Performance of Older Adults'. *Perceptual and Motor Skills* 53: 183–186.

Ventura, J., Liberman, R. P., Green, M. F., Shaner, A., and Mintz, J. (1998). 'Training and Quality Assurance with the Structured Clinical Interview for DSM-IV (SCID-I/P)'. *Psychiatry Research* 79: 163–173.

Vida, S., Monks, R. C., and Des Rosiers, P. (2002). 'Prevalence and Correlates of Elder Abuse and Neglect in a Geriatric Psychiatry Service'. *Canadian Journal of Psychiatry* 47: 459–467.

Wetherell, J. L., Le Roux, H., and Gatz, M. (2003). 'DSM-IV Criteria for Generalized Anxiety Disorder in Older Adults: Distinguishing the Worried from the Well'. *Psychology and Aging* 18: 622–627.

World Blind Union (2011). 'Ageing and Visual Impairment: A Report by the Elderly Working Group of the World Blind Union'. http://www.worldblindunion.org/English/resources/Pages/General-Documents.aspx.

World Health Organization (2011). 'Suicide Prevention (SUPRE)'. http://www.who.int/mental_health/prevention/suicide/suicideprevent/en/index.html.

World Health Organization (2013). 'Deafness and Hearing Loss'. http://who.int/mediacentre/factsheets/fs300/en/index.html.

Yoon, C., May, C. P., and Hasher, L. (1999). 'Aging, Circadian Arousal Patterns, and Cognition'. In N. Schwartz, D. Park, B. Knauper, and S. Sudman (eds), *Cognition, Aging, and Self-reports* (pp. 117–143). Philadelphia: Psychology Press.

Zarit, S. H. and Zarit, J. M. (2007). *Mental Disorders in Older Adults: Fundamentals of Assessment and Treatment* (2nd edn). New York: Guilford Press.

Zweig, R. A. (2008). 'Personality Disorders in Older Adults: Assessment Challenges and Strategies'. *Professional Psychology: Research and Practice* 39: 298–305.

CHAPTER 10

GEROPSYCHOLOGICAL ASSESSMENT

ROCÍO FERNÁNDEZ-BALLESTEROS, MARÍA OLIVA MÁRQUEZ, AND MARTA SANTACREU

INTRODUCTION

THE history of psychology shows that when scientific psychology came into being in the last third of the nineteenth century, societies were younger, with a higher proportion of under-16s than of over-60s. Therefore, most assessment tools developed at this time were designed for the assessment of children and young adults. At the beginning of the twenty-first century, a high proportion of individuals are living in ageing societies with more older than young individuals. Consequently, psychologists must address the areas of ageing, age and the aged, given the priority goal of improving well-being and quality of life throughout the lifespan.

As Birren (1996) proposed, three models can be distinguished for geropsychology: (1) the psychology of *ageing* deals with changes in average functioning of individuals across the lifespan; (2) the psychology of *age* is devoted to age differences, comparing groups of people of different ages; and finally, (3) the psychology of *the aged* is concerned with the thematic study of older individuals with and without clinical disorders (see also Schroots, Fernández-Ballesteros, and Rudinger 1995). As this chapter is devoted to assessment in clinical geropsychology—based on knowledge from the psychology of ageing and age—we are focusing on the aged, which means that our object of study is older persons in clinical settings.

The importance of *clinical geropsychology* is reflected in the results of a study with experts on geropsychology from thirty European countries. Key persons were asked to identify the three most important fields of application of geropsychology in their country (Pinquart, Fernández-Ballesteros, and Torpdahl 2007). Geropsychology most often concerned the clinical field (in 70% of the countries studied). Specialists in the field of clinical psychology provide assessment, consultation, and intervention services related to psychological adaptations in later life, psychopathology, behavioural problems, problems in daily living, medical and legal decision-making capacity, independent living arrangements, and behavioural competencies.

Moreover, *assessing older persons* is one of the most extensive fields in geropsychology, as reported by Fernández-Ballesteros and Pinquart (2011). A search of the most prominent topics in applied geropsychology on the PsycInfo database revealed that the most frequently cited topic was the assessment of older adults (accounting for about one-third of identified citations) (n = 2,500). Other fields identified were psychotherapy/counselling (1,000 papers), quality of life, adult education (around 800 papers each), prevention/health promotion (about 700 papers), care-giving and rehabilitation (respectively, 700 and 650), and older workers (about 550). Other topics were less common, such as problems of older drivers, cognitive training, or ageing in the workplace (in total no more than 200 papers).

Assessing older adults takes into consideration several *theoretical concepts about life development* that are relevant for clinical geropsychology work (e.g. Baltes, Lindenberger, and Staudinger 2006). First of all, from a phylogenetic point of view, the human being is a *historical and interactive organism*; at the same time, from an ontogenetic perspective, human psychological development must be considered as a *lifelong process*, so that changes, stability, the losses and gains of a human being throughout their lifetime depend on the historical and environmental circumstances interacting with their behavioural systems (Gould 1981).

Therefore, the diversity of life circumstances in interaction with idiosyncratic individual bio-behavioural systems shapes this lifelong process. On the basis of this perspective of the ageing process, at a given point in the lifespan, individuals may present gains in one area of functioning and losses in another (Schaie 2005a, 2005b). In sum, from a theoretical point of view, *multidimensionality* and *multidirectionality* are principles within the ageing process that explain the broader inter-individual variability of human characteristics over the lifespan and in old age.

In addition to inter-individual variability, taking into consideration cross-sectional, longitudinal, and experimental studies we can also find within-person variability in psychological development. In other words, *plasticity* is an inherent human characteristic, so that individuals have a broad capacity for change over the lifespan; both natural environmental changes and effective interventions optimize human characteristics, promote positive change, and compensate losses, maintaining or improving biopsychosocial functioning and reversing negative changes, or at least delaying age-associated negative changes. In sum, over the lifespan and throughout old age, *positive change is always possible*.

It is important to point out that these principles about ageing, well established in geropsychology, may clash with the nihilistic attitudes regarding the aged held by the general population and by some professionals. As Fernández-Ballesteros, Reig, and Zamarrón (2008) have stressed, geropsychologists must start out from the basis that even though age is an important biological factor per se, it cannot explain psychological functioning. Our goal here is to emphasize the need for careful multidimensional assessment before making any explanatory judgments based on age.

Finally, as Fernández-Ballesteros and Pinquart (2011) have pointed out, geropsychologists—over and above the general guidelines of their respective countries—should take into account a set of principles, norms, or guidelines for psychological practice with older adults. The American Psychological Association (APA) (2004) published a set of twenty *Guidelines for Psychological Practice with Older Adults*, whose main goal was to 'develop criteria to define the expertise necessary for working with older adults and their families and for evaluating competencies at both the generalist and specialist levels' (238). These Guidelines are developed in the following sections: Attitudes (2); General Knowledge about Adult Development, Aging, and Older Adults (4); Clinical Issues (3); Assessment (3); Intervention, Consultation, and Other Services Provision (7); and Education (1).

We summarize the first four guidelines due to their importance for assessing older adults: *Attitudes* refers to general guidelines dealing with the required competence of the psychologist; a second set of guidelines refers to the importance of considering psychologists' stereotypes and images about ageing and older individuals. The *Knowledge about Adult Development* section refers to continuing education and training in theory and research in ageing, the dynamic of the ageing process, the relevance of sociocultural factors, and biological and health-related aspects of ageing. *Clinical Issues* guidelines refer to knowledge about pathological changes regarding cognitive competence, functional abilities, and the prevalence and nature of psychopathology. *Assessment* contains the following guidelines: to be familiar with the theory, research, and practice of various methods of assessment with older adults and knowledgeable about assessment instruments that are psychometrically suitable for use with them; to understand the problem of using assessment instruments created for younger individuals when assessing older adults and to develop skills for tailoring assessments to accommodate older adults' specific characteristics and contexts; and to develop skills for recognizing cognitive changes in older adults, and conducting and interpreting cognitive screening and functional ability evaluations.

In conclusion, although there are certain screening tools for preliminary assessment, geropsychological assessment must be carried out by appropriately trained psychologists who take professional responsibility for older patients.

ASSESSING OLDER ADULTS: MAIN COMPONENTS AND CHARACTERISTICS

The demand

Psychological assessment is a subdiscipline of scientific psychology concerned with 'the decision-making process that includes various tasks, operations and actions—conducted in a given sequence—in order to answer the client's demand (the client being the individual, the institution, family members, and so forth, as appropriate) requiring basic psychological knowledge and professional abilities' (Fernández-Ballesteros et al. 2001: 188). This process, which depends on the requirements of the client/patient, requires information from multiple data sources (interviews, observations, medical history, etc.) and the administration of a diversity of instruments (scales, tests, etc.), and, finally, the integration of all collected information in order to meet the demand. In other words, assessment is dependent upon the case's demand.

In science, description, classification, prediction/prognosis, explanation, and/or control and evaluation are the most common objectives. The most frequent assessment demands in geropsychology refer to the diagnosis, prognosis, placement, treatment, and evaluation of the older adult. Since diagnosis is the condition for treatment inclusion and for programme or services eligibility, diagnosis is one of the most frequent demands. Nevertheless, clinical problems require tailored treatment or interventions; in those cases, a comprehensive assessment must be performed in order to describe problematic conditions as well as those individual resources needed for designing a given treatment. Finally, assessment is sometimes performed to evaluate treatment effects; usually treatment evaluation is performed through pre-post testing designs, so that baseline assessment measures are taken prior to the treatment (Nezu and Nezu 2008). However, other treatment and/or intervention programmes may be evaluated through a 'goal attainment' strategy (e.g. Kiresuk and Lund 1977). In sum, assessment is required for any type of behavioural change through treatment, and all treatment requires evaluation and follow-up.

COMPREHENSIVE, MULTIDIMENSIONAL, AND MULTILEVEL ASSESSMENT

Assessing older adults from a clinical perspective requires a broad outlook that takes into account *multidimensional components* (biopsychosocial characteristics) assessed from a *multilevel perspective* (from the individual to the environment and the community). From a geriatric point of view, Gallo, Reichel, and Andersen (1988), Fletcher (1998), and Rubinstein and Rubinstein (1991) emphasize the need for multidimensional assessment of the older patient (sensory functions, mobility, mental and physical conditions, use of medicine and social environment). Also, geropsychologists (Fernández-Ballesteros and Pinquart 2011; Kane and Kane 1981; Wahl and Lehr 2002) consider that psychological assessment must be *comprehensive, multidimensional*, and performed from a *multilevel* perspective. Comprehensive, multidimensional and multilevel assessment is based on the three characteristics of the psychology of ageing already highlighted:

1. The multidirectionality of psychological change across the ageing process—that is, the impairment of certain behaviours and growth in others–is usually present in the same individual; therefore, the geropsychologist must assess not only psychopathological functioning but also potential competences and assets (e.g. Baltes et al. 2006; Heckhausen, Dixon, and Baltes 1989).
2. The three most prevalent problems in old age—dementia, depression, and dependency—are not only broad and complex, but also closely associated with one another (see chapters in this Handbook on Functional Sequelae of Cognitive Decline in Later Life; Late-life Depression; and Late-life Anxiety); therefore, older adults in the clinical context must be assessed considering the possibility of chronic multi-pathologies (e.g. Kane and Kane 2000).
3. Age is not the most important or the only determinant of psychopathology in old age, with personal and socio-environmental circumstances playing an important role in healthy and pathological processes (Wahl and Gitlin 2007). Therefore, the assessment of an older adult must cover the examination of contextual conditions at the family, community, and social levels in order to arrive at a comprehensive diagnosis, and, in turn, the best intervention.

The main content areas for assessment can be grouped as follows: Functionality and Activities of Daily Living (ADL), Physical Fitness and Health, Cognitive Functioning, Mental Health, Affect and Control, Social Functioning, Environmental Resources, and Quality of Life.

Assessment instruments

The APA guidelines for psychological practice with older adults state that 'psychologists strive to be familiar with theory, research, and practice of various methods of assessment with older adults, and knowledgeable of assessment instruments that are psychometrically suitable for use with them' (Art. 11, APA 2004: 237). These guidelines imply that multidimensional components must be assessed through a diversity of assessment tools developed on the basis of certain methods with a series of psychometric or statistical guarantees.

As stressed by several authors, assessment tools can be based on several methods for data collection: observation, objective tasks, self-report, other-relative reports, and subjective methods (see Fernández-Ballesteros 1992, 2003, 2004). To consider some examples, in the field of ADL, the *Assessment of Living Skills and Resources* (ALSAR; Clemson et al. 2008; Drinka et al. 2000; Williams et al. 1991), focuses on the accomplishment of tasks, and is therefore based on the assessor's observation of the patient's skills in performing ADLs. The Lawton *Instrumental Activities of Daily Living* (IADL) is a self-report assessment procedure, while the *Katz Index* of Independence in Activities of Daily Living (ADL) is a clinical scale to be scored by an expert. It can be concluded that since methodological categories usually have similar sources of errors (e.g. all self-reports have similar sets of bias, such as social desirability or faking either good or bad, depending on circumstances; and self-monitoring and observation are threatened, for example, by reactivity), the use of several instruments based on different methods should improve the quality of results through a process of 'triangulation'.

Moreover, the use of several methods is not only recommended from a methodological point of view, it is also supported from a theoretical perspective. Thus, most assessment content comprises complex constructs (such as health, quality of life, or memory) whose empirical definition is also difficult. As recommended from a *multiplism* perspective, complex constructs should be assessed through a set of selected *methods/instruments/measures*. Thus, Cook (1985) suggests a multiplism perspective from a post-positivist position: multiple dimensions assessed through multiple methods and multiple instruments/measures is the only possibility for conducting a scientifically sound assessment. For example, in the assessment of cognitive impairment, a set of questions in a mental examination cannot be sufficient: it is also necessary to consider the assessment of cognitive functioning through the administration of cognitive ability tests (memory, learning, language), neuropsychological tools and other medical examinations. In addition, for the assessment of ADL, self-reported scales must be complemented with expert observations in order to avoid the self-report bias frequently found in older adults (see Fernández-Ballesteros and Zamarrón 1996). Therefore, following the multiplism perspective, multidimension/multimethod/multi-instrument assessment is recommended in order to triangulate all the variables involved in a given case.

Psychometric properties

Geropsychology guidelines suggest that instruments must be selected on the basis of their *psychometric properties* or the proven scientific guarantees they offer for responding to the demands of the assessment. When a set of questions, problems, or items is drawn up in order to obtain a score and make comparisons among individuals, from the classical theory of tests (e.g. APA 1999), reliability and validity are the most important scientific properties it should show.

Reliability refers to the extent to which a score on a certain test is free from *measurement errors*. Three sources of error are usually considered: the degree of diversity of items included in the test; the extent to which test administration at different times and on different occasions yields different results; and, finally, the extent to which different raters, observers, interviewers, or test administrators obtain different results. These three sources of error are tested in terms of *internal consistency, test-retest reliability*, and *inter-rater reliability*. It must be borne in mind that the most appropriate reliability property of a given instrument depends on its nature (in an objective test in which administrators have no influence on the score yielded, inter-rater reliability would make no sense). In sum, on deciding which instrument to select for assessing a given older patient with a given set of issues, these three ways of evaluating reliability must be taken into consideration.

From a very simplistic perspective, the *validity* of an instrument or measurement tool is defined as the degree to which it measures what it claims to measure. Nevertheless, the concept of validity is a highly complex scientific property, referring not to a given instrument or test but to the *inference* made from it; in other words, we cannot look for *valid instruments*, but we can seek tools that will help us to arrive at a *valid inference* or conclusion. This is not the place to address this methodological issue; here we shall briefly describe those types of validity frequently covered in the field of geropsychological assessment.

It is important to start with the type of inference required in our assessment demand. If the demand is to arrive at a clinical diagnosis, the best validity indicator is one with high sensitivity and specificity. Being sensitive means detecting the relevant clinical problem if present (very few *false negative* results), while being specific means not detecting other diagnoses (very few *false positive* results). A prerequisite of many measurement instruments is *content validity* or 'the systematic examination of the test content to determine whether it covers a representative sample of the behaviour domain to be measured' (Anastasi and Urbina 1997: 114). Other types of demand require concurrent or predictive power or, in other words, the assessment of the extent to which a given measure can be associated with other measures (of the same conceptual network) at present (*concurrent validity*) or in the future (*predictive validity*). When a very high-level construct—such as extraversion or memory ability—is to be assessed, the *convergent* validity (to what extent the test is associated with other theoretically sound measures) and *discriminant* validity (to what extent a test is *not* associated with other theoretically sound measures) provide bases for selecting an instrument.

However, when the assessment tool is required for the evaluation of a certain programme (e.g. in psycho-stimulation training), *experimental validity* is necessary. Messick (1984, 1989, 1995) proposed that validity be judged relative to the extent to which scores can be changed as a consequence of a given treatment or training programme. This type of validity can be understood as the concept of consequential validity and utility proposed by Messick, but the appropriateness of a measure for use in the evaluation of a given treatment or intervention programme is also called *sensitivity* or *responsiveness*, defined as the ability to detect change over time.

Finally, it must be stated that the properties mentioned endorse the quality of a given method/instrument/measure, but this is irrelevant if there is no previous information about their *appropriateness for older adults*. In other words, there is an extensive body of literature regarding the psychometric properties of instruments with which the geropsychologist should be familiar (for a review, see APA 1999).

Up to now, we have dealt only with the scientific properties required in normative instruments, but there are also idiographic methods and measures that can be helpful for assessing the more idiosyncratic characteristics of older adults. For example, Antonucci and Akiyama (1987) developed an open protocol for assessing number and proximity of social contacts; Birren and Deutchman (1991; see also Birren and Schroots 2006) and Svensson and Randall (2003) introduced the autobiography as a critical resource in between psychological assessment and psychotherapy. Finally, Neimeyer and Hagans (2002) developed a series of narrative procedures and an adaptation of the Repertory Grid technique for assessing how older adults give meaning to their experiences. For example, constructs such as 'friendliness' or 'madness' yielded as relevant constructs by a given person can be explored through such narrative techniques (see http://www.wiley.com//legacy/wileychi/easyguide/ for more information about repertory grids).

Thus, as emphasized by Fernández-Ballesteros and Pinquart (2011), an important aspect of the assessment of older persons is that it should cover both the idiographic examination of subjective functioning and also nomothetic assessment, with comparisons between individuals, criteria, or cut-off for diagnosis, using normative samples of older adults.

The process of assessment–intervention–evaluation

As has been pointed out by the European Association of Psychological Assessment (EAPA) Guidelines for the Assessment Process (GAP; Fernández-Ballesteros et al. 2001), psychological assessment is a long process of decision-making and problem-solving starting when a given person/institution (client) asks a certified geropsychologist a question about a single case, in our case an older adult with a clinical problem. This question can involve operations such as description, classification (or diagnosis), prediction, intervention, and evaluation. GAPs consist of ninety-six guidelines organized in four main steps: (1) analysing the case (descriptive assessment); (2) organizing and reporting results; (3) planning the intervention (and carrying it out); and (4) intervention evaluation and follow-up.

Although some authors use 'assessment' and 'evaluation' as interchangeable terms, Cronbach (1990) has emphasized that assessment refers to an individual (or group of individuals), whereas evaluation is concerned with treatments or interventions. In the evaluation literature, there are commonly general recommendations about how to select sensitive, efficient, reliable, and valid targets for evaluating change (dependent variables) and which are the most suitable designs (e.g. Nezu and Nezu 2008).

As suggested by Fernández-Ballesteros and Pinquart (2011), three main recommendations regarding treatment evaluation in old age can be highlighted: (1) As has already been stressed, the use of multiple measures and multiple informants is required. (2) 'Maturation' is an important threat to treatment validity in older adults because 'maturation'—in our case it could be 'decline' or 'deterioration'—is one of the internal validity threats defined as changes in participants over time (age) and confounded with treatment effects. (3) In common practice, use of a multiple-baseline design can help target multiple measures from multiple informants assessed over time.

Finally, it must be pointed out that this assessment–intervention–evaluation process takes place through the *interaction of geropsychologist-assessor and the older adult-assessee*. As already pointed out, from the assessor perspective, APA guideline 2 states that assessors must be aware that their stereotypes and attitudes about ageing, age, and the aged could be influencing their professional behaviour, as extensively tested by social psychologists. Fiske et al. (2002) point out, from an international perspective, that professionals' views about older people involve 'low competence' and 'high kindness' and that these components lead to paternalistic prejudice. Furthermore, Bustillos and Fernández-Ballesteros (2011) found that in contexts where personnel reported more positive images of competence, older adults showed more positive functioning in accordance with the professionals' behaviours. Geropsychologists should be aware of their own images about the assessee.

Finally, since there is usually a cohort distance between assessor and client, some clients' historical and personal characteristics could be neglected by the assessor. For example, the assessor needs to be aware that the older client could have a low educational level, or be less accustomed to psychological consultation, and unused to being assessed. Likewise, the assessor should take into account sensory conditions (such as the need for help with hearing or vision), as well as the fact that older clients tire more easily than others, before starting the assessment sessions—or even before deciding the most suitable time for the assessment sessions and the number of sessions.

MAIN DOMAINS OF ASSESSMENT: INSTRUMENTS AND MEASURES

If we enter 'older adults' ('old people', 'the elderly') 'assessment' ('tools', 'measurement devices', 'instruments', 'psychological tests') in Google Scholar, we find over three million entries. Consequently, we can state that there are a very large number of assessment tools for older adults. Given the limitations of space in a chapter devoted to assessment in the international context of clinical geropsychology, the goal here was to select the best instruments and measures, taking an international view and with the previously outlined theoretical perspectives in mind.

The procedure followed for selecting the domains, and in turn, the instruments and measures, was: (1) examination of the main psychology databases: PSYCINFO, PSYCARTICLES PSICODOC; CSI ISOC; PSYCBOOKS; PSYCCRITIQUES; (2) examination of biomedical databases: MEDLINE (EBSCO); PUBMED (National Library of Medicine); CSIC IME; (3) examination of WEB Knowledge (ISI), WEB of Science; Journal Citation Reports. The inclusion criterion for an instrument or measure is that it was present in at least two of the three database groups. Finally, the instruments were classified in the following domains: (1) Functionality and Activities of Daily Living; (2) Physical Functioning and

Health; (3) Cognitive Functioning; (4) Mental Health, Affect, and Satisfaction; (5) Social Functioning; (6) The Environment; and (7) Quality of Life.

Functionality and activities of daily living

The most widely studied domain in the assessment of older adults is functionality for Activities of Daily Living (ADL), or the person's ability to perform activities in order to have an independent life. ADLs can refer to performing *basic* (walking, eating, etc.) or *instrumental* activities (IADLs) (shopping, cleaning the house, etc.) (e.g. Pearson 2000; Spector 1990). This domain is usually assessed through the level of difficulty in performing basic or instrumental activities reported by the older person (or by a relative or care-giver), or by observing performance. The ADL assessment is close to the disability evaluation of the International Classification of Impairments, Disabilities, and Handicaps (ICIDH) proposed by the World Health Organization (2001).

An annotated selection of the assessment instruments and measures from this domain is described, including four instruments for assessing activities of daily living (see Table 10.1). Different forms of assessment and the activities most commonly included in this domain are presented.

Physical functioning and health status

ADLs depend on and are based on physical functioning and health, which is especially relevant for predicting several health problems associated with ageing, as well as providing significant data for the evaluation of rehabilitation programmes. Therefore, physical functioning can be assessed for description, diagnostic, prognosis, and evaluation purposes. The assessment of physical functioning usually includes objective measures (peak flow, grip strength, etc.). Sometimes these are assessed by self-report ('how do you feel after walking a mile'), converting this domain into a subjective condition. Basic physical measures such as balance, strength and vital capacity are shown in Table 10.2.

In addition, disability and dependency are the results of illness, so health is one of the most commonly assessed domains in older people, not only on the part of medical doctors but also on the part of others, such as social workers, psychologists, and other healthcare providers. Although medical examinations, clinical records and other types of evaluation are required for accurate diagnosis, reported health is also an important source of information. This broad area includes perceived health, symptoms, diagnoses, health resources available, healthy life styles, and so on.

Due to limitations of space in this chapter, only two general health assessment instruments will be presented here. The first one, shown in Table 10.3, is the Medical Outcome Study 36-Item Short Form Survey (SF-36), which was designed to measure general health status in different contexts: clinical, research, and gerontological services. This survey is usually considered to be a health-related quality-of-life questionnaire reporting relevant information about health. Second, the Mini Nutritional Assessment (MNA) is included in Table 10.3. We consider nutritional status to be especially important, with regard to health since nutrition is significantly related to several health problems, including being overweight, having poor

Table 10.1 Functionality and activities of daily living (ADL)

Instruments	Authors	Objective	Description	Administration	Population	Score and Norms	Statistical properties	Use
Katz Index of Independence in Activities of Daily Living (ADL)	S. Katz, A. B. Ford, A. W. Moskowitz, B. A. Jackson, M. W. Jaffe (1963).	Functional assessment of the health status and assistance received.	6 items: bathe, dress, toilet, transfer, feed self, and continence.	Self-report/ trained observers.	Ill or disabled old people.	3-point scale/item. 8-point hierarchical overall score from A: independent to G: total dependent.	Several reports of: (1) construct, content, concurrent and predictive (health status and mortality) validity, and (2) scale reliability and internal consistency ($\alpha > .87$). (Wallace 1998).	Treatment changes and prognosis.
Assessment of Living Skills and Resources (ALSAR)	J. Williams, T. Drinka, J. Greenberg, J. Farrell-Holtan, R. Euhardy, and P. Schram (1991).	Rate people's skills and available resources for each IADL task.	11 items: reading, telephone, medication, money, meals, laundry, housekeeping, maintenance, transportation, shopping, and leisure.	An interview, supplemented with observation of skills by an expert.	Over 60 years old.	3-point scale (0–2) is obtained for Skill level, Resource level, and a combination of the two, which is called Risk for each IADL. There is also a Total Risk Score 'R-score' (0–44): over 20 = moderate risk, over 30 = high risk.	Internal consistency ($\alpha = .90$). Construct validity: correlates significantly ($r = .58$) with Barthel Index. Predictive validity of R-score for negative outcomes.	Classification, prognosis and treatment design.

(Continued)

Table 10.1 Continued

Instruments	Authors	Objective	Description	Administration	Population	Score and Norms	Statistical properties	Use
Assessment of Motor and Process Skills (AMPS)	A.G. Fisher (1997).	Rate quality of effort, efficiency, safety, and independence.	16 ADL motor and 20 ADL process skill items, within the context of performing the chosen.	Interview to determine which tasks are familiar, relevant and of sufficient challenge to the person being evaluated. Then, the person performs each self-chosen task in a familiar environment the way he or she usually does it.	Over 3 years old.	4-point scale/item. AMPS software reports normalized standard scores, standardized z-scores, and percentile rank.	Several studies report intra-rater, inter-rater, and test-retest reliability and validity across age, gender, ethnic group, and world region. (Fisher and Bernspång 2007; Fisher and Bray Jones 2010; Hayase et al. 2004).	Cross-cultural. Treatment design.

| Functional Independence Measure (FIM) | B. B. Hamilton, C. V. Granger, F. S. Sherwin, M. Zielezny, and J. S. Tashman (1987). | Physical and cognitive disability, rating by the level of care burden. | 6 scales: Self-care (Eating, Grooming, Bathing/showering, Dressing upper body, Dressing lower body and Toileting); Sphincters (Bladder management and Bowel management); Mobility (Transfers: bed/chair/wheelchair, Transfers: toilet, Transfers: bathtub/shower, Locomotion: walking/wheelchair and Locomotion: stairs); Communication (Expression and Comprehension); Psychosocial (Social interaction), Cognition (Problem-solving and Memory). | Trained observers. It takes 30 minutes. | Older adults, clinical samples, at-risk samples. | 7-point scale/item. Total score from 18 = dependent to 126 = independent. | Good test-retest reliability of motor subscale (ICC = .9) and cognitive subscale (ICC = .8). Kappa > .45 Construct validity of the motor and cognitive subscales. | Research, clinical, and administrative purposes. |

Table 10.2 Physical functioning

Instruments	Authors	Objective	Description	Administration	Population	Score and Norms	Statistical properties	Use
Hand Grip Strength Test	T. Rantanen J. M. Guralnik, D. Foley, K. Masaki, S. Leveille, J. D. Curb, et al. (1999).	Measure the maximum isometric strength of the hand and forearm muscles.	The person has to press a dynamometer hard with the hands.	The subject holds the dynamometer in the hand to be tested.	30–85 yrs old, from 7 European countries (Fernández-Ballesteros et al. 2004).	Strength is measured by kilogrammes moved. Several studies rate the scores according to age and gender.	Predictive validity: disability, mortality. Dynamometer may need to be calibrated regularly, therefore is difficult to have normative data.	Physical fitness. Ageing process.
Berg Balance Scale	K. O. Berg, S. L Wood-Dauphinee, J. T. Williams, and D. Gayton, (1989).	Measure of Balance.	13 items: Sitting to standing, Standing unsupported, Sitting unsupported, Standing to sitting, Transfers, Standing with eyes closed, Standing with feet together, Reaching forward with an outstretched arm, Retrieving object from floor, Turning to look behind, Turning 360°, Placing alternate foot on stool and Standing with one foot in front of the other foot and Standing on one foot.	Observation of the task performance. The equipment needed is: step stool, mat table, chair with arms, tape measure, stopwatch, pen, and table.	Older adults.	5-point scale/ item (0–4) rating by the quality of the performance or the time taken to complete the task. Total score 56. A score over 45 means impaired and risk for falling.	Poor sensitivity and high specificity for falling status and assistive device use. Inter-rater reliability ICC = .98 (Thorbahn, L. D. and Newton, R. A. 1996)	Predict risk of falling.

Modified Gait Abnormality Rating Scale (GARSm)	J. M. Van Swearingen, K. A. Paschal, P. Bonino, J. F. Yang. (1996).	Measure risk of falling by rating the gait.	7 items: variability, guardedness, staggering, foot contact, hip ROM, shoulder extension, and arm-heel-strike synchrony.	Observation of gait.	Community dwelling, frail older adults.	4-point scale/item (0–3). The total score is the sum of the 7 individual items. It represents a rate of risk for falling based on gait abnormalities documented and the abnormality severity.	Intra-rater and inter-rater reliability: Kappa > .6; ICCs >. 9. Concurrent (stride lengths $r = -.754$; walking speed $r = -.679$) and construct (discriminates between subjects with and without a fall history) validity.	Prognosis.
Peak Expiratory Flow	B. M. Wright. (1959).	Measure person's maximum speed of expiration and the degree of obstruction in the airways.	The person has to blow through a meter, which reads between 60 and 800 litres per minute.	Trained interviewer.	Populations 30–85, from 7 European countries (Fernández-Ballesteros et al. 2004).	Measured by litres per minute or centimetres. There are normative rating scores for the EU attending to age and gender.	High predictive reliability of total mortality in elderly. Correlations with pulmonary symptoms and other indices of chronic disease. (Cook et al. 1989, 1991)	Asthma and breath problems monitoring, prognosis.

Table 10.3 Health

Instruments	Authors	Objective	Description	Administration	Population	Score and Norms	Statistical properties	Use
The Medical Outcome Study 36-Item Short Form Survey (SF-36)	J. E. Ware, C. D. Sherbourne (1992).	General health status.	8 domains: physical functioning, role-physical, bodily pain, general health, vitality, social functioning, role-emotional, and mental health.	High variety, including: self-administration, interview in person or by telephone and computerized adaptive testing. It takes approximately 10 minutes.	Over 14 yrs.	100-point scale (mean= 50; SD = 10). Higher scores mean better health.	Several studies report construct, criterion, content validity, and reliability: prediction of mortality; internal-consistency reliability from .67 to .90; high subscales test-retest reliability.	Clinical and research demand.
Mini Nutritional Assessment (MNA)	Nestle Research Center/ Clintec.	Person's nutrition status.	4 domains: Anthropometric Assessment, Global Evaluation, Dietetic Assessment, and Subjective Assessment.	Trained interviewer.	Frail older adults.	30-point scale. 24–30 = well-nourished; 17–23.5 = at risk of malnutrition; 0–17 = under-nutrition.	Sensitivity = 96%; Specificity = 98%; predictive value = 97% (mortality and hospital cost). Kappa = .51.	Part of a comprehensive geriatric assessment.

mobility, and cardiovascular diseases. MNA relates general health to anthropometric and dietetic assessment, potentially important components of a geropsychological assessment (Vellas et al. 1999).

Cognitive functioning

Cognitive functioning is one of the most important domains for assessment in older adults both because in normal ageing cognitive decline is common, and because of the prevalence of cognitive impairment due to some kind of dementia (see Langley 2000). As Rabbitt (2005) points out, through cognitive assessment, three main questions must be answered: when mental problems appeared and advanced rapidly; whether all mental abilities changed at the same rate; and to what extent cognitive decline can be considered significantly impaired. The relevance of cognitive functioning and mental status assessment in older adults is high, and there are three main objectives: (1) to detect and measure potential cognitive decline over time, identifying mental aptitudes profiles; (2) to detect, measure, and diagnose potential cognitive impairment due to some type of CNS illness; and (3) in case of decline or impairment, to be able to design an intervention programme to optimize cognitive functioning, to compensate decline and/or to slow the impairment process.

Three types of instruments can be used for assessing cognitive functioning and detecting the presence of potential cognitive decline and/or impairment: mental examinations, intelligence tests, and tests of learning. Among the first of these, the most internationally used are the Mini Mental State Examination (MMSE; Folstein et al. 1975), the Short Portable Mental Status Questionnaire (SPMSQ; Pfeiffer 1975; see Langley 2000), and the Montreal Cognitive Assessment (MoCa; Nasreddine et al. 2005), which are shown in Table 10.4. These are screening scales, with quick and easy administration.

However, in order to arrive at a diagnosis of cognitive impairment, much more sophisticated instruments are required to assess intelligence, memory, executive functioning, and learning. Table 10.5 shows five internationally used instruments including the Wechsler Adult Intelligence Scale (WAIS-IV) and the Reynolds Intellectual Assessment Scales (RIAS), measuring intelligence; the Rivermead Behavioral Memory Test (RBMT-3), assessing memory functioning; and the Delis–Kaplan Executive Function System™ (D–KEFS™), evaluating cognitive functioning. These four tests are useful not only to evaluate cognitive decline and memory problems, but also to identify preserved capacities that are important to consider on designing cognitive intervention. The fifth test, the AVLT (Auditory Verbal Learning Test), is a learning test which provides a learning profile useful for assessing cognitive plasticity, learning potential, as well as predicting cognitive modifiability (Fernández-Ballesteros et al. 2003, 2005; Lezak 2000; Van der Elst, Van Boxtel Van Breukelen, and Jolles 2005; Zamarrón, Tarrága, and Fernández-Ballesteros 2009).

Mental health, affect, and satisfaction

In the field of gerontology, there is a large body of work about mood and emotions. Within this domain, several instruments and measures have been developed with three different

Table 10.4 Cognitive functioning: mental status

Instruments	Authors	Objective	Description	Administration	Population	Score and Norms	Statistical properties	Use
Mini Mental State Examination (MMSE)	M. F. Folstein, S. Folstein, P. R. McHugh (1975).	Screening for cognitive impairment and dementia.	11 items: orientation, immediate and delayed episodic recall, working memory, language and visuospatial abilities.	Trained examiner. It takes approximately 10 minutes.	Clinical and national samples by age, gender, education, and context.	30-point scale based on sum of correct answers. Cut-off for level of severity of cognitive impairment by age and educational level.	Several studies report: sensitivity and specificity, reliability (test-retest, inter-rater, and internal consistency) and construct validity (correlates with other screening, intelligence and memory test).	Widely used for research and clinical demands.
Short Portable Mental Status Questionnaire (SPMSQ)	E. Pfeiffer (1975).	Screening cognitive impairment.	10 items about recent and past memory, memory for well-rehearsed and non-well-rehearsed information, orientation in place and time, and simple arithmetical abilities.	Trained interviewer. It takes approximately 5 minutes.	Clinical and general population by age, gender, education, and context.	10-point scale based on sum of errors. 0–2 errors = normal mental functioning; 3–4 errors = mild cognitive impairment; 5–7 errors = moderate cognitive impairment; 8–10 errors: severe cognitive impairment.	Using a cut-off of 3 errors: sensitivity and specificity are over 84% for detecting cognitive impairment.	Research and clinical demands.

| Montreal Cognitive Assessment (MoCa) | Z. Nasreddine et al. (2005) http://www.mocatest.org/default.asp. | It is a cognitive screening test to assess mild cognitive impairment | 11 items that assess: attention and concentration, executive functions, memory, language, visuoconstructional skills, conceptual thinking, calculations, and orientation. | Time to administer is approximately 10 minutes. | Clinical and general population by education. | 30-point scale based on sum of correct answers; a score of 26 or above is considered normal. Add one point for an individual who has 12 years or fewer of formal education | Detected MCI with 90–96% range sensitivity and specificity of 87% with 95% confidence interval and detected 100% of Alzheimer's dementia with a specificity of 87%. (Nasreddine et al. 2005). | Research and clinical demands. |

Table 10.5 Cognitive functioning: intelligence, memory, and learning

Instruments	Authors	Objective	Description	Administration	Population	Score and Norms	Statistical properties	Use
Wechsler Adult Intelligence Scale (WAIS–IV)	D. Wechsler (2008).	Rate intelligence and quality of cognitive processes.	15 subtests divided into 4 scales: Verbal Comprehension Index, Perceptual Reasoning Index, Working Memory Index, and Processing Speed Index.	Trained examiner.	People 16–90 yrs old.	Scale scores and total score are obtained (Mean = 100 SD = 15). Normative scores rating by age.	High reliability and validity data are reported by several studies.	Classification, description, prediction, or planning of interventions.
Reynolds Intellectual Assessment Scales (RIAS)	C. R. Reynolds, R. W. Kamphaus. (2003).	Measure general intelligence.	6 subtests: 2 Verbal intelligence, 2 Nonverbal intelligence, and 2 General memory.	Trained examiner. It takes approximately 25 minutes.	People 3–94 years old.	Provide a verbal and nonverbal intelligence score, whose resulting combination is the Composite Intelligence Index (CIX). Manual explains how to calculate scores and provides a range of scores (T and Z scores).	Several studies report high different validity coefficients. Reliability coefficients between .83 and 1.	

Rivermead Behavioral Memory Test—Third Edition (RBMT-3)	First edition: B. A. Wilson, J. Cockburn, and A. Baddeley (1985).	It was designed to predict everyday memory problems in people with acquired, non-progressive brain injury, and to monitor change over time.	14 scored subtests which assess memory for names and objects, design recognition, orientation, faces, appointments, routes, messages, dates, and stories.	Trained interviewer. It takes 30 minutes. There are 2 versions that allow retesting.	People 16–89 yrs old.	Provides subtests and total score (GMI), which is standardized to have mean = 100 and SD = 15.	Sensitive to memory deficits. Third edition manual reports: subtest reliability coefficients ranged from 0.57 to 0.86 and GMI reliability coefficient = .87. Several studies report good index of validity and reliability (.67–1).	Rehabilitation and treatment changes.
Auditory Verbal Learning Test (AVLT)	List of words A. Rey (1964). Training design (see: Lezak 2000; Fernández-Ballesteros et al. 2003, 2005)	Measures recent memory, verbal learning, susceptibility to (proactive and retroactive) interference, retention of information after a certain period of time during which other activities are performed, and recognition memory.	It consists of 2 lists of 15 words. 6 trials: pre-test and 5 trials with different learning resources: repetition, feedback, and reinforcement. After an interference task: a free recall trial.	Trained interviewer. It takes approximately 40 minutes.	Over-55s, Alzheimer's disease patients, mild cognitive impairment older adults.	Score from 6 Trials; Gain score (T6–T1); Free recall after interference (T7). Normative data by age (55–102 years old) and pathology. Fernández-Ballesteros et al. (2012).	Sensitivity (89%) to classify healthy older adults, mild cognitive impaired (MCI) individuals, and Alzheimer's disease patients.	Assessment of learning potential, cognitive plasticity, and modifiability (Zamarrón et al. 2010).

(Continued)

Table 10.5 Continued

Instruments	Authors	Objective	Description	Administration	Population	Score and Norms	Statistical properties	Use
Delis–Kaplan Executive Function System™ (D-KEFS™)	D.C. Delis, E. Kaplan, and J.H. Kramer (2001).	Developed to evaluate executive functions believed to be mediated by the frontal lobe, such as: flexibility of thinking, inhibition, problem-solving, planning, impulse control, concept formation, abstract thinking, and creativity.	9 subtests which assess: Trail Making, Verbal Fluency, Design Fluency, Colour–Word Interference, Sorting, Twenty Questions, Word Context, Tower, and Proverb.	Trained examiner. Variable depending on subtest selected to apply, full battery takes 90 minutes. It includes alternate versions of: Verbal Fluency, Sorting, Twenty Questions	People 8–89 years old.	Record and score the nine D-KEFS subtests as a complete battery or as individual subtests	Normed data on stratified sample of 1,750. Reliability and Validity completed for individual subtests vs aggregate for entire battery deemed adequate.	Classification, description, prediction, or planning of interventions.

aims: (1) to measure mental disorders such as anxiety and depression; (2) to measure positive mental health; and (3) to assess affect and control.

With regard to mental disorders, special attention must be paid to certain psychopathological problems, which differ from the symptoms presented by younger populations and can be confounded with other disorders. For example, depressed older adults may present memory problems or somatic symptoms that may be confounded with dementia. In Table 10.6, we describe the Geriatric Depression Scale (Yesevage et al. 1983), which does not include somatic symptoms, to assess depression in later life. Moreover, although anxiety seems to be less prevalent than depression in older adults, anxiety can be difficult to diagnose because it is hard to distinguish whether or not the symptoms might in fact be due to a medical condition or to medication.

As in depression, the anxiety symptoms described for adolescents and adults (wobbliness in legs, hands trembling, and fear of losing control) can be confounded by symptoms of diseases prevalent in later life and normal age-related decline (Parkinson's, dementia, decline in muscle strength). Therefore, it is recommended that anxiety is measured on the basis of normative data for older adults, including those suffering from any illness. Thus, Table 10.6 also describes the Geriatric Anxiety Inventory, which was developed for the purpose of accurately classifying whether normal older people and psychogeriatric patients suffer from anxiety.

On the other hand, within geropsychological assessment, particular attention must be paid to mental health (from a positive point of view), life satisfaction, and positive and negative emotions. Keyes (2005) has reported that affect seems not to be a continuum from negative to positive, but rather two different factors that correlate, which means that the opposite of mental health is not the lack of any disorders. Therefore, measures of positive affect are considered as important as measures of negative affect because they can show positive aspects and resources of the individual as expressions of (mental) health. Thus, Table 10.7 describes three instruments widely used in older adult populations: the Mental Health Continuum Short Form (MHC-SF), the Positive Affect and Negative Affect Scale (PANAS), and the Philadelphia Geriatric Morale Scale (PGCMS).

Social functioning

Throughout the history of gerontology, social functioning has been a basic domain affecting many other older adult conditions, such as disability, health, life satisfaction, and positive mood, and is an indicator for healthy or active ageing (see Antonucci and Akiyama 1987; Fernández-Ballesteros 2008; Fiori, Smith, and Antonucci 2007; Levin 2000).

Social functioning is also a broad domain, requiring the assessment of a range of variables: family and social network (e.g. number of members in the network, contact frequency), family and social support (e.g. instrumental and affective support, satisfaction), social resources (e.g. availability, use, satisfaction), social roles (e.g. receiving care, providing care), social activity, and social productivity. This broad variety of social factors includes objective measures (number of friends and family members, number of contacts, availability of social resources, frequency of unpaid productive activities, etc.) and subjective measures (satisfaction with family and social relationships, closeness, etc.).

Table 10.6 Mental health

Instruments	Authors	Objective	Description	Administration	Population	Score and Norms	Statistical properties	Use
Geriatric Depression Scale (GDS)	J. A. Yesevage, T. L Brink, T. L. Rose, O. Lum, V. Huang, M. D. Adey, M. D. Leirer (1983). J. I. Sheikh, and J. A. Yesavage (1986).	Assess depression in older adults.	30 items. The scale includes a list of depressive symptoms avoiding somatic aspects that can lead to diagnosing false positives in this population.	Self-report. It takes between 5–10 minutes.	Older adults (it seems not to work accurately with cognitively impaired people).	Dichotomous items (yes or no). Cut-off for different depression severity.	Specificity: 95% Studies report that the GDS constitutes a reliable and valid screening device for measuring depression in the elderly.	Assessing dimensional depression.
Geriatric Anxiety Inventory (GAI)	N. A. Pachana, G. J. Byrne, H. Siddle, N. Koloski, E. Harley, E. Arnold (2007).	Measure common symptoms of anxiety in older adults.	20 describing general clinical symptoms and subsyndromal expressions of anxiety.	Self-report or interview.	Normal older people and psychogeriatric people.	Yes/no response. Total score is the sum of 'yes' responses. Cut-off = 10/11.	Reliability: Cronbach'α = 0.91 for normal older people and 0.93 in a psychogeriatric simple. Inter-rater and test-retest reliability were found to be excellent. Sensitivity of 75% and specificity of 84%. Concurrent validity measured by correlation with other tools.	Assessing dimensional anxiety.

Table 10.7 Positive mental health, affect, and satisfaction

Instruments	Authors	Objective	Description	Administration	Population	Score and Norms	Statistical properties	Use
Mental Health Continuum Short Form (MHC–SF)	C. L. M. Keyes (2005).	Measure mental health as flourishing.	14 items, organized in 3 domains: emotional well-being (happy, interested in life, and satisfied), psychological well-being (self-acceptance, personal growth, purpose in life, environmental mastery, autonomy, and positive relations with others), and social well-being (social acceptance, social actualization, social contribution, social coherence, and social integration).	Self-report, interview in person or by telephone.	Adolescents and adults.	6-point scale, indicating frequency of experienced symptoms of mental health.	Internal consistency > .80 and discriminant validity in adolescents and adults. Test-retest reliability from .57 to .71, depending on the subscale and the time elapsed between the 2 assessments. The 3-factor structure has been confirmed in adolescents and adults.	Assessment of positive mental health.
Positive Affect and Negative Affect Scale (PANAS)	D. Watson, L. A. Clark, A. Tellegen (1988).	Measure mood status: negative (NA) and positive (PA) affect independently.	A list of 10 positive and 10 negative adjectives. The person has to report about the feeling intensity or frequency for a period of time (at this moment, today, the past few days, the past week, the past few weeks, the past year, and generally).	Self-report.	General population.	5-point scale per adjective. The result is an average of the score on each list.	Reliability: Cronbach's α range for PA = .86–.90 and for NA = .84–.87. Test-retest correlations for an 8-week period range for PA = .47–.68 and for NA = .39–.71; for the general time period, PA =.68 and NA = .71. Construct validity is reported by correlation with depression and anxiety scales (negative with PA and positive with NA).	Assessing positive and negative emotion and assessing balance.

(Continued)

Table 10.7 Continued

Instruments	Authors	Objective	Description	Administration	Population	Score and Norms	Statistical properties	Use
Philadelphia Geriatric Morale Scale (PGCMS)	M. P. Lawton (1975).	It measures perceived morale in elderly people through 3 factors: agitation, attitude toward own ageing, and lonely dissatisfaction.	17 items.	Self-report or interviewer.	People aged 70 to 90.	Dichotomous items (agree or disagree). Total score is the sum of high-morale responses (0–17). Scores ranged from 13–17 = high scores on the morale scale; 10–12 = mid-range; and 0–9 = lower end.	Factor analysis of the scale identified the 3 main factors: agitation, dissatisfaction, and attitudes towards one's own ageing with Cronbach's α of 0.85, 0.81 and 0.85, respectively. Construct validity reported by correlation with other well-being measures.	Assessing life satisfaction.

Table 10.8 Social functioning

The Lubben Social Network Scale—Revised (LSNS-R)

Authors	J. E. Lubben (1988, 2002).
Objective	Gauge social isolation in older adults by measuring perceived social support from family and friends.
Description	12 items which measure size, closeness, and frequency of contacts of a respondent's social network; number of family members and friends the older adult contacts and how frequently; they also inquire about helping others, having confidants, being a confidant, and current living arrangements.
Administration	Self-administered questionnaire with health professionals as informants. Takes 5–10 minutes to complete.
Population	Older people in any context.
Score and Norms	6-points scale/item ranging from 0 to 5. Total score is the sum of the item scores, and ranges from 0 to 60. The higher the score, the greater the social integration. Score < 20 = isolated; 21–25 = high risk for isolation; 26–30 = moderate risk for isolation; > 30 low risk for isolation.
Statistical properties	Mean internal consistency: Cronbach's α = .78.
Use	Clinical and research demands.

Due to the complexity of social functioning, assessment procedures usually cover no more than a few of these factors. It is very difficult to find instruments embracing all of them, and several authors recommend qualitative procedures for assessing social functioning. One of the most widely used instruments is the *Lubben Social Network Scale— revised* (LSNS-R; Lubben 1988), which is a short and quite complete instrument that measures social functioning accurately, and is briefly described in Table 10.8.

Finally, in an effort to cover both qualitative and quantitative social functioning information, we also consider the *Convoy of Social Relations* based on the Kahn and Antonucci Convoy Model (1980). The instrument was developed by Antonucci and Akiyama (1987) and has been widely used across the lifespan and internationally (Antonucci, Akiyama, and Takahashi 2004). The format protocol consists in a diagram showing in the middle 'the subject' ('you') surrounded by three concentric circles, as shown in Figure 10.1. The examiner asks the respondent/s to place in the first circle of the diagram the names of the people 'whom it was hard to imagine life without'; in the middle circle of the network diagram to place those to 'whom you may not feel quite that close'; and, finally, in the outer circle, to place those 'whom you have not already mentioned but who are close enough and important enough in your life that they should be placed in your personal network'. Respondents are instructed that the overall network size was the count of the total number of people mentioned in the diagram, and more questions follow on the structural (e.g. age, sex, closeness, years known, proximity, and frequency of contact) and functional (number and types of support provided and received) characteristics of their social networks.

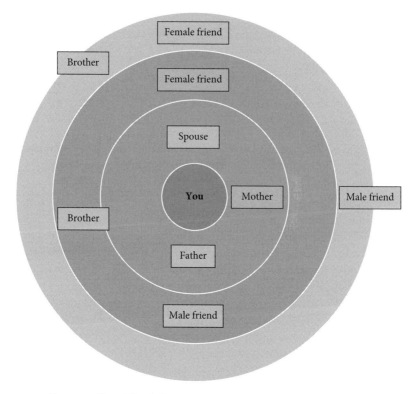

FIGURE 10.1 Convoy of social relations.

Reproduced from Attachment and close relationships across the life span, Toni Antonucci, Hiroko Akiyama, and Keiko Takahashi, *Attachment & Human Development*, 6(4), pp. 353–70, (c) 2004, Taylor and Francis. Reprinted by permission of the publisher (Taylor & Francis Ltd, http://www.tandf.co.uk/journals).

The environment

This domain refers to the person's environmental quality. It includes not only the place where the person lives (house, room, nursing home, residence, etc.) and the neighbourhood or surroundings (facilities available, safety, accessibility, etc.), but also social and political variables. Cutler (2000) defines four characteristics to define a successful universal environment: (1) supportive, referring to the possibility of providing substitutes for a loss of functioning, with the aim of promoting independence; (2) accessibility, regarding possible access, for example, by a person using a wheelchair; (3) adaptability, such as the possibility to modify the environment to adjust to different levels of disability; and (4) safety, with regard to being protected against hazards.

The importance of environmental assessment derives from the required person–environment fit (see Wahl and Iwarsson 2007; Fernandez-Ballesteros 2001). In other words, the environment must be assessed in order to arrive at an adjustment between environmental pressure and the person's demands. For example, people who cannot walk will be able to continue going out and enjoying life if the environment where they live can provide a wheelchair and is accessible to it. In contrast, people with greater levels of competence want to maintain or even improve their environmental pressure, with a view to optimizing their functioning.

For assessing the environment, two instruments have been selected for evaluating older adults living in the community or in institutions. Their respective relevance depends on the context of the assessment and where the people assessed are living. *The Housing Enabler* (Iwarsson 1999) is an assessment tool for community-dwelling older adults, and measures the accessibility of the environment, taking into account personal disabilities and environmental barriers. The *Multiphasic Environmental Assessment Procedure* was developed by Moos and Lemke (1984, 1996) to measure different aspects of the residential setting (both personal and environmental) for older adults living in institutions: physical and architectural traits, organization and policy characteristics, social climate scales, and residents' and personnel characteristics. Fernández-Ballesteros (1996) developed a Spanish version—*Sistema de Evaluación de Residencias de Ancianos* (SERA)—adding three more residential characteristics: satisfaction, needs, and environment–behaviour interactions. The SERA has been widely used in Spanish-speaking countries and has also been translated into Portuguese. Both instruments are described in Table 10.9.

Quality of life

Quality of life (QoL) is the summit of the assessment pyramid, which means that it involves the qualification of most of the areas we have already addressed. This is why it has been considered an extremely complex, abstract, and scattered concept that is difficult to define (Fernández-Ballesteros 1997; Walker 2005). Indeed, some researchers have reduced it to health and subjective variables, which could be considered a poor and limited definition. In any case, it has great impact on research and practice, and is commonly included in ageing-assessment protocols.

Fernández-Ballesteros (1993, 2011) proposed an integration of this broad concept considering two dimensions: (1) personal or internal (physical functioning, social status, etc.) vs socio-environmental or external (residential comfort, health system, etc.) and (2) subjective (e.g. well-being or perceived health) vs objective (income, physical environment, etc.). Unfortunately, most of the available instruments for assessing QoL involve the subjective assessment of personal conditions, which converts QoL into a subjective concept closely akin to subjective health or/and personal well-being.

For the assessment of this domain, three instruments are selected and described in Table 10.10. The first is one of the most widely used, and has been translated into several languages: the *World Health Organization Quality of Life* (WHOQOL) assessment. It focuses on the subjective perception of different components of QoL. The second is the *Short Quality of Life Questionnaire* (CUBRECAVI), based on Fernández-Ballesteros' QoL concept (1993), and therefore including objective and subjective questions on the most important life aspects, which has been used in Latin American countries. Finally, the *Schedule for Evaluation of Individual QoL* (SEIQoL) is an idiographic instrument which allows the individual to name and weigh those domains of greatest relevance for their quality of life.

Table 10.9 The environment

Instruments	Authors	Objective	Description	Administration	Population	Score and Norms	Statistical properties	Use
The Housing Enabler	S. Iwarsson (1999).	Analyse accessibility problems by relating functional limitations and dependence on mobility devices to environmental barriers.	3 subscales: (1) P: Functional limitations (13 items) and dependence on mobility devices (2 items), (2) E: Physical environmental barriers: outdoor environment (33 items), entrances (49 items), indoor environment (100 items), and communication features (6 items), and (3) Calculation of accessibility score: combining scores on subscales 1 and 2.	Subscales 1 combines observation and interview, 2 uses observation, and 3 is a calculation of the results in subscales 1 and 2.	Older adults living at home.	For reliable and valid data collection and analysis, instrument-specific software is recommended. The degree of objective, norm-based person–environment fit problems in the home is calculated; higher scores mean more P–E fit problems.	Inter-rater reliability, content and construct validity have been reported (Iwarsson et al. 2005)	Research, teaching, and practice. It is also relevant for disciplines such as architecture, rehabilitation, occupational therapy, societal planning, and environmental gerontology.

| Multiphasic Environmental Assessment Procedure (MEAP/ SERA) | R. H. Moos and S. Lemke. (1984, 1996); R. Fernández-Ballesteros (1996); Fernández-Ballesteros et al. (1991) | Comprehensive assessment of person–environment adjustment: physical, organizational, social climate, and personal (residents' and personnel characteristics). | MEAP: 5 Scales: (1) Physical and architectural features (8 dimensions), (2) Policy and Organizational Characteristics (9 dimensions), (3) Residents and Staff Resources (7 dimensions), (4) Social Climate (7 dimensions). Also available is a (5) Rating scale (4 dimensions and 24 items). SERA: Adding to the MEAP 5 Environmental instruments the following: (6) Needs Schedule (open-ended self-report), (7) Satisfaction Questionnaire (7 items to residents and staff), (8) Behavioural, maps behaviour–environment. | Direct observation by trained raters, interview with staff and residents and self-reports individually or in groups depending on the scale. In total, it takes around 6–7 hours. | Nursing homes, residential facilities, and apartments. Community dwellings situation are not included. | Each subtest/ item is measured on scales with different numbers of points. They most require dichotomous answer (0/1) by item. Raw scores are in percentages. Both versions are standardized, providing T scores. | Subtest Internal reliability range between .47 and .99; inter-rater reliability runs from .69 to .99. | Assessment of facilities for older adults, planning changes and evaluation. Design of new residential settings. Relevant also for disciplines such as architecture, rehabilitation, occupational therapy, societal planning, and environmental gerontology. |

Table 10.10 Quality of life

Instruments	Authors	Objective	Description	Administration	Population	Score and Norms	Statistical properties	Use
The World Health Organization Quality of Life assessment (WHOQOL)	WHOQOL Group (1998).	General QoL instrument developed cross-culturally and systematically, and with different forms for different purposes.	WHOQOL-100 items divided into: subjective overall QoL and health (4 items), the individual's appraisal in 6 domains of QoL (Physical health, Psychological, Bodily image and appearance, Level of Independence/Mobility, Social relationships, Environment, and Spirituality/Religion/Personal beliefs), which cover 24 facets (4 items for each facet). WHOQOL-Brief (26), which is reduced to 1 item for each of the 24 facets.	Self-report or interview.	Different populations (healthy and with different illnesses) and countries to be compared.	All items are rated on a 5-point scale (1–5). Score relating to facets, domains, and overall QoL and general health.	Discriminant validity, content validity, test-retest reliability, and sensitivity to change.	In medical practice, improving the doctor–patient relationship, in assessing the effectiveness and relative merits of different treatments, in health services evaluation, in research, in policy-making

Instrument	Authors	Aim	Description	Administration	Population	Norms	Reliability	Uses
Short Quality of Life Questionnaire (CUBRECAVI)	R. F. Fernández-Ballesteros, M. D. Zamarrón (2007).	Measure QoL assessed through objective and subjective questions.	9 domains and 21 items: Physical and mental health, Social integration, Activity and leisure, Life satisfaction, Functional abilities, Social and health services, Environmental quality, Education and Income. Plus a question asking for appraisal of general QoL and a list of the most important quality of life domains which the person must rank; therefore CUBRECAVI can be used as an idiographic instrument, weighting standard domains.	Interviewer. It takes approximately 20 minutes.	Older adults living in the community and in residences. It is broadly used all over Latin America, Spain, and Portugal.	Numbers of scale points vary per item. For reliable and valid data analysis, instrument-specific software is recommended. The results provided are QoL profiles including the different domains and a total score (combination of the domain scores). Norms for Spanish elders as well as for elders from Latin America. There are no norms.	Reliability (Cronbach'sα range .47–.92) and construct validity have been reported by studies in Spain and in several Latin American countries. It has been used for evaluating intervention programmes.	Description, Research, Treatment changes.
Schedule for Evaluation of Individual QoL (SEIQoL)	C. A. O'Boyle, H. M. McGee, A. Hickey, C. R. B. Joyce, J. Browne, K. O'Malley, B. Hiltbrunner. (1993).	Idiographic instrument which allows the individual to name and weight those domains of greatest relevance for his/her quality of life.	3 elements in which the individual has to name the 5 aspects of life considered crucial to his/her QoL and to rate current functioning and satisfaction for each aspect. Finally, the relative importance of each aspect of QoL is measured through the weight the individual assigns to each in judging overall QoL.	Semi-structured interview, following 5 steps. It takes between 10 and 20 minutes.	Older adults.	There are no norms.	Internal validity > .70.	Research and clinical use.

IMPLICATIONS FOR PRACTICE

Assessment is the spinal cord of clinical practice: diagnosis, counselling, treatment planning, treatment evaluation, and follow-up are all supported by assessment tasks. Therefore, clinical geropsychologists must have deep knowledge and skills about the process of assessment, intervention, and evaluation in clinical practice as well as sizeable skills in selection, administration, evaluation, interpretation, and reporting of all assessment instruments. Finally, the clinical geropsychologist must be aware of his/her own attitudes about ageing, age, and the aged, and should following specific guidelines for assessing older adults.

SUMMARY

The objective of this chapter was to introduce the main issues concerning clinical geropsychological assessment. First of all, assessment of older adults must be based on several theoretical concepts about lifespan and development, which have been reviewed. In addition, data supporting the importance of assessment in clinical geropsychology has been reviewed. Psychological assessment is conducted through a decision-making process across which instruments and measures are administered for testing hypotheses about the case. In relation to this assessment process, ethical and methodological recommendations published by national and international organizations have been described and recommended. Psychological assessment of older adults has some specific characteristics, which have been reviewed. Finally, in this chapter, an overview of thirty instruments and measures classified into seven domains were briefly described. We believe that these instruments allow the reader to select a psychological battery for assessing older adults, taking into consideration the most important theoretical requirements already described in the earlier sections of this chapter: that is, to use multidimensional, multimethod, multilevel assessment approaches.

KEY REFERENCES AND SOURCES FOR FURTHER READING

Fernández-Ballesteros, R. (2004). 'Psychological Assessment'. In C. D. Spielberger (ed), *Encyclopedia of Applied Psychology*. New York: Elsevier.

Fernández-Ballesteros, R., De Bruyn, E. E. E., Godoy, A., Hornke, L. F., TerLaak, J., Vizcarro, C., et al. (2001). 'Guidelines for the Assessment Process (GAP): A Proposal for Discussion'. *European Journal of Psychological Assessment* 17(3): 187–200.

Jankowicz, D. (2003). *The Easy Guide to Repertory Grids*. Chichester: Wiley.

Kane, R. A. and Kane, R. L. (eds) (2000). *Assessing Older Persons: Measures, Meaning, and Practical Applications*. New York: Oxford University Press.

Nezu, A. M. and Nezu, C. M. (eds) (2008). *Evidenced-based Outcome Research: A Practical Guide to Conducting Randomized Clinical Trials for Psychosocial Interventions*. New York: Oxford University Press.

Schaie, K. W. (2005). *Developmental Influences on Adult Intelligence: The Seattle Longitudinal Study*. New York: Oxford University Press.

REFERENCES

Anastasi, A. and Urbina, S. (1997). *Psychological Testing* (7th edn). Upper Saddle River: Prentice Hall.

Antonucci, T. C. and Akiyama, H. (1987). 'Social Networks in Adult Life and a Preliminary Examination of the Convoy Model'. *Journal of Gerontology* 42: 519–527.

Antonucci, T. C. Akiyama, H., and Takahashi, K. (2004). 'Attachment and Close Relationships across the Life Span'. *Attachment and Human Development* 6: 353–370.

American Psychological Association (1999). *Standards for Educational and Psychological Testing*. Washington, DC: American Psychological Association.

American Psychological Association (2004). *Guidelines for Psychological Practice with Older Adults*. Washington, DC: American Psychological Association.

Baltes, P. B., Lindenberger, U., and Staudinge, U. M. (2006). 'Life Span Theory in Developmental Psychology'. In R. Lerner (ed), *Handbook of Child Psychology* (6th edn, Vol. 1, pp. 569–664). Hoboken, NJ: Wiley.

Berg, K. O., Wood-Dauphinee, S. L., Williams, J. T., and Gayton, D. (1989). 'Measuring Balance in the Elderly: Preliminary Development of an Instrument'. *Psychotherapy Canada* 41: 304–311.

Birren, J. E. and Deutchman, D. E. (1991). *Guiding Autobiographical Groups for Older Adults*. Baltimore: Johns Hopkins University Press.

Birren, J. (1996). 'The History of Gerontology'. In J. Birren (ed), *The Encyclopedia of Gerontology. Ageing, Age and the Aged* (pp. 655–665). New York: Academic Press.

Birren, J. E. and Schroots, J. J. F. (2006). 'Autobiographical Memory and the Narrative Self over the Life Span'. In J. E. Birren and W. Schaie (eds), *Handbook of the Psychology of Aging* (pp. 477–498). New York: Academic Press.

Bustillos, A. and Fernández-Ballesteros, R. (submitted). 'Is Older Adults' Functioning Effect of the Stereotypes Held by Caregivers?' *GeroPsychology*.

Clemson, L. Bundy, A., Unsworth, C., and Fiatatone Singh, M. (2008). *ALSAR-R2 Assessment of Living Skills and Resources*. http://sydney.edu.au/health-sciences/documents/assessment-living-skills.pdf

Cook, N. R., Evans, D. A., Scherr, F. E., Speizer, F. E., Vedal, S., and Branch, L. G., et al. (1989). 'Peak Expiratory Flow Rate in an Elderly Population'. *American Journal of Epidemiology* 130: 66–78. http://www.peakflow.com.

Cook, N. R., Evans, D. A., Scherr, P. A., Speizer, F. E., Taylor, J. O., and Hennekens, C. H. (1991). 'Peak Expiratory Flow Rate and 5 Year Mortality in an Elderly Population'. *American Journal of Epidemiology* 133: 784–794.

Cook, T. D. (1985). 'Postpositivist Critical Multiplism'. In R. L. Shotland and M. M. Mark (eds), *Social Science and Social Policy* (pp. 21–62), Beverly Hills, CA: Sage.

Cronbach, L. J. (1990). *Essentials of Psychological Testing* (5th edn). New York: Harper and Row.

Cutler, L. J. (2000). 'Assessment of Physical Environment of Older Adults'. In R. A. Kane and R. L. Kane (eds), *Assessing Older Persons: Measures, Meaning, and Practical Applications* (pp. 360–379). New York: Oxford.

Delis, D. C., Kaplan, E., and Kramer, J. H. (2001). *Delis-Kaplan Executive Function System (D-KEFS)*. San Antonio, TX: The Psychological Corporation.

Drinka, T. J. K., Williams, J., Schram, M., Farrell-Holtan, J., and Euhardy, M. (2000). 'Assessment of Living Skills and Resources (ALSAR©), an Instrumental Activities of Daily Living Assessment Instrument'. In D. Osterweil, K., Brummel-Smith, and J. Beck (eds), *Comprehensive Geriatric Assessment* (pp. 726–729). New York: McGraw-Hill.

Fernández-Ballesteros, R., Izal, M., Hernández, J. M., Montorio, I., and Llorente, G. (1991). 'Evaluation of Residential Programs for the Elderly in Spain and the United States'. *Evaluation Practice* 12: 159–164. [In *Sociological Abstracts* 1992.]

Fernández-Ballesteros, R. (ed) (1992). *Introducción a la evaluación psicológica*. Vols 1–2. Madrid: Pirámide. [50th edn, 1996].

Fernández-Ballesteros, R. (1993). 'The Construct of Quality of Life among the Elderly'. In E. Bergi, I. A. Gergely, and K. Rajzi (eds), *Recent Advances in Aging and Science*. Milan: Moduzzi.

Fernández-Ballesteros, R. and Zamarrón, M. D. (1996). 'New Findings in Social Desirability and Faking'. *Psychological Reports* 78: 1–3.

Fernández-Ballesteros, R. and Zamarrón, M. D. (2007) *CUBRECAVI Cuestionario Breve de Calidad de Vida*. Madrid: TEA Ediciones.

Fernández-Ballesteros, R. (Dir) (1996): *Sistema de Evaluación de Residencias de Ancianos (SERA)*. Madrid: INSERSO.

Fernández-Ballesteros, R. (1997). 'Quality of Life: Concept and Assessment'. In J. Adair, D. Belanger, and K. Dion (eds), *Advances in Psychological Science: Vol. 1: Social, Personal and Cultural Aspects*. Montreal: Psychological Press.

Fernández-Ballesteros, R. (2001). 'Environmental Conditions, Health and Satisfaction among the Elderly: Some Empirical Results'. *Psicothema* 13(1): 40–49.

Fernández-Ballesteros, R., De Bruyn, E. E. E., Godoy, A., Hornke, L. F., TerLaak, J., Vizcarro, C., et al. (2001). 'Guidelines for the Assessment Process (GAP): A Proposal for Discussion'. *European Journal of Psychological Assessment* 17(3): 187–200.

Fernández-Ballesteros, R. (2003). 'Self-report Questionnaires'. In S. Haynes and E. Heiby (eds), *Behavioral Assessment*. New York: Wiley.

Fernández-Ballesteros, R. Zamarrón, M. D., Tárraga, L., Moya, R., and Iñiguez, J. (2003). 'Learning Potential in Healthy, Mild Cognitive Impairment Subjects and in Alzheimer Patients'. *European Psychologist* 8: 148–160.

Fernández-Ballesteros, R. (2004). 'Psychological Assessment'. In C. D. Spielberger (ed.), *Encyclopedia of Applied Psychology*. New York: Elsevier.

Fernández-Ballesteros, R., Zamarrón, M. D., Rudinger, G. Schroots, F. J., Heikinen, E., Drusini, A., et al. (2004). 'Assessing Competence: The European Survey on Aging Protocol (ESAP)'. *Gerontology* 50: 330–347.

Fernández-Ballesteros, R., Zamarrón, M. D., and Tarraga, L. (2005). 'Learning Potential: A New Method for Assessing Cognitive Impairment'. *International Psychogeriatrics* 17: 119–128.

Fernández-Ballesteros, R. (2008). 'Active Aging'. *The Contribution of Psychology*. Gottingën: Hogrefe and Huber.

Fernández-Ballesteros, R. Reig, A., and Zamarrón, M. D. (2008). 'Evaluación'. In R. Fernández-Ballesteros (ed), *Psicología de la vejez. Una Psicogerontología aplicada*. Madrid: Pirámide.

Fernández-Ballesteros, R. (2011). 'Quality of Life in Older Life. Some Problematic Issues'. *Applied Research in Quality of Life* 11: 21–40.

Fernández-Ballesteros, R., and Pinquart, M. (2011). 'Geropsychology'. In P. Martin, F. Cheung, M. Kyrios, L. Littlefield, M. Knowles, J. M. Prieto, et al. (eds), *IAAP Handbook of Applied Psychology*. Chichcster: Wiley-Blackwell.

Fernández-Ballesteros, R., Botella, J., Zamarrón, M. D., Molina, M. A., Cabras, E., Tárraga, L., et al. (2012). 'Cognitive Plasticity in Normal and Pathological Aging'. *Clinical Intervention on Aging* 7: 15–25.

Fiori, K. L., Smith J., and Antonucci, T. (2007). 'Social Network Types among Older Adults: A Multidimensional Approach'. *Journal of Gerontology* 62: P322–P330.

Fisher, A. G. (1997). *Assessment of motor and process skills* (2nd edn). Fort Collins, Colorado: Three Star Press.

Fisher, A. G. and Bernspång, B. (2007). 'Response to: A Critique of the Assessment of Motor and Process Skills (AMPS) in Mental Health Practice'. *Mental Health Occupational Therapy* 12: 10–11. http://www.ampsintl.com/AMPS/documents/MHOT%20March%202007.pdf.

Fisher, A. G. and Bray Jones, K. (2010). *Assessment of Motor and Process Skills: Vol. 1: Development, Standardization, and Administration Manual* (7th edn). Fort Collins, CO: Three Star Press.

Fiske, S. T., Cuddy, A. C., Glick, P., and Xu, L. (2002). 'A Model of Often Mixed Stereotype Content: Competence and Warmth Respectively Follow from Perceived Status and Competition'. *Journal of Personality and Social Psychology* 82: 878–902.

Fletcher, A. (1998). 'Multidimensional Assessment of Elderly People in the Community'. *British Bulletin* 54: 945–960.

Folstein, M. F., Folstein, S., and McHugh, P. R. (1975). 'Mini-Mental State: A Practical Method for Grading the Cogntive State of Patients for the Clinicians'. *Journal of Psychiatric Research* 12(3): 189–198.

Gallo, J. J., Reichel, W., and Andersen, L. (1988). *Handbook of Geriatric Assessment*. Rockville, MD: Aspen.

Gould, J. G. (1981). *The Mismeasure of Man*. New York: Norton.

Hamilton, B. B, Granger, C. V., Sherwin, F. S., Zielezny, M., and Tashman, J. S. (1987). 'A Uniform National Data System for Medical Rehabilitation'. In M. J. Fuhrer (ed), *Rehabilitation Outcomes: Analysis and Measurement* (pp. 137–147). Baltimore, MD: Brookes.

Hayase, D., Mosenteen, D. A., Thimmaiah, D., Zemke, S., Atler, K., and Fisher, A. G. (2004). 'Age-related Changes in Activities of Daily Living (ADL) Ability'. *Australian Occupational Therapy Journal* 51: 192–198.

Heckhausen, J., Dixon, R. A., and Baltes, P. B. (1989). 'Gains and Losses in Development throughout Adulthood as Perceived by Different Age Groups'. *Developmental Psychology* 25: 109–121.

Iwarsson, S. (1999). 'The Housing Enabler: An Objective Tool for Assessing Accessibility'. *British Journal of Occupational Therapy* 62: 491–497.

Iwarsson, S., Sixsmith, J., Oswald, F., Wahl, H.-W., Nygren, C., Sixsmith, A., et al. (2005). 'The ENABLE–AGE Project: Multi-dimensional Methodology for European Housing Research'. In N. Wilkinson and Y. Hurol (eds), *Housing Research Methodologies*. Mersin: Urban International Press.

Kane, R. A. and Kane, R. L. (1981). *Assessing the Elderly: A Practical Guide to Measurement*. Lexington, MA: Lexington Books.

Kane, R. A. and Kane, R. L. (eds) (2000). *Assessing Older Persons: Measures, Meaning, and Practical Applications*. New York: Oxford University Press.

Katz S. C., Ford A. B., Moskowitz R. W., and Jaffe, M. W. (1963). 'Studies of Illness in the Aged. The Index of ADL: A Standardized Measure of Biological and Psychosocial Function'. *Journal of the American Medical Association* 185: 914–919.

Keyes, C. L. M. (2005). 'Mental Illness and/or Mental Health? Investigating Axioms of the Complete State Model of Health'. *Journal of Consulting and Clinical Psychology* 73(3): 539–548.

Kahn, R. L. and Antonucci, T. C. (1980). 'Convoys over the Life Course: Attachment, Roles, and Social Support'. In P. B. Baltes and O. Brim (eds), *Life-span Development and Behavior* (Vol. 3, pp. 253–268). New York: Academic Press.

Kiresuk, T. J. and Lund, S. H. (1977). 'Program Evaluation and the Management of Organizations'. In W. F. Anderson, B. J. Frieden, and M. J. Murphy (eds), *Managing Human Services* (pp. 280–317). Washington, DC: International City Management Association.

Langley, L. K. (2000). 'Cognitive Assessment of Older Adults'. In R. L. Kane and R. A. Kane (eds), *Assessing Older Persons* (2nd edn, pp. 65–128). New York: Oxford University Press.

Lawton, M. P. (1975). 'The Philadelphia Geriatric Center Morale Scale: A Revision'. *Journal of Gerontology* 30: 85–89.

Levin, C. (2000). 'Social Functioning'. In R. L. Kane and R. A. Kane (eds), *Assessing Older Persons* (pp. 170–199). New York: Oxford University Press.

Lezak, M. (2000). *Neuropsychological Assessment* (3rd edn). New York: Oxford University Press.

Lubben, J. E. (1988). 'Assessing Social Networks among Elderly Populations'. *Journal of Family and Community Health* 11: 42–52. http://www.bc.edu/schools/gssw/lubben/.

Lubben, J. E. (2002). Centrality of Social Ties to Vitality among Older Adults. In *The 130th Annual Meeting of APHA*.

Messick, S. (1984). 'Assessment in Context: Appraising Student Performance in Relation to Instructional Quality'. *Educational Researcher* 13(3): 3–8.

Messick, S. (1989). 'Validity'. In R. L. Linn (ed.), *Educational Measurement* (pp. 13–103). New York: Macmillan.

Messick, S. (1995). 'Validity of Psychological Assessment: Validation of Inferences from Persons' Responses and Performances as Scientific Inquiry into Score Meaning'. *American Psychologist* 50: 741–749.

Moos, R. and Lemke, S. (1984). 'Supportive Residential Settings for Older People'. In I. Altman, M. P. Lawton, and J. Wohlwill (eds), *Elderly People and the Environment: Human Behavior and Environment* (pp. 159–190). New York: Plenum.

Moos, R. and Lemke, S. (1996). *The Multiphasic Environment Assessment Procedure MEAP*. Palo Alto, CA: Sage.

Nasreddine, Z. S., Phillips, N. A., Bédirian, V., Charbonneau, S., Whitehead, V., Collin, I., et al. (2005). 'The Montreal Cognitive Assessment, MoCA: A Brief Screening Tool for Mild Cognitive Impairment'. *Journal of the American Geriatrics Society* 53: 695–699.

Neimeyer, G. J. and Hagans, C. L. (2002). 'More Madness in our Method? The Effects of Repertory Grid Variations on Construct Differentiation'. *Journal of Constructivist Psychology* 15: 139–160.

Nezu, A. M. and Nezu, C. M. (eds) (2008). *Evidenced-based Outcome Research: A Practical Guide to Conducting Randomized Clinical Trials for Psychosocial Interventions*. New York: Oxford University Press.

O'Boyle, C. A., McGee, H. M., Hickey, A., Joyce, C. R. B., Browne, J., O'Malley, K. and Hiltbrunner, B. (1993). *The Schedule for the Evaluation of Individual Quality of Life (SEIQoL). Administration Manual*. Dublin: Royal College of Surgeons in Ireland.

Pachana, N. A., Byrne, G. J., Siddle, H., Koloski, N., Harley, E., and Arnold, E. (2007). 'Development and Validation of the Geriatric Anxiety Inventory'. *International Psychogeriatrics* 19: 103–114.

Pearson, V. L. (2000). 'Assessment of Function in Older Adults'. In R. L. Kane and R. A. Kane (eds), *Assessing Older Persons* (pp. 17–48). New York: Oxford University Press.

Pfeiffer E. (1975). 'Short Portable Mental Status Questionnaire'. *Journal of the American Geriatric Society* 23: 433–441.

Pinquart, M., Fernández-Ballesteros, R., and Torpdahl, P. (2007). 'Teaching, Research, and Application of Geropsychology in Europe'. *European Psychologist* 12: 229–234.

Rabbitt, P. (2005). 'Cognitive Changes across Lifespan'. In M. L. Johnson (ed), *Age and Ageing* (pp. 190–199). Cambridge: Cambridge University Press.

Rantanen T., Guralnik, J. M., Foley, D., Masaki, K., Leveille, S., Curb, J. D., et al. (1999). 'Midlife Hand Grip Strength as a Predictor of Old Age Disability'. *Journal of the American Medical Association* 281(6): 558–560.

Rey, A. (1964). *L'examen Clinique en psicologie*. Paris: Presses Universitaires de France.

Reynolds, C. R. and Kamphaus, R. W. (2003). *Reynolds intellectual assessment scales*. Lutz, FL: Psychological Assessment Resources Inc.

Rubinstein, L. and Rubinstein, L. V. (1991). 'Multidimensional Assessment of Elderly Patients'. *Advances in Internal Medicine* 36: 81–108.

Schaie, K. W. (2005a). *Developmental Influences on Adult Intelligence: The Seattle Longitudinal Study*. New York: Oxford University Press.

Schaie, K. W. (2005b). 'What Can We Learn from Longitudinal Studies of Adult Development?' *Research on Human Development* 2: 133–158.

Schroots, J. J. F., Fernández-Ballesteros, R., and Rudinger, G. (eds) (1995). '*Eugeron: Aging, Health and Competence. Report 1. Rationale and Concepts*'. Amsterdam: University of Amsterdam, ERGO/University.

Sheikh, J. I. and Yesavage, J. A. (1986). 'Geriatric Depression Scale (GDS): Recent Evidence and Development of a Shorter Version'. *Clinical Gerontologist: The Journal of Aging and Mental Health* 5(1–2): 165–173.

Spector, W. D. (1990). 'Functional Disability Scales'. In R. Spilker (ed), *Quality of Life Assessment in Clinical Trials* (pp. 115–129). New York: Raven Press.

Svensson, T. and Randall, M. (2003). 'Autobiography'. In R. Fernández-Ballesteros (ed), *Encyclopedia of Psychological Assessment*. (Vol 1, pp. 120–123). London: Sage.

Thorbahn, L. D. and Newton, R. A. (1996). 'Use of the Berg Balance Test to Predict Falls in Elderly Persons'. *Physical Therapy* 76: 576–583.

Van der Elst, W., Van Boxtel M. P., Van Breukelen, G. J., and Jolles, J. (2005). 'Rey's Verbal Learning Test: Normative Data for 1855 Healthy Participants Aged 24–81 Years and the Influence of Age, Sex, Education, and Mode of Presentation'. *Journal of the International Neuropsychological Society* 11(3): 290–302.

Van Swearingen, J. M., Paschal, K. A., Bonino, P., and Yang, J. F. (1996). 'The Modified Gait Abnormality Rating Scale for Recognizing the Risk of Recurrent Falls in Community-dwelling Elderly Adults'. *Physical Therapy* 76: 994–1002.

Vellas, B., Guigoz, Y., Garry, P. J., Nourhashemi, F., Bennahum, D., Laugue, S., et al. (1999). 'The Mini Nutritional Assessment (MNA) and its Use in Grading the Nutritional State of Elderly Patients'. *Nutrition* 15: 116–122.

Wahl, H.-W. and U. Lehr (2002). 'Applied Fields in Psychological Assessment: Gerontology'. In R. Fernandez-Ballesteros (ed), *Encyclopedia of Psychological Assessment* (Vol. 1, pp. 63–69). London: Sage.

Wahl, H.-W. and Gitlin, L. N. (2007). 'Environmental Gerontology'. In J. E. Birren (ed), *Encyclopedia of Gerontology*. Oxford: Elsevier.

Wahl, H.-W. and Iwarsson, S. (2007). 'Person–environment Relations in Old Age'. In R. Fernandez-Ballesteros (ed), *Geropsychology. European Perspectives for an Ageing World* (pp. 49–66). Göttingen: Hogrefe.

Walker, A. (2005). 'A European Perspective on Quality of Life in Old Age'. *European Journal of Aging* 2: 2–13.

Wallace, M. (1998). 'Katz Index of Independence in Activities of Daily Living (ADL)'. http://www.hartfordign.org/publications/trythis/issue02.pdf.

Ware J.E. and Sherbourne C.D. (1992). 'The MOS 36-item short form health survey (SF-36) I'. *Medical Care* 30: 473–483.

Watson, D., Clark, L. A., and Tellegen, A. (1988). 'Development and Validation of Brief Measures of Positive and Negative Affect: The PANAS Scales'. *Journal of Personality and Social Psychology* 54(6): 1063–1070.

Wechsler Adult Intelligence Scale (4th edition). (2008). NCS Pearson, Inc.

WHOQOL Group (1998). 'The World Health Organization Quality of Life Assessment (WHOQOL): Development and General Psychometric Properties'. *Social Science & Medicine* 46: 1569–1585.

World Health Organization (2001): *International Classification of Functioning, Disability and Health (ICF)*. Geneva: WHO.

Williams, J., Drinka, T., Greenberg, J. Farrell-Holtan, J., Euhardy, R., and Schram, P. (1991). 'Development and Testing of the Assessment of Living Skills and Resources (ALSAR) in Elderly Community-dwelling Veterans'. *The Gerontologist* 31(1): 84–91.

Wilson, B. A. Cockburn, J., and Baddeley, A. D. (1985). *The Rivermead Behavioural Memory Test*. London. Pearson Assessment.

Wright, B. M. and McKerrow, C. B. (1959). Maximum Forced Expiratory Flow Rate as a Measure of Ventilatory Capacity. *British Medical Journal* 21(2): 1041–1047.

Yesevage, J. A., Brink, T. L. Rose, T. L., Lum, O. Huang, V., Adey, M. D., et al. (1983). 'Development and Validation of a Geriatric Depression Screening Scale'. *Journal of Psychiatric Research* 17: 37–49.

Zamarrón, M. D., Tárraga, L., and Fernández-Ballesteros, R. (2009). 'Changes in Reserve Capacity in Alzheimer's Disease Patients Receiving Cognitive Stimulation Programs'. *Psychology in Spain* 13: 48–54.

....

CHAPTER 11

ASSESSING CHANGE OF COGNITIVE TRAJECTORIES OVER TIME IN LATER LIFE

....

DUSTIN B. HAMMERS, KEVIN DUFF, AND GORDON J.CHELUNE

ASSESSING CHANGE IN COGNITIVE TRAJECTORIES IN LATER LIFE

....

SUPPOSE an 82-year-old female has subjectively experienced changes in her memory skills over the past one to two years and begins commenting to her friends and family about her increased difficulties. During these conversations, suppose also that one of her family members recommends that she speak with her doctor about her memory challenges, and that she makes an appointment with her primary care physician (PCP). What is the optimal manner in which we, as a field, can assess changes in cognitive functioning as this individual ages over time? Is this best done at the PCP's office, or in a specialty clinic? Should her cognitive abilities be assessed once or multiple times? Against what standard do we compare her current performance and abilities and how do we follow her over time?

The following chapter will describe methods of evaluating cognitive change over time using evidence-based practices in the field of clinical neuropsychology (Chelune 2010). While doing so, a description of cognitive changes during the 'normal' ageing process will be initially undertaken, followed by a brief review of cognitive trajectories for a few syndromes associated with abnormal decline. A discussion of the practice of clinical neuropsychology will ensue, accompanied by concerns arising when using traditional single time-point assessments. The benefits of and challenges to using serial assessments will also be discussed, as well as a basic review of the statistical methods available to identify reliable change over time. The chapter concludes with proposed research directions for the field to better tailor the use of cognitive trajectories to monitor predicted decline in the individual patient.

'Normal' Cognitive Ageing

Generally speaking, cognition is not considered to remain stable across the lifespan, but is often characterized as a trajectory of growth from birth through the first two to three decades of life, leading to a period of relative stability for most individuals until the fifth or sixth decade of life (Salthouse 2009). Following this time period, however, a phase of senescence or a loss of function and adaptability occurs for many individuals, such that many researchers consider cognitive decline to be an 'inevitable' part of advancing age (Schaie 1994). While some types of cognitive function, such as crystallized abilities like vocabulary and fund-of-knowledge skills, tend to accumulate across time until at least the age of 70, other cognitive abilities often show an accelerated decline after the ages of 50 to 60. Speed of information processing has been termed a 'foundational cognitive ability' (Vance et al. 2012), as a number of cognitive abilities rely on intact processing speed. In fact, the reduction in mental processing speed tends to be a hallmark of primary cognitive ageing, with a number of lines of research, including longitudinal data from the Swedish Adoption/Twin Study of Ageing (Finkel et al. 2007), suggesting that reduced speed of processing is the leading indicator of associated declines over time in cognitive domains such as reasoning, memory, mental flexibility, and visual-spatial skills. For example, as processing speed abilities decline, the ability to rapidly attend to and retain incoming information becomes compromised. Losses in the ability to rapidly and efficiently process information have also been associated with declines in daily functioning (Marcotte et al. 2010), particularly in relation to complex tasks such as automobile driving (Marcotte and Scott 2009; Uc et al. 2006). Researchers have also suggested that sensory changes in vision and hearing may be a significant contributor to this slowed processing (Salthouse 2009).

While general trends exist when considering the average trajectory of individuals as they age, it should be noted that a large degree of heterogeneity exists when considering individual trajectories (Hayden et al. 2011; Wilson et al. 2002). In his work *Positive Aging* (Hill 2005), Hill conceptualized four distinct patterns of ageing, including 'successful aging' (those who do not decline appreciably over time), 'normal ageing' (whose decline is typical as described above), 'impaired ageing' (progressive decline due to physiological impairment), and 'diseased ageing' (substantial decline in functional impairment). These categorizations contrast with the simple notion of 'Normal vs Abnormal' ageing; moreover, the findings that a substantial minority of the overall population tends to display only minimal cognitive declines over time (Hill et al. 1995) argues against the 'inevitability' of cognitive declines for all older individuals. For example, in their research on a cohort of priests, nuns, and brothers from the Religious Orders Study (Bennett et al. 2002), Hayden and colleagues (2011) observed that of the approximately 1000 participants (mean age 75) followed with annual cognitive evaluations, two-thirds belonged to a subgroup experiencing very slow global cognitive decline, whereas only 8% of the sample belonged to what could be categorized as an 'impaired ageing' or 'diseased ageing' group.

A number of causes have been proposed to explain the average course of cognitive change associated with ageing, including changes as a result of medical/physical factors, environmental factors, or neuro-anatomical alterations. Briefly, as individuals age, the frequency of medical conditions that may compromise cognitive function increases (see Houston and Bondi 2006 for a more comprehensive review). Such conditions may range from simple primary sensory processing to those related to known or suspected medical conditions that affect brain functioning, such as normal pressure hydrocephalus, hypothyroidism, hypertension, insulin resistance/metabolic syndrome, nutritional or vitamin deficiencies (e.g. B_{12} or thiamine), traumatic brain injury, and obstructive sleep apnoea. Each of these conditions possesses a unique profile of cognitive weakness. In response to increased medical complications in older adults in general, ageing individuals are often prescribed an increased number of medications, many of which may have cognitive side-effects above and beyond those attributable to the conditions themselves, including reductions in attention, processing speed, and memory (Houston and Bondi 2006). Additionally, changes in hearing or vision can interfere with the capacity to attend to auditory or visual stimuli respectively, thus reducing an individual's overall cognitive functioning. Further, reductions in mobility or general health may result in increased social withdrawal and/or decreased physical exercise, thereby limiting the level of social engagement and/or cognitive and physical stimulation, which have also been individually associated with age-related cognitive declines (Ertel, Glymour, and Berkman 2008; Larson et al. 2006).

As a result of these and other medical/environmental influences on the ageing individual, research suggests that neuronal atrophy, the accumulation of white-matter lesions, and decreased frontal connectivity are involved in the anatomical sequelae of normal ageing (Buckner 2004). Research evaluating individuals without dementia across the lifespan has identified a mostly linear decline between the ages of 60 and 95 related to total brain volume, total gray matter, total white matter, hippocampal volume, orbitofrontal volume, dorsolateral prefrontal cortex, and primary motor and somatosensory cortices using magnetic resonance imaging (MRI; Driscoll et al. 2009; Kennedy and Raz 2009). In addition, using high-resolution diffusion tensor imaging (DTI), Kennedy and Raz (2009) found that regional white-matter integrity differentially influenced cognitive performance, with degradation of anterior brain areas being associated with reduced working memory and processing speed skills, while posterior degradation was associated with reduced executive functioning (e.g. inhibition and task switching). Poorer episodic memory was related to age differences in central white-matter regions. Specifically regarding memory functioning, loss of integrity of the frontal-striatal circuitry was associated with abnormalities in executive retrieval strategies and the medial temporal lobe system (Hedden and Gabrieli 2004). Similar DTI studies have suggested that frontal white matter may be preferentially vulnerable to changes over time, regardless of cause (Salat et al. 2005). Finally, alterations in the availability or distribution of the neurotransmitter dopamine, which have been observed over time using positron emission tomography (PET) imaging and biochemical studies (Antonini et al. 1993; Goldman-Rakic and Brown 1981; Rinne et al. 1993; Wenk et al. 1989), are associated with cognitive functions such as executive functioning and speed of processing. In general, whether as a consequence of a number of known or unknown medical/anatomical or environmental factors, several lines of research have indicated that age-related cognitive declines frequently occur and affect a number of cognitive and functional domains in a large proportion of the general population.

Abnormal Cognitive Changes
in Later Life

While typical cognitive ageing is often associated with the aforementioned profiles and influences, individual cognitive trajectories can be modified by the presence of neurodegenerative disease states and result in abnormal cognitive profiles. Such individuals would often be categorized by the 'diseased ageing' conceptualization as described previously (Hill 2005). The cognitive processes associated with learning and delayed retention of information, as well as information processing/verbal fluency, have been suggested as particularly sensitive indicators of early conversion from normal to abnormal ageing in the presence of disease states (Masur et al. 1994; Monsch et al. 1992; Petersen et al. 1994). A number of so-called boundary conditions have been defined to characterize a transition stage from normal to abnormal cognitive ageing, the details of which are beyond the scope of this chapter, with the term mild cognitive impairment (MCI; Petersen 2004) gaining the widest acceptance at the current time. Dementia, a clinical syndrome used to describe severe declines in cognition and impairment of daily functioning according to the fourth edition of the *Diagnostic and Statistical Manual of Mental Disorders* (*DSM-IV-TR*; American Psychiatric Association 2000), is an overarching term with a number of prominent aetiologies characterizing the syndrome. Also beyond the scope of this chapter, it should be noted that while the use of such diagnostic criteria for dementia has been advanced with the recent National Institutes of Health-Alzheimer's Association (NIA-AA) research criteria and guidelines for diagnosing dementia due to Alzheimer's disease (McKhann et al. 2011), the recently released fifth edition of the *Diagnostic and Statistical Manual of Mental Disorders* (*DSM-5*; American Psychiatric Association 2013) has transitioned from the use of the term 'dementia' to 'major neurocognitive disorder'; as the vast majority of clinicians and researchers continue to use 'dementia' in accordance with NIA-AA guidelines, this book chapter will do the same. Large-scale international consensus studies have found that dementia increases in prevalence across the age spectrum from less than 4% before the age of 75 to approximately 13% for ages 80 to 84; for individuals in developed countries beyond the age of 85, the prevalence of dementia rises to approximately 30% (Ferri et al. 2005). As the longevity of the global population increases, it has been proposed that the number of people living with dementia will almost double every twenty years.

While a multitude of aetiologies exist that may result in dementia, a few are notably prominent and thus warrant a description of their typical prevalence rates and cognitive trajectories. Alzheimer's disease (AD), identified by the accumulation of beta amyloid plaques and neurofibrillary tangles in the brain, is the most common cause of dementia globally, accounting for approximately 35% of believed 'pure' cases and 50% of all cases when 'mixed' AD and vascular pathology is included (Mendez and Cummings 2003). Early-onset AD (prior to 65 years of age) is characterized by a rapid decline, whereas late-onset AD (after age 65) typically presents with a more insidious onset and gradual progression. The cognitive deficits associated with AD are significantly associated with early episodic impairments of learning and memory, as well as loss of semantic knowledge and general language impairment, visual spatial impairments, and executive dysfunction (Smith and Bondi 2008). Simple attention and motor functions are typically preserved early in the disease progression; however, as AD progresses, global cognitive impairment is common. Vascular dementia (VaD) is considered the second most common form of dementia, with at least 10–15% of dementia cases considered 'purely' vascular. As VaD typically results from cerebrovascular insults secondary to vascular risk factors like atherosclerosis, hypertension, and diabetes mellitus type II, onset is most often between 60 and 75 years of age (Mendez and Cummings 2003). The course of VaD displays a high degree of variability depending on the nature of the aetiology. VaD associated with multiple infarcts will often progress in a stepwise fashion, with intermittent stable periods followed by declines related to ischaemic events (e.g. stroke), and early deficits observed in processing speed, attention, executive functions, and visual-spatial skills; alternatively, large cerebral infarcts will lead to neuropsychological impairments in domains associated with compromised anatomical locations (Schoenberg and Duff 2011). When vascular risk factors are present and believed to be resulting in cognitive declines not severe enough to warrant a diagnosis of dementia, the spectrum of disorders known as 'vascular cognitive impairment' (VCI; Chui 2006; Hachinski et al. 2006) is now more commonly being applied.

Two additional common aetiologies of dementia are Dementia with Lewy Bodies (DLB) and Frontotemporal dementia (FTD). DLB accounts for 10–30% of all new cases of dementia, and is characterized by the presence of Lewy bodies (neurotoxic inclusions made of the protein alpha-synuclein) throughout the cerebral cortex. The age of onset typically ranges from 50 to 70 years of age, and while the course is gradual, similar to AD, the progression is slightly more rapid (five to seven years from diagnosis to death; Mendez and Cummings 2003). The presence of visual hallucinations, Parkinsonism, fluctuations in cognition, and REM sleep behaviour disorder symptoms are highly diagnostic for DLB, and early deficits in visual-spatial skills, learning and attention, and executive skills are typically observed (Levy and Chelune 2007; Schoenberg and Duff 2011). While delayed retention is often preserved early in DLB, over time memory skills also severely decline. Similar to DLB, FTD has an age of onset earlier than is typical for AD (i.e. 50 to 60 years of age), and accounts for 5–10% of all forms of dementia. A number of diagnoses are grouped into the FTD classification given their associated degeneration of the frontal and temporal lobes, including frontal/behavioural-variant FTD (predominant executive dysfunction and disinhibited personality change), and primary progressive aphasia (predominant language impairment; fluent primary progressive aphasia, non-fluent primary progressive aphasia, or semantic dementia; Mendez and Cummings 2003; Schoenberg and Duff 2011).

Research has suggested that there is typically a non-linear relationship between cognitive decline and neuropathological insult in individuals with various forms of dementia (amyloid plaques and neurofibrillary tangles for AD, Lewy bodies for DLB, etc.). As such, neuropathological abnormalities and cognitive decline need not occur contemporaneously; specifically, while AD pathological changes may be present during preclinical phases, the dementia typically develops at a later time point. For example, histopathological studies have found the presence of early neurofibrillary tangle formations in transentorhinal cortex early in adulthood (Braak and Del Tredici 2011; Ohm et al. 1995) for individuals eventually developing dementia associated with AD. It has been suggested that these neural changes accumulate at a very slow rate over time and result in an eventual diagnosis of dementia. Frank changes in cognitive trajectory may not be expected until various neuropathological processes (plaques and tangles) have reached a threshold (Backman, Small, and Fratiglioni 2001). Similarly, mild declines in cognitive functioning (predominantly memory and executive functioning) have been observed across a number of studies in the years preceding an eventual diagnosis of AD, ranging from 2 to 6+ years pre-diagnosis (Backman et al. 2001; Chen et al. 2001; Lange et al. 2002); a more recent study observed mild changes in cognitive trajectory up to nine years prior to diagnosis (Laukka et al. 2012). A model for cognitive decline in preclinical dementia has been proposed (Smith and Bondi 2008) such that initial declines are followed by a period of stabilization, as a result of the recruitment of alternative brain structures that temporarily attenuate cognitive decline (primarily frontal and temporal cortex). However, as neuropathological abnormalities accumulate, a threshold is reached such that cognitive trajectories decline rapidly as compensatory processes are no longer able to support the cognitive process in the face of repeated neuropathological insult. These declines lead to a subsequent diagnosis of dementia. Support for such a proposal can be found in neuroimaging studies suggesting compensatory activation (Reuter-Lorenz 2002) and increased laterality (Reuter-Lorenz et al. 2000) of the frontal lobes of individuals of advanced age.

Assessing Normal and Abnormal Changes in Cognition

The practice of clinical neuropsychology involves the evaluation of brain-behaviour relationships for the assessment, diagnosis, and treatment of patients across a wide array of conditions, including medical, neurological, psychiatric, and developmental presentations. As such, a clinical neuropsychologist uses psychological, neurological, cognitive, behavioural, and physiological principles and methods to evaluate patients' cognitive, behavioural, and emotional profiles, and their relationship to normal and abnormal central nervous system functioning (Barth et al. 2003). A neuropsychological assessment typically consists of an in-depth clinical interview followed by an evaluation of specific cognitive domains relevant to a referral question. Neuropsychological tests are selected to comprise a battery that ideally has appropriate validity and reliability, as well as having adequate sensitivity and specificity for a particular condition at hand (Lezak, Howieson, and Loring 2004). Neuropsychological tasks are administered in an objective and consistent fashion, after which each test performance is scored and compared to an external reference group.

While neuropsychological evaluations may be used to derive descriptive statements about an individual's cognitive skills, they are most commonly used for diagnostic purposes where the central purpose is to determine whether the patient's neurocognitive status has changed either from a presumed premorbid level or in comparison to a baseline assessment (Busch, Chelune, and Suchy 2006). In both situations, the emphasis is on the assessment of *change*. In the case of single-point assessments, the clinician uses normative information to determine where the patient is currently performing within the reference population and then must determine whether this is significantly discrepant from where s/he is likely to have been performing prior to his/her illness or injury (i.e. has there been a change in trajectory?). Increasingly, neuropsychologists are using demographically corrected norms (e.g. the fourth edition of the Wechsler Scales) more specifically to identify a presumed premorbid level of functioning for a given individual. In the case of our 82-year-old woman with whom we began this chapter, if she obtained an age-adjusted memory score of 96, we might dismiss her memory complaints since her score falls in the 'average' range for the general population in her age group. However, if we factor in that she was a successful university professor with a PhD, we would find that her 'average' performance was more than two standard deviations below demographic expectations, a score that would be expected to occur among less than 3% of those in her demographic cohort.

Consideration of a patient's individual performances on the various norm-referenced test procedures in the neuropsychological battery allows the practitioner to construct a patient-specific profile of cognitive strengths and weaknesses—virtually a 'snapshot' in time. This profile can then be compared to those prototypic cognitive profiles that characterize known medical, neurological, or psychiatric conditions. For example, patients with AD typically present with deficits in semantic knowledge and difficulties with episodic memory affecting both retrieval and recognition memory. On the other hand, patients with FTD have disproportionate difficulties with executive functions and, while they may have difficulties with memory, this is typically more apparent on tasks of retrieval than recognition. While neuropsychologists often make diagnostic inferences based on norm-referenced cognitive profiles derived from single-point assessments, it is most often the changes in cognitive profiles over time that best distinguish normal from abnormal cognitive trajectories among older populations (Chelune and Duff 2012). The evaluation of meaningful change in cognitive trajectories requires the clinician to be able empirically to distinguish whether changes in test performance are a function of normal variations in individual performance and the fidelity of the test instruments, or whether they represent statistically significant and clinically meaningful changes that have diagnostic value.

CONCERNS REGARDING SINGLE ASSESSMENTS

While single assessments are a practical necessity when a patient presents for an initial neuropsychological evaluation, a few areas of concern arise that may interfere with the interpretation of test results from single-point assessments. First, single-point assessments frequently lack objective knowledge about a patient's premorbid functioning and must rely solely on normative comparisons with a comparison group to provide a context to the patient's scores. As most patients do not present with medical records thoroughly documenting their level of childhood abilities, the examiner typically relies on patient self-report and collateral reports to ascertain premorbid capacities. Such information is vulnerable to biases based on the patient's or collateral's mood or subjective perceptions. For example, patients with decreased awareness may be unable to clearly identify past functional capacities and under-report real-world deficits (Cahn-Weiner, Ready, and Malloy 2003). Similarly, if the collateral for a patient is a nurse or family friend with limited knowledge of the patient's premorbid functioning, then accurate insight into change from previous levels cannot fully be gathered. An alternative situation, one which neuropsychologists often encounter, is how to interpret 'normal' results in a patient who has been reported by family or care-givers to have previously been high achieving for his/her level of education. As 'high achieving' is a rather subjective notion, there is often little evidence to support such a claim other than utilizing demographic- or reading-based measures to estimate premorbid status

(Duff, Chelune, and Dennett 2011a), though such practices still rely on using an inferred discrepancy between current results and an estimated baseline in clinical decision-making.

A second notable limitation of single-point evaluations is that a 'snapshot' in time provides limited information about the patient's cognition. In the example above of our 'high-achieving' patient, it is possible that while still performing within expectations given age and education corrections, a decline may have occurred in the patient's cognition such that the patient should have performed in the high-average or superior range if a neurodegenerative process had not interfered with cognitive functioning. Given that single-point evaluations provide limited context into trajectories over time, the clinician is left only to hypothesize about initial levels of cognition and subsequent decline.

THE USE OF SERIAL ASSESSMENTS

In response to a number of these concerns regarding single-point assessments, neuropsychologists are increasingly embracing the practice of serial assessments (Busch et al. 2006; Chelune 2003; Duff et al. 2010a; Howieson et al. 2008). Unlike the use of an inferred discrepancy between the patient's performance and that of a normative sample, serial assessments allow for the identification of observed changes or discrepancies between a baseline and second assessment to provide information about a patient's cognitive trajectory over time. Although using serial assessments does not eliminate certain concerns arising from the assessment process that may compromise the interpretation of test findings, repeated assessments act as a collection of measurements that provide a more dynamic view of the patient's cognitive trajectory. It should be emphasized that interpreting the results from serial neuropsychological assessments is not necessarily easier than for single assessments, for in some ways serial assessments multiply the complexity of clinical interpretation and the vulnerability to factors such as patient characteristics (medical/psychiatric/sleep conditions affecting concentration), setting characteristics (room too hot/cold; loud noises; anxiety resulting from testing setting), or the use of appropriate normative samples. The dynamic nature of serial assessments, however, allows for greater understanding of a patient's course when assessing diagnostically meaningful change.

OBSTACLES TO OVERCOME WITH SERIAL ASSESSMENTS

While conducting serial assessments is highly advantageous for evaluating changes in cognitive trajectories, the astute clinician must do so with a sound appreciation of the methodological and patient factors that are unique to repeat assessments.

Consider our 82-year-old female patient in a further example. Following her initial evaluation, which suggested memory skills within normal limits, she undergoes a second evaluation a year later. Her performance has remained within normal limits, but declined by 6 standard score points (let's say from a standard score of 102 to 96). The clinician faces certain issues when interpreting this 6-point discrepancy: should this be viewed as a stable memory performance over time or does this represent a decline? Under ideal conditions tests should yield the same score at baseline as at retest in the absence of a significant intervening variable such as disease progression or a surgical/medical intervention. In the absence of perfect stability and reliability, clinicians need to appreciate and account for *bias* and *error*. Bias can be systematic (e.g. disease progression, practice effects, demographic influences) or random (e.g. bereavement, health issues, time of day). Error may take the form of measurement error, regression to the mean, or floor/ceiling effects.

The first cause for concern is bias, or sources of systematic change in test performance (Lineweaver and Chelune 2003) that do not reflect true changes in cognition. A number of factors related to bias can influence serial assessments, including the impact of practice effects. It is well known that cognitive test performance in the aggregate improves from one assessment to the next due to familiarity and repeated exposure to the test stimuli. Performance typically improves when testing is repeated, even among older adults. This can lead to faulty conclusions being drawn if such factors are not accounted for when evaluating for slow deterioration of cognition over time (as in monitoring the conversion from MCI to dementia) or for mild improvements as a result of a drug intervention (Calamia, Markon, and Tranel 2012). Domains such as executive functioning and learning/memory tend to be most susceptible to practice effects (Bartels et al. 2010), with the greatest amount of practice or improvement occurring between the first and the second assessments (Ivnik et al. 1999). Executive tasks often rely on logic or problem-solving, such that once the patient has 'figured out' the concept of the problem, performance during a successive evaluation will not be as challenging (Lezak et al. 2012). Similarly, for memory tests there is the obvious concern that patients who have been exposed to certain word lists, stories, or geometric figures in the past may recognize or retain the content more easily when the test is repeated. In addition, research has suggested that some practice effects exist even when utilizing alternate forms of many neuropsychological tests (Beglinger et al. 2005; Hinton-Bayre and Geffen 2005), suggesting that the experience of learning 'how' to take tests will improve repeated performance in the future (i.e. test sophistication; Ronnlund, Lovden, and Nilsson 2008). However, in a recent meta-analysis evaluating the literature on practice effects in repeat neuropsychological assessments, Calamia and colleagues (2012) found that practice effects consistently occur with repeat testing, but vary as a function of several factors, including ageing, test-retest intervals, and use of alternate forms.

Additional sources of systematic or random bias may include intervening variables and demographic considerations (Lineweaver and Chelune 2003). Intervening variables may include factors that can alter the trajectory of natural cognitive change over time, such as intervention effects (in a systematic fashion) or unplanned/extraneous events (in a random fashion). For example, pharmacological interventions such as the prescription of cholinesterase inhibitors or NMDA-receptor antagonists between two neuropsychological evaluations may lead to a stabilization or mild improvement in cognition, thus systematically and predictably altering trajectories of decline. Alternatively, extraneous events may present in the form of the passing of a loved one shortly before a repeat evaluation, resulting in grief and random/unpredicted declines in mood and cognition.

Further, demographic factors such as age, education, gender, ethnicity, and premorbid functioning may also act as sources of bias (Lineweaver and Chelune 2003) insofar as these factors may influence cognitive trajectories. In general, age has been considered the 'least equivocal risk factor' for cognitive decline and dementia (Smith and Rush 2006). A myriad of longitudinal studies have suggested that the prevalence of dementia and cognitive decline increases across the age spectrum, continuing into the early 90s (Cache County Study; Miech et al. 2002) and beyond (Framingham Study; Bachman et al. 1993). Rates of cognitive decline and dementia are reportedly slightly higher for women than men in several studies (Stockholm, Sweden Study, Fratiglioni et al. 1997; Cache County Study, Breitner et al. 1999). However, other large-scale studies have indicated inconsistent results (Framingham Study, Bachman et al. 1993; Mayo Clinic Study, Edland et al. 2002), and suggest that the difference in prevalence rates may be misleading due to the discrepancy in survival rates between men and women above the age of 60. Higher levels of education and premorbid functioning have been considered to have a buffering effect on cognitive decline, such that these factors can mask or compensate for the effects of neurological insult for a longer period of time than lower levels of education and premorbid functioning. As such, these elements collectively comprise the notion of 'cognitive reserve', which is considered to be a buffering factor that alters the threshold of neurological damage attainable prior to the manifestation of clinical declines (Stern 2002). Interestingly, however, once individuals with higher levels of reserve eventually reach the threshold for cognitive decline, their rates of decline are faster than individuals with less education and prior functioning (and thus, reserve; Stern 2009). Finally, genetics have also been shown to be a source of systematic change regarding cognitive trajectories, including genetic mutations with a causative link with various forms of dementia (amyloid precursor protein gene, presenilin 1 and 2), and genes known to increase susceptibility to developing dementia (apolipoprotein ε gene; Rocchi et al. 2003).

While bias is a major source of concern, an equal concern when using multiple time-point evaluations is error, or sources of random change not associated with true change in cognitive ability. Sources of error include measurement error and regression to the mean, and statistical considerations like ceiling/floor effects. Regression to the mean is the notion that extreme scores will tend to change, or regress, to less extreme scores when assessed repeatedly, based on base rates and the inconsistency of random influences during an evaluation (Duff 2012). When an individual performs in the extremes, whether high or low, of the normative distribution of scores for a particular task during their first evaluation, it is statistically more likely on retesting that this individual's follow-up score will more closely approximate the population's mean. Similarly, floor and ceiling effects can influence the results during a serial evaluation in that they may artificially restrict the range of possible scores for a second evaluation. A ceiling effect occurs when tests are so easy that the typical respondent scores near or at the top of the possible scoring range, though this may also occur when test performance by an individual is exceptionally strong. The opposite is true for floor effects, in that tests are so difficult that the average performance is near or at the bottom of the range of possible scores, or that the individual is severely impaired. For example, when ceiling effects occur at Time 1, significant improvements in ability at Time 2 cannot be as easily evaluated because the respondent has already 'maxed out' the test score during the initial evaluation, consequently leaving no opportunity for measurable improvement.

Additional causes for concern can be related to the compounding effects of measurement error due to repeat assessments. Psychological tests lack perfect precision and each act of measurement introduces some level of measurement error into the system (Lineweaver and Chelune 2003). Standard Error of Measurement (SEM) is a function of the reliability of a test and the standard deviation of the testing sample. More specifically, SEM is a measure of the variance of obtained scores around the true score for each patient performance (Slick 2006). With each additional neuropsychological assessment, additional measurement error will be introduced into the evaluation; as error is, by definition, not systematic, it becomes increasingly difficult to predict how statistical error is impacting the trajectory of performance. For example, if measurement error caused an observed score to be a value of 53 at Time 1 and a value of 47 at Time 2, despite the true score being 50 each time, a clinician may incorrectly interpret a decline in performance over time, which is actually just a function of the measurement error. Consequently, each additional evaluation raises the possibility of statistical error interfering with accuracy and diagnostic conclusions, adding to the increased complexity when making interpretations from serial assessments.

ASSESSING RELIABLE CHANGE

Let us return to the example of the 82-year-old woman presenting with memory complaints. Her neuropsychologist administers the Ideal Memory Test (IMT) and she obtains a standard score of 96. A year later she returns and obtains a score of 92 on the IMT. How should the neuropsychologist interpret the patient's 4-point performance decrement? Could this simply be test-retest variability? Could it be the result of normal ageing? Or, within the context of memory complaints, could it be a clinically meaningful sign of cognitive deterioration? These questions have vexed psychologists for years. Fortunately, a family of related statistical procedures has been developed that can assist the clinician to sort through the various issues involved in serial assessment, and determine whether observed changes in a patient's performances are clinically meaningful.

The procedures, collectively referred to as *reliable change methods* (Chelune 2003; Hinton-Bayre 2010), attempt differentially to take into account the impact of differential practice effects and other systematic biases, measurement error, and regression to the mean on the interpretation of change scores. There are two general approaches: the *simple difference* method and the *predicted difference* method. Taking their lead from Matarazzo and Herman (1984), both approaches consider difference scores not simply in terms of their magnitude but, importantly, their frequency or base rate in a reference population such as a standardization sample or another patient group.

SIMPLE DIFFERENCE APPROACHES

Simple-difference approaches begin by obtaining the observed difference between scores at Time 1 and Time 2 (T2–T1). In our example of the 82-year-old tested with the IMT, the difference reflects a decline of –4 points. The meaning of this difference will depend on how frequently other people in a reference population such as a normal standardization sample also obtain such test-retest difference scores. If we were able to look at the psychometric data in the IMT manual we might find that the mean test-retest difference score for a sample of 400 individuals was not 0 points but +4.51, reflecting a positive retest bias or practice effect. Being the 'ideal' memory test, we might also find that the authors report that the standard deviation (SD) of the test-retest difference scores is 4.77 (note: the SD of difference scores is not the same as the SD of the test, which in the case of a test using a Standard Score metric would be 15). To estimate the relative frequency of individuals scoring −4 or less on the IMT, we would first calculate the difference between the person's observed retest score (92) and their expected retest score including the practice effect (baseline + practice effect: 96 + 4.51 = 100.51). This would yield a simple difference score of −8.51 (92−100.51). We can now determine where this simple difference score lies in the distribution of difference scores in the reference population by dividing it by the SD of differences to obtain a z-score (−8.51/ 4.77 = −1.78). Comparing this z-score to the area under the normal curve, we find that only 3.75% of the reference population would be expected to obtain z-scores this extreme, suggesting that our patient's decline of 4 points on retesting is a rare occurrence. So, perhaps our patient is showing signs of progressive memory loss and might benefit from medication and behavioural intervention.

Unfortunately, most test manuals and many publications presenting the results of serial assessments do not report the observed test-retest SD of differences. To circumvent this limitation, investigators have devised a number of simple difference methods to *estimate* the SD of differences based on the test-retest summary statistics (i.e. Means, SDs, and test-retest correlation coefficient) so that Reliable Change Index (RCI) scores can be computed. It is beyond the scope of this chapter to review these in depth here, and we will present only an overview. See Table 11.1 for a listing of Reliable Change formulas. The earliest RCI method was advanced by Jacobson and Truax (1991). Using the SD of test scores at baseline and the test-retest reliability coefficient, they computed an SEM at Time 1, multiplied it by 2 to account for measurement error in the retest scores, and then computed a Standard Error of the Difference (SED), an estimate of the SD of the difference scores. Chelune and colleagues (Chelune et al. 1993) offered a practice-effect-adjusted RCI modification by suggesting that the mean practice effect for the reference population be incorporated in the calculation of the simple difference. Iverson (Iverson 2001) further modified

Table 11.1 Reliable change scores and their formula

Reliable Change Score	Formula
Simple discrepancy score	$T_2 - T_1$
Standard deviation index	$T_2 - T_1/S_1$
Reliable Change Index (RCI)	$T_2 - T_1/SED$
	$SED = \sqrt{2(S_1[\sqrt{1 - r_{12}}])^2 2S_1^2(1 - r_{12})}$
RCI controlling for practice effects (RCI+PE)—and alternate calculation of SED by Iverson	$(T_2 - T_1) - (M_2 - M_1)/SED$
	$SED_{Iverson} = \sqrt{(S_1\sqrt{1 - r_{12}})^2 + (S_2\sqrt{1 - r_{12}})^2}$
	$(T_2 - T_1) - (M_2 - M_1)/SED_{Iverson}$
Standardized Regression Based formula (SRB)	$Y' = bT_1 + c$
	$RCI_{SRB} = T_2 - T_2'/SEE$

T_1 = score at Time 1; T_2 = score at Time 2; S_1 = standard deviation at Time 1; S_2 = standard deviation at Time 2; SED = standard error of the difference; r_{12} = correlation between Time 1 and 2 scores; M_1 = control group mean at Time 1; M_2 = control group mean at Time 2; b = slope of the regression model (beta coefficient); c = intercept of the regression model (constant); SEE = standard error of the estimate of the regression model; Y' = predicted score at Time 2 based on regression model.

this practice-adjusted RCI by computing separate SEMs for baseline and retest scores and pooling these to compute an estimate of the standard deviation of differences. Further refinements have been made to methods of estimating the distribution of test-retest difference scores, the mean of the difference scores (Blasi et al. 2009), and the relative merits of these approaches have been reviewed and debated in the literature (Hinton-Bayre and Geffen 2005; Hinton-Bayre 2010; Lineweaver and Chelune 2003; Maassen 2000; Stein et al. 2010). Although differences among the RCI procedures have generally been small (Hinton-Bayre and Geffen 2005; Hinton-Bayre 2010), the simple-difference approach itself has some major limitations. First, the approach treats practice as invariant, adding mean practice effect as a constant to everyone regardless of their baseline performance. It also does not take into account the effects of regression to the mean, which may be sizeable when the baseline score is very high or very low and the test has modest reliability. Finally, the simple difference approach relies on only the observed test-retest scores and does not take into consideration other factors that might differentially influence or bias the rate of test-retest change at the individual level (e.g. age, education, gender, level of baseline performance, medical factors, etc.). For these reasons, there is a growing preference to use the predicted difference method of evaluating test-retest changes, and these are beginning to make their appearance in test manuals (Pearson 2009).

Predicted Difference Approaches

The predicted difference method uses linear regression to generate predicted retest scores (Y_p) for individuals based on their specific baseline performances (X) and then subtracts this predicted score from their observed retest scores (Y_o) to obtain their personal *change score* discrepancy ($Y_o - Y_p$). Additional sources of potential bias (e.g. age, education, gender) can be added to the regression equation in a multivariate manner (McSweeny et al. 1993). This approach allows practice effects to be modelled as a function of individual baseline performance as well as accounting for regression to the mean. Akin to the simple difference approach where the standard error term used to obtain the z-score reflects the dispersion of difference scores around the mean of the *difference scores*, the predicted difference approach uses the *Standard Error of the Estimate* (SEE) for the regression equation to reflect the dispersion of scores around the regression line.

In our case example with the IMT memory test, the test's author found the regression equation for predicting retest scores was given as: $Y' = (1.036 \times$ Baseline score) + ($-0.04155 \times$ Age) + 3.064, with an SEE of 4.6478. If we enter our patient's baseline score of 96 and age of 82 into the equation, and compare their observed (92) vs predicted retest scores (99.11), we get a *change score* discrepancy ($Y_o - Y_p$) of -7.11. Note that *Age* has a negative beta weight, suggesting that as people age they show less of a practice effect on the IMT. If we divide this difference by the SEE (7.11/4.6478), we obtain a z-score of -1.53, indicating that only 6.3% of cases would obtain a retest score this low given the patient's age and original baseline. The difference between the z-score obtained via the simple difference method (-1.78) and the predicted difference method (-1.53) highlights the potential benefits of the predicted difference method where factors such as age can influence clinical expectations of meaningfulness.

While there is a growing body of predicted difference equations for a variety of tests commonly used with older adults (Attix et al. 2009; Duff 2010; Duff et al. 2010a; Duff et al. 2005; Stein et al. 2010), and some tests such as the fourth edition of the Wechsler Adult Intelligence and Memory Scales are incorporating predicted difference algorithms into their scoring software (Pearson 2009), there is still a paucity of published longitudinal regression-based data on test-retest performance. Crawford and colleagues (Crawford and Garthwaite 2007; Crawford et al. 2012) have been able to demonstrate that it is possible to construct both bivariate and multivariate regression equations based on simple summary statistics (sample size, test-retest means and standard deviations, and zero-order correlations) that are almost invariably available in test manuals and published reports on serial assessment. Using simple calculators provided free of charge on Crawford's website (see RegBuild_MR.exe in Downloads at http://homepages.abdn.ac.uk/j.crawford/pages/dept/), clinicians can easily compute predicted difference equations that can be applied to the individual case for determining the relative frequency of a given patient's test-retest difference scores without actual access to the raw test-retest standardization data. Given the ease of access and use of these calculators for developing predicted difference equations, there is virtually no further need for clinicians or researchers to use simple difference methods based on estimates of the dispersion of test-retest change scores.

AIMS FOR FUTURE RESEARCH

Shift from recording change to predicting change

While we have argued that the use of serial assessments displays benefits over single-time-period clinical neuropsychology evaluations, the current model of assessment is predominantly characterized by clinicians assessing individuals across two time periods and observing the change over time. A number of issues can be raised with this practice. First, plotting two performance values on a graph may imply a linear progression of improvement or decline over time. For example, evaluations in two consecutive years do not allow us to identify possible fluctuations in performance between those two evaluations, as we tend to think of improvement or decline as consistent. In addition, should declines be observed, we learn little about the slope or severity of the declines; an individual may have displayed an initial gradual decline between the two evaluations, a rapid decline immediately after Time 1 followed by stability until Time 2, or they may have remained relatively stable throughout most of the interim between evaluations and experienced a rapid decline in the period immediately preceding the second evaluation. While these current practices are beneficial to *document* change over time and assist with differential diagnosis, the results do not necessarily provide us with meaningful information as to whether the individual will continue to decline in the future. An area of improvement in the field of clinical neuropsychology lies in our capacity to *predict* future performance based on past results. Instead of simply chronicling past change, future prediction of change would allow us to consider cognitive interventions at an earlier time period. Early detection and intervention of cognitive impairments will have a serious impact on society, given that delaying AD onset by one year would reduce the number of these cases in 2050 by 9.2 million (Brookmeyer et al. 2007), and delaying both AD onset and disease progression by two years would reduce burden by more than 22.8 million cases, with most of that decrease among late-stage cases that require the most intensive care. These findings highlight the impact that predictive models can have on treatment interventions.

Deriving Ipsative Trajectories of Cognitive Change

A second aim of future research should be to focus on deriving ipsative trajectories for cognitive change. Currently, cognitive performance is considered in the context of normative data, which may become problematic when an individual declines over time but still falls within expectation given the appropriate normative sample. For example, a patient that performs at the upper end of the average range at Time 1 but near the lower limit of the average range at Time 2 is often considered cause for concern, but not yet appropriate for treatment intervention as the patient likely does not meet criteria for MCI or dementia. Should we as a field shift more towards considering individual trajectories and how they differ from normal decline over time, intervention methods would likely be implemented much earlier in the disease process. In the example above, waiting until the individual declines to the point of normative impairment (1.5 to 2 standard deviations below the mean) prior to treatment intervention would mean that individuals with high premorbid functioning would have to decline for a longer period of time prior to being considered appropriate for intervention (Stern 2009). Such a shift would require a focus on individual rates of change, as compared to absolute declines. The development and advancement of regression-based models as suggested above would allow researchers and clinicians to evaluate change over time using slopes of cognitive change. This could make it possible to detect meaningful changes in an individual cognitive trajectory, even when cognitive performance appears normal compared to the average performance of others. Data derived from the completed Cache County Study of Memory, Health, and Aging (Welsh-Bohmer et al. 2006) is currently in the process of developing individual, standardized regression-based trajectories of cognitive change over serial assessments to identify those who are deviating from their expected personal cognitive trajectory of retest performance, which will likely provide earlier interventions and increased clinical benefit.

Utilization of Practice Effects in Clinical Practice

The capacity to profit from experience (learning) and to apply this information to prospective situations (memory) has biological and functional advantages. As alluded to previously, practice effects are often observed during repeat or serial assessments; however, these effects are often not taken into consideration during screening for dementia, and previous observations are not utilized, even when longitudinal data are available. At the level of the individual, the *absence* of cognitive change is typically interpreted as demonstrating stability when in fact the absence of an *expected* change may reflect a meaningful decrement in ability. The problem is further compounded when an individual's retest scores are compared to cross-sectional group normative expectations without consideration that the individual has been repeatedly exposed to the test material and is not showing the expected improvements with practice. Taken together, the typical interpretation of longitudinal screening data fails to capitalize on the potential sensitivity of serial neuropsychological assessment to detect the earliest signs of cognitive decline in AD. Research on practice effects at the University of Utah has demonstrated the importance of identifying practice effects as a potential behavioural marker for early decline.

Despite prior studies finding minimal practice effects in MCI (Cooper et al. 2004), our patients classified as amnestic MCI displayed similar levels of practice compared to cognitively healthy adults when retested with a brief cognitive battery after one week (Duff et al. 2008). Even more paradoxical was that these patients showed *greater* levels of practice than their intact peers on two memory measures. We hypothesized about a number of potentials reasons for this unexpected finding, including the fact that ceiling effects in the healthy group limited their practice effects as well as the heterogeneity of the MCI group. With respect to this latter explanation, we did appear to identify two subgroups within our MCI sample: those that benefited from practice and those that did not. Regardless of the interpretation of these findings, they clearly have clinical implications. For example, does someone really have amnestic MCI if s/he benefits so much from repeated exposure to testing materials that s/he is reclassified as 'intact' after one week? That is, should repeat testing be used to clarify questionable diagnoses of MCI? From a treatment standpoint, if some individuals with amnestic MCI benefit from practice, repetition, or additional learning trials, then should cognitive rehabilitation be indicated for these patients? Additionally, might cholinesterase inhibitors and other cognitive enhancing medications work optimally in those patients who demonstrate the capacity to learn? A final clinical question might be: what is the prognostic value of practice effects in these patients? To start to address this question, we followed these participants across one year and repeated their cognitive evaluations. As shown in Figure 11.1, those patients that showed large practice effects after one week (MCI + PE; dotted line) remained cognitively stable across one year, whereas those patients that showed minimal practice effects (MCI-PE; solid line) significantly declined on a measure of delayed memory (Duff et al. 2011b). These findings, coupled with the earlier ones, highlight the clinical utility of practice effects in the diagnosis and prognosis of patients with MCI.

In other studies using similar practice effects paradigms in older adults, we have observed that:

1. Practice effects relate to dementia severity in patients with Alzheimer's disease and other types of dementias (Duff, Chelune, and Dennett 2012b). These findings might also force us to re-examine the 'learning potential' of patients with Alzheimer's disease.
2. Practice effects were negatively correlated with cerebral amyloid deposition (via ^{18}F-flutemetamol), such that higher practice effects were associated with lower amyloid deposition and lower practice effects were associated with higher amyloid deposits (Duff et al. 2012c).

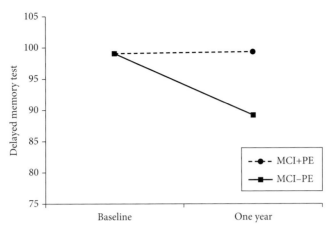

FIGURE 11.1 Practice effects (PE) and cognitive outcomes in Mild Cognitive Impairment (MCI).

3. Within-session practice effects predicted response to a cognitive training programme in community-dwelling older adults (Duff et al. 2010b). From a research standpoint, it might be possible to use practice effects to enrich samples for clinical trials.
4. Practice effects add to the prediction of future cognitive functioning, above and beyond baseline levels of cognition (Duff et al. 2010a).
5. Practice effects do not seem to vary as a function of age, education, premorbid intellect, or depression, which may make them a unique and useful clinical tool (Duff et al. 2012a).

Overall, practice effects from repeated cognitive testing are still primarily considered a 'nuisance' variable that distorts findings of longitudinal evaluations. However, our work (as well as that of others) indicates that they provide some very valuable information about cerebral integrity and brain plasticity.

CASE EXAMPLE AND IMPLICATIONS FOR PRACTICE

Please consider a final case example to illustrate the benefit of using serial assessments for tracking cognitive trajectories. In our example throughout this chapter, an 82-year-old, right-handed female sought the services of a neuropsychologist due to declining memory over the previous one to two years. She has a PhD in accounting and has worked as a university professor. Her past medical history is significant for peripheral neuropathy and bilateral cataract surgery, and she was not receiving any medications at the time of her initial evaluation. An assessment was undertaken and the patient obtained a Mini Mental Status Examination (MMSE) score of 27/30 and an intact

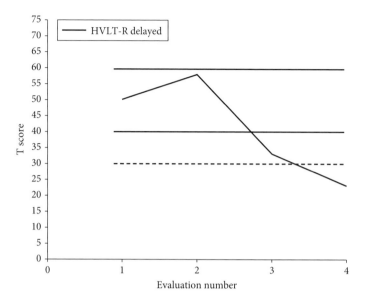

FIGURE 11.2 Performance of case example on the Hopkins Verbal Learning Test (HVLT) Delayed Recall task across four neuropsychological evaluations. Solid horizontal lines reflect 1 standard deviation above and below the mean, and the dotted horizontal line reflects impairment (T-score of 31).

memory profile (age-normed T-score of 50; see Figure 11.2 for her memory profile over time) using the Hopkins Verbal Learning Test-Revised (HVLT-R; Brandt and Benedict 2001) delayed recall variable. Given that no declines in functioning were reported, no diagnosis of memory impairment or dementia was appropriate at that time. After an additional twelve months of similar cognitive concerns, the patient was re-evaluated to assess for change over time. At that time a MMSE score of 28 was obtained and her memory abilities via the HVLT-R improved from the average to the high-average range (age-normed T-score of 58); at the time of the second evaluation, the patient in hindsight acknowledged past difficulty with depression at the first evaluation that had since resolved. Ten months later the patient was re-referred due to report of increased memory loss, at which point her MMSE remained 27/30 but her memory scores on the HVLT-R notably declined. As the solid horizontal lines in Figure 11.2 reflect 1 standard deviation variation in scores above and below the mean (T-scores of 40–60; 16–84th percentiles) and the dashed horizontal line reflects impairment (T-score of 31; 3rd percentile), the patient's delayed memory performance declined to the borderline impaired range, which would be consistent with Mild Cognitive Impairment (MCI), Amnestic Subtype based on Petersen criteria (Petersen 2004). As the literature suggests that these patients have an increased risk of showing further decline and developing a dementia, a fourth evaluation was recommended in twelve months to track her rate of change. At the fourth testing session, the patient's MMSE score had declined to 23/30 and her memory deficits were more progressed, falling in the impaired range of functioning (T-score of 23). At this time, a serious consideration for conversion from MCI to dementia was considered with respect to her functional abilities.

While not all patients have the luxury of being evaluated on four separate occasions, spanning across three years, the above example highlights a number of important issues. First, initial memory complaints may predate clinical impairment by a number of years, particularly in individuals with high premorbid functioning. It took two years to identify borderline levels of impairment in this patient, and three full years to eventually detect impairment. Her high level of education and occupational status (and as such premorbid functioning and cognitive reserve) may have protected her from the cumulative effects of neurological insult during the first two evaluations, until a threshold was reached between Time 2 and Time 3, at which period her cognitive abilities notably declined. Second, this case identifies the role of practice effects and extraneous patient factors. In this case, the improvement between Time 1 and Time 2 may have reflected an improvement in mood (a change in patient characteristics) that the patient previously did not consider a problem, as well as the observation of benefit from being exposed to the materials previously (a practice effect). As discussed previously, such an improvement is likely dually influenced by previous exposure to test materials, formulation of test-taking strategies, and in some cases a reduction in apprehension or nervousness that may occur as a result of increased familiarity with the testing environment. While mild practice effects may have existed at Time 3 or Time 4, it is more likely that delayed memory recall abilities had declined to the point that she was not capable of benefiting from her prior testing experiences, which is also suggestive of poor overall prognosis (Duff et al. 2010a). Third, her decline from Time 2 to Time 3 may have resulted from the combined contribution of true declines in cognition and regression to the mean in response to her previously above average performance. Fourth, while the decline from Time 2 to Time 3 was fairly notable in this example, having the prior performances on the HVLT-R allowed the examiners to make determinations of the level of decline based on base rates using methods such as Reliable Change Indices. Finally, it is clear that a single-point assessment at any stage of the process would not be able to contribute to capturing the dynamic nature of the patient's cognitive trajectory as well as the series of evaluations that she underwent; consequently, repeated assessment via subspecialty consultation was beneficial for this patient.

SUMMARY

This chapter provides information to the reader regarding methods used in the practice of clinical neuropsychology when evaluating cognitive change over time. While typical cognitive changes may be associated with the 'normal' ageing process, in a growing proportion of patients cognitive declines may arise based on particular syndromes such as neurodegenerative disease that result in abnormalities to normal cognitive trajectories. Although single-time-point neuropsychological assessments may frequently be necessary to derive clinical conclusions, particularly when no prior information is known about a patient, we have attempted to highlight the benefits of utilizing serial assessments over time, in order to gain a dynamic view of test performance, as well as the statistical methods available to identify reliable change over time. Finally, while applying ipsative trajectories and practice effects to clinical practice would aid clinicians in better understanding cognitive trajectories for individual patients, additional research is necessary to best utilize such factors clinically.

REFERENCES

American Psychiatric Association (2000). *Diagnostic and Statistical Manual of Mental Disorders* (4th edn, text rev.). Washington, DC: American Psychiatric Association.

American Psychiatric Association (2013). *Diagnostic and Statistical Manual of Mental Disorders* (5th edn). Washington, DC: American Psychiatric Association.

Antonini, A., Leenders, K. L., Reist, H., Thomann, R., Beer, H. F., and Locher, J. (1993). 'Effect of Age on D2 Dopamine Receptors in Normal Human Brain Measured by Positron Emission Tomography and 11C-raclopride'. *Archives of Neurology* 50(5): 474–480.

Attix, D. K., Story, T. J., Chelune, G. J., Ball, J. D., Stutts, M. L., Hart, R. P., et al. (2009). 'The Prediction of Change: Normative Neuropsychological Trajectories'. *Clinical Neuropsychologist* 23(1): 21–38. doi:10.1080/13854040801945078.

Bachman, D. L., Wolf, P. A., Linn, R. T., Knoefel, J. E., Cobb, J. L., Belanger, A. J., et al. (1993). 'Incidence of Dementia and Probable Alzheimer's Disease in a General Population: The Framingham Study'. *Neurology* 43(3Pt1): 515–519.

Backman, L., Small, B. J., and Fratiglioni, L. (2001). 'Stability of the Preclinical Episodic Memory Deficit in Alzheimer's Disease'. *Brain* 124(Pt1): 96–102.

Bartels, C., Wegrzyn, M., Wiedl, A., Ackermann, V., and Ehrenreich, H. (2010). 'Practice Effects in Healthy Adults: A Longitudinal Study on Frequent Repetitive Cognitive Testing'. *BMC Neuroscience* 11: 118.

Barth, J. T., Pliskin, N., Axelrod, B., Faust, D., Fisher, J., Harley, J. P., et al. (2003). 'Introduction to the NAN 2001 Definition of a Clinical Neuropsychologist. NAN Policy and Planning Committee' [Review]. *Archives of Clinical Neuropsychology* 18(5): 551–555.

Beglinger, L. J., Gaydos, B., Tangphao-Daniels, O., Duff, K., Kareken, D. A., Crawford, J., et al. (2005). 'Practice Effects and the Use of Alternate Forms in Serial Neuropsychological Testing'. *Archives of Clinical Neuropsychology* 20(4): 517–529.

Bennett, D. A., Wilson, R. S., Schneider, J. A., Evans, D. A., Beckett, L. A., Aggarwal, N. T., et al. (2002). 'Natural History of Mild Cognitive Impairment in Older Persons' [Research Support, US Govt, PHS]. *Neurology* 59(2): 198–205.

Blasi, S., Zehnder, A. E., Berres, M., Taylor, K. I., Spiegel, R., and Monsch, A. U. (2009). 'Norms for Change in Episodic Memory as a Prerequisite for the Diagnosis of Mild Cognitive Impairment (MCI)'. *Neuropsychology* 23(2): 189–200.

Braak, H. and Del Tredici, K. (2011). 'The Pathological Process Underlying Alzheimer's Disease in Individuals under Thirty'. *Acta Neuropathologica* 121(2): 171–181.

Brandt, J. and Benedict, R. (2001). *Hopkins Verbal Learning Test—Revised*. Odessa, FL: PAR.

Breitner, J. C., Wyse, B. W., Anthony, J. C., Welsh-Bohmer, K. A., Steffens, D. C., Norton, M. C., et al. (1999). 'APOE-epsilon4 Count Predicts Age When Prevalence of AD Increases, Then Declines: The Cache County Study'. *Neurology* 53(2): 321–331.

Brookmeyer, R., Johnson, E., Ziegler-Graham, K., and Arrighi, H. M. (2007). 'Forecasting the Global Burden of Alzheimer's Disease'. *Alzheimer's & Dementia* 3(3): 186–191.

Buckner, R. L. (2004). 'Memory and Executive Function in Aging and AD: Multiple Factors that Cause Decline and Reserve Factors that Compensate'. *Neuron* 44(1): 195–208.

Busch, R., Chelune, G., and Suchy, Y. (2006). 'Using Norms in Neuropsychological Assessment of the Elderly'. In K.-A. D. Welsh-Bohmer and K. Welsh-Bohmer (eds), *Geriatric Neuropsychology: Assessment and Intervention* (pp. 141–165). New York: Gilford.

Cahn-Weiner, D. A., Ready, R. E., and Malloy, P. F. (2003). 'Neuropsychological Predictors of Everyday Memory and Everyday Functioning in Patients with Mild Alzheimer's Disease'. *Journal of Geriatric Psychiatry and Neurology* 16(2): 84–89.

Calamia, M., Markon, K., and Tranel, D. (2012). 'Scoring Higher the Second Time Around: Meta-analyses of Practice Effects in Neuropsychological Assessment'. *Clinical Neuropsychologist* 26(4): 543–570.

Chelune, G., Naugle, R., Lüders, H., Sedlak, J., and Awad, I. (1993). 'Individual Change Following Epilepsy Surgery: Practice Effects and Base-rate Information'. *Neuropsychology* 1: 41–52.

Chelune, G. (2003). 'Assessing Reliable Neuropsychological Change'. In R. Franklin (ed), *Prediction in Forensic and Neuropsychology: New Approaches to Psychometrically Sound Assessment*. Nahwah, NJ: Erlbaum.

Chelune, G. J. (2010). 'Evidence-based Research and Practice in Clinical Neuropsychology'. *Clinical Neuropsychologist* 24(3): 454–467.

Chelune, G. and Duff, K. (2012). *The Assessment of Change: Serial Assessments in Dementia Evaluation*. New York: Springer.

Chen, P., Ratcliff, G., Belle, S. H., Cauley, J. A., DeKosky, S. T., and Ganguli, M. (2001). 'Patterns of Cognitive Decline in Presymptomatic Alzheimer Disease: A Prospective Community Study'. *Archives of General Psychiatry* 58(9): 853–858.

Chui, H. C. (2006). 'Vascular Cognitive Impairment: Today and Tomorrow'. *Alzheimer's & Dementia* 2(3): 185–194.

Cooper, D. B., Lacritz, L. H., Weiner, M. F., Rosenberg, R. N., and Cullum, C. M. (2004). 'Category Fluency in Mild Cognitive Impairment: Reduced Effect of Practice in Test-retest Conditions'. *Alzheimer Disease and Associated Disorders* 18(3): 120–122.

Crawford, J. R. and Garthwaite, P. H. (2007). 'Using Regression Equations Built from Summary Data in the Neuropsychological Assessment of the Individual Case'. *Neuropsychology* 21(5): 611–620. doi:10.1037/0894-4105.21.5.611.

Crawford, J. R., Garthwaite, P. H., Denham, A. K., and Chelune, G. J. (2012). 'Using Regression Equations Built from Summary Data in the Psychological Assessment of the Individual Case: Extension to Multiple Regression'. *Psychological Assessment* 24(4): 801–814.

Driscoll, I., Davatzikos, C., An, Y., Wu, X., Shen, D., Kraut, M., et al. (2009). 'Longitudinal Pattern of Regional Brain Volume Change Differentiates Normal Aging from MCI'. *Neurology* 72(22): 1906–1913.

Duff, K., Schoenberg, M. R., Patton, D., Paulsen, J. S., Bayless, J. D., Mold, J., et al. (2005). 'Regression-based Formulas for Predicting Change in RBANS Subtests with Older Adults'. *Archives of Clinical Neuropsychology* 20(3): 281–290.

Duff, K., Beglinger, L., Van Der Heiden, S., Moser, D., Arndt, S., Schultz, S., et al. (2008). 'Short-term Practice Effects in Amnestic Mild Cognitive Impairment: Implications for Diagnosis and Treatment'. *International Psychogeriatrics* 20(5): 986–999.

Duff, K. (2010). 'Predicting Premorbid Memory Functioning in Older Adults'. *Applied Neuropsychology* 17(4): 278–282.

Duff, K., Beglinger, L. J., Moser, D. J., Paulsen, J. S., Schultz, S. K., and Arndt, S. (2010a). 'Predicting Cognitive Change in Older Adults: The Relative Contribution of Practice Effects'. *Archives of Clinical Neuropsychology* 25(2): 81–88.

Duff, K., Beglinger, L. J., Moser, D. J., Schultz, S. K., and Paulsen, J. S. (2010b). 'Practice Effects and Outcome of Cognitive Training: Preliminary Evidence from a Memory Training Course'. *American Journal of Geriatric Psychiatry* 18(1): 91.

Duff, K., Chelune, G. J., and Dennett, K. (2011a). 'Predicting Estimates of Premorbid Memory Functioning: Validation in a Dementia Sample'. *Archives of Clinical Neuropsychology* 26(8): 701–705.

Duff, K., Lyketsos, C. G., Beglinger, L. J., Chelune, G., Moser, D. J., Arndt, S., et al. (2011b). 'Practice Effects Predict Cognitive Outcome in Amnestic Mild Cognitive Impairment'. *American Journal of Geriatric Psychiatry* 19(11): 932–939.

Duff, K. (2012). 'Evidence-based Indicators of Neuropsychological Change in the Individual Patient: Relevant Concepts and Methods'. *Archives of Clinical Neuropsychology* 27(3): 248–261.

Duff, K., Callister, C., Dennett, K., and Tometich, D. (2012a). 'Practice Effects: A Unique Cognitive Variable'. *Clinical Neuropsychologist* 26(7): 1117–1127.

Duff, K., Chelune, G., and Dennett, K. (2012b). 'Within-session Practice Effects in Patients Referred for Suspected Dementia'. *Dementia and Geriatric Cognitive Disorders* 33(4): 245–249.

Duff, K., Hoffman, J., Foster, N., Dennett, K., Thurfjell, L., Wang, A., et al. (2012c). *Flutemetamol is Related to Practice Effects on Cognitive Testing*. Paper presented at the Human Amyloid Imaging, Miami Beach, FL.

Edland, S. D., Rocca, W. A., Petersen, R. C., Cha, R. H., and Kokmen, E. (2002). 'Dementia and Alzheimer Disease Incidence Rates Do Not Vary by Sex in Rochester, Minn'. *Archives of Neurology* 59(10): 1589–1593.

Ertel, K. A., Glymour, M. M., and Berkman, L. F. (2008). 'Effects of Social Integration on Preserving Memory Function in a Nationally Representative US Elderly Population'. *American Journal of Public Health* 98(7): 1215–1220.

Ferri, C. P., Prince, M., Brayne, C., Brodaty, H., Fratiglioni, L., Ganguli, M., et al. (2005). 'Global Prevalence of Dementia: A Delphi Consensus Study'. *The Lancet* 366(9503): 2112–2117.

Finkel, D., Reynolds, C. A., McArdle, J. J., and Pedersen, N. L. (2007). 'Age Changes in Processing Speed as a Leading Indicator of Cognitive Aging'. *Psychology and Aging* 22(3): 558–568.

Fratiglioni, L., Viitanen, M., von Strauss, E., Tontodonati, V., Herlitz, A., and Winblad, B. (1997). 'Very Old Women at Highest Risk of Dementia and Alzheimer's Disease: Incidence Data from the Kungsholmen Project, Stockholm'. *Neurology* 48(1): 132–138.

Goldman-Rakic, P. S. and Brown, R. M. (1981). 'Regional Changes of Monoamines in Cerebral Cortex and Subcortical Structures of Aging Rhesus Monkeys'. *Neuroscience* 6(2): 177–187.

Hachinski, V., Iadecola, C., Petersen, R. C., Breteler, M. M., Nyenhuis, D. L., Black, S. E., et al. (2006). 'National Institute of Neurological Disorders and Stroke-Canadian Stroke Network Vascular Cognitive Impairment Harmonization Standards'. *Stroke* 37(9): 2220–2241.

Hayden, K. M., Reed, B. R., Manly, J. J., Tommet, D., Pietrzak, R. H., Chelune, G. J., et al. (2011). 'Cognitive Decline in the Elderly: An Analysis of Population Heterogeneity'. *Age and Ageing* 40(6): 684–689. doi:10.1093/ageing/afr101.

Hedden, T. and Gabrieli, J. D. (2004). 'Insights into the Ageing Mind: A View from Cognitive Neuroscience'. *Nature Reviews Neuroscience* 5(2): 87–96.

Hill, R. D. (2005). *Positive Aging*. New York: W. W. Norton.

Hill, R. D., Wahlin, A., Winblad, B., and Backman, L. (1995). 'The Role of Demographic and Life Style Variables in Utilizing Cognitive Support for Episodic Remembering among Very Old Adults'. *Journals of Gerontology Series B: Psychological Sciences and Social Sciences* 50(4): 219–227.

Hinton-Bayre, A. and Geffen, G. (2005). 'Comparability, Reliability, and Practice Effects on Alternate Forms of the Digit Symbol Substitution and Symbol Digit Modalities Tests'. *Psychological Assessment* 17(2): 237–241.

Hinton-Bayre, A. D. (2010). 'Deriving Reliable Change Statistics from Test-retest Normative Data: Comparison of Models and Mathematical Expressions'. *Archives of Clinical Neuropsychology* 25(3): 244–256.

Houston, W. and Bondi, M. (2006). 'Potentially Reversible Cognitive Symptoms in Older Adults'. In D. Attix and K. Welsh-Bohmer (eds), *Geriatric Neuropsychology: Assessment and Intervention* (pp. 103–130). New York: Guilford Press.

Howieson, D. B., Carlson, N. E., Moore, M. M., Wasserman, D., Abendroth, C. D., Payne-Murphy, J., et al. (2008). 'Trajectory of Mild Cognitive Impairment Onset'. *Journal of the International Neuropsychological Society* 14(2): 192–198.

Iverson, G. L. (2001). 'Interpreting Change on the WAIS-III/WMS-III in Clinical Samples'. *Archives of Clinical Neuropsychology* 16(2): 183–191.

Ivnik, R. J., Smith, G. E., Lucas, J. A., Petersen, R. C., Boeve, B. F., Kokmen, E., et al. (1999). 'Testing Normal Older People Three or Four Times at 1- to 2-year Intervals: Defining Normal Variance'. *Neuropsychology* 13(1): 121–127.

Jacobson, N. S. and Truax, P. (1991). 'Clinical Significance: A Statistical Approach to Defining Meaningful Change in Psychotherapy Research'. *Journal of Consulting and Clinical Psychology* 59(1): 12–19.

Kennedy, K. M. and Raz, N. (2009). 'Aging White Matter and Cognition: Differential Effects of Regional Variations in Diffusion Properties on Memory, Executive Functions, and Speed'. *Neuropsychologia* 47(3): 916–927.

Lange, K. L., Bondi, M. W., Salmon, D. P., Galasko, D., Delis, D. C., Thomas, R. G., et al. (2002). 'Decline in Verbal Memory during Preclinical Alzheimer's Disease: Examination of the Effect of APOE Genotype'. *Journal of the International Neuropsychological Society* 8(7): 943–955.

Larson, E. B., Wang, L., Bowen, J. D., McCormick, W. C., Teri, L., Crane, P., et al. (2006). 'Exercise is Associated with Reduced Risk for Incident Dementia among Persons 65 Years of Age and Older'. *Annals of Internal Medicine* 144(2): 73–81.

Laukka, E. J., Macdonald, S. W., Fratiglioni, L., and Backman, L. (2012). 'Preclinical Cognitive Trajectories Differ for Alzheimer's Disease and Vascular Dementia'. *Journal of the International Neuropsychological Society* 18(2): 191–199.

Levy, J. A. and Chelune, G. J. (2007). 'Cognitive-behavioral Profiles of Neurodegenerative Dementias: Beyond Alzheimer's Disease'. *Journal of Geriatric Psychiatry and Neurology* 20(4): 227–238.

Lezak, M., Howieson, D., and Loring, D. (2004). *Neuropsychological Assessment* (4th edn). New York: Oxford University Press.

Lezak, M., Howieson, D., Bigler, E., and Tranel, D. (2012). *Neuropsychological Assessment* (5th edn). New York: Oxford University Press.

Lineweaver, T. and Chelune, G. J. (2003). 'Use of the WAIS-III and WMS-III in the Context of Serial Assessments: Interpreting Reliable and Meaningful Change'. In D. Tulsky, D. Saklofske, G. J. Chelune, R. Heaton, R. J. Ivnik, R. Bornstein, et al. (eds), *Clinical Interpretation of the WAIS-III and WMS-III* (pp. 303–337). New York: Academic Press.

Maassen, G. H. (2000). 'Principles of Defining Reliable Change Indices'. *Journal of Clinical and Experimental Neuropsychology* 22(5): 622–632.

McKhann, G., Kopman, D., Chertkow, H., Hyman, B., Jack, C., Kawas, C., et al. (2011). 'The Diagnosis of Dementia due to Alzheimer's Disease: Recommendations from the National Institute on Aging—Alzheimer's Association Workgroups on Diagnostic Guidelines for Alzheimer's Disease'. *Alzheimer's and Dementia* 7(3): 263–269.

McSweeny, A., Naugle, R. I., Chelune, G. J., and Luders, H. (1993). '"T-scores for Change:" An Illustration of a Regression Approach to Depicting Change in Clinical Neuropsychology'. *Clinical Neuropsychologist* 7: 300–312.

Marcotte, T. and Scott, J. (2009). 'Neuropsychological Performance and the Assessment of Driving Behavior'. In I. Grant and K. Adams (eds), *Neuropsychological Assessment of Neuropsychiatric Disorders* (3rd edn, pp. 652–687). New York: Oxford University Press.

Marcotte, T., Scott, J., Kamat, R., and Heaton, R. (2010). 'Neuropsychology and the Prediction of Everyday Functioning'. In T. I. G. Marcotte (ed.), *Neuropsychology of Everyday Functioning* (pp. 5–38). New York: Guilford Press.

Masur, D. M., Sliwinski, M., Lipton, R. B., Blau, A. D., and Crystal, H. A. (1994). 'Neuropsychological Prediction of Dementia and the Absence of Dementia in Healthy Elderly Persons'. *Neurology* 44(8): 1427–1432.

Matarazzo, J. D. and Herman, D. O. (1984). 'Base Rate Data for the WAIS-R: Test-retest Stability and VIQ-PIQ Differences'. *Journal of Clinical Neuropsychology* 6(4): 351–366.

Mendez, M. and Cummings, J. (2003). *Dementia: A Clinical Approach* (3rd edn). Philadelphia: Butterworth Heinemann.

Miech, R. A., Breitner, J. C., Zandi, P. P., Khachaturian, A. S., Anthony, J. C., and Mayer, L. (2002). 'Incidence of AD May Decline in the Early 90s for Men, Later for Women: The Cache County Study'. *Neurology* 58(2): 209–218.

Monsch, A. U., Bondi, M. W., Butters, N., Salmon, D. P., Katzman, R., and Thal, L. J. (1992). 'Comparisons of Verbal Fluency Tasks in the Detection of Dementia of the Alzheimer Type'. *Archives of Neurology* 49(12): 1253–1258.

Ohm, T. G., Kirca, M., Bohl, J., Scharnagl, H., Gross, W., and Marz, W. (1995). 'Apolipoprotein E Polymorphism Influences not only Cerebral Senile Plaque Load but also Alzheimer-type Neurofibrillary Tangle Formation'. *Neuroscience* 66(3): 583–587.

Pearson. (2009). *Advanced Clinical Solutions For WAIS-IV and WMS-IV Clinical and Interpretative Manual*. San Antonio, TX: Pearson.

Petersen, R. C., Smith, G. E., Ivnik, R. J., Kokmen, E., and Tangalos, E. G. (1994). 'Memory Function in Very Early Alzheimer's Disease'. *Neurology* 44(5): 867–872.

Petersen, R. C. (2004). 'Mild Cognitive Impairment as a Diagnostic Entity'. *Journal of Internal Medicine* 256(3): 183–194.

Reuter-Lorenz, P., Jonides, J., Smith, E. E., Hartley, A., Miller, A., Marshuetz, C., and Koeppe, R. A. (2000). 'Age Differences in the Frontal Lateralization of Verbal and Spatial Working Memory Revealed by PET'. *Journal of Cognitive Neuroscience* 12(1): 174–187.

Reuter-Lorenz, P. (2002). 'New Visions of the Aging Mind and Brain'. *Trends in Cognitive Sciences* 6(9): 394.

Rinne, J. O., Hietala, J., Ruotsalainen, U., Sako, E., Laihinen, A., Nagren, K., et al. (1993). 'Decrease in Human Striatal Dopamine D2 Receptor Density with Age: A PET Study with [11C]raclopride'. *Journal of Cerebral Blood Flow & Metabolism* 13(2): 310–314.

Rocchi, A., Pellegrini, S., Siciliano, G., and Murri, L. (2003). 'Causative and Susceptibility Genes for Alzheimer's Disease: A Review'. *Brain Research Bulletin* 61(1): 1–24.

Ronnlund, M., Lovden, M., and Nilsson, L. G. (2008). 'Cross-sectional versus Longitudinal Age Gradients of Tower of Hanoi Performance: The Role of Practice Effects and Cohort Differences in Education'. *Neuropsychology, Development, and Cognition. Section B, Aging, Neuropsychology and Cognition* 15(1): 40–67.

Salat, D. H., Tuch, D. S., Greve, D. N., van der Kouwe, A. J., Hevelone, N. D., Zaleta, A. K., et al. (2005). 'Age-related Alterations in White Matter Microstructure Measured by Diffusion Tensor Imaging'. *Neurobiology and Aging* 26(8): 1215–1227.

Salthouse, T. A. (2009). 'Decomposing Age Correlations on Neuropsychological and Cognitive Variables'. *Journal of the International Neuropsychological Society* 15(5): 650–661.

Schaie, K. W. (1994). 'The Course of Adult Intellectual Development'. *American Psychologist* 49(4): 304–313.

Schoenberg, M. and Duff, K. (2011). 'Dementias and Mild Cognitive Impairment in Adults'. In M. Schoenberg and J. Scott (eds), *The Little Black Book of Neuropsychology* (1st edn, pp. 357–404). New York: Springer.

Slick, D. (2006). 'Psychometrics in Neuropsychological Assessment'. In E. Strauss, E. Sherman, and O. Spreen (eds), *A Compendium of Neuropsychological Tests* (pp. 1–43). New York: Oxford University Press.

Smith, G. and Rush, B. (2006). 'Normal Aging and Mild Cognitive Impairment'. In D. Attix and K. Welsh-Bohmer (eds), *Geriatric Neuropsychology: Assessment and Intervention* (pp. 27–55). New York: Guilford Press.

Smith, G. and Bondi, M. (2008). 'Normal Aging, Mild Cognitive Impairment, and Alzheimer's Disease'. In J. Morgan and J. Ricker (eds), *Textbook of Clinical Neuropsychology* (1st edn, pp. 762–780). New York: Taylor and Francis.

Stein, J., Luppa, M., Brahler, E., Konig, H. H., and Riedel-Heller, S. G. (2010). 'The Assessment of Changes in Cognitive Functioning: Reliable Change Indices for Neuropsychological Instruments in the Elderly—A Systematic Review'. *Dementia and Geriatric Cognitive Disorders* 29(3): 275–286.

Stern, Y. (2002). 'What is Cognitive Reserve? Theory and Research Application of the Reserve Concept'. *Journal of the International Neuropsychological Society* 8(3): 448–460.

Stern, Y. (2009). 'Cognitive Reserve'. *Neuropsychologia* 47(10): 2015–2028.

Uc, E. Y., Rizzo, M., Anderson, S. W., Sparks, J., Rodnitzky, R. L., and Dawson, J. D. (2006). 'Impaired Visual Search in Drivers with Parkinson's Disease'. *Annals of Neurology* 60(4): 407–413.

Vance, D. E., Graham, M. A., Fazeli, P. L., Heaton, K., and Moneyham, L. (2012). 'An Overview of Nonpathological Geroneuropsychology: Implications for Nursing Practice and Research'. *Journal of Neuroscience Nursing* 44(1): 43–53.

Welsh-Bohmer, K. A., Breitner, J. C., Hayden, K. M., Lyketsos, C., Zandi, P. P., Tschanz, J. T., et al. (2006). 'Modifying Dementia Risk and Trajectories of Cognitive Decline in Aging: The Cache County Memory Study'. *Alzheimer's & Dementia* 2(3): 257–260.

Wenk, G. L., Pierce, D. J., Struble, R. G., Price, D. L., and Cork, L. C. (1989). 'Age-related Changes in Multiple Neurotransmitter Systems in the Monkey Brain'. *Neurobiology of Aging* 10(1): 11–19.

Wilson, R. S., Beckett, L. A., Barnes, L. L., Schneider, J. A., Bach, J., Evans, D. A., et al. (2002). 'Individual Differences in Rates of Change in Cognitive Abilities of Older Persons' [Research Support, US Govt, PHS]. *Psychology and Aging* 17(2): 179–193.

CHAPTER 12

INTERNATIONAL PERSPECTIVES ON CAPACITY ASSESSMENT

MARYBETH BAILAR-HEATH AND JENNIFER MOYE

INTRODUCTION

CIVIL capacity assessments of older adults are increasingly prevalent across all sectors of society (Marson and Zebley 2001; Moye and Marson 2007). Civil capacity assessment refers to evaluations used to determine an individual's ability to make decisions, manage funds, live independently, and drive. Healthcare professionals, attorneys, financial planners, home-care agencies, families, and older adults themselves struggle with how to provide decisional support, when needed, respecting the individual's autonomy while protecting the individual from harm. In most situations, issues of the need for support are handled informally, with collaboration of the older adult, family, and professionals (Qualls and Smyer 2007; Smyer, Schaie, and Kapp 1996). Assessments of capacity come to light particularly when there is a disagreement between a patient and a care-giver: for example, when a patient refuses a treatment that a physician is recommending or when a patient is spending money differently than an adult child care-giver feels is appropriate. Assessments of capacity also occur when an older adult has come to endure considerable harm (e.g. been exploited out of large sums of money), but lacks insight and does not wish to accept supports. In such cases, professionals and family members are often unsure whether to respect the adult's decision regardless of associated risk, or to protect the individual through an appointment of a surrogate decision-maker. The goals of this chapter are to review the concept of capacity from international legal perspectives, and to then apply those perspectives to the assessment task.

WHAT IS CAPACITY?

Capacity is a term that is used differently across settings, jurisdictions, and certainly between countries. To make matters even more complicated, the term 'competency' is used interchangeably with 'capacity' in some areas, while other jurisdictions deline-ate conceptual differences between the two terms. For example, in the US, historically the term 'competency' is more often used in legal settings, whereas 'capacity' is used in clinical settings. But more recently, the term capacity appears in the law, because it con-veys the idea of functioning within a specific area (American Bar Association (ABA) and American Psychological Association (APA) Assessment of Capacity in Older Adults Project Working Group 2005). While there is variability in usage across countries, other countries such as Canada, the UK, and Portugal have evolved to use the term 'incapacity' to describe a person incapable of caring for person or property (Alvaro 2012; Bielby 2005; Borges et al. 2008).

In this chapter, we will use the term 'capacity' to refer to an individual's requisite cogni-tive and functional abilities to complete a specific task (e.g. manage their finances) or make a specific decision (e.g. refuse a recommended medical treatment). In healthcare settings, a clinician (e.g. a geropsychologist) may be called upon to evaluate an older adult and offer a professional opinion concerning an individual's capacity to adequately complete a specific task or make a specific decision. It is important to note that if the clinician finds the indi-vidual to lack capacity, this does not alter the individual's legal status, but may permit certain actions such as the activation of a durable power of attorney for healthcare.

In a legal setting, a judge or other legal decision-maker determines legal capacity of a person, most often as raised in the context of a hearing or dispute. The legal decision-maker considers a legal standard and determines whether an individual meets the requirements for incapacity based on that standard. Depending on the jurisdiction, the input of a clinician or others may be sought in order to assist with the decision.

Questions of capacity may arise in a variety of populations, including those with severe mental or medical illness. With increasing numbers of adults living longer and the asso-ciated rise in the prevalence of dementia, which often poses questions related to capacity, there may be increased need for capacity evaluations (Alzheimer's Association 2011). There also has been increased attention internationally on the prevalence of elder abuse and finan-cial exploitation (Acierno et al. 2010; Cooper, Selwood, and Livingston 2008; Lowenstein et al. 2009). Finally, families are increasingly living at a geographical distance, meaning that older adults may have less familial support in navigating their own care and placements of support as they age.

DIFFERENT TYPES OF CAPACITY

'Capacity' pertains to an ability to complete a *specific* task or make a *specific* decision. Hence, there are multiple types of capacity. In healthcare settings, questions of capacity are most often related to the following types of capacity:

- medical consent
- sexual consent
- financial management
- independent living
- driving.

Additional civil capacities that may be encountered in other settings include testamentary capacity (i.e. capacity to execute a will), donative capacity, and contractual capacity (ABA and APA Assessment of Capacity in Older Adults Project Working Group 2005).

GUARDIANSHIP LAW AS A LENS TO COMPARE INTERNATIONAL PERSPECTIVES ON CAPACITY

Although many situations involving impaired capacity do not proceed to legal adjudication, because assessments of capacity are ultimately psycho-legal in nature, they should begin with a consideration of the legal standard for capacity in the jurisdiction (ABA and APA Assessment of Capacity in Older Adults Project Working Group 2008). Questions of civil capacity of older adults most often come to the court in the form of guardianship proceedings (also called conservatorship or curatorship in other countries (Convention on the International Protection of Adults 2000; Quinn 2004)). Therefore, guardianship law may be used as a lens through which to view legal approaches to capacity, as well as the outcomes of a finding of incapacity. Guardianship is a relationship created by state law in which a court gives one person, the guardian, the duty and power to make personal and/or property decisions for an individual determined by the court to be incapacitated (ABA and APA Assessment of Capacity in Older Adults Project Working Group 2006). Guardians are often empowered to make medical decisions on behalf of adults who lack capacity to consent. In this chapter we begin by discussing guardianship law in the US. Then we discuss approaches within the United Nations and internationally.

US perspectives on guardianship

In the US, the concept of guardianship has been inherited from English law, and historically from Roman law based on the doctrine of 'parens patriae'—the responsibility and power of the state to act as parent in protecting the individual, and also the assets of an individual (Sabatino and Basinger 2000).

The process of guardianship appointment in the US has drawn criticism since at least the 1970s. Specifically, there have been concerns regarding limited due process, lack of protection of rights, poor interface between medical providers and the court, overly intrusive interventions leading to the loss of all decision-making rights, and the potential for guardianship to hasten institutionalization (Horstman 1975; Mitchell 1978; Reynolds 2002; Zimny and Grossberg 1998).

The past twenty years have witnessed an explosion of statutory reform in adult guardianship within the US with 261 separate laws passed governing adult guardianship, including comprehensive reform bills in thirty-two states (Wingspan Conferees 2001; Wood 1988–2010–2010). A major focus of the guardianship legal reform has been to shift definitions of capacity away from global diagnostic-based concepts (e.g. the individual is incompetent due to schizophrenia) to a more complex, functional definition. The Uniform Guardianship and Protective Proceedings Act (National Conference of Commissioners on Uniform State

Laws 1997), an act drafted by a council of legal commissioners to serve as a model, defines an incapacitated person as 'an individual...unable to receive and evaluate information or make or communicate decisions to such an extent that the individual lacks the ability to meet essential requirements for physical health, safety, or self-care, even with appropriate technological assistance' (Article 1, Section 102(5): 7). The 1997 model act adds an emphasis on decision-making and de-emphasizes a diagnostic standard. A number of states (Colorado, Massachusetts, Minnesota, Hawaii) have statutes based on the 1997 model act, while others are based on an earlier 1982 version; still other states have incapacity standards that are particular to statutory evolution within their respective state (Wood 1988–2010).

A useful analysis of incapacity standards in state guardianship law finds that states may include one or more of the following tests or elements to define incapacity: (1) a disease or disorder; (2) cognitive or decisional impairment; (3) functional disabilities (i.e. 'inability to care for self'); and (4) exceeding an essential needs threshold such that there is an unacceptable risk to the person or society (Anderer 1990; Sabatino and Basinger 2000).

Implications of evolving US law on clinical practice

The changing legal definition of capacity in US guardianship law, as well as legal reforms addressing due process protections, directly impact the clinical process of capacity evaluation.

Limited guardianship and functional evaluation

As courts have moved away from findings of incompetency to consider capacity, the notion of 'limited' guardianship has arisen. Previously, courts found persons 'incompetent' and appointed a plenary or full guardian—with the authority to make all decisions for the incapacitated person (except for those excluded by statute), and with the incapacitated person (formerly called 'the ward') losing all decisional rights.

In recent years courts have moved away from the practice of full guardianship to favour (or in some states *require*) 'limited' guardianship (ABA and APA Assessment of Capacity in Older Adults Project Working Group 2006). Limited guardianship means that the judge considers the clinical evidence and other case facts to create a judicial order that limits the guardian's authority to make decisions in only those areas where the individual requires assistance, and preserves rights in any area where the individual still has the capacity to make decisions (Moye and Naik 2011; Quinn 2004). Limited guardianship seeks to attain an optimal balance of care and protection with autonomy and dignity. This practice is consistent with a contemporary scientific understanding of neurologic and psychiatric illness in which a person may have strengths and weaknesses in cognitive functioning translating to intact or impaired specific capacities.

As such, this has shifted the process of clinical evaluation of capacity for guardianship to evaluation and opinions about discrete areas of function to support limited guardianship. While not all states require clinical evaluations for guardianship, most (more than thirty) do (Mayhew 2005). Some states specifically require 'functional' assessment; others, while not mandating the form of assessment, do require (through procedural rules) information about functional abilities (Commission on National Probate Court Standards and Advisory

Committee on Interstate Guardianships 1993). Therefore, the practice of capacity evaluation has shifted away from a focus on establishing a diagnosis to describing specific decisional and functional strengths and weaknesses.

Diversion to less restrictive alternatives

Within the US, all states have enacted provisions for the older adult, while capable, to appoint an agent to make healthcare or financial decisions. Durable power of attorney and other related instruments are favoured because they provide a clear record of the individual's choice of surrogate, and sometimes offer additional directions (Sabatino 1994). They also avoid the intrusive and costly intervention of the courts. In the US guardianship reform movement, many reform bills acknowledge these less restrictive alternatives by providing that the petition should state what alternatives had been examined and that the court should find that no less restrictive alternatives would suffice before the appointment of a guardian (Quinn 2004; Wilber and Reynolds 1995).

This practice also informs clinical work. The Patient Self Determination Act (US General Accounting Office 1995) requires that all adults be offered the opportunity to execute an advance directive upon admission to a hospital. Of course, the completion of an advance directive does not need to wait for an admission, and is probably best accomplished outside of an urgent medical situation. As such, clinicians working with older adults in the early stages of neurocognitive illness may encourage the older adult to execute durable powers of attorney for healthcare or finances to avoid later guardianship should the older adult become incapacitated. Even in situations where there is no previously executed formal document, many areas of functional decline can be managed outside of legal mechanisms, such as shared bank accounts when financial management is difficult or providing transportation when driving becomes unsafe. As such, the clinical evaluation becomes an opportunity to identify resources for the patient and family, especially those outside of guardianship.

Encourage presence of the alleged incapacitated person at the hearing

Another component of US guardianship reform is to encourage the alleged incapacitated person to be at the hearing by requiring the presence unless good cause be shown and accommodating the individual through provisions such as hearings at convenient locations (Hurme and Wood 2006). Accordingly, in addition to evaluating capacity, courts may ask clinicians for an opinion on whether it is possible vs harmful for the individual to attend the hearing, and if the person does attend, what accommodations may be necessary (e.g. hearing amplification).

International perspectives on guardianship

Similarly to the US, concerns surrounding guardianship of older adults have been on the legal agenda in various countries since the 1960s. As in the US, guardianship procedures in other countries have historically often viewed capacity as 'all or nothing', and rules defining the determination of capacity were vague and overly simplistic, with a finding of incapacity leading to complete loss of legal status and rights. In the past several decades, a broad wave of legal reform has swept developed countries in this field of law. Developing nations are also evidencing increased attention to this issue (Faunce 2005; Hamid et al. 2008).

Convention on the Rights of Persons with Disabilities

A major international milestone occurred in December 2006, when the UN General Assembly adopted the Convention on the Rights of Persons with Disabilities (CRPD; Convention on the Rights of Persons with Disabilities 2008). The CRPD 'marks an important step towards equality, dignity and access to society for elderly people, with and without disabilities' (Kanter 2009: 527–28). As of January 2013, the CPRD has been signed by 155 countries (including both developed and developing nations). Broadly speaking, the CRPD represents a conceptual shift from a medical model of disability (which focuses on diagnosis and inability) to a human rights model (which focuses on capability and inclusion). Of note, it is the first international law to combine human, civil, political, social, and economic rights into the same document (Kanter 2009). It seeks to correct previous manifestations of 'protection' for disabled persons that removed personal rights.

While the document addresses a group of people more expansive than just older adults, a specific section of the document is particularly relevant to this population. This section is Article 12, entitled 'Equal recognition before the law'. Article 12 challenges paternalistic approaches to people who lack capacity. It is in opposition to historic guardianship procedures that have deprived individuals of their rights to make decisions about aspects of their lives and instead implement provision of supports. One of the reasons for this change is to encourage people who are considered incapacitated to seek assistance, which they may have been reluctant to do in the past, for fear of being subjected to guardianship or worse (Kanter 2009).

Article 12 also emphasizes the necessity of a supportive decision-making model as an alternative to imposed guardianship (or substitute decision-making). Essentially, instead of enacting laws that substitute a guardian's decision for the decision of the individual, the CRPD's proposed model states that, (1) all people have the right to make decisions and choices about their own lives, and that, (2) everyone at times may seek and need help from family and friends, so those lacking capacity should be entitled to that same right. The document recognizes that some persons do need assistance to exercise their legal capacity, but the onus of responsibility for providing support and safeguards is placed on the state (Kanter 2009).

Guardianship across the globe

Many nations have changed their guardianship laws in recent years in a manner consistent with the CRPD (i.e. preserving the legal rights, status, and independence of those found to be incapacitated). For example, in Japan, an 'advisory' system has been implemented in which the family court may appoint a helper. When a helper is appointed to an older adult, the adult does not lose his or her legal status or independence. Instead, specific acts are decided on jointly by the person and his/her helper in order to be valid (Arai 2000; Doron 2002; Maeda 2000; Mizuno and Namba 2001). In Germany, there has been a paradigm shift from traditional guardianship to 'care and assistance'. The court in Germany may appoint a 'caretaker' for an incapacitated person, and the court must tailor the specific tasks which the caretaker has the responsibility to fulfil. The incapacitated person does not lose legal status or any other legal rights (Doron 2002; Schlüter and Liemeier 1990; Valdes-Stauber, Deinert, and Kilian 2011; Youngs 2002; Zenz 1989).

Interestingly, Sweden has two different forms of assistance that may be employed for incapacitated persons. In one, an administrator or trustee is appointed, and there is a loss of legal capacity, but only in a circumscribed area or areas. In the second form, a mentor is appointed to act on behalf of the adult but there is no loss of legal capacities (Doron 2002; Herr 1995). The mentor is often a relative, and the appointment of the mentor does not necessitate a court hearing (Björkstén 2008). If the individual understands the concept of having a mentor, and wishes to have one, he or she may sign a form to this effect. If he or she does not understand the concept, a physician may complete a medical certificate requesting a mentor for the individual (Björkstén 2008). Israel, until recently, was employing full guardianship in which the incapacitated person lost all legal rights in all spheres of life (Doron 2004). The court is now increasing its tendency to appoint a guardian without declaring legal incompetence (i.e. the ward retains his/her legal rights) (Melamed, Yaron-Melamed, and Heinik 2010).

In addition to shifts in the role of the guardian and the movement to support decision-making without removing rights, countries have also modified procedural approaches to guardianship recognizing the important psycho-legal nature of capacity, i.e. capacity as a concept with both clinical and legal referents, and one in which clinical and legal professionals need to work together. For example, in Hong Kong, courts that manage guardianship are instead 'tribunals' that are 'quasi-judicial' and multidisciplinary, and consist of three panels: lawyers, physicians/psychologists/social workers, and persons who have personal experience with mentally incapacitated persons (Wong and Scully 2003). Guardianship tribunals are also utilized in Australia, with similarly assigned panels consisting of legal, professional, and community members (Ferres 2007). Various boards throughout the provinces of Canada, such as in Ontario and Alberta, also show an appreciation for collaboration among legal and clinical professionals in assisting with guardianship cases.

As has been described, guardianship law has evolved significantly across the world in the past several decades. In a useful review of international guardianship perspectives Doron (2002) synthesizes the several commonalities among legal reform in many countries. He concludes that guardianship law reform among many nations demonstrates: (1) greater emphasis on autonomy and independence; (2) an evolution from paternalism to partnership; (3) improved due process; (4) implementation of least restrictive alternatives; (5) increased flexibility; and (6) sensitivity to cultural and legal tradition. Given these international shifts to reduce absolute capacity judgments to a provision of more supports only in the specific domains in which support is needed, clinical capacity assessment is more crucial than ever in order to guide the exploration and provision of necessary supports.

ASSESSMENT OF CAPACITY

When to assess capacity

Geropsychologists and other mental health professionals may be retained by the court or other governing body to perform a capacity evaluation in the context of a guardianship petition or other hearing. Capacity assessments are also commonly requested and performed in a variety of clinical settings, including outpatient mental practice, outpatient neuropsychological evaluation practice, inpatient psychiatry or medical hospitals, nursing homes, assisted-living facilities, and home-based care settings. There are a number of scenarios in such clinical settings in which the question of capacity may arise, triggering a request for capacity assessment. In general, it may be important to assess capacity when:

- a patient's stated decision will likely result in harm that the patient does not anticipate or appreciate;
- a patient's behaviour or decision is not consistent with established patterns or known values;
- a patient does not appear to be implementing sound reasoning when considering treatment options;
- a patient possesses risk factors for impaired decision-making. Such risk factors may include organic brain disease (e.g. dementia, delirium, brain injury) or serious mental illness (e.g. schizophrenia, severe depression, bipolar disorder).

Regarding the last point above, it is imperative to emphasize that diagnosis alone is *not* sufficient evidence of incapacity. Research has shown that individuals with mild neurocognitive or mental disorders such as early Alzheimer's disease and schizophrenia may retain capacity (Moye et al. 2004a; Palmer et al. 2004; Palmer et al. 2005). The presence of a cognitive or psychiatric disorder, then, should be viewed as a risk factor that may trigger an assessment.

Capacity assessment is frequently requested by providers when a patient makes a decision that does not coincide with the provider's recommendation. In such a case, it is important to keep in mind that individuals are allowed to make what a clinician views as a 'bad' decision, and this alone does not indicate that they are incapacitated. Instead of basing a conclusion about capacity on whether the individual's decision is good or bad in the eyes of the provider, an evaluation must assess the *process* that the individual uses to make the decision (Moye et al. 2011). In other words, capacity does not necessarily equal good decision-making; it instead is characterized by a process of knowledgeable and internally consistent decision-making informed by the individual's values.

A framework for assessment

As legal frameworks for capacity have shifted, clinical and legal practitioners have increasingly sought to enhance their expertise in understanding and evaluating capacity. One such example of this is the joint effort of the American Bar Association (ABA) and American Psychological Association (APA) to develop educational handbooks for their membership regarding capacity evaluation of older adults (ABA and APA Assessment of Capacity in Older Adults Project Working Group 2005, 2006, 2008). Similarly, other disciplines have worked within their professional organizations to enhance professional readiness to tackle issues of capacity. The ABA-APA effort was driven by the concerns of the organizations' membership to provide professional guidance to their members (lawyers, judges, and psychologists). The National College of Probate Judges (NCPJ) in the US also joined the effort when the group focused on guidance to legal professionals in the US who are judges.

The working group developed a framework to guide assessment of capacity by psychologists that may be useful to psychologists and other disciplines (ABA and APA Assessment of Capacity in Older Adults Project Working Group 2008). The framework consists of nine elements: legal, functional, diagnostic, cognitive, psychiatric/emotional, values, risks, enhancing capacity, and the clinical judgment. This framework is discussed in detail in the handbook for psychologists with applications across the domains of medical consent, sexual consent, financial management, testamentary capacity, driving, and independent living.

The framework begins with the 'legal standard' to orient the assessment process to consideration of the legal standard for the specific capacity in question. The legal standard informs the functional elements on which the evaluation must focus. A capacity evaluation that only describes the diagnosis and cognitive abilities, and perhaps only infers functional abilities, misses the opportunity to directly assess function and place it at the centre of the capacity evaluation process. However, a capacity evaluation must also consider the diagnosis (element 3) that is causing the functional impairments and how these are expressed in cognitive (element 4) and psychiatric (element 5) symptomatology.

The ABA-APA framework built on the seminal work by Grisso (2003), who articulated that a capacity assessment is never merely an assessment of abilities but a consideration of these within context. As such, the ABA-APA framework includes an assessment of values (element 6), risks facing the individual (element 7), and interventions that may enhance capacity (element 8).

The last element of the ABA-APA framework is the professional clinical judgment. A capacity evaluation report must offer a clear opinion about the issue at hand—integrating the clinical data and the value, risks, and interventional elements. There is no single equation or score used to arrive at the clinical judgment, but instead the clinical judgment is a process of arriving at a decision in view of all the elements. Generally, when all the data is at hand, a clinical decision can emerge and can be substantiated by sound data. Although the ABA-APA framework was based in part on the elements of incapacity found in the US Uniform Guardianship and Protective Proceedings Act, the framework sets out a broad set of clinical criteria that are likely to be relevant across countries.

Consideration of values and multicultural differences

Legal standards for capacity in guardianship law have evolved to emphasize discrete strengths and weaknesses, but also an emphasis on the choices of the person, partnership with the person, and cultural and historical referents (ABA 2003). An emphasis on individual choice reflecting personal reasons is present in US legal standards for healthcare consent, defined by the abilities to: understand diagnostic and treatment information, appreciate the personal significance of this information relative to the individual's situation, reason about the risks and benefits of treatment alternatives in light of personal consequences, and evidence a choice (Berg et al. 2001; Grisso and Appelbaum 1998a). Similarly, in Hong Kong, England and Wales, common law for decision-making capacity requires that the individual understand and retain the relevant information, believe that information, reason adequately, and express a choice (Johnston and Liddle 2007; Wong and Scully 2003). In Australia, the individual must demonstrate knowledge of the context of the decision at hand and the choices available, appreciate the risks and benefits of the choices, communicate a decision, and remember that decision and be consistent with it (Bennett and Hallen 2005). Inherent in this model is the ability to reason about risks and benefits of treatment in view of consequences as they apply to the individual's life.

A critical aspect of assessment of capacity, in any jurisdiction, state, or country, is sensitivity to individual differences, including those related to race, ethnicity, religion, generational/age cohort, or other cultural factors. Cultural attitudes, values, beliefs, and practices play a significant role in an individual's approach to medical decision-making (Karel 2000) and other decisions about independent living, management of funds, and so on. For example, with regard to healthcare, some cultural traditions emphasize the importance of spiritual issues for health and healing or value interventions from a community healer, whereas generally speaking the western biomedical view of health is based on a mechanistic model of the human body and discounts the spirit or soul (Karel 2007). Cultural differences also influence decisions about life-sustaining treatments, end-of-life care, advance directives, and even whether or not the patient should be informed of serious medical conditions and actively participate in treatment decisions (Thompson, Pitts, and Schwankovsky 1993). For example, some cultural groups believe that informing a patient of a terminal condition causes unnecessary distress, burden, and hopelessness for the patient preferences (Kagawa-Singer and Blackhall 2001). In addition, many older adults (of varying ethnic backgrounds) believe medical treatment decisions should be made by the treating physician and family, and therefore may not wish to participate in questioning about their personal preferences (Moye, Armesto, and Karel 2005).

If a question arises about an individual's capacity to make a decision or complete a task, the influence of cultural factors must be examined as part of the capacity evaluation. The first step for the evaluator is to engage in an ongoing process of self-evaluation of his or her own cultural and personal values and biases and how these may affect clinical judgments (APA 2002). In particular, it is important that evaluators be especially sensitive to situations in which they do not agree with a patient's decision. Clinicians vary in how they determine capacity. Some clinicians weigh certain abilities, such as memory, more heavily than other abilities such as understanding (Marson et al. 1997) or may be influenced by the clinician's own emotional reactions to the patient (Braun et al. 2009). Therefore, it is important to direct the capacity evaluation to the consistency of the choice with the patient's values, not the evaluator's values.

It is useful, then, to begin a capacity evaluation by understanding the individual's values (Karel, Powell, and Cantor 2004; Lambert, Gibson and Nathanson 1990; Pearlman et al. 1998). Patients with neurocognitive and neuropsychiatric disorders may still be able to express values even if they cannot manage technical aspects of certain decisions or tasks (Karel et al. 2010). Consideration of reasoning in terms of values is explicitly recognized in some legal procedures. For example, in England and Wales, a checklist of factors is provided that must be considered, including past and present wishes, and feelings, beliefs, and values of the individual (Johnston and Liddle 2007). Values-related discussions with patients can be embedded in the capacity assessment interview (Moye et al. 2008).

If possible, it can be helpful to interview a family member or individual close to the patient in order to assist in gleaning this information about the patient. Having this information assists the evaluator in assessing whether the patient's decisions or actions are in line with past values if the patient cannot state it him or herself and the source is reliable. The extent to which decisions appear consistent with personal values and beliefs can be an important indicator of intact reasoning ability (Moye et al. 2004b, 2004a) vs focusing overly on 'rational' reasoning.

Finally, as in all types of standardized psychological and/or cognitive evaluation, assessment tools must be used with great caution in a cross-cultural context. For example, in the US, neuropsychological tests are known to have poor specificity with ethnic minority populations, despite the use of separate test norms for ethnic minorities, such that 'cognitively normal ethnic minorities are more likely than whites to be misdiagnosed as impaired' (Manly 2006 204–5). In her comprehensive review of cultural factors in neuropsychological assessment, Manly (2006) posits that 'acculturation, quality of education, literacy and racial socialization are more meaningful and useful background variables to help adjust expectations for neuropsychological test scores and improve specificity of cognitive tests, regardless of race/ethnicity' (200). Examples of such background variables to consider include the patient's native language, level of exposure to the mainstream culture, years *and* quality of schooling (e.g. teacher–student ratio, length of school year), and stereotype threat. Stereotype threat refers to a fear that one's performance will substantiate a negative stereotype about one's ethnic or cultural group, and this fear leads to reduced attention to the task at hand, which may in turn lead to attenuated performance. Writing from a US perspective, Levy (2009) also discusses the evidence of stereotype threat behaviour in older adults. As such, older adults' performance on testing may be influenced by a fear of substantiating ageist stereotypes.

These cross-cultural factors are likely to be relevant across countries. The reader is directed to Manly's (2006) text for helpful and practical recommendations in considering such factors. Briefly, some recommendations include (1) cautiously using the best available norms from the appropriate population; (2) assessing language proficiency of bilingual or multilingual patients (in each language); and (3) avoiding the use of an interpreter simply to translate and administer items from a test that is written in, and normed in, a different language.

Using empirically supported assessment tools for evaluation of function

As the practice of clinical assessment of capacity has grown, so too has the availability of assessment instruments that aim to operationalize legal standards of capacity into clinical tools. Such tools, described by Grisso (2003) as Forensic Assessment Instruments (FAI) may assist in standardizing the assessment of capacity and to focus the assessment on functional abilities vs using only self or care-giver reports, or trying to infer from cognitive tests alone.

These tools vary in nature. They may consist of a set of questions for structuring a clinical interview, such as the MacArthur Competence Assessment Tool for Treatment (MacCAT-T; Grisso and Appelbaum 1998b), which provides a set of questions in a format for evaluating consent to medical treatment, as well as guidelines for interpreting responses. Other tools are more skill-based, such as the Financial Capacity Instrument (FCI; Marson et al. 2000), which provides direct assessment of financial skills and judgment. Many of these tools are described in the ABA-APA psychologist handbook (ABA and APA Assessment of Capacity in Older Adults Project Working Group 2008), which can be downloaded for free at www. apa.org/pi/aging for readers interested in learning more about available instruments.

Forensic Assessment Instruments for capacity assessment of older adults have developed in numerous countries and languages (e.g. Kitamura et al. 1998; Pinsker et al. 2006; Sousa, Simões, and Firmino 2010). While the outcome of a capacity assessment will always be based on the professional's clinical judgment, these tools are an important step in enhancing the reliability and validity of the functional assessment element of capacity evaluation. Additional research is needed to further establish the normative properties and empirical basis of these tools.

The Science of Capacity and Decision-making

There is an emerging body of scientific literature on capacity, enabled in large part by the development of FAIs, as valid research is predicated on reliable data. This research has established that healthcare and research consent is diminished in dementia (Kim, Karlawish, and Caine 2002; Marson et al. 1996; Moye et al. 2004a) and more variably in psychiatric illnesses (Appelbaum and Grisso 1995; Palmer et al. 2004; Palmer et al. 2005). Although individuals with mild impairment may retain the ability to understand information and express choices and values, support may be needed for reasoning (Moye et al. 2004b). Capacities involving complex procedural skills and judgment, such as financial management, driving, and independent living, are more cognitively complex and similarly impaired in dementia (Ball et al. 2006; Barbas and Wilde 2001; Griffith et al. 2003; Sherod et al. 2009; Skelton et al. 2010), sometimes in subtle ways that may open a person to exploitation or risk. Other capacities such as testamentary capacity have seen very little research.

This important but nascent body of research in the area of capacity is not well integrated into the scientific study of decision-making outside the concept of capacity. For example, cognitive decisional science has revealed the important role of affective and intuitive components of decision-making that are not represented in traditional models of legal capacity (Beisecker 1988; Blanchard-Fields and Camp 1990; Kahneman 2003; Tversky and Kahneman 1981). Capacity research is quite challenging, therefore, because it must be built upon the legal definitions of capacity—which are not empirically founded but instead more rational (that is, what a person or persons thinks are the appropriate definitions) in consideration of societal norms and justice. At the same time, capacity research must build on this legal structure but bridge to what decisional science offers in terms of how we as humans arrive at decisions. This work remains to be done.

Capacity assessment is built upon many of the same principles and techniques of comprehensive psychological assessment, such as the selection of reliable and valid assessment tools appropriate to the task and individual. Future research that enhances the reliability and validity of forensic assessment instruments, and our understanding of how to integrate results of these with careful consideration of the factual data concerning the individual's diagnosis, cognitive, and psychiatric status, and sensitive consideration of the individuals values and risks is needed. Such information will assist clinicians in the important tasks of capacity assessment to balance the critical roles of protecting vulnerable individuals from harm while we promote decisional autonomy.

SUMMARY

The issue of capacity is clearly an important one for those who work with older adults. As longevity increases, so does the risk for physical and cognitive disorders, and retaining autonomy must be carefully balanced with risks to one's safety. Capacity is a complex construct with multiple components and determinants. Its roots are in law rather than in a scientifically based theoretical framework, and therefore the legal standard defining capacity in a given jurisdiction, state, or nation informs the assessment of capacity. In recent decades, there has been an enormous evolution in guardianship law internationally, and guardianship law may be used as a lens to view and define capacity. While individual jurisdictions each have their own unique legal standards, guardianship law has generally seen a shift from paternalism to partnership, with greater emphasis on autonomy and independence, improved due process, and implementation of least restrictive alternatives. In addition, increased flexibility is apparent in the general shift from a dichotomy of complete incompetency vs competency to a model incorporating strengths and weaknesses, and delineating specific areas of capacity.

This evolution in guardianship law among many nations increases the importance of specialized and thorough assessment of capacity by clinicians. For example, the assessment needs to target specific capacities and integrate the individual's unique values and cultural background. Fortunately, various organizations and professionals have begun the work of developing helpful frameworks for approaching the assessment of capacity as well as tools that can be used in such an assessment, but there is obviously a great need for ongoing research in this area.

ACKNOWLEDGEMENTS

This chapter draws from material developed by one of the authors (JM) for the *Assessment of Older Adults with Diminished Capacity: A Handbook for Psychologists*, a work product of the American Bar Association and American Psychological Association Assessment of Capacity in Older Adults Project Working Group. We thank Liliana Sousa and Douglas Olsen for their assistance in locating international sources.

KEY REFERENCES AND SOURCES FOR FURTHER READING

American Bar Association and American Psychological Association Assessment of Capacity in Older Adults Project Working Group (2005). *Assessment of Older Adults with Diminished Capacity: A Handbook for Lawyers*. Washington, DC: American Bar Association and American Psychological Association.

Grisso, T. and Appelbaum, P. S. (1998a). *Assessing Competence to Consent to Treatment*. New York: Oxford University Press.

Qualls, S. H. and Smyer, M. A. (eds) (2007). *Aging and Decision-Making Capacity: Clinical, Family, and Legal Issues*. New York: Wiley.

Quinn, M. J. (2004). *Guardianships of Adults: Achieving Justice, Autonomy, and Safety.* New York: Springer.

Sabatino, C. P. and Basinger, S. L. (2000). 'Competency: Reforming our Legal Fictions'. *Journal of Mental Health and Aging* 6(2): 119–143.

REFERENCES

Acierno, R., Hernandez, M. A., Amstadter, A. B., Resnick, H. S., Steve, K., Muzzy, W., et al. (2010). 'Prevalence and Correlates of Emotional, Physical, Sexual, and Financial Abuse and Potential Neglect in the United States: The National Elder Mistreatment Study'. *American Journal of Public Health* 100(2): 292–297.

Alvaro, L. C. (2012). 'Competencia: conceptos generales y aplicacion en la demencia' [Competency: General Principles and Applicability in Dementia]. *Neurologia* 27(5): 290–300.

Alzheimer's Association (2011). *2011 Alzheimer's Disease Facts and Figures.* Chicago: Alzheimer's Association.

American Bar Association (2003). *Model Rules of Professional Conduct.* Washington, DC: American Bar Association.

American Bar Association and American Psychological Association Assessment of Capacity in Older Adults Project Working Group (2005). *Assessment of Older Adults with Diminished Capacity: A Handbook for Lawyers.* Washington, DC: American Bar Association and American Psychological Association.

American Bar Association and American Psychological Association Assessment of Capacity in Older Adults Project Working Group (2006). *Judicial Determination of Capacity of Older Adults in Guardianship Proceedings: A Handbook for Judges.* Washington, DC: American Bar Association and American Psychological Association.

American Bar Association and American Psychological Association Assessment of Capacity in Older Adults Project Working Group (2008). *Assessment of Older Adults with Diminished Capacity: A Handbook for Psychologists.* Washington, DC: American Bar Association and American Psychological Association.

American Psychological Association (2002). *Ethical Principles of Psychologists and Code of Conduct.* Washington, DC: American Psychological Association.

Anderer, S. J. (1990). *Determining Competency in Guardianship Proceedings.* Washington, DC: American Bar Association.

Appelbaum, P. S. and Grisso, T. (1995). 'The MacArthur Treatment Competency Study 1: Mental Illness and Competence to Consent to Treatment'. *Law and Human Behavior* 19: 105–126.

Arai, M. (2000). 'Japan's New Safety Net: Reform of Statutory Guardianships and the Creation of Voluntary Guardianship'. *NAELA Quarterly* 13(4): 5–8.

Ball, K. K., Roenker, D. L., Wadley, V. G., Edwards, J. B., Roth, D. L., McGwin, G., et al. (2006). 'Can High-risk Older Drivers be Identified through Performance-based Measures in a Department of Motor Vehicles Setting?' *Journal of the American Geriatrics Society* 54: 77–84.

Barbas, N. R. and Wilde, E. A. (2001). 'Competency issues in Dementia: Medical Decision Making, Driving and Independent Living'. *Journal of Geriatric Psychiatry and Neurology* 14: 199–212.

Beisecker, A. (1988). 'Aging and the Desire for Information and Input in Medical Decisions: Patient Consumerism in Medical Encounters'. *The Gerontologist* 28: 330–335.

Bennett, H. and Hallen, P. (2005). 'Guardianship and Financial Management Legislation: What Doctors in Aged Care Need to Know'. *Internal Medicine Journal* 35: 482–487.

Berg, J. W., Appelbaum, P. S., Lidz, C. W., and Parker, L. S. (2001). *Informed Consent: Legal Theory and Clinical Practice*. New York: Oxford University Press.

Bielby, P. (2005). 'The Conflation of Competence and Capacity in English Medical Law: A Philosophical Critique'. *Medicine, Healthcare, and Philosophy* 8(3): 357–369.

Björkstén, S. K. (2008). 'Practice of Competence Assessment in Sweden'. In G. Stoppe (ed.), *Competence Assessment in Dementia* (pp. 161–163). New York: Springer.

Blanchard-Fields, F. and Camp, C. (1990). 'Affect, Individual Differences, and Real World Problem Solving across the Adult Life Span'. In T. Hess (ed.), *Aging and Cognition: Knowledge Organization and Utilization* (pp. 461–497). Amsterdam: North Holland.

Borges, S. C., Colón, M. F., Silva Marques, A., and Vieira, N. (2008). 'Perfil dos indivíduos periciados no âmbito de processos de inabilitação e interdição na delegação do centro do INML' [Profiling of the Persons Evaluated in Interdiction/Disqualification Processes in Medico-Legal National Institute from Region Centre]. *Psiquiatria Clínica* 29: 117–125.

Braun, M., Gurrera, R. J., Karel, M. J., Armesto, J. C., and Moye, J. (2009). 'Are Clinicians ever Biased in their Judgments of the Capacity of Older Adults to make Medical Decisions?' *Generations* 33: 78–81.

Commission on National Probate Court Standards and Advisory Committee on Interstate Guardianships (1993). *National Probate Court Standards*. Williamsburg, VA: National College of Probate Judges and National Center for State Courts.

Convention on the International Protection of Adults (2000). Convention on the International Protection of Adults, Hague Conference on Private International Law (Vol. 35). Netherlands.

Convention on the Rights of Persons with Disabilities (2008). Convention on the Rights of Persons with Disabilities (Vol. Chapter IV(15)). New York: United Nations.

Cooper, C., Selwood, A., and Livingston, G. (2008). 'The Prevalence of Elder Abuse and Neglect: A Systematic Review'. *Age and Ageing* 37(2): 151–160.

Doron, I. (2002). 'Elder Guardianship Kaleidoscope—A Comparative Perspective'. *International Journal of Law, Policy and the Family* 16: 368–398.

Doron, I. (2004). 'Aging in the Shadow of the Law'. *Journal of Aging and Social Policy* 16(4): 59–77.

Faunce, T. A. (2005). 'Collaborative Research Trials: A Strategy for Fostering Mental Health Protections in Developing Nations'. *International Journal of Law and Psychiatry* 28: 171–181.

Ferres, B. (2007). 'Personal Reflections of a Tribunal Member—The Interface between Medical Practice and Legal Decision Making in Guardianship'. *Medicine and Law* 26(1): 15–22.

Griffith, H. R., Belue, K., Sicola, A., Krzywanski, S., Zamrini, E., Harrell, L., et al. (2003). 'Impaired Financial Abilities in Mild Cognitive Impairment: A Direct Assessment Approach'. *Neurology* 60: 449–457.

Grisso, T. (2003). *Evaluating Competences* (2nd edn). New York: Plenum.

Grisso, T. and Appelbaum, P. S. (1998a). *Assessing Competence to Consent to Treatment*. New York: Oxford University Press.

Grisso, T. and Appelbaum, P. S. (1998b). *MacArthur Competency Assessment Tool for Treatment (MacCAT-T)*. Sarasota, FL: Professional Resource Press.

Hamid, H., Abanilla, K., Bauta, B., and Huang, K. (2008). 'Evaluating the WHO Assessment Instrument for Mental Health Systems by Comparing Mental Health Policies in Four Countries'. *Bulletin of the World Health Organization* 86: 467–473.

Herr, S. S. (1995). 'Maximizing Autonomy: Reforming Personal Support Laws in Sweden and the United States'. *Journal of the Association for Persons with Severe Handicaps* 20(3): 213–223.

Horstman, P. (1975). 'Protective Services for the Elderly: The Limits of Parens Patriae'. *Missouri Law Review* 40: 215–236.

Hurme, S. and Wood, E. (2006). *Then and Now—2006, Guardianship Statutory Reform Factoids*. Washington, DC: American Bar Association.

Johnston, C. and Liddle, J. (2007). 'The Mental Capacity Act 2005: A New Framework for Healthcare Decision Making'. *Law, Ethics and Medicine* 33: 94–97.

Kagawa-Singer, M. and Blackhall, L. J. (2001). 'Negotiating Cross-cultural Issues at the End of Life'. *Journal of the American Medical Association* 286(23): 2993–3001.

Kahneman, D. (2003). 'A Perspective on Judgment and Choice: Mapping Bounded Rationality'. *American Psychologist* 58: 697–720.

Kanter, A. (2009). 'The United Nations Convention on the Rights of Persons with Disabilities and its Implications for the Rights of Elderly People under International Law'. *Georgia State University Law Review* 25(3): 526–573.

Karel, M. J. (2000). 'The Assessment of Values in Medical Decision Making'. *Journal of Aging Studies* 14: 403–422.

Karel, M. J., Powell, J., and Cantor, M. (2004). 'Using a Values Discussion Guide to Facilitate Communication in Advance Care Planning'. *Patient Education and Counseling* 55: 22–31.

Karel, M. J. (2007). 'Culture and Medical Decision Making: Assessment and Intervention'. In S. H. Qualls and M. Smyer (eds), *Changes in Decision-making Capacities in Older Adults: Assessment and Intervention* (pp. 145–174). Hoboken, NJ: Wiley.

Karel, M. J., Gurrera, R. J., Hicken, B., and Moye, J. (2010). 'Reasoning in Medical Consent Capacity: The Consideration of Values'. *Journal of Clinical Ethics* 21: 58–71.

Kim, S. Y. H., Karlawish, J. H. T., and Caine, E. D. (2002). 'Current State of Research on Decision-making Competence of Cognitively Impaired Elderly Persons'. *American Journal of Geriatric Psychiatry* 10: 151–165.

Kitamura, F., Tomoda, A., Tsukada, K., Tanaka, M., Kawakami, I., Mishima, S., et al. (1998). 'Method of Assessment of Competency to Consent in the Mentally Ill: Rationale, Development, and Comparison with the Medically Ill'. *International Journal of Law and Psychiatry* 21(3): 223.

Lambert, P., Gibson, J. M., and Nathanson, P. (1990). 'The Values History: An Innovation in Surrogate Medical Decision Making'. *Law, Medicine and Health Care* 18: 202–212.

Levy, B. R. (2009). 'Stereotype Embodiment: A Psychosocial Approach to Aging'. *Current Directions in Psychological Science* 18: 332–336.

Lowenstein, A., Eisikovits, Z., Band-Winterstein, T., and Enos, H. G. (2009). 'Is Elder Abuse and Neglect a Social Phenomenon? Data from the First National Prevalence Survey in Israel'. *Journal of Elder Abuse and Neglect* 21(3): 253–277.

Maeda, D. (2000). 'Social Security, Health Care, and Social Services for the Elderly in Japan'. In S. Yoshida (ed.), *Aging in Japan* (pp. 105–142). Tokyo: Japan Aging Research Center.

Manly, J. J. (2006). 'Cultural Issues'. In D. K. Attix and K. A. Welsh-Bohmer (eds), *Geriatric Neuropsychology: Assessment and Intervention* (pp. 198–222). New York: Guilford Press.

Marson, D. C., Chatterjee, A., Ingram, K. K., and Harrell, L. E. (1996). 'Toward a Neurologic Model of Competency: Cognitive Predictors of Capacity to Consent in Alzheimer's Disease Using Three Different Legal Standards'. *Neurology* 46: 666–672.

Marson, D. C., Hawkins, L., McInturff, B., and Harrell, L. E. (1997). 'Cognitive Models that Predict Physician Judgments of Capacity to Consent in mild Alzheimer's Disease'. *Journal of the American Geriatrics Society* 45: 458–464.

Marson, D. C., Sawrie, S., McInturff, B., Snyder, S., Chatterjee, A., Stalvey, T., et al. (2000). 'Assessing Financial Capacity in Patients with Alzheimer's Disease: A Conceptual Model and Prototype Instrument'. *Archives of Neurology* 57: 877–884.

Marson, D. C. and Zebley, L. (2001). 'The Other Side of the Retirement Years: Cognitive Decline, Dementia and Loss of Financial Capacity'. *Journal of Retirement Planning* 4(1): 30–38.

Mayhew, M. (2005). 'Survey of State Guardianship Laws: Statutory Provisions for Clinical Evaluations'. *Bifocal* 26: 1–19.

Melamed, Y., Yaron-Melamed, L., and Heinik, J. (2010). 'Guardianship Appointment: Current Status in Israel'. *Israel Journal of Psychiatry and Related Sciences* 47(4): 260–268.

Mitchell, A. (1978). 'Involuntary Guardianship for Incompetents: A Strategy for Legal Services Advocates'. *Clearinghouse Review* 12: 451–468.

Mizuno, Y. and Namba, Y. (2001). 'Aging Society and an Adult Guardianship System'. *Japanese Journal of Geriatrics* 38(5): 591–599.

Moye, J., Karel, M. J., Azar, A., R., and Gurrera, R. J. (2004a). 'Capacity to Consent to Treatment: Empirical Comparison of Three Instruments in Older Adults with and without Dementia'. *Gerontologist* 44: 166–175.

Moye, J., Karel, M. J., Azar, A. R., and Gurrera, R. J. (2004b). 'Hopes and Cautions for Instrument-based Evaluations of Consent Capacity: Results of a Construct Validity Study of Three Instruments'. *Ethics, Law, and Aging Review* 10: 39–61.

Moye, J., Armesto, J. C., and Karel, M. J. (2005). 'Evaluating Capacity of Older Adults in Rehabilitation Settings: Conceptual Models and Clinical Challenges'. *Rehabilitation Psychology* 50(3): 207–214.

Moye, J. and Marson, D. C. (2007). 'Assessment of Decision Making Capacity in Older Adults: An Emerging Area of Research and Practice'. *Journal of Gerontology* 62: 3–11.

Moye, J., Karel, M. J., Edelstein, B., Hicken, B., Armesto, J. C., and Gurrera, R. J. (2008). 'Assessment of Capacity to Consent to Treatment: Current Research, the "ACCT" Approach, Future Directions'. *Clinical Gerontologist* 31: 37–66.

Moye, J., Marson, D., Edelstein, B., Wood, S., and Saldivar, A. (2011). 'Decision Making Capacity'. In K. Warner Schaie and S. L. Willis (eds), *Handbook of the Psychology of Aging* (7th edn, pp. 367–379). London: Academic Press.

Moye, J. and Naik, A. (2011). 'Physician Evaluations Are Key to Preserving Rights for Individuals Facing Guardianship'. *Journal of the American Medical Association* 305: 936–937.

National Conference of Commissioners on Uniform State Laws (1997). *Uniform Guardianship and Protective Proceedings Act*. http://www.law.upenn.edu/bll/ulc/fnact99/1990s/ugppa97.htm.

Palmer, B. W., Dunn, L. B., Appelbaum, P. S., and Jeste, D. V. (2004). 'Correlates of Treatment-related Decision-making Capacity among Middle-aged and Older Patients with Schizophrenia'. *Archives of General Psychiatry* 61(3): 230–236.

Palmer, B. W., Dunn, L. B., Appelbaum, P. S., Mudaliar, S., Thal, L., Henry, R., et al. (2005). 'Assessment of Capacity to Consent to Research among Older Persons with Schizophrenia, Alzheimer Disease, or Diabetes Mellitus: Comparison of a 3-Item Questionnaire with a Comprehensive Standardized Capacity Instrument'. *Archives of General Psychiatry* 62(7): 726–733.

Pearlman, R., Starks, H., Cain, K., Rosengreen, D., and Patrick, D. (1998). *Your Life, Your Choices—Planning for Future Medical Decisions: How to Prepare a Personalized Living Will* (No. PB#98159437). Springfield, VA: US Department of Commerce, National Technical Information Service.

Pinsker, D. M., Stone, V. E., Pachana, N. A., and Greenspan, S. (2006). 'Social Vulnerability Scale for Older Adults: A Validation Study'. *Clinical Psychologist* 10: 109–119.

Qualls, S. H. and Smyer, M. A. (eds) (2007). *Aging and Decision-making Capacity: Clinical, Family, and Legal Issues*. New York: Wiley.

Quinn, M. J. (2004). *Guardianships of Adults: Achieving Justice, Autonomy, and Safety.* New York: Springer.

Reynolds, S. L. (2002). 'Guardianship Primavera: A First Look at Factors Associated with Having a Legal Guardian Using a Nationally Representative Sample of Community-dwelling Adults'. *Aging & Mental Health* 6(2): 109–120.

Sabatino, C. P. (1994). 'Ten Legal Myths about Advance Medical Directives'. *Clearinghouse Review* 28(6): 653–656.

Sabatino, C. P. and Basinger, S. L. (2000). 'Competency: Reforming our Legal Fictions'. *Journal of Mental Health and Aging* 6(2): 119–143.

Schlüter, W. and Liedmeier, N. (1990). 'Reform of the Guardianship and Health Care Right—A Contribution of Government to the Protection of the Elderly'. *Zeitschrift fur Gerontologie* [European Journal of Geriatrics] 23(2): 68–78.

Sherod, M. G., Griffith, H. R., Copeland, J., Belue, K., Krzywanski, S., Zamrini, E. Y., et al. (2009). 'Neurocognitive Predictors of Financial Capacity across the Dementia Spectrum: Normal Aging, MCI, and Alzheimer's Disease'. *Journal of the International Neuropsychological Society* 15: 258–267.

Skelton, F., Kunik, M., Regev, T., and Naik, A. (2010). 'Determining if an Older Adult Can Make and Execute Decisions to Live Safely at Home: A Capacity Assessment and Intervention Model'. *Archives of Gerontology and Geriatrics* 50: 300–305.

Smyer, M. A., Schaie, K. W., and Kapp, M. B. (eds) (1996). *Older Adults Decision-making and the Law*. New York: Springer.

Sousa, L. B., Simões, M. R., and Firmino, H. (2010). *Instrumento de Avaliação da Capacidade Financeira (IACFin)* [Financial Capacity Assessment Instrument]. Coimbra: Faculdade de Psicologia e de Ciências da Educação da Universidade de Coimbra.

Thompson, S. C., Pitts, J. S., and Schwankovsky, L. (1993). 'Preferences for Involvement in Medical Decision-making: Situational and Demographic Influences'. *Patient Education and Counseling* 22: 133–140.

Tversky, A. and Kahneman, D. (1981). 'The Framing of Decisions and the Psychology of Choice'. *Science* 211: 453–458.

US General Accounting Office (1995). *Patient Self-Determination Act of 1990*. Washington, DC: General Accounting Office.

Valdes-Stauber, J., Deinert, H., and Kilian, R. (2011). 'Consequences of the German Federal Guardianship Law after Reunification'. http://www.ncbi.nlm.nih.gov/pubmed/21744178. Retrieved 1 November 2011.

Wilber, K. H. and Reynolds, S. L. (1995). 'Rethinking Alternatives to Guardianship'. *Gerontologist* 35(2): 248–257.

Wingspan Conferees (2001). 'Wingspan: The Second National Guardianship Conference, Recommendations'. www.naela.com. Retrieved 29 December 2006.

Wong, J. G. and Scully, P. (2003). 'A Practical Guide to Capacity Assessment and Patient Consent in Hong Kong'. *Hong Kong Medical Journal* 9: 284–289.

Wood, E. (1988–2010). 'Directions of Reform'. http://www.abanet.org/aging/legislativeupdates/home.shtml. Retrieved 15 Januay 2010.

Youngs, R. (2002). *Sourcebook on German Law* (2nd edn). London: Cavendish.

Zenz, G. A. (1989). 'The End of Guardianship for the Elderly? Facts and Objectives in Current Discussions on the Proposed Reform Legislation in the Federal Republic of Germany'. In J. Eekelaar and D. Pearl (eds), *An Aging World: Dilemmas and Challenges for Law and Social Policy*. Oxford: Clarendon Press.

Zimny, G. H. and Grossberg, G. T. (1998). *Guardianship of the Elderly*. New York: Springer.

CHAPTER 13

SUICIDAL IDEATION IN LATE LIFE

ALISA A. O'RILEY, KIMBERLY VAN ORDEN, AND YEATES CONWELL

INTRODUCTION

MANAGING older patients with suicidal ideation (SI) represents one of the most difficult challenges facing clinicians and mental health providers (Jobes et al. 2008). Whenever a patient reports thoughts of harming him or herself, clinicians must cope with increased anxiety about the patient's safety, the inevitable anxieties involved in attempting to predict future behaviour, and fears about potential liability (Jobes et al. 2008). Patients with SI also inevitably require the allocation of additional resources due to the need for additional monitoring and, in some cases, more intensive treatment (Jobes et al. 2008). Finally, evidence suggests that SI is associated with negative health outcomes among older adults, including more severe distress (Szanto et al. 2007), less favourable responses to mental health treatment (Szanto et al. 2003), a higher chance of relapsing after mental health treatment (De Leo et al. 2005; Szanto et al. 2001), and increased all-cause mortality (Dewey et al. 1993; Maier and Smith 1999).

SI in later life may also increase risk for suicide deaths, as it is associated with suicide attempts (Miret et al. 2010). The association between SI and death by suicide in older adults is less clear, as only one study has examined the correlation between SI and death by suicide, and this study was not case controlled (Waern et al. 1999). Although the association between SI and death by suicide has not been empirically established, it is important to note that assessing SI is one of the most important components to assessing suicide risk across all age groups (Beck, Kovacs, and Weissman 1979). In many countries, including Mauritius, Zimbabwe, Argentina, Belize, Brazil, Canada, Chile, Columbia, Costa Rica, Barbados, Cuba, Ecuador, El Salvador, Guyana, Mexico, Paraguay, Puerto Rico, Trinidad and Tobago, the US, Uruguay, Venezuela, Albania, Armenia, Austria, Belarus, Belgium, Bosnia and Herzegovina, Bulgaria, Croatia, Czech Republic, Denmark, Estonia, Finland, France, Georgia, Germany, Hungary, Israel, Italy, Kazakhstan, Latvia, Lithuania, Luxembourg, Netherlands, Norway, Poland, Portugal, Romania, the Russian

Federation, Serbia, Slovakia, Slovenia, Spain, Sweden, Switzerland, Macedonia FYR, Ukraine, India, Sri Lanka, Australia, China, Japan, New Zealand, and the Republic of Korea, older adults have disproportionately high rates of death by suicide (World Health Organization Suicide Prevention and Special Programmes (WHO SUPRE) 2013). A common viewpoint is to conceptualize suicidal behaviour as operating on a continuum where SI leads to suicide attempt(s), which ultimately may lead to death by suicide (O'Carroll et al. 1996). However, it is important to note that the evidence behind this assumption is mixed. First, rates of SI are much higher than suicide attempts or death by suicide (e.g. Casey et al. 2008), and further, some studies suggest that risk factors for SI may differ in some respects from risk factors for death by suicide (e.g. Useda et al. 2007). These findings suggest that SI does not perfectly predict death by suicide. On the other hand, in past studies of older adults, research has demonstrated that SI may be a valid surrogate endpoint for death by suicide (Links, Heisel, and Quastel 2005). These findings suggest that increasing our understanding of SI in late-life may improve our ability to prevent deaths by suicide. For all of these reasons, SI in late-life represents a major public health concern. This chapter will set out to examine the definition of SI, how SI is measured, the prevalence of SI among older adults, risk and protective factors for SI in late-life, and what is currently known about treatment of SI in late-life.

DEFINITION OF SI

One of the major difficulties in summarizing and clarifying what is currently known about SI in late-life centres on the fact that there is little agreement about how best to define thoughts of suicide (O'Carroll et al. 1996). Several attempts have been made to create a standard definition of SI (Silverman et al. 2007a). For example, the US Centers for Disease Control defines SI very broadly as 'thinking about, considering, or planning for suicide' (Centers for Disease Control 2011). Thus, in this definition, individuals with SI may or may not have suicidal intent. Other nomenclatures have attempted to more specifically characterize SI. In 1996, a group of internationally renowned suicide prevention experts set out to create a nomenclature for suicide; these experts defined SI as 'any self-reported thoughts of engaging in suicide related behavior' (O'Carroll et al. 1996: 247). This group differentiated between 'casual' and 'serious' ideation, and further differentiated between individuals with persistent and transient serious ideation. In 2007, the nomenclature developed by O'Carroll and colleagues was revised (Silverman et al. 2007b). This group further characterized SI by the frequency (casual, transient, persistent), the level of intent (with no intent, with undetermined degree of suicidal intent, and with intent), and the level of motivation (passive vs active) behind thoughts of suicide.

Largely because of the difficulties inherent in conducting research on behaviours with very low base rates, in the interest of maximizing sample sizes, most research studies do not utilize any of the nomenclatures developed to define suicidal behaviour; however, many researchers have differentiated between passive (thoughts of death or wishing for death) and active (thinking or planning on taking one's life) SI (e.g. Bartels et al. 2002). Passive ideation is also sometimes referred to as death ideation.

At the current time, our understanding of the differences between passive and active SI is limited. Some evidence clearly suggests that passive and active SI are distinctly different categories. For example, prevalence studies suggest that frequencies of passive ideation are much higher than frequencies of active ideation (see prevalence section below), and that older adults are more likely to endorse passive ideation than active ideation (see, for example, Ayalon et al. 2007). Some researchers have suggested that passive ideation may even be normative at the end of life (see, for example, Chochinov 2003). In addition, researchers and clinicians have argued that passive ideation indicates a lower level of suicide risk than active SI (Raue et al. 2006), but studies examining the validity of this assumption have yielded mixed results. For example, some research with both older adults who have experienced chronic Major Depressive Disorder and older adults with late-onset depression suggests that the distinction between passive and active ideation may be arbitrary (Szanto et al. 1996). Specifically, depressed older adults with passive and active ideation are similar in terms of demographics, levels of hopelessness, and personality traits (Szanto et al. 1996). In addition, when depressed individuals with passive and active ideation are followed over time, it appears that the type of ideation (active or passive) depressed older adults experience often changes; that is, depressed individuals who experience passive ideation at one point may experience active ideation at another point and vice versa. While these findings about depressed older adults are interesting, it is important to note that, while depression is strongly associated with both passive and active SI, not everyone who exhibits SI is depressed (Conwell and Thompson 2008). Currently, little is known about older adults with SI in the absence of depression, and more research is needed examining this unique group.

The need to better understand the meaning behind passive SI and whether it differs from active suicidal thinking has been particularly relevant in discussions about physician assisted suicide and euthanasia (Chochinov et al. 1998). Although the debate about suicide at the end of life is beyond the scope of the current chapter, work examining passive SI in terminally ill patients may help to clarify our understanding of passive ideation in late-life more generally. Research indicates that passive SI is common in terminally ill patients (point prevalence is 17–45%; Breitbart et al. 2000; Chochinov et al. 1998). As is the case with the general population, passive ideation among the terminally ill is associated with depressive symptoms, poor social support, and pain (Chochinov et al.); however, depression and other psychiatric symptoms do not fully characterize the distress experienced by some terminally ill patients with passive SI (Chochinov 2003). Researchers who focus on existential distress in the terminally ill have developed models to explain passive ideation in this population based on the notion that severe distress at the end of life may be indicative of a loss of dignity and a loss of meaning in life (Breitbart and Heller 2003; Chochinov 2003). Further, they have demonstrated that treatments designed to increase meaningfulness and dignity result in decreased passive SI among terminally ill patients (Breitbart and Heller 2003; Chochinov 2003). Currently, we do not know how models of passive ideation in the terminally ill apply to the general population of older adults; however, the results of research examining thoughts of death in individuals at the end of life provide some evidence that passive ideation may indicate an important and unique clinical marker of distress. Overall, more research is needed examining the experience of older adults who demonstrate passive SI or prominent thoughts of death.

Measuring SI in Older Adults

Because it is not yet clear that the benefits of suicide risk screening outweigh the costs, many public health organizations (including the US Preventive Services Task Force (USPSTF)) do not currently recommend large-scale screening programmes for SI in primary care (Gaynes et al. 2004). However, systematic depression screening is recommended, typically including one or more items that capture suicidal thoughts. For example, many studies have examined SI using single items from the Patient Health Questionnaire (PHQ-9; Kroenke, Spitzer, and Williams 2001; Spitzer, Kroenke, and Williams 1999) and the Hamilton Depression Scale (HAM-D; Hamilton 1960). Although the use of single items from depression screening instruments is often useful because such data is widely available and accessible, there are limitations to this method of assessing SI. First, we are not aware of any research examining the reliability or validity of these single-item measures of SI. Second, these items often do not differentiate between different types of SI. For example, the PHQ-9 suicide item (item 9: 'Over the last 2 weeks, how often have you been bothered by any thoughts that you would be better off dead or of hurting yourself in some way?') consists of a double-barrelled question assessing both thoughts of death (passive ideation) and thoughts of taking one's life (active ideation, Kroenke et al. 2001). Thus, when a patient or participant endorses this item, it is impossible to know the level of intent behind the SI the individual is experiencing without further follow-up and clarification.

Although universal screening for SI is not recommended in primary care, use of instruments specifically designed to assess SI may be indicated for select subgroups where the risk may be elevated and interventions available, or in research. Several such instruments are available. One of the most widely used instruments to assess SI is Beck and colleagues' Scale for Suicide Ideation (SSI; Beck et al. 1979). The SSI assesses active and passive ideation as well as intent. It has been used in several studies examining SI in older adults (e.g. Szanto et al. 1996); however, this instrument has not been validated for use in late-life. Similarly, two other instruments originally designed for use with younger adults, the Paykel Suicide Scale (Paykel et al. 1974), which assesses passive and active ideation over the past year, and the Columbia-Suicide Severity Rating Scale (Posner et al. 2011), which is mandated by the Federal Drug Administration for use in clinical drug trials (including dementia drug trials), have also been used in several studies examining SI in older adults; however, these measures were not originally designed for this purpose.

Researchers have noted that the use of SI measures designed and validated for use with younger adults may not be valid for use with older adults (Heisel and Flett 2006), in part because evidence suggests that risk factors for suicide in older adults differ significantly from risk factors for suicide in younger adults (Conwell and Thompson 2008). For example, evidence suggests that older adults who die by suicide are more likely to be depressed, are more likely to use a firearm, are less likely to have substance abuse problems, are more likely to be socially isolated, are less likely to have previous suicide attempts, and are more likely to have physical illness or functional impairment than younger adults who die by suicide (Conwell and Thompson 2008). There is currently one measure designed specifically to assess SI in older adults. The Geriatric Suicide Ideation Scale (GSIS; Heisel and Flett 2006) was designed to assess risk factors for suicide specific to late-life. Although the GSIS is a relatively new measure, it has been normed and validated on a variety of samples of older adults (including community-dwelling older adults, older adults receiving psychiatric care, and older adults residing in long-term care facilities; Heisel and Flett 2006) and is increasingly used in studies examining SI in late-life.

How common are passive and active SI in late-life?

Studies examining frequency of SI in older adults have reported widely varying prevalence rates. Among community-dwelling older adults, frequencies of passive ideation range from 3.4% to 27.3% (Ayalon and Litwin 2009; Ayalon et al. 2007; Cohen et al. 2008; Rurup et al. 2011). Of interest because of racial differences in suicide deaths, one study examining racial differences in frequency of passive ideation found no differences between frequency of ideation in European Americans and African Americans (Cohen et al. 2008). Fewer studies have been conducted examining frequency of active ideation in community-dwelling older adults; however, one study found that 0.6% of community-dwelling older adults had current active SI (Ayalon et al. 2007). A handful of studies have examined the frequency of ideation in older adults seeking care in primary care clinics. Frequencies of passive ideation in these studies range from 15% to 27.5% (Bartels et al. 2002; Raue et al. 2010), and frequencies of active SI range from 1% to 10.4% (Bartels et al. 2002; Pfaff et al. 2007; Raue et al. 2010). Prevalence of SI appears to be slightly higher among frail older adults. For example, in one study of residents of long term care facilities, 43% of older adults reported passive ideation and 11% of older adults reported active ideation (Malfent et al. 2009). In another study examining homebound older adults, Sirey and colleagues found that 13% of older adult reported passive ideation (Sirey et al. 2008). Finally, numerous studies have examined the prevalence of SI among older adults with depressive symptoms. In these studies, frequencies of active SI range from 3% to 58% (Alexopoulous et al. 1999; Britton et al. 2008; Bruce et al. 2004; Lynch et al. 1999; Raue et al. 2010; Szanto et al. 2001; Tan and Wong 2008; Vannoy et al. 2007).

The wide range of frequency of SI in these studies of older adults may be attributed to two factors. First, the samples examined in the studies differ significantly in terms of psychiatric history and symptom severity. It is possible, for example, that depressed older adults recruited from mental health clinics and psychiatric hospitals (e.g. Alexopoulos et al., 1999) may demonstrate more significant levels of SI than depressed older adults recruited from primary care offices (e.g. Bruce et al. 2004). Second, studies vary significantly in how SI is measured and operationalized. As was mentioned earlier in the section on measurement, operationalizing SI by a single item from a depressive screener may yield different results than operationalizing SI by an instrument specifically designed to assess that construct. Future research, using more precise measures, is needed to determine why estimates of prevalence of SI in older adults vary so widely.

Risk and protective factors for SI in older adults

Numerous studies have been conducted examining correlates of SI in older adults. These studies suggest several possible risk and protective factors for SI in late-life. Interestingly, many of the risk factors described below are also risk factors for death by suicide in older adults, including: depressive symptoms, anxiety symptoms, social disconnectedness, physical health problems, and certain personality traits (Conwell and Thompson 2008; Van Orden and Conwell 2011). These findings suggest that addressing risk factors for SI among older adults may also prevent deaths by suicide in late-life.

Demographic variables

Research examining the association between SI in older adults and demographic variables has frequently produced mixed results. For example,, several studies have demonstrated that increased age is associated with more passive SI and less active SI (Ayalon et al. 2007; Duberstein et al. 1999; Gallo, Anthony, and Muthén 1994; Lynch et al. 1999); however, other studies have demonstrated that increased age is associated with higher levels of both passive and active ideation (Edwards et al. 2006; Vannoy et al. 2007). Similarly, some research has demonstrated that older women report more SI than older men (Ayalon et al. 2007), but other studies have shown that older men experience more SI than older women (Szanto et al. 2003; Tan and Wong 2008). One study that may explain these discrepant findings demonstrated that older women experience more passive SI and older men report more active SI (Bartels et al. 2002). Finally, research has consistently shown that older adults with lower SES have higher levels of SI (Chen et al. 2011; Cohen et al. 2009; Cohen et al. 2010).

Psychiatric problems

Several studies have demonstrated a very strong association between severity of depressive symptoms and both passive and active SI in older adults (Alexopoulos et al. 1999; Ayalon and Litwin 2009; Ayalon et al. 2007; Bartels et al. 2002; Chen et al. 2011; Cohen et al. 2008; Cukrowicz et al. 2009; Edwards et al. 2006; Heisel and Flett 2008; Kim et al. 2006; Lynch et al. 1999; Pfaff and Almeida 2004; Rurup et al. 2011; Szanto et al. 2001; Szanto et al. 2007; Tan and Wong 2008; Witte et al. 2006). These studies suggest that SI is associated with depressive symptoms, and, when older adults with depression and no SI are compared to older adults with depression and SI, individuals with depression and SI tend to have more severe depressive symptoms. A handful of studies have also demonstrated a significant, positive association between anxiety symptoms and SI in late-life (Bartels et al. 2002; Lenze et al. 2000; Szanto et al. 2003; Tan and Wong 2008). In addition to symptoms of depression and anxiety, strong evidence suggests that older adults with SI are more likely to have a history of suicide attempts than older adults without SI (Alexopoulos et al. 1999; Bartels et al. 2002; Pfaff and Almeida 2004; Szanto et al. 2001; Tan and Wong 2008; Witte et al. 2006). Finally, several studies have demonstrated an association between SI and general cognitive impairment (Ayalon and Litwin 2009; Ayalon et al. 2007; Heisel, Flett, and Besser 2002).

Social disconnectedness

Numerous studies have also demonstrated an association between both passive and active SI in older adults and poor social support, which is one form of social disconnectedness (Alexopoulos et al. 1999; Ayalon and Litwin 2009; Bartels et al. 2002; Kim et al. 2006; Rowe et al. 2006; Rurup et al. 2011; Vanderhorst and McLaren 2005). Interestingly, in one study examining differences between European American and African American older adults with SI, poor social support was only associated with SI in European Americans (Cohen et al. 2008). In addition to findings about social support, research has also demonstrated that feeling like a burden on those around you is associated with SI in older adults (Britton et al. 2008; Jahn et al. 2011). Finally, research has demonstrated that a higher sense of belonging is protective against SI in late-life (McLaren et al. 2007).

Physical health, pain, and disability

Physical health problems (both subjective and objective) have consistently been found to increase risk for SI in older adults (Ayalon and Litwin 2009; Ayalon et al. 2007; Bartels et al. 2002; Cohen et al. 2008; Heisel and Flett 2008; Pfaff and Almeida 2004). Interestingly, however, several studies have demonstrated that both objective and subjective measures of physical health is more strongly associated with passive SI than with active SI (Ayalon and Litwin 2009; Ayalon et al. 2007). In addition to physical health, pain has also been found to increase risk for SI in older adults and especially for older men (Edwards et al. 2006; Sirey et al. 2008; Tang and Crane 2006). Finally, functional impairment has also been associated with SI in late-life (Edwards et al. 2006; Kim et al. 2006).

Personality, cognition, and coping

Research has demonstrated an association between SI in late-life and several different personality traits. Duberstein and colleagues demonstrated that depressed older adults with SI have higher neuroticism and higher openness to experience than depressed older adults without SI (Duberstein et al. 2000). Other research has also found that SI in older adults is associated with higher levels of neuroticism (Segal et al. 2011; Vannoy et al. 2007). Finally, research has demonstrated an association between SI in older adults and symptoms of narcissistic, borderline, and histrionic personality disorders (Heisel et al. 2007; Segal et al. 2011). In terms of cognitive patterns and patterns of coping, SI in older adults has been associated with a loss of a sense of agency in older men (Hobbs and McLaren 2009), a lower sense of mastery in both men and women (Rurup et al. 2011), and a tendency to use emotional coping, avoidance coping, and thought suppression techniques (Cukrowicz et al. 2008; Lynch et al. 2004). Similarly, some studies have shown that older adults with SI have more hopelessness (measured in different ways) than older adults without SI (Britton et al. 2008; Kim et al. 2006; Szanto et al. 2001; Witte et al. 2006).

Protective factors

In terms of factors that may protect against SI in older adults, research has demonstrated that older adults with more psychological well-being (Heisel and Flett 2008), more meaning in life (Heisel and Flett 2008), more future orientation (Hirsch et al. 2006), more positive affect (Hirsch et al. 2007), and more reasons for living (Britton et al. 2008) tend to have lower levels of SI.

Behavioural Treatment of SI in Late-life

In this section, we attempt to answer the question, 'what are the best interventions to help older adults with SI?' However, scant data are available that speak to this question. Given differences in clinical presentations and risk factors, we cannot assume that treatments shown to help suicidal younger adults will help older adults. Intervening with suicidal older adults is thus an area in great need of research attention.

Turning to data that are available, collaborative care models (CCMs) for depression in late-life have been proposed as a means of addressing late-life suicide risk, resting on the assumption that treating depression will address one of the strongest risk factors for suicide in later life (Bruce 1999). CCMs are effective in improving depression outcomes by augmenting depression treatment in primary care (or other settings, such as social service agencies) with psychiatric consultation and medication recommendations, psychoeducation for patients, symptom monitoring, and the option of brief psychotherapy that can be delivered by non-mental-health specialists (Gilbody et al. 2006). Two collaborative care models have been examined among older adults samples with regards to their effectiveness for SI (discussed below), and both have shown promise with regards to the reduction or prevention of SI.

The Improving Mood–Promoting Access to Collaborative Treatment (IMPACT) trial examined the effectiveness of a collaborative care management programme for late-life depression delivered in primary care (Unützer et al. 2002). Adults aged 60 or older who were receiving primary care services at one of eighteen participating clinics were screened for depression; those who met criteria for major depression or dysthymia (and consented) were randomly assigned to either the intervention condition or usual care. The intervention consisted of access to a depression care manager (i.e. a nurse or psychologist) over twelve months, who provided psychoeducation on late-life depression and coordinated the patient's depression treatment with the primary care physician, including input from the supervising psychiatrist and the provision of algorithm-based recommendations. The first step in the algorithm was prescription of an anti-depressant (typically an SSRI) or a course of problem-solving therapy (PST) delivered by the care manager. Assessments were conducted over one year and included measurements of depression, satisfaction with care, functional impairment, and quality of life. The older adults assigned to the intervention condition demonstrated lower depressive symptom severity, greater satisfaction with their care, lower functional impairment, and greater quality of life at the end of the twelve-month intervention. Further, fewer patients assigned to the intervention condition endorsed death/SI at the end of the intervention period (twelve months post-baseline) and at eighteen-month follow-up (Unützer et al. 2006). However, at the end of the intervention, 10% of patients in the intervention condition reported SI, indicating a significant proportion of patients for whom the IMPACT CCM was not effective with regards to eliminating SI, though the proportion was significantly less than in the Usual Care condition (16%).

The primary outcome of the second trial, the Prevention of Suicide in Primary Care Elderly: Collaborative Trial (PROSPECT) was SI (Bruce 1999; Bruce et al. 2004), although depression severity was also measured. The design of PROSPECT involved the random assignment of twenty primary care practices to usual care or the PROSPECT intervention.

The intervention consisted of depression care management (by nurses, social workers, or psychologists) for two years for patients who met criteria for Major Depression or Minor Depression. The presence of SI at baseline was not a requirement for inclusion in the trial. Care management activities included helping physicians recognize depression, monitoring depressive symptoms, providing algorithm-based medication recommendations (the first step was prescription of citalopram at the target daily dose of 30 mg), managing treatment adherence, and providing interpersonal psychotherapy (IPT) for those patients who refused medication (and agreed to IPT). Care managers received weekly group supervision from psychiatrists (and as-needed phone consultation). At twenty-four months follow-up, among those patients with Major Depression at baseline, a significantly lower proportion of patients reported death or suicidal ideation in the intervention condition (i.e. 11.3%) compared to those assigned to the usual care condition (i.e. 14.7%; Alexopoulos et al. 2009). Similarly, depression severity was significantly reduced for those assigned to the intervention condition compared to usual care for those patients with Major Depression at baseline. A beneficial intervention effect was not demonstrated for those with Minor Depression at baseline for either SI or depressive symptom severity. Results of the PROSPECT trial suggest that CCMs in primary care settings that target depression may help reduce or prevent death or suicidal ideation among older adults with Major Depression.

Strengths of the IMPACT and PROSPECT trials include the use of multisite randomized designs, inclusion of both psychopharmacological and behavioural treatments, and specific evaluation of SI. However, the lack of an effect on SI among those PROSPECT patients with Minor Depression should be kept in mind given that Minor Depression among older adults is associated with increased risk of suicide death (Conwell and Thompson 2008). Further, among those with Major Depression in the PROSPECT trial, not all were free from SI at twenty-four months; rather, 11% of those in the intervention condition with Major Depression at baseline reported death or suicidal ideation at twenty-four months (Alexopoulos et al. 2009)—a comparable proportion to the 10% in IMPACT trial (Unützer et al. 2006)—indicating that a substantial number of those patients who received either the IMPACT or PROSPECT interventions either developed or continued to present with death or suicidal ideation after ongoing depression care management. These findings suggest that targeting depression may not be sufficient among all older adults, even those with Major Depression, to eliminate SI. One reason for an incomplete response regarding SI may be that in these trials depression was not treated to remission; in the PROSPECT trial, at twenty-four months follow-up, fewer than half of the patients with Major Depression at baseline were in remission in the Intervention Group (45.4%) compared to 31.5% in the Usual Care group. It may also be the case, however, that targeting other key risk factors for late-life suicide in trials to reduce suicidal ideation, including social disconnectedness and functional impairment, could improve suicide-related outcomes. Another possible modification that could potentially increase the effectiveness of the PROSPECT design is a greater emphasis on the behavioural intervention (i.e. IPT). In the PROSPECT trial, patients were offered IPT if they declined medication (Bruce 1999). It could be that a treatment in which IPT is offered jointly with medication would be maximally effective in reducing SI.

One reason that placing a greater emphasis on IPT might have improved the CCM in the PROSPECT trial is that IPT is especially conducive to targeting both depression and social disconnectedness. The rationale behind IPT is that interpersonal problems are both causes and consequences of depression and, when these problems are addressed, depression will resolve (see Hinrichsen and Iselin, this volume; Weissman et al. 2000). Marnin Heisel and his colleagues proposed that IPT is ideally suited to treat older adults with SI because these older adults often present with social problem-solving deficits and difficulties with interpersonal functioning, both of which are associated with SI among older adults and are key treatment targets in IPT (Heisel et al. 2009). Thus, available empirical data indicate a good match between risk factors for late-life SI and the proposed targets and mechanisms in IPT. Preliminary (uncontrolled) data from Heisel and colleagues indicate that IPT is a promising approach to the treatment of death and SI in later life as the treatment was acceptable to a small sample of suicidal older adults and resulted in significant pre-post reductions in death and SI, as well as reductions in depression symptom severity (Heisel et al. 2009). Further, data indicate that IPT is useful in preventing relapse and maintaining gains in social functioning among older adults with depression (Lenze et al. 2002; Reynolds et al. 1999). There are also treatment manuals specifically describing the implementation of IPT with older adults (Hinrichsen and Clougherty 2006), including a modification for older adults with cognitive impairment (Miller 2009), thereby assisting clinicians in translating research findings into clinical practice.

Another intervention that was designed to target social problem-solving skills and is effective in treating depression is problem-solving therapy (PST; Bell and D'Zurilla 2009). This was the behavioural intervention used in the IMPACT trial (Arean et al. 2008). PST is a skills-based form of psychotherapy that focuses on solving problems that are contributing to depression. The core of PST is teaching—and helping the patient utilize—a structured process for problem-solving (Arean and Huh 2006). This process involves a sequence of seven steps, including such tasks as defining the problem, formulating a goal, and brainstorming solutions. The rationale behind PST is that unsolved problems cause depression; further, when people become depressed, they lose energy and motivation to solve problems, which compounds depression. Thus, to treat depression, a structured process for problem-solving is implemented that helps patients re-engage skills they already possess or learn skills that were missing in their behavioural repertoires. There are two forms of PST that are researched and used in clinical practice. The first, associated with the work of D'Zurilla and Nezu (2007), is designed for mental health outpatient clinics. This form of PST teaches the seven skills sequentially, adding new skills as the patient demonstrates mastery. The majority of the research on PST with older adults has been conducted with the form of PST designed to be delivered in non-mental-health settings, such as primary care offices. This form of PST is associated with the work of Patricia Arean and Mark Hegel and is typically referred to as PST-PC (for primary care; Arean et al. 2008). PST-PC has been shown to be effective at treating Major Depression and Dysthymia (Arean et al. 2008), including depressive symptoms with comorbid executive dysfunction (Alexopoulos et al. 2003). The delivery of PST by social service agencies has also been shown to be effective at treating Minor Depression in older adults (Ciechanowski et al. 2004). Behavioural interventions that included problem-solving have been shown to decrease SI in middle-aged and younger adults (Rudd et al. 1996; Salkovskis, Artha, and Storer 1990). Thus, research could examine the effectiveness of PST for suicidal older adults, especially given the ease with which PST can be taught and implemented. PST-PC can be successfully implemented by non-mental-health professionals (Arean and Huh 2006) and symptom relief is often evident in patients after only four sessions (Ciechanowski et al. 2004). However, as with any psychotherapy implemented with suicidal patients, additional treatment components would be needed, including thorough risk assessments and safety planning, and potentially concurrent use of case management, per the protocol of Brown and colleagues (2005).

The form of CBT that has strong support for preventing suicide attempts among middle-aged and younger adults is dialectical behaviour therapy (DBT; Linehan et al. 2007). Developed by Marsha Linehan (1993), DBT has been shown in several trials to reduce the likelihood of suicide attempts, hospitalizations associated with SI, and non-suicidal self-injury (Linehan et al. 2006; Linehan et al. 1999; Linehan et al. 1991). The rationale of DBT is that emotion dysregulation results in dysregulation in other domains, resulting in negative outcomes such as interpersonal problems and suicidal thoughts and behaviours. Standard DBT involves weekly individual therapy, phone-skills coaching available twenty-four hours per day, weekly group skills training, and a consultation team for DBT therapists. An adaptation of DBT for depressed older adults with personality disorders was compared to anti-depressant medication in a randomized trial (Lynch et al. 2007). This adaptation involved providing fourteen weeks of DBT skills training in a group format as well as weekly scheduled phone coaching sessions (thirty minutes in duration). Individual therapy was not provided. The DBT adaptation combined with anti-depressant medication was superior to medication alone with regards to reducing depression symptom severity and remission from Major Depression; however, no effects on SI were reported. Similarly, Cognitive Therapy has been shown to prevent suicide attempts, without an effect on SI, among middle-aged adults (Brown et al. 2005). A randomized trial with older men with previous suicide attempts is under way (as of the writing of this chapter). All in all, these data suggest that DBT and CT may be useful in the prevention of repeat suicide attempts and in the treatment of conditions comorbid with SI, including depression and personality disorders, but their effectiveness with older adults in the reduction or prevention of SI is unclear.

IMPLICATIONS FOR PRACTICE

SI in late-life is an important public health concern and a major problem facing clinicians working with older adults. Currently, our understanding of SI in late-life is incomplete. For example, more research is needed examining potentially important differences between passive and active SI. Similarly, although numerous studies have been conducted examining risk and protective factors for SI in late-life, much more research is needed examining how effectively to treat SI in this population. Despite this paucity of research, there are some promising studies that suggest that SI in older adults will respond to behavioural treatments. These studies provide hope that we will eventually have established, evidence-based interventions that will effectively treat SI in this population.

SUMMARY

SI in late-life represents a major public health concern and a critical problem for clinicians working with older adults. Much more research is needed examining the aetiology, course, and treatment of SI in late-life. Despite our need for more research, the evidence we have clearly suggests that every older adult experiencing SI (passive or active) is in pain (physically and/or emotionally), and that the pain associated with SI in older adults is treatable. Clinicians working with older adults experiencing SI are charged with working collaboratively with the older adults they are treating to find solutions that will reduce their patients' pain in ways that will both help their patients maintain their autonomy and live out meaningful lives.

Acknowledgements

This research was supported in part by Grant No. T32MH20061 from the National Institute of Mental Health.

Key References and Sources for Further Reading

American Association of Suicidology (AAS). http://www.suicidology.org/home.

Conwell, Y., Van Orden, K., and Caine, E. (2011). 'Suicide in Older Adults'. *Psychiatric Clinics of North America* 34(2): 451–468.

Erlangsen, A., Nordentoft, M., Conwell, Y., Waern, M., De Leo, D., Lindner, R., et al. (2011). 'Key Considerations for Preventing Suicide in Older Adults: Consensus Opinions of an Expert Panel'. *Crisis* 32(2): 106–109.

International Association for Suicide Prevention (IASP). http://www.iasp.info/.

Lapierre, S., Erlangsen, A., Waern, M., De Leo, D., Oyama, H., Scocco, P., et al. (2011). 'A Systematic Review of Elderly Suicide Prevention Programs'. *Crisis* 32(2): 88–98.

United States Centers for Disease Control and Prevention (CDC) Injury Prevention and Control. http://www.cdc.gov/violenceprevention/suicide/.

World Health Organization Suicide Prevention and Special Programmes (WHO SUPRE). http://www.who.int/mental_health/prevention/suicide/supresuicideprevent/en/.

References

Alexopoulos, G. S., Bruce, M. L., Hull, J., Sirey, J. A., and Kakuma, T. (1999). 'Clinical Determinants of Suicidal Ideation and Behavior in Geriatric Depression'. *Archives of General Psychiatry* 56: 1048–1053.

Alexopoulos, G. S., Raue, P., and Arean, P. (2003). 'Problem-solving Therapy versus Supportive Therapy in Geriatric Major Depression with Executive Dysfunction'. *American Journal of Geriatric Psychiatry* 11(1): 46–52.

Alexopoulos, G. S., Reynolds, C. F., Bruce, M. L., Katz, I. R., Raue, P. J., Mulsant, B. H., et al. (2009). 'Reducing Suicidal Ideation and Depression in Older Primary Care Patients: 24-month Outcomes of the PROSPECT Study'. *American Journal of Psychiatry* 166(8): 882–890.

Arean, P. and Huh, T. (2006). 'Problem-Solving Therapy with Older Adults'. In S. H. Qualls and B. Knight (eds), *Psychotherapy for Depression in Older Adults* (pp. 133–149). New York: Wiley.

Arean, P., Hegel, M., Vannoy, S., Fan, M. Y., and Unützer, J. (2008). 'Effectiveness of Problem-solving Therapy for Older, Primary Care Patients with Depression: Results from the IMPACT Project'. *The Gerontologist* 48(3): 311–323.

Ayalon, L., Mackin, S., Arean P. A., Chen, H., and Herr, E. C. M. (2007). 'The Role of Cognitive Functioning and Distress in Suicidal Ideation in Older Adults'. *Journal of the American Geriatrics Society* 55: 1090–1094.

Ayalon, L. and Litwin, H. (2009). 'What Cognitive Functions are Associated with Passive Suicidal Ideation? Findings from a National Sample of Community Dwelling Israelis'. *International Journal of Geriatric Psychiatry* 24(5): 472–478.

Bartels, S. J., Coakley, E., Oxman, T. E., Constantino, G., Oslin, D., Chen, H., et al. (2002). 'Suicidal and Death Ideation in Older Primary Care Patients with Depression, Anxiety, and At-risk Alcohol Use'. *American Journal of Geriatric Psychiatry* 10(4): 417–427.

Beck, A. T., Kovacs, M., and Weissman, A. (1979). 'Assessment of Suicidal Ideation: The Scale for Suicide Ideation'. *Journal of Consulting and Clinical Psychology* 47(2): 343–352.

Bell, A. C. and D'Zurilla, T. J. (2009). 'Problem-solving Therapy for Depression: A Meta-analysis'. *Clinical Psychology Review* 29: 348–353.

Breitbart, W., Rosenfeld, B., Pessin, H., Kaim, M., Funesti-Esch, J., Galietta, M., et al. (2000). 'Depression, Hopelessness, and Desire for Hastened Death in Terminally Ill Patents with Cancer'. *Journal of the American Medical Association* 284: 2907–2911.

Breitbart, W. and Heller, K. S. (2003). 'Reframing Hope: Meaning-centered Care for Patients Near the End of Life'. *Journal of Palliative Medicine* 6(6): 979–988.

Britton, P. C., Duberstein, P. R., Conner, K. R., Heisel, M. J., Hirsch, J. K., and Conwell, Y. (2008). 'Reasons for Living, Hopelessness, and Suicide Ideation among Depressed Adults 50 Years or Older'. *American Journal of Geriatric Psychiatry* 16(9): 736–741.

Brown, G. K., Ten, H. T., Henriques, G. R., Xie, S. X., Hollander, J. E., and Beck, A. T. (2005). 'Cognitive Therapy for the Prevention of Suicide Attempts: A Randomized Controlled Trial'. *Journal of the American Medical Association* 294(5): 563–570.

Bruce, M. L. (1999). 'Designing an Intervention to Prevent Suicide: PROSPECT (Prevention of Suicide in Primary Care Elderly: Collaborative Trial)'. *Dialogues in Clinical Neuroscience* 1(2): 100–110.

Bruce, M. L., Ten Have, T. R., Reynolds, C. F., Katz, I. I., Schulberg, H. C., Mulsant, B. H., et al. (2004). 'Reducing Suicidal Ideation and Depressive Symptoms in Depressed Older Primary Care Patients: A Randomized Control Trial'. *Journal of the American Medical Association* 291(9): 1081–1091.

Casey, P., Dunn, G., Kelly, B. D., Lehtinen, V., Dalgard, O. S., Dorwick, C., et al. (2008). 'The Prevalence of Suicidal Ideation in the General Population: Results from the Outcome of Depression International Network (ODIN) Study'. *Social Psychiatry and Psychiatric Epidemiology* 43: 299–304.

Centers for Disease Control (CDC) (2011). 'Definitions: Self-directed Violence'. *Centers for Disease Control and Prevention.* 11 November. http://www.cdc.gov/violenceprevention/sui cide/definitions.html. Retrieved 19 January 2012.

Chen, W., Chen, C., Ho, C., Chou, F. H., Lee, M. B., Lung, F., et al. (2011). 'The Relationship between Quality of Life, Psychiatric Illness, and Suicidal Ideation in Geriatric Veterans Living in a Veterans' Home: A Structural Equation Modeling Approach'. *American Journal of Geriatric Psychiatry* 19(6): 597–601.

Chochinov, H. M., Wilson, K. G., Enns, M., Mowchun, N., Lander, S., Levitt, M., et al. (1998). 'Desire for Death in the Terminally Ill'. *American Journal of Psychiatry* 152(8): 1185–1191.

Chochinov, H. M. (2003). 'Thinking outside the Box: Depression, Hope, and Meaning at the End of Life'. *Journal of Palliative Medicine* 6(6): 973–977.

Ciechanowski, P., Wagner, E., Schmaling, K., Schwartz, S., Williams, B., Diehr, P., et al. (2004). 'Community-integrated Home-based Depression Treatment in Older Adults: A Randomized Controlled Trial'. *Journal of the American Medical Association* 291(13): 1569–1577.

Cohen, C. I., Colemon, Y., Yaffee, R. and Casimir, G. J. (2008). 'Racial Differences in Suicidality in an Older Urban Population'. *The Gerontologist* 48(1): 71–78.

Cohen, A., Gilman, S. E., Houck, P. R., Szanto, K. and Reynolds, C. F. (2009). 'Socioeconomic Status and Anxiety as Predictors of Antidepressant Treatment Response and Suicidal Ideation in Older Adults'. *Social Psychiatry and Psychiatric Epidemiology* 44: 272–277.

Cohen, A., Chapman, B. P., Gilman, S. E., Delmerico, A. M., Wieczorek, W., Duberstein, P. R. et al. (2010). 'Social Inequalities in the Occurrence of Suicidal Ideation among Older Primary Care Patients'. *American Journal of Geriatric Psychiatry* 18(12): 1146–1154.

Conwell, Y. and Thompson, C. (2008). 'Suicidal Behavior in Elders'. *Psychiatric Clinics of North America* 31: 333–356.

Cukrowicz, K. C., Ekblad, A. G., Cheavems, J. S., Rosenthal, M. Z., and Lynch, T. R. (2008). 'Coping and Thought Suppression as Predictors of Suicidal Ideation in Depressed Older Adults with Personality Disorders'. *Aging & Mental Health* 12(1): 149–157.

Cukrowicz, K. C., Duberstein, P. R., Vannoy, S. D., Lynch, T. R., McQuoid, D. R., and Steffens, D. C. (2009). 'Course of Suicidal Ideation and Predictors of Change in Depressed Older Adults'. *Journal of Affective Disorders* 113: 30–36.

De Leo, D., Ester, C., Spathonis, K., and Burgis, S. (2005). 'Lifetime Risk of Suicide Ideation and Attempts in an Australian Community: Prevalence, Suicidal Process, and Help-seeking Behaviour'. *Journal of Affective Disorders* 86: 215–224.

Dewey, M. E., Davidson, I. A., and Copeland, J. R. M. (1993). 'Expressed Wish to Die and Mortality in Older People: A Community Replication'. *Age and Ageing* 22: 109–113.

Duberstein, P. R., Conwell, Y., Seidlitz, L., Lyness, J. M., Cox, C., and Caine, E. D. (1999). 'Age and Suicide Ideation in Older Depressed Inpatients'. *American Journal of Geriatric Psychiatry* 7: 289–296.

Duberstein, P. R., Conwell, Y., Seidlitz, L., Denning, D. G., Cox, C., and Caine, E. D. (2000). 'Personality Traits and Suicidal Behavior and Ideation in Depressed Inpatients 50 Years of Age and Older'. *Journals of Gerontology Series B: Psychological Sciences* 55(1): 18–26.

D'Zurilla, T. J. and Nezu, A. M. (2007). *Problem-Solving Therapy: A Positive Approach to Clinical Intervention*. New York: Springer.

Edwards, R. R., Smith, M. T., Kudel, I., and Haythornthwaite, J. (2006). 'Pain-related Catastrophizing as a Risk Factor for Suicidal Ideation in Chronic Pain'. *Pain* 126: 272–279.

Gallo, J. J., Anthony, J. C., and Muthén, B. O. (1994). 'Age Differences in the Symptoms of Depression: A Latent Trait Analysis'. *Journal of Gerontology: Psychological Sciences* 49(6): 251–264.

Gaynes, B. N., West, S. L., Ford, C. A., Frame, P., Klein, J., and Lohr, K. N. (2004). 'Screening for Suicide Risk in Adults: A Summary of the Evidence for the U.S. Preventive Services Task Force'. *Annals of Internal Medicine* 140: 822–835.

Gilbody, S., Bower, P., Fletcher, J., Richards, D., and Sutton, A. J. (2006). 'Collaborative Care for Depression: A Cumulative Meta-analysis and Review of Longer-term Outcomes'. *Archives of Internal Medicine* 166(21): 2314–2321.

Hamilton, M. (1960). 'A Rating Scale for Depression'. *Journal of Neurology, Neurosurgery, and Psychiatry* 23: 56–62.

Heisel, M. J., Flett, G. L., and Besser, A. (2002). 'Cognitive Functioning and Geriatric Suicide Ideation: Testing a Meditational Model'. *American Journal of Geriatric Psychiatry* 10(4): 428–436.

Heisel, M. J. and Flett, G. L. (2006). 'The Development and Initial Validation of the Geriatric Suicide Ideation Scale'. *American Journal of Geriatric Psychiatry* 14(9): 742–751.

Heisel, M. J., Links, P. S., Conn, D., van Reekum, R., and Flett, G. L. (2007). 'Narcissistic Personality and Vulnerability to Late-life Suicidality'. *American Journal of Geriatric Psychiatry* 15: 734–741.

Heisel, M. J. and Flett, G. L. (2008). 'Psychological Resilience to Suicide Ideation among Older Adults'. *Clinical Gerontologist* 31(4): 51–70.

Heisel, M. J., Duberstein, P. R., Talbot, N. L., King, D. A., and Tu, X. M. (2009). 'Adapting Interpersonal Psychotherapy for Older Adults at Risk for Suicide: Preliminary Findings'. *Professional Psychology: Research and Practice* 40(2): 156–164.

Hinrichsen, G. A. and Clougherty, K. F. (2006). *Interpersonal Psychotherapy for Depressed Older Adults*. Washington, DC: American Psychological Association.

Hirsch, J. K., Duberstein, P. R., Conner, K. R., Heisel, M. J., Beckman, A., Franus, N. et al. (2006). 'Future Orientation and Suicide Ideation and Attempts in Depressed Adults Age 50 and over'. *American Journal of Geriatric Psychiatry* 14: 752–757.

Hirsch, J. K., Duberstein, P. R., Chapman, B., and Lyness, J. M. (2007). 'Positive Affect and Suicide Ideation in Older Adult Primary Care Patients'. *Psychology and Aging* 22: 380–385.

Hobbs, M. and McLaren, S. (2009). 'The Interrelations of Agency, Depression, and Suicidal Ideation among Older Adults'. *Suicide and Life Threatening Behavior* 39(2): 161–171.

Jahn, D. R., Cukrowicz, K. C., Linton, K., and Prabhu, F. (2011). 'The Mediating Effect of Perceived Burdensomeness on the Relation between Depressive Symptoms and Suicide Ideation in a Community Sample of Older Adults'. *Aging & Mental Health* 15: 214–220.

Jobes, D. A., Rudd, M. D., Overhosler, J. C., and Joiner, T. E. (2008). 'Ethical and Competent Care of Suicidal Patients: Contemporary Challenges, New Developments, and Considerations for Clinical Practice'. *Professional Psychology: Research and Practice* 39(4): 405–413.

Kim, Y. A., Bogner, H. R., Brown, G. K., and Gallo, J. J. (2006). 'Chronic Medical Conditions and Wishes to Die among Older Primary Care Patients'. *International Journal of Psychiatry in Medicine* 36(2): 183–198.

Kroenke, K., Spitzer, R., and Williams, J. B. (2001). 'The PHQ-9: Validity of a Brief Depression Severity Measure'. *Journal of General Internal Medicine* 16(9): 606–613.

Lenze, E. J., Mulsant, B. H., Shear, M. K., Schulberg, H. C., Dew, M. A., Begley, A. E., et al. (2000). 'Comorbid Anxiety Disorders in Depressed Elderly Patients'. *American Journal of Psychiatry* 157(5): 722–728.

Lenze, E. J., Dew, M. A., Mazumdar, S., Begley, A. E., Cornes, C., Miller, M. D., et al. (2002). 'Combined Pharmacotherapy and Psychotherapy as Maintenance Treatment for Late-life Depression: Effects on Social Adjustment'. *American Journal of Psychiatry* 159(3): 466–468.

Linehan, M. M., Armstrong, H. E., Suarez, A., Allmon, D., and Heard, H. L. (1991). 'Cognitive-behavioral Treatment of Chronically Parasuicidal Borderline Patients'. *Archives of General Psychiatry* 48(12): 1060–1064.

Linehan, M. M. (1993). *Cognitive-behavioral Treatment of Borderline Personality Disorder*. New York: Guilford Press.

Linehan, M. M., Schmidt, H., Dimeff, L. A., Craft, J. C., Kanter, J., and Comtois, K. A. (1999). 'Dialectical Behavior Therapy for Patients with Borderline Personality Disorder and Drug-dependence'. *American Journal of Addictions* 8(4): 279–292.

Linehan, M. M., Comtois, K. A., Murray, A. M., Brown, M. Z., Gallop, R. J., Heard, H. L., et al. (2006). 'Two-Year Randomized Controlled Trial and Follow-up of Dialectical Behavior Therapy vs Therapy by Experts for Suicidal Behaviors and Borderline Personality Disorder'. *Archives of General Psychiatry* 63(7): 757–766.

Linehan, M. M., Bohus, M., and Lynch, T. R. (2007). 'Dialectical Behavior Therapy for Pervasive Emotion Dysregulation: Theoretical and Practical Underpinnings'. In J. Gross (ed.), *Handbook of Emotion Regulation* (pp. 581–605). New York: Guilford Press.

Links, P. S., Heisel, M. J., and Quastel, A. (2005). 'Is Suicide Ideation a Surrogate Endpoint for Geriatric Suicide?' *Suicide and Life-threatening Behavior* 35(2): 193–205.

Lynch, T. R., Johnson, C. S., Mendelson, T., Robins, C. J., Krishnan, K. R., and Blazer, D. G. (1999). 'Correlates of Suicidal Ideation among an Elderly Depressed Sample'. *Journal of Affective Disorders* 56: 9–15.

Lynch, T. R., Cheavens, J. S., Morse, J. Q., and Rosenthal, M. Z. (2004). 'A Model Predicting Suicidal Ideation and Hopelessness in Depressed Older Adults: The Impact of Emotion Inhibition and Affect Intensity'. *Aging & Mental Health* 8(6): 486–497.

Lynch, T. R., Cheavens, J. S., Cukrowicz, K. C., Thorp, S. R., Bronner, L., and Beyer, J. (2007). 'Treatment of Older Adults with Co-morbid Personality Disorder and Depression: A Dialectical Behavior Therapy Approach'. *International Journal of Geriatric Psychiatry* 22(2): 131–143.

McLaren, S., Gomez, R., Bailey, M., and Van Der Horst, R. K. (2007). 'The Association of Depression and Sense of Belonging and Suicidal Ideation among Older Adults: Applicability of Resiliency Models'. *Suicide and Life-threatening Behavior* 37(1): 89–103.

Maier, H. and Smith, J. (1999). 'Psychological Predictors of Mortality'. *Journal of Gerontology: Psychological Sciences* 54B: 44–54.

Malfent, D., Wondrak, T., Kapusta, N. D., and Sonneck, G. (2009). 'Suicidal Ideation and its Correlates among Elderly in Residential Care Homes'. *International Journal of Geriatric Psychiatry* 25: 843–849.

Miller, M.D. (2009). *Clinician's Guide to Interpersonal Psychotherapy in Late Life*. New York: Oxford University Press.

Miret, M., Nuevo, R., Morant, C., Sainz-Cortón, Jiménez-Arriero, M. A., López-Ibor, J. J., et al. (2010). 'Difference between Younger and Older Adults in the Structure of Suicidal Intent and its Correlates'. *American Journal of Geriatric Psychiatry* 18: 839–847.

O'Carroll, P. W., Berman, A. L., Maris, R. W., Moscicki, E. K., Tanney, B. L., and Silverman, M. M. (1996). 'Beyond the Tower of Babel: A Nomenclature for Suicidology'. *Suicide and Life-threatening Behavior* 26: 237–252.

Paykel, E. S., Myers, J. K., Lindenthal, J. J., and Tanner, J. (1974). 'Suicidal Feelings in the General Population: A Prevalence Study'. *British Journal of Psychiatry* 124: 460–469.

Pfaff, J. J. and Almeida, O. (2004). 'Identifying Suicidal Ideation among Older Adults in a General Practice Setting'. *Journal of Affective Disorders* 83: 73–77.

Pfaff, J. J., Almeida, O. P., Witte, T. K., Waesche, M. C., and Joiner, T. E. (2007). 'Relationship between Quantity and Frequency of Alcohol Use and Indices of Suicidal Behavior in an Elderly Australian Sample'. *Suicide and Life-threatening Behavior* 37(6): 616–626.

Posner, K., Brown, G. K., and Stanley, B., Brent, D. A., Yershova, K. V., Oquendo, M. A., et al. (2011). 'The Columbia-Suicide Severity Rating Scale: Initial Validity and Internal Consistency Findings from Three Multisite Studies with Adolescents and Adults'. *American Journal of Psychiatry* 168: 1266–1277.

Raue, P. J., Brown, E., Meyers, B. S., Schulberg, H. C., and Bruce, M. L. (2006). 'Does Every Allusion to Possible Suicide Require the Same Response?: A Structured Method of Assessing and Managing Risk'. *Journal of Family Practice* 55(7): 605–612.

Raue, P. J., Morales, K. H., Post, E. P., Bogner, H. R., Ten Have, T., and Bruce, M. L. (2010). 'The Wish to Die and 5-year Mortality in Elderly Primary Care Patients'. *American Journal of Geriatric Psychiatry* 18: 341–350.

Reynolds, C. F., Frank, E., Perel, J. M., Imber, S. D., Cornes, C., Miller, M. D., et al. (1999). 'Nortriptyline and Interpersonal Psychotherapy as Maintenance Therapies for Recurrent Major Depression: A Randomized Controlled Trial in Patients Older than 59 Years'. *Journal of the American Medical Association* 281(1): 39–45.

Rowe, J. L., Conwell, Y., Schulberg, H. C., and Bruce, M. L. (2006). 'Social Support and Suicidal Ideation in Older Adults Using Home Healthcare Services'. *American Journal of Geriatric Psychiatry* 14: 758–766.

Rudd, M. D., Rajab, M. H., Orman, D. T., Joiner, T., Stulman, D. A., and Dixon, W. (1996). 'Effectiveness of an Outpatient Intervention Targeting Suicidal Young Adults: Preliminary Results'. *Journal of Consulting and Clinical Psychology* 64(1): 179–190.

Rurup, M. L., Deeg, D. J.., Poppelaars, J. L., Kerkhof, A. J. F. M., and Onwuteaka-Philipsen, B. D. (2011). 'Wish to Die in Older People: A Quantitative Study of Prevalence and Associated Factors'. *Crisis* 32(4): 194–203.

Salkovskis, P. M., Atha, C., and Storer, D. (1990). 'Cognitive-behavioural Problem Solving in the Treatment of Patients who Repeatedly Attempt Suicide: A Controlled Trial'. *British Journal of Psychiatry* 157: 871–876.

Segal, D. L., Marty, M. A., Meyer, W. J., and Coolidge, F. L. (2011). 'Personality, Suicidal Ideation, and Reasons for Living among Older Adults'. *Journal of Gerontology Series B: Psychological and Social Sciences*. Advance online publication.

Silverman, M. M., Berman, A. L., Sanddal, N. D., O'Carroll, P. W., and Joiner, T. E. J. (2007a). 'Rebuilding the Tower of Babel: A Revised Nomenclature for the Study of Suicide and Suicidal Behavior Part 1: Background, Rationale, and Methodology'. *Suicide and Life-Threatening Behavior* 37(3): 248–263.

Silverman, M. M., Berman, A. L., Sanddal, N. D., O'Carroll, P. W., and Joiner, T. E. J. (2007b). 'Rebuilding the Tower of Babel: A Revised Nomenclature for the Study of Suicide and Suicidal Behavior Part 2: Suicide-related Ideations, Communications, and Behaviors'. *Suicide and Life-threatening Behavior* 37(3): 264–277.

Sirey, J. A., Bruce, M. L., Carpenter, M., Booker, D., Reid, M. C., Newell, K. A., et al. (2008). 'Depressive Symptoms and Suicidal Ideation among Older Adults Receiving Home Delivered Meals'. *International Journal of Geriatric Psychiatry* 23: 1306–1311.

Spitzer, R., Kroenke, K., and Williams, J. (1999). 'Validation and Utility of a Self-report Version of PRIME-MD: The PHQ Primary Care Study'. *Journal of the American Medical Association* 282: 1737–1744.

Szanto, K., Reynolds, C. F., and Frank, E., Stack, J., Fasiczka, A. L., Miller, M., et al. (1996). 'Suicide in Elderly Depressed Patients: Is Active vs. Passive Suicidal Ideation a Clinically Valid Distinction?' *American Journal of Geriatric Psychiatry* 4(3): 197–207.

Szanto, K., Mulsant, B.H., Houck, P.R., Miller, M., Mazumdar, S., and Reynolds, C.F. (2001). 'Treatment Outcome in Suicidal vs. Non-suicidal Elderly Patients'. *American Journal of Geriatric Psychiatry* 9: 261–268.

Szanto, K., Mulsant, B. H., Houck, P., Dew, M. A., and Reynolds, C. F. (2003). 'Occurrence and Course of Suicidality during Short-term Treatment of Late-life Depression'. *Archives of General Psychiatry* 60: 610–617.

Szanto, K., Mulsant, B. H., Houck, P. R., Dew, M. A., Dombrovski, A., Pollock, B. G., et al. (2007). 'Emergence, Persistence, and Resolution of Suicidal Ideation during Treatment of Depression in Old Age'. *Journal of Affective Disorders* 98: 153–161.

Tan, L. L. and Wong, H. B. (2008). 'Severity of Depression and Suicidal Ideations among Elderly People in Singapore'. *International Psychogeratrics* 20(2): 338–346.

Tang, N. K. and Crane, C. (2006). 'Suicidality in Chronic Pain: A Review of the Prevalence, Risk Factors and Psychological Links'. *Psychological Medicine* 36: 575–586.

Unützer, J., Katon, W., Callahan, C. M., Williams, J. W., Jr, Hunkeler, E., Harpole, L., et al. (2002). 'Collaborative Care Management of Late-life Depression in the Primary Care Setting: A Randomized Controlled Trial'. *Journal of the American Medical Association* 288(22): 2836–2845.

Unützer, J., Tang, L., Oishi, S., Katon, W., Williams, J. W., Jr, Hunkeler, E., et al. (2006). 'Reducing Suicidal Ideation in Depressed Older Primary Care Patients'. *Journal of the American Geriatrics Society* 54: 1550–1556.

Useda, J. D., Duberstein, P. R., Conner, K. R., Beckman, A., Franus, N., Tu, X., et al. (2007). 'Personality Differences in Attempted Suicide versus Suicide in Adults 50 Years of Age or Older'. *Journal of Consulting and Clinical Psychology* 75: 126–133.

Van Orden, K. and Conwell, Y. (2011). 'Suicides in Late Life'. *Current Psychiatry Reports* 13(3): 234–241.

Vanderhorst, R. K. and McLaren, S. (2005). 'Social Relationships as Predictors of Depression and Suicidal Ideation in Older Adults'. *Aging & Mental Health* 9(6): 517–525.

Vannoy, S. D., Duberstein, P., Cukrowicz, K., Lin, E., Fan, M., Unützer, J. (2007). 'The Relationship between Suicide Ideation and Late-life Depression'. *American Journal of Geriatric Psychiatry* 15: 1024–1033.

Waern, M., Beskow, J., Runeson, B., and Skoog, I. (1999). 'Suicidal Feelings in the Last Year of Life in Elderly People who Commit Suicide'. *Lancet* 354: 917–918.

Weissman, M. M., Markowitz, J. C., and Klerman, G. L. (2000). *Comprehensive Guide to Interpersonal Psychotherapy*. New York: Basic Books.

Witte, T. K., Joiner, T. E., Brown, G. K., Beck, A. T., Beckman, A., Duberstein, P., et al. (2006). 'Factors of Suicide Ideation and their Relation to Clinical and Other Indicators in Older Adults'. *Journal of Affective Disorders* 94: 165–172.

World Health Organization Suicide Prevention and Special Programmes (2013). *Country Reports and Charts Available*. http://www.who.int/mental_health/prevention/suicide/coun try_reports/en/index.html. Retrieved 5 April 2013.

....

CHAPTER 14

EVALUATION AND TREATMENT OF GERIATRIC NEUROCOGNITIVE DISORDERS

....

PHILLIP D. RUPPERT AND DEBORAH K. ATTIX

INTRODUCTION

....

IT is well known that we live in an ageing population. The percentage of the US population aged 65 or older is projected to increase from 15% in 2015 to 20% in 2030 (United States Census Bureau 2012). Similarly, the percentage of the world population aged 65 or older is expected to increase from 10% in 2015 to 14% in 2030 (United Nations Population Division 2010). Of course, there is a range of non-pathological cognitive changes that attend 'normal ageing' (Story and Attix 2010). However, cognitive impairments extending beyond normal ageing are common in older adults. For example, it has been estimated that 14% of Americans over the age of 70 have dementia and that 22% of this cohort have some form of mild cognitive impairment (MCI; Plassman et al. 2007, 2008). Furthermore, the risk of cognitive impairment increases dramatically after age 70 (Plassman et al. 2007). Global prevalence for dementia was recently estimated at twenty-four million people, and this number is expected to nearly double every twenty years, to forty-two million in 2020 and eighty-one million in 2040 (Ferri et al. 2005). At the time of that survey, regions with highest prevalence included China (five million), the European Union (five million), USA (three million), India (1.5 million), Japan (one million), Russia (one million), and Indonesia (one million). In addition to the primary cognitive deficits that are caused by dementia and MCI, concurrent problems related to these conditions are prevalent and have considerable individual, family, and societal impact, including functional deficits in daily activities, neuropsychiatric symptoms, and economic burden (Hill et al. 2002; Lyketsos et al. 2002; Wimo, Winblad, and Jönsson 2010). Multiple disciplines work in concert to meet the needs of this ageing population, including geropsychologists, neuropsychologists, geriatricians, geriatric psychiatrists, and family physicians.

Given the prevalence of cognitive impairment in older adults and the potential for significant functional and financial costs to patients and families, it is essential that psychologists are aware of the best practices for identifying, characterizing, and treating such compromises. Specifically, psychologists working with older adults will benefit from understanding the more common aetiologies for cognitive impairment as well as knowledge of methods for assessing cognition and a framework for providing neuropsychological interventions with these patients.

In this chapter, we first provide a brief review of the most common causes of cognitive impairment in later life. We then discuss methods for assessing cognition in older adults. This includes a review of the more commonly used screening measures, as well as a discussion of factors relevant to referral for comprehensive neuropsychological assessment. We then present a brief summary of the purposes and recommended practices for providing feedback on cognitive test results to patients and care-givers. Finally, we close the chapter with a section that addresses the provision of neuropsychological interventions to older adults with cognitive impairments and their care-givers.

Causes of Cognitive Dysfunction in Later Life

Dementia and MCI are phenotypes with a vast number of aetiologies, and a proper discussion of all possible causes is beyond the scope of this chapter. Interested readers may refer to more comprehensive texts for detailed review of conditions that cause dementia (Attix and Welsh-Bohmer 2006). However, these conditions can be broadly classified into one of three categories: degenerative, stable, and reversible. Some of the more commonly encountered aetiologies from these three categories are as follows.

Degenerative dementias are those that are characterized by progressive deterioration of cognitive status, resulting in functional disability. Often, these dementias involve cortical structures, as well as subcortical systems. Some of the more common neurodegenerative conditions include Alzheimer's disease, subtypes of fronto-temporal dementia, and Lewy body dementia. Together, degenerative conditions constitute the majority of dementia aetiologies, with Alzheimer's disease being the single most common cause of dementia (Breitner et al. 1999; Qiu et al. 2007; Van der Flier and Scheltens 2005).

Stable or slowly progressive dementias are those conditions that are characterized by cognitive and functional deficits that are relatively stable or that are typically slowly progressive in severity over time. Common causes of this type of dementia include, stroke, cerebrovascular disease, Parkinson's disease, and chronic encephalopathies.

The terms 'reversible dementia' or 'treatable dementia' are frequently used to refer to conditions causing cognitive deficits which are treatable and for which cognitive deficits may improve or remediate with treatment of the underlying condition. Some common examples of such conditions in older persons include normal-pressure hydrocephalus, hypothyroidism, vitamin deficiencies, obstructive sleep apnoea, medication side effects, and depression.

Table 14.1 outlines some features of common neurological disorders. This table includes but a few of the many possible sources of cognitive dysfunction in elders, but illustrates how

Table 14.1 Common neurobehavioural features of select neurological conditions

Cognitive syndrome	Course	Neuropsychological features
Mild cognitive impairment	Variable	• Cognitive compromise extending beyond normal ageing as reflected in deficits on tests correcting for age and education • Multiple subtypes (amnestic single domain, amnestic multiple-domain, non-amnestic single domain, non-amnestic multiple domain • Essentially normal functional status • Stability varies, with longitudinal studies demonstrating progression to AD, stability, or improvement, reflecting heterogeneous aetiologies
Alzheimer's disease	Progressive	• Early deficits in memory retrieval and rapid forgetting of information • Limited benefit from recognition cueing • Slowed processing speed • Later deficits in executive function, language, and visual-perceptual skills
Fronto-temporal dementia	Progressive	• Behavioural variant presents with pronounced executive dysfunction and less obvious difficulties with memory • Language variants present with prominent early dysnomia or semantic processing deficits • Motor variants may present with progressive apraxia or motor neuron disease
Lewy body dementia	Progressive	• Cognitive symptoms precede or have concurrent onset with Parkinsonism • Deficits in executive function, visual-perceptual skills, and speed of processing • Memory deficits less prominent early
Vascular dementia	Stable/ step-wise/ slowly progressive	• Typical presentation involves deficits in 'subcortical' functions, such as processing speed, executive efficiency, and memory encoding/retrieval deficits • Memory typically improves with cueing
Parkinson's disease dementia	Stable/slowly progressive	• Prominent cognitive and psychomotor slowing • Deficits in 'subcortical' functions, such as executive efficiency and memory encoding/retrieval • Memory typically improves with cueing
Normal pressure hydrocephalus	Stable/reversible	• Deficits in attention, processing, speed, executive efficiency, memory encoding/retrieval, and visual-spatial abilities
Obstructive sleep apnoea	Stable	• Weaknesses in attention, concentration, and vigilance
Geriatric depression	Stable/variable with mood episodes	• Weaknesses in attention, concentration, processing speed, and effortful processing • Psychomotor slowing • Memory retrieval difficulty that improves with cueing

neurobehavioural constellations reflect various conditions. Clinicians must be familiar with and consistently update their knowledge of the neurobehavioural presentation and course, neuro-anatomical, and genetic features of disorders related to the populations in which they practise.

EVALUATION

Whether a patient presents with frank cognitive and behavioural impairments or the patient and family are just beginning to suspect subtle cognitive change, objective psychometric assessment of cognition is usually informative for diagnostic and treatment planning purposes. In this section, we will discuss the situations in which objective assessment of cognitive function can be beneficial. We review common psychometric methods for assessing cognition, including screening measures and more formal neuropsychological evaluation. We also discuss factors critical in the assessment of cognition in older adults. For a more general overview, refer to the chapter on 'Geropsychological Assessment' in this Handbook.

There are a number of situations in which objective assessment of cognition is beneficial. Rabin, Barr, and Burton (2005) surveyed neuropsychologists about a number of practice issues, including common reasons for referral. This survey found that neuropsychological evaluations are most commonly requested to aid in differential diagnosis or to attain a cognitive profile that would assist the referral source in treatment planning. Other common referral questions included forensic determination, educational planning, assessing capacity to work, establishing a baseline for subsequent testing, and assessing capacity for independent living. Less commonly cited reasons for referral included evaluations before and after a medical intervention and the localization of brain lesions.

Once it is apparent that a formal assessment of the patient's cognition would be helpful, the clinician has the option of conducting a brief evaluation, possibly by using one of the screening measures described below, or referring the patient to a neuropsychologist to obtain a comprehensive and detailed evaluation of cognitive and emotional functioning. The decision to use screening measures vs a more comprehensive evaluation will depend on the specific needs of each case. However, some of the more common factors that influence this decision include: the amount of information needed, need for differential diagnosis, severity of the cognitive impairment, estimated level of pre-morbid cognition due to insensitivity of screening measures to subtle changes in previously high-functioning patients, weighing the effects of depression vs cognitive dysfunction, and ability of the patient to participate in a comprehensive neuropsychological exam.

If screening assessment is appropriate, a number of measures are available. Some of these measures are described below. When available, citations are provided for notable normative sets for these screening measures. Additionally, comprehensive reviews of the available normative sets for many of these screening measures can be found in Busch and Chapin (2008) and in Strauss, Sherman, and Spreen (2006). As with any clinical test, the clinician should be familiar with the psychometric properties (e.g. reliability and validity) and diagnostic accuracy statistics of the test and cut scores. These issues are discussed in a recent review of cognitive screening measures (Lonic, Tierney, and Ebmeier 2009). The authors of that review point out that, unfortunately, such data is limited for many cognitive screening measures.

Consideration of such instrumentation variables should guide not only test selection, but also interpretation of obtained results.

The *Mini-mental State Examination* (MMSE) has become one of the most widely administered cognitive tests (Folstein, Folstein, and McHugh 1975). The MMSE is a screening test of global level of cognitive function, with items assessing orientation, registration, attention and calculation, recall, naming, repetition, reading and comprehension, writing, and drawing. The test can be administered and scored in as little as five to ten minutes. The maximum possible score is 30. There have been several hundred studies that have examined the properties, utility, and limitations of the MMSE. A number of these studies have specifically examined the utility of the MMSE for identifying patients with dementia or MCI. Reviews of recent literature can be found in Strauss et al. (2006) and in Mitchell (2009). In most clinical settings, performance is usually evaluated by comparing the patient's total score to an empirically derived cut score. However, recommended cut scores vary by study. Clinicians using the MMSE should be well versed in cut score sensitivities and specificities for conditions under evaluation. Importantly, demographic factors such as age, level of education, and occupation have been shown to influence performance (Frisoni et al. 1993; Iverson 1998).

The *Montreal Cognitive Assessment* (MoCA) is a relatively new measure gaining popularity in clinical and research use. It too was developed as a quick tool for screening for MCI (Nasreddine et al. 2005). It is a 30-point test that samples orientation, attention/working memory, aspects of executive functioning, short-term memory, language, and visuospatial ability. The entire test can be administered in approximately ten minutes. As the MoCA is a relatively new test, normative and validity studies are just now emerging, but the test shows promise as a screening instrument with several research studies employing it for such purposes. Notably, a number of emerging studies have suggested that the MoCA has superior sensitivity and sensitivity to the MMSE for a wide range of neuropathological conditions (Dong et al. 2012; Freitas et al. 2012; Markwick, Zamboni, and de Jager 2012; Phabphal and Kanjanasatien 2011; Whitney et al. 2012). Normative data stratified by age and education are available (Rossetti et al. 2011). The MoCA has also been translated for use in a number of other languages.

The original version of the *Dementia Rating Scale-2* (DRS-2) was developed to determine the magnitude of cognitive impairment in patients with known or suspected dementia that were too impaired to participate in more formal cognitive testing (Coblentz et al. 1973; Mattis 1988). This measure was updated with the publication of the Dementia Rating Scale-2 (DRS-2) in 2001 (Jurica, Leitten, and Mattis 2001). While the test content remained the same, new normative data were published as well as an updated manual, scoring book, and introduction of an alternate form. This measure can typically be administered to healthy older persons in ten to fifteen minutes, but administration time can take as long as thirty to forty-five minutes in a patient with dementia. The test yields five subscale scores that measure attention, initiation/perseveration, construction, conceptualization, and memory, which combine to produce a DRS-2 Total Score. Normative data were collected as part of Mayo's Older Americans Normative Studies (MOANS) and are available in the DRS-2 manual and in an article by Lucas and colleagues (1998). As for the MMSE, performance on the DRS-2 has been shown to be moderated by demographic variables, such as age, education, and ethnicity (Lucas et al. 1998; Rilling et al. 2005). For this reason, there have been efforts at collecting norms that take these demographic variables into account (Rilling et al. 2005).

The *Repeatable Battery for the Assessment of Neuropsychological Status* (RBANS; Randolph 1998) is a brief battery of neuropsychological tests developed to assess cognition in adults. The RBANS is comprised of twelve sub-tests that are grouped into the following five indices: Immediate Memory, Visuospatial/Constructional, Language, Attention, and Delayed Memory. A total score is also calculated. The test battery can be administered in approximately twenty to thirty minutes, and an alternate form is available for retest purposes. As with many neuropsychological tests, performance on the RBANS has been shown to be correlated with age, education, and ethnicity (Beatty et al. 2003; Duff et al. 2003; Patton et al. 2003). While the normative tables included in the RBANS stimulus booklets correct for age, they do not account for the effects of education or ethnicity. However, education corrections for older adults have subsequently been published (Duff et al. 2003; Gontkovsky, Mold, and Beatty 2002), and Patton et al. (2003) have reported RBANS norms for a sample of healthy older African Americans.

The *Consortium to Establish a Registry for Alzheimer's Disease Neuropsychological Battery* (CERAD-NB) was originally developed to provide a brief, reliable, and standardized neuropsychological assessment of Alzheimer's disease (AD) for research purposes (Morris et al. 1989). However, since its introduction, the CERAD-NB has been used in clinical settings as well. The CERAD-NB is comprised of tests measuring the cognitive domains typically affected in AD (e.g. memory, language, and praxis). The battery can be administered in twenty to thirty minutes. Norms were originally published by Morris et al. (1989). However, multiple additional normative sets have since been published (Beeri et al. 2006; Fillenbaum et al. 2001; Ganguli et al. 1991; Unverzagt et al. 1996; Welsh et al. 1994). As with most measures, performance on the CERAD-NB is correlated with demographic variables (e.g. education, ethnicity), and thus a number of these normative sets account for these factors.

Finally, in reflection of emerging trends, use of computerized testing warrants discussion. Clinicians and researchers have seemingly been interested in using computers as cognitive assessment tools since the introduction of the personal computer (Perez et al. 1978). Proponents cite several advantages over traditional (i.e. paper and pencil) neuropsychological tests, including highly standardized administration, more precise measurement of certain abilities (e.g. reaction time, processing speed), ease of administration, randomization of trials and stimuli to minimize practice effects upon repeated testing, and automatic scoring and reporting (Schatz and Browndyke 2002; Schatz and Zillmer 2003). Additionally, such tests have the potential for internet administration to facilitate widespread screening and detection of cognitive decline in elders. Given these potential advantages, a number of computerized screening instruments have been developed or adapted for assessing cognition. A recent review examined the status of several batteries in terms of access to normative data, evidence for reliability and validity, and overall usability (Wild et al. 2008). They identified some of the more well-known computerized batteries for assessing cognitive ageing, including the Automated Neuropsychological Assessment Metrics (ANAM), the Computer Administered Neuropsychological Screen for Mild Cognitive Impairment (CANS-MCI), the Cambridge Neuropsychological Test Automated Battery (CANTAB), the CNS Vital Signs, Computerized Neuropsychological Test Battery (CNTB), the Cognitive Drug Research Computerized Assessment System (COGDRAS), CogState, the Cognitive Stability Index (CSI), MCI Screen, MicroCog, and Mindstreams (Neurotrax). This review concluded that while empirical support for test validity was available for most of these batteries, other criteria were less satisfactorily met. For instance, about half of these batteries were judged as having less than adequate normative data for older populations. There were also limited reliability data available for most batteries. Finally, the authors also noted that differences in computer literacy in older persons have been largely ignored as a contributing factor to the performance of older adults on computerized test batteries. Clearly, the utility of these measures as clinical tools would be enhanced by additional studies.

Screening measures often provide a clinician with basic information that can inform further referrals and treatment-planning questions. While they confer several advantages such as brevity and logistical ease, clinicians should be aware of the potential drawbacks of these measures. The greatest limitation pertains to the often limited classification accuracy of these measures. Specifically, because screening measures contain relatively fewer items than traditional neuropsychological tests, these measures are inherently less reliable, which consequently impacts validity (Nunnally and Bernstein 1994). As a result, case identification accuracy (e.g. sensitivity and specificity) is impacted, as is the ability to conduct differential diagnosis. The restricted range of possible scores on screening measures also biases these measures towards lower levels of cognitive ability, which results in a ceiling effect on some measures.

Comprehensive neuropsychological evaluation yields nuanced information, with the following advantages:

- greater reliability due to a greater number of test items
- typically greater construct and content validity due to more comprehensive assessment of abilities than is possible by screening measures
- greater criterion validity allowing for greater diagnostic and prognostic confidence
- greater sensitivity and specificity, especially for individuals at the extremes of the normal distribution of cognitive ability (i.e. very high-functioning or very low-functioning individuals)
- availability of more robust and diverse normative sets. In addition to thorough test manuals and normative data on individual manuals, four normative volumes reflecting research and clinical normative data on standardized measures exist for consultation (Heaton et al. 2004; Lezak et al. 2012; Mitrushina, Boone, and D'Elia 2005; Strauss et al. 2006).

Comprehensive neuropsychological testing is particularly relevant in cases where differential diagnosis is needed and when patients differ from the average population (e.g. in age, education, ethnicity/cultural background, psychological status). Comprehensive testing typically yields scores in the domains of general intellect, memory, language, perception and attention, visuo-construction, psychomotor and psychosensory functions, and executive function (Tranel 2008). The evaluation also typically involves an assessment of the patient's mood, as depression and anxiety can impact cognition and function. Finally, independent and embedded measures of performance and symptom validity are often administered throughout the evaluation to ensure the validity of results.

Once performance is measured, scores are compared to normative datasets, which correct for demographic variables that have been shown to moderate performance on some cognitive measures, such as age, education, and ethnicity. Such corrections allow for interpretation of cognitive strengths and weaknesses relative to groups of healthy peers. The patient's cognitive profile can also be examined for consistency with the typical cognitive profiles for various neuropathological conditions (e.g. Alzheimer's disease, Lewy body disease, cerebrovascular disease, etc.). It is this comparison of patient performances to both healthy and known clinical groups in tandem with consideration of the patient's history, a clinical interview, and behavioural observations that allows the neuropsychologist to draw informed conclusions that can aid differential diagnosis.

FEEDBACK

In clinical cases, once a screening or comprehensive cognitive evaluation has been conducted and a report summarizing the evaluation findings has been completed, it is customary to provide the patient with the opportunity to receive feedback on the evaluation results and recommendations. Patients and families are usually interested in feedback to address questions of cognition, behaviour, function, and other concerns that likely prompted the evaluation.

The purposes for feedback and guidelines for provision of feedback were recently outlined by the American Psychological Association's Taskforce on Dementia Assessment (American Psychological Association 2012). These topics are also discussed in detail in a thoughtful, informative chapter by Green (2006). One of the primary purposes of feedback is to inform the patient and family about the cognitive strengths and weaknesses that were observed on testing and to explain how these performances relate to functional changes that have been noticed in the patient. Feedback also provides a forum for the clinician to discuss possible aetiologies (e.g. neuropathological, psychiatric) for the observed changes. However, discussion of possible medical aetiologies by a neuropsychologist is typically conservative, as there is often overlap in the neuropsychological presentation of different neuropathologies. Thus, another common objective of feedback is to recommend follow-up with other healthcare providers, such as a neurologist or other physician, for complementary testing such as neuroimaging, electroencephalogram (EEG), and/or laboratory workup that can assist in identifying an underlying neuropathological condition. If deficits are identified on testing, patients and families frequently ask about potential treatments and interventions. In such cases, the feedback can involve discussion of techniques that the patient may find helpful for compensating for functional deficits. Sometimes, referral for neuropsychological intervention (as discussed below) may be appropriate. Because functional changes often elicit strong emotional responses such as grief and frustration for patients and families, treatment recommendations also commonly include referral for psychotherapy. Additionally, therapeutic recommendation may be made specifically for care-givers (e.g. support groups), as this population has been shown to be at increased risk for psychological distress and other health outcomes; Torti et al. (2004) provides a nice multinational/multicultural review of this literature. Finally, referral can also be made to a physician for discussion of potential medical and pharmacological interventions for behavioural symptoms.

Typically, feedback is provided directly to the patient; however, it is also common for family members or care-givers to be present so that they are informed of the evaluation findings and recommendations. Clear communication with the patient and family about the plan for feedback is essential. In-person feedback is almost always more appropriate than phone or letter feedback, as it allows processing of nonverbal information, provides a therapeutic setting, and often minimizes misinterpretation. However, there are occasionally situations in which in-person feedback is less feasible, namely in cases where the patient lives in a remote rural area or if obtaining transportation is difficult. In such cases, it may be possible to provide feedback over the phone or using videoconferencing software. However, the clinical appropriateness of such feedback methods will need to be judged on a case-by-case basis. Finally, feedback should be conducted in a way that maximizes patient understanding of the findings. Some practices that support this include reviewing the purpose of the assessment; asking at the outset of the feedback session if the patient and family have specific questions to be addressed; querying the patient and family throughout the feedback session to gauge understanding of the findings; allowing the patient and family to take notes during feedback; providing written materials such as brochures or a copy of the report for review; limiting the feedback to the most essential points and repeating and reviewing these points throughout the session; and finally providing the patient and family with the opportunity to contact the clinician afterwards should additional questions arise.

Intervention

Once clinical evaluation has been conducted and feedback of the test results has occurred, patients and care-givers often ask if there is anything that can be done to remediate and/ or cope with any identified cognitive impairments. In this section, we address this question with a discussion of interventions that have been shown to be effective with cognitively impaired older adults. While a variety of pharmacological agents exist for alleviating some of the cognitive deficits in some forms of dementia (Saddichha and Pandey 2008), we will focus here on behavioural interventions for individuals with cognitive compromise. In this section, we introduce the concept of neuropsychological interventions and outline a model that can be used in the treatment planning of such interventions. We close with two case examples to illustrate the use of this model in providing neuropsychological interventions to cognitively impaired older adults.

   We use the term 'neuropsychological interventions' to refer to interventions or techniques designed to promote coping and adjustment to cognitive and functional deficits through the use of compensatory strategies and residual abilities. A large variety of such interventions have been introduced and investigated in the literature. In general, the more widely used and studied techniques involve use of visual imagery, association, categorization, spaced retrieval, formal computerized training programs, or training in the use of external aides (e.g. calendars, notebooks, smartphones). It is beyond the scope of this chapter to provide an overview or comparison of individual intervention techniques. However, the reader is encouraged to explore the extant literature to learn more about specific techniques. An excellent place to begin would be one of the many systematic reviews of neuropsychological interventions that have been published in recent years (Aguirre et al. 2013; Gates et al. 2011; Olazarán et al. 2004; Teixeira et al. 2012). Once a clinician has learned a set of specific neuropsychological interventions relevant to his/her patient population, these can be implemented in the context of a well-considered treatment plan using a model such as that described below.

As in psychotherapy and other intervention modalities, therapeutic success is more likely to occur in the context of a carefully considered treatment plan that is formulated at the outset of intervention. With this in mind, we review an intervention model to facilitate planning. This particular model was initially presented and is discussed in greater detail in a previous book chapter by one of the authors of the current chapter (Attix 2006). Using this approach, the initial session with the patient and care-givers serves as an intervention evaluation, the purpose of which is to provide the clinician with the necessary information to identify treatment *targets* and *strategies*. Information sources include records, reports of the patient and any available care-givers, and behavioural observations made by the clinician during the evaluation. Essential variables to review in the intervention evaluation include:

- goals
- motivation
- neuropsychological evaluation
- insight
- affective status
- current compensatory methods and activities
- unique patient and environmental factors.

Within the context of neuropsychological intervention, goals refer to desired functional outcomes that are amenable to treatment. The identification of treatment goals usually springs directly from the patient and/or care-giver's report of functional deficits during the intervention evaluation. Complaints may include cognitive errors that are frequently made by the patient, but can also include the negative emotional reactions (i.e. frustration) that often occur in response to such errors. Both the patient's and a care-giver's perspective on the most notable cognitive, affective, and functional deficits should be obtained, as at times these will be discrepant. In these situations, the reasons for this discrepancy will need to be explored. For example, the patient may have reduced insight into deficits (as discussed below); or in contrast, the care-giver may be over-pathologizing benign errors. Of course, different people also have different priorities. Once functional deficits have been identified, the clinician can then work towards identifying their cognitive antecedents (e.g. memory deficit, executive dysfunction) in order to identify how best to intervene. Goals should be tempered by realism. If patients are referred in the early stages of a neurodegenerative condition or after natural recovery from an acute insult, it is essential to communicate that the overarching goal of neuropsychological intervention will be to manage and compensate for cognitive deficits rather than to 'cure' or remediate them.

Motivation refers to the patient's interest in and ability for effortful participation in the intervention process, which involves regular attendance of sessions and engagement in between-session assignments. Some patients present with less than optimal motivation for participation in intervention. In such cases, the reason for diminished motivation should be addressed, ideally prior to initiation of the intervention plan. Some of the more common sources of reduced motivation include depression and/or personality factors. However, certain types of brain injury (e.g. medial frontal lobe damage) can also result in organic 'disorders of diminished motivation' such as apathy, abulia, and, in severe cases, akinetic mutism (Marin and Wilkosz 2005). While depression and personality factors are potentially modifiable through techniques such as motivational interviewing, motivational deficits secondary to central nervous system dysfunction may be more immutable. In such cases, neuropsychological intervention may still proceed; however, the treatment plan will need to incorporate techniques requiring minimal to no patient effort (e.g. spaced-retrieval, behavioural conditioning).

When available, neuropsychological test data provide a valuable resource for intervention planning. These results guide both the identification of realistic targets and strategy selection. In its crudest application, a comprehensive neuropsychological evaluation can provide information about the patient's general level of cognitive function (e.g. is there a mild, moderate, or severe degree of overall impairment?). Such a broad level of classification is useful in that it can quickly provide the clinician with a sense of the range of interventions that may be useful with the client. For example, a patient with only mild memory impairment can be expected to learn and utilize a greater range of interventions than a patient with a moderate level of dementia, affecting both memory and executive functions. When more detailed data are available, the profile can inform the intervention in a fine-grained manner. For example, if there is a memory deficit, is it more attributable to poor encoding, storage, or retrieval processes? If there is executive dysfunction, are some executive processes (e.g. working memory, cognitive flexibility, processing speed, etc.) more impaired or preserved than others? For patients with primarily lateralized brain dysfunction, are there modality-specific processing weaknesses (i.e. verbal vs nonverbal)? The answers to these questions will help the clinician to design the intervention approach in a manner that utilizes relative strengths to compensate for relative weaknesses. Finally, the diagnostic impressions resulting from such data can inform the clinician about the underlying neuropathology and allow for incorporating the expected progression of cognitive, behavioural, and affective symptoms into the treatment plan. Here again, this information aids the clinician in selecting optimal intervention techniques and in setting relevant and appropriate goals with the patient and care-givers.

Insight is another important patient factor critical to the development of the intervention treatment plan. The essential question with regard to insight is: to what degree does the patient demonstrate awareness into both the presence and magnitude of cognitive deficits? Reduced insight into deficits occurs fairly often in older adults with cognitive deficits, particularly in patients with neurodegenerative conditions such as behavioural variant fronto-temporal dementia or Alzheimer's disease. Certainly, lack of insight will impact treatment outcome (Clare et al. 2004; Koltai, Welsh-Bohmer, and Schmechel 2001). The clinical term for this phenomenon is 'anosognosia', and it occurs with greater frequency as the severity of cognitive impairment increases (Rosen 2011). The primary complication of anosognosia in neuropsychological intervention occurs when a patient with reduced insight into deficits may be less motivated to learn or practise compensatory techniques. However, another reason to assess for anosognosia is because this phenomenon typically co-occurs with deficits in reasoning and judgment, so that actual ability to learn and utilize techniques can be hindered. Typically, insight can be quickly and easily assessed by informally comparing the patient's report of cognitive and functional deficits to the report of care-givers and objective data. If more formal assessment of insight is needed, brief assessment instruments are available (Buckley et al. 2010; Migliorelli et al. 1995).

Mood disorders occur with enough frequency in older adults, and particularly with patients having cognitive impairment, that a thorough assessment of affective status should always be conducted (Evans et al. 2005; Steffens et al. 2009). Assessment of emotional status incorporates the report of the patient and family as well as objective data. In the context of neuropsychological intervention, the clinician should specifically assess for the presence of affective symptoms that can undermine the patient's ability effectively to participate (e.g. depression, apathy, anhedonia, anxiety, irritability). For cases in which the affective distress is of sufficient magnitude that it would be expected to inhibit motivation and/or participation in the intervention process, it is preferable to treat the affective distress first in order to maximize subsequent benefit from intervention. However, for cases in which there are only milder affective symptoms that are mostly occurring secondary to cognitive failures and loss of cognitive ability (e.g. frustration, grief), these issues can usually be addressed directly during the course of neuropsychological intervention. One final point is that patients with mood disorders, such as depression or anxiety, may be more prone to making negative self-appraisals of their cognitive abilities than non-depressed patients (Bartley et al. 2012). Objective cognitive data can thus be particularly helpful when working with such patients to address actual level of ability.

While the overarching goal of neuropsychological intervention is to teach the patient techniques to compensate for cognitive, behavioural, and functional deficits, often patients and families presenting for neuropsychological intervention will have already developed some type of behavioural adaptations to compensate for these deficits. Thus, careful review of the patient's current compensatory methods and activities is prudent. This review often includes questioning the patient and family about how the patient currently keeps track of important information such as appointments and medication information, as well as querying how well these existing systems are working for the patient. Sometimes the systems that are currently used work well, while other times these systems may be improved with modifications. Another reason for reviewing existing compensatory techniques is so that the clinician does not inadvertently make recommendations that counter existing functional adaptions.

Finally, aside from the specific factors listed above, the clinician should make note of any unique patient and environmental factors that may arise during the intervention evaluation or during the course of the intervention sessions. Specifically, the clinician is interested in factors that might, for better or worse, modify the intervention process. Common issues include unique patient medical or personality factors, composition of the household and the ability of the family system to support intervention approaches, and the conduciveness of the physical environment to functioning.

Careful review of the variables discussed above should allow for development of a treatment plan that identifies clear targets for intervention and enables the clinician to select optimal intervention methods for each patient. Two case examples are presented below to illustrate the use of such a model. Across patient populations there may be common factors that moderate the approach and typical results intervention. Outcome monitoring is essential to informed, ethical and responsible practice. Clinical observation and judgment should be supplemented with formal measures where appropriate. Here too, utilization of objective tests and rating scales should be employed with awareness of validity for the relevant geriatric population. Ideally, outcomes can be demonstrated in three areas: objective performance, subjective well-being, and functional gains. In this manner, patient perception, function, and ability are all captured to best illustrate the benefit of intervention.

CASE EXAMPLES

Below, two case examples illustrate the process of treatment planning as a function of the variables described in this model and how they can interrelate.

Case 1: Mr R, depression with memory complaints

Mr R was a 58-year-old man with fourteen years of education who presented for treatment of memory deficits. He reported a one-year history of relatively new memory difficulties.

Goals and motivation

Mr R expressed strong interest in learning methods to alleviate his memory problems.

Neuropsychological profile and insight

The patient had never had comprehensive neuropsychological testing, but cognitive screening had recently been completed by the patient's primary-care doctor (MMSE = 30/30). As described above, Mr R reported significant memory problems during the intervention evaluation. Because many studies have found a weak association between memory complaints and actual memory ability in depressed patients, we wanted to obtain a more detailed assessment of the patient's cognitive abilities. Therefore, in the second intervention session, we administered a brief battery of neuropsychological tests that primarily assessed executive functioning, learning, and memory. Results of this testing revealed occasional relative inefficiencies on tests of processing speed, but all other performances, including his performance on tests of learning and memory, were within expectation for his age and level of education. Mr R's initial description of cognitive deficits suggested that he had adequate insight.

Affective status

As noted, Mr R reported significant symptoms of depression in the evaluation interview and endorsed a moderate degree of depression symptoms on a mood questionnaire (Beck Depression Inventory-II = 22). He detailed feelings of isolation and grief, and he cited the death of his ailing mother in the past year, for whom he had been the primary care-giver, as a significant stressor.

Unique factors and current compensatory methods and activities

Mr R was single and living alone. He reported that he had minimal social supports. He was not currently using any compensatory methods or activities for his self-reported memory problems.

Intervention

1 Delineation of variables impacting memory functioning.
2 Therapeutic intervention.

This case illustrates the importance of objective data in symptom characterization and treatment. Absent this data, it would seem reasonable to target the patient's concern with memory functioning. However, in this case grief and affective distress were the underpinning of the perceived memory disorder. Treatment of memory without attention to these would not likely alleviate symptoms.

Objective quantification of cognition facilitated the accurate characterization of symptoms and helped to define the therapeutic targets and approach. Intervention thus began with therapeutic feedback using the results of testing and facilitation of treatment of depression. Feedback included reviewing the test results of normal memory functioning relative to age and education-matched peers and the significance of the isolated weakness on tests of processing speed. The frequency of such findings among those with depression was reviewed as well as the body of research which has consistently found a strong relationship between affective distress and negative self-appraisals. Because Mr R's perception or experience of memory deficits was felt to be related to his depressed mood, we referred him for psychotherapy. We also recommended that he consider consulting with his primary care doctor or with a psychiatrist regarding possible pharmacological treatment of depression.

Case 2: Ms D, mild cognitive impairment

Ms D was a 71-year-old woman with eighteen years of education who was referred for intervention by her neurologist in the context of concern for cognitive decline by the patient and her family.

Goals and motivation

Ms D was interested in getting help for problems with increasing forgetfulness that she had experienced over the previous year. She identified three specific functional goals: (1) to increase her ability to learn and retain information that her family tells her; (2) to better remember her appointments, as there had been a few incidents when she missed an appointment because she had forgotten about it; and (3) to enhance her ability to remember names, as she was embarrassed with her difficulty remembering the names of acquaintances.

Neuropsychological profile and insight

Cognitive screening was performed by Ms D's neurologist and did not reveal significant deficits (MoCA = 29/30). However, comprehensive neuropsychological testing identified deficits that were not evident on cognitive screening. Specifically, her neuropsychological profile was notable for borderline performance on aspects of executive function and on multiple tests of learning and memory. With specific regard to memory, encoding and retrieval appeared to be more affected than storage of information. Upon feedback, Ms D demonstrated good insight into the nature and severity of these deficits.

Affective status

Ms D described her mood as 'good' and did not endorse significant mood symptoms on formal testing. However, she did report mild distress and frustration in response to her cognitive difficulties. She was particularly bothered by her occasional difficulty in recalling names.

Unique factors and current compensatory methods and activities

Ms D lived with her husband, who was in good physical and cognitive health. She also had a number of children who lived nearby. She described her husband and family as being very supportive. With regard to current strategies, she was using a few different written systems to track information (e.g. separate appointment, contact, grocery, and to-do lists).

Intervention

Treatment focused on the goals that were identified in the intervention evaluation. All had to do with learning and memory, with a specific focus on retention of important information, appointments, and names. The *target* of intervention was thus memory. The *strategies*, based upon Ms D's standing, included two approaches:

1 *External aids*: First, Ms D entered treatment using multiple notes and lists to attempt to track information. Because she had difficulty tracking multiple systems, these external aids were failing. Both her input and extraction of information was inconsistent. Intervention focused upon (1) reducing her total number of calendars from four to one, with this single calendar being large enough to contain sufficient information for appointment details but small enough to fit easily into Ms D's purse for transport; (2) establishing a routine (with initial reminding from her family) of reviewing her calendar every morning after she had eaten breakfast and every evening to enter any appointments not already recorded. Furthermore, note pads were placed by home phones to record phone calls or important content of conversations.

2 *Memory strategies*: Memory strategies designed to enhance learning and consolidation of target information were based on repetition and association. These techniques were modelled and practised, and real world applications were reviewed. First, Ms D was taught a simplified version of a face-name recall strategy involving use of mental images of the face of the person to be remembered coupled with images representing the person's name or something that would help her to later recall the name (Clare et al. 2002). For example, she found it helpful to remember her neighbour's name (Jim) by creating a mental image of him working out in a gym (e.g. Jim from the gym). Second, key family members were taught to use spaced retrieval, which uses active supported repetition of target information to enhance attention and learning of the target stimuli (Camp, Bird, and Cherry 2000).

IMPLICATIONS FOR PRACTICE

The most important implications for clinical practice that were presented in this chapter centre around the methods for identification and treatment of cognitive symptoms in older adults. There are a variety of cognitive screening measures available that enable clinicians to obtain a fairly quick assessment of a patient's cognitive ability. However, clinicians need to be aware that screening measures provide limited information and are not typically appropriate for use as diagnostic instruments. Detailed cognitive appraisal can be obtained through referral for comprehensive neuropsychological evaluation. If cognitive or functional deficits are present, the clinician may consider use of or referral to a specialist using intervention techniques that are discussed in the neuropsychological literature. Such techniques are often best presented in the context of a carefully considered treatment plan that is specific to the individual patient.

SUMMARY

In this chapter, we have reviewed the prevalence of cognitive compromise in older adults and the disorders of ageing commonly giving rise to cognitive deficits and related emotional and functional compromises. Screening approaches were reviewed, as well as the utility of comprehensive neuropsychological evaluation. The importance of therapeutic feedback was considered, and a model for treatment planning in neuropsychological intervention was discussed.

It has been our experience that each of these components (assessment, feedback, intervention) are greatly valued by patients and their care-givers. From assessment and feedback, the patient and family can gain greater awareness about the nature of compromises, as well as potential aetiologies and possible course of the cognitive and functional deficits. Interventions then provide the patient with a means to cope with the practical implications of these deficits as well as larger existential issues such as grief, independence, and quality of life.

KEY REFERENCES AND SOURCES FOR FURTHER READING

American Psychological Association (2012). 'Guidelines for the Evaluation of Dementia and Age-related Cognitive Change'. *American Psychologist* 67(1): 1–9.

Attix, D. K. and Welsh-Bohmer, K. A. (eds) (2006). *Geriatric Neuropsychology: Assessment and Intervention*. New York: Guilford Press.

Busch, R. M. and Chapin, J. S. (2008). 'Review of Normative Data for Common Screening Measures Used to Evaluate Cognitive Functioning in Elderly Individuals'. *Clinical Neuropsychologist* 22(4): 620–650.

Heaton, R. K., Miller, S. W., Taylor, M. J., and Grant, I. (2004). *Revised Comprehensive Norms for an Expanded Halstead-Reitan Battery: Demographically Adjusted Neuropsychological Norms for African American and Caucasian Adults*. Lutz, FL: PAR.

Lezak, M. D., Howieson, D. B., Bigler, E. D., and Tranel, D. (2012). *Neuropsychological Assessment* (5th edn). New York: Oxford University Press.

Mitrushina, M. N., Boone, K. B., and D'Elia, L. F. (2005). *Handbook of Normative Data for Neuropsychological Assessment* (2nd edn). New York: Oxford University Press.

References

Aguirre, E., Woods, R. T., Spector, A. and Orrell, M. (2013). 'Cognitive Stimulation for Dementia: A Systematic Review of the Evidence of Effectiveness from Randomised Controlled Trials'. *Ageing Research Reviews* 12(1): 253–262.

American Psychological Association (2012). 'Guidelines for the Evaluation of Dementia and Age-related Cognitive Change'. *American Psychologist* 67(1): 1–9.

Attix, D. K. (2006). 'An Integrated Model for Geriatric Neuropsychological Intervention'. In D. K. Attix and K. Welsh-Bohmer (eds), *Geriatric Neuropsychology: Assessment and Intervention* (pp. 241–260). New York: Guildford Press.

Attix, D. K. and Welsh-Bohmer, K. A. (eds) (2006). *Geriatric Neuropsychology: Assessment and Intervention*. New York: Guildford Press.

Bartley, M., Bokde, A. L., and Ewers, M., Faluyi, Y. O., Tobon, W. O., et al. (2012). 'Subjective Memory Complaints in Community Dwelling Healthy Older People: The Influence of Brain and Psychopathology'. *International Journal of Geriatric Psychiatry* 27(8): 836–43.

Beatty, W. W., Mold, J. W., and Gontkovsky, S. T. (2003). 'RBANS Performance: Influences of Sex and Education'. *Journal of Clinical and Experimental Neuropsychology* 25(8): 1065–1069.

Beeri, M. S., Schmeidler, J., Sano, M., Wang, J., Lally, R., et al. (2006). 'Age, Gender, and Education Norms on the CERAD Neuropsychological Battery in the Oldest Old'. *Neurology* 67(6): 1006–1010.

Breitner, J. C., Wyse, B. W., Anthony, J. C., Welsh-Bohmer, K. A., Steffens, D. C., et al. (1999). 'APOE-epsilon4 Count Predicts Age when Prevalence of AD Increases, then Declines: the Cache County Study'. *Neurology* 53(2): 321–331.

Buckley, T., Norton, M. C., Deberard, M. S., Welsh-Bohmer, K. A., and Tschanz, J. T. (2010). 'A Brief Metacognition Questionnaire for the Elderly: Comparison with Cognitive Performance and Informant Ratings the Cache County Study'. *International Journal of Geriatric Psychiatry* 25(7): 739–747.

Busch, R. M. and Chapin, J. S. (2008). 'Review of Normative Data for Common Screening Measures Used to Evaluate Cognitive Functioning in Elderly Individuals'. *Clinical Neuropsychologist* 22(4): 620–650.

Camp, C. J., Bird, M. J., and Cherry, K. E. (2000). 'Retrieval Strategies as a Rehabilitation Aid for Cognitive Loss in Pathological Aging'. In R. D. Hill, L. Bäckman, and A. S. Neely (eds), *Cognitive Rehabilitation in Old Age* (pp. 224–248). New York: Oxford University Press.

Clare, L., Wilson, B. A., Carter, G., Roth, I. and Hodges, J. R. (2002). 'Relearning Face-name Associations in Early Alzheimer's Disease'. *Neuropsychology* 16(4): 538–547.

Clare, L., Wilson, B. A., Carter, G., Roth, I., and Hodges, J. R. (2004). 'Awareness in Early-stage Alzheimer's Disease: Relationship to Outcome of Cognitive Rehabilitation'. *Journal of Clinical and Experimental Neuropsychology* 26(2): 215–226.

Coblentz, J. M., Mattis, S., Zingesser, L. H., Kasoff, S. S., Wiśniewski, H. M., et al. (1973). 'Presenile Dementia: Clinical Aspects and Evaluation of Cerebrospinal Fluid Dynamics'. *Archives of Neurology* 29(5): 299–308.

Dong, Y., Lee, W. Y., Basri, N. A., Collinson, S. L., Merchant, R. A., et al. (2012). 'The Montreal Cognitive Assessment is Superior to the Mini-Mental State Examination in Detecting Patients at Higher Risk of Dementia'. *International Psychogeriatrics/IPA* 24(11): 1749–1755.

Duff, K., Patton, D., Schoenberg, M. R., Mold, J., Scott, J. G., et al. (2003). 'Age- and Education-corrected Independent Normative Data for the RBANS in a Community dwelling Elderly Sample'. *The Clinical Neuropsychologist* 17(3): 351–366.

Evans, D. L., Charney, D. S., and Lewis, L., Golden, R. M., Gorman, J. M., et al. (2005). 'Mood Disorders in the Medically Ill: Scientific Review and Recommendations'. *Biological Psychiatry* 58(3): 175–189.

Ferri, C. P., Prince, M., Brayne, C., Brodaty, H., Fratiglioni, L., et al. (2005). 'Global Prevalence of Dementia: A Delphi Consensus Study'. *Lancet* 366(9503): 2112–2117.

Fillenbaum, G. G., Heyman, A., Huber, M. S., Ganguli, M., and Unverzagt, F. W. (2001). 'Performance of Elderly African American and White Community Residents on the CERAD Neuropsychological Battery'. *Journal of the International Neuropsychological Society* 7(4): 502–9.

Folstein, M. F., Folstein, S. E., and McHugh, P. R. (1975). '"Mini-mental State". A Practical Method for Grading the Cognitive State of Patients for the Clinician'. *Journal of Psychiatric Research* 12(3): 189–98.

Freitas, S., Simões, M. R., Alves, L., Duro, D., and Santana, I. (2012). 'Montreal Cognitive Assessment (MoCA): Validation Study for Frontotemporal Dementia'. *Journal of Geriatric Psychiatry and Neurology* 25(3): 146–154.

Frisoni, G. B., Rozzini, R., Bianchetti, A., and Trabucchi, M. (1993). 'Principal Lifetime Occupation and MMSE Score in Elderly Persons'. *Journal of Gerontology* 48(6): S310–S314.

Ganguli, M., Ratcliff, G., Huff, F. J., Belle, S., Kancel, M. J., et al. (1991). 'Effects of Age, Gender, and Education on Cognitive Tests in a Rural Elderly Community Sample: Norms from the Monongahela Valley Independent Elders Survey'. *Neuroepidemiology* 10(1): 42–52.

Gates, N. J., Sachdev, P. S., Fiatarone Singh, M. A., and Valenzuela, M. (2011). 'Cognitive and Memory Training in Adults at Risk of Dementia: A Systematic Review'. *BMC Geriatrics* 11: 55.

Gontkovsky, S. T., Mold, J. W., and Beatty, W. W. (2002). 'Age and Educational Influences on RBANS Index Scores in a Nondemented Geriatric Sample'. *Clinical Neuropsychologist* 16(3): 258–263.

Green, J. (2006). 'Feedback'. In D. K. Attix and K. Welsh-Bohmer (eds), *Geriatric Neuropsychology: Assessment and Intervention* (pp. 223–236). New York: Guildford Press.

Heaton, R. K., Miller, S. W., Taylor, M. J., and Grant, I. (2004). *Revised Comprehensive Norms for an Expanded Halstead-Reitan Battery: Demographically Adjusted Neuropsychological Norms for African American and Caucasian Adults.* Lutz, FL: PAR.

Hill, J. W., Futterman, R., Duttagupta, S., Mastey, V., Lloyd, J. R., et al. (2002). 'Alzheimer's Disease and Related Dementias Increase Costs of Comorbidities in Managed Medicare'. *Neurology* 58(1): 62–70.

Iverson, G. L. (1998). 'Interpretation of Mini-Mental State Examination Scores in Community-dwelling Elderly and Geriatric Neuropsychiatry Patients'. *International Journal of Geriatric Psychiatry* 13(10): 661–666.

Jurica, P. J., Leitten, C. L., and Mattis, S. (2001). *Dementia Rating Scale–2.* Odessa, FL: Psychological Assessment Resources.

Koltai, D. C., Welsh-Bohmer, K. A., and Schmechel, D. E. (2001). 'Influence of Anosognosia on Treatment Outcome among Dementia Patients'. *Neuropsychological Rehabilitation* 11(3–4): 455–475.

Lezak, M. D., Howieson, D. B., Bigler, E. D., and Tranel, D. (2012). *Neuropsychological Assessment* (5th edn). New York: Oxford University Press.

Lonie, J. A., Tierney, K. M., and Ebmeier, K. P. (2009). 'Screening for Mild Cognitive Impairment: A Systematic Review'. *International Journal of Geriatric Psychiatry* 24(9): 902–915.

Lucas, J. A., Ivnik, R. J., Smith, G. E., Bohac, D. L., Tangalos, E. G., et al. (1998). 'Normative Data for the Mattis Dementia Rating Scale'. *Journal of Clinical and Experimental Neuropsychology* 20(4): 536–547.

Lyketsos, C. G., Lopez, O., Jones, B., Fitzpatrick, A. L., Breitner, J., et al. (2002). 'Prevalence of Neuropsychiatric Symptoms in Dementia and Mild Cognitive Impairment'. *Journal of the American Medical Association* 288(12): 1475–1483.

Marin, R. S. and Wilkosz, P. A. (2005). 'Disorders of Diminished Motivation'. *Journal of Head Trauma Rehabilitation* 20(4): 377–388.

Markwick, A., Zamboni, G., and de Jager, C. A. (2012). 'Profiles of Cognitive Subtest Impairment in the Montreal Cognitive Assessment (MoCA) in a Research Cohort with Normal Mini-Mental State Examination (MMSE) Scores'. *Journal of Clinical and Experimental Neuropsychology* 34(7): 750–757.

Mattis, S. (1988). *Dementia Rating Scale: Professional Manual*. Odessa, FL: Psychological Assessment Resources.

Migliorelli, R., Tesón, A., Sabe, L., Petracca, G., Petracchi, M., et al. (1995). 'Anosognosia in Alzheimer's Disease: A Study of Associated Factors'. *Journal of Neuropsychiatry and Clinical Neurosciences* 7(3): 338–44.

Mitchell, A. J. (2009). 'A Meta-analysis of the Accuracy of the Mini-mental State Examination in the Detection of Dementia and Mild Cognitive Impairment'. *Journal of Psychiatric Research* 43(4): 411–431.

Mitrushina, M. N., Boone, K. B., and D'Elia, L. F. (2005). *Handbook of Normative Data for Neuropsychological Assessment* (2nd edn). New York: Oxford University Press.

Morris, J. C., Heyman, A., Mohs, R. C., Hughes, J. P., van Belle, G., et al. (1989). 'The Consortium to Establish a Registry for Alzheimer's Disease (CERAD). Part I. Clinical and Neuropsychological Assessment of Alzheimer's Disease'. *Neurology* 39(9): 1159–1165.

Nasreddine, Z. S., Phillips, N. A., Bédirian, V., Charbonneau, S., Whitehead, V., et al. (2005). 'The Montreal Cognitive Assessment, MoCA: A Brief Screening Tool for Mild Cognitive Impairment'. *Journal of the American Geriatrics Society* 53(4): 695–699.

Nunnally, J. C. and Bernstein, I. H. (1994). *Psychometric Theory*. New York: McGraw-Hill.

Olazarán, J., Muñiz, R., Reisberg, B., Peña-Casanova, J., del Ser, T., et al. (2004). 'Benefits of Cognitive-motor Intervention in MCI and Mild to Moderate Alzheimer Disease'. *Neurology* 63(12): 2348–2353.

Patton, D. E., Duff, K., Schoenberg, M. R., Mold, J., Scott, J. G., et al. (2003). 'Performance of Cognitively Normal African Americans on the RBANS in Community Dwelling Older Adults'. *Clinical Neuropsychologist* 17(4): 515–530.

Perez, F. I., Hruska, N. A., Stell, R. L., and Rivera, V. M. (1978). 'Computerized Assessment of Memory Performance in Dementia'. *Canadian Journal of Neurological Sciences* 5(3): 307–312.

Phabphal, K. and Kanjanasatien, J. (2011). 'Montreal Cognitive Assessment in Cryptogenic Epilepsy Patients with Normal Mini-Mental State Examination Scores'. *Epileptic Disorders: International Epilepsy Journal with Videotape* 13(4): 375–381.

Plassman, B. L., Langa, K. M., Fisher, G. G., Heeringa, S. G., Weir, D. R., et al. (2007). 'Prevalence of Dementia in the United States: The Aging, Demographics, and Memory Study'. *Neuroepidemiology* 29(1–2): 125–32.

Plassman, B. L., Langa, K. M., Fisher, G. G., Heeringa, S. G., Weir, D. R., et al. (2008). 'Prevalence of Cognitive Impairment without Dementia in the United States'. *Annals of Internal Medicine* 148(6): 427–434.

Qiu, C., De Ronchi, D., and Fratiglioni, L. (2007). 'The Epidemiology of the Dementias: An Update'. *Current Opinion in Psychiatry* 20(4): 380–385.

Rabin, L. A., Barr, W. B., and Burton, L. A. (2005). 'Assessment Practices of Clinical Neuropsychologists in the United States and Canada: A Survey of INS, NAN, and APA Division 40 Members'. *Archives of Clinical Neuropsychology* 20(1): 33–65.

Randolph, C. (1998). *RBANS Manual*. San Antonio, TX: The Psychological Corporation.

Rilling, L. M., Lucas, J. A., Ivnik, R. J., Smith, G. E., Willis, F. B., et al. (2005). 'Mayo's Older African American Normative Studies: Norms for the Mattis Dementia Rating Scale'. *Clinical Neuropsychologist* 19(2): 229–242.

Rosen, H. J. (2011). 'Anosognosia in Neurodegenerative Disease'. *Neurocase* 17(3): 231–241.

Rossetti, H. C., Lacritz, L. H., Cullum, C. M., and Weiner, M. F. (2011). 'Normative Data for the Montreal Cognitive Assessment (MoCA) in a Population-based Sample'. *Neurology* 77(13): 1272–1275.

Saddichha, S. and Pandey, V. (2008). 'Alzheimer's and Non-Alzheimer's Dementia: A Critical Review of Pharmacological and Nonpharmacological Strategies'. *American Journal of Alzheimer's Disease and Other Dementias* 23(2): 150–161.

Schatz, P. and Browndyke, J. (2002). 'Applications of Computer-based Neuropsychological Assessment'. *Journal of Head Trauma Rehabilitation* 17(5): 395–410.

Schatz, P. and Zillmer, E. A. (2003). 'Computer-based Assessment Of Sports-related Concussion'. *Applied Neuropsychology* 10(1): 42–47.

Steffens, D. C., Fisher, G. G., Langa, K. M., Potter, G. G., et al. (2009). 'Prevalence of Depression among Older Americans: The Aging, Demographics and Memory Study'. *International Psychogeriatrics/IPA* 21(5): 879–888.

Story, T. and Attix, D. K. (2010). 'Models of Developmental Neuropsychology: Adult and Geriatric'. In S. Hunter and J. Donders (eds), *Principles and Practice of Lifespan Developmental Neuropsychology* (pp. 41–54). Cambridge: Cambridge University Press.

Strauss, E., Sherman, E., and Spreen, O. (eds) (2006). *A Compendium of Neuropsychological Tests: Administration, Norms, and Commentary* (3rd edn). Oxford: Oxford University Press.

Teixeira, C. V., Gobbi, L. T., Corazza, D. I., Stella, F., Costa, J. L., et al. (2012). 'Non-pharmacological Interventions on Cognitive Functions in Older People with Mild Cognitive Impairment (MCI)'. *Archives of Gerontology and Geriatrics* 54(1): 175–180.

Torti, F. M., Gwyther, L. P., Reed, S. D., Friedman, J. Y., and Schulman, K. A. (2004). 'A Multinational Review of Recent Trends and Reports in Dementia Caregiver Burden'. *Alzheimer Disease and Associated Disorders* 18(2): 99–109.

Tranel, D. (2008). 'Theories of Clinical Neuropsychology and Brain-Behavior Relationships'. In J. Morgan and J. Ricker (eds), *Textbook of Clinical Neuropsychology* (pp. 25–37). New York: Taylor and Francis.

United Nations Population Division (2010). 'World Population Prospects: The 2010 Revision'. (updated 28 June 2011). http://esa.un.org/wpp/Excel-Data/population.htm.

United States Census Bureau (2012). '2012 National Population Projections: Summary Tables'. (updated 15 May 2013). http://www.census.gov/population/projections/data/national/2012/summarytables.html.

Unverzagt, F. W., Hall, K. S., Torke, A. M., Rediger, J. D., Mercado, N., et al. (1996). 'Effects of Age, Education, and Gender on CERAD Neuropsychological Test Performance in an African American Sample'. *Clinical Neuropsychologist* 10(2): 180–190.

Van der Flier, W. M. and Scheltens, P. (2005). 'Epidemiology and Risk Factors of Dementia'. *Journal of Neurology, Neurosurgery and Psychiatry* 76(suppl. 5): v2–V7.

Welsh, K. A., Butters, N., Mohs, R. C., Beekly, D., Edland, S., et al. (1994). 'The Consortium to Establish a Registry for Alzheimer's Disease (CERAD). Part V. A Normative Study of the Neuropsychological Battery'. *Neurology* 44(4): 609–614.

Whitney, K. A., Mossbarger, B., Herman, S. M., and Ibarra, S. L. (2012). 'Is the Montreal Cognitive Assessment Superior to the Mini-mental State Examination in Detecting Subtle Cognitive Impairment among Middle-aged Outpatient U.S. Military Veterans?' *Archives of Clinical Neuropsychology* 27(7): 742–748.

Wild, K., Howieson, D., Webbe, F., Seelye, A., and Kaye, J. (2008). 'Status of Computerized Cognitive Testing in Aging: A Systematic Review'. *Alzheimer's and Dementia* 4(6): 428–437.

Wimo, A., Winblad, B., and Jönsson, L. (2010). 'The Worldwide Societal Costs of Dementia: Estimates for 2009'. *Alzheimer's and Dementia* 6(2): 98–103.

....

CHAPTER 15

FUNCTIONAL SEQUELAE OF COGNITIVE DECLINE IN LATER LIFE

....

HOLLY A. TUOKKO AND COLETTE M. SMART

FUNCTIONAL EVERYDAY BEHAVIOURS

Functional impairment typically refers to limitations in a person's ability to carry out certain functions in their daily lives. In the context of the International Statistical Classification of Diseases and Related Problems (ICD-10; World Health Organization (WHO) 1993), difficulties performing everyday activities and work-related activities are characterized as 'disability' (the final consequences of the disablement process; Verbrugge and Jette 1994). As a companion to the ICD, the International Classification of Functioning, Disability and Health (ICF; WHO 2001) shifts the focus from cause to impact, conceptualizing disability as more than medical or biological dysfunction, and taking into account the social and contextual factors that affect a person's functioning. In the ICF framework, every human being can experience decrements in health, and experience some degree of disability. The ICF addresses a broad range of activities including self-care, engagement in domestic life, and interpersonal interactions and relationships. The functional impairments to be examined in this chapter, then, involve those affecting everyday behaviours or competencies including limitations in social and occupational spheres of life, as well as limitations in interpersonal interactions and relationships. Everyday competence refers to the effective management of daily life that requires the orchestration of a broad range of skills including those required for personal care through to leisure activities, and their implementation throughout the day (Baltes et al. 1993).

Approaches proposed to organize and develop the concept of functional, everyday behaviours and competencies, and disability (e.g. ICF; WHO 2001) specifically within the context of ageing have recognized the importance of engagement in daily self-care activities that promote independent functioning and incorporated these into evaluations of the health status of older adults. The term activities of daily living (ADLs) is typically used to describe basic personal care, and includes activities such as feeding, bathing, and grooming that are survival-oriented and critical to independent life (Katz et al. 1963). To capture more complex levels of functioning required for independence, Lawton and Brody (1969) proposed the term instrumental activities of daily living (IADLs), which includes activities such as telephone use, shopping, financial management, food preparation, housework, transportation, and medication management. Numerous scales, checklists and other instruments to measure these domains have been developed and vary in content depending on the setting and circumstances in question.

These basic constructs (ADLs and IADLs) serve as the foundation for conceptualizing, more broadly, the construct of everyday competence. Everyday competence is generally considered to involve multiple domains and multiple components (Baltes et al. 1993; Diehl 1998; Willis 1991). Diehl (1998) argues that everyday competence involves physical, psychological, and social functioning, which all interact to produce everyday behaviour. Within each of these domains are multiple components. For example, the psychological domain might include basic cognitive function such as attention and memory, *as well as* feelings of control, self-efficacy, styles of coping, and regulation of affect.

Probably the most comprehensive model of everyday competence is that conceptualized by Willis (1991). Willis conceives of everyday competence in terms of *antecedents, components, mechanisms*, and *outcomes*. *Antecedents* refer to both individual factors (such as physical health and cognition), and sociocultural factors (such as cultural stereotypes of ageing and social healthcare policies). The antecedents are thought to be active across all domains of everyday competence and across various contexts. Unlike the antecedents, *components* are both domain-and context-specific. Willis breaks this section of the model into intra-individual (including both physical and mental abilities) and contextual (including social and physical contexts) components. For example, the physical, mental, and contextual components of driving a vehicle are quite different than the components required for cooking a meal. Thus, components may be quite variable across individuals and situations. *Mechanisms* refer to factors that moderate the actual expression of everyday competence, given that competence in a particular area does not guarantee that essential behaviours will be performed when necessary. Mechanisms can be either related to attributions and control (e.g. poor feelings of self-efficacy can influence medication compliance; Rodin, Timko, and Harris 1985), or to functional behaviours (e.g. maintaining a vehicle so it is ready and available to meet transportation needs). *Outcomes* refer to psychological and physical well-being, which, as noted by Diehl (1998), are also included as antecedents. If one maintains a high level of everyday competence through the antecedent, component, and mechanism stages of the model, positive well-being would likely ensue, thus contributing to future competence in everyday situations, and vice versa. This speaks to the recursive nature of the model and highlights how either a cascade of decline in everyday competence could occur, or how an initially competent person in the right context could continue to be relatively competent throughout their life.

Although not specified by Willis (1991), this model is consistent with Selective Optimization with Compensation theory (SOC; Baltes and Baltes 1990). This theory proposes that these three processes of developmental regulation are essential for the maintenance of successful functioning in everyday life. Selection refers to developing and committing to personal goals or the *selection* of functional domains on which to focus one's resources. Optimization refers to the means through which developmental potential is maximized and includes the investment of time and energy into the selected goal (e.g. practice of goal-relevant skills). Compensation, in contrast to optimization, refers to counteracting or avoiding losses, rather than achieving positive states (e.g. activating unused resources for alternative means of realizing a goal). Freund (2008), building on the SOC model, views successful ageing as the management of internal and external resources throughout one's lifespan and notes that, due to ageing-related changes in the availability and efficiency of resources, the ratio of gains (optimization) to losses (compensation) shifts in the pursuit of personal goals (selection). With increasing age, resource losses caused by declining heath and cognitive functioning result in an orientation toward loss avoidance or maintenance of function rather than toward optimizing gains as observed for younger adults. This shift in goal orientation is viewed as adaptive in terms of subjective well-being.

Diehl (1998) identified awareness as a key potential motivator of compensatory behaviour, where those who are more aware of their own deficits are more likely to compensate for them and find alternative methods of completing desired tasks. Diehl (1998) notes that other factors have been identified as potential motivators, such as positive relations between feelings of self-efficacy and perceived competence (Baltes, Wahl, and Schmid-Furstoss 1990). Locus of control was also found to be associated with perceived everyday competence, where those with an external locus of control (i.e. attribute events to factors outside their control) needed more assistance when performing everyday activities than those who perceive events to be under their own internal control (i.e. internal locus of control; Duffy and MacDonald 1990).

Willis (1991) recognizes that her model is primarily of heuristic value and cannot elaborate on all aspects of everyday competence. Yet it remains the most comprehensive model to date and is the only model that adequately considers how person and context transact to produce varying levels of everyday competence. The application of this approach within a clinical context would be dependent on the specific purpose of the specific application with the specific clinical population under specific conditions. For example, the application of this approach to examining driving as an everyday competence (Lindstrom-Forneri et al. 2010) would entail taking into consideration health, sensory, and physical factors, cognitive, social cognitive, and emotional factors, as well as driving experience, and other environmental factors (e.g. conditions under which driving takes place) and may form the basis of a comprehensive or team assessment process (Korner-Bitensky, et al. 2005).

Measurement

There are a number of measurement tools and strategies used to assess functional, everyday behaviours and competencies that differ with respect to *content* and *method* (see Table 15.1).

As indicated in Table 15.1, the *content* of measures used to collect information about everyday functioning using subjective or objective *methods* may be global or specific. To date, most subjective measures have been global in nature. Typically, questions relevant to each domain are evaluated on a 3- or 4-point scale. For example, a question relevant to the ability to transport oneself outside of walking distance might read, 'can you use public transportation: a) without help, b) with some help, c) not at all?' (Willis 1996).

Objective measures are becoming more common and overcome some of the disadvantages of subjective measures (see Table 15.2). One example of a *global objective* measure is the Everyday Problems Test (EPT; Diehl, Willis, and Schaie 1995; Marsiske and Willis 1995; Willis and Marsiske 1993), which examines one's ability to solve problems within the typical

Table 15.1 Description of the *content* and *method* for measures of everyday behaviours

Content of the measure (type of information collected)	Method (manner in which information is collected from participants)
Global measure <ul><li>fewer questions per domain</li><li>spans a number of domains (e.g. many ADL/IADL scales contain a few questions or tasks for each of many domains such as telephone use, shopping, food preparation, housekeeping, laundry, transportation, medication, and financial management)</li><li>fail to describe the domains with much detail</li></ul>Specific measure<ul><li>many questions per domain, usually focusing on only one domain</li><li>probe a single domain in detail, but cannot speak to a person's overall level of everyday competence</li></ul>	Subjective measures<ul><li>self-report of functioning</li><li>knowledgeable informant's report of participant functioning; employed when there is reason to believe participants may overestimate their level of competence, or cannot accurately self-report, or when a researcher or clinician wishes to compare self- to informant-report; discrepancy between informant- and self-reports is often used as a measure of awareness, with caution, given the numerous factors that could affect reporting by each party</li></ul>Objective measures<ul><li>performance-based</li><li>typically administered to a participant by a trained observer</li><li>stimuli are relevant to everyday life</li></ul>

seven IADL domains. With regard to medication, for example, a participant is shown the label of an over-the-counter cough medicine and asked to tell how many times per day it should be taken. For financial management, participants are asked to complete a specified portion of a tax return form. Diehl et al. (1995) developed an in-home version of the EPT, which has good ecological validity, but is time-consuming and thus enables only a limited view of performance on different tasks. Another example of a *global, objective* measure is the Texas Functional Living Scale (Cullum et al. 2001), which contains twenty-one items organized into five subscales—Dressing, Time, Money, Communication, and Memory—and requires fifteen to twenty minutes to administer.

An example of a *specific objective* measure is the Measure of Awareness of Financial Skills (MAFS; Cramer et al. 2004; Van Wielingen et al. 2004), which assesses abilities such as identifying and counting currency, completing cash transactions, writing cheques, balancing a cheque book, understanding a credit card bill. A standardized scoring procedure is employed, which clearly delineates what constitutes acceptable performances to facilitate interpretation.

Advantages and disadvantages of subjective and objective measures are shown in Table 15.2. To overcome many of the current limitations of subjective and objective approaches, Diehl (1998) recommends a triangulation-of-method approach, which incorporates performance-based measures as well as self- and informant-report data in a comprehensive assessment of everyday competence. Having all three sources of data also allows for comparisons between them. Discrepancies between self- and other-report are commonly used as measures of awareness (Fleming, Strong, and Ashton 1996). Similarly, discrepancies

Table 15.2 Advantages and disadvantages of subjective and objective methods for assessing everyday competence

Methods of measurement	
Subjective (self-report)	Objective (performance-based)
Advantages: • can be administered in a short period of time • technicians can be trained to administer tests in the place of professionals	Advantages: • has high face validity relative to subjective assessment, since objective tasks can be designed to mimic real-world situations • circumvents the over- or underestimation of competence in self- and informant-report.
Disadvantages: • provide minimal information on concomitants and causes of incapacities in particular domains. Asking an older adult whether they can transport themselves does not provide information as to why that may be the case. • focus on what is happening rather than why.	Disadvantages: • the amount of time required for tester training and administration. • Depending on the domain, it may not be possible to examine the full breadth of tasks involved (e.g. ability to handle complex investment portfolios) • safety/liability concerns may preclude objective assessment (e.g. complex on-road driving or flying) without involving experts in the specific field.

between self-report and performance can also be used in this way. Comparisons between other-report and performance may lend support to the validity of the other's report. This is the approach taken in developing the MAFS, a three-part instrument that includes a questionnaire to be administered to the client/participant, a parallel informant questionnaire to be completed by a supportive family member or friend, and a performance measure. Comparison of the reports (self and other) and with information derived from the performance measure provides a comprehensive examination within the domain of financial management. Diehl (1998) speculates that if the data sources converge, researchers and practitioners can be confident that competency evaluations are not due to assessment errors; alternatively, if data sources are divergent, more information should then be gathered before everyday competencies are determined.

One particularly notable disadvantage to both subjective and objective assessment is that most measures examine what one can do, not whether one can get it done. That is, the majority of extant measures do not consider the context in which an older adult is situated. Theory on person–environment fit holds that context can have substantial effects on one's everyday competence (Lawton 1989). There are a number of ways context can be measured (Schaie and Willis 1999): looking at technical descriptors such as the architectural design and placement of social spaces in older adults' environments (Campo and Chadhury 2012); measuring indicators of support such as what resources are available and accessible for those in independent living situations (Iwarsson 2012); measuring the degree to which dependence or independence is fostered by social and physical context within institutional settings (Aranda et al. 2011); and describing specific situations where older adults are required to display competence (Nygård et al. 2012). To date, no measure of context has been established as the gold standard in everyday competence research.

Factors Affecting Everyday Behaviours

As indicated, a number of factors have been identified that influence functional everyday behaviour. These include individual factors such as physical health and cognition, and factors external to the individual such as physical and sociocultural environmental contexts. It is beyond the scope of this chapter to address all of these factors. With respect to physical health, suffice it to say that many health problems, including those that are age-associated, may influence independent functioning. In a study examining attributable risk for functional disability associated with chronic conditions in older adults, five chronic conditions (i.e. foot problems, arthritis, cognitive impairment, heart problems, and vision) made the largest contributions to ADL and IADL-related functional disabilities (Griffith et al. 2010). That said, it is rarely the mere presence of the health condition itself but the symptoms associated with the condition that may limit functional everyday behaviours. Certainly, musculo-skeletal symptoms such as pain, stiffness, and numbness may affect a person's mobility and limit his/her abilities to perform housework, go shopping, and may perhaps affect dressing, self-feeding, and functional transfers. Sensory deficits (e.g. vision, hearing) may impinge upon one's ability to perform everyday tasks requiring the use of these senses, such as the use of technology, the telephone, or tasks requiring sensory feedback (e.g. personal hygiene and grooming). Often, assistive devices can be very helpful in offsetting the impact of these physical and sensory conditions, allowing the individual to maximize their functional independence, albeit with some limitations.

As already noted, cognition and social cognition (e.g. self-efficacy, locus of control) can also affect the performance of functional everyday tasks, and in some circumstance this can be profound. Although cognitive functions change as a consequence of normal ageing, these changes are typically insufficient to affect basic activities of daily living. In contrast, as noted by Baltes et al. (1993), IADLs are more susceptible to changes in cognition. A clear co-occurrence of cognitive and functional losses has been shown in a number of studies using general population samples (Black and Rush 2002; Njegovan et al. 2001) or other samples without frank cognitive impairment (Barberger-Gateau et al. 1999; Steen et al. 2001). In a cohort of 5874 community-dwelling adults aged 65 years and older, Njegovan et al (2001) observed a clear hierarchy of functional loss associated with cognitive decline. Using global measures of cognition (i.e. Modified Mini-mental State Examination; 3MS) and functional status (i.e. Older American Resources and Services items; OARS), persons who did and did not lose independence over the five-year period were compared on the 3MS. For each functional domain (i.e. eating, dressing, grooming, walking, transferring into and out of bed, taking a bath or shower, going to the bathroom, telephone use, transportation out of walking distance, shopping, preparing meals, doing housework, taking medication), greater cognitive decline was seen for those who lost independence in comparison with those who remained independent. To identify the hierarchy of functional loss, mean 3MS scores (time 1 and time 2) were examined in relation to the emergence of loss within each domain. The order of loss of independence from least to most cognitive loss was: housework, shopping, bathing, walking, transportation, meal preparation, toileting, telephone use, finances, trans-ferring, medication use, dressing, grooming, and eating. As anticipated, IADLs were lost at higher levels of cognitive functioning than ADLs, though there was some overlap.

The temporal sequencing of losses in cognition and functional everyday behaviours has also been examined in longitudinal studies (e.g. Artero, Touchon, and Ritchie 2001; Black and Rush 2002; Steen et al. 2001), with some studies suggesting that cognitive loss occurs first (e.g. Steen et al. 2001) while others suggesting that both cognitive and functional losses show roughly parallel progression (e.g. Barberger-Gateau, Dartigues, and Letenneur 1993). It is important to consider, particularly in the context of population-based or general popu-lation samples, that necessarily attributing everyday functioning losses to cognitive status neglects the roles other factors, such as physical health status, may play.

Another way in which the relations between cognition and functional everyday behav-iour have been examined is through the studies of identified cognitive impairment. The most common condition considered to typify pathological cognitive ageing is dementia, which affects approximately 5–10% of people aged 65 years and older (e.g. Canadian Study of Health and Aging Working Group 1994; Lobo et al. 2000). The prevalence of dementia increases continuously with age from a small percentage (1–2%) in those aged 65 to 69 to over 20% in those 85 years of age and older. Most existing literature has defined demen-tia according to the Diagnostic and Statistical Manual (*DSM-IV*; American Psychiatric Association (APA) 2000); dementia is characterized by multiple cognitive deficits includ-ing impairment in memory and one or more other areas of cognition (i.e. aphasia/language disturbance; apraxia/impaired ability to carry out motor activities despite intact motor function; agnosia/failure to recognize or identify objects despite intact sensory function; disturbance in executive functioning such as planning, organizing, sequencing, abstract-ing). According to the diagnostic criteria, these cognitive deficits are seen to cause signifi-cant impairment in social or occupational functioning and represent a significant decline from a previous level of functioning. The exact nature of the social and occupational func-tioning is not clearly defined and typically has been interpreted to refer to IADL/ADL loss with the hierarchy of loss in functional everyday behaviours similar to that described by Njegovan et al. (2001).

In the *DSM-5* (APA 2013), dementia is no longer identified as such. Instead, the diagnos-tic criteria for Major Neurocognitive Disorders specify the presence of significant cognitive decline from a previous level of performance. This decline must be evident in one or more cognitive domains, including complex attention, executive function, learning and memory, perceptual motor, or social cognition, based on concern expressed by the individual them-selves, a knowledgeable informant, or a clinician, and preferably documented by stand-ardized neuropsychological testing or other quantified clinical assessment. The cognitive deficits *must* interfere with everyday activities with, at minimum, assistance being required with complex activities of daily living (e.g. paying bills or managing medications). Similar criteria are used to identify Mild Neurocognitive Disorder with the cognitive decline being characterized as modest (instead of significant) and *not* interfering with everyday activities.

Even prior to the *DSM-5* (APA 2013) inclusion of diagnostic criteria for Mild Neurocognitive Disorder, much attention was focused on cognitive difficulties occurring in the transitional stage prior to the emergence of dementia. The prevalence of this form of cognitive impairment, though differing by exact definition, has been estimated to be double that of dementia in adults aged 65 years and older (16.6%; Graham et al. 1997). Various terms have been used to identify this transitional stage such as Mild Cognitive Impairment (MCI; Petersen et al. 1999) and Cognitive Impairment, no Dementia (CIND; Graham et al. 1997), all of which are defined somewhat differently and may capture different segments of the group of people with some cognitive impairment (see Ritchie and Tuokko 2010 for a comparison of groups differing in definition). In some definitions, performance on basic ADL and IADL tasks is addressed (i.e. no deficits on ADL but may have minimal disturbance on IADLs) but little guidance is provided as to how to apply this criterion (Petersen 2004). Groups identified with definitions that do not specify ADL/IADL performance, have shown deficits in IADLs, presumably as a consequence of the cognitive impairment. The application of the *DSM-5* criteria is likely to change our understanding of the interplay between cognition and functional everyday behaviours. In a recent review of the literature examining IADLs and MCI in older adults, Gold (2012) drew the conclusion that healthy older adults, those with some form of cognitive impairment (i.e. non-dementia) and those with dementia were distinguishable on IADL tasks (e.g. Barberger-Gateau et al. 1999; Doble, Fisk, and Rockwood 1998; Ebly, Hogan, and Parhad 1995). It was also noted that individuals with cognitive impairment in multiple domains were more impaired on IADL tasks than those with single cognitive domain impairments (Aretouli and Brandt 2009; Burton et al. 2009; Farias et al. 2008), but showed less IADL impairment than those with dementia (e.g. Farias et al. 2006; Tam et al. 2007). From longitudinal investigations, Gold summarized that IADL changes can be predictive of future cognitive decline and those with both cognitive and IADL impairment are at greater risk of future cognitive decline than those with impairment in only one (e.g. Peres et al. 2008; Purser et al. 2005; Wadley, Crowe, and Marsiske 2007). In addition, it appeared that financial management may be a particularly early change associated with cognitive impairment (Tuokko, Morris, and Ebert 2005) and may be a strong predictor of future decline to dementia (Peres et al. 2008).

Relations between *specific domains of cognitive function* and IADL are complex and multifactorial. Different cognitive domains may play a greater or lesser role at different points in the trajectories of normal and pathological ageing, and different everyday competencies likely draw on specific cognitive domains. In the following sections, we review the literature pertaining to cognitive domains related to everyday functioning, how such cognitive domains are measured, and how deficits in daily functioning may be remediated or avoided altogether. We preface this review by noting that relationships between cognitive processes and IADL function are often moderate at best. Additionally, unless otherwise specified, studies tend to conceptualize IADLs as a global construct rather than specific competencies and their requisite cognitive processes.

SPECIFIC COGNITIVE FUNCTIONS RELATED TO EVERYDAY BEHAVIOUR

A preponderance of research on older adults focuses on memory processes, specifically episodic memory (EM), presumably because of the imperative towards early detection and differential diagnosis of dementia, particularly dementia of the Alzheimer's type (DAT). However, empirical evidence suggests that EM is not the cognitive process most strongly associated with IADL performance. Rather, evidence suggests that general intellectual (or 'general cognitive') functioning and executive functioning (EF) are most strongly related to everyday competence (Loewenstein and Acevedo 2009; Royall et al. 2007). The theory of cognitive reserve attempts to explain why there is not a one-to-one relationship between degree of brain pathology and observed dysfunction, postulating that there are several moderating variables that may promote adaptation and protect the individual against behavioural difficulties in the face of brain pathology. General intellectual function is frequently correlated with educational attainment, which serves as one such proxy for cognitive reserve (Stern 2002). Thus, intellectual function may allow access to a repertoire of potential solutions and compensations for functional difficulties, allowing individuals with higher reserve to tolerate relatively higher degrees of objective pathology (Loewenstein and Acevedo 2009). While debate abounds regarding the precise definition of EF, it can be construed most broadly as the ability to respond creatively to novel problems (Norman and Shallice 1986). It is not difficult to see why EF might be related to everyday competence—many of the high-level tasks we associate with IADLs involve both knowledge and the ability flexibly and creatively to solve problems in the face of changing circumstances, such as managing a new medication regimen or dealing with an unexpectedly overdrawn bank account.

Several studies have explored the associations between intellectual function, EF, and everyday competence or functional status. EF in particular is of interest because it is a domain that may be targeted for enhancement or remediation, unlike intellectual function, which is unlikely to change over time. For example, Bell-McGinty et al. (2002) found that neuropsychological measures of EF accounted for 54% of the variance in both observed and self-reported IADL status even after controlling for demographic variables such as age, gender, and education. Cahn-Weiner et al. (2007) assessed the association between informant-reported IADLs and EM, EF, and MRI brain volumes in a group of 124 older adults ranging from normal to moderate dementia. While both EM and EF were associated with baseline IADLs, only EF was significantly associated with a decline in IADL performance over time. Perhaps EF is necessary for developing novel methods of adaptation and compensation as decline in memory occurs; at the point where EF itself begins to decline, these compensations can no longer occur, and effective IADL performance can no longer be maintained. Johnson, Lui and Yaffe (2007) followed a large (i.e. >7000) prospective sample of community-dwelling older women and examined cross-sectional and longitudinal predictors of functional impairment, specifically focusing on general cognitive function and EF. After controlling for age, education, medical burden, depression, and baseline functional status, they found that women with impaired EF, as measured by Trails Part B, had a higher rate of cross-sectional and longitudinal ADL and IADL impairment, and also had increased risk of mortality as compared to women with impairment in general cognitive function (as measured by the MMSE).

As noted above, historically the relationship between EM and everyday competence has been somewhat unclear, although recent research has begun to clarify this relationship. For example, Royall et al. (2005) followed older adults over a three-year period and found that the relationship between EM and everyday competence was largely explained by EF. In contrast, Farias et al. (2009) used random-effects models to examine the relative contribution of EM and EF in stability in IADL function over time, finding that EM and EF were independent in their relative contributions. In explaining the discrepancy, they posit that key differences may include their use of memory and EF measures with similar psychometric properties and a cognitively diverse sample including individuals with varying degrees of dementia. By extension, EM and EF may offer different relative contributions dependent on the baseline cognitive status of the individual in question. The potential role for memory in IADLs has been supported in recent studies on individuals with MCI. Evidence suggests that individuals with MCI (including single-domain, amnestic MCI) may have mild IADL dysfunction (while still retaining overall independence), which is now reflected in the updated criteria on MCI diagnosis (Albert et al. 2011). A recent study by Bangen et al. (2010) indicated that individuals with amnestic MCI (i.e. only impaired in memory, aMCI) showed decrements in finance management, whereas individuals with non-amnestic MCI were more impaired in the domains of health and safety, using a performance-based IADL measure. Hughes et al. (2012) conducted a large cross-sectional examination of community-dwelling seniors including those with and without significant cognitive impairment. Individuals who met neuropsychological criteria for MCI were more likely than healthy seniors to be dependent in at least one IADL task such as shopping, meal preparation, housework, and handling finances. Across the sample, better memory and EF performance were associated with a lower risk of IADL impairment. Unsurprisingly, individuals with multi-domain amnestic MCI were most likely to be grossly dependent in all IADL tasks, mitigated by the degree of EF impairment manifested.

Prospective memory (PM) is becoming increasingly recognized as an important domain of interest for older adults, albeit one that garners comparatively less attention in standardized clinical neuropsychological assessment (Fish, Wilson, and Manly 2010). PM, sometimes referred to as memory for intentions, involves setting an intention and then remembering that that intention has to be executed in the future, or 'remembering to remember' (McDaniel and Einstein 2000). PM can be either time-based (e.g. remembering something that needs to occur at a set time) or event-based (e.g. remembering someone's birthday). A focus on future intentions sets PM apart from most other types of declarative memory, which tend to be retrospective in nature. Additionally, while PM is considered a type of memory, it is a complex process that involves retrospective memory, attention, and EF. Older adults perform worse in PM tasks that require strategic/controlled vs automatic processing, which often transpire in event-based rather than time-based tasks (Henry et al. 2004). Considering the evidence for relationships between retrospective memory, EF, and IADLs, it is unsurprising then that PM would also be related to IADL performance.

Anecdotal evidence indicates that complaints related to PM are among some of the most common reported by older adults in clinical practice (as well as in the general population) and have a clear relationship to IADL performance, such as remembering to take medications, attend doctor's appointments, and manage bill payment (Baddeley 1997). A limited amount of research has been conducted on the relationship between PM and IADL function in older adults, despite their clear theoretical relationship. Schmitter-Edgecombe, Woo, and Greeley (2009) examined multiple memory processes and their relationship to everyday functional impairment in individuals with diagnosed MCI. While aMCI individuals predictably showed more impairment in content memory measures compared to those with non-amnestic MCI and healthy controls, both MCI groups showed impairment on PM (as well as temporal order and source memory) compared to the control group. Importantly, these non-content memory measures independently predicted IADL function over and above content measures. Recent work by Woods et al. (2012) examined the relationship between PM and IADLs in fifty community-dwelling healthy older adults. Participants completed the IADLQ (a self-report measure of IADL functioning), the Prospective and Retrospective Memory Questionnaire (PRMQ), and the Memory for Intentions Screening Test (MIST, a performance-based measure of PM), in addition to measures of general cognitive function, EF, and mood. Regression analyses indicated that event-based scores from the MIST and self-reported PM on the PRMQ both contributed to self-reported IADLs on the IADLQ, even after controlling for age, education, gender, medical and psychiatric comorbidities, general cognition, EF, and self-reported retrospective memory on the PRMQ. Other recent research suggests that changes in PM may represent the earliest and most subtle signs of non-normative cognitive decline, perhaps occurring even before EM deficits, which tend to be the focus of clinical-diagnostic evaluation (e.g. Huppert and Beardsall 1993; Troyer and Murphy 2007).

Finally, while the majority of research has examined IADLs at the global level, some studies have attempted to isolate cognitive processes related to specific IADLs. For example, working memory has been shown to be an important process related to finance management (Earnst et al. 2001; Hoskin, Jackson, and Crowe 2005). Memory, attention, and concept formation have been associated with medication adherence and management (Hinkin et al. 2002; Jeste et al. 2003; Putzke et al. 2000). Driving is a particular example that has garnered much interest, a uniquely complex activity that requires many cognitive abilities simultaneously, including attention, visuoperception, memory, motor functions, EF, and metacognitive awareness, in addition to personality and motivational factors (Rizzo and Kellison 2009).

Assessment of relevant cognitive functions

Knowing which cognitive domains contribute to everyday competence, the challenge then becomes finding reliable and valid measures with adequate predictive ability. Synthesizing the breadth of research in this area is beyond the scope of this chapter. For current purposes, we summarize major findings and limitations of different types of assessment of cognitive functions and their predictive ability with respect to everyday functioning. Although we have noted that IADLs have been shown to be related to EM, PM, and EF, the preponderance of research has tended to focus on EF tests with significant predictive validity.

Standardized neuropsychometric tests

Most traditional clinical-neuropsychological tests were designed with a focus on lesion identification and localization, and as such may have a tenuous relationship at best with everyday functional abilities (Chaytor and Schmitter-Edgecombe 2003). Taking the case of EF in particular, neuropsychological tests have been notoriously limited in capturing an individual's real-world deficits, and anecdotal evidence abounds of individuals with significant EF impairment evident in daily life who nevertheless perform within normal limits on formal neuropsychometric measures (Burgess et al. 2006; Sohlberg and Mateer 2001). One reason for this may be that the testing situation is often highly structured and involves minimal or no competing demands, which is very unlike the real world in which novel problem-solving occurs in complex and unpredictable contexts (Norman and Shallice 1986). As such, traditional clinical neuropsychometric tests have demonstrated a moderate level of predictive validity regarding functional status (Marcotte et al. 2009).

Of the studies that conceptualize IADLs as a global construct, the strongest predictors tend to be measures of EF (see Table 15.3 for examples of EF measures by domain). More specifically, one of the tests with the most robust relationship to overall IADL functioning is the Trail Making Test part B. Bell-McGinty et al. (2002) found that, of a battery of five standardized EF measures used, only Trails B and the Wisconsin Card Sorting Test (WCST) independently predicted functional status over and above demographic variables. Similarly, Cahn-Weiner et al. (2002) used Trails B, WCST, and letter fluency to predict IADL performance. Trails B was the only measure significantly to predict scores on a performance-based IADL measure, while both Trails B and letter fluency predicted informant ratings of IADL performance. Limitations of the study include a small sample (thirty-two participants) and the absence of any information on clinical characterization (e.g. cognitively normal, MCI). Mitchell and Miller (2008) recruited a group of community-dwelling older adults (65 years and older) and measured EF using several subtests of the D-KEFS, including condition 4 of the Trail Making Test (similar to the original Trails Part B), in addition to letter fluency, design fluency, and the Tower test. In a linear regression model, Trails condition 4 was the only significant IADL predictor above and beyond depression score, years of education, and the other executive measures.

Other executive measures have also been found to predict global IADL status. Jefferson et al. (2006) administered a comprehensive EF battery to nondemented older adults with

Table 15.3 Selected neuropsychological measures related to everyday functions

Measurement type	Example measures
EF domains	
Working Memory	Digits Backward
Inhibitory Control	Colour-Word Test, e.g. from the Delis-Kaplan Executive Function System (D-KEFS; Delis et al. 2001)
Planning	Tower of London
	Porteus Maze
Cognitive Flexibility	Trails B
	Wisconsin Card Sorting Test
Cognitive Fluency	Letter Fluency (e.g. FAS)
	Design Fluency
Ecologically Valid Tests	Rivermead Behavioural Memory Test (RBMT; Wilson, Cockburn, and Baddeley 1985)
	Test of Everyday Attention (TEA; Robertson et al. 1996),
	Behavioral Assessment of the Dysexecutive Syndrome (BADS; Wilson et al. 1996)
	Memory for Intentions Test (MIST; Raskin and Buckheit 2010)
Self-report and Semi-structured Interviews	Frontal Systems Behavior Inventory (FrSBe; Grace and Molloy 2001)
	Dysexecutive Questionnaire from the BADS
	Test of Practical Judgment (TOP-J; Rabin et al. 2007a)

stable cardiovascular disease who were at risk for cognitive decline. Their analyses indicated that inhibitory control, as measured by the Interference trial from the D-KEFS Color Word Test, had the greatest predictive value with regards to informant-rated IADLs as compared to measures of working memory, generativity, planning, and sequencing. Lewis and Miller (2007) recruited older adults with average EF performance as well as mild, moderate, and severe EF deficits as classified by the Executive Functions Interview (EXIT), and tested them on a battery of EF measures and a performance-based measure of IADLs. While each of the EF domains probed (i.e. working memory, planning, cognitive flexibility, and cognitive fluency) were correlated with IADL performance, planning ability (as measured by the Tower of London and Porteus Mazes) was the only significant predictor.

In summary, evidence exists that standard neuropsychometric tests can predict with a moderate degree of significance an individual's global IADL status. Our discussion of some of the most pertinent findings, however, belies the fact that specific IADLs can differ greatly in their task demands and requisite cognitive abilities. While various tests often predict global rating scales of self- and informant-report or even performance-based measures, it stands to reason that different tests may predict very specific functions, and individuals may be able to perform some IADLs but not others (Hall et al. 2011; Loewenstein and Acevedo 2009). This is very much akin to the literature examining neuropsychological predictors of competency which indicates that assessment needs to occur at the level of specific domains (e.g. health, finance) and is not meaningful at a global level (Willis 1996). Additionally, different individuals may perform poorly on the same task (e.g. finance management) due to failure in a variety of different processes (e.g. organization, planning, prospective memory), emphasizing that the process is just as important as the completion of the task (Loewenstein and Acevedo 2009; Milberg, Hebben, and Kaplan 2009). Thus, further research is required to examine which tests (and therefore which domains) best predict specific IADL functions, contingent on why the process is breaking down for the particular individual.

Ecologically valid tests

To address the modest relationship between traditional neuropsychological tests and daily functioning, there has been a growing movement toward development and use of what are referred to as 'ecologically valid' tests (Burgess et al. 2006; Spooner and Pachana 2006). More specifically, ecologically valid tests represent conditions under which one can generalize from the results of controlled experimental procedures to naturally occurring events in real-world situations (Brunswik 1956). An important aspect of such tests is verisimilitude, or the degree to which the methods of data collection and component processes required of a task mimic how the behaviour unfolds in the real world (Rabin, Burton, and Barr 2007b). See Table 15.3 for prominent examples of such tests. Unfortunately, clinical neuropsychologists vary widely in their use of such tests, and they are most commonly used in rehabilitation settings where there is a clear focus on remediation and restoration of independent daily function (Rabin et al. 2007b). Occupational therapists are more likely to use tests that have apparent ecological relevance to their clientele, but these tests may not be constructed with underlying cognitive processes in mind in the same manner as neuropsychometric tests.

Self-report questionnaires and semi-structured interviews

There are various questionnaires and clinician-administered interviews that have been used to predict daily function, many of which fall under the domain of EF. For example, the Frontal Systems Behaviour Inventory (FrSBe; Grace and Molloy 2001) is a forty-six-item scale that examines three components of EF: cognitive-executive functions, apathy, and disinhibition. It has parallel respondent and informant versions, and asks for ratings on the three subscales before the injury or illness, and at the current time. The initial scale was normed and developed with healthy individuals, with additional data provided on several neurological samples including various types of dementia. Boyle et al. (2003) examined a group of individuals with diagnosed DAT, and found that the cognitive-executive and apathy subscales predicted a significant amount of variance (17% and 24%, respectively) on the Lawton-Brody ADL scale (Lawton and Brody 1969). In a similar study, Stout et al. (2003) administered the FrSBe to a sample of individuals with mild, moderate, and severe DAT, finding that apathy was significantly related to basic ADL functions, whereas cognitive-executive dysfunction was related to IADL functioning. Zahodne and Tremont (2012) found that, among individuals with aMCI, FrSBe-apathy, but not depression, was associated with greater functional impairment on the Lawton-Brody IADL scale.

The Test of Practical Judgment (TOP-J; Rabin et al. 2007a), a nine- or fifteen-item semi-structured interview that asks for open-ended responses regarding everyday problems in the safety, medical, social/ethical, and financial aspects of EF, has been developed recently for specific use with older adults. Judgment is a highly complex process that involves not only EF, but also memory and language, and is therefore a domain sensitive to decline. In their measure development paper, Rabin et al. (2007a) compared the TOP-J to the only two previously existing measures of judgment—the Judgment subtest of the Neurobehavioural Cognitive Status Exam (Northern California Neurobehavioral Group 1988) and the Judgment subscale of the Neuropsychological Assessment Battery (Stern and White 2003)—and found that their measure had the greater reliability and internal consistency of the three measures. They also demonstrated the TOP-J to have convergent validity with other EF tests and discriminant validity with tests of other cognitive functions such as attention and visuo-construction. Importantly, individuals with no cognitive impairment, MCI, and mild AD showed increasingly poorer performance on the TOP-J. While the measure shows promise, several factors should be taken into consideration with its use. First, when using such a test clinically, one must establish whether any apparent deficit represents a true decline in function instead of a longstanding weakness due to pre-morbid cognitive limitations or a simple lack of opportunity to practise such skills. Additionally, the authors themselves note that responses to hypothetical scenarios may or may not predict actual real-world behaviour, no objective measure of which was used in the development study. Particularly if the individual has any kind of awareness deficit, it is possible to have intellectual knowledge for appropriate problem-solving yet lack the ability to implement such knowledge (Crosson et al. 1989), highlighting the need for corroborating informant report and/or objective measures of real-world behaviour.

In summary, evidence suggests that various types of neuropsychometric tests hold a moderate level of predictive validity with respect to functional status, varying as a function of patient population and diagnosis. Efforts are being made to develop more ecologically valid tests, although research is still forthcoming on their particular ability to predict everyday function. Self-report questionnaires and semi-structured interviews, particularly those related to EF, can often prove quite informative in predicting everyday function in older adults.

Interventions Addressing Everyday Behaviour

For the last three decades, the field of cognitive rehabilitation for acquired brain injury has demonstrated that it is possible to intervene in the lives of individuals with neurocognitive impairment and produce meaningful change not only in cognition but also in everyday function (e.g. Cicerone et al. 2011). Given the psychosocial and economic impact of loss of IADL function (and therefore independence) in older adults, there is an imperative to investigate similar types of cognitive intervention methods in this age group. These efforts are further supported by a growing body of research in basic neuroscience indicating that experience-dependent structural and functional neuroplasticity are possible across the lifespan. Such advances have been made possible through two major avenues: translational work using animal models and the advent of advanced neuroimaging techniques such as functional magnetic resonance imaging (fMRI) (Greenwood 2007). Accordingly, the field of cognitive intervention with older adults is now garnering strong interest, although the work varies widely based on patient population, theoretical orientation, and target behaviours. Summarizing the entirety of this field is beyond the scope of this chapter; here we will focus on differences in the focus and the timing of intervention in older adults. It is important to note from the outset that one major limitation of much of the literature conducted on cognitive intervention in older adults has been a focus on improving basic cognitive processes, with comparatively less attention paid to real-world, functional outcomes. We also note that sometimes there is confusion in the literature as to the terminology used for intervention with seniors. Specifically, some authors refer to cognitive training as standardized, group-based interventions for specific cognitive processes that are disseminated to healthy older adults, whereas cognitive rehabilitation is highly individualized, delivered to one person at a time, and targeted toward individuals already showing significant cognitive impairment (e.g. dementia) (Clare et al. 2005). However, this distinction is not always maintained. To avoid further confusion, we use the term cognitive intervention to refer to any type of intervention used in older adults to enhance or remediate some aspect of cognitive function.

Task-specific vs process-specific interventions

A major theoretical distinction exists in the approach to IADL intervention for seniors: focus directly on the target behaviour (e.g. meal preparation), or focus on cognitive processes that are thought to underlie and support execution of the target behaviour (e.g. EF). In the first approach, where a task is repeated and routinized, task-specific training can be of great benefit (Loewenstein and Acevedo 2009). Controlling for processing speed demands, evidence suggests, that procedural memory may be relatively robust against age-related decline (Kester et al. 2002). Relying on non-declarative memory systems, it can be used to facilitate skill or habit acquisition and strengthening while bypassing any pre-existing impairments in EM or executive functions (EF). More specifically, using this approach would involve specification and sequencing of relevant steps in which the patient would train using behavioural practice and errorless learning to ensure encoding only of accurate steps and not off-task behaviours (Wilson et al. 1994). Reinforcing improvements and successes are also an important motivating factor for successful implementation of task-specific routines. Orellano, Colon, and Arbesman (2012) conducted a systematic review of the occupational therapy literature for evidence-based practice in IADL for older adults, concluding that there was strong evidence in favour of multicomponent interventions to improve and maintain IADL in community-dwelling older adults. This suggests that effective training methods exist whereby older adults can acquire task-specific routines of functional relevance, such as remembering to take medication, preparing meals, and keeping track of finances. The trade-off is that training effects are specific to the task in question and tend not to generalize to other tasks (Lustig et al. 2009). Furthermore, training in procedural memory would not necessarily equip the individual with the requisite skills to manage a situation where there is a deviation from the usual routine, such as overdrawing one's bank account unexpectedly.

The second approach to intervention is to focus on cognitive processes that are thought to underlie successful IADL execution, which would include EF as well as prospective and retrospective memory. EF presents a particularly important target for intervention, as there are normative declines in cognitive control processes even for older adults without signs of pathologic ageing (Braver and Barch 2002). Therefore, it is likely that most older adults could benefit from remediation in certain aspects of EF. Important advances have been made in the field of EF rehabilitation (e.g. Cicerone et al. 2011, 2006), and recent years have seen a crossover of such approaches from brain injury rehabilitation to intervention with older adults. A good example of this is goal management training (GMT; Levine et al. 2000; Levine et al. 2011), one of the most well-known and empirically supported interventions for EF rehabilitation. This is a five-stage process (see Table 15.4), where the stages are repeated in an iterative fashion wherever there is a mismatch between the current action and the goal to be accomplished (Levine et al. 2000). While the patient learns a series of predefined steps as described, these are not task-specific and can be applied to any novel problem-solving situation, greatly increasing the likelihood of transfer of training to different contexts and problem spaces.

Table 15.4 Stages in goal management training

Stage	Action
Stage 1	directing attention toward a goal,
Stage 2	selection of a particular goal,
Stage 3	parsing that goal into subcomponents or subgoals,
Stage 4	encoding and retention of subgoals, and
Stage 5	monitoring to determine whether the outcome of action matches the desired goal.

Levine et al. (2007) published a test of GMT in older adults in a special issue of the *Journal of the International Neuropsychological Society* focused on cognitive rehabilitation in older adults. Using a randomized controlled trial (RCT) intervention vs waitlist control design, a modified form of GMT (four weeks, four sessions) was administered to healthy older adults aged 71–87 years. While the participants underwent an extensive neuropsychological evaluation, measurement of intervention outcomes focused on self-reported dysexecutive symptoms (using the Dysexecutive Questionnaire, DEX) and experimental paradigms meant to simulate real-life tasks (SRLTs). More specifically, of interest was the processes that participants used to approach such tasks as opposed to the absolute scores per se. Examples of such tasks included setting up a carpool and assigning people to a schedule of swimming lessons. A statistically significant improvement on use of task strategies, checking one's progress, and engagement with the task, as well as a decrease in self-reported dysexecutive symptoms was observed. Gains made by the first treatment group were maintained over the follow-up period during which the waitlist group crossed over into the active intervention condition, and both groups maintained gains at six-month follow-up. A strength of this study was the use of naturalistic tasks to assess outcome of the intervention. One limitation, however, is that GMT was administered as part of a larger rehabilitation programme including modules on memory and psychosocial training, and while the changes in the measures reported pertain to hypothesized changes due to GMT, the impact of the other interventions cannot be ruled out. Additionally, as these were healthy older adults with no frank neuropsychological impairment, there may have been a ceiling effect with regard to ascertaining impact on real-world functions. This is an important point where the application of rehabilitation programmes in older adults does not directly parallel that in individuals with acquired brain injury. In the latter group, the purpose is restitution of function in a group of individuals with measured impairment who are not expected to decline further. In the former group, the approach would seem to be one of prevention, where the optimal time for intervention is while the individual has enough cognitive reserve to adopt functional strategies before significant decline begins to manifest. Thus, in order to evaluate the efficacy of this type of application of cognitive rehabilitation in older adults, it is necessary to pursue longitudinal studies tracking the relative trajectories of function in those who have and who have not received intervention. Given the wealth of literature demonstrating the relationship between EF and IADL performance, GMT holds promise as one of the few (or perhaps only) empirically supported interventions for EF. However, in GMT, individuals must have a certain level of awareness of their deficits and be motivated to implement behavioural changes. This may preclude implementation with individuals with more advanced cognitive impairment such as dementia or MCI-EF domain.

An obvious target for cognitive intervention with seniors has been memory, although as the literature indicates, there is mixed evidence for its relationship to daily functioning. Belleville (2008) reviewed the current literature on memory-based interventions in MCI. She surveyed seven published studies examining the effects of cognitive training (primarily memory), many of which demonstrated significant improvements in subjective and/or objective memory measures with moderate to large effect sizes. However, the studies surveyed had several limitations: often there was no comparable control group, sample sizes were small thereby limiting power, there was minimal longitudinal follow-up and, most importantly, there was no subjective or objective evidence of improvement in functional status as a result of memory training.

Finally, Ball, Edwards, and Ross (2007) provide evidence for transfer of training following a processing speed intervention in older adults. Specifically, they reviewed evidence for six studies using the same processing speed intervention and its impact on both basic cognitive and everyday abilities. The intervention consisted of trainer-guided practice on computerized training exercises involving target detection, identification, discrimination, and localization, with the aim of increasing mental processing speed as opposed to psychomotor reaction time. Training provided post-test gains on the Useful Field of View (UFOV) test, a computerized measure of selective and divided attention (Ball et al. 1988; Sims et al. 1998) previously noted to hold predictive validity for driving ability (Clay et al. 2005) as well as other everyday abilities as measured by the Timed Instrumental Activities of Daily Living test. Most impressively, gains were maintained for at least two years post-intervention, with more efficient performance of IADLs and safer driving behaviours.

Timing of the intervention

Considering the work on cognitive reserve (Stern 2002; Suchy, Kraybill, and Franchow 2010), one might assume that the best time to intervene is when the individual can harness and strengthen existing skills and work on prevention of decline rather than restitution or compensation for already manifest impairment. Given that decline in IADLs is taken as one important diagnostic marker in the transition from normal to pathologic ageing (Gold 2012), preventing such decline could have dramatic consequences. Several decades of research have examined the use of cognitive intervention with healthy older adults. Lustig et al. (2009) surveyed the cognitive intervention literature with older adults, classifying interventions into strategy training, cognitive process training, multimodal programmes (i.e. cognitive plus psychosocial), and cardiovascular programmes. They concluded that multimodal programmes and those with the greatest variety in training exposures produced the greatest transfer of training effects. One such example, the Advanced Cognitive Training for Independent and Vital Elderly (ACTIVE) study was a large, multisite study conducted at six major ageing centres across the US, and involved close to 3000 healthy older American adults. In this RCT, seniors were randomized to one of three cognitive interventions (memory, processing speed, or reasoning training) or a no-contact control group. The intervention groups had ten sessions of treatment, approximately sixty to seventy-five minutes per session, with a proportion receiving four booster sessions approximately one year after the active intervention. A proportion of each group showed statistically significant, domain-specific improvement immediately after the intervention, with further gains made in the processing speed and reasoning groups following the booster sessions. While the cognitive gains were maintained at two years post-training (Ball et al. 2002) and maintained at five-year follow-up (Willis et al. 2006), no impact on everyday function was ascertained at two years, and all participants showed significant functional decline at five years, although less pronounced in the group that received training in reasoning and problem-solving.

In a more focal intervention, Troyer (2001) reported on a five-session, ten-hour memory intervention developed for cognitively intact seniors. The intervention was designed to provide psychoeducation about normal ageing and memory functions, increase use of compensatory strategies, and enhance memory self-efficacy. Pre/post-test comparisons indicated an improvement in knowledge about ageing, as well as an increased repertoire of available compensatory strategies, self-reported satisfaction with memory, and everyday memory ability. On objective testing, there was an improvement on a measure of prospective memory (PM) but not list learning. As noted previously, to the extent that PM is involved in everyday functioning, this intervention may hold promise in helping seniors institute strategies that may preserve current levels of function and delay decline.

A limitation of interventions with healthy individuals is that by definition they lack significant functional impairment. Thus, there is a ceiling effect limiting detection of improvement, unless individuals are followed longitudinally and there is comparison of relative rates of IADL decline between those who did and did not receive intervention. By contrast, individuals with MCI may present a unique group to target for intervention, as they may be showing some mild functional impairment but clearly not to the degree of that observed in individuals with diagnosed dementia (Albert et al. 2011). Thus, such intervention may delay the progression of functional decline and associated dementia. Again, this highlights the need for longitudinal studies that demonstrate that intervention reduces the rate and/or severity of decline in individuals with MCI as measured by self-report/informant and objective IADL measures, which unfortunately is often lacking (Belleville 2008).

Sitzer, Twamely, and Jeste (2006) performed a meta-analysis of the literature on cognitive training with individuals already diagnosed with Alzheimer's disease. They included seventeen high-quality studies in their analysis, fourteen of which used an RCT design. The greatest overall effect size for any one domain was observed for performance-based ADLs (Cohen's d = .69), based on two studies that used compensatory procedural memory strategies for performance of specific ADLs. However, these studies did not examine performance of untrained ADLs; thus, no evidence was available regarding transfer of training. While there was a moderate effect size for cognitive training on specific cognitive domains (d = .50), no studies that focused specifically on cognition provided evidence of improvement in performance-based ADLs, again raising the question of transfer of training from basic cognitive processes.

IMPLICATIONS FOR PRACTICE

In this chapter we have illuminated the complex relationship between cognitive decline and everyday functioning in older adults. Functional impairment can result in financial and social burden for the individual as well as impact the older adult's immediate support network, and has diagnostic and prognostic implications regarding impending dementia. Several important points bear emphasizing for the practising clinician:

Assessment considerations

A true picture of functional status can be difficult to ascertain based on self-report alone, given that performance is often influenced by contextual and intrapersonal (e.g. emotional state) factors. Where there is concern from the individual or an informant regarding a specific functional impairment, the clinician would be best served to conduct a targeted assessment on that specific domain of interest (e.g. finances), rather than to look at global functional status. In such an assessment, a convergence of evidence across multiple testing methods – i.e., standard neuropsychometric tests, relevant ecologically valid measures, performance-based measures, and informant report – is likely to portray a more accurate picture of functional status than using either method in isolation.

Intervention Considerations

Research supports the idea that older adults at various levels of cognitive compromise can engage in and benefit from cognitive intervention. That said, the level of functional impairment observed will provide specific guidance to the clinician regarding the type of intervention most likely to be beneficial. More specifically, where marked impairment already exists, task-specific routines acquired through procedural memory are likely to be most beneficial. If, however, significant impairment is not yet manifest, a preventative approach can be taken through multimodal rehabilitation training in EF that would transfer across a variety of complex IADLs. As noted, while general intellectual function correlates significantly with global IADL status, it also provides a proxy for cognitive reserve, which further speaks to the likelihood that an individual will be able to benefit from more complex intervention. Finally, it bears mentioning that one rate-limiting factor of the success of any intervention is an individual's level of motivation. Any intervention strategy will require the individual to engage actively in sustained practice at home in order to acquire new skills. Late-life depression can be associated with anhedonia and amotivation, and can significantly impact individual's ability to engage in cognitive intervention. Thus, it will be important to assess for any mood disorders and whether these warrant concurrent treatment. If not medically contraindicated, the individual might be considered for a trial of an atypical or 'activating' anti-depressant (e.g. Buproprion). The primary mechanism of action for such pharmacological agents is dopamine reuptake inhibition, particularly relevant in this context given that dopaminergic activation is associated with reward and reinforcement learning (Düzel et al. 2010; Wise 2004). Consultation with a geriatric psychiatrist or behavioural neurologist is likely to be instructive in this regard. As a further adjunct, the individual may benefit from a trial of cognitive-behaviour therapy (CBT) to examine automatic thoughts and core beliefs that could interfere with new skill acquisition. Specifically, it will be important to attend to the individual's beliefs regarding anticipated benefits (again related to motivation), as well as their sense of self-efficacy or their beliefs about their own ability to learn and make change—the latter in particular has been shown to be a significant predictor in who benefits from cognitive rehabilitation (Cicerone and Azulay 2007). The older adult can be referred for a separate course of CBT concurrent with cognitive intervention, or CBT strategies can be woven directly into the intervention itself.

SUMMARY

In summary, there appear to be hierarchical relations within ADL/IADL tasks, at least when global measures are considered, with complex IADL tasks such as shopping and financial management often affected early in the course of cognitive decline. There is ample evidence to indicate that specific cognitive functions are associated with successful

IADL performance over and above physical health status. Strong relations are seen with general intellectual function, EF, processing speed, and, more recently, PM. The literature on EM and IADLs is mixed, with some studies indicating a unique contribution while others suggest that the association is mediated by EF integrity. IADL deficits may begin in subtle degrees while older adults are relatively cognitively intact, and continue to progress as they advance along a continuum of pathological ageing to MCI and dementia. Given both the psychosocial impact on the individual and care-givers and the financial impact of loss of functional independence, there is an imperative to find means to intervene in the lives of older adults to promote IADL function and independent living as long as is possible. Encouragingly, a growing body of literature indicates that older adults at various levels of cognitive health or impairment can benefit from cognitive training. Given the relationship between cognition and IADL performance, one would expect that such training could show measurable benefit in independent functioning. Unfortunately, it is a major limitation of many, or even most, of the studies on cognitive intervention in older adults that they fail to use ecologically relevant assessment methods related to either cognition or IADL performance. Two major theoretical approaches to intervention exist: one focuses on targeting a specific activity and training that activity using procedural memory, while the other focuses on targeting strategic processes that may underlie execution of IADLs. While activity-specific interventions seem effective across varying degrees of cognitive impairment, there is typically no transfer of training beyond the specific task, and no strategies provided in managing deviations from the typical task routine. Studies focusing on processes such as processing speed and EF seem promising, but are often limited by failure to use performance-based or real-world measures of daily functioning. Finally, intervention can occur at different points in the continuum of cognitive decline; with studies on healthy older adults, in particular, there is a need for better longitudinal follow-up for a stronger proof of principle that training does, in fact, prevent or delay decline in everyday functioning. It is important to remember that cognition is only one determinant of everyday functional behaviours, albeit a very important one. Teasing apart the physical, cognitive, social cognitive, and other factors that affect performance on everyday tasks is an important challenge both in research investigations and in clinical practice.

Key References and Sources for Further Reading:

'Activities of Daily Living', *International Encyclopedia of Rehabilitation*. http://cirrie.buffalo. edu/encyclopedia/en/article/37/.

Alzheimer's Association (2012). *What We Know Today about Alzheimer's Disease*. http://www. alz.org/research/science/alzheimers_research.asp.

The American Congress on Rehabilitation Medicine (ACRM) has a recently formed special interest group (SIG) on geriatric rehabilitation. More information can be found at http:// www.acrm.org/acrm-communities/geriatrics.

Rotman Research Institute at Baycrest, Centre for Brain Fitness contains information on Goal Management Training and the Memory and Aging program. http://www.baycrest.org/ research/rotman-research-institute/centre-for-brain-fitness/.

REFERENCES

Albert, M. S. DeKosky, S. T., Dickson, D., Dubois, B., Feldman, H. H., et al. (2011). 'The Diagnosis of Mild Cognitive Impairment due to Alzheimer's Disease: Recommendations from the National Institute on Aging-Alzheimer Association Workgroups on Diagnostic Guidelines for Alzheimer's Disease'. *Alzheimer's & Dementia* 7: 270–279.

American Psychiatric Association (2000). *Diagnostic and Statistical Manual of Mental Disorders* (4th edn, text revision). Washington, DC: American Psychiatric Association.

American Psychiatric Association (2013). *Diagnostic and Statistical Manual of Mental Disorders*, (5th edn). Arlington, VA: American Psychiatric Association.

Aranda, M. P., Ray, L. A., Snih, S. A., Ottenbacher, K. J., and Markides, K. S. (2011). 'The Protective Effect of Neighborhood Composition on Increasing Frailty among Older Mexican Americans: A Barrio Advantage?' *Journal of Aging and Health* 23: 1189–1217.

Aretouli, E. and Brandt, J. (2009). 'Everyday Functioning in Mild Cognitive Impairment and its Relationship with Executive Cognition'. *International Journal of Geriatric Psychiatry* 25: 224–233.

Artero, S., Touchon, J., and Ritchie, K. (2001). 'Disability and Mild Cognitive Impairment: A Longitudinal Population-based Study'. *International Journal of Geriatric Psychiatry* 16: 1092–1097.

Baddeley, A. D. (1997). *Human Memory: Theory and Practice*. Hove: Psychology Press.

Ball, K., Beard, B. L., Roenker, D. L., Miller, R. L., and Griggs, D. S. (1988). 'Age and Visual Search: Expanding the Useful Field of View'. *Optics, Image Science, and Vision* 5: 2210–19.

Ball, K., Berch, D. B., Helmers, K. F., Jobe, J. D., Leveck, M. D., et al. (2002). 'Advanced Cognitive Training for Independent and Vital Elderly Study Group. Effects of Cognitive Training Interventions with Older Adults: A Randomized Controlled Trial'. *Journal of the American Medical Association* 288: 2271–81.

Ball, K., Edwards, J. D., and Ross, L. A. (2007). 'The Impact of Speed of Processing Training on Cognitive and Everyday Functions'. *Journals of Gerontology, Series B: Psychological Sciences and Social Sciences* 62(special issue 1): 19–31.

Baltes, P. B. and Baltes, M. M. (1990). 'Psychological Perspectives on Successful Aging: The Model of Selective Optimization with Compensation'. In P. B. Baltes and M. M. Baltes (eds), *Successful Aging: Perspectives from the Behavioral Sciences* (pp. 1–34). New York: Cambridge University Press.

Baltes, M. M., Wahl, H.-W., and Schmid-Furstoss, U. (1990). 'The Daily Life of Elderly Germans: Activity Patterns, Personal Control, and Functional Health'. *Journals of Gerontology, Series B: Psychological Sciences* 45: P173–P179.

Baltes, M. M., Mayr, U., Borchelt, M., Maas, I., and Wilms, H.-U. (1993). 'Everyday Competence in Old and Very Old Age: An Inter-disciplinary Perspective'. *Ageing and Society* 13: 657–80.

Bangen, K. J., Jak, A. J., Schiehser, D. M., Delano-Wood, L., Tuminello, E., et al. (2010). 'Complex Activities of Daily Living Vary by Mild Cognitive Impairment Subtype'. *Journal of the International Neuropsychological Society* 16(4): 630–639.

Barberger-Gateau, P., Dartigues, J.-F., and Letenneur, L. (1993). 'Four Instrumental Activities of Daily Living Score as a Predictor of One-year Incident Dementia'. *Age and Ageing* 22: 457–463.

Barberger-Gateau, P., Fabrigoule, C., Rouch, I., Letenneur, L., and Dartigues, J.-F. (1999). 'Neuropsychological Correlates of Self-reported Performance in Instrumental Activities of Daily Living and Prediction of Dementia'. *Journals of Gerontology, Series B: Psychological and Social Sciences* 54: P293–P303.

Belleville, S. (2008). 'Cognitive Training for Persons with Mild Cognitive Impairment'. *International Psychogeriatrics* 20: 57–66.

Bell-McGinty, S., Podell, K., Franzen, M., Baird, A. D., and Williams, M. J. (2002). 'Standard Measures of Executive Function in Predicting Instrumental Activities of Daily Living in Older Adults'. *International Journal of Geriatric Psychiatry* 17: 828–834.

Black, S. A. and Rush, R. D. (2002). 'Cognitive and Functional Decline in Adults Aged 75 and Older'. *Journal of the American Geriatrics Society* 50: 1978–1986.

Boyle, P. A., Malloy, P. F., Salloway, S., Cahn-Weiner, D., Cohen, R., et al. (2003). 'Executive Dysfunction and Apathy Predict Functional Impairment in Alzheimer Disease'. *American Journal of Geriatric Psychiatry* 11: 214–221.

Braver, T. S. and Barch, D. M. (2002). 'A Theory of Cognitive Control, Aging Cognition, and Neuromodulation'. *Neuroscience and Biobehavioral Reviews* 26: 809–817.

Brunswik, E. (1956). *Perception and the Representative Design of Psychological Experiments* (2nd edn). Berkeley: University of California Press.

Burgess, P. W., Alderman, N., Forbes, C., Costello, A., Coates, L. M., et al. (2006). 'The Case for Development and Use of 'Ecologically Valid' Measures of Executive Function in Experimental and Clinical Neuropsychology'. *Journal of the International Neuropsychological Society* 12: 194–209.

Burton, C. L., Strauss, E., Bunce, D., Hunter, M. A., and Hultsch, D. F. (2009). 'Functional Abilities in Older Adults with Mild Cognitive Impairment'. *Gerontology* 55: 570–581.

Cahn-Weiner, D. A., Boyle, P. A., and Malloy, P. F. (2002). 'Tests of Executive Function Predict Instrumental Activities of Daily Living in Community Dwelling Older Individuals'. *Applied Neuropsychology* 9: 187–191.

Cahn-Weiner, D. A., Farias, S. T., Julian, L., Harvey, D. J., Kramer, J. H., et al. (2007). 'Cognitive and Neuroimaging Predictors of Instrumental Activities of Daily Living'. *Journal of the International Neuropsychological Society* 13: 747–757.

Campo, M. and Chaudhury, H. (2012). 'Informal Social Interaction among Residents with Dementia in Special Care Units: Exploring the Role of Physical and Social Environments'. *Dementia* 11: 401–423.

Canadian Study of Health and Aging Working Group (1994). 'Canadian Study of Health and Aging: Study Methods and Prevalence of Dementia'. *Canadian Medical Association Journal* 150: 899–913.

Chaytor, N. and Schmitter-Edgecombe, M. (2003). 'The Ecological Validity of Neuropsychological Tests: A Review of the Literature on Everyday Cognitive Skills'. *Neuropsychology Review* 13: 181–197.

Cicerone, K. D., Levin, H., Malec, J., Stuss, D., and Whyte, J. (2006). 'Cognitive Rehabilitation Interventions for Executive Function: Moving from Bench to Bedside in Patients with Traumatic Brain Injury'. *Journal of Cognitive Neuroscience* 18: 1212–1222.

Cicerone, K. D. and Azulay, J. (2007). 'Perceived Self-efficacy and Life Satisfaction after Traumatic Brain Injury'. *Journal of Head Trauma Rehabilitation* 22: 257–266.

Cicerone, K. D., Langenbahn, D. M., Braden, C., Malec, J. F., Kalmar, K., et al. (2011). 'Evidence-based Cognitive Rehabilitation: Updated Review of the Literature from 2003–2008'. *Archives of Physical Medicine and Rehabilitation* 92: 519–30.

Clare, L., Woods, R. T., Moniz Cook, E. D., Orrell, M., and Spector, A. (2005). 'Cognitive Rehabilitation and Cognitive Training for Early-stage Alzheimer's Disease and Vascular Dementia'. *Cochrane Review* 2.

Clay, O. J., Wadley, V. G., Edwards, J. D., Roth, D. L., Roenker, D. L., et al. (2005). 'Cumulative Meta-analysis of the Relationship between Useful Field of View and Driving Performance in Older Adults: Current and Future Implications'. *Optometry and Vision Sciences* 82: 724–731.

Cramer, K., Tuokko, H., Mateer, C. A., and Hultsch, D. F. (2004). 'Measuring Awareness of Financial Skills: Reliability and Validity of a New Measure'. *Aging & Mental Health* 8: 161–171.

Crosson, B., Poeschel Barco, P., Velozo, C. A., Bolesta, M. M., Cooper, P. V., et al. (1989). 'Awareness and Compensation in Postacute Head Injury Rehabilitation'. *Journal of Head Trauma Rehabilitation* 4: 46–54.

Cullum, C. M., Saine, K., Chan, L., Martin-Cook, K., Gray, K. F., et al. (2001). 'Performance-based Instrument to Assess Functional Capacity in Dementia: The Texas Functional Living Scale'. *Neuropsychiatry, Neuropsychology, and Behavioral Neurology* 14: 103–108.

Delis, D. C., Kaplan, E., and Kramer, J. H. (2001). *Delis-Kaplan Executive Function System: Technical Manual*. San Antonio, TX: Harcourt Assessment Company.

Diehl, M., Willis, S. L., and Schaie, K. W. (1995). 'Everyday Problem Solving in Older Adults: Observational Assessment and Cognitive Correlates'. *Psychology & Aging* 10: 478.

Diehl, M. (1998). 'Everyday Competence in Later Life: Current Status and Future Directions'. *Gerontologist* 38: 422–433.

Doble, S. E., Fisk, J. D., and Rockwood, K. (1998). 'Identifying ADL Changes in the Early Stages of Cognitive Impairment'. *Gerontologist* 38: 114–115.

Duffy, M. E. and MacDonald, E. (1990). 'Determinants of Functional Health of Older Persons'. *Gerontologist* 30: 503–509.

Düzel, E., Bunzeck, N., Guitart-Masip, M., and Düzel, S. (2010). 'Novelty-related Motivation of Anticipation and Exploration by Dopamine (NOMAD): Implications for Healthy Aging'. *Neuroscience & Biobehavioral Reviews* 34: 660–669.

Earnst, K. S., Wadley, V. G., Aldridge, T. M., Steenwyk, A. B., Hammond, A. E., et al. (2001). 'Loss of Financial Capacity in Alzheimer's Disease: The Role of Working Memory'. *Aging and Neuropsychology* 8: 109–119.

Ebly, E. M., Hogan, D. B., and Parhad, I. M. (1995). 'Cognitive Impairment in the Non-demented Elderly. Results from the Canadian Study of Health and Aging'. *Archives of Neurology* 52: 612–619.

Farias, S. T., Mungas, D., Reed, B. R., Harvey, D., Cahn-Weiner, D., et al. (2006). 'MCI is Associated with Deficits in Everyday Functioning'. *Alzheimer Disease and Associated Disorders* 20: 217–223.

Farias, S. T., Mungas, D., Reed, B. R., Cahn-Weiner, D., Jagust, W., et al. (2008). 'The Measurement of Everyday Cognition (ECog): Scale Development and Psychometric Properties'. *Neuropsychology* 22: 531–544.

Farias, S. T., Cahn-Weiner, D. A., Harvey, D. J., Reed, B. R., Mungas, D., et al. (2009). 'Longitudinal Changes in Memory and Executive Functioning are Associated with Longitudinal Change in Instrumental Activities of Daily Living in Older Adults'. *Applied Neuropsychology* 23: 446–461.

Fish, J., Wilson, B. A., and Manly, T. (2010). 'The Assessment and Rehabilitation of Prospective Memory Problems in People with Neurological Disorders: A Review'. *Neuropsychological Rehabilitation* 20: 161–179.

Fleming, J. M., Strong, J., and Ashton, R. (1996). 'Self-awareness of Deficits in Adults with Traumatic Brain Injury: How Best to Measure?' *Brain Injury* 10: 1–15.

Freund, A. (2008). 'Successful Aging as Management of Resources: The Role of Selection, Optimization, and Compensation'. *Research in Human Development* 5: 94–106.

Gold, D. A. (2012). 'An Examination of Instrumental Activities of Daily Living Assessment in Older Adults and Mild Cognitive Impairment'. *Journal of Clinical and Experimental Neuropsychology* 34: 11–34.

Grace, J. and Molloy, P. F. (2001). *Frontal Systems Behavior Scale (FrSBe)*. Lutz, FL: Psychological Assessment Resources.

Graham, J. E., Rockwood, K., Beattie, B. L., Eastwood, R., Gauthier, S., et al. (1997). 'Prevalence and Severity of Cognitive Impairment with and without Dementia in an Elderly Population'. *Lancet* 349: 1793–1796.

Greenwood, P. M. (2007). 'Functional Plasticity in Cognitive Aging: Review and Hypothesis'. *Neuropsychology* 21: 657–673.

Griffith, L., Raina, P., Wu, H., Zhu, B., and Stathokostas, L. (2010). 'Population Attributable Risk for Functional Disability Associated with Chronic Conditions in Canadian Older Adults'. *Age and Ageing* 39: 738–745.

Hall, J. R., Vo, H. T. Johnson, L. A., Barber, R. C., and O'Bryant, S. E. (2011). 'The Link between Cognitive Measures and ADLs and IADL Functioning in Mild Alzheimer's: What Has Gender Got to Do with it?' *International Journal of Alzheimer's Disease.* doi:10.4061/2011/276734.

Henry, J. D., MacLeod, M. S., Phillips, L. H., and Crawford, J. R. (2004). 'A Meta-analytic Review of Prospective Memory and Aging'. *Psychology and Aging* 19: 27–39.

Hinkin, C. H., Castellon, S. A., Durvasula, R. S., Barber, R. C., and O'Bryant, S. E. (2002). 'Medication Adherence among HIV+ Adults: Effects of Cognitive Dysfunction and Regimen'. *Neurology* 59: 1944–1950.

Hoskin, K. M., Jackson, M., and Crowe, S. F. (2005). 'Can Neuropsychological Assessment Predict Capacity to Manage Personal Finances? A Comparison between Brain Impaired Individuals with and without Administrators'. *Psychiatry, Psychology, and the Law* 12: 56–67.

Hughes, T. F., Chang, C. C., Bilt, J. V., Snitz, B. E., and Ganguli, M. (2012). 'Mild Cognitive Deficits and Everyday Functioning among Older Adults in the Community: The Monongahela-Youghiogheny Healthy Aging Team Study'. *American Journal of Geriatric Psychiatry* (epub ahead of print).

Huppert, F. A. and Beardsall, L. (1993). 'Prospective Memory Impairment as an Early Indicator of Dementia'. *Journal of Clinical and Experimental Neuropsychology* 15: 805–821.

Iwarsson, S. (2012). 'Implementation of Research-based Strategies to Foster Person-environment Fit in Housing Environments: Challenges and Experiences during 20 Years'. *Journal of Housing for the Elderly* 26: 62–71.

Jefferson, A. L., Paul, R. H., Ozonoff, A., and Cohen, R. A. (2006). 'Evaluating Elements of Executive Functioning as Predictors of Instrumental Activities of Daily Living (IADLs)'. *Archives of Clinical Neuropsychology* 21: 311–320.

Jeste, D. V., Dunn, L. B., Palmer, B. W., Saks, E., Halpain, M., et al. (2003). 'A Collaborative Model for Research on Decisional Capacity and Informed Consent in Older Patients with Schizophrenia: Bioethics Unit of a Geriatric Psychiatry Intervention Research Center'. *Psychopharmacology* 171: 68–74.

Johnson, J. K., Lui, L.-Y., and Yaffe, K. (2007). 'Executive Function, More than Global Cognition, Predicts Functional Decline and Mortality in Elderly Women'. *Journals of Gerontology, Series A: Biological Sciences and Medical Sciences* 62: 1134–1141.

Katz, S., Ford, A. B., Moskowitz, R. W., Jackson, B. A., and Jaffee, M. W. (1963). 'Studies of Illness in the Aged. The Index of ADL: A Standardized Measure of Biological and Psychological Function'. *Journal of the American Medical Association* 185: 94–101.

Kester, J. D., Benjamin, A. S., Castel, A. D., and Craik, F. I. M. (2002). 'Memory in Elderly People'. In A. Baddeley, B. Wilson, and M. Kopelman (eds), *Handbook of Memory Disorder* (pp. 543–567). Chichester: Wiley.

Korner-Bitensky, N., Gelinas, I., Man-Son-Hing, M., and Marshall, S. (2005). 'Recommendations of the Canadian Consensus Conference on Driving Evaluation in Older Drivers'. *Physical and Occupational Therapy in Geriatrics* 23: 123–144.

Lawton, M. P. (1989). 'Behavior-relevant Ecological Factors'. In K. W. Schaie and C. Schooler (eds), *Social Structure and Aging: Psychological Processes* (pp. 57–78). Hillsdale, NJ: Erlbaum.

Lawton, M. P. and Brody, E. M. (1969). 'Assessment of Older People: Self-maintaining and Instrumental Activities of Daily Living'. *Gerontologist* 9: 179–185.

Levine, B., Robertson, I. H., Clare, L., Carter, G., Hong, J., et al. (2000). 'Rehabilitation of Executive Function: An Experimental-clinical Validation of Goal Management Training'. *Journal of the International Neuropsychological Society* 6: 299–312.

Levine, B., Stuss, D. T., Winocur, G., Binns, M. A., Fahy, L., et al. (2007). 'Cognitive Rehabilitation in the Elderly: Effects on Strategic Behavior in Relation to Goal Management'. *Journal of the International Neuropsychological Society* 13: 143–52.

Levine, B., Schweizer, T. A., O'Connor, C., Turner, G., Gillingham, S., et al. (2011). 'Rehabilitation of Executive Functioning in Patients with Frontal Lobe Brain Damage with Goal Management Training'. *Frontiers in Human Neuroscience* 5(9). doi: 10.3389/fnhum.2011.00009.

Lewis, M. S. and Miller, L. S.(2007). 'Executive Control Functioning and Functional Ability in Older Adults'. *The Clinical Neuropsychologist* 21: 274–285.

Lindstrom-Forneri, W., Tuokko, H., Garrett, D., and Molnar, F. (2010). 'Driving as an Everyday Competence: A Model of Driving Competence and Behavior'. *Clinical Gerontologist* 33: 283–297.

Lobo, A., Launer, L. J., Fratigliono, L., Andersen, K., Di Carlo, A., et al. (2000). 'Prevalence of Dementia and Major Subtypes in Europe: A Collaborative Study of Population-based Cohorts. Neurologic Disease in the Elderly Research Group'. *Neurology* 54: S4–S9.

Loewenstein, D. and Acevedo, A. (2009). 'The Relationship between Instrumental Activities of Daily Living and Neuropsychological Performance'. In T. D. Marcotte and I. Grant (eds), *Neuropsychology of Everyday Functioning* (pp. 93–112). New York: Guilford Press.

Lustig, C., Shah, P., Seidler, R., and Reuter-Lorenz, P. (2009). 'Aging, Training, and the Brain: A Review and Future Directions'. *Neuropsychology Review* 19: 504–522.

McDaniel, M. A. and Einstein, G. O. (2000). 'Strategic and Automatic Processes in Prospective Memory Retrieval: A Multiprocess Framework'. *Applied Cognitive Psychology* 14: S127–S144.

Marcotte, T. D., Scott, J. C., Kamat, R., and Heaton, R. K. (2009). 'Neuropsychology and the Prediction of Everyday Functioning'. In T. D. Marcotte and I. Grant (eds), *Neuropsychology of Everyday Functioning* (pp. 5–38). New York: Guilford Press.

Marsiske, M. and Willis, S. L. (1995). 'Dimensionality of Everyday Problem Solving in Older Adults'. *Psychology & Aging* 10: 269–283.

Milberg, W. P., Hebben, N., and Kaplan, E. (2009). 'The Boston Process Approach to Neuropsychological Assessment'. In I. Grant and K. M. Adams (eds), *Neuropsychological Assessment of Neuropsychiatric and Neuromedical Disorders* (3rd edn; pp. 42–65). New York: Oxford University Press.

Mitchell, M. and Miller, L. S. (2008). 'Prediction of Functional Status in Older Adults: The Ecological Validity of Four Delis-Kaplan Executive Function System Subtests'. *Journal of Clinical and Experimental Neuropsychology* 30: 683–690.

Njegovan, V., Man-Son-Hing, M., Mitchell, S. L., and Molnar, F. J. (2001). 'The Hierarchy of Functional Loss Associated with Cognitive Decline in Older Persons'. *Journals of Gerontology, Series A: Biological and Medical Sciences* 56: M638–M643.

Norman, D. A. and Shallice, T. (1986). 'Attention to Action: Willed and Automatic Control of Behavior'. In R. J. Davidson, G. E. Schwarts, and D. Shapiro (eds), *Consciousness and Self-regulation: Advances in Research and Therapy* (pp. 1–18). New York: Plenum.

Northern California Neurobehavioral Group (1988). *Manual for the Neurobehavioral Cognitive Status Exam*. Fairfax, CA: Northern California Neurobehavioral Group.

Nygård, L., Pantzar, M., Uppgard, B., and Kottorp, A. (2012). 'Detection of Activity Limitations in Older Adults with MCI or Alzheimer's Disease through Evaluation of Perceived Difficulty in Use of Everyday Technology: A Replication Study'. *Aging & Mental Health* 16: 3612–3371.

Orellano, E., Colon, W. I., and Arbesman, M. (2012). 'Effect of Occupation and Activity-based Interventions on Instrumental Activities of Daily Living Performance among Community-dwelling Older Adults: A Systematic Review'. *American Journal of Occupational Therapy* 66: 292–300.

Peres, K., Helmer, C., Amiela, H., Orgogozo, J. M., Rouch, I., et al. (2008). 'Natural History of Decline in Instrumental Activities of Daily Living Performance over the 10 Years Preceding Clinical Diagnosis of Dementia: A Prospective Population-based Study'. *Journal of the American Geriatrics Society* 56: 37–44.

Petersen, R. C., Smith, G. E., Waring, S. C., Ivnik, R. J., Kokmen, E., et al. (1997). 'Aging, Memory, and Mild Cognitive Impairment'. *International Psychogeriatrics* 9(suppl. 1): 65–9.

Petersen, R. C., Smith, G. E., Waring, S. C., Ivnik, R. J., Tangalos, E. G., et al. (1999). 'Mild Cognitive Impairment: Clinical Characterization and Outcome'. *Archives of Neurology* 56: 303–308.

Petersen, R. C. (2004). 'Mild Cognitive Impairment as a Diagnostic Entity'. *Journal of Internal Medicine* 256: 183–194.

Purser, J. L., Fillenbaum, G. G., Pieper, C. F., and Wallace, R. B. (2005). 'Mild Cognitive Impairment and 10 Year Trajectories of Disability in the Iowa Established Populations for Epidemiologic Studies in the Elderly Cohort'. *Journal of the American Geriatrics Society* 53: 1966–1972.

Putzke, J. D., Williams, M. A., Daniel, F., Bourge, R. C., and Boll, T. J. (2000). 'Activities of Daily Living among Heart Transplant Candidates: Neuropsychological and Cardiac Function Predictors'. *Journal of Heart and Lung Transplantation* 19: 995–1006.

Rabin, L. A., Borgos, M. J., Saykin, A. J., Wishart, H. A., Crane, P. K., et al. (2007a). 'Judgment in Older Adults: Development and Psychometric Evaluation of the Test of Practical Judgment (TOP-J)'. *Journal of Clinical and Experimental Neuropsychology* 29: 752–767.

Rabin, L. A., Burton, L. A., and Barr, W. B. (2007b). 'Utilization Rates of Ecologically Oriented Instruments among Clinical Neuropsychologists'. *Clinical Neuropsychologist* 21: 727–743.

Raskin, S. and Buckheit, C. (2010). *Memory for Intentions Test*. Lutz, FL: Psychological Assessment Resources.

Ritchie, L. J. and Tuokko, H. (2010). 'Patterns of Cognitive Decline, Conversion Rates, & Predictive Validity for Three Models of MCI'. *American Journal of Alzheimer's Disease and Other Dementias* 25(7): 592–603.

Rizzo, M. and Kellison, I. (2009). 'The Brain on the Road'. In T. D. Marcotte and I. Grant (eds), *Neuropsychology of Everyday Functioning* (pp. 168–208). New York: Guilford Press.

Robertson, I. H., Ward, T., Ridgeway, V., and Nimmo-Smith, I. (1996). 'The Structure of Normal Human Attention: The Test of Everyday Attention'. *Journal of the International Neuropsychological Society* 2: 525–534.

Rodin, J., Timko, C., and Harris, S. (1985). 'The Construct of Control'. In M. P. Lawton (ed.), *Annual Review of Gerontology and Geriatrics* (vol. 6; pp. 3–55). New York: Springer.

Royall, D. R., Palmer, R., Chiodo, L. K., and Polk, M. J. (2005). 'Executive Control Mediates Memory's Association with Change in Instrumental Activities of Daily Living: The Freedom House Study'. *Journal of the American Geriatrics Society* 53: 11–17.

Royall, D. R., Lauterbach, E. C., Kaufer, D., Malloy, P., Coburn, K. L., et al. (2007). 'The Cognitive Correlates of Functional Status: A Review from the Committee on Research of the

American Neuropsychiatric Association'. *Journal of Neuropsychiatry & Clinical Neurosciences* 19: 249–265.

Schaie, K. W. and Willis, S. L. (1999). 'Theories of Everyday Competence and Aging'. In V. L. Bengtson and K. W. Schaie (eds), *Handbook of Theories of Aging* (pp. 174–195). New York: Springer.

Schmitter-Edgecombe, M., Woo, E., and Greeley, D. R. (2009). 'Characterizing Multiple Memory Deficits and their Relation to Everyday Functioning in Individuals with Mild Cognitive Impairment'. *Neuropsychology* 23: 168–177.

Sims, R. V., Owsley, C., Allman, R. M., Ball, K., and Smoot, T. M. (1998). 'A Preliminary Assessment of the Medical and Functional Factors Associated with Vehicle Crashes by Older Adults'. *Journal of the American Geriatrics Society* 46: 556–561.

Sitzer, D. I., Twamley, E. W., and Jeste, D. V. (2006). 'Cognitive Training in Alzheimer's Disease: A Meta-analysis of the Literature'. *Acta Psychiatrica Scandinavica* 114: 75–90.

Sohlberg, M. M. and Mateer, C. A. (2001). 'Management of Dysexecutive Symptoms'. In *Cognitive Rehabilitation: An Integrative Neuropsychological Approach* (2nd edn; pp. 230–268). New York: Guilford Press.

Spooner, D. M. and Pachana, N. A. (2006). 'Ecological Validity in Neuropsychological Assessment: A Case for Greater Consideration in Research with Neurologically Intact Populations'. *Archives of Clinical Neuropsychology* 21: 326–337.

Steen, G, Sonn, U., Hanson, A. B., and Steen, B. (2001). 'Cognitive Function and Functional Ability. A Cross-sectional and Longitudinal Study at Ages 85 and 95 in a Non-demented Population'. *Aging: Clinical and Experimental Research* 13: 68–77.

Stern, R. A. and White, T. (2003). *Neuropsychological Assessment Battery: Administration, Scoring, and Interpretation Manual*. Lutz, FL: Psychological Assessment Resources.

Stern, Y. (2002). 'What is Cognitive Reserve? Theory and Research Application of the Reserve Concept'. *Journal of the International Neuropsychological Society* 8: 448–460.

Stout, J., Wyman, M., Johnson, S., Peavy, G., and Salmon, D. (2003). 'Frontal Behavioral Syndromes and Functional Status in Probable Alzheimer Disease'. *American Journal of Geriatric Psychiatry* 11: 683–686.

Stuss, D. T., Robertson, I. H., Craik, F. I. M., Levine, B., Alexander, M. P., et al. (2007). 'Cognitive Rehabilitation in the Elderly: A Randomized Trial to Evaluate a New Protocol'. *Journal of the International Neuropsychological Society* 13: 120–131.

Suchy, Y., Kraybill, M. L., and Franchow, E. (2010). 'Instrumental Activities of Daily Living among Community-dwelling Older Adults: Discrepancies between Self-report and Performance are Mediated by Cognitive Reserve'. *Journal of Clinical and Experimental Neuropsychology* 33: 92–100.

Tam, C. W. C., Lam, L. C. W., Chiu, H. F. K., and Lui, V. W. C. (2007). 'Characteristic Profiles of Instrumental Activities of Daily Living in Chinese Older Persons with Mild Cognitive Impairment'. *American Journal of Alzheimer's Disease and Other Dementias* 22: 211–217.

Troyer, A. K. (2001). 'Improving Memory Knowledge, Satisfaction, and Functioning via an Education and Intervention Program for Older Adults'. *Aging, Neuropsychology, & Cognition* 8: 256–268.

Troyer, A. K. and Murphy, K. J. (2007). 'Memory for Intentions in Amnestic Mild Cognitive Impairment: Time and Event-based Prospective Memory'. *Journal of the International Neuropsychological Society* 13: 365–369.

Tuokko, H., Morris, C., and Ebert, P. (2005). 'Mild Cognitive Impairment and Everyday Functioning in Older Adults'. *Neurocase* 11: 40–47.

Van Wielingen, L., Tuokko, H., Cramer, K., Mateer, C., and Hultsch, D. (2004). 'Awareness of Financial Skills in Dementia'. *Aging & Mental Health* 8: 374–380.

Verbrugge, L. M. and Jette, A. M. (1994). 'The Disablement Process'. *Social Science & Medicine* 38: 1–14.

Wadley, V. G., Crowe, M., Marsiske, M., Cook, S. E., Unverzagt, F. W., et al. (2007). 'Changes in Everyday Functioning among Individuals with Psychometrically Defined Mild Cognitive Impairment in the Advanced Cognitive Training for Independent and Vital Elderly Study'. *Journal of the American Geriatrics Society* 55(8): 1192–1198.

Willis, S. L. (1991). 'Cognition and Everyday Competence'. In K. W. Schaie and M. P. Lawton (eds), *Annual Review of Gerontology and Geriatrics* (vol. 11; pp. 80–109). New York: Springer.

Willis, S. L. and Marsiske, M. (1993). *Manual for the Everyday Problems Test*. University Park, PA: The Pennsylvania State University.

Willis, S. L. (1996). 'Assessing Everyday Competence in the Cognitively Challenged Elderly'. In M. A. Smyer and K. W. Schaie (eds), *Older Adults' Decision-making and the Law* (pp. 87–127). New York: Springer.

Willis, S. L., Tennstedt, S. L., Marsiske, M., Ball, K., Elias, J., et al. (2006). 'ACTIVE Study Group: Long-term Effects of Cognitive Training on Everyday Functional Outcomes in Older Adults'. *Journal of the American Medical Association* 296: 2805–2814.

Wilson, B. A., Cockburn, J., and Baddeley, A. D. (1985). *The Rivermead Behavioural Memory Test*. Reading: Thames Valley Test.

Wilson, B. A., Baddeley, A., Evans, J. J., and Shiel, A. J. (1994). 'Errorless Learning in the Rehabilitation of Memory Impaired People'. *Neuropsychological Rehabilitation* 4: 307–326.

Wilson, B. A., Alderman, N., Burgess, P. W., Emslie, H., and Evans, J. J. (1996). *Behavioral Assessment of the Dysexecutive Syndrome (BADS)*. Bury St. Edmunds: Thames Valley Test Company.

Wise, R. A. (2004). 'Dopamine, Learning and Motivation'. *Nature Reviews Neuroscience* 5: 483–494.

Woods, S. P., Weinborn, M., Velnoweth, A., Rooney, A., and Bucks, R. S. (2012). 'Memory for Intentions is Uniquely Associated with Instrumental Activities of Daily Living in Healthy Older Adults'. *Journal of the International Neuropsychological Society* 18: 134–138.

World Health Organization (1993). *The ICD-10 Classification of Mental and Behavioural Disorders: Diagnostic Criteria for Research*. Geneva: WHO.

World Health Organization (2001). *International Classification of Functioning, Disability and Health: ICF*. Geneva: WHO.

Zahodne, L. B. and Tremont, G. (2012). 'Unique Effects of Apathy and Depression Signs on Cognition and Function in Amnestic Mild Cognitive Impairment'. *International Journal of Geriatric Psychiatry* 28(1): 50–56. doi: 10.1002/gps.3789.

CHAPTER 16

OLDER ADULTS AND LONG-TERM CARE

Trends and Challenges in Mental Health Treatment

ELIZABETH VONGXAIBURANA, VICTOR MOLINARI, AND KATHRYN HYER

INTRODUCTION

THIS chapter addresses the challenges faced by the international community in planning to satisfy the mental health needs of the long-term care (LTC) population, especially those living in nursing homes. We first discuss international trends in LTC, followed by segments on financial considerations, general barriers to quality mental healthcare, and LTC staffing issues. Given the high prevalence of mental health problems in nursing homes documented over the years (Bartels, Moak, and Dums 2002; Burns et al. 1993), these sections then set the stage for a discussion of how best to provide quality mental healthcare in LTC institutional settings, particularly the necessity of employing adequately trained staff to conduct mental health screening as the basis for proper treatment. Comprehensive person-centered biopsychosocial care must be a guiding framework for true 'culture change' that promotes quality of life and personal growth rather than mere survival for our oldest and most frail adults. Irrespective of citizenship or culture, people prefer to live out their lives in their own home and in the manner to which they are accustomed. Frequently termed 'ageing in place', the concept highlights the idea that despite some limitations, older adults prefer to continue to be part of a community and/or family group, and follow usual routines and life-style preferences for as long as possible. However, when circumstances arise necessitating assistive care, such as physical limitation due to age-related illness, injury, or cognitive decline, those services may be provided in the individual's home or in a variety of other settings.

As defined by the World Health Organization (WHO) in *Lessons for Long-term Care Policy* (2002a: 15), LTC is 'personal care (e.g. bathing and grooming)' provided to people 'not fully capable of self-care on a long-term basis'. For our purposes, LTC is defined as care delivered to frail older adults because of their need for assistance in activities of daily living

(ADLs), which include toileting, transferring, and eating. While most of this type of care is delivered at home, institutionalized care is often viewed as synonymous with the term LTC. Institutionalized care is indeed an important component of LTC because it addresses the multiple needs of the most frail and often impoverished older adults. Known by several names, including residential aged care facilities (RACFs), assisted living facilities (ALFs), nursing homes (NHs), care homes, and care homes with nursing, LTC settings may be government-sponsored or private entities that are largely unregulated. Depending on severity of resident condition, service provision, and regulation of the facilities, payment for those services will vary by type of facility and government reimbursement policies. For the purposes of discussion, we will use the term 'LTC facilities' to encompass all types of care homes.

Alzheimer's disease (AD) has risen from the eighth leading cause of death in 2002 (Anderson and Smith 2005) to the sixth in 2009 (Kochanek et al. 2011). Recognizing the challenge of rising life expectancy amidst escalating dementia-related impairment in old age, the G8 Public Health Ministers held a dementia summit in December 2013 (Alzheimer's Disease International, 2013) to coincide with the G8 economic conference. Noting the rising prevalence for those at risk of dementia which outpaces resources allocated to cope with the epidemic the G8 countries agreed to work together to approach the epidemic. An earlier Alzheimer's Disease International World Alzheimer Report (2010) on the global economic impact of dementia calls attention to the financial urgency associated with increasing frailty: in 2010, the approximate overall dementia-related expenditures were $604 billion USD, with nearly 70% of this price tag borne by Western European and North American nations. In fact, 'if dementia were a company, it would be the world's largest by annual revenue exceeding Wal-Mart (US $414 billion) and Exxon Mobil (US $311 billion)' (2010: 5). The Report further underscores the impact of dementia worldwide, as the immense cost to society already adversely affects worldwide health and social care institutions and individual families, yet remains wholly under-appreciated. Although a recent article suggests a projected decline in dementia due to the reduced risk of later born cohorts in England and Wales, major societal concerns will continue for the foreseeable future (Matthews et al. 2013).

Panza et al. (2011) note the connection between frailty, an overall increased state of weakened defences representative of system decline, and unfavourable health outcomes and cognition. Current understanding of frailty entails a broader conceptualization than previously considered, encompassing not only the physical, but psychosocial spheres as well (711). As such, the authors state that cognitive decline is an element of frailty, and that there is a connection between physical frailty and dementia (711). Occurrence of AD and mild cognitive impairment indeed is associated with physical frailty (in Panza et al. 2011; respectively, Buchman et al. 2008; Boyle et al. 2010). A positive link between nutritional status and cognitive functioning has also been found, even among a 'well-nourished' community sample (La Rue et al. 1997). The need for increasing degrees of assistive care arises and only intensifies from this confluence. Reasons for supported care can range from assistance with instrumental ADLs such as preparing meals or driving to the need for continuous supervision and complete personal care. As the personal care needs of individuals increase, these needs may be met through informal care, or a range of formal community or institutional LTC services scattered throughout varied physical locations commensurate with those needs.

The increase in longevity and in numbers of older people presents many challenges to LTC and mental health service providers. A UN report on *World Population Aging, 1950–2050* notes that the global trend of population ageing is 'unprecedented, pervasive, and enduring', with the oldest old (those aged 80 and older) being the fastest-growing demographic worldwide (WHO 2001). *An Aging World: 2008* by Kinsella and Wan (2009) further affirms worldwide population ageing concerns. The UN Population Fund and HelpAge International (2012) highlight that individuals aged 60 plus will increase from 11% to 20% of the population by 2050; this group cautions that this unprecedented longevity bears multiple challenges. Yet how are the mental health needs of this burgeoning, vulnerable population addressed? This chapter examines older adults' mental health and quality of life in the current LTC environment. We will discuss how regardless of culture, there are some recurring themes concerning the important role of family and financing in promoting the quality of life for LTC residents of all nations.

Availability and provision of LTC services vary substantially by country. It is short-sighted to believe that only industrialized countries need LTC policies: A 2002 WHO report, *Lessons for Long-term Care Policy*, notes that requirements for LTC in developing nations will soon outpace their industrialized counterparts (WHO 2002a). We acknowledge and provide evidence throughout the chapter that this decade-old prediction is indeed coming to pass. Katz (2011) notes that NHs are a staple of LTC in developed countries; this trend is expected to be maintained in developing countries. The WHO (2002a) details developing countries' need for LTC as determined by the degree of care required and by whether informal unpaid care-givers are available. Furthermore, the report speaks to the importance of promoting care strategies tailored specifically to a country's existing resources, regardless of income (WHO 2002a: 55). Worldwide, experts agree on the essential elements of care-giving, i.e. patient-centred care that meets individuals' needs, honours patient preference, and exhibits compassion. Tolson et al. (2011) described a 2010 international workshop convened to address the wide range of LTC environments and experiences. Assembled by the International Association of Gerontology and Geriatrics in collaboration with WHO, this gathering sought concordance on patient-centred strategies of care. Consensus statements on LTC highlighted person-centred care that is mindful of individuals' medical needs, preferences, and placed within the larger context framework of care-givers, families, communities, and society (Tolson et al. 2011: 185–188). We will discuss/develop this theme of biopsychosocial models of care in this chapter, as well as offer a view to the future of LTC with a focus on the most vulnerable LTC population, NH residents.

International Long-term Care Trends

'Ageing in place' is preferable to (and usually less expensive) than being uprooted from one's home and placed in a care facility; supports (such as in-home care) to extend community living are thereby encouraged. Informal care services can be provided by family or friends, regardless of payment. However, a constellation of factors have reduced the availability of informal care. Gibson et al. (2010) note that shifting family structures, the preference to have fewer children, and the tendency to live further away from one's family all have an effect on informal care provision, and/or contribute to its uncertainty.

In addition, individuals tapped to provide such care themselves may require informal emotional and physical support. Sinunu, Yount, and El Afify (2009) conducted a study of informal and formal LTC for frail Egyptians. These authors comment that the public healthcare system in the Middle East is poorly equipped to manage LTC. Demographic changes have caused families to adopt new strategies to manage the care of older adult family members related to competing economic demands and changes in the role of women in the workforce. Thus, the authors maintain that dependence on informal care cannot continue in the long term. Furthermore, trends in service delivery vary from nation to nation. Different priorities, customs, and accessibilities add to the challenges of service delivery (Gibson et al. 2010).

Considerations factored into the LTC equation are reflected in trends in service delivery for developing countries, as summarized in the WHO report (2002a). Ranging from absence of any official LTC programmes (Indonesia), to accelerated availability of home health services due to high rates of ageing (Shanghai and Beijing), to countries that have made home healthcare a main concern (Costa Rica), to others that are just in the early stages of such planning (Thailand, Mexico), varying priorities and resources are in play. For example, South Africa has had a unique development of community-based care as a reaction to the HIV/AIDS epidemic, exemplifying how the burden of a chronic, communicable disease intensifies the LTC challenge. WHO (2002a) further details broad trends seen in international LTC. Efforts to make home-based care available can be seen across the board: certain countries such as Lithuania, South Korea, and Ukraine offer a broad menu of options including 'home health, personal care, and homemaking' (WHO 2002a: 47). Extant home health is tied to the overall health system, on a monetary and administrative level; Costa Rica and South Korea have incorporated home health into 'primary care', as have to a lesser degree China, Lithuania, Mexico and Ukraine. NGOs (Non-Governmental Organizations) are assuming a significant role in expanding LTC in some countries, such as Mexico and Ukraine. This snapshot of LTC issues and concerns in developing countries underscores the need for cultural sensitivity and awareness of national/regional issues when organizing, planning, and executing LTC.

The 2010 World Bank report on LTC needs in European countries (Croatia, and more recent EU member states such as Bulgaria, Latvia, and Poland) also speaks of LTC struggles. Growing demand for LTC services by an increasingly dependent ageing population has resulted in steady growth in home/community-based care (2010: 2). Although supply has been increasing to meet the growing need for LTC availability, low financing nationwide for LTC will directly affect long-term sustainability. Building databases on LTC coverage to analyse overarching facts and trends will be helpful to guide international LTC public policy reform (World Bank 2010). Unfortunately, limited international data on LTC policy has emerged since the 2002 WHO report.

FINANCING

A common international theme in LTC financing is expenditures expressed as a proportion of one's gross domestic product (GDP): despite varying sources of payment and structure of reimbursement, many countries have comparable LTC spending (Katz 2011: 489). A 2011 report on supplying care-giving needs in OECD (The Organisation for Economic Co-operation and Development) countries (Colombo et al. 2011: 46–47) discusses the cost of LTC across twenty-nine countries, and makes recommendations for policy and approaches to address LTC in a cost-sustainable way. OECD countries share information on several fronts, including health and social policy, and are a useful comparative source of LTC resources and utilization. Although care funding and delivery vary internationally, data show public LTC spending outweighs private: in 2008, an average 1.5% of OECD countries' GDP was spent on LTC. See Table 16.1.

Switzerland's privately funded LTC stands out as the lone exception, weighing in at 60%; the US is at 40%, and Germany at 31%. Typically, the private segment of overall LTC spending is just about 15%; the overall private stake of healthcare expenditures weighs in at 25%. Public funding continues to be the primary source of LTC financial support in nearly all OECD nations (Huber et al. 2005), with private sources typically predominantly supportive of institutional, rather than at-home care-giving. Although countries may be comprised of differing age structures and utilize different public/private formats, cost containment and spending trends remain similar, with informal care continuing as a main resource of existing support.

What factors contribute to the high cost of public LTC provision? As populations get older and family care-giving resources diminish, demand for LTC services is increasing due to public demand for first-rate care, thereby raising pressure for public expenditures for LTC (Colombo et al. 2011). Though several variables are at play, Katz (2011: 489) suggests rising costs are a consequence of administrative overhead. Organizational and administrative expenses in the US and Canada illustrate the inconsistent prices of LTC: for NHs, $62 per capita and $29 per capita, respectively; for home care, $42 per capita and $13 per capita, respectively (Katz 2011; Woolhandler, Campbell, and Himmelstein 2003).

The public policy domain does not usually highlight LTC issues, save examples of public outrage, such as neglect or abuse (Nadash and Ahrens 2005); however, the swelling older adult population and its increasing burden of illness, disability, and healthcare cost will render these issues unavoidable (Nadash and Ahrens 2005; The World Bank 2010). Though longstanding, such matters will eventually reach a critical mass, emerging to the forefront of policy and legislation.

Barriers to Quality Mental Healthcare in General LTC

Many issues complicate mental health service provision in older people; as such, the challenge of delivering necessary care and services is of particular concern. Through the last decade, several assessments of geriatric mental health quality have been carried out via governing bodies, presidential commissions, and professional expert panels. At the heart of these inquiries is a genuine push to improve mental healthcare for older adults.

In 1999, a working group of the American Association for Geriatric Psychiatry issued a statement promoting the elevation of research on geriatric mental health services utilization into a formal scientific field (Borson et al. 2001: 192). Strategic issues involving mental

Table 16.1 The share of public LTC expenditure is higher than that of private LTC expenditure in OECD countries

Percentage of GDP 2008*

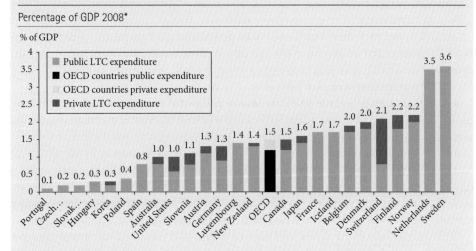

The share of public LTC expenditure is higher than that of private LTC expenditure in OECD countries
Percentage of GDP, 2008

Country	Public LTC expenditure (% GDP)	Private LTC expenditure (% GDP)	Total LTC expenditure (% GDP)	Year	Comments
Portugal			0.1	2006	nursing LTC only
Czech Republic	0.2		0.2	2008	nursing LTC only
Slovak Republic	0.2		0.2	2006	
Hungary	0.3		0.3	2008	nursing LTC only
Korea	0.2	0.1	0.3	2008	
Poland	0.4		0.4	2008	
Spain	0.6	0.2	0.8	2008	
Australia	0.8	0.2	1	2005	
United States	0.6	0.4	1	2008	nursing LTC only
Slovenia	0.8	0.3	1.1	2008	
Austria	1.1	0.2	1.3	2008	nursing LTC only
Germany	0.9	0.4	1.3	2008	
Luxembourg	1.4		1.4	2005	
New Zealand	1.3	0.1	1.4	2008	
OECD	1.2	0.3	1.5	2008	
Canada	1.2	0.3	1.5	2008	nursing LTC only
Japan	1.4	0.2	1.6	2008	
France	1.7		1.7	2008	
Iceland	1.7		1.7	2008	nursing LTC only
Belgium	1.7	0.2	2	2008	nursing LTC only
Denmark	1.8	0.2	2	2007	nursing LTC only
Switzerland	0.8	1.3	2.1	2007	nursing LTC only
Finland	1.8	0.4	2.2	2008	
Norway	2	0.2	2.2	2008	nursing LTC only
Netherlands	3.5		3.5	2008	
Sweden	3.6		3.6	2008	

health service delivery were emphasized, key concerns addressed, and vulnerable populations identified. Recommendations included promoting translational research, incorporating multimodal approaches within mental health treatment to span the LTC continuum, and introducing systems research in the healthcare arena.

In the US, the 2002 President's New Freedom Commission on Mental Health assessed the state of mental health for older Americans, evaluating efficiency, identifying unsatisfied areas, and determining what is lacking (Bartels 2003: 486). Four main areas were targeted for improvement: the disconnection between research and practice in mental healthcare; financial disincentives and the dearth of resources directed specifically at geriatric mental health; insufficient focus on psychiatric treatments that support full recovery; and lack of attention to interventions and services that prevent the mental health problems of older adults (Bartels 2003). Proposals for action were discussed to foster accessibility of older adults to the full spectrum of mental healthcare. Issues related to care-giver staff retention, and support for care-givers were also reviewed (Bartels 2003: 492–495). Despite a decade elapsing since this report, it is clear that much more work needs to be done to fulfil these goals.

In their consensus statement on how to enhance quality mental healthcare, the American Geriatrics Society and the American Association for Geriatric Psychiatry Expert Panel on Quality Mental Health Care in Nursing Homes issued policy recommendations emphasizing the management of depression and how to address dementia-related behavioural symptoms (2003a). Policy proposals to sustain valuable mental health services in LTC facilities were also issued by these organizations to reduce mental health problems in the targeted populations (2003a), and to influence LTC policies to promote access to services (2003b).

Staffing

Staffing and training of an LTC workforce are issues of global concern. The paucity of healthcare providers trained in geriatrics is one major issue in low quality care (Institute of Medicine 2008). Research indicates that despite a growing need for practitioners,

---

Note: Data for Austria, Belgium, Canada, the Czech Republic, Denmark, Hungary, Iceland, Norway, Portugal, Switzerland and the US refer only to health-related long-term care expenditure. In other cases, expenditure relates to both health-related (nursing) and social LTC expenditure. Social expenditures on LTC in the Czech Republic are estimated at 1% of GDP (Source: Czech Ministry of Health 2009). Data for Iceland and the US refer only to nursing LTC in institutions. Data for the US underestimate expenditure on fully private LTC arrangements. Data for Poland exclude infrastructure expenditure, amounting to about 0.25% of GDP in 2007. Data for the Netherlands do not reflect user co-payments, estimated at 8% of total AWBZ expenditure in 2007. Data for Australia refer to 2005; data for the Slovak Republic and Portugal refer to 2006; data for Denmark, Japan and Switzerland refer to 2007.

Source: Colombo, F. et al (2011), *Help Wanted? Providing and Paying for Long-Term Care*, OECD Publishing, http://www.oecd.org/health/longtermcare/helpwanted.

respect for geriatrics as a discipline has been slow in developing. Surveys of physicians have found that geriatrics is perceived to have less professional stature, while specialties such as neurosurgery and cardiology are at the top of the 'prestige hierarchy' (Album and Westin 2008; Norredam and Album 2007). The link between undesirability and choice of specialty has translated into a shortage of geriatricians: the current LTC environment is vastly underserved. In the US alone, 36 000 geriatricians will be needed by 2030 to care for the anticipated ageing boom, yet current numbers fall far short of this goal (Institute of Medicine 2008). Part of the problem emanates from the relatively low pay of geriatrics vis-à-vis other specialties, probably stemming from difficulties making diagnoses and formulating treatment plans based on lengthy medical histories, including multiple comorbid medical conditions and concomitant medications, all within the designated fifteen-minute insurance payment time frames. Thomas (2011) asserts that this disparity reflects overt ageism. Medina-Walpole et al. (2002) describe the shortage of geriatric medicine specialists, and note this disparity has persisted for decades. To address the grave lack of geriatricians and underserved presence of geriatrics in academia, English and Vanschagen (2011) argue the need for formation of added geriatric medicine fellowships. In a similar vein, the specialty of gerontological nursing also faces a shortage, with less than 1% of registered nurses having special training with older adults leading to certification in geriatrics (Hartford Institute for Geriatric Nursing 2012).

Regarding the specific need for psychological expertise, the field of geropsychology is not training enough specialists to remedy the dearth of psychologists trained in LTC (Molinari and Edelstein 2011); indeed, estimated need far exceeds projected availability of competent geropsychologists skilled at delivering optimal mental healthcare for older adults in general, a persistent problem for decades (Karel, Gatz, and Smyer 2012; Knight et al. 2009; Qualls et al. 2002).

Similar challenges facing geriatric social work await resolution, including disincentives for geriatric social work specialization, retention of extant staff, and satisfying the need to fill openings left by retirees (National Association of Social Workers 2006). Geriatric social workers are in demand, not only to serve older adults in a counselling capacity and to coordinate interdisciplinary care, but also to mitigate care-giver burden often seen in LTC (Lee et al. 2009). A study tracking social work graduates specialized in geriatrics showed that a focused training programme such as the Hartford Partnership Program for Aging Education (HPPAE) excels at preparing and retaining geriatric social workers in the field of ageing; this underscores the potential to counteract current trends of few graduates having training in ageing (Lee et al. 2009). Such outcomes are encouraging and have implications for workers involved in geriatric mental health across the board. Focused preparation and retention programmes should extend beyond social work and are needed for other professionals involved in geriatric and mental healthcare. Furthermore, the importance of building respect for the institution of care-giving in society is critical: unless key players of policy and administration collaborate to reverse the extremely negative, underpaid, overworked image of formal LTC care-givers, the gap between the need for and the availability of services will persist (Colombo et al. 2011).

Mental Illness Prevalence Rates
in Institutional Care

Long-standing data speak to the challenges of coordination and delivery of mental health services in LTC settings. At some point nearly 40% of older adults will reside in an LTC setting (Seperson 2002) for some period of time, including those admitted for acute rehabilitation and expected to be short-stay. The majority (60–90%) of NH residents have mental health problems that meet diagnostic criteria (Li 2010; Mechanic and McAlpine 2000; Reichman and Katz 1996). Currently there are more people with mental illness in NHs than in all other institutional settings combined (Fullerton et al. 2009; Grabowski et al. 2009). Besides declines in ADL function, mental health symptoms are influential predictors of NH placement (Black et al. 1999). However, the last ten years have seen an increasing shift in mental illness composition in varied LTC settings. Whereas dementia used to be more prevalent, a detailed review of NHs by Grabowski et al. (2010) indicates that residents with dementia are now outnumbered by those admissions with significant mental health symptoms. In ALFs, over 67% of the residents were found to have dementia based on *DSM* criteria (Rosenblatt et al. 2004).

The implications of this seismic shift in LTC admissions reveal a growing unmet need especially for managing those with behavioural problems. Yet, NHs are often ill-equipped to handle this specialized population. Given the severe nature of the medical problems required for admission, NHs have focused on addressing physical health issues and are not staffed to deal with mental health problems. However, in recent years, it appears that there has been more attunement to mental health and quality of life issues of NH residents in the US. NH administrators and staff are well aware of the mental health concerns of their residents, are creative in their attempts to address behavioural issues, document accordingly, and generally feel satisfied with resident mental healthcare (Molinari et al. 2011; Molinari et al. 2009; Molinari et al. 2008). Unfortunately, despite well-publicized concerns over medication side-effects of psychiatric medications given to frail older adults in LTC facilities, psychopharmacology remains the first line of treatment for those with mental health problems (Molinari et al. 2010). NHs appear hamstrung by systemic and reimbursement hurdles that hinder them from employing mental health professionals and instituting ongoing staff training to manage those with more severe mental health problems via non-psychopharmacological behavioural health protocols.

Mental Health Screening

A group of international scholars, including members of the International Psychogeriatric Association Task Force on Mental Health Services in Long-term Care Facilities, recently collaborated to review key concerns regarding administration of mental health screening assessments in LTC. According to Pachana et al. (2010: 1107–1108), use of suitable and precise screening assessments are integral to effective care delivery in NHs. However, in their examination of concerns surrounding mental health assessment in the institutional LTC setting, no international consensus among mental health screening tools or RACF-specific guidelines were found. However, attention has been drawn to this issue, and it is hoped that future guidelines are forthcoming. Pachana et al. (2010) do note that effective, accurate screening involves consideration of several factors, including not only the unique patient evaluated on a case-by-case basis, but also the particular individual administering the screening tool; adequate resources in an LTC facility so that trained staff exist to administer the instrument; knowledge and insight of mental health issues in the LTC resident population; and obstacles posed by differing levels of frailty and cognitive impairment of older adults.

In the US, the Preadmission Screening and Resident Review (PASRR) is required of all incoming NH residents to safeguard against improper admission of individuals with Serious Mental Illness (SMI) whose mental health needs are beyond the scope of the NH setting, and to ensure those residents who are in need of mental health resources are able to receive them (Li 2010). Should the initial PASRR screen identify an individual with SMI, a more extensive PASRR2 evaluation is required to develop a detailed treatment plan to address the person's mental health issues. Unfortunately, at this point, the bulk of those with mental health problems in NHs are not necessarily screened upon admission, because those residents with dementia as well as those with adjustment problems to communal living who do not meet the full criteria for SMI are excluded from the PASRR process.

BIOPSYCHOSOCIAL APPROACHES
TO MENTAL HEALTH

Twenty-five years after its introduction, Borrell-Carrió et al. (2004) reviewed the biopsychosocial model. Originally a reaction to the reductionist tendencies of medicine discounting the patient's subjective report as scientifically viable, thereby objectifying the patient, this perspective maintains that an effective response to a patient's burden of illness requires multifaceted consideration of the individual's 'biological, psychological, and social' components of illness (576). Though variously interpreted, executed and criticized since its inception, the underlying goal of this methodology has remained the same: to maintain the human element in medicine, thereby preserving patient dignity and autonomy in medical encounters.

Application of biopsychosocial models to patient care has been pertinent especially for painful conditions (Weiner et al. 1998). Given the unique parameters of geriatric mental healthcare and the need for more effective mental health incorporative strategies, addressing mental health challenges via a biopsychosocial framework holds promise for improving quality of care in NHs. This patient-centred emphasis is highlighted in approaches such as narrative medicine, an innovative methodology which incorporates in the clinical practice setting active listening, clear and effective communication, and attempts to verbalize the patient's experiences of their sickness, thereby fostering patient–practitioner connectivity and patient autonomy via strengthening the practitioner–patient relationship (Charon 2007). Such a sensitive approach would be particularly useful in serving the psychological needs of this vulnerable population. International interest in training for this method has been on the rise, reflecting a desire within medicine for a more genuine utilization of the practitioner as an agent of personal change via attention to the illness narrative. Greenhalgh and Hurwitz (1999) note that attention to the patient's story promotes empathy and appreciation between the patient and medical practitioner, permits meaning to be built from the illness experience, and yields a narrative that itself is inherently therapeutic. Swift and Dieppe (2005) have stressed the importance of shared written illness narratives of patients who 'feel they are flourishing despite their condition' (115) as a helpful resource.

The biopsychosocial model implies application of such strategies from LTC to end of life (EOL). 'When based on a person's need instead of illness, palliative and end-of-life care should also include the frail elderly' (Östlund, Brown, and Johnston 2012). Maintaining comfort measures to soothe the individual should be part and parcel of care. Despite this obvious application, extant literature on EOL care in NHs is scarce; what there is primarily highlights deficiencies (Oliver, Porock, and Zweig 2005). The latter authors note that the predominant focus of NHs is reparative and curative care; this is often at odds with the needs of the dying, and the result is often poorly managed symptoms and suffering at EOL. These authors note that further research into improving EOL care is needed. In the US alone, it is anticipated that nearly 40% of all deaths will take place in an NH (Brock and Foley 1998). Han, Tiggle, and Remsburg (2008) note that the form of EOL care known as hospice underscores the individual's comfort, remission of pain symptoms, and addresses the individual's emotional and spiritual needs. Location of such care is not limited to independent hospice facilities, but can occur at one's residence, hospital, or LTC setting. With such flexibility in a programme designed to alleviate suffering at EOL, implementation in NHs must become a reality.

The palliative care movement echoes narrative medicine in its focus on preservation of dignity. Lothian and Philp (2001: 668) define dignity as 'an individual maintaining self respect and being valued by others', whereas autonomy relates to 'an individual's control of decision making'. WHO affirms that protecting the dignity of the human being is essential to human rights (2002b). Östlund et al. (2012) reviewed the literature and determined that clinical practices stemming from WHO's concept of dignity and the European Parliament's emphasis on preserving dignity at EOL might include listening closely to those dying and treating them with respect; symptom control; proffering assistance in daily coping strategies; and urging family member engagement. Proulx and Jacelon (2004: 115) define dying with dignity as acknowledging not only one's inherent and immutable self-worth as a human being, but also other central characteristics such as freedom from physical discomfort; promoting independence, functionality, connectivity to other people; and encouraging overall feelings of significance. Inherent in upholding dignity is the ethical principle of respect for persons. Unless the personal narrative of each patient is taken into consideration, the definition of dying with dignity cannot truly be upheld nor carried out in practice. Respecting the unique narrative of each patient, which entails mutual exploration of a biography shaped by individual experiences and ideals, means that there is no 'universal best way to die' (116). A time commitment to continuous, open dialogue and awareness of individual preferences and sensitivity of care as fostered via a narrative approach are key in truly understanding what death with dignity entails, on a patient-by-patient basis. These EOL care principles are precepts of care for all LTC residents.

'CULTURE CHANGE' IN NHs: GETTING BEYOND 'BLAMING' THE INDIVIDUAL

The connection between disability, environment and outcome is well established. Wahl and Weisman (2003) note the seminal work by Lawton (1977, 1999), a chief advocate for environmental gerontology as an emerging specialized field; evolving derivatives include environmental modification and socio-physical considerations (Wahl and Weisman 2003: 616). Lawton's environmental docility hypothesis (1974: 258) postulates that one's degree of disability is strongly correlated with the degree to which one's capabilities are limited or enhanced by the environment. This recognition of behavioural change as affected by the physical environment also has implications for environment-influenced mental health outcomes. Such insight remains a theme which guides current 'culture change' thinking.

Begun as a grassroots concept nearly a decade ago, Miller et al. (2010: S65–S67) describe 'culture change' as a movement geared away from the traditional NH structure—in the philosophical, environmental, and organizational sense. This involves stepping away from the format by which the majority of NHs are currently organized and operate, characterized by institutionalized care practice, in favour of a model that focuses on the individual NH resident. Forward-thinking care moves beyond institutionalization norms to make resident-focused care a priority: individual residents' needs are addressed in a familial context.

The term 'culture change' is often used synonymously with resident-centred care (Miller et al. 2010). Jones (2011: 18–19) suggests that the 'heart of culture change' is the link between frontline staff and patients, influencing their daily care interactions. Person-centred care entails staff respecting the patient's wishes as a core component of care. Person-centred care links the biopsychosocial model with narrative medicine and the 'culture change' movement.

Harris, Poulsen, and Vlangas (2006: 7) identified six 'culture change' constructs in the literature, including resident-directed activities; home-like, rather than institutional-looking living environments; promoting contact between residents, family, NH staff, and society; a staff-empowering environment that fosters supportive resident-directed activities; administration that encourages teamwork and local decision-making; management that enables collaborative and decentralized decision-making; and regular monitoring via quality assessment measures to guide improvement. In all, the 'culture change' movement represents a deliberate focus on the creation of residences that look and feel more like home, and foster an environment that is a site for personal growth, rather than a stereotypical place of illness and death.

Examples of 'culture change' models include the Adards Community Model (Tasmania, Australia) (Cohen-Mansfield and Bester 2006), the small group home model in the Netherlands (Verbeek et al. 2009), Eden Alternative (2011) (US, Australia, New Zealand, Europe, Canada, and South Africa), Green House (2011) (US), the Empira Collaborative (Arling et al. 2011) (US), and the Wellspring Model (Stone et al. 2002) (US). For example, Bill Thomas's Eden Alternative began in 1991 as a non-profit organization focused on 'alleviating the plagues of loneliness, helplessness, and boredom' he perceived as rampant in traditional NH settings (Eden Alternative 2011) and modelled 'culture change' consultation to guide LTC. Aimed at improving relationships between residents, staff, and management, as well as the greater community, the Eden Alternative sought to create a more home-like environment via introduction of live plants, pets, and visiting neighbourhood groups, facilitating human companionship and socialization. Provision of worthwhile activities of interest to raise the spirits of residents was also emphasized (Eden Alternative 2011; Green House Project 2011).

Thomas's Green House Project further extends the Eden Alternative principles, and aims to improve quality of life for NH residents via deliberately small, welcoming, home-like facilities that lack the feel of institutions. In addition to including residents in food preparation, conflict resolution, and governance of their unique communities, these living arrangements also foster close-knit relationships between staff and residents with altered staffing and care delivery modalities, seeking to preserve residents' independence, autonomy, and satisfaction with living arrangements (Green House Project 2011). Unique to this model of care is the re-thinking of specific roles for residents and job descriptions for particular disciplines in the traditional NH. This modification is also reflected in usage of different LTC terminology for workers in an effort to leave no vestige of institutional roots or negative connotations. For example, Green House residents are not referred to as patients, but as Elders; assistants once referred to as certified nurse assistants are now known as Shahbaz (plural: Shahbazim), encompassing varied personal care and activity-facilitating tasks to support and nurture residents. This creates a distinct community setting evocative of family (Shapiro 2005).

In discussing a related culture change model, Lustbader (2000) decried current LTC norms addressing only the physical component of care. Widespread use of the acute care model, even outside of short-stay care, is used to drive care delivery and maintain control of patients' routines in LTC. This narrow focus has sacrificed quality of life for a constricted view of quality of care, steadily eroding individual control over their lives (Lustbader 2000: 185–186). The author details an ongoing response to this disenfranchisement of patients. Known as the Pioneer Network, this professional network of 'game-changers' in the LTC field seeks to return locus of control back to residents. Though recognizing no set single strategy for this 'culture change', Lustbader (2000: 186) describes the following elements as key to the Pioneer efforts: facilitating and promoting the individual's customized schedules; providing choices for mealtimes and eating; offering various options for keeping clean beyond just tub bath/shower; maintaining and facilitating continence for as long as possible; and, encouraging all remaining abilities for an individual's self-care and mobility.

Harris and colleagues (2006: 6) note that the existence of several different 'culture change' approaches, models, and procedures currently operative in LTC, combined with a lack of standardized definition, has resulted in diverse tools developed for evaluation, yet no 'universally agreed upon method to measure the extent of implementation of culture change practices in nursing homes'. Indeed, instruments in use are in need of validation and cross-validation, with a varied range of approaches called for, including 'surveys, interviews, and/or observations' (15). Recently, efforts have been made to develop more rigorous instrumentation to quantify criteria for 'culture change'. Lum et al. (2008–2009: 35) reported increased family satisfaction with their loved one's care, and 'with their own experience' of Green House NHs. However, empirical research findings regarding the effects of 'culture change' on resident and family outcomes remains thin. This is surprising given the pervasive 'culture change' buzzword that has permeated the NH industry over the last decade.

Further studies are needed to identify and measure quality of life components operative in such models, as measurement difficulties persist.

FLOURISHING, NOT JUST SURVIVING: HOW TO PROMOTE MENTAL HEALTH AND QUALITY OF LIFE IN NH RESIDENTS

In nations such as Canada, Austria, and some Scandinavian countries, LTC is regulated by regional governments; in contrast, national standards for LTC exist in Australia, Germany, Ireland, Japan, New Zealand, the UK and the US (Huber et al. 2005). Upon close examination of quality of care assessment in NHs, it becomes apparent that quality indicators focus on physical, rather than psychological aspects of care. For example, NH deficiency citations appear to be the sole way of determining if NHs in the US are actually adhering to federal regulations (Kim et al. 2009). While appropriate attention must be paid to the prevention of medical problems by assurance of adequate sanitation, attention to dietary needs, and prevention of pressure ulcers, a comprehensive evaluation of NH residents' needs should consider the entire biopsychosocial spectrum. Regulations must be attuned not only to the letter, but to the spirit of patient-centred care. Promotion of positive creative initiatives to incentivize overall quality of care should be considered. Grabowski et al. (2010) point out that the unique needs of NH residents with mental illnesses must be reflected in specific quality indicators. Indeed, quality of life parameters may be more sensitive mental health indicators than what is currently examined at the facility level. Further and ongoing inquiry into the problem of underserved geriatric mental health needs and the promotion of a positive psychology (Hill 2011) is a moral mandate. Health may not be guaranteed, but flourishing is a potential throughout the lifespan and must not be disregarded at any developmental stage. Supporting the potential for personal growth throughout life in any setting is a worthwhile endeavour in every country of the world, and requires the coordinated scientific efforts of the international community to keep the person front and centre in person-centred care.

PRACTICE IMPLICATIONS

This chapter yields a variety of implications for practice. On a systemic level, geriatric mental health professionals should advocate for the expansion of LTC living settings that promote less restrictive environments to buttress the older adult's own decision-making, generate meaning, and assure a better quality of life. Mental health professionals must recognize that working with older adults in LTC is a challenging enterprise that requires specialized skills honed by advanced training. They must be flexible regarding leaving their tidy offices and providing services in non-traditional community (e.g. home; senior centre, etc.) or institutional environments. With the right planning and staffing, LTC environments can foster psychological health. However, mental health problems occur under even seemingly ideal circumstances, and the LTC mental health professional must be ready and properly trained to assess aggressively and treat appropriately complicated geriatric cases with multiple medical and psychological comorbidities. For instance, a person with mild dementia and a heart condition may have both cognitive and physical reasons to become socially isolated and depressed. Advocating for the biopsychosocial model of care, the competent geriatric mental health professional must be diagnostically able to tease out the varied components of the presenting problem and to treat with state-of-the-art evidence-based protocols. Geriatric mental health professionals must be aware of the primary role that informal care, especially from families, plays in long-term healthcare, and how to enlist and nurture support via family meetings and counselling. To assure the best outcomes, they must keep up with the latest research advances and be able to consult, as concerned geriatric interdisciplinary team members, with other disciplines to promote integrated healthcare. They must be willing to navigate the formidable system of healthcare to obtain the services necessary to nurture the person's mental health and quality of life during their most vulnerable years.

Summary

This chapter takes an international focus, and provides a review of the trends and challenges in mental health treatment for older adults in LTC. Across cultures, there are some recurring themes. At the familial level, there are insufficient resources and training to manage and cope with worsening symptoms of illness, amplified financial hardship, and overall strain due to increased care-giving duties. At the institutional level, inadequate/insufficient training for staff persists despite such a high prevalence of mental health disorders. Mental health needs therefore often remain undetected, with financial disincentives (Li 2010: 349) for trained geriatric professionals further downgrading their priority in healthcare. There is the obvious need for an international biopsychosocial person-centred framework in LTC to be integrated within the unique fabric of each country's healthcare system. Research must evaluate public policy initiatives that attempt to foster effective public/private financial arrangements, and explore the common ingredients of quality care for frail older adults that render optimal LTC for those of varied cultural backgrounds living in different countries and being provided services in diverse geriatric settings.

Key References and Sources for Further Reading

Alzheimer's Association (2013). *Alzheimer's Disease Facts and Figures*. http://www.alz.org/downloads/facts_figures_2013.pdf.

Alzheimer's Disease International (2012). *World Alzheimer Report 2012: Overcoming the Stigma of Dementia*. http://www.alz.co.uk/research/WorldAlzheimerReport2012.pdf.

Hurd, M. D., Martorell, P., Delavande, A., Mullen, K. J., and Langa, K. M. (2013). 'Monetary Costs of Dementia in the United States'. *New England Journal of Medicine* 368: 1326–1334.

References

Album, D., and Westin, S. (2008). 'Do Diseases have a Prestige Hierarchy? A Survey among Physicians and Medical Students'. *Social Science & Medicine* 66: 182–188.

Alzheimer's Disease International (December 2013) *The Policy Brief for Heads of Government: The Global Impact of Dementia 2013-2050*. http://www.alz.co.uk/research/GlobalImpactDementia2013.pdf

Alzheimer's Disease International (2010). *World Alzheimer Report 2010: The Global Economic Impact of Dementia*. (Executive summary.) http://www.alz.co.uk/research/files/WorldAlzheimerReport2010ExecutiveSummary.pdf.

American Geriatrics Society, American Association for Geriatric Psychiatry (2003a). 'Consensus Statement on Improving the Quality of Mental Health Care in U.S. Nursing Homes: Management of Depression and Behavioral Symptoms Associated with Dementia'. *Journal of the American Geriatrics Society* 51: 1287–1298.

American Geriatrics Society, American Association for Geriatric Psychiatry (2003b). 'The American Geriatrics Society and American Association for Geriatric Psychiatry Recommendations for Policies in Support of Quality Mental Health Care in U.S. Nursing Homes'. *Journal of the American Geriatrics Society* 51: 1299–1304.

Anderson, R. N. and Smith, B. L. (2005). Deaths: leading causes for 2002. *National Vital Statistics Reports* 53:1–89.

Arling, P., Arling, G., Inui, T., Abrahamson, K., Mueller, et al. (2011). 'A Case Study of a Highly Effective Nursing Home Quality Improvement Collaborative: The Empira Fall Prevention Project'. Paper presented at the Gerontological Society of America's 64th Annual Scientific Meeting, Boston, MA.

Bartels, S. J., Moak, G. S., and Dums, A. R. (2002). 'Models of Mental Health Services in Nursing Homes: A Review of the Literature'. *Psychiatric Services* 53: 1390–1396.

Bartels, S. J. (2003). 'Improving the System of Care for Older Adults with Mental Illness in the United States'. *American Journal of Geriatric Psychiatry* 11: 486–497.

Black, B. S., Rabins, P. V., and German, P. S. (1999). 'Predictors of Nursing Home Placement Among Elderly Public Housing Residents'. *The Gerontologist* 39: 559–568.

Borrell-Carrió, F., Suchman, A. L., and Epstein, R. M. (2004). 'The Biopsychosocial model 25 Years Later: Principles, Practice and Scientific Inquiry'. *Annals of Family Medicine* 2: 576–582.

Borson, S., Bartels, S. J., Colenda, C. C., Gottlieb, G. L., and Meyers, B. (2001). 'Geriatric Mental Health Services Research: Strategic Plan for an Aging Population'. *American Journal of Geriatric Psychiatry* 9: 191–204.

Boyle, P. A., Buchman, A. S., Wilson, R. S., Leurgans, S. E., and Bennett, D. A. (2010). 'Physical Frailty is Associated with Incident Mild Cognitive Impairment in Community-based Older Persons'. *Journal of the American Geriatrics Society* 58: 248–255.

Brock D. B. and Foley, D. J. (1998). 'Demography and Epidemiology of Dying in the U.S. with Emphasis on Deaths of Older Persons'. *Hospice Journal* 13: 49–60.

Buchman, A. S., Schneider, J. A., Leurgans, S., and Bennett, D. A. (2008). 'Physical Frailty in Older Persons is Associated with Alzheimer Disease Pathology'. *Neurology* 71: 499–504.

Burns, B. J., Wagner, H. R., Taube, J. E., Magaziner, J., Permyutt, T., et al. (1993). 'Mental Health Service Use by the Elderly in Nursing Homes'. *American Journal of Public Health* 83: 331–337.

Charon, R. (2007). 'What To Do with Stories: The Sciences of Narrative Medicine'. *Canadian Family Physician* 53. 1265–7.

Cohen-Mansfield, J. and Bester, A. (2006). 'Flexibility as a Management Principle in Dementia Care: The Adards Example'. *The Gerontologist* 46: 540–544.

Colombo, F., et al. (2011). *Help Wanted? Providing and Paying for Long-Term Care*. OECD Health Policy Studies. Paris: OECD. http://dx.doi.org/10.1787/9789264097759-en.

Eden Alternative (2011). *About the Eden Alternative*. http://www.edenalt.org/about-the-eden-alternative.

English, S. K. and Vanschagen, J. E. (2011). 'Creating a Geriatric Medicine Fellowship Program in 10 "Easy" Steps'. *Journal of the American Geriatrics Society* 59: 1934–40.

Fullerton, C. A., McGuire, T. G., Feng, Z., Mor, V., and Grabowski, D. C. (2009). 'Trends in Mental Health Admissions to Nursing Homes: 1999–2005'. *Psychiatric Services* 60: 965–971.

Gibson, M. C., Carter, M. W., Helmes, E., and Edberg, A. K. (2010). 'Principles of Good Care for Long-term Care Facilities'. *International Psychogeriatrics* 22: 1072–1083.

Grabowski, D. C., Aschbrenner, K. A., Feng, Z., and Mor, V. (2009). 'Mental Illness in Nursing Homes: Variations Across States'. *Health Affairs* 28: 689–700.

Grabowski, D. C., Aschbrenner, K. A., Rome, V. F., and Bartels, S. J. (2010). 'Quality of Mental Health Care for Nursing Home Residents: A Literature Review'. *Medical Care Research Review* 67: 627–56.

Green House Project (2011). *Mission and Vision*. http://thegreenhouseproject.org/about-us.

Greenhalgh, T. and Hurwitz, B. (1999). 'Why Study Narrative?' *British Medical Journal* 318: 48–50.

Han, B., Tiggle, R. B., and Remsburg, R. E. (2008). 'Characteristics of Patients Receiving Hospice Care at Home versus in Nursing Homes: Results from the National Home and Hospice Care Survey and the National Nursing Home Survey'. *American Journal of Hospice and Palliative Medicine* 24: 479–486.

Harris, Y., Poulsen, R., and Vlangas, G. (2006). *Measuring Culture Change: Literature Review*. Englewood, CO: Colorado Foundation for Medical Care.

Hartford Institute for Geriatric Nursing (2012). *Geriatric Trends and Statistics*. http://hartfordign.org/About.

Hill, R. D. (2011). 'A Positive Aging Framework for Guiding Geropsychology Interventions'. *Behavior Therapy* 42: 66–77.

Huber, M., Hennessey, P., Izumi, J., Kim, W., and Lundsgaard, J. (2005). *Long Term Care For Older People: The OECD Health Project*. Paris: OECD.

Institute of Medicine (2008). *Retooling for an Aging America: Building the Health Care Workforce*. Washington, DC: National Academies.

Jones C. S. (2011). 'Person-centered Care. The Heart of Culture Change'. *Journal of Gerontological Nursing* 37: 18–25.

Karel, M. J., Gatz, M., and Smyer, M. A. (2012). 'Aging and Mental Health in the Decade Ahead: What Psychologists Need to Know'. *American Psychologist* 67: 184–198.

Katz, P. (2011). 'An International Perspective on Long Term Care: Focus on Nursing Homes'. *Journal of the American Medical Directors Association* 12: 487–492.

Kim, H., Kovner, C., Harrington, C., Greene, W., and Mezey, M. (2009). 'A Panel Data Analysis of the Relationships of Nursing Home Staffing Levels and Standards to Regulatory Deficiencies'. *Journal of Gerontology: Social Sciences* 64B: 269–278.

Kinsella, K. and Wan, H. (2009). *An Aging World: 2008*. US Census Bureau, International Population Reports, P95/09-1. Washington, DC: US Government Printing Office.

Knight, B., Karel, M. G., Hinrichsen, G. A., Qualls, S. H., and Duffy, M. (2009). 'Pikes Peak Model for Training in Professional Geropyschology'. *American Psychologist* 64: 205–214.

Kochanek, K. D., Xu, J., Murphy, S. L., Miniño, A. M., and Kung, H. C. (2011). 'Deaths: Preliminary Data for 2009'. *National Vital Statistics Reports* 59: 1–51.

La Rue, A., Koehler, K. M., Wayne, S. J., Chiulli, S. J., Haaland, K. Y., et al. (1997). 'Nutritional Status and Cognitive Functioning in a Normally Aging Sample: A 6-y Reassessment'. *American Journal of Clinical Nutrition* 65: 20–29.

Lawton, M. P. (1974). 'Social Ecology and the Health of Older People'. *American Journal of Public Health* 64: 257–260.

Lawton, M. P. (1977). 'The Impact of the Environment on Aging and Behavior'. In J. E. Birren and K. W. Shaie (eds), *Handbook on the Psychology of Aging* (pp. 276–301). New York: Van Nostrand.

Lawton, M. P. (1999). 'Environmental Taxonomy: Generalizations from Research with Older Adults'. In S. L. Friedman and T. D. Wachs (eds), *Measuring Environment across the Lifespan* (pp. 91–124). Washington, DC: American Psychological Association.

Lee, S. E. Damron-Rodriguez, J., Lawrance, F. P., and Volland, P. J. (2009). 'Geriatric Social Work Career Tracking: Graduates of the Hartford Partnership Program for Aging Education (HPPAE)'. *Journal of Gerontological Social Work* 52: 336–353.

Li, Y. (2010). 'Provision of Mental Health Services in U.S. Nursing Homes 1995–2004'. *Psychiatric Services* 61: 349–355.

Lothian, K. and Philp, I. (2001). 'Maintaining the Dignity and Autonomy of Older People in the Healthcare Setting'. *British Medical Journal* 322: 668–670.

Lum, T. Y., Kane, R. A., Cutler, L. J., and Yu, T. C. (2008–2009). 'Effects of Green House® Nursing Homes on Residents' Families'. *Health Care Financing Review* 3: 35–51.

Lustbader, W. (2000). 'The Pioneer Challenge: A Radical Change in the Culture of Nursing Homes'. In L. S. Noelker and Z. Harel (eds), *Linking Quality of Long-term Care and Quality of Life* (pp. 185–203). New York: Springer.

Matthews, F. E., Arthur, A., Barnes, L. E., Bond, J., Jagger, C., et al. (2013). 'A Two-decade Comparison of Prevalence of Dementia in Individuals aged 65 Years and Older from Three Geographical Areas of England: Results of the Cognitive Function and Ageing Study I and II'. *Lancet* 382(9902): 1405–1412.

Mechanic, D. and McAlpine, D. D. (2000). 'Use of Nursing Homes in the Care of Persons with Severe Mental Illness: 1985 to 1995'. *Psychiatric Services* 51: 354–358.

Medina-Walpole, A., Barker, W. H., Katz, P. R., Karuza, J., Williams, T. F., et al. (2002). 'The Current State of Geriatric Medicine: A National Survey of Fellowship-trained Geriatricians 1990 to 1998'. *Journal of the American Geriatrics Society* 50: 949–955.

Miller, S. C., Miller, E. A., Jung, H. Y., Sterns, S., Clark, M., et al. (2010). 'Nursing Home Organizational Change: The "Culture Change" Movement as Viewed by Long-term Care Specialists'. *Medical Care Research and Review* 67(4)(suppl.): S65S–S81.

Molinari, V., Merritt, S., Mills, W., Chiriboga, D., Conboy, A., et al. (2008). 'Serious Mental Illness in Florida Nursing Homes: Need for Training'. *Gerontology and Geriatrics Education* 29: 66–83.

Molinari, V., Hedgecock, D., Branch, L. Brown, L., and Hyer, K. (2009). 'Mental Health Services in Nursing Homes: A Survey of Florida Nursing Home Administrative Personnel'. *Aging & Mental Health* 13: 477–486.

Molinari, V., Chiriboga, D., Branch, L., Cho, S., Turner, K., et al. (2010). 'Provision of Psychopharmacological Services in Nursing Homes'. *Journals of Gerontology: Psychological Sciences and Social Sciences* 65: 57–60.

Molinari, V. and Edelstein, B. (2011). 'Commentary on the Current Status and the Future of Behavior Therapy in Long-term Care Settings'. *Behavior Therapy* 42: 59–65.

Molinari, V. Chiriboga, D. A., Branch, L. G., Schinka, J., Schonfeld, L., et al. (2011). 'Reasons for Psychiatric Prescription for New Nursing Home Residents'. *Aging & Mental Health* 15(7) 904–912.

Nadash, P. and Ahrens, J. (2005). *Long-term Care: An Overview*: Policy Brief (Center for Home Care Policy and Research). http://www.vnsny.org/research/publications/pdf/n022_ltc_brief_final.pdf.

National Association of Social Workers (2006). *Assuring the Sufficiency of a Frontline Workforce: A National Study of Licensed Social Workers*. Executive summary. http://workforce.socialworkers.org/studies/nasw_06_execsummary.pdf.

Norredam, M. and Album, D. (2007). 'Prestige and its Significance for Medical Specialties and Diseases'. *Scandinavian Journal of Public Health* 35: 655–661.

Oliver, D. P., Porock, D., and Zweig, S. (2005). 'End-of-life Care in U.S. Nursing Homes: A Review of the Evidence'. *Journal of the American Medical Directors Association* 6: S21–S30.

Östlund, U., Brown, H., and Johnston, B. (2012). 'Dignity Conserving Care at End-of-life: A Narrative Review'. *European Journal of Oncology Nursing* 16: 353–367.

Pachana, N. A., Helmes, E., Byrne, Edelstein, B. A., Konnert, C. A., et al (2010). 'Screening for Mental Disorders in Residential Aged Care Facilities'. *International Psychogeriatrics* 22: 1107–1120.

Panza, F., Solfrizzi, V., Frisardi, V., Maggi, S., Sancarlo, D., et al (2011). 'Different Models of Frailty in Predementia and Dementia Syndromes'. *Journal of Nutrition, Health and Aging* 15: 711–9.

Proulx, K. and Jacelon, C. (2004). 'Dying with Dignity: The Good Patient versus the Good Death'. *American Journal of Hospital and Palliative Care* 21: 116–120.

Qualls, S. H., Segal, D. L., Norman, S., Niederehe, G., and Gallagher-Thompson, D. (2002). 'Psychologists in Practice with Older Adults: Current Patterns, Sources of Training, and Need for Continuing Education'. *Professional Psychology* 33: 435–442.

Reichman, W. E. and Katz, P. R. (1996). *Psychiatric Care in the Nursing Home*. New York: Oxford.

Rosenblatt, A., Samus, Q. M., Steele, C. D., Baker, A. S., Harper, M. G., et al. (2004). 'The Maryland Assisted Living Study: Prevalence, Recognition, and Treatment of Dementia and Other Psychiatric Disorders in the Assisted Living Population of Central Maryland'. *Journal of the American Geriatrics Society* 52: 1618–1625.

Seperson, S. B. (2002). 'Demographics about Aging'. In S. B. Seperson and C. Hegemann (eds), *Elder Care and Service Learning: A Handbook* (pp. 17–30). Westport, CT: Auburn House.

Shapiro, J. (2005). 'Reformers Seek to Reinvent Nursing Homes'. *National Public Radio*. http://www.npr.org/templates/story/story.php?storyId=4713566.

Sinunu, M., Yount, K. M., and El Afify, N. A. W. (2009). 'Informal and Formal Long-term Care for Frail Older Adults in Cairo, Egypt: Family Caregiving Decisions in a Context of Social Change'. *Journal of Cross Cultural Gerontology* 24: 63–76.

Stone, R. I., Reinhard. S. C., Bowers, B., et al. (2002). '*Evaluation of the Wellspring Model for Improving Nursing Home Quality*'. New York: Commonwealth Fund.

Swift, T. L. and Dieppe, P. A. (2005). 'Using Expert Patients' Narratives as an Educational Resource'. *Patient Education and Counseling* 57: 115–121.

Thomas, B. (2011). 'Learn to Value Life in Elderhood'. *San Francisco Chronicle*. http://www.sfgate.com/cgi-bin/article.cgi?f=/c/a/2011/06/02/EDMM1JOKCO.DTL.

Tolson, D., Rolland, Y., Andrieu, S., Aquino, J. P., Beard, J., et al. (2011). 'International Association of Gerontology and Geriatrics: A Global Agenda for Clinical Research and Quality of Care in Nursing Homes'. *Journal of the American Medical Directors Association* 12: 184–189.

United Nations Population Fund and HelpAge International (2012). *Ageing in the Twenty-first Century: A Celebration and a Challenge*. http://www.helpage.org/download/50af6e052ed68.

Verbeek, H., Van Rossum, E., Zwakhalen, S. M. G., Kempen G. I. J. M., and Hamers, J. P. H. (2009). 'Small, Homelike Care Environments for Older People with Dementia: A Literature Review'. *International Psychogeriatrics* 21: 252–264.

Wahl, H. W. and Weisman, G. D. (2003). 'Environmental Gerontology at the Beginning of the New Millennium: Reflections on its Historical, Empirical, and Theoretical Development'. *Gerontologist* 43: 616–627.

Weiner, D. K., Peterson, B. L., Logue, P., and Keefe, F. J. (1998). 'Predictors of Pain Self-report in Nursing Home Residents'. *Aging (Milano)* 10: 411–20.

Woolhandler, S., Campbell, T., and Himmelstein, D. (2003). 'Costs of Health Care Administration in the United States and Canada'. *New England Journal of Medicine* 349: 768–775.

World Bank (2010). *Long Term Care Policies for Older Populations in New EU Member States and Croatia: Challenges and Opportunities*. Washington, DC: World Bank. http://siteresources. worldbank.org/ECAEXT/Resources/LTC_full_summary_final.pdf.

World Health Organization (2001). *World Population Ageing: 1950–2050*. Geneva: WHO. http:// www.un.org/esa/population/publications/worldageing19502050/.

World Health Organization (2002a). *Lessons for Long-term Care Policy*. No. WHO/NMH/ CCL/02.1. Geneva: Cross-Cluster Initiative on Long-Term Care: Noncommunicable Diseases and Mental Health Cluster, WHO, and WHO Collaborating Centre for Research on Health of the Elderly, JDC-Brookdale Institute. http://www.who.int/chp/knowledge/publi cations/ltc_policy_lessons.pdf.

World Health Organization (2002b). '*25 Questions and Answers on Health and Human Rights*'. Geneva: WHO. http://whqlibdoc.who.int/hq/2002/9241545690.pdf.

....

CHAPTER 17

ADVANCED ILLNESS
AND THE END OF LIFE

....

JULIA E. KASL-GODLEY AND KYSA M. CHRISTIE

INTRODUCTION

....

> To shy away from death is to shy away from living.
>
> Halpern 2004: 194

Older adults may live years with chronic, progressive and often comorbid, debilitating illnesses (Anderson and Horvath 2004), with the incidence of chronic and terminal illnesses increasing with age. Among middle- and high-income countries (e.g. Australia, Brazil, China, Japan, South Africa, the UK, the US), four of the five leading causes of death are chronic diseases: ischaemic heart disease, cerebrovascular disease, trachea/bronchus/lung cancers, and chronic obstructive pulmonary disease (WHO 2008). Thus, end of life is more often an extended process for which people usually have time to prepare rather than a sudden event. Yet individuals often feel unprepared for dying which can create a disconnect between preferences and actual care at end of life (Bell, Somogyi-Zalud, and Masaki 2010). Moreover, family members and professional healthcare providers may be equally unprepared.

Being familiar with issues related to chronic, advanced, and terminal illness, that is, issues inherent to palliative and hospice care work, is a professional necessity when working with older adults. Increasingly, geropsychologists will be expected to provide basic elements of palliative care (e.g. pain and symptom assessment and management, advance care planning, basic psychosocial and spiritual support). To this end, this chapter offers a description of hospice or end-of-life care as a subgroup of the larger field of palliative care, a discussion of the transition from 'living with' to 'dying from' a serious illness, clinical issues commonly seen in the ill person as well as family members, and the ways in which geropsychologists can be helpful with these issues.

As you read, we invite you to notice your own assumptions and reactions to illness and dying. Because dying is such a personal experience, we all carry memories, emotions, and assumptions about the end of life. Awareness of reactions to death and dying is necessary for self-care and the care of your patients. In addition, we hope that you not only gain knowledge that allows you to integrate palliative care into your practice but an appreciation for what makes working with patients and families with advanced and terminal illness such a unique and meaningful endeavour.

To provide a context for many of the challenges and rewards that arise when working with individuals with advanced illness and at end of life, this chapter includes a case example of an older adult with chronic, complex medical conditions. We begin with his visit to the emergency room and will return to his story throughout the chapter.

Mr Ben Alberts, an 81-year-old Caucasian man with a history of congestive heart failure, diabetes, colitis, kidney disease, and depression, presented to the emergency room with difficulty breathing, extreme fatigue and weakness, sudden weight gain, and swelling in his legs. After being diagnosed with an exacerbation of heart disease and kidney failure, the Palliative Care team was consulted to discuss goals of care with Mr Alberts and his family. After several conversations, Mr Alberts and his family decided that he would transition to inpatient hospice for end-of-life care. The medical team estimated that he had 'weeks to months' to live, though because of his significant heart disease, he was also at risk of dying suddenly.

On the inpatient hospice and palliative care unit, Mr Alberts spent his days and nights in bed. He was easily fatigued, to the point of having difficulty even holding his head up in bed. His voice was weak and soft, but he enjoyed talking with his family and the hospice care team. Grace, his wife of sixty years, was a petite, talkative woman with a strong presence. She had been his primary care-giver for years, and their children described her care and commitment to his health as the reason their father was still alive.

Although Mr Alberts had been living with multiple serious medical problems for years, the transition to hospice marked a change in how he and his family viewed their time together. The family seemed acutely aware that their time was limited and, during the first few weeks, his wife spent all day at Mr Alberts' bedside and he received phone calls and cards from family and friends.

As part of the standard care on the hospice unit, the team psychologist met with Mr Alberts and his wife for an initial assessment of their coping and adjustment. When the conversation shifted to Mr Alberts' experience of being in the hospital for end-of-life care, Mrs Alberts excused herself 'to give Ben some privacy'. As she left, Mr Alberts said, 'Grace always does that, she always leaves. She won't talk about me dying. I'm worried about her. How can I know she's going to be okay when I'm gone if we can't talk about it?'

What Is Palliative Care and Where Might it Occur?

Many misconceptions exist about the definition of palliative care and its relationship to hospice or end-of-life care. 'Palliative care' is a broad term that refers to care provided at *any point* in the trajectory of a serious illness for the purpose of alleviating physical and psycho-social-spiritual suffering, enhancing quality of life, effectively managing

Box 17.1 Who is appropriate for palliative care?

Any one of the following situations may be sufficient to consult palliative care.

- *Surprise.* You would not be surprised if the patient died within twelve months
- *Frequent admissions.* Repeated admissions for the same condition within several months
- *Complex symptoms.* Admission for difficult symptoms or psychological need
- *Complex care requirement.* Functional dependence or complex home support needed
- *Failure to thrive.* Decline in functional status, weight, or ability to care for self
- *Advance care need.* No history of completing an advance care directive, or having a discussion about end-of-life care preferences (e.g. do not resuscitate, do not intubate (DNR/DNI)
- *Limited social support.* Family stress, chronic mental illness, lack of care-givers
- *Limited prognosis.* Metastatic or locally advanced cancer, hip fracture with cognitive impairment, or out-of-hospital cardiac arrest

Data from Weissman, D. E., & Meier, D. E., Identifying patients in need of a palliative care assessment in the hospital setting: A consensus report from the Center to Advance Palliative Care. *Journal of Palliative Medicine*, 14, pp. 17–23, 2011, Mary Ann Liebert, Inc.

symptoms, and offering comprehensive, interdisciplinary support to the patient and family throughout the course of illness, regardless of stage of disease (National Consensus Project for Quality Palliative Care 2013; WHO 2007). Palliative care also helps patients and families make difficult medical decisions that enable them to work towards their goals, especially as outcomes become more uncertain. Palliative care ideally begins at the point of initial diagnosis of a serious, potentially life-limiting illness, and can be delivered concurrently with other therapies that are intended to cure a disease or prolong life (see Box 17.1 Who is appropriate for palliative care?). Palliative care can occur across the entire continuum of care: the treatment-intensive hospital setting; assisted living or long-term care facilities; ambulatory care medical clinics and home-care programmes. If disease-directed therapy stops working, palliative care can become the main focus of care. Although the primary focus is enhancing quality of life, palliative care may even extend life (Temel et al. 2010).

Palliative care also includes 'end-of-life care', which might involve referral to a formal hospice programme, as well as support of the family through the bereavement period. Hospice services can be provided in the home, nursing homes, residential facilities, or on inpatient units. In the US, hospice care is often linked to the specific programmes offered under the Medicare Hospice Benefit. Individuals receiving hospice care must typically forgo active disease-directed therapy for the terminal illness, though interventions intended to maximize quality of life are continued. However, individuals can receive disease-directed treatment for medical problems other than the terminal illness under Medicare. Furthermore, if an individual's condition stabilizes or improves, he or she can disenrol from hospice care and return to regular Medicare coverage.

How Do We Know When it Is the End of Life?

A significant challenge in end-of-life care is how to conceptualize when the process of dying begins. For many people, death will occur years or decades following a diagnosis of a serious illness. In these cases, death is the final event of a gradual process of decline caused by an underlying illness such as heart disease. For other people, even within the context of a serious illness, death may occur hours to days following an acute event such as a fall or infection. 'How long do I have left to live?' is often an explicit or implicit question. Despite its salience, a clear answer can be difficult for physicians to give, and for patients and families to hear. While providers can offer estimates of time such as 'hours to days', 'days to weeks', 'weeks to months', 'months to years', many physicians overestimate patients' survival time (Glare et al. 2003).

Regardless of the time frame, providers, patients, and/or family members often delay acknowledging that someone is dying until death seems unavoidable or imminent (i.e. in days to weeks). This delay creates practical and emotional challenges for what people can accomplish before death, including managing symptoms well, addressing unfinished business, saying goodbyes, and having time to reflect on one's life and one's legacy. Much of the work with individuals with serious illness is about tolerating and managing the uncertainty inherent in this stage of life and striving for balance between preparing for death and focusing on how they want to live in the time they have left, however long it may be.

Physicians often avoid difficult conversations because they fear patients will become overwhelmed, distraught, and ask for futile care (Wright et al. 2008). However, this outcome seems to depend on a patient's ability to process the information. For example, if end-of-life discussions occur among patients who are psychologically numb, this discussion can 'backfire' and result in the receipt of more aggressive care (Maciejewski and Prigerson 2012). However, clear communication about end-of-life preferences helps a person's vision, hopes, and preferences align with actual care received. For example, the congruence of preferred vs actual place of death ranges widely (30–91%) (Bell et al. 2010). Factors that increase congruence include good patient understanding of the illness, physician support, a do-not-resuscitate advance directive, and family support. In contrast, lower patient/care-giver education levels, a need for twenty-four-hour nursing care, unclear prognosis, and perceived family inability to cope all decrease congruence (Bell et al. 2010). Ideally, discussions about goals of care and treatment preferences at the end of life are ongoing, involve patients, family members, and medical teams, and occur during non-crises.

Common Clinical Issues

In this section, we review physical symptoms common in advanced and terminal illness, then discuss psycho-social-spiritual reactions. For many people who are approaching the end of life, an important intervention is to anticipate their symptoms and strengthen their ability to cope with them.

Physical symptoms

A working knowledge of common illnesses and related physical symptoms can help geropsychologists appreciate the physical symptoms with which their patients are living, and how such symptoms influence quality of life. Additionally, physical symptoms can be a significant source of psycho-social-spiritual distress.

Pain

Pain can occur anywhere in the body and take various forms. It can be muscular, neuropathic, or originate in the skin, organs, or bones. It may be acute, chronic, and/or intermittent. It may be related to the disease and/or its treatment. Assessment should include pain location, quality, intensity, duration, factors that exacerbate or alleviate pain, and the impact on the person. Adequate pain control is one of the greatest concerns of seriously and terminally ill patients and, fortunately, effective pharmacological interventions exist (Steinhauser et al. 2000). However, despite concerns about unmanaged pain, it is not uncommon for patients to be hesitant about pain control. Individuals with advanced or terminal illness may have particular beliefs about pain that affect its management, such as that it should be experienced and tolerated because it is retribution for past misdeeds, a characterological deficit if one cannot bear it, or simply an indication of if/how the illness is progressing. Individuals also may be reluctant to report pain for fear of burdening family or providers, of seeming too demanding, or of reprisals for complaining. They may believe that the pain cannot be alleviated or improved, or make assumptions about possible side-effects (e.g. 'If I take this medication, I will be too lethargic or confused'). Individuals may fear 'addiction', often confusing it with dependence or tolerance, which can feed into physicians' own misunderstandings about the use of pain medications and the likelihood of addiction. Individuals themselves, especially those with addiction histories now in recovery, may fear susceptibility to re-addiction or ostracism from supportive others. In addition, physicians may underestimate pain, if there is a history of pain and/or substance use which can increase medication tolerance. Alternatively, physicians may overestimate the contribution of psychological factors to pain and thus under-treat pain. Geropsychologists can elucidate these factors and their role in pain management, in addition to providing effective psychological interventions to manage pain as adjunctive treatment to pharmacological approaches. Pain management at the end of life should be aggressive and not be withheld for concerns related to developing an addiction to pain medication (Dalal and Bruera 2011).

Dyspnoea

Dyspnoea means difficulty breathing or breathlessness. It is a symptom of chronic lung diseases (COPD), heart failure, and advanced cancer, as well as diseases with significant muscle loss such as multiple sclerosis and amyotrophic lateral sclerosis. Patients with dyspnoea describe feeling like they are being smothered or suffocated, that their chest feels tight, their breathing is rapid, and they cannot get enough air or stop thinking about their breathing (Kamal et al. 2011). The course of dyspnoea fluctuates such that patients can have periods of increased or decreased difficulty breathing (Campbell 2012).

Dyspnoea typically occurs in conjunction with other medical symptoms, as well as psychosocial and spiritual distress. Not surprisingly, feeling as though one is suffocating is frightening and anxiety provoking, for the patient as well as for family members and professional care-givers. Periods of dyspnoea also can be powerful reminders of the patient's serious health problems and elicit existential concerns about meaning, suffering, and dying.

Opioids are the most well studied and used pharmacological treatment to manage dyspnoea and the evidence is largely supportive of their efficacy (Kamal et al. 2011). Non-pharmacologic interventions also are effective. Using a fan to provide a cool breeze on a person's face reduces dyspnoea. Psychoeducation about the feeling of suffocation, compared to physiological risk of suffocating can be helpful. Cognitive interventions aimed at identifying and managing automatic thoughts related to suffocation that arise during periods of dyspnoea, as well as relaxation strategies, particularly breathing retraining, can reduce the distress caused by breathlessness (Corner et al. 1996).

Fatigue, decreased energy, weakness

Fatigue is characterized by weariness or exhaustion resulting from physical or mental exertion. Fatigue can result from dyspnoea, the direct effects of cancer or anti-cancer treatment, as well as cancer-related symptoms, deconditioning, co-existing infections, or nutrition/appetite loss (Okuyama et al. 2008). Fatigue may also co-occur with pain and depression (Rao and Cohen 2004; Ross and Alexander 2001).

Fatigue often results in emotional distress both from the significant functional changes and limited ability to engage in daily activities but also from the meaning attributed to the symptom—i.e. that one's disease is progressing, that one is helpless and useless and no longer capable of doing anything one once did. Although it may be accurate that the disease is progressing, geropsychologists can encourage individuals to reconsider how they approach tasks and activities. For example, individuals can be encouraged to pace activity, alternating physical activity with rest, and try to reduce the demands of everyday living. Individuals may also modify pleasurable activities or identify new ones that can provide the same function with less physical demands, and set priorities to ensure that valued or important activities can be continued and less important activities let go.

Returning to the case of Mr Alberts, although his heart disease and physical deconditioning left him fatigued and weak, after a month in hospice care he was stronger and more medically stable than he had been at admission. In part, these improvements were due to having full-time nursing care, which helped him conserve his energy and ensured that he took his medications regularly. However, the team began to notice fluctuations in Mr Alberts' behaviour. To one physician he would describe feeling fine, but later in the day would say he felt very depressed. He cried often, but was unable to explain why. While Mr Alberts had a history of depression, which increased the likelihood that the physical and emotional stress of being ill would lead to a depressive episode, it was unclear the extent to which his heart disease may be mimicking depression or exacerbating depressive symptoms (e.g. fatigue, low energy, physical slowing). The hospice psychologist was tasked with determining whether his reactions reflected normative adjustment or a clinical diagnosis of Major Depressive Disorder.

During a clinical interview that included the Geriatric Depression Scale-Short Form and follow-up questions that probed items Mr Alberts endorsed, it became clear that Mr

Alberts' mood varied with his energy level, and this variation accounted for the differing reports of his mood. In the mornings when physicians made their rounds, Mr Alberts was rested and relatively positive. However, as he tired over the course of the day, he expressed more depressed affect. When tired, he was irritable and equated his fatigue with being useless and a burden. He described thinking he was a burden because his family spent much of their time visiting him rather than living their own lives. Mr Alberts cried during the interview, sharing 'I'm tired of living like this, it's too much for me and it's too much for my family.' In addition to low energy and fatigue, Mr Alberts endorsed feeling sad, worthless, guilty, and hopeless that life could be worth living even when sick. While concurrent changes in mood and energy are normative, the presence of these cognitive and emotional symptoms (e.g. worthlessness, guilt, hopelessness) reflected a clinical depression.

Loss of appetite

Loss of appetite frequently occurs during the terminal phase of many illnesses, particularly cancer. Eating is such an integral part of daily life, and indeed is life-sustaining prior to the terminal phase of illness. Moreover, given the nurturing significance of food across cultures, not being able to feed a loved one can elicit confusion, frustration, and helplessness in family members and care-givers. Family members may be concerned that their loved one is 'starving to death' or suffering with hunger pains. This perception can be exacerbated by visible weight loss or cachexia, which often occurs towards the end of life. However, loss of appetite towards the end of life is truly a *loss* of appetite, in which the patient rarely feels hungry and has little desire for food. Loss of appetite and weight loss are generally products of the underlying disease process.

As disease progresses and appetite decreases, questions about artificial nutrition and artificial hydration often occur. Decisions to administer or withdraw artificial nutrition should centre on the patient's goals of care, as well as conversations about the benefits and risks (informed consent) and patient preferences. Geropsychologists can encourage patients and family members to explore and discuss nutrition and hydration preferences in the context of goals of care (Del Rio et al. 2012). For example, if a person is unable to eat because a tumour is interfering with the ability to swallow, artificial nutrition may be helpful. This intervention may be especially helpful if the person still feels hungry or thirsty, and a feeding tube could alleviate suffering or discomfort related to hunger. In general, if the patient enjoys the taste, feel, or experience of the food, eating may still be possible. However, pressuring patients to eat when they are not hungry, or the forced feeding of someone who is not hungry is unlikely to be beneficial for either the patient or family, despite the loving and nurturing intentions.

Delirium

Delirium is a disorder of consciousness which presents as hyperactivity (increased arousal, agitation, hallucinations, day-night reversal), hypoactivity (withdrawal, lethargy, reduced arousal), or a mix of the two. Hallucinations can be pleasant (dead relatives, guardian beings, young children, or babies) or unpleasant (bugs are common).

Delirium can be very distressing for the individuals themselves, their family members, and treatment providers. For families, delirium can be frightening to witness, evoke fear and helplessness, and is associated with generalized anxiety in the care-giver (Buss et al. 2007). Agitation can be particularly troubling to families, yet they may feel ambivalent about aggressively managing this symptom if it means sedating individuals and eliminating the possibility of meaningful communication. In addition, families often misinterpret the causes of delirium, attributing the behaviour to opioids, pain, psychosis, or even death anxiety. Geropsychologists can help families by normalizing delirium as a common, manageable experience, as well as by providing psychoeducation (i.e. explanations of the putative causes, expected course) and reviewing management strategies.

Terminal delirium is highly prevalent in the advanced stages of dying and is typically refractory to intervention, which may be a function of nonreversible causes such as tumour burden, renal/hepatic failure, or vascular complications. However, the aetiology of delirium is often multifactorial, and potentially reversible causes should be considered such as urinary tract infections, constipation, pain, medications (e.g. opioid toxicities) or vitamin deficiencies. Even in terminal delirium, delirious individuals may continue to have periods of relative lucidity, and family should be encouraged to take advantage of that time (Namba et al. 2007).

Non-pharmacological interventions include maintenance of structure/routine, presence of familiar belongings or people, reduction or elimination of noise or excess stimulation, and reassurance (e.g. that the patient is safe, being well-cared for, not challenging or minimizing delusions or hallucinations). In addition, geropsychologists will want to look for potentially meaningful clues to unfinished life tasks, as well as to current unmet needs, in the behaviour of delirious individuals.

Psycho-social-spiritual reactions

Up until this point, we have focused on physical changes and symptoms associated with advanced illness and end of life. Patients and families also experience many psycho-social-spiritual responses. These responses may be normative or non-normative, even clinically significant, such as diagnosable psychiatric disorders. Though much can be learned from framing death as a normative event within lifespan development, many individuals are emotionally distressed at the end of life. Distress is treated most effectively when both the underlying causes and meaning/significance of the symptoms are considered. Equally important, however, is identifying and facilitating positive emotions and a sense of well-being that many individuals experience, including gratitude, compassion, forgiveness, spiritual comfort, and post-traumatic growth.

Stress associated with treatment decisions

Individuals with advanced or terminal illness can face a myriad of treatment decisions such as choosing not to start life-prolonging interventions, withdrawing or discontinuing life-prolonging treatments, or completing advance directives. Individuals may be overwhelmed with the entire process and need a sounding board. Geropsychologists can listen, offer basic information about illness and the dying process, identify medically ill persons' and their families' values and goals for living and dying, clarify treatment options, obtain advanced directives, and evaluate factors that can influence decision-making and decisional capacity (e.g. depression, pain, religiosity, value of quality of life, fear of the dying process, cognitive impairment, and the influence of family members).

Strain in interpersonal relationships and unfinished business

Illness impacts families along the disease continuum, from diagnosis to death, and members must integrate the experience of the patient's illness into their ongoing lives. Illness can trigger changes in roles, relationships, communication, and finances (Stenberg, Ruland, and Miaskowski 2010), and family members may experience conflict over these changes. Families may struggle to communicate effectively and make decisions collaboratively, particularly in families with long-standing, conflictual patterns of relating (King and Quill 2006). Geropsychologists can discuss ways to modulate conflictual patterns and discern the family's ability to tolerate and resolve conflict.

Families may also be stressed by unfinished business, both practical—such as wills that are not updated, final arrangements that are incomplete—or emotional—such as unrepaired relationships or limited legacy-building activities. Geropsychologists can assist individuals with advanced, life-limiting, or terminal illness and their families with saying what they still need to say and doing what is important to them. Byock (2004) offers a helpful framework for this work, building on the fundamental tenet that while people cannot undo the past, they can express forgiveness, gratitude, and affection, thereby increasing the likelihood of healing and reconciliation.

In the case of Mr Alberts, the family followed an unspoken rule that they would not talk about him dying, despite the obvious fact that Mr Alberts was living in the inpatient hospice unit. His family was close and supportive, but unable to talk about him dying, particularly when his wife Grace was in the room. In response to Mrs Alberts' avoidance and Mr Alberts' frustration that he could not talk with his wife about dying, the psychologist met individually with Mrs Alberts about how she was coping with Ben's hospitalization and physical decline. She seemed overwhelmed as she talked about her feelings, 'It feels like a roller coaster. One minute I'm having good memories of Ben and me, but then I get sad when I remember he's dying…I'm going to miss him so much.' The psychologist normalized Mrs Alberts' experiences and the unpredictability and intensity of her love, loss, and grief, and also reflected the amount of effort Grace spent avoiding feeling sad. When the psychologist noted how exhausting and lonely it sounded, Mrs Alberts responded that despite doing everything she could imagine not to feel overwhelmed and sad, she remained scared and sad. She explained that she saw herself as a strong woman, and took pride in her ability to care for herself and her husband. She indicated that she wanted to have a different kind of conversation with Ben in which she could discuss her emotions but did not know how. The psychologist offered to meet jointly with the couple, and also offered hope and encouragement that they could learn how to have these different conversations.

The psychologist met with the couple at bedside, and initially was more active through redirecting, interrupting, and encouraging them to talk about how Ben's illness affected them. Mr Alberts talked about the difficulty of living with a serious illness and explained 'how tired I am of being sick and tired' and that he felt ready to die. This statement was painful for Grace to hear. She shared feeling angry because she believed that Ben was giving up the little time they had left together. The psychologist created space for the couple to share their difficulties and experiences, and explored their assumptions about what it meant to be 'ready to die'. As the couple talked, they expressed a range of thoughts that initially seemed contradictory to them (i.e., feeling ready to die and still loving his wife deeply).

This conversation was the first of many conversations about dying (and living) between the psychologist and Mr and Mrs Alberts. The conversations became easier to facilitate and within weeks, the couple started sharing conversations they had had on their own. Even after sixty years of marriage, the couple discovered new things about each other. They talked about how each of them wanted to be remembered, as well as Mr Alberts' hopes and concerns about what his wife's life would look like after he died. The couple began including other family members in these conversations, which provided opportunities for everyone to consider and share their own hopes for life, dying and death. These discussions also rewrote the family's unspoken rule that conversations about death and dying were too painful or difficult to have.

Grief

Individuals with advanced or terminal illness often experience a myriad of losses: loss of health, function, independence, autonomy, control, predictability, mental clarity, sense of purpose or meaning, status in the family, future hopes and dreams, and a sense of normalcy. Grief over these losses is normative, and can manifest in waves of emotion, including anger, sadness, irritability, and distractibility (Casarett, Kutner, and Abrahm 2001). How individuals make sense of loss is critical to adjustment. Geropsychologists can provide opportunities for medically ill individuals and their families to explore the meaning and impact of current or anticipated losses in order to help them create new meaning in the face of adversity (Nadeau 2001). Even if new meaning cannot be found easily, sharing one's sorrow and loss lessens the isolation of the experience.

Geropsychologists will want to be able to identify normal grief and distinguish it from complicated grief or Prolonged Grief Disorder (Dillen, Fontaine, and Verhofstadt-Denève 2008). Prolonged Grief Disorder is characterized by distressing and functionally disabling symptoms including intrusive thoughts and images of the deceased person, painful yearning for his/her presence, and some combination of shock and emotional numbing, mistrust, anger, diminished sense of self and meaning in life, and difficulty accepting the loss or avoidance of reminders of the loss (Prigerson et al. 2009). Geropsychologists will also want to be aware of the factors that put family members at risk for complications in the bereavement process as well as those factors that are protective, in the hopes of being able to intervene on modifiable factors prior to bereavement. Risk factors for prolonged grief include secondary stressors (e.g. financial strains); multiple, concurrent losses (Tomarken et al. 2008); circumstances of the death such as lack of preparation (Barry, Kasl, and Prigerson 2002) or hospital death (Wright et al. 2010); interpersonal factors and psychological vulnerabilities. Interpersonal factors encompass the degree to which family members feel close to or dependent on (Johnson et al. 2007) or define themselves by their relationship to the ill person (Mancini et al. 2009) or experience unresolved family issues (Kissane et al. 1996; Kissane and Bloch 2008). Psychological vulnerabilities include depression and perceived burden (Schulz et al. 2006); experiential or behavioural avoidance (Shear 2010); intolerance of uncertainty (Boelen, Van den Bout, and Van den Hout 2003); and rumination (Stroebe et al. 2007). Factors that can be protective against complications in bereavement include an ability to make sense of loss, find personal meaning or compensatory benefit in the experience, an ability to regulate one's emotional state, spirituality, and general resiliency characteristics such as self-esteem, hardiness, and positive expectancies (Bonanno 2004; Neimeyer, Baldwin, and Gillies 2006).

Geropsychologists can provide psychoeducation and support for normative grief (for those individuals seeking support) and make referrals for specialized treatment when individuals experience complications in bereavement (Wittouck et al. 2011). Approaches include Complicated Grief Disorder treatment (Shear et al. 2005), narrative-based interventions (Neimeyer 2001), cognitive-behavioural therapy (Boelen et al. 2007), grief therapy (Worden 2008), and family-focused grief therapy (Kissane and Bloch 2008).

Existential issues

Often as a result of the multitude of losses, individuals' basic sense of who they are is threatened. Many individuals at the end of life report a diminished sense of dignity, believe they are a burden to others, or express a waning will to live and a growing desire for death (Chochinov et al. 2002). Perceived burden is associated with loss of dignity, suffering, depression, and a desire for hastened death (McPherson, Wilson, and Murray 2007).

Individuals can experience spiritual or existential angst, a crisis of faith or hopelessness, questions of meaning, or guilt. Geropsychologists' and medically ill individuals' tasks include identifying aspects of the individuals' identity that transcend the illness or physical decline and seeing them for the individuals they have been, rather than the disease with which they live. Fruitful areas to explore are religious/spiritual beliefs, evaluations of self-worth, sources of meaning and purpose, ways to continue to contribute that accommodate the illness, things that the ill individuals value, and their legacy. Ethical wills or legacy documents—a document in which the individual communicates personal values and beliefs, life stories and lessons and advice with the intention of passing them on to another generation—can be particularly useful to this end.

Geropsychologists may find themselves needing to sit with and validate individuals' suffering while raising the possibility that life still can have meaning in the midst of suffering. Sometimes a geropsychologist's greatest intervention is to bear witness to the suffering, validate the experience, and affirm the individual's humanity—complete with flaws, regrets, failings, goodness, resiliencies, and fundamental worth to others. Trying to 'fix' or lessen the feeling can be invalidating in many circumstances. Therapeutic approaches such as life review (Butler 1963), acceptance and commitment therapy (Hayes, Strosahl, and Wilson 1999), meaning-centred GROUP PSYCHOTHERAPY (e.g. Breitbart et al. 2010), and dignity therapy (Chochinov 2012) are particularly useful to this end. See LeMay and Wilson (2008) for a comprehensive review of treatments for existential distress in advanced illness.

Psychiatric Disorders

As mentioned earlier, individuals with advanced and terminal illness may experience psychiatric symptoms, often elevated to the point of diagnosable disorders. In the following section, we review three of the more common psychiatric disorders: depression, anxiety, and post-traumatic stress disorder (PTSD). See Kasl-Godley (2011) for a broader discussion of psychiatric disorders at the end of life.

Depression

Prevalence of Major Depressive Disorder among persons with advanced disease ranges from 5% to 15% and varies depending on the patient population, type and severity of physical illness, and method and timing of assessment (Hotopf et al. 2002; Kadan-Lottick et al. 2005; Reeve, Lloyd-Willams, and Dowrick 2008; Wilson et al. 2007). When including clinically significant depressive symptoms or Adjustment Disorders, the rates increase to 20–50% among patients in palliative and hospice settings (Derogatis et al. 1983; Rayner et al. 2011).

Certain medical illnesses, disease complications, and/or treatment are associated with depression. These conditions include cancer (particularly pancreatic, oropharynx, breast, brain tumours or metastases), hypercalcaemia, anaemia, corticosteroids, chemotherapy, whole brain radiation, CNS complications, and thyroid disorders (Miovic and Block 2007). Additional risk factors include functional dependence and loss of control, poor pain control, a diminished sense of meaning or purpose, a history of depression, perception of oneself as a burden, poor support, and concurrent stressors such as financial strain and younger age (Wilson, Lander, and Chochinov 2009).

Ideally, all individuals should be screened for depression at the time of referral to palliative care. Assessment should include a comprehensive review of possible risk factors, behavioural observation, proxy reports when possible and, clinical interview/self-report screening measures such as the Geriatric Depression Scale or Hospital Anxiety and Depression Scale. Geropsychologists may also need to monitor any tendency within themselves or other providers to minimize symptoms of depression—rationalizing them away by saying, 'I'd feel that way too if I had advanced cancer.'

One key issue during assessment is to consider the overlap of symptoms associated with advanced or terminal illness, medication, and depression. For example, decreased appetite, weight loss, sleep disturbances, and fatigue or decreased energy can be a function of depression, disease, and/or medication. Furthermore, symptoms can represent Major Depression, Adjustment Disorder with Depressed Mood, grief and complicated bereavement, and/or subsyndromal symptoms. When developing differential diagnoses, it is useful to consider not only the severity, pervasiveness, and/or duration of symptoms but the presence of particular cognitive symptoms—namely dysphoria, anhedonia, hopelessness, negative self-image, guilt, helplessness, worthlessness, and goal-directed suicidal ideation.

Another salient issue among people with terminal illness is normative thoughts of death. Although terminally ill individuals may hope that death comes quickly and even desire hastening their dying process, most do not have plans to hasten their death nor exhibit goal-directed suicidal ideation (SI) which is more typical of severe depression and hopelessness. Typically, thoughts of death are transient and associated with feelings of loss of control and anxiety about the future. Some individuals may be afraid to share thoughts about wishing to die for fear that they will be seen as suicidal. If individuals endorse thoughts of death, geropsychologists will want to explore the person's reasons for wanting to end life now and the meanings of the desire to die; presence of physical symptoms and their degree of management, particularly pain; religious, spiritual, and existential concerns; and reasons for living (Spencer et al. 2012). Risk for goal-directed SI increases in the presence of suffering, poor prognosis, poor communication with healthcare providers, difficulties with making treatment decisions and with everyday living, hopelessness, helplessness, substance use, personal and family history of suicide, lack of social support, and diminished control (Leung et al. 2013).

For Mr Alberts, the aetiology of his depression was multifactorial. His mood was influenced by his medical problems (heart failure, weakness, fatigue), his history of depression, and the constrained communication with his family about death and dying. When the psychologist highlighted the ways in which these physical and emotional issues were contributing to his depressed mood, Mr Alberts expressed relief. He also felt encouraged when he heard about available treatment options. After consultation with the medical team, the psychologist recommended a combination of interventions, including restarting an anti-depressant, taking a low-dose stimulant in the afternoon to improve his energy, and individual and couple psychotherapy at bedside. The psychotherapy focused on helping the couple become less emotionally isolated from each other and come to terms with Mr Alberts' decline, identifying and challenging Mr Alberts' automatic thoughts about being a burden, and reinforcing the values and legacy Mr Alberts exemplified in his life, and transmitted to his family.

Mr Alberts' mood improved with treatment. His relationships with his wife and adult children became closer, and the family developed the strength to talk when sad or crying, rather than turning away from each other or changing the subject. Their closeness was palpable and created a quiet strength that each member of the family could draw upon when needed.

Treatment of mood disorders at the end of life should include aggressive management of the underlying medical illness and associated physical symptoms as well as the mood disorder. The overarching goals are to manage the psychiatric symptoms, strengthen coping with the disease and associated changes, reduce helplessness and hopelessness, promote meaning making, and improve quality of life. There are very few studies examining the effectiveness of psychological treatment for depression in hospice and palliative care patients but the findings are encouraging. CBT has been found to reduce depressive symptoms in patients with advanced cancer (Williams and Dale 2006) as has supportive-expressive therapy (Kissane et al. 2007). Cognitive therapy has also been found to reduce depressive symptoms as well as fatigue, insomnia, and anxiety in women with metastatic breast cancer (Savard et al. 2006). Mindfulness-based stress reduction seems to be a useful approach in managing depressive symptoms in people with cancer (Garland et al. 2007). Life review, which is an explicit focus of hospice and palliative care, is effective in treating depression in older adults (Serrano et al. 2004), but it has not been examined as a means of reducing depression in terminally ill patients.

Anxiety

Prevalence of anxiety disorders in individuals with advanced and terminal illness ranges from 2% to 30% (Kadan-Lottick et al. 2005; Miovic and Block 2007; Roth and Massie 2007; Spencer et al. 2010). Risk factors include physical performance status, underlying disease, particularly for those diseases that cause shortness of breath and hypoxia (e.g. pneumonia, pulmonary embolism, lung cancer, pleural effusion, COPD, and cardiac disease), endocrine disorders (diabetes, hyper/hypothyroidism), neurological diseases (Parkinson's), metabolic disorders (hypo/hypercalcaemia, hyperkalaemia, dehydration, hyponatraemia), sepsis, or impending cardiac or respiratory arrest. Anxiety can also be associated with medications (e.g. corticosteroids, stimulants, anti-emetics, bronchodilators) and withdrawal from medication (e.g. opioids, benzodiazepines) or alcohol.

Anxiety may represent a conditioned response to treatment (e.g. chemotherapy, radiation) or a reaction to poorly controlled symptoms such as pain. Procedures such as wound care or personal care that may exacerbate discomfort can result in conditioned anxiety (Roth and Massie 2007). A prior history of anxiety disorder also may increase risk for anxiety at the end of life.

Medically ill individuals often experience anxiety in response to uncertainties and fears inherent in living with life-limiting or terminal illness. They may fear medical interventions, treatment, or particular symptoms and may worry about their capacity to cope with those symptoms. They may fear incapacity, dependency, or disfigurement, and may have specific fears about dying, engendered in part from past experiences of the death of significant others. They may fear past transgressions and being rejected or abandoned. They may be concerned about how their loved ones will cope after they are gone. They may worry about financial, legal, and practical matters and fear not having time to complete their affairs. They may fear non-existence or the afterlife.

Assessment of anxiety in individuals with advanced or terminal illness is complicated by the fact that physical causes of anxiety can be difficult to distinguish from psychological ones. Physical symptoms used to diagnose anxiety and panic may be present as a part of the normal dying process. In addition, anxiety symptoms may reflect a diagnosable disorder, normative fears, or existential suffering and are likely to co-occur with depression and/ or delirium. As with depression, it may be helpful to focus on cognitive symptoms such as de-realization, de-personalization, and fears of going crazy, generalized worries, or worries about a future panic attack (Periyakoil, Skultety, and Sheikh 2005). As part of an assessment, geropsychologists will want to explore the nature of patients' and involved family members' fears. Common shared fears include that the medically ill person will suffer, that the care-giver will not be available when the person needs him/her, that the care-giver will not know what to do in the event of a medical crisis, or that the person's treatment preferences will not be honoured (Bambauer et al. 2006).

Treatment of anxiety disorders includes aggressive management of symptoms associated with the underlying physical illness as well as anxiety. Very few studies have examined the effectiveness of psychotherapeutic interventions for anxiety in hospice and palliative care patients. Cognitive restructuring, relaxation training, and coping skills rehearsal have been associated with reduced anxiety and psychological distress in individuals with advanced cancer (Moorey et al. 1998). Supportive therapy and psychoeducation are also effective in reducing anxiety symptoms.

Acute stress response and post-traumatic stress disorder (PTSD)

Individuals diagnosed with a life-threatening illness may be at increased risk for developing acute stress responses and PTSD, with estimates ranging from 0% to 33% (Kangas, Henry, and Bryant 2002; McGarvey et al. 1998). Risk factors include prior negative life stressors, female gender, younger age at diagnosis, avoidant coping, poor social support, reduced physical functioning, poor provider–patient communication, prior trauma history, and psychological problems and elevated distress subsequent to diagnosis (Butler et al. 1999; Kangas, Henry, and Bryant 2005, 2007).

To what extent the life-threatening or terminal illness is the instigating trauma vs a trigger for pre-existing PTSD is unclear. Deterioration of health may create a sense of vulnerability or loss of control similar to that experienced during the original trauma (Buffum and Wolfe 1995). The threat to life and body integrity inherent in terminal illness, to both personal and physical integrity, may mimic the original trauma, exacerbating previous PTSD (Feldman and Periyakoil 2006). Post-treatment scars or physical limitations can be persistent reminders of the disease and evoke perceived threat. Pain may trigger PTSD symptoms or be a co-occurring condition (Gold et al. 2012). Diagnostic tests, medical procedures, or even personal care can also trigger overwhelming anxiety if they reproduce the trauma experience (e.g. colonoscopy mimicking sexual abuse, cleaning of genitals during personal care). Tests and procedures that evoke prior trauma experiences may result in the individual with PTSD avoiding or ignoring problems or refusing care.

PTSD can impinge on factors important to hospice and palliative care, namely emotional and practical support, communication, life review, and unfinished business (Feldman 2011). Many individuals with PTSD are used to being isolated and detached and are wary of interpersonal relationships, particularly those with people in positions of authority. They have a high need for control and are avoidant of trauma reminders. They may have difficulty communicating with care providers, as direct, clear communication requires effective affect regulation and trust of others, both of which are difficult for persons with PTSD. The normal process of life review and attending to unfinished business for persons with PTSD at the end of life may induce anxiety, guilt, anger, or sadness when key memories are trauma related. Thus, individuals with PTSD may avoid the life review process in order to avoid or suppress reminders or feelings.

Standard treatments for PTSD have limitations for individuals at the end of life, particularly length of time, both in terms of duration of treatment and length of individual sessions (e.g. prolonged exposure) and the likelihood of increasing distress in the short term when individuals may have only a relatively short time to live. Pilot studies of prolonged exposure with older adults look promising but they have not been replicated with individuals with advanced illness (Thorpe 2009). A model proposed by Hyer and Woods (1998) for treatment of PTSD in older adults also has potential application to the treatment of PTSD at the end of life. In this multistage model, treatment begins by addressing short-term concerns, then proceeds to longer-range concerns should the medically ill persons live long enough to benefit from addressing such issues. Supportive-expressive therapy in combination with psychoeducation has been associated with reductions in traumatic stress symptoms and mood disturbance in women with advanced breast cancer (Classen et al. 2001).

What is Different about Hospice and Palliative Care Work?

Psychotherapy with individuals with advanced and terminal illness typically demands cognitive flexibility, high distress tolerance, and a high tolerance for ambiguity. The pace can be rapid and the manner in which issues unfold can be unpredictable. Geropsychologists need to be comfortable 'seizing the moment' and tackling difficult issues, even when one has no prior relationship, rather than waiting 'to develop a therapeutic rapport'. They need to be able to evaluate critically and modify their practice to accommodate their patients' medical status (e.g. fatigue, cognitive impairment, pain) and to help colleagues of other disciplines do the same.

Like other forms of psychotherapy in medical settings, psychotherapy as part of palliative care will rarely follow the typical, fifty-minute outpatient model in which individuals are self-referred and requesting assistance. Geropsychologists must be comfortable checking in with individuals, unsolicited, and learn how to engage individuals and family members who may not conceptualize their symptoms in psychological terms and/or who are sceptical about mental healthcare. Psychologists are often working with emotions and reactions that are normative but distressing (e.g. fear, sadness, anticipatory grief, existential distress). When feelings are normalized, validated, and supported, patients and families often welcome conversations with psychologists. Psychotherapy also requires flexibility, as treatment rarely matches standardized protocols (e.g. twelve sessions of CBT for depression) and the empirical literature guiding psychological treatment approaches is limited. This limited empirical base necessitates extrapolating from existing relevant literature with appropriate modifications. Therapy goals may need to be very focused and time-limited, with the expectation that every session may need to stand on its own.

Psychotherapy may also involve more self-disclosure on the part of the therapist, although the guidelines for appropriate self-disclosure in the service of the patient still apply, and the potential for stronger emotional and counter-transference responses is important to recognize (see Katz and Johnson 2006). Psychotherapy in this setting necessitates reflective practice and a high degree of self-awareness, particularly because dying and death is a universal experience that evokes complex feelings in patients, families, and providers alike. See Kastenbaum (2000) for additional discussion of psychotherapy with dying persons.

Working in the field of palliative care offers unique opportunities to change lives for the better, including our own. By helping seriously ill patients and their families find connection and healing in the midst of medical suffering, we ourselves are privileged to find deeper meaning in our own lives. In the words of a recent geropsychology student engaged in palliative care, 'It reinforces my identity as a clinical psychologist and reminds me of the privileges of this career' (Lee, personal communication).

IMPLICATIONS FOR PRACTICE

Developing competence to work with individuals and families coping with serious illness and death is a professional necessity of working with older adults. The following principles summarize the key points of the chapter with respect to clinical practice:

- Older adults may live for years with chronic, progressive, and often comorbid, debilitating illnesses. Thus, dying is more often an extended process for which people have time to prepare, rather than a sudden event. Yet individuals often feel unprepared for dying. Geropsychologists play a key role in helping patients and families prepare for and navigate the transition of 'living with' to 'dying from' a serious illness.

- Palliative care is specialized care for people with a serious illness. It can be provided at any point in the trajectory of a serious illness and ideally begins when a serious illness is diagnosed. The focus of palliative care is to alleviate physical and psycho-social-spiritual suffering, enhance quality of life, manage symptoms, and offer comprehensive, interdisciplinary support to the patient and family throughout the course of illness.
- Geropsychologists must be aware of physical symptoms and disease trajectories of common diseases and symptoms experienced by palliative care patients (e.g. pain, fatigue, dyspnoea, delirium) and be aware of approaches to symptom management, both medical and psychological.
- Geropsychologists must be aware of psychosocial and spiritual challenges that occur during advanced illness and dying, from normative sadness about loss and change to existential angst about meaning and purpose, to development or exacerbation of psychopathology, including major depression or anxiety.
- Geropsychologists also need to be aware of evidence-based methods for differentiating and then working with anticipatory grief, typical and prolonged grief, and distinguishing these conditions from major depression and anxiety or PTSD.
- Living with serious illness and even dying are often times of incredible growth, healing, meaning, and closeness for individuals and families. Geropsychologists need to be mindful of the positive emotions and sense of well-being that individuals can experience. In addition, geropsychologists can reflect and maintain the essence and uniqueness of someone coping with advanced illness or death.
- See Key References below for websites and additional clinical resources.

Summary

Familiarity with issues related to chronic, advanced and terminal illness, that is, issues inherent to palliative care, are professional necessities when working with older adults. This chapter described palliative care, including clinical issues commonly experienced by a person with a serious or advanced illness, and the ways in which geropsychologists can be helpful with these issues. We outlined common physical and psychosocial concerns and reviewed psychological assessment and management techniques for pain, dyspnoea, fatigue, loss of appetite, and delirium, as well as stress associated with treatment decisions, strain in interpersonal relationships, unfinished business, grief, existential issues, depression, anxiety, and PTSD. Although living with and dying from a serious illness present physical and psychosocial concerns, we also encouraged geropsychologists to consider the ways in which facing advanced illness provides opportunities for growth, meaning making, and closeness.

Key References and Sources for Further Reading

Byock, I. (2004). *The Four Things That Matter Most. A Book about Living*. New York: Free Press.

Callanan, M. (2008). *Final Journeys. A Practical Guide for Bringing Care and Comfort at the End of Life*. New York: Bantam Books.

Education for Palliative and End-of-Life Care (http://www.epec.net/). Provides educational materials designed to educate all healthcare professionals in the essential clinical competencies of palliative care. Curriculum include EPEC for caregivers, emergency medicine, long-term care, oncology, paediatrics and veterans.

Emanuel, L. L. and Librach, S. L. (2007). *Palliative Care: Core Skills and Clinical Competencies.* Philadelphia, PA: Saunders.

Feldman, D. B. and Lasher, S. A. (2007). *The End-of-Life Handbook. A Compassionate Guide to Connecting with and Caring for a Dying Loved One.* Oakland, CA: New Harbinger Publications.

Halifax, J. (2008). *Being with Dying: Cultivating Compassion and Fearlessness in the Presence of Death.* Boston, MA: Shambhala Publications.

Hallenbeck, J. L. (2003). *Palliative Care Perspective.* New York: Oxford University Press.

Katz, R. S. and Johnson, T. A. (2006). *When Professionals Weep. Emotional and Counter transference Responses in End-of-life Care.* New York: Routledge.

National Hospice and Palliative Care Organization (http://www.nhpco.org/). Largest nonprofit membership organization representing hospice and palliative care programmes and professionals in US. Develops educational programmes to enhance understanding and availability of hospice and palliative care.

Qualls, S. H. and Kasl-Godley, J. E. (eds) (2011). *End-of-Life Issues, Grief, and Bereavement: What Clinicians Need to Know.* Hoboken, NJ: Wiley.

Speck, P. (2009). *Teamwork in Palliative Care. Fulfilling or Frustrating?* New York: Oxford University Press.

Werth, J. L. and Blevins, D. (eds) (2006). *Psychosocial Issues Near the End of Life. A Resource for Professional Care Providers.* Washington, DC: American Psychological Association.

Yalom, I. (2008). *Staring at the Sun. Overcoming the Terror of Death.* San Francisco, CA: Jossey-Bass.

REFERENCES

Anderson, G. and Horvath, J. (2004). 'The Growing Burden of Chronic Disease in America'. *Public Health Reports* 119: 263–270.

Bambauer, K. Z., Zhang, B., Maciejewski, P. K., Sahay, N., Pirl, W. F., et al. (2006). 'Mutuality and Specificity of Mental Disorders in Advanced Cancer Patients and Caregivers'. *Social Psychiatry and Psychiatric Epidemiology* 41: 819–824.

Barry L. C., Kasl S. V., and Prigerson H. G. (2002). 'Psychiatric Disorders among Bereaved Persons: The Role of Perceived Circumstances of Death and Preparedness for Death'. *American Journal of Geriatric Psychiatry* 10: 447–457.

Bell, C. L., Somogyi-Zalud, E., and Masaki, K. H. (2010). 'Factors Associated with Congruence between Preferred and Actual Place of Death'. *Journal of Pain and Symptom Management* 39: 591–604.

Boelen, P. A., Van den Bout, J., and Van den Hout, M. A. (2003). 'The Role of Negative Interpretations of Grief Reactions in Emotional Problems after Bereavement'. *Journal of Behavior Therapy and Experimental Psychiatry* 34: 225–238.

Boelen, P. A., De Keijser, J., Van den Hout, M. A., and Van den Bout, J. (2007). 'Treatment of Complicated Grief: A Comparison between Cognitive-Behavioral Therapy and Supportive Counseling'. *Journal of Consulting and Clinical Psychology* 75: 277–284.

Bonanno, G. A. (2004). 'Loss, Trauma, and Human Resilience: Have We Underestimated the Human Capacity to Thrive after Extremely Aversive Events?' *American Psychologist* 59: 20–28.

Breitbart, W., Rosenfeld, B., Gibson, C., Pessin, H., Poppito, S., et al. (2010). 'Meaning-centered Group Psychotherapy for Patients with Advanced Cancer: A Pilot Randomized Controlled Trial'. *Psycho-Oncology* 19: 21–28.

Buffum, M. D. and Wolfe, N. S. (1995). 'Posttraumatic Stress Disorder and the World War II Veteran'. *Geriatric Nursing* 16: 264–270.

Buss, M. K., Vanderwerker, L. C., Inouye, S. K., Zhang, B., Block, S. D., et al. (2007). 'Associations between Caregiver-perceived Delirium in Patients with Cancer and Generalized Anxiety in their Caregivers'. *Journal of Palliative Medicine* 10: 1083–1092.

Butler, L. D., Koopman, C., Classen, C., and Spiegel, D. (1999). 'Traumatic Stress, Life Events, and Emotional Support in Women with Metastatic Breast Cancer: Cancer-related Traumatic Stress Symptoms Associated with Past and Current Stressors'. *Health Psychology* 18: 555–560.

Butler, R. N. (1963). 'The Life Review: An Interpretation of Reminiscence in the Aged'. *Psychiatry* 26: 65–76.

Byock, I. (2004). *The Four Things That Matter Most: A Book About Living*. New York: Free Press.

Campbell, M. L. (2012). 'Dyspnea Prevalence, Trajectories, and Measurement in Critical Care and at Life's End'. *Current Opinion in Supportive and Palliative Care* 6: 168–171.

Casarett, D., Kutner, J. S., and Abrahm, J. (2001). 'Life after Death: A Practical Approach to Grief and Bereavement'. *Annals of Internal Medicine* 134: 208–215.

Chochinov, H. M., Hack, T., Hassard, T., Kristjanson, L. J., McClement, S., et al. (2002). 'Dignity in the Terminally Ill: A Cross-sectional, Cohort Study'. *Lancet* 360: 2026–2030.

Chochinov, H. M. (2012). *Dignity Therapy: Final Words for Final Days*. New York: Oxford University Press.

Classen, C., Butler, L. D., Koopman, C., Miller, E., DiMiceli, S., et al. (2001). 'Supportive-expressive Group Therapy and Distress in Patients with Metastatic Breast Cancer: A Randomized Clinical Intervention Trial'. *Archives of General Psychiatry* 58: 494–501.

Corner, J., Plant, H., A'Hern, R., and Bailey, C. (1996). 'Non-pharmacological Intervention for Breathlessness in Lung Cancer'. *Palliative Medicine* 10: 299–305.

Dalal, S. and Bruera, E. (2011). 'Assessment and Management of Pain in the Terminally Ill'. *Primary Care* 38: 195–223.

Del Rio, M. I., Shand, B., Bonati, P., Palma, A., Maldonado, A., et al. (2012). 'Hydration and Nutrition at the End of Life: A Systematic Review of Emotional Impact, Perceptions, and Decision-making among Patients, Family, and Health Care Staff'. *Psycho-Oncology* 21: 913–921.

Derogatis, L. R., Morrow, G. R., Fetting, J., Penman, D., Piasetsky, S., et al. (1983). 'The Prevalence of Psychiatric Disorders among Cancer Patients'. *Journal of the American Medical Association* 249: 751–757.

Dillen, L., Fontaine, J. R. J., and Verhofstadt-Denève, L. (2008). 'Are Normal and Complicated Grief Different Constructs? A Confirmatory Factor Analytic Test'. *Clinical Psychology and Psychotherapy* 15: 386–395.

Feldman, D. B. and Periyakoil, V. S. (2006). 'Posttraumatic Stress Disorder at the End of Life'. *Journal of Palliative Medicine* 9: 213–218.

Feldman, D. B. (2011). 'Posttraumatic Stress Disorder at the End of Life: Extant Research and Proposed Psychosocial Treatment Approach'. *Palliative and Supportive Care* 9: 407–418.

Garland, S. N., Carlson, L. E., Cook, S., Lansdell, L., and Speca, M. (2007). 'A Non-randomized Comparison of Mindfulness-based Stress Reduction and Healing Arts Programs for

Facilitating Post-traumatic Growth and Spirituality in Cancer Outpatients'. *Supportive Care in Cancer* 15: 949–961.

Glare, P., Virik, K., Jones, M., Hudson, M., Eychmuller, S., et al. (2003). 'A Systematic Review of Physicians' Survival Predictions in Terminally Ill Cancer Patients'. *British Medical Journal* 327: 195–198.

Gold, J. I., Douglas, M. K., Thomas, M. L., Elliott, J. E., Rao, S. M., et al. (2012). 'The Relationship between Posttraumatic Stress Disorder, Mood States, Functional Status, and Quality of Life in Oncology Outpatients'. *Journal of Pain and Symptom Management* 44(4): 520–531.

Halpern, S. P. (2004). *The Etiquette of Illness: What to Say When You Can't Find the Words*. New York: Bloomsbury.

Hayes, S. C., Strosahl, K. D., and Wilson, K. G. (1999). *Acceptance and Commitment Therapy: An Experiential Approach to Behavior Change*. New York: Guilford Press.

Hotopf, M., Chidgey, J., Addington-Hall, J., and Ly, K. L. (2002). 'Depression in Advanced Disease: A Systematic Review Part 1. Prevalence and Case Finding'. *Palliative Medicine* 16: 81–97.

Hyer, L. and Woods, M. (1998). 'Phenomenology and Treatment of Trauma in Later Life'. *Cognitive-behavioral Therapies for Trauma* (pp. 383–414). New York: Guilford Press.

Johnson J. G., Zhang B., Greer J. A., and Prigerson H. G. (2007). 'Parental Control, Partner Dependency, and Complicated Grief among Widowed Adults in the Community'. *Journal of Nervous and Mental Disorders* 195: 26–30.

Kadan-Lottick, N. S., Vanderwerker, L. C., Block, S. D., Zhang, B., and Prigerson, H. G. (2005). 'Psychiatric Disorders and Mental Health Service Use in Patients with Advanced Cancer: A Report from the Coping with Cancer Study'. *Cancer* 104: 2872–2881.

Kamal, A. H., Maguire, J. M., Wheeler, J. L., Currow, D. C., and Abernethy, A. P. (2011). 'Dyspnea Review for the Palliative Care Professional: Assessment, Burdens, and Etiologies'. *Journal of Palliative Medicine* 14: 1167–1172.

Kangas, M., Henry, J. L., and Bryant, R. A. (2002). 'Posttraumatic Stress Disorder Following Cancer. A Conceptual and Empirical Review'. *Clinical Psychology Review* 22: 499–524.

Kangas, M., Henry, J. L., and Bryant, R. A. (2005). 'Predictors of Posttraumatic Stress Disorder Following Cancer'. *Health Psychology* 24: 579–585.

Kangas, M., Henry, J. L., and Bryant, R. A. (2007). 'Correlates of Acute Stress Disorder in Cancer Patients'. *Journal of Traumatic Stress* 20: 325–334.

Kasl-Godley, J. E. (2011). 'Serious Mental Illness'. In S. H. Qualls and J. E. Kasl-Godley (eds), *End-of-life Issues, Grief, and Bereavement: What Clinicians Need to Know*. Hoboken, NJ: Wiley.

Kastenbaum, R. (2000). 'Counseling the Elderly Dying Patient'. *Professional Psychology in Long Term Care: A Comprehensive Guide* (pp. 201–226). New York: Hatherleigh Press.

Katz, R. S. and Johnson, T. A. (2006). *When Professionals Weep: Emotional and Countertransference Responses in End-of-life Care*. London: CRC Press.

King, D. A. and Quill, T. (2006). 'Working with Families in Palliative Care: One Size Does Not Fit All'. *Journal of Palliative Medicine* 9: 704–715.

Kissane, D. W., Bloch, S., Onghena, P., McKenzie, D. P., Snyder, R. D., et al. (1996). 'The Melbourne Family Grief Study, II: Psychosocial Morbidity and Grief in Bereaved Families'. *American Journal of Psychiatry* 153: 659–666.

Kissane, D. W., Grabsch, B., Clarke, D. M., Smith, G. C., Love, A. W., et al. (2007). 'Supportive-expressive Group Therapy for Women with Metastatic Breast Cancer: Survival and Psychosocial Outcome from a Randomized Controlled Trial'. *Psycho-Oncology* 16: 277–286.

Kissane, D. W. and Bloch, S. (2008). *Family Focused Grief Therapy: A Model of Family-Centred Care during Palliative Care and Bereavement*. Philadelphia: Open University Press.

LeMay, K. and Wilson, K. G. (2008). 'Treatment of Existential Distress in Life Threatening Illness: A Review of Manualized Interventions'. *Clinical Psychology Review* 28: 472–493.

Leung, Y. W., Li, M., Devins, G., Zimmermann, C., Rydall, A., et al. (2013). 'Routine Screening for Suicidal Intention in Patients with Cancer'. *Psycho-Oncology* 22(11): 2537–2545. doi:10.10002/pon3319.

McGarvey, E. L., Canterbury, R. J., Koopman, C., Clavet, G. J., Cohen, R., et al. (1998). 'Acute Stress Disorder Following Diagnosis of Cancer'. *International Journal of Rehabilitation and Health* 4: 1–15.

Maciejewski, P. K. and Prigerson, H. G. (2013). 'Emotional Numbness Modifies the Effect of End-of-Life (EOL) Discussions on EOL Care'. *Journal of Pain and Symptom Management* 45: 841–847.

McPherson, C. J., Wilson, K. G., and Murray, M. A. (2007). 'Feeling Like a Burden to Others: A Systematic Review Focusing on the End of Life'. *Palliative Medicine* 21: 115–128.

Mancini, A. D., Robinaugh, D., Shear, K., and Bonanno, G. A. (2009). 'Does Attachment Avoidance Help People Cope with Loss? The Moderating Effects of Relationship Quality'. *Journal of Clinical Psychology* 65: 1127–1136.

Miovic, M. and Block, S. (2007). 'Psychiatric Disorders in Advanced Cancer'. *Cancer* 110: 1665–1676.

Moorey, S., Greer, S., Bliss, J., and Law, M. (1998). 'A Comparison Of Adjuvant Psychological Therapy and Supportive Counselling in Patients with Cancer'. *Psycho-Oncology* 7: 218–228.

Nadeau, J. W. (2001). 'Meaning Making in Family Bereavement: A Family Systems Approach'. In M. S. Stroebe, R. O. Hansson, W. Stroebe, and H. Schut (eds), *Handbook of Bereavement Research: Consequences, Coping, and Care* (pp. 329–347). Washington, DC: American Psychological Association.

Namba, M., Morita, T., Imura, C., Kiyohara, E., Ishikawa, S., et al. (2007). 'Terminal Delirium: Families' Experience'. *Palliative Medicine* 21: 587–594.

National Consensus Project for Quality Palliative Care (2013). *Clinical Practice Guidelines for Quality Palliative Care* (3rd edn). Pittsburgh, PA: National Consensus Project for Quality Palliative Care. http://www.nationalconsensusproject.org.

Neimeyer, R. A. (ed.). (2001). *Meaning Reconstruction and the Experience of Loss* (vol. 8). Washington, DC: American Psychological Association.

Neimeyer, R. A., Baldwin, S. A., and Gillies, J. (2006). 'Continuing Bonds and Reconstructing Meaning: Mitigating Complications in Bereavement'. *Death Studies* 30: 715–738.

Okuyama, T., Akechi, T., Shima, Y., Sugahara, Y., Okamura, H., et al. (2008). 'Factors Correlated with Fatigue in Terminally Ill Cancer Patients: A Longitudinal Study'. *Journal of Pain and Symptom Management* 35: 515–523.

Periyakoil, V. S., Skultety, K., and Sheikh, J. (2005). 'Panic, Anxiety, and Chronic Dyspnea'. *Journal of Palliative Medicine* 8: 453–459.

Prigerson, H. G., Horowitz, M. J., Jacobs, S. C., Parkes, C. M., Aslan, M., et al. (2009). 'Prolonged Grief Disorder: Psychometric Validation Of Criteria Proposed for DSM-V and ICD-11'. *PLoS Medicine* 6: e1000121.

Rao, A. and Cohen, H. J. (2004). 'Symptom Management in the Elderly Cancer Patient: Fatigue, Pain, and Depression'. *Journal of the National Cancer Institute Monographs* 32: 150–157.

Rayner, L., Lee, W., Price, A., Monroe, B., Sykes, N., et al. (2011). 'The Clinical Epidemiology of Depression in Palliative Care and the Predictive Value of Somatic Symptoms: Cross-sectional Survey with Four-week Follow-up'. *Palliative Medicine* 25: 229–241.

Reeve, J. L., Lloyd-Williams, M., and Dowrick, C. (2008). 'Revisiting Depression in Palliative Care Settings: The Need to Focus on Clinical Utility over Validity'. *Palliative Medicine* 22: 383–391.

Ross, D. D. and Alexander, C. S. (2001). 'Management of Common Symptoms in Terminally Ill Patients: Part I. Fatigue, Anorexia, Cachexia, Nausea and Vomiting'. *American Family Physician* 64: 807–815.

Roth, A. J. and Massie, M. J. (2007). 'Anxiety and Its Management in Advanced Cancer'. *Current Opinion in Supportive and Palliative Care* 1: 50–56.

Savard, J., Simard, S., Giguère, I., Ivers, H., Morin, C. M., et al. (2006). 'Randomized Clinical Trial on Cognitive Therapy for Depression in Women with Metastatic Breast Cancer: Psychological and Immunological Effects'. *Palliative and Supportive Care* 4: 219–237.

Schulz, R., Boerner, K., Shear, K., Zhang, S., and Gitlin, L. N. (2006). 'Predictors of Complicated Grief among Dementia Caregivers: A Prospective Study of Bereavement'. *American Journal of Geriatric Psychiatry* 14: 650–658.

Serrano, J. P., Latorre, J. M., Gatz, M., and Montanes, J. (2004). 'Life Review Therapy Using Autobiographical Retrieval Practice for Older Adults with Depressive Symptomatology'. *Psychology and Aging* 19: 270–277.

Shear, K., Frank, E., Houck, P. R., and Reynolds, C. F. III (2005). 'Treatment of complicated Grief: A Randomized Controlled Trial'. *Journal of the American Medical Association* 293: 2601–2608.

Shear, M. K. (2010). 'Exploring the Role of Experiential Avoidance from the Perspective of Attachment Theory and the Dual Process Model'. *Omega* 61: 357–369.

Spencer, R., Nilsson M., Wright A., Pirl W., and Prigerson H. (2010). 'Anxiety Disorders in Advanced Cancer Patients: Correlates and Predictors of End-of-life Outcomes'. *Cancer* 116: 1810–1819.

Spencer, R. J, Ray, A., Pirl, W. F., and Prigerson, H. G. (2012). 'Clinical Correlates of Suicidal Thoughts in Patients with Advanced Cancer'. *American Journal of Geriatric Psychiatry* 20: 327–336.

Steinhauser, K. E., Christakis, N. A., Clipp, E. C., McNeilly, M., McIntyre, L., et al. (2000). 'Factors Considered Important at the End of Life by Patients, Family, Physicians, and Other Care Providers'. *Journal of the American Medical Association* 284: 2476–2482.

Stenberg, U., Ruland, C. M., and Miaskowski, C. (2010). 'Review of the Literature on the Effects of Caring for a Patient with Cancer'. *Psycho-Oncology* 19: 1013–1025.

Stroebe, M., Boelen, P. A., Van den Hout, M., Stroebe, W., Salemink, E., et al. (2007). 'Ruminative Coping as Avoidance: A Reinterpretation of its Function in Adjustment to Bereavement'. *European Archives of Psychiatry and Clinical Neuroscience* 257: 462–472.

Temel, J. S., Greer, J. A., Muzikansky, A., Gallagher, E. R., Admane, S., et al. (2010). 'Early Palliative Care for Patients with Metastatic Non-small-cell Lung Cancer'. *New England Journal of Medicine* 363: 733–742.

Thorpe, S. (2009). 'Addressing PTSD among Older Veterans'. Paper presented at the Meeting the Challenges of the Uniform Mental Health Services Handbook Conference, Palo Alto, CA.

Tomarken, A., Holland, J., Schachter, S., Vanderwerker, L., Zuckerman, E., et al. (2008). 'Factors of Complicated Grief Pre-death in Caregivers of Cancer Patients'. *Psycho-Oncology* 17: 105–111.

Weissman, D. E. and Meier, D. E. (2011). 'Identifying Patients in Need of a Palliative Care Assessment in the Hospital Setting: A Consensus Report from the Center to Advance Palliative Care'. *Journal of Palliative Medicine* 14: 17–23.

World Health Organization (2007). *Palliative Care*. Geneva: WHO. http://www.who.int/cancer/palliative/en/.

World Health Organization (2008). *The Global Burden of Disease: 2004 Update*. Geneva: WHO.

Williams, S. and Dale, J. (2006). 'The Effectiveness of Treatment for Depression/Depressive Symptoms in Adults with Cancer: A Systematic Review'. *British Journal of Cancer* 94: 372–390.

Wilson, K. G., Chochinov, H. M., Skirko, M. G., Allard, P., Chary, S., et al. (2007). 'Depression and Anxiety Disorders in Palliative Cancer Care'. *Journal of Pain and Symptom Management* 33: 118–129.

Wilson, K. G., Lander, M., and Chochinov, H. M. (2009). 'Diagnosis and Management of Depression in Palliative Care'. *Handbook of Psychiatry in Palliative Medicine* (pp. 39–68). Oxford: Oxford University Press.

Wittouck, C., Van Autreve, S., De Jaegere, E., Portzky, G., and Van Heeringen, K. (2011). 'The Prevention and Treatment of Complicated Grief: A Meta-analysis'. *Clinical Psychology Review* 31: 69–78.

Worden, J. W. (2008). *Grief Counseling and Grief Therapy: A Handbook for the Mental Health Practitioner* (4th edn). New York: Springer.

Wright, A. A., Keating, N. L., Balboni, T. A., Matulonis, U. A., Block, S. D., et al. (2010). 'Place of Death: Correlations with Quality of Life of Patients with Cancer and Predictors of Bereaved Caregivers' Mental Health'. *Journal of Clinical Oncology* 28: 4457–4464.

Wright, A. A., Zhang, B., Ray, A., Mack, J. W., Trice, E., et al. (2008). 'Associations between End-of-life Discussions, Patient Mental Health, Medical Care near Death, and Caregiver Bereavement Adjustment'. *Journal of the American Medical Association* 300: 1655–1673.

PART III

SOURCES OF PSYCHOLOGICAL DISTRESS

CHAPTER 18

LONELINESS AND HEALTH IN LATER LIFE

CONSTANÇA PAÚL

INTRODUCTION

LONELINESS is a major issue in the ageing literature, but more importantly is a negative experience for human beings, contributing to poor quality of life across the globe. The experience of loneliness appears to be a very relevant issue from a social as well as a psychological point of view, and assumes particular relevance in old age. Beside the objective conditions that contribute to loneliness, the subjective experience is somehow universal and independent from an individual's socio-economic conditions; this constitutes a challenge for those working in the ageing field. From a psychological perspective, in addition to investigating the causes of loneliness, one should devote time to understanding the consequences of loneliness for subjective well-being as well as physical and mental health. Withdrawing from work contexts, increasing loss of friends and family members due to death, and other age-related losses may lead to strong feelings of loneliness. Considering that loneliness may be a modifiable factor of distress in old age, it is crucial clearly to understand its determinants and consequences in order to organize interventions to prevent or buffer negative outcomes during the ageing process.

There is no universal definition of loneliness, although it is generally described as a perceived deprivation of social contact, the lack of people available or willing to share social and emotional experiences, a state where an individual has the potential to interact with others but is not doing so, or a discrepancy between the actual and desired interaction and intimacy with others (Gierveld 1998; Victor et al 2000). Whether loneliness is considered a social or a psychological problem, intervention will focus on facilitating social networks or working on emotional problems that contribute to feelings of loneliness and depression.

While loneliness describes the subjective feeling of living in the absence of social contacts or support, it can be contrasted with objective social isolation (Wenger et al 1996). This differentiation is widely recognized, and according to Gierveld (1987) there would be several cognitive processes that mediate between characteristics of the social network and the experience of loneliness. Several recent investigations show that it is the respondent's evaluation of their relationship rather than the number of social contacts in a person's social network that is important (Routasalo et al. 2006; Victor et al. 2000). A slightly different way of looking at this issue is to consider that loneliness may comprise two primary dimensions, both recognized as negative experiences: emotional and social isolation. The first refers to a lack of others to whom the individual can be emotionally attached and a lack of the experience of social bonding that is intuitively desired, whereas the second, social isolation, describes the actual number of people in a person's social structure, referring to the lack of an acceptable social network (Weiss 1973).

Within emotional loneliness, Ditommaso et al. (2004) have proposed the concept of romantic loneliness. When the loss of an intimate relationship occurs—for example widowhood—older people became more vulnerable to loneliness, despite other conditions and circumstances. The simplest form of a network is a social dyad (e.g. spouse relationship), and the impact of losing a loved one, particularly in the case of a long-lasting marital relationship, is enormous. Not only may there be the loss of a partner to share intimate thoughts and feelings, but also the loss of a partner who may have given crucial support and encouragement in facing the challenges of the ageing process. Even when normal grief occurs people will probably have a lasting longing feeling of loneliness that makes the restoration process difficult, as well as potentially inhibiting re-engagement in daily activities and relationships with others. This is true even when the death of the spouse reduces the perceived burden due to a long period of care-giving. Most of the literature on bereavement in later life (e.g. Gallagher-Thompson et al. 2011) focuses mainly on the traumatic event of the death of a spouse and fails to look at loneliness as a negative outcome that deserves particular attention. The loss of a spouse cannot be treated only by reinterpretation of experience but requires a redefinition of the self and life, to discover a new meaning to invest in within the context of a reduced time in which to live.

Loneliness is a popular issue in the media, which frequently reports loneliness in later life, mostly in relation to a negative stereotype of older people. Dykstra (2009) writes about three loneliness myths: (1) loneliness is common only among the very old; (2) people in northern, more individualistic countries are more lonely than those in family-oriented, southern countries; and (3) loneliness has increased over the past decades. With regard to the first myth, it would appear that loneliness in later life is overestimated by others, and when reviewing the literature we can observe a U-shaped curve, with loneliness higher in the young-adult age group (ages 15–24), decreasing in middle age and increasing again among the oldest old, aged 80+ years. With regard to the second myth, concerning differential prevalence of loneliness along north–south lines, there is a general consensus about the higher rates of reported loneliness in southern and eastern European countries, thus negating the idea that people in individualistic countries from the north of Europe are lonelier (Dykstra 2009). Probable explanations are different individual characteristics, country differences, or some interaction of the two. The final myth about increasing loneliness was also not confirmed by existing data (e.g. Victor et al. 2002). In the subsequent examination of loneliness, myths will be debunked by the scientific literature reviewed in the next section of this chapter.

Recently Rokach (2012) has recognized loneliness as a social stigma. This author characterizes three different types of experiences of loneliness: (1) loneliness as a universal phenomenon, that is, fundamental to being human; (2) loneliness as a subjective experience influenced by personal and situational variables; and (3) loneliness as a complex and multifaceted experience, painful, severely distressing, and personal. Concerning explanations of loneliness, Dykstra (2009) points to three types of argument: social characteristics of the network; relationship standards and expectations; and poor self-esteem, which inhibits the individual from interacting with others or causes others to withdraw. While the first two

---

Box 18.1 Main findings about loneliness

The main findings about loneliness are:

1 It is a common subjective experience.
2 It is a negative condition for human beings.
3 The prevalence of loneliness is higher in southern European countries compared to northern European countries.
4 Loneliness is more prevalent in young and older cohorts than in middle-aged adults.
5 Loneliness is associated with several variables although the direction of the association, as cause or consequences, is far from clear.
6 Most probably, personal and contextual variables have a bidirectional relationship with respect to loneliness.

---

arguments are more sociological in nature, the last is more psychological and appeals to personal characteristics as well as life history that may condition the experience of loneliness. This corroborates Rokach's viewpoint on stigma, as people consider it a personal failure not to have an adequate social network and the intimacy they desire during the life course, reaching the end of life with few significant interpersonal connections.

There is a well established although not very clear association between loneliness, health outcomes, and mortality (e.g. Cacioppo et al. 2006; Momtaz et al. 2012) on the one hand, and social support and loneliness on the other (e.g. Routasalo et al. 2006). Uchino (2004) presents a comprehensive model relating social integration and social support with physical health, in which he introduced loneliness as a direct pathway by which social integration may influence mortality, something that has not been studied so far. This is a challenge that persists nowadays and we still need to establish clearly the difference between the concepts of loneliness and social isolation to reach a clear hypothesis with respect to the association of loneliness with physical health. The main findings from the revision of the literature on loneliness can be seen in Box 18.1.

This chapter begins by looking at the prevalence and major trends of loneliness in old age, with a commentary on the theoretical status of loneliness in causal networks. Next the variables associated with loneliness as predictors and as outcomes are reviewed, paying particular attention to physical and mental health issues. Finally, possible interventions to address deleterious effects of loneliness in old age are discussed.

PREVALENCE AND MAJOR TRENDS OF LONELINESS

The prevalence of loneliness varies widely between studies due to different conceptions of loneliness and methods of assessment, but overall findings suggest the importance of studying the determinants of both social isolation and perceived social isolation throughout the ageing process in culturally distinct community samples (Rokach, Orzeck, and Neto 2004).

The percentage of older people who often feel lonely in European countries as described by Walker and Maltby (1997) ranged from 5% in Denmark to 36% in Greece. Northern countries, including the UK, showed a lower rate of loneliness than Mediterranean countries, despite lower levels of social contact and a higher percentage of old people living alone. Similar findings were presented in a review by Dykstra (2009) that showed northern European countries reporting less loneliness than people in southern countries. Nevertheless, Mediterranean countries seem to have larger and stronger families from which one could expect closer relationships that might prevent loneliness. This discrepancy between people from the north and the south of Europe may be due to a different self-evaluation of loneliness, different expectations towards the role of family members or friends during the ageing process, or being more prone to complain about the availability of people in the network.

In a recent study on cross-national differences in old people's loneliness, from a large cross-national project on ageing issues, the Survey of Health, Ageing and Retirement in Europe (SHARE), Fokkema, Gierveld, and Dykstra (2012) corroborate the Dykstra (2009) north–south division in Europe by reporting lower rates of loneliness in Denmark, Switzerland, and the Netherlands, and higher rates in Greece, Spain, and Italy but also France. Central European countries such as the Czech Republic and Poland also show a higher prevalence of loneliness, joining the south with poor results.

All over the world studies report a high prevalence of loneliness in older people. Perissinotto, Cenzer, and Covinsky (2012) reported 43% of older people (60+ years) who participated in the longitudinal Health and Retirement Study in the USA to be feeling lonely. Park, Yang, Lee, Haley and Chiriboga (2012) found more than 50% of older Korean Americans experiencing loneliness. Momtaz et al. (2012) reported 29.3% experienced loneliness in a representative sample of older Malaysians. Theeke (2009) reported 20% of an older cohort feeling lonely in the US, ranging from 12% to 38%; and finally the estimated prevalence of loneliness in older people in China is 29.6% (Yang and Victor 2008).

There is a common perception that loneliness and isolation have become more prevalent, namely in Britain, as a result of the changes in the family structure, particularly post-Second World War. To confirm the veracity of this presumption, Victor et al. (2002) compared historical data with contemporary ones. The overall prevalence of loneliness ranged from 5% to 9% and showed no increase. The rates for specific age or gender groups were also stable. Reported loneliness among those living alone decreased from 32% in 1945 to 14% in 1999; similar results were also found in Dykstra's (2009) research. According to Victor et al. (2002), rates of loneliness presented in others major British studies ranged between 5% and 16% in people 65 years and over, although it is recognized that a perceived stigma associated with admitting loneliness can result in the underestimation of these rates of loneliness. Paúl et al. (2006) found in a representative UK sample that feelings of loneliness were reported by 7% of older people, ranging from 3% in the group aged 65–69 years to 13% in the group aged 80+ years. More females (8%) than males (5%) reported feeling lonely. According to Dykstra (2009), loneliness seems to be common only in the group 75+ years old.

In Portugal the prevalence of people feeling lonely all of the time was 4.6% with 11.7% reported feeling lonely on a regular basis within an overall total of 16.3% people reporting loneliness, although only 7% of people presented with a limited social network (Lubben 1988, score <20). Loneliness varied by gender with more women feeling lonely (20.4%) than men (7.3%), and by educational level with more illiterate people (25.8%) reporting loneliness. The amount of people feeling lonely increased with age: 9.9% in the 50–64 years age group, 16.3% in the group aged 65–74 years, 20.9% in the group aged 75–84 years, and 26.8% in people aged 85 and over (Paúl and Ribeiro 2009).

A prevalence study on loneliness in the UK using data from the European Social Survey, including people aged 15 years and older, again showed a U-shaped distribution, confirming higher rates of loneliness in people under 25 years old and in people 65 years and over. Depression appears associated with loneliness for all age groups but physical health is associated with loneliness in young and middle-aged people, but not in older people. Curiously, for older people the quality of social relations is protective for loneliness, while for young people it is the quantity of social relationships that matters (Victor and Yang 2012). This study corroborates with that reported by Pinquart and Sörensen (2001), who also report a U-shaped association between age and loneliness, where the quality rather than the quantity of the social network is strongly correlated with loneliness. Friends and neighbours seem more effective in dealing with loneliness than family members. Gender (being a woman), having low socio-economic status and low competence, and living in nursing homes were also associated with higher loneliness. A growing tendency for developing feelings of loneliness in late-life was observed in a 28-year prospective study of Aartsen and Jylhä (2011) based on data from Tampere, Finland (TamELSA). Approximately one-third of people that did not experience loneliness at baseline later developed feelings of loneliness.

In a meta-analysis of research findings on loneliness in older adults, Pinquart and Sörensen (2001) concluded that 5–15% of older adults report frequent loneliness. Jones, Victor, and Vetter (1985) compared loneliness in rural and urban communities, finding a prevalence of 2% and 5% respectively. Females felt lonelier then men, and loneliness increased with age. An extensive study of Finns aged 74+ years found that 39.4% of the sample suffered from loneliness not associated with the frequency of contacts with children and friends, but rather with the satisfaction with these contacts (Routasalo et al. 2006). Some previous researchers suggested that the feeling of loneliness is more common among people aged 75+ than younger adults, but that the prevalence of loneliness levels off after the age of 90 years (Andersson 1998).

Considering the differentiation between social and emotional loneliness, Drennan et al. (2008) found that social and family loneliness were low among older people in Ireland but that a specific form of loneliness concerning close relationships with a partner or friends was relatively high. These authors used the SELSA-S scale (Ditommaso et al. 2004) to measure loneliness, and that instrument introduced a second dimension to emotional loneliness related to attachment and intimate relationships called 'romantic loneliness' as mentioned earlier.

The explanation of loneliness varies if we consider individual vs country level loneliness and also loneliness levels between countries. Authors report that cross-national loneliness is attributable to marital status (greater among those not married), lower socio-economic status, and poor health. Other variables in some countries (e.g. Spain) are the proportion of people that do not have living parents, or that are informal care-givers, or people that depend on informal family care (e.g. Czech Republic). Financial and health problems seem to be strong predictors of loneliness, although the most generally accepted association is between loneliness and social relationships. According to Fokkema et al. (2012), living alone is one of the main risk factors for loneliness.

Most of the studies on loneliness are cross-sectional, preventing the establishment of causal relations between loneliness and associated variables. The associations seem to follow expected trends with older people, women, those who have lost their spouse/partner, those

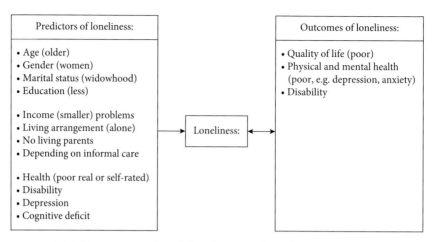

FIGURE 18.1 Variables associated with loneliness in hypothetical causal networks.

with less education and income, those living alone, with poor health and a disability, being more prone to loneliness (see Figure 18.1). Although loneliness is more frequently viewed as an outcome of adverse conditions, it can also be looked at as a causal variable of deleterious outcomes on health and well-being. In the first hypothesis we have to consider which are the predictive variables associated with loneliness; in the second hypothesis we have to check which are the outcomes of loneliness, namely those concerning physical and mental health. Those reporting loneliness may have a less active life style and poor self-care, becoming more prone to disability and illness. Older persons with poor health may experience difficulties in maintaining social relationships because they cannot communicate properly, want to hide their condition, or simply because social contacts become more difficult, and thus they become socially isolated and lonely. In any event, loneliness appears a vulnerability factor in later life and according to Cacioppo, Hawkley, and Bernston (2003) loneliness is a powerful but little understood risk factor for broad-based morbidity and mortality.

Loneliness, in addition to being an objective condition, appears also to encompass subjective feelings accompanying the ageing process for a significant percentage of old people, independent of their social network and living arrangements. Moreover, alongside the macro socio-economic determinants of loneliness, which other variables may be associated with negative feelings of loneliness? The predictors of loneliness in a UK study were being divorced/separated or widowed and not having good quality of life (Paúl et al. 2006). Data confirmed the expected associations between loneliness, widowhood, self-perceived poor health, psychological distress, and cognitive deficit, but failed to show, when controlling for all the other variables in the model, the association with gender, age, living arrangements, social network, or the number of health problems, as found in other studies (e.g. Prince et al. 1997; Routasalo and Pitkala 2003). Some relevant associations between loneliness and usual predictors of social isolation (living arrangements, namely living alone and social network) became non-significant in the adjusted model of loneliness, with the exception of being a widow/widower that goes on being a predictor of loneliness, which is relevant both from a theoretical as well as a practical point of view. This finding suggests, on the one hand, the independence of both concepts of emotional and social isolation, and, on the other hand, the subjective and affective nature of loneliness in old age. A similar perspective was reported by Hughes et al. (2004), who found that objective and subjective isolation are modestly related, which reinforces the idea that the quantitative and qualitative aspects of social relationships are quite distinct.

According to Routasalo and Pitkala (2003), demographic factors (age, widowhood, institutional care, and living alone) appeared in a large number of cross-sectional studies, whereas social factors (low number of social contacts or lack of friends) appeared in only a few population-based studies or studies with small samples. In a subsequent paper Routasalo et al. (2006) showed that in addition to living alone, being depressed, reporting a feeling of being misunderstood, and the presence of unfulfilled expectations towards contacts with others are relevant predictors of loneliness.

In a Portuguese sample of older community dwellers, Paúl and Ribeiro (2009) show that being widowed, perceiving one's own health as poor or very poor, having psychological distress, and cognitive decline were associated with loneliness. Other predictors of social loneliness were greater age, poorer health, living in rural areas, and lack of contact with friends. Family loneliness was predicted by rural setting, being male, having a lower income, being widowed, having no access to transportation, infrequent contact with children and relatives, and being a care-giver at home. Marital status, particularly being widowed, never married, or divorced, predicted romantic loneliness. The authors concluded that the quality of social and family relations might not buffer the older person from the experience of romantic loneliness, which means that loneliness is clearly a multifaceted and complex experience that can affect old people both socially and emotionally.

According to Prince et al. (1997), loneliness was more common among people living alone; lacking supportive neighbours, or contact with friends; upset with their relationship with a child; and for women older than 82 years. Better-quality housing was associated with less loneliness. They did not find any association between loneliness and not having children, or frequency of contact with relatives. The correlation of depressive symptoms seemed similar over the life course, although their prevalence could be different across age (Nolen-Hoeksema and Ahrens 2002). These authors showed a decreasing level of depression and loneliness in people aged 65–75 compared with younger subjects (25–35 or 45–55 years), although loneliness correlates significantly with depression in all age groups.

In short, most of the studies reviewed here report an increasing risk of loneliness in older people and in women (e.g. Jones et al. 1985; Prince et al. 1997; Routasalo et al. 2006; Uchino 2004). Other variables, such as widowhood, education, or income, are less consensual.

LONELINESS AND HEALTH

As mentioned previously, loneliness is associated with both subjective and objective health outcomes (Andersson 1998; Tomaka, Thompson, and Palacios 2006). In a revision of a large number of cross-sectional studies conducted to determine the correlates of loneliness, Routasalo and Pitkala (2003) presented the strength of association between loneliness and health factors in older people. According to these authors, the most closely associated factors, as shown in several population-based studies, were the impairment of physical functioning, poor health, anxiety, sensory impairment, depression, and mortality. Illness and disability may limit social interaction and foster the feeling of loneliness, which seems particularly likely during older age. Recently, a special issue of the *Journal of Psychology* presented several papers linking loneliness to various health conditions such as rheumatic disease, fibromyalgia, and depression, among others (Rokach 2012).

More recently, in another revision of relevant studies on loneliness with the purpose of showing the medical impact and biological effects of loneliness, Luanaigh and Lawlor (2008) concluded that loneliness has been negatively associated with physical health (e.g. poor sleep, systolic hypertension, heart disease), depression, and poorer cognition. Additionally, social isolation predicts morbidity and mortality from cancer, cardiovascular disease, and a host of other causes (Hawkley and Cacioppo 2003). In a study of the effects of types of social network, perceived social support, and loneliness on the health of older people, Stephens et al. (2011) concluded that loneliness was moderately related to total social support but strongly predicted mental and physical health.

As for the number of health problems, Mullins et al. (1996), though utilizing a more objective measure of disability in their study, reported no relationship between health concerns and feelings of loneliness. These authors suggested that functionally disabled people generally receive more care and attention than those whose poor health status is self-perceived, but not necessarily manifest; it may also indicate that formal services are more accessible to disabled people, permitting greater social contact. A face-value interpretation of the findings is that attitudes about health may be a more important variable in loneliness than actual health conditions.

Overall, the association between loneliness and health outcomes is widely accepted (e.g. Cacioppo et al. 2003; Hawkley et al. 2003; Hawkley and Cacioppo 2003; Uchino 2004). Cacioppo and Hawkley (2003) identified three pathways linking loneliness to disease: health behaviour and life styles, excessive stress reactivity, and inadequate or inefficient physiological repair and maintenance processes.

Perissinotto et al. (2012) studied the association between loneliness as a predictor of functional decline and death. Based on the results of a multivariate analysis adjusted for demographic variables, socio-economic status, living situation, depression, and various medical conditions, the authors concluded that subjects feeling loneliness were more likely to experience a decline in activities of daily living, develop difficulties with upper extremity tasks, experience decline in mobility, or experience difficulty in climbing stairs. Loneliness was associated with a 1.45 increase in the risk of death compared with people who were not lonely. The association of loneliness with the rate of motor decline in older people living in the community was studied by Buchman et al. (2010), who found that for each 1-point increase in the level of loneliness at baseline, motor decline was 40% more rapid. So they found that loneliness and being alone were independent predictors of motor decline. The association between loneliness and motor decline persisted, even after controlling for depressive symptoms, cognition, and baseline disability, among other factors.

It seems that the association of disability with loneliness varies with gender. Korporaal, van Groenou, and van Tilburg (2008) found that one's own disability as well as spousal disability were related to higher levels of social loneliness. For men only, their wives' disability was related to higher levels of social loneliness, whereas for women their own disability was related to higher levels of social loneliness. These findings suggest that we must be attentive not only to the effect of disability in social loneliness but also to differential effects in partners, particularly for men that are at elevated risk when their wife is disabled. Thus marriage may not be a protective factor for loneliness when one of the partners is disabled. Golden et al. (2009) also found higher rates of loneliness in women, widows, and people with a physical disability. Loneliness increases with age whenever explanatory models are not adjusted for variables related to age, such as gender or poor health. Jones et al. (1985) found a highly significant association between loneliness and disability in rural as well as in urban older people, independently of age. El-Mansoury et al. (2008) studied loneliness in women with rheumatoid arthritis in the Netherlands and Egypt and concluded that loneliness was higher in Egypt than in the Netherlands. Affection is the variable that better explains loneliness in both countries, and the authors suggest that family is important in Egypt but perhaps not as important in the Netherlands, where lower social support is more common.

In regard to mental health, loneliness has been identified as a primary issue affecting seniors, and numerous studies have confirmed the close relationship between loneliness and depression in old age (Alpass and Neville 2003; Cacioppo et al. 2006; Cheng, Fung, and Chan 2008), particularly among very old women (Paúl and Ribeiro 2008). In several study findings, the main consequences of loneliness are described as decreased well-being and depression. Heikkinen and Kauppinen (2004) reported that loneliness, together with other variables including a large number of chronic diseases, poor self-rated health, poor functional capacity, poor vision, and perceived negative changes in life, predicted depressive symptomatology. In a study focused on the association between loneliness, psychological distress, and disability in later life, Paúl et al. (2006) found that those older people feeling lonely had the highest percentage of psychological disturbance (55%). In a later study Paúl and Ribeiro (2008) found that women feeling loneliness had the highest percentage of psychological disturbance (65.8%). Greater loneliness was also related to increased psychiatric morbidity, increased physical impairment, low life satisfaction, small social networks, and the lack of a confidant. According to the findings of Bowling et al. (1989), the two variables most likely to distinguish between lonely and non-lonely older people were increased psychiatric morbidity and decreased life satisfaction. The consequences of loneliness are mainly decreased well-being and depression. The associations between disease, disability, and demographic variables and loneliness, as well as its mental health consequences, are not completely understood.

When questioning the association between loneliness and health/disability, one cannot omit depression from the equation due to a strong association between both conditions. Evidence shows that loneliness is a powerful predictor of depression but both constructs are clearly different and explained by different sets of determinants; as for loneliness, the predictors are marital status (divorced/separated and widowed) and poor self-perceived quality of life. For depression, the single most important predictor is loneliness and the number of health problems, limitations due to illness, not knowing the neighbours, and poor quality of life (Paúl, Ayis, and Ebrahim 2007).

Research has revealed poorer self-rated health as being related to greater loneliness among older people, as well as a close relationship between depression and loneliness (Mullins et al. 1996). People with poor physical and mental health may restrict their social contacts and activities outside their homes, or people feeling lonely may become more careless (Routasalo and Pitkala 2003). In either case, this finding may have important indicators for health and social professionals who assist older people in the community in adjusting to health-related changes, depression resulting from loneliness, or both. As for cognitive deficits, they appear to be associated with loneliness but again we cannot assume it as a cause or consequence of experiencing loneliness. Alpass and Neville (2003) stress the association between loneliness and chronic illness and self-rated health in older adults and depression. They found no relation between diagnosis of illness and depression but a clear association of loneliness and depression.

IMPLICATIONS FOR PRACTICE

Huge changes in the conception of work and retirement, new familial arrangements that extend to diverse networks, the compression of morbidity, the massive use of new technologies of information and communication, and the encouragement of social participation of ever more active people will all probably contribute to a lessening of social isolation contributing to loneliness. Will this hinder loneliness and its impact? Probably not and so the remaining variables of a more individual nature associated with loneliness need to be addressed from a psychological point of view.

Policies and programmes to prevent loneliness and prevent or delay disability among older people are needed to foster positive outcomes of the ageing process. Several possible psychosocial interventions to diminish loneliness and to promote well-being in later life will be discussed. According to Masi et al. (2010), there are four primary intervention strategies to cope with loneliness: (1) improving social skills; (2) enhancing social support; (3) increasing opportunities for social contact; and (4) addressing maladaptive social cognition. So mostly social interventions are envisaged for loneliness, again probably targeting more social isolation than loneliness. Community intervention promoting sociability between older people, inter-generational solidarity, and avoiding social isolation enhance the quality of life of old people, and diminish feelings of loneliness to some extent. Stevens (2001) presents an educational programme on friendship enrichment for older women to combat loneliness. The main goal was empowerment: by helping women clarify their needs in friendship, analyse their current social network, set goals in friendship, and develop strategies to achieve goals, loneliness might be averted. There was some evidence in improving existing friendships and reducing loneliness. With a similar perspective, Andrews et al. (2003) assessed the satisfaction of users of a local home-visiting befriending service in the UK that provided the opportunity to develop a new social bond. Users reported friendly reciprocity between themselves and the volunteers that visited them weekly. Evidence from this study attests to the value of befriending in ameliorating the effects of social isolation even though some operational aspects (e.g. matching volunteer with user) could be improved. Fostering solidarity between generations by all available means, as encouraged by the World Health Association (2002) and recently the EY2012EC initiative (EY2012 Coalition 2012), will result in lessening loneliness among older people.

Cattan, White, and Learmouth (2005) reviewed studies between 1970 and 2002 to check the efficacy of interventions targeting social isolation and loneliness among older people. They found thirty studies classified according to (1) 'group interventions' (n = 17); (2) face-to-face interventions (n = 10); (3) 'service provision' (n = 3); and (4) 'community development' (n = 1). Only a third of the studies were effective; these utilized group activities with an educational or support input. The literature review supports educational and social activity group interventions to alleviate social isolation and loneliness among older people.

The effectiveness of home visiting and befriending was not clearly demonstrated. The integrative meta-analysis revealed that single-group pre-post and non-randomized comparison studies were the most successful interventions in reduction of loneliness and focused maladaptive social cognition. Fokkema and van Tilburg (2007) reviewed several interventions in the Netherlands and concluded that the effect of loneliness reduction is not clear, although some seem to have at least a preventive effect, avoiding increased feelings of loneliness as observed in control groups.

Although some major studies in the field of loneliness (e.g. ENRICHD Investigators 2001; National Institute of Health 2001) did not find a reduction in mortality after intervention to reduce patient depression and increase social support levels, the authors believe that post-intervention measurement periods of weeks or months allow little time for observing any pathophysiological or health outcome, as loneliness may unfold over several years (Cacioppo and Hawkley 2003).

Interventions oriented to people at risk of emotional isolation (particularly widows) should be more available (Paúl and Ribeiro 2009). Along with social interventions that focus mostly on social isolation, older people will benefit from psychological interventions helping them to cope with widowhood, psychological distress (mainly depression), and the challenges of declines associated with ageing (see Christensen et al. 2009, for a review) that are in turn associated with feelings of loneliness. The stress model can help in understanding the deleterious effect of loneliness. We have to be attentive to psychological signs of helplessness and low self-esteem that frequently coexist with loneliness, provoking double burden and deleterious consequences for the ageing process.

From a psychological point of view, intervention should focus on coping mechanisms used by those community-dwelling individuals who feel significant levels of loneliness to enhance its effects. As pointed out earlier, one possible explanation of loneliness is lower self-esteem that could lead to avoidance or inhibition of social contacts and difficulties in close relationships, resulting in poor social networks. Psychological interventions in face-to-face or group settings may help people to raise self-esteem and learn to deal with others, thereby enlarging their social networks; this in turn will help their ability to cope with loneliness. Reminiscence therapy is reported to be effective in lessening the feeling of loneliness (Chiang et al 2010). The authors explain that memory is used as a therapeutic intervention to help validate a sense of self. The authors demonstrated that the group therapy built a strong sense of belonging and cohesion among participants that decreased the feelings of loneliness in another study, a follow up study of institutionalized males.

Although there is an abundant literature on loneliness, a deeper and more systematic knowledge about it from a psychological perspective will help to develop and implement more specific interventions to deal with the problem and increase quality of life in older adults.

REFERENCES

Aartsen, M. and Jylhä, M. (2011). 'Onset of Loneliness in Older Adults: Results of a 28 Year Prospective Study'. *European Journal of Ageing* 8(1): 31–38.

Alpass, F. M. and Neville, S. (2003). 'Loneliness, Health and Depression in Older Males'. *Aging & Mental Health* 7: 212–216.

Andersson L. (1998). 'Loneliness Research and Interventions: A Review of the Literature'. *Aging & Mental Health* 2: 264–274.

Andrews, G., Gavin, N., Begley, S., and Brodie, D. (2003). 'Assisting Friendships, Combating Loneliness: Users' Views on a "Befriending" Scheme'. *Ageing & Society* 23: 349–362.

Bowling, A., Edelmann, R., Leaver, J., and Oekel, T. (1989). 'Loneliness, Mobility, Well-being and Social Support in a Sample of Over 85 Year Olds'. *Personality and Individual Differences* 10: 1189–1192.

Buchman, A. S., Boyle, P. A., Wilson, R. S., James, B. D., Leurgans, S. E., Arnold, S. E., et al. (2010). 'Loneliness and the Rate of Motor Decline in Old Age: The Rush Memory and Aging Project, a Community-based Cohort Study'. *BMC Geriatrics* 10: 77.

Cacioppo, J. and Hawkley, L. (2003). 'Social Isolation and Health, with an Emphasis on Underlying Mechanisms'. *Perspectives in Biology and Medicine* 46(3): S39–S52.

Cacioppo, J., Hawkley L., and Bernston, G. (2003). 'The Anatomy of Loneliness'. *Current Directions in Psychological Science* 12(3): 71–74.

Cacioppo, J., Hughes. M., Waite, L., Hawkley, L., and Thisted, R. (2006). 'Loneliness as a Specific Risk Factor for Depressive Symptoms: Cross-Sectional and Longitudinal Analyses'. *Psychology and Aging* 21(1): 140–151.

Cattan, M., White, M., and Learmouth, A. (2005). 'Preventing Social Isolation and Loneliness among Older People: A Systematic Review of Health Promotion Interventions'. *Ageing & Society* 25: 41–67.

Cheng, S., Fung, H., and Chan, A. (2008). 'Living Status and Psychological Well-being: Social Comparison as a Moderator in Later Life'. *Aging & Mental Health* 12: 654–661.

Chiang, K.-J., Chu, H., Chang, H.-J., Chung, M.-H., Chen, C.-H., Chiou, H.-Y., et al. (2010). 'The Effects of Reminiscence Therapy on Psychological Well-being, Depression, and Loneliness among the Institutionalized Aged'. *International Journal of Geriatric Psychiatry* 25: 380–388.

Christensen, K., Doblhammer, G., Rau, R., and Vupel, J. (2009). 'Ageing Populations: The Challenges Ahead'. *Lancet* 374: 1196–1208.

Ditommaso, E., Brannen, C., and Best, L. (2004). 'Measurement and Validity Characteristics of the Short Version of the Social and Emotional Scale for Adults'. *Educational and Psychological Measurement* 64: 99–119.

Drennan, J., Treacy, M., Butler, M., Byrne, A., Fealy, G., Frazer, K., et al. (2008). 'The Experience of Social and Emotional Loneliness among Older People in Ireland'. *Ageing & Society* 28: 1113–1132.

Dykstra, P. (2009). 'Older Adult Loneliness: Myths and Realities'. *European Journal of Ageing* 6(2): 91–100. doi:10.1007/s10433-099-0110-3.

El-Mansoury, T. M., Taal, E., Abdel-Nasser, A. M., Riemsa, R. P., Mahfouz, R., Mahmoud, J. A., et al. (2008). 'Loneliness among Women with Rheumatoid Arthritis: A Cross-cultural Study in the Netherlands and Egypt'. *Clinical Rheumatology* 27: 1109–1118.

ENRICHD Investigators (2001). 'Enhancing Recovery in Coronary Heart Disease (ENRICHD) Study Intervention: Rationale and Design'. *Psychosomatic Medicine* 63: 747–755.

EY2012 Coalition (2012). European Programme for Employment and Social Solidarity (PROGRESS), European Year for Active Ageing and Solidarity Between Generations.

Fokkema, C. M. and van Tilburg, T. G. (2007). 'Loneliness Interventions among Older Adults: Sense or Nonsense?' *Tijdschroft voor Gerontologie en Geriatrie* 38(4): 185–203.

Fokkema, T., Gierveld, J., and Dykstra, P. (2012). 'Cross-National Differences in Older Adult Loneliness'. *Journal of Psychology* 46(1–2): 201–228.

Gallagher-Thompson, D., Dupart, T., Liu, W., Gray, H., Eto, T., and Thompson, L. (2011). 'Assessment and Treatment Issues in Bereavement in Later Life'. In K. Laidlaw and B. Knight (eds), *Handbook of Emotional Disorders in Later Life: Assessment and Treatment* (pp. 287–307). Oxford: Oxford University Press.

Gierveld J. (1987). 'Developing and Testing a Model of Loneliness'. *Journal of Personality and Social Psychology* 53: 119–128.

Gierveld, J. (1998). 'A Review of Loneliness: Concept and Definitions Determinants and Consequences'. *Reviews in Clinical Gerontology* 8: 73–80.

Golden, J., Conroy, R., Bruce, I., Denihan, A., Greene, E., Kirby, M., et al. (2009). 'Loneliness, Social Support Networks, Mood and Wellbeing in Community-dwelling Elderly'. *International Journal of Geriatric Psychiatry* 24: 694–700.

Hawkley, L., Burleson, M., Bernston, G., and Cacioppo, J. (2003). 'Loneliness in Everyday Life: Cardiovascular Activity, Psychosocial Context and Health Behaviours'. *Journal of Personality and Social Psychology* 85(1): 105–120.

Hawkley, L. and Cacioppo, J. (2003). 'Loneliness and Pathways to Disease'. *Brain, Behavior, and Immunity* 17: 98–105.

Heikkinen, R. and Kauppinen, M. (2004). 'Depressive Symptoms in Late Life: A 10-years Follow-up'. *Archives of Gerontology and Geriatrics* 38: 239–250.

Hughes, M., Waite, L., Hawkley, L., and Cacciopo, J. (2004). 'A Short Scale for Measuring Loneliness in Large Surveys: Results from Two Population-based Studies'. *Journal of Aging Research* 26: 655–672.

Jones, D. A., Victor, C. R., and Vetter, N. J. (1985). 'The Problem of Loneliness in the Elderly in the Community: Characteristics of those who are Lonely and the Factors Related to Loneliness'. *Journal of the Royal College of General Practice* 35: 136–139.

Korporaal, M., van Groenou, M., and van Tilburg, T. (2008). 'Effects of Own and Spousal Disability on Loneliness among Older Adults'. *Journal of Aging and Health* 20(3): 306–325.

Luanaigh, C. and Lawlor, B. (2008). 'Loneliness and Health of Older People'. *International Journal of Geriatric Psychiatry* 23: 1213–1221.

Lubben, J. E. (1988). 'Assessing Social Networks among Elderly Populations'. *Family and Community Health* 11(3): 42–52.

Masi, C., Chen, H.-Y., Hawkley, L., and Cacioppo, J. (2010). 'A Meta-analysis of Interventions to Reduce Loneliness'. *Personality and Social Psychology Review* 15(3): 219–266. doi:10.1177/1088868310377394.

Momtaz, Y., Hamid, T., Yusoff, S., Ibrahim, R., Chai, S., Yahaya, N., et al. (2012). 'Loneliness as a Risk Factor for Hypertension in Later Life'. *Journal of Aging and Health* 24(4): 696–710.

Mullins, L., Smith, R., Colquitt, R., and Mushel, M. (1996). 'An Examination of the Effects of Self-rated and Objective Indicators of Health Condition and Economic Condition on the Loneliness of Older Persons'. *Journal of Applied Gerontology* 15: 23–37.

National Institute of Health (NIH) News Release (2001). http://www.nhlbi.nih.gov/new/press/01-11-13.htm.

Nolen-Hoeksema, S. and Ahrens C. (2002). 'Age Differences and Similarities in Correlates of Depressive Symptoms'. *Psychology and Aging* 17(1): 116–124.

Park, N., Yang, Y., Lee, B., Haley, W., and Chiriboga, D. (2012). 'The Mediating Role of Loneliness in the Relation between Social Engagement and Depressive Symptoms among Older Korean Americans: Do Men and Women Differ?' *Journals of Gerontology, Series B: Psychological Sciences and Social Sciences* 68(2): 193–201. doi:10.1093/geronb/gbs062.

Paúl, C., Ayis, S., and Ebrahim, S. (2006). 'Psychological Distress, Loneliness and Disability in Old Age'. *Psychology, Health & Medicine* 11: 221–232.

Paúl, C., Ayis, S., and Ebrahim, S. (2007). 'Disability and Psychosocial Outcomes in Old Age'. *Journal of Aging and Health* 19(5): 723–741.

Paúl, C. and Ribeiro, O. (2008). 'Psychological Distress in Very Old Women'. In W. Hansson and E. Olsson (eds), *New Perspectives on Women and Depression* (pp. 183–99). New York: Nova Science.

Paúl, C. and Ribeiro, O. (2009). 'Predicting Loneliness in Old People Living in the Community'. *Reviews in Clinical Gerontology* 19: 53–60.

Perissinotto, C., Cenzer, I., and Covinsky, K. (2012). 'Loneliness in Older Persons: A Predictor of Functional Decline and Death'. *Archives of Internal Medicine* 172(14): 1078–1084.

Pinquart, M. and Sörensen, S. (2001). 'Influences on Loneliness in Older Adults: A Meta-analysis'. *Basic and Applied Social Psychology* 23: 245–266.

Prince, M., Harwood, R., Blizard, R., Thomas, A., and Mann, A. (1997). 'Social Support Deficits, Loneliness and Life Events as Risk Factors for Depression in Old Age. The Gospel Oak Project VI'. *Psychological Medicine* 27: 323–332.

Rokach A. (2012). 'Loneliness Updated: An Introduction'. *Journal of Psychology* 146(1–2): 1–6.

Rokach, A., Orzeck, A., and Neto, F. (2004). 'Coping with Loneliness in Old Age: A Cross cultural Comparison. *Current Psychology* 23: 124–137.

Routasalo, P. and Pitkala, K. (2003). 'Loneliness among Older People'. *Reviews in Clinical Gerontology* 13: 303–311.

Routasalo, P., Savikko, N., Tilvis, R., Standberg, T., and Pitkala, K. (2006). 'Social Contacts and their Relationship to Loneliness among Aged People—a Population-based Study'. *Gerontology* 52(3): 181–187.

Stephens, C., Alpass, F., Twers, A., and Stevenson, B. (2011). 'The Effects of Types of Social Networks, Perceived Social Support, and Loneliness on the Health of Older People: Accounting for the Social Context'. *Journal of Aging and Health* 23(6): 887–911).

Stevens, N. (2001). 'Combating Loneliness: A Friendship Enrichment Programme'. *Ageing & Society* 21: 183–202.

Theeke, L. A. (2009). 'Predictors of Loneliness in US Adults over Age Sixty-five'. *Archives of Psychiatric Nursing* 23: 387–396. doi:10.1016/j.apnu.2008.11.002.

Tomaka, J., Thompson, S., and Palacios, R. (2006). 'The Relation of Social Isolation, Loneliness and Social Support to Disease Outcomes among the Elderly'. *Journal of Aging and Health* 18: 359–384.

Uchino, B. (2004). *Social Support and Physical Health*. New Haven, CT: Yale University Press.

Victor, C., Scambler, S., Bond, J., and Bowling, A. (2000). 'Being Alone in Later Life: Loneliness, Social Isolation and Living Alone'. *Reviews in Clinical Gerontology* 10: 407–417.

Victor, C., Scambler, S., Shah, S., Cook, D., Harris, T., Rink, E., et al. (2002). 'Has Loneliness amongst Older People Increased? An Investigation into Variations Between Cohorts'. *Ageing & Society* 22: 585–587.

Victor, C. and Yang, K. (2012). 'The Prevalence of Loneliness among Adults: A Case Study of the United Kingdom'. *Journal of Psychology* 146(1–2): 85–104.

Walker, A. and Maltby, T. (1997). *Ageing Europe*. Buckingham: Open University Press.

Weiss R. (1973). *Loneliness: the Experience of Emotional and Social Isolation*. Cambridge, MA: MIT Press.

Wenger, G., Davies, R., Shahtahmasebi, S., and Scott, A. (1996). 'Social Isolation and Loneliness in Old Age: Review and Model'. *Ageing & Society* 16: 333–143.

World Health Organization (2002). *Active Ageing: A Policy Framework*. Geneva: WHO.

Yang, K. and Victor, C. R. (2008). 'The Prevalence and Risk Factors for Loneliness among Older People in China'. *Ageing & Society* 28(3): 305–327.

CHAPTER 19

NEUROPSYCHIATRIC APPROACHES TO WORKING WITH DEPRESSED OLDER PEOPLE

SERGIO E. STARKSTEIN AND SIMONE BROCKMAN

INTRODUCTION

NEURODEGENERATIVE disorders such as Parkinson's disease (PD) and Alzheimer's disease (AD), as well as acute brain lesions, such as strokes, are frequent events in old age. The neuropsychiatry approach to working with older people has to consider psychiatric comorbidities that are frequently found in these conditions. Depression is among the most prevalent psychiatric disorders in people with PD, AD, and stroke, with a negative impact on both patients and care-givers. This chapter will focus on the diagnosis, epidemiology, clinical correlates, and management of depression in PD, AD, and stroke.

DEPRESSION IN STROKE

Cross-sectional studies report that about 20% of patients with acute stroke suffer from major depression, while an additional 20% develop minor depression (Robinson 2006). One of the most challenging problems in neuropsychiatry is how to diagnose depression when the symptoms of the neurological illness overlap with those of the affective disorder. Four strategies have been proposed to deal with this problem: (1) the 'inclusive approach' in which symptoms of depression are counted as present regardless of whether they may be related to the physical illness (Cohen-Cole and Stoudemire 1987); (2) the 'exclusive approach' in which symptoms are removed from the diagnostic criteria whenever there is a potential overlap between depression and the neurological condition (Gallo et al. 1997); (3) the 'substitutive approach' in which somatic symptoms of depression are replaced with psychiatric symptoms (Olin et al. 2002b); and finally, (4) the 'aetiological approach' in which symptoms of depression are included only when the examiner considers the symptom not to be related to the neurological disorder

(Chemerinski et al. 2001). Most research studies have used the inclusive approach, with the aim of increasing the sensitivity of the study, while accepting the risk of lower specificity.

Diagnosis and epidemiology of depression in stroke

The prevalence of post-stroke depression (PSD) is highly related to the method used to arrive at the diagnosis of the psychiatric condition. Most studies have used appropriate standardized interviews, such as the Present State Exam (Wing, Cooper, and Sartorius 1974), the Structured Clinical Interview for DSM (Spitzer et al. 1992), or the Mini International Neuropsychiatric Inventory (Sheehan et al. 1998). Based on information provided by these instruments, diagnoses were often generated based on DSM criteria for either major or minor depression (Robinson 2006). The specificity of syndromal depression has been examined in several studies (Cumming et al. 2010; Paradiso, Chikubo, and Robinson 1997). Summarizing the literature, Spalletta and Robinson (2010) concluded there is no need to modify the DSM-IV criteria for the diagnosis of PSD. Pompili and co-workers (Pompili et al. 2012) summarized the literature on suicide among patients with PSD and found that stroke was a significant risk factor for suicide. Most stroke patients who committed suicide were depressed, and this combination was most frequent among women and young adults.

Other relevant variables with an influence on the frequency of PSD are assessment methods, time since stroke, lesion side, and sample characteristics (Robinson 2006). Studies using structured psychiatric interviews and standardized diagnostic criteria for mood disorders reported rates between 11% and 15% for post-stroke major depression and between 8% and 12% for minor depression in community settings, which increase to 16–27% for major depression and 13–20% for minor depression in acute hospital settings (Robinson 2006). Ayerbe and colleagues (2013) examined the cumulative incidence, prevalence, and duration of PSD up to fifteen years after stroke among patients recruited from a population-based stroke register. During the fifteen years after the stroke, the annual incidence of PSD ranged from 7% to 21%. Most episodes of depression started within a year of stroke, with 33% of patients becoming depressed within the first three months after stroke. The authors concluded that stroke patients needed periodic assessments for depression.

Lesion location may play a significant role in the duration of PSD, with patients having cortical lesions suffering longer lasting depressions compared to patients with subcortical lesions (Starkstein, Robinson, and Price 1988). This study also demonstrated a significant association between distance of the lesion to the frontal pole and severity of depression (i.e. the closer the lesion to the frontal pole, the more severe the depression).

In conclusion, for research studies and, where possible, in clinical practice, PSD should be diagnosed using structured interviews and standardized diagnostic criteria to improve reliability and specificity. In the acute stage about 20% of patients will suffer from major depression and another 20% will have minor depression. PSD is not a fleeting condition and tends to last for months or years after the acute event.

Clinical correlates of PSD

The association between PSD and lesion location remains a debated issue. Starkstein and co-workers found a significant association between PSD and both cortical and subcortical left hemisphere lesions (Starkstein, Robinson, and Price 1987). Moreover, they also showed a significant association between depression severity and proximity of the lesion to the frontal pole (i.e. more anterior lesions were associated with more severe depressions) (Starkstein et al. 1987). However, this correlation was true for left but not right hemisphere strokes (Starkstein et al. 1987). While these findings were partially or fully replicated by other authors, other studies failed to replicate these results (Carson et al. 2000). Reasons for these discrepancies have been addressed by Robinson (Robinson 2006) and include assessing depression at different times since stroke and recruitment biases (e.g. acute in-patients vs patients living in the community). An important limitation to all these studies is that patients with severe aphasia were not assessed for depression. Nevertheless, Robinson (2006) demonstrated that patients with left hemisphere anterior lesions with or without aphasia had more severe depression than patients with right anterior lesions.

A significant association between more severe physical and functional deficits and more severe depression has been consistently demonstrated (Robinson 2006), although the direction of this association remains unclear. Some studies have demonstrated that depression predicts worse recovery while other studies have shown that poor functioning and more severe motor problems are significant predictors of depression (Robinson 2006).

A significant association between PSD and more severe cognitive deficits has been demonstrated for patients with left (but not right) hemisphere lesions (Bolla-Wilson et al. 1989). Kimura and co-workers (Kimura, Robinson, and Kosier 2000) demonstrated that patients with PSD who responded to the anti-depressant nortriptyline had greater improvement in cognitive functioning as reflected by higher Mini-Mental State Examination (MMSE) scores than non-responders.

An association between PSD and increased mortality has been repeatedly demonstrated (Williams, Ghose, and Swindle 2004). An interesting study by Jorge and co-workers (Jorge et al. 2003) showed that patients with PSD who received anti-depressants had significantly lower mortality than placebo-treated patients, suggesting that treatment with anti-depressants within the first six months after stroke is associated with increased survival.

In conclusion, while the association between PSD and lesion location remains to be clarified, there is strong converging evidence that PSD has a negative impact on the patient's activities of daily living (ADLs), cognitive function, and mortality.

Treatment of PSD

Pharmacological interventions

Several small-scale randomized controlled trials (RCTs) have demonstrated the efficacy of tricyclic anti-depressants and selective serotonergic reuptake inhibitors (SSRIs) for PSD (Robinson 2006). The efficacy of anti-depressants was examined in two independent meta-analyses. Chen and co-workers (Chen et al. 2006) reported on sixteen RCTs with a total of 1320 patients who met inclusion criteria, and found a significantly greater improvement of depression with active treatment as compared to placebo. Positive effects were observed after four weeks of treatment, and longer duration of treatment was associated with greater response. Hackett and co-workers (Hackett et al. 2004) reported on sixteen trials (seventeen interventions) with 1655 participants who met inclusion criteria, and found a small effect in favour of active treatment on response rates and reduction in depression scores. Nevertheless, outcomes were quite heterogeneous (e.g. due to sampling bias, differential efficacy of anti-depressants, duration of treatment and sample size), and active treatment was associated with increased frequency of adverse events.

Psychosocial interventions

Few studies have examined the efficacy of psychosocial interventions to treat PSD. Lincoln and co-workers (Lincoln and Flannaghan 2003) showed cognitive-behavioural treatment to be no more effective than a standard care or attention control. A recent RCT (Smith et al. 2012) examined the efficacy of a Web-based intervention for PSD in men with a recent stroke and with spouses providing care. The main finding was that one month after the intervention care-givers but not patients showed significantly lower depression scores.

One meta-analysis (already mentioned above) included examination of the efficacy of psychotherapy for PSD (Hackett et al. 2004). Four trials of psychotherapy were included in this review; the forms of psychotherapy included problem-solving therapy with counselling delivered by social workers, structured cognitive-behavioural therapy delivered by nurses, motivational interviewing delivered by nurses and non-clinical psychologists, and a supportive psychological intervention including educational components, delivered by a variety of healthcare workers. The frequency and duration of sessions was individually tailored to patient needs in three of the four interventions, and three trials used standard care as the control comparison. Depression data were available for three trials (445 participants) with only piecemeal data available from the fourth trial. Across the studies included, no significant effect for active treatment against control was shown. However, the authors did note that there was good evidence that efficacy was linked to providing the patient with an adequate exposure to the intervention, and so the use of a standardized, pre-specified framework for therapy was recommended in future psychotherapy studies on this population.

In conclusion, the efficacy of both tricyclic anti-depressants and SSRIs has been demonstrated in several RCTs. It is important to stress that tricyclic drugs have several contraindications and important adverse effects which may impact frail older individuals. While less frequent, side effects have also been reported with the use of SSRIs. Few studies examined the efficacy of psychosocial interventions, and these treatments deserve further study.

Prevention of PSD

Several RCTs have examined the efficacy of pharmacological interventions to prevent PSD. Robinson and co-workers (Robinson et al. 2008) conducted a multi-centre RCT that included 176 non-depressed patients who were randomized to escitalopram (an SSRI anti-depressant), a non-blinded problem-solving therapy, or placebo (tablet). The main finding was that both active treatments were superior to placebo in preventing PSD. A meta-analysis on the efficacy of fluoxetine for the prophylaxis of PSD (Yi, Liu, and Zhai 2010) demonstrated a significant reduction in the frequency of PSD, increased recovery of neurological function and improved independence on ADLs with treatment. It is important to note that nausea, insomnia, and seizures were significantly more frequent in the fluoxetine treatment group as compared to the placebo group.

Psychotherapy interventions to prevent PSD have been less frequently carried out. A meta-analysis of problem-solving therapy, motivational interventions and multidisciplinary home-based therapy targeting psychosocial stressors showed a significant improvement in psychological distress but not in depression outcome (Hackett et al. 2004). The authors suggested that future trials of psychotherapy in PSD should include better outcome measures, have an adequate sample size, and carefully specify the type of psychotherapy intervention.

In conclusion, there is promising evidence that anti-depressants may be effective in preventing PSD. Nevertheless, these medications have potential side effects that may impact on this frail population, and further supporting evidence for their usefulness is needed. More research should be conducted on the potential utility of psychosocial interventions for preventing PSD.

Depression in Alzheimer's Disease

Depression is among the most frequent emotional disorders in AD. Many studies have examined the epidemiology, phenomenology, mechanism, clinical correlates, and management of depression in AD (Lyketsos and Olin 2002). As discussed already, one of the main limitations in this field is how to make a valid diagnosis of depression in the context of an illness that features loss of interest, psychic retardation, loss of energy and restricted social interests, and dependence on others for most living arrangements and daily activities. Lyketsos and colleagues (2001) suggested that the individual symptom approach may ignore the high overlap of symptoms and should not be used for diagnostic purposes. Using latent class analysis, they identified a group with affective symptoms of depression as well as symptoms of anxiety and apathy.

In 2002, the National Institutes of Mental Health (NIMH) organized a work group that proposed standardized diagnostic criteria for depression in AD (Olin et al. 2002a, Olin et al. 2002b). These criteria are similar to the DSM-IV criteria for major depression, but with the addition of irritability and social isolation, and the replacement of loss of interest with loss of pleasure in response to social contact. Other modifications included the requirement of three rather than five symptoms for the diagnosis of depression and that symptoms did not have to be present nearly every day (Table 19.1).

Starkstein and co-workers (Starkstein et al. 2011b) recently validated a set of diagnostic criteria for major depression in AD. The study included 971 patients with mild, moderate or severe AD that were assessed with a structured psychiatric interview. A latent class analysis showed that all nine DSM-IV diagnostic criteria for major depression identified a cluster with high statistical significance. A second cluster identified patients with an intermediate frequency of depressive symptoms, most of whom met DSM-IV criteria for minor depression (see Figure 19.1). Another relevant finding was that both anxiety and apathy were significantly associated with depression, while irritability was not. These findings provide validity to the DSM-IV criteria for major depression for use in AD. They further suggest that anxiety is a common comorbid condition of major depression in AD, and that irritability is no more frequent than in non-depressed individuals.

Table 19.1 Provisional diagnostic criteria for depression of Alzheimer's disease

A. Three or more of the following symptoms have been present during the same two-week period and represent a change from previous functioning: at least one of the symptoms is either depressed mood or decreased positive affect or pleasure.
  (1) Clinically significant depressed mood
  (2) Decreased positive affect or pleasure in response to social contacts and usual activities
  (3) Social isolation or withdrawal
  (4) Disruption in appetite
  (5) Disruption in sleep
  (6) Psychomotor changes
  (7) Irritability
  (8) Fatigue or loss of energy
  (9) Feelings of worthlessness, hopelessness, or excessive or inappropriate guilt
  (10) Recurrent thoughts of death, suicidal ideation, plan or attempt
B. All criteria met for dementia of the Alzheimer Type
C. The symptoms cause clinically significant distress or disruption in functioning
D. The symptoms do not occur exclusively during the course of a delirium
E. The symptoms are not due to the direct physiological effects of a substance
F. The symptoms are not better accounted for by other psychiatric conditions

Specify if: **Co-occurring Onset**: If onset antedates or co-occurs with the AD symptoms.

Post-AD Onset: if onset occurs after AD symptoms.

Specify: **With Psychosis of AD.**

With other significant behavioural signs or symptoms.

With past history of mood disorders.

Adapted from *The American Journal of Geriatric Psychiatry*, 10 (2), Jason T. Olin, Lon S. Schneider, Ira R. Katz, Barnett S. Meyers, George S. Alexopoulos, John C. Breitner, Martha L. Bruce, Eric D. Caine, Jeffrey L. Cummings, Davangere P. Devanand, K. Ranga Rama Krishnan, Constantine G. Lyketsos, Jeffrey M. Lyness, et al., Provisional Diagnostic Criteria for Depression of Alzheimer Disease, pp. 125–8, Copyright (2002), with permission from Elsevier.

Prevalence of depression in AD

The prevalence of depression in AD has been reported to range from 10% to more than 80% (Migliorelli et al. 1995). This wide variability may reflect some of the diagnostic biases discussed above. Other important confounders in the extant research may be the proportion of men/women with AD and the severity of dementia in various study populations. Population studies reported a prevalence of 'dysphoria' of 20%, and an eighteen-month incidence of 18% (Lyketsos and Olin 2002).

Among a consecutive series of patients attending a memory clinic, Migliorelli and co-workers (Migliorelli et al. 1995) reported a frequency of major depression of 23% and minor depression of 28%. Women were more likely than men to be depressed. The incidence of major depression was reported to be of about 20% in an eighteen-month follow-up study (Starkstein et al. 1997), and when left untreated, major depression in AD may last for eighteen months or more (Starkstein et al. 1997). A personal history of depression was

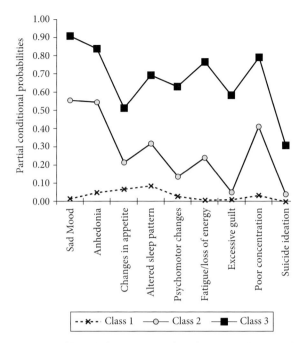

FIGURE 19.1 Symptom profiles of the three (ordered) latent class model for Alzheimer's disease. Figure showing partial conditional probabilities for a three-class model, indicating how presence of each diagnostic symptom for depression relates to the depression latent classes.

Reprinted from *The American Journal of Geriatric Psychiatry*, 16(6), Sergio E. Starkstein, Milan Dragovic, Ricardo Jorge, Simone Brockman, and Robert G. Robinson, Diagnostic Criteria for Depression in Alzheimer Disease: A Study of Symptom Patterns Using Latent Class Analysis, pp. 551–58, Copyright (2011), with permission from Elsevier.

reported to be a significant predictor of depression in AD (Migliorelli et al. 1995). Levy and co-workers (Levy et al. 1996) reported a high recurrence rate of depression during a one-year period.

In conclusion, depression is a frequent finding even in the early stages of AD. A longitudinal study has demonstrated that most patients with AD will suffer from depression at some stage during the evolution of the illness (Starkstein et al. 1997).

Comorbidity of depression in AD

Depression in AD has been associated with worse quality of life, greater disability in ADLs, a faster cognitive decline, and relatively higher mortality (Kales et al. 2005; Lee and Lyketsos 2003). Moreover, patients with dementia with comorbid depression have significantly higher rates of requiring nursing home placement than non-depressed patients with dementia (Kales et al. 2005).

Starkstein and co-workers (Starkstein et al. 2005) reported that depressed AD patients had more severe social dysfunction and greater impairment in ADLs than AD patients without depression. Moreover, depressed AD patients also showed more severe anxiety, delusions and Parkinsonism than AD patients without depression. Given that loss of inter-est and motivation is a cardinal symptom for both apathy and depression, these psychiatric syndromes frequently coexist in AD (Starkstein et al. 2005). An eighteen-month longitu-dinal study showed that the presence of apathy at baseline was a significant predictor of increasing depression during follow-up, suggesting that apathy may be an early marker or a prodromal stage of depression in AD (Starkstein et al. 2006).

Patients with dementia may present with sudden episodes of crying that they are unable to suppress. Sudden crying episodes are termed 'emotional lability' whenever they occur in mood congruent situations, whilst 'pathological crying' is defined as the sudden onset of crying episodes that do not correspond to an underlying congruent emotional change. Starkstein and co-workers (Starkstein et al. 1995; Arbus et al. 2010) reported that patologi-cal affective display crying was significantly related to higher depression and anxiety scores, and may constitute a marker of an underlying depression.

Treatment of depression in AD

Pharmacological treatment

Arbus and co-workers (2010) examined the prevalence of anti-depressant use in AD in the context of a multi-centre, four-year prospective study. The main finding was that only 60% of depressed patients with dementia (most of them in their first depressive episode) were prescribed anti-depressants (Arbus et al. 2010). Early RCTs as well as a relatively recent meta-analysis (Thompson et al. 2007) suggested significant efficacy for anti-depressants over placebo for both treatment response and remission of depression. Lyketsos and co-workers (Lyketsos et al. 2003) carried out an RCT using the SSRI sertraline in a study that included forty-four patients with AD and major depression. Full response (i.e. no longer meeting diagnostic criteria for depression) was present in 38% of the sertraline group as compared to 20% of the placebo group. The sertraline group showed a significantly greater improvement on the Cornell Scale for Depression in Dementia (CSDD) than the placebo group. Twice as many participants dropped out of the placebo-treated group as compared to the sertraline-treated group. Most side effects of sertraline were mild and consisted of diz-ziness and gastrointestinal symptoms. On the other hand, there was no evidence that mood improvement was associated with cognitive improvement (Munro et al. 2004).

Sertraline was used in a more recent and larger RCT (Rosenberg et al. 2010) which enrolled 131 patients with mild-moderate AD meeting the NIMH criteria for depression in AD. The main finding was that neither remission rate nor scores on the CSDD were sig-nificantly different between sertraline and placebo groups after twelve weeks of treatment. Sertraline-treated patients suffered more frequent gastrointestinal and respiratory side effects than the placebo group. Interestingly, depression severity improved by an aver-age of 50%, and 40% of the participants were judged to be either 'better' or 'much better' in their mood. The different outcome with the previous sertraline study may be explained by the use of different criteria for diagnosing depression and the larger sample size. A twenty-four-week study extension again failed to show a significant benefit of sertraline over placebo (Weintraub et al. 2010).

A recent multi-centre RCT recruited 326 AD patients diagnosed with depression based on CSDD scores of 8 or more (Banerjee et al. 2011) rather than a diagnostic interview.

Participants were allocated to receive sertraline (target dose 150 mg/day), mirtazapine (target dose 45 mg/day) or placebo. After thirteen weeks of follow-up there were no significant differences between the two active treatment and placebo groups. Moreover, side effects were more frequent among patients treated with sertraline or mirtazapine as compared to those treated with placebo.

The impact of discontinuing anti-depressants among individuals with dementia was examined in a recent RCT that included 128 patients with dementia who had been prescribed escitalopram, citalopram, sertraline, or paroxetine for three months or more (Bergh, Selbaek, and Engedal 2012). The main finding was that patients who discontinued anti-depressant treatment had significantly higher depression scores after twenty-five weeks than the continuation group, although mean scores were within the non-depressed range. On the other hand, there were no significant between-group differences on scores assessing cognitive functions, Parkinsonism, quality of life, or impairments in ADLs. The authors suggested that while anti-depressants could be discontinued in most patients with dementia, follow-up assessments were important to identify depression relapse.

In conclusion, the role of anti-depressants in AD is unclear. Two RCTs showed lack of efficacy for sertraline as compared to placebo, and a recent study showed a lack of efficacy for mirtazapine. Future studies using validated diagnosis for depression may clarify the role of anti-depressants in AD.

Psychotherapy

Guetin and co-workers (Guetin et al. 2009) carried out an RCT of receptive music therapy for anxiety and depression in thirty patients with AD. They found a significant improvement in both anxiety and depression for the music therapy group as compared to the placebo group, and the benefits of music therapy were sustained for up to eight weeks after the discontinuation of sessions. However, the study was limited by a small sample size, and findings have yet to be replicated. Stanley and co-workers have recently examined the efficacy of 'Peaceful Mind', a cognitive-behavioural-based therapy for anxiety in dementia (Stanley et al. 2013). Thirty-two patients with mild or moderate dementia were randomized to active treatment or usual care and were followed for three and six months. The intervention included up to twelve weekly sessions during the first three months, and up to eight brief telephone sessions between months three to six. The main finding was that patients who received active treatment reported less anxiety and higher quality of life than the control group.

DEPRESSION IN PARKINSON'S DISEASE

Patients with PD show many symptoms in common with depression. Both patients with PD and patients with depression frequently show a stooped posture, shuffling gait, hypophonic speech, blunted facial expression, and motor and cognitive slowness (i.e. bradykinesia and bradyphrenia, respectively). This overlap makes a reliable and valid diagnosis of depression in PD quite challenging. Therefore, the first issue to examine is the validity of depression syndromes in PD. In one of the first studies in this area, Starkstein and co-workers

(Starkstein et al. 1990b) separated a series of 103 patients into groups who reported or denied the presence of sad mood, respectively. When items of the Hamilton Depression Scale (HAM-D) were compared between groups, there were no significant differences for early-morning awakening and concentration difficulties, demonstrating that all the other psychological and somatic symptoms of depression in the HAM-D may be used to diagnose depression in PD.

A NINDS/NIMH work group examined the phenomenology of depression in PD and provided important recommendations (Marsh et al. 2006). First, they stressed that anxiety should be included as part of the psychiatric assessment of depression in PD, and that the association between depression and apathy should be further investigated. Second, the work group suggested that symptoms of psychomotor changes, diminished concentration, and loss of interest may be omitted from the depression diagnostic criteria.

In a more recent study, Starkstein and co-workers (Starkstein et al. 2011a) examined the validity of symptoms of depression in a consecutive series of 259 patients with PD using latent class analysis (LCA). This statistical technique assesses the symptom profile of individual patients and produces classes of patients in terms of their pattern of symptoms. The main finding was that all nine DSM-IV diagnostic criteria for major depression identify a depressive class with high statistical significance. All the twenty-eight patients included in this class met DSM-IV criteria for major depression. There was another class that included patients with an intermediate frequency of depressive symptoms, with about two-thirds of them meeting DSM-IV criteria for either dysthymia, major, or minor depression. Finally, there was a third class with low probabilities of depressive symptoms and 81% of them met no DSM-IV criteria for any depression. Interestingly, both apathy and anxiety were present in most patients in the class with severe depression.

Brown and co-workers (Brown et al. 2011) used LCA in a large study that included 513 PD patients and found four classes with symptoms of depression and anxiety, depression only, anxiety only and neither depression nor anxiety.

In conclusion, empirical studies suggest that DSM-IV criteria for major depression should be used unmodified in PD, and this will likely remain unchanged with the DSM-5. Both apathy and anxiety may be included as additional symptoms for the diagnosis of depression in PD. Finally, there is a subgroup of patients with PD with mild or subsyndromal depression whose clinical relevance should be further investigated.

Frequency of depression in PD

The frequency of depression in PD was reported to range from 8% in community studies to 40% among patients attending specialized movement disorders clinics (Cummings 1992). Leentjens and co-workers (Leentjens et al. 2003) reported that 9% of patients with PD had depression at the time of diagnosis, as compared to 4% among age-comparable healthy controls. Starkstein and co-workers (Starkstein et al. 1990a) reported that 17% of a series of 103 patients with PD had major depression, 22% had minor depression, and 13% had dysthymia. Several confounders should be considered, such as type of assessment (prevalence of depression is higher in studies using structured interviews) and sampling characteristics (depression frequency is usually lower in epidemiological studies).

Longitudinal evolution of depression in PD

The longitudinal course of depression in PD has been examined in several studies. Starkstein and co-workers (Starkstein et al. 1990a) reported that 29% of PD patients with major depression were depressed before the onset of motor symptoms. A one-year follow-up study showed that 89% of patients with major depression at baseline were still depressed at follow-up, as compared to 37% of patients with minor depression at baseline and 18% of patients with no depression at baseline (Starkstein et al. 1992a). Most depressed patients were untreated for the mood disorder.

Clinical correlates of depression in PD

Palhagen and co-workers (Palhagen et al. 2008) reported that PD patients with depression were more disabled, had more severe dyskinesias, and reported more insomnia than non-depressed patients with PD. Starkstein and co-workers (Starkstein et al. 1992b) found that PD patients with depression had a significant decline of MMSE scores over time and more severe deficits on activities of daily living as compared to PD patients without depression. Moreover, patients with major depression had a faster progression along the Hohen and Yahr stages of the illness (Goetz et al. 2004), suggesting that major depression in PD is a marker of a more malignant type of illness. Starkstein and co-workers (Starkstein, Preziosis, and Robinson 1991) also showed a significant association between major depression and increased pain and sleep problems.

Treatment of depression in PD

Pharmacological studies

Recent RCTs have clarified the efficacy of anti-depressant medication in PD. Devos and co-workers (Devos et al. 2008) carried out an RCT using the tricyclic drug desipramine (up to 75 mg/day) and the SSRI citalopram (up to 20 mg/day). The main finding was that desipramine had higher efficacy than citalopram and placebo during the first two weeks of treatment, but that there were no significant differences between both active drugs after thirty days of treatment. Side effects, albeit mild, were more frequent in the desipramine group.

Menza and co-workers (Menza et al. 2009) compared the efficacy of the tricyclic anti-depressant nortriptyline and the SSRI paroxetine in a National Institute of Health (NIH)-funded RCT with fifty-two patients with PD and depression. The main finding was that patients on nortriptyline had a significantly greater reduction in depression scores than patients on paroxetine, while the latter were no different from patients treated with placebo.

A recent randomized, double-blind, placebo controlled study by Richard and co-workers (Richard et al. 2012) examined the efficacy and safety of paroxetine as compared to the selective norepinephrine reuptake inhibitor (SNRI) venlafaxine to treat depression in PD. A total of 115 subjects participated across twenty sites in the USA. They found that both active compounds were significantly better than placebo as reflected in reduced Hamilton (HAM-D) depression scores. Both medications were generally safe and well tolerated as compared to placebo.

In conclusion, pharmacological studies suggest that both tricyclics and SSRIs may be effective treatments of depression in PD. However, there are discrepant findings such as the efficacy of SSRIs in some but not most studies, which should be further examined in large-scale studies. It is also important to note that anti-depressants have contraindications, relevant drug interactions, and side effects which should all be considered before starting treatment.

Psychotherapy

A recent study demonstrated the feasibility of using CBT for depression in PD (Dobkin et al. 2011). These authors carried out an RCT of individually administered CBT as compared to clinical monitoring that included eighty patients with PD meeting DSM-IV criteria for major depression. Patients were randomized to a controlled trial of CBT relative to clinical monitoring. CBT was tailored to the needs of individuals with PD. Modifications included emphasis on behavioural and anxiety management, and a supplemental care-giver education programme. Patients received ten weekly individual sessions of manualized CBT, and treatment included exercise, behavioural activation, thought monitoring and restructuring, relaxation training, worry control, and sleep hygiene. Therapists were an experienced psychologist and two doctoral-level psychologists. The group treated with CBT had greater reductions in depression scores than the clinical monitoring group. There were also improvements on relevant secondary outcome measures, such as anxiety, quality of life, and Parkinsonism. While this study is the largest RCT to date, treatment follow-up was only at one-month, therefore future research should focus on the durability of treatment effects of CBT at both six- and twelve-month follow-ups. Interventions aimed at comorbid anxiety and depression in PD are also lacking (Pachana et al. 2013).

In conclusion, both tricyclic anti-depressants and SSRIs demonstrated utility in treating depression in PD. Nevertheless, it is important to note several discrepancies between some studies, such as paroxetine showing significant benefits in some but not all studies. Both tricyclic and SSRI compounds have formal contraindications and relevant side effects in PD, and these medications should be used with care in this frail population. CBT may be a useful option for patients unable to tolerate anti-depressant medication, but further replication studies are needed.

IMPLICATIONS FOR PRACTICE

Depression in neurological disorders is clearly underdiagnosed, and efforts should be made to improve the screening of affective and anxiety disorders in this population. Once diagnosed, depression may be successfully treated with pharmacotherapy, psychotherapy, or both. Treatment modality will depend on patients: preference, severity of depression, and contraindications to psychotropic medication.

We reviewed evidence demonstrating that most patients with acute or chronic neurological disorders will suffer depression at some stage of their illness. Depression has a negative impact on patients' quality of life and mortality, and on care-giver burden. Treatment studies are providing strong evidence that different treatment modalities may improve patients' emotional status.

SUMMARY

Given the high comorbidity between depressive and neurological symptoms, the psychiatric diagnosis and treatment of affective disorders in neuropsychiatry remains challenging. Depression is highly prevalent in both chronic and acute neurological conditions, and has a negative impact on quality of life. Response to anti-depressant medication remains variable, and preliminary psychological interventions have been demonstrated to be beneficial.

ACKNOWLEDGEMENTS

This study was partially supported by grants from the University of Western Australia, and the National Health and Medical Research Council.

Send correspondence to: Prof. Sergio E. Starkstein, Education Building T-7, Fremantle Hospital, Fremantle, 6959 WA, Australia, e-mail: sergio.starkstein@uwa.edu.au, phone: (08)-9431-2013.

KEY REFERENCES AND SOURCES FOR FURTHER READING

Dobkin, R. D., Menza, M., Allen, L. A., Gara, M. A., Mark, M. H., et al. (2011). 'Cognitive-behavioral Therapy for Depression in Parkinson's Disease: A Randomized, Controlled Trial'. *American Journal of Psychiatry* 168: 1066–1074.

Hackett, M. L., Anderson, C. S., and House, A. O. (2004). 'Interventions for Treating Depression after Stroke'. *Cochrane Database of Systematic Reviews* 4.

Jorge, R. E., Robinson, R. G., Arndt, S., and Starkstein, S. (2003). 'Mortality and Poststroke Depression: A Placebo-controlled Trial of Antidepressants'. *American Journal of Psychiatry* 160: 1823–1829.

Olin, J. T., Schneider, L. S., Katz, I. R., Meyers, B. S., Alexopoulos, G. S., et al. (2002). 'Provisional Diagnostic Criteria for Depression of Alzheimer Disease'. *American Journal of Geriatric Psychiatry* 10: 125–128.

Pachana, N. A., Egan, S. J., Laidlaw, K., Dissanayaka, N., Byrne, G. J., Brockman, S., Marsh, R., and Starkstein, S. (2013). 'Clinical Issues in the Treatment of Anxiety and Depression in Older Adults with Parkinson's Disease'. *Movement Disorders* 28(14): 1930–1934.

Richard, I. H., McDermott, M. P., Kurlan, R., Lyness, J. M., Como, P. G., et al. (2012). 'A Randomized, Double-blind, Placebo-controlled Trial of Antidepressants in Parkinson Disease'. *Neurology* 78: 1229–1236.

Robinson, R. G. (2006). *The Clinical Neuropsychiatry of Stroke*. Cambridge, Cambridge University Press.

Starkstein, S. E., Dragovic, M., Jorge, R., Brockman, S., and Robinson, R. G. (2011). 'Diagnostic Criteria for Depression in Alzheimer Disease: A Study of Symptom Patterns Using Latent Class Analysis'. *American Journal of Geriatric Psychiatry* 19: 551–558.

References

Arbus, C., Gardette, V., Bui, E., Cantet, C., Andrieu, S., et al. (2010). 'Antidepressant Use in Alzheimer's Disease Patients: Results of the REAL.FR Cohort'. *International Psychogeriatrics* 22: 120–128.

Ayerbe, L., Ayis, S., Crichton, S., Wolfe, C. D., and Rudd, A. G. (2013). 'The Natural History of Depression up to 15 Years after Stroke: The South London Stroke Register'. *Stroke* 44: 1105–1110.

Banerjee, S., Hellier, J., Dewey, M., Romeo, R., Ballard, C., et al. (2011). 'Sertraline or Mirtazapine for Depression in Dementia (HTA-SADD): A Randomised, Multicentre, Double-blind, Placebo-controlled Trial'. *Lancet* 378: 403–411.

Bergh, S., Selbaek, G., and Engedal, K. (2012). 'Discontinuation of Antidepressants in People with Dementia and Neuropsychiatric Symptoms (DESEP Study): Double Blind, Randomised, Parallel Group, Placebo Controlled Trial'. *British Medical Journal* 344: e1566.

Bolla-Wilson, K., Robinson, R. G., Starkstein, S. E., Boston, J., and Price, T. R. (1989). 'Lateralization of Dementia of Depression in Stroke Patients'. *American Journal of Psychiatry* 146: 627–634.

Brown, R. G., Landau, S., Hindle, J. V., Playfer, J., Samuel, M., et al. (2011). 'Depression and Anxiety Related Subtypes in Parkinson's Disease'. *Journal of Neurology, Neurosurgery & Psychiatry* 82: 803–809.

Carson, A. J., MacHale, S., Allen, K., Lawrie, S. M., Dennis, M., et al. (2000). 'Depression after Stroke and Lesion Location: A Systematic Review'. *Lancet* 356: 122–126.

Chemerinski, E., Petracca, G., Sabe, L., Kremer, J., and Starkstein, S. E. (2001). 'The Specificity of Depressive Symptoms in Patients with Alzheimer's Disease'. *American Journal of Psychiatry* 158: 68–72.

Chen, Y., Guo, J. J., Zhan, S., and Patel, N. C. (2006). 'Treatment Effects of Antidepressants in Patients with Post-stroke Depression: A Meta-analysis'. *Annals of Pharmacotherapy* 40: 2115–2122.

Cohen-Cole, S. A. and Stoudemire, A. (1987). 'Major Depression and Physical Illness'. *Psychiatric Clinics of North America* 10: 1–17.

Cumming, T. B., Churilov, L., Skoog, I., Blomstrand, C., and Linden, T. (2010). 'Little Evidence for Different Phenomenology in Poststroke Depression'. *Acta Psychiatrica Scandinavica* 121: 424–430.

Cummings, J. L. (1992). 'Depression and Parkinson's Disease: A Review'. *American Journal of Psychiatry* 149: 443–454.

Devos, D., Dujardin, K., Poirot, I., Moreau, C., Cottencin, O., et al. (2008). 'Comparison of Desipramine and Citalopram Treatments for Depression in Parkinson's Disease: A Double-blind, Randomized, Placebo-controlled Study'. *Movement Disorders* 23: 850–857.

Dobkin, R. D., Menza, M., Allen, L. A., Gara, M. A., Mark, M. H., et al. (2011). 'Cognitive-behavioral Therapy for Depression in Parkinson's Disease: A Randomized, Controlled Trial'. *American Journal of Psychiatry* 168: 1066–1074.

Gallo, J. J., Rabins, P. V., Lyketsos, C. G., Tien, A. Y., and Anthony, J. C. (1997). 'Depression without Sadness: Functional Outcomes of Nondysphoric Depression in Later Life'. *Journal of the American Geriatrics Society* 45: 570–578.

Goetz, C. G., Poewe, W., Rascol, O., Sampaio, C., Stebbins, G. T., et al. (2004). 'Movement Disorder Society Task Force Report on the Hoehn and Yahr Staging Scale: Status and Recommendations. The Movement Disorder Society Task Force on Rating Scales for Parkinson's Disease.' *Movement Disorders* 19 (9): 1020–1028.

Guetin, S., Portet, F., Picot, M. C., Pommie, C., Messaoudi, M., et al. (2009). 'Effect of Music Therapy on Anxiety and Depression in Patients with Alzheimer's Type Dementia: Randomised, Controlled Study'. *Dementia and Geriatric Cognitive Disorders* 28: 36–46.

Hackett, M. L., Anderson, C. S., and House, A. O. (2004). 'Interventions for Treating Depression after Stroke'. *Cochrane Database of Systematic Reviews* 4.

Jorge, R. E., Robinson, R. G., Arndt, S., and Starkstein, S. (2003). 'Mortality and Poststroke Depression: A Placebo-controlled Trial of Antidepressants'. *American Journal of Psychiatry* 160: 1823–1829.

Kales, H. C., Chen, P., Blow, F. C., Welsh, D. E., and Mellow, A. M. (2005). 'Rates of Clinical Depression Diagnosis, Functional Impairment, and Nursing Home Placement in Coexisting Dementia and Depression'. *American Journal of Geriatric Psychiatry* 13: 441–449.

Kimura, M., Robinson, R. G., and Kosier, J. T. (2000). 'Treatment of Cognitive Impairment after Poststroke Depression: A Double-blind Treatment Trial'. *Stroke* 31: 1482–1486.

Lee, H. B. and Lyketsos, C. G. (2003). 'Depression in Alzheimer's Disease: Heterogeneity and Related Issues'. *Biological Psychiatry* 54: 353–362.

Leentjens, A. F., Van Den Akker, M., Metsemakers, J. F., and Troost, J. (2003). 'The Incidence of Parkinson's Disease in the Netherlands: Results from a Longitudinal General Practice-based Registration'. *Neuroepidemiology* 22: 311–312.

Levy, M. L., Cummings, J. L., Fairbanks, L. A., Bravi, D., Calvani, M, et al. (1996). 'Longitudinal Assessment of Symptoms of Depression, Agitation, and Psychosis in 181 Patients with Alzheimer's Disease'. *American Journal of Psychiatry* 153: 1438–1443.

Lincoln, N. B. and Flannaghan, T. (2003). 'Cognitive Behavioral Psychotherapy for Depression Following Stroke: A Randomized Controlled Trial'. *Stroke* 34: 111–115.

Lyketsos, C. G., Breitner, J. C., and Rabins, P. V. (2001). 'An Evidence-based Proposal for the Classification of Neuropsychiatric Disturbance in Alzheimer's Disease'. *International Journal of Geriatric Psychiatry* 16: 1037–1042.

Lyketsos, C. G. and Olin, J. (2002). 'Depression in Alzheimer's Disease: Overview and Treatment'. *Biological Psychiatry* 52: 243–252.

Lyketsos, C. G., Delcampo, L., Steinberg, M., Miles, Q., Steele, C. D., et al. (2003). 'Treating Depression in Alzheimer Disease: Efficacy and Safety of Sertraline Therapy, and the Benefits of Depression Reduction: The DIADS'. *Archives of General Psychiatry* 60: 737–746.

Marsh, L., McDonald, W. M., Cummings, J., and Ravina, B. (2006). 'Provisional Diagnostic Criteria for Depression in Parkinson's Disease: Report of an NINDS/NIMH Work Group'. *Movement Disorders* 21: 148–158.

Menza, M., Dobkin, R. D., Marin, H., Mark, M. H., Gara, M., et al. (2009). 'A Controlled Trial of Antidepressants in Patients with Parkinson's Disease and Depression'. *Neurology* 72: 886–892.

Migliorelli, R., Teson, A., Sabe, L., Petrachi, M., Leiguarda, R., et al. (1995). 'Prevalence and Correlates of Dysthymia and Major Depression among Patients with Alzheimer's Disease'. *American Journal of Psychiatry* 152: 37–44.

Munro, C. A., Brandt, J., Sheppard, J. M., Steele, C. D., Samus, Q. M., et al. (2004). 'Cognitive Response to Pharmacological Treatment for Depression in Alzheimer Disease: Secondary Outcomes from the Depression in Alzheimer's Disease Study (DIADS)'. *American Journal of Geriatric Psychiatry* 12: 491–498.

Olin, J. T., Katz, I. R., Meyers, B. S., Schneider, L. S., and Lebowitz, B. D. (2002a). 'Provisional Diagnostic Criteria for Depression of Alzheimer Disease: Rationale and Background'. *American Journal of Geriatric Psychiatry* 10: 129–141.

Olin, J. T., Schneider, L. S., Katz, I. R., Meyers, B. S., Alexopoulos, G. S., et al. (2002b). 'Provisional Diagnostic Criteria for Depression of Alzheimer Disease'. *American Journal of Geriatric Psychiatry* 10: 125–128.

Pachana, N. A., Egan, S. J., Laidlaw, K., Dissanayaka, N., Byrne, G. J., Brockman, S., Marsh, R., and Starkstein, S. (2013). 'Clinical Issues in the Treatment of Anxiety and Depression in Older Adults with Parkinson's Disease'. *Movement Disorders* 28(14): 1930–1934.

Palhagen, S. E., Carlsson, M., Curman, E., Walinder, J., et al. (2008). 'Depressive Illness in Parkinson's Disease: Indication of a More Advanced and Widespread Neurodegenerative Process?' *Acta Neurologica Scandinavica* 117: 295–304.

Paradiso, S., Ohkubo, T., and Robinson, R. G. (1997). 'Vegetative and Psychological Symptoms Associated with Depressed Mood over the First Two Years after Stroke'. *International Journal of Psychiatry in Medicine* 27: 137–157.

Pompili, M., Venturini, P., Campi, S., Seretti, M. E., Montebovi, F., et al. (2012). 'Do Stroke Patients Have an Increased Risk of Developing Suicidal Ideation or Dying by Suicide? An Overview of the Current Literature'. *CNS Neuroscience and Therapeutics* 18: 711–721.

Richard, I. H., McDermott, M. P., Kurlan, R., Lyness, J. M., Como, P. G., et al. (2012). 'A Randomized, Double-blind, Placebo-controlled Trial of Antidepressants in Parkinson Disease'. *Neurology* 78: 1229–1236.

Robinson, R. G. (2006). *The Clinical Neuropsychiatry of Stroke*. Cambridge: Cambridge University Press.

Robinson, R. G., Jorge, R., Moser, D., Acion, L., Solodkin, A., et al. (2008). 'Escitalopram and Problem-solving Therapy for Prevention of Poststroke Depression: A Randomized Controlled Trial'. *Journal of the American Medical Association* 28: 2391–2400.

Rosenberg, P. B., Drye, L. T., Martin, B. K., Frangakis, C., Mintzer, J. E., et al. (2010). 'Sertraline for the Treatment of Depression in Alzheimer Disease'. *American Journal of Geriatric Psychiatry* 18: 136–145.

Sheehan, D. V., Lecrubier, Y., Sheehan, K. H., Amorim, P., Janavs, J., et al. (1998). 'The Mini-International Neuropsychiatric Interview (M.I.N.I.): The Development and Validation of a Structured Diagnostic Psychiatric Interview for DSM-IV and ICD-10'. *Journal of Clinical Psychiatry* 59(Suppl 20): 22–33; quiz 34–57.

Smith, G. C., Egbert, N., Dellman-Jenkins, M., Nanna, K., and Palmieri, P. A. (2012). 'Reducing Depression in Stroke Survivors and their Informal Caregivers: A Randomized Clinical Trial of a Web-based Intervention'. *Rehabilitation Psychology* 57: 196–206.

Spalletta, G. and Robinson, R. G. (2010). 'How Should Depression be Diagnosed in Patients with Stroke?' *Acta Psychiatrica Scandinavica* 121: 401–403.

Spitzer, R. L., Williams, J. B., Gibbon, M., and First, M. B. (1992). 'The Structured Clinical Interview for DSM-III-R (SCID). I: History, Rationale, and Description'. *Archives of General Psychiatry* 49: 624–629.

Stanley, M. A., Calleo, J., Bush, A. L., Wilson, N., Snow, A. L., et al. (2013). 'The Peaceful Mind Program: A Pilot Test of a Cognitive-behavioral Therapy-based Intervention for Anxious Patients with Dementia'. *American Journal of Geriatric Psychiatry* 21: 696–708.

Starkstein, S. E., Robinson, R. G., and Price, T. R. (1987). 'Comparison of Cortical and Subcortical Lesions in the Production of Poststroke Mood Disorders'. *Brain* 110(Pt 4): 1045–1059.

Starkstein, S. E., Preziosi, T. J., Bolduc, P. L., and Robinson, R. G. (1990a). 'Depression in Parkinson's Disease'. *Journal of Nervous and Mental Disease* 178: 27–31.

Starkstein, S. E., Preziosi, T. J., Forrester, A. W., and Robinson, R. G. (1990b). 'Specificity of Affective and Autonomic Symptoms of Depression in Parkinson's Disease'. *Journal of Neurology, Neurosurgery and Psychiatry* 53: 869–873.

Starkstein, S. E., Preziosi, T. J., and Robinson, R. G. (1991). 'Sleep Disorders, Pain, and Depression in Parkinson's Disease'. *European Neurology* 31: 352–355.

Starkstein, S. E., Mayberg, H. S., Leiguarda, R., Preziosi, T. J., and Robinson, R. G. (1992a). 'A Prospective Longitudinal Study of Depression, Cognitive Decline, and Physical Impairments in Patients with Parkinson's Disease'. *Journal of Neurology, Neurosurgery and Psychiatry* 55: 377–382.

Starkstein, S. E., Mayberg, H. S., Leiguarda, R., Preziosi, T. J., and Robinson, R. G. (1992b). 'A Prospective Longitudinal Study of Depression, Cognitive Decline, and Physical Impairments in Patients with Parkinson's Disease'. *Journal of Neurology, Neurosurgery, and Psychiatry* 55: 377–382.

Starkstein, S. E., Migliorelli, R., Teson, A., Petracca, G., Chemerinsky, E., et al. (1995). 'Prevalence and Clinical Correlates of Pathological Affective Display in Alzheimer's Disease'. *Journal of Neurology, Neurosurgery and Psychiatry* 59: 55–60.

Starkstein, S. E., Chemerinski, E., Sabe, L., Kuzis, G., Petracca, G., et al. (1997). 'Prospective Longitudinal Study of Depression and Anosognosia in Alzheimer's Disease'. *British Journal of Psychiatry* 171: 47–52.

Starkstein, S. E., Jorge, R., Mizrahi, R., and Robinson, R. G. (2005). 'The Construct of Minor and Major Depression in Alzheimer's Disease'. *American Journal of Psychiatry* 162: 2086–2093.

Starkstein, S. E., Jorge, R., Mizrahi, R., and Robinson, R. G. (2006). 'A Prospective Longitudinal Study of Apathy in Alzheimer's Disease'. *Journal of Neurology, Neurosurgery and Psychiatry* 77: 8–11.

Starkstein, S. E., Dragovic, M., Jorge, R., Brockman, S., Merello, M., et al. (2011a). 'Diagnostic Criteria for Depression in Parkinson's Disease: A Study of Symptom Patterns Using Latent Class Analysis'. *Movement Disorders* 26: 2239–2245.

Starkstein, S. E., Dragovic, M., Jorge, R., Brockman, S., and Robinson, R. G. (2011b). 'Diagnostic Criteria for Depression in Alzheimer Disease: A Study of Symptom Patterns Using Latent Class Analysis'. *American Journal of Geriatric Psychiatry* 19: 551–558.

Starkstein, S. E., Robinson, R. G., and Price, T. R. (1988). 'Comparison of Spontaneously Recovered versus Nonrecovered Patients with Poststroke Depression'. *Stroke: A Journal of Cerebral Circulation* 19: 1491–1496.

Thompson, S., Herrmann, N., Rapoport, M. J., and Lanctot, K. L. (2007). 'Efficacy and Safety of Antidepressants for Treatment of Depression in Alzheimer's Disease: A Metaanalysis'. *Canadian Journal of Psychiatry—Revue Canadienne de Psychiatrie* 52: 248–255.

Weintraub, D., Rosenberg, P. B., Drye, L. T., Martin, B. K., Frangakis, C., et al. (2010). 'Sertraline for the Treatment of Depression in Alzheimer Disease: Week-24 Outcomes'. *American Journal of Geriatric Psychiatry* 18: 332–340.

Williams, L. S., Ghose, S. S., and Swindle, R. W. (2004). 'Depression and Other Mental Health Diagnoses Increase Mortality Risk after Ischemic Stroke'. *American Journal of Psychiatry* 161: 1090–1095.

Wing, J. K., Cooper, J. E., and Sartorius, N. (1974). *Measurement and Classification of Psychiatric Symptoms*. Cambridge: Cambridge University Press.

Yi, Z. M., Liu, F., and Zhai, S. D. (2010). 'Fluoxetine for the Prophylaxis of Poststroke Depression in Patients with Stroke: A Meta-analysis'. *International Journal Of Clinical Practice* 64: 1310–1317.

CHAPTER 20

....

LATE-LIFE DEPRESSION

....

ELIZABETH A. DINAPOLI AND FORREST R. SCOGIN

INTRODUCTION

AGE can substantially influence the presentation of depression, including its symptomatology, prevalence, aetiology, and treatment response. Thus, data obtained on depression in one age group is unlikely to translate completely to another age group. The global population is ageing at a rapid rate and by 2030 it is estimated that older adults will comprise 13% of the total worldwide population (Lopez et al. 2006). Consequently, there has been great interest in studying depression in this population. Late-life depression often goes unrecognized, which is particularly concerning because it can have serious consequences (e.g. morbidity and mortality). Therefore, identifying factors associated with onset and maintenance of late-life depression is critical to improving preventative and interventive practices.

EPIDEMIOLOGY OF LATE-LIFE DEPRESSION

Many symptoms of late-life depression (e.g. low energy, loss of appetite, and sleep difficulties) can be mistakenly thought to be caused by other medical illnesses or age-related changes. Depression in late-life may become evident only after these symptoms do not meet criteria for bereavement and are not direct effects of a medical illness or medication (American Psychiatric Association (APA) 2000). To have a diagnosis of major depression, an older adult must have five or more of the following symptoms for at least two weeks: depressed mood, loss of interest or pleasure in usual activities, significant weight loss or weight gain, insomnia or hypersomnia, psychomotor agitation or retardation, fatigue or loss of energy, feelings of worthlessness or guilt, diminished ability to think or concentrate, and recurrent thoughts of death or suicide (APA 2000). The depressive symptoms must cause clinically significant distress or impairment in social, occupational, or other important areas of functioning. Older adults that do not fulfil the duration criteria or show the required number of symptoms (i.e. at least two but fewer than five symptoms) to make the diagnosis of major depression can be given an unofficial diagnosis of minor depression. In contrast to minor and major depression, dysthymia is a chronic disturbance of mood that is present nearly every day for two or more years. Older adults with dysthymia have symptoms similar to major depression, only they tend to be mild to moderate in severity and may include low self-esteem (APA 2000). Another distinction can be made by at least one episode of depression occurring prior to late-life (i.e. early onset) vs not occurring until old age (i.e. late onset; Roth 1955).

Unfortunately, late-life depression is under-recognized and thus undertreated (Simon and VonKorff 1995). This is partially due to older adults sometimes presenting complaints to clinicians that do not typically signal late-life depression, such as concerns about physical health, social relationships, or economic burdens. For example, many older adults focus on physical or somatic symptoms (e.g. fatigue, sleep disturbance, chronic pain, appetite loss, etc.) of depression (Balsis and Cully 2008; Hegeman et al. 2012). It is thought that this differential presentation of symptoms is due to depression being expressed differently across the lifespan (Balsis and Cully 2008). For example, depression in older adults is more commonly associated with sleep disturbances, agitation, hypochondriasis, subjective cognitive complaints (e.g. poor concentration and memory) and vegetative symptoms (e.g. fatigue, psychomotor retardation) than depression in younger adults (Hegeman et al. 2012; Husain et al. 2005; Teper and Thomas 2006). On the other hand, emotional symptoms (e.g. worthlessness and guilt), as well as suicidal ideation, are less common in older adults than in younger adults (Hegeman et al. 2012; Husain et al. 2005). Additionally, older adults tend to be more severely depressed (i.e. greater number of major depressive episodes with longer durations) and have more psychomotor disturbance and psychosis (both hallucinations and delusions; Brodaty et al. 1997; Husain et al. 2005).

Depression is one of the most commonly occurring mental health disorders in late-life. In fact, depressive symptoms are present in 6% to 15% of community-dwelling older adults (Akincigil et al. 2011; Blazer 2003; Gallagher et al. 2010; Mojtabai and Olfson 2004). However, these rates begin to decline as the severity level of depression increases. For example, in community-dwelling older adults, prevalence of major depressive disorder ranges from approximately 1% to 6%, whereas prevalence of dysthymia is 1% to 2% and prevalence of minor depression is 4% to 18.6% (Meeks et al. 2011; Mojtabai and Olfson 2004; Østbye et al. 2005; Päivärinta et al. 1999; Zisook and Downs 1998). Among selected samples of depressed older adults, 38% can be categorized as having early-onset depression and 62% as having late-onset depression (Gallagher et al. 2010). Depression in older adults is more prevalent among women than men and this trend persists through very old age (i.e. 85 years and older; Bergdahl et al. 2007). Findings on race/ethnicity differences have been inconsistent, with some studies suggesting that African Americans and other minorities experience higher levels of depressive symptoms compared to non-Hispanic whites (Li 2008; Skarupski et al. 2005), and others finding the reverse (Dunlop et al. 2003; Gallo, Cooper-Patrick, and Lesikar 1998).

Rates of depressive symptoms generally increase in clinical populations of older adults. The prevalence of depression is lowest in community-dwelling older adults and continues to increase as settings become more restrictive (e.g. primary care to inpatient hospitals), with the highest rates in institutionalized residents. For example, the North Carolina Epidemiologic Catchment Area study estimated the prevalence of subsyndromal depressive symptoms of hospitalized older adults (25–33%), nonpsychiatric outpatients (10–15%) and long-term care residents (30–40%; as reported in Edelstein, Shreve-Neiger, and Scheck

2004). A systematic review of epidemiological studies of late-life depression (Meeks et al. 2011) found similar results for prevalence of major depression in primary care settings (4–3.7%; Aranda, Lee, and Wilson 2001; Licht-Strunk et al. 2005), medical inpatients (13.3–21.6%; Koenig et al. 1991; Koenig 1997), and long-term care settings (6–15.7%; Morrow-Howell et al. 2008; Parmelee, Katz, and Lawton 1992).

The risk of older adults developing depression is predicted to increase with time and age (Kessler et al. 2003). Annual rates of depression diagnosis in community-dwelling older adults have nearly doubled, from 3.2% to 6.3% between 1992 to 2005 (Akincigil et al. 2011). In 1989, the estimated incidence of major depression in the US was 3 per 1000 person-years (Eaton et al. 1989). More recently, incidence rates for major depressive disorder have significantly increased and range from 7 to 104.3 per 1000 person-years (Gureje, Oladeji, and Abiona 2011; Luijendijk et al. 2008). Furthermore, Luijendijk et al. (2008) found that incidence rates more than double when episodes of clinically relevant depressive symptoms (e.g. core symptoms of major depression during psychiatric interview, self-reported depression, or initiation of anti-depressant drug treatment) are included. The increase in incidence of depression with time likely reflects a cultural shift in mental healthcare (e.g. more open to seeking help/medication and greater recognition of depression; Kessler et al. 2003). Incidence of depression also increases with age, with over 10% of new cases in older adults 70–74 years old and approximately 15% in adults over 75 years old (Solhaug et al. 2012). Another clinical concern is recurrence rates of depression for older adults. Recurrence rates of late-life depression range from 13% to 88%, depending on the duration of follow-up and whether they received maintenance treatment (as reported in Luijendijk et al. 2008).

These statistics (e.g. prevalence, incidence and recurrence) are particularly concerning because late-life depression can have devastating effects on a variety of domains, including cognitive performance (McBride and Abeles 2000), life satisfaction (Lue, Chen, and Wu 2010), and quality of life (Chachamovich et al. 2008), as well as social and physical functioning (Lenze et al. 2001; Liu, Leung, and Chi 2011). In addition, depressive symptoms predict lower levels of personal health satisfaction and greater medical care use (Han 2002; Himelhoch et al. 2004; Rowan et al. 2002), with total median medical costs of late-life depressive symptoms being approximately $2147 over a one-year period (Unützer et al. 1996). Furthermore, depressive disorders accelerate the disease process in older adults (Van Gool et al. 2005), as well as increase the risk of hospitalization (Rumsfeld et al. 2005), nursing home dependence (Harris 2007), and mortality (St. John and Montgomery 2009). Late-life depression is also one of the most common risk factors for suicide in older adults, which in 2005 had rates of 14.7 per 100 000 persons (Centers for Disease Control and Prevention 2008).

AETIOLOGY OF LATE-LIFE DEPRESSION

It is recognized that most behaviour is due to an interaction of many factors. Similarly, late-life depression is caused by a combination of biological, psychological, and social factors (Blazer 2010). Therefore, the development of late-life depression is likely a multifaceted interaction among possibilities such as genetic vulnerabilities, comorbid medical and

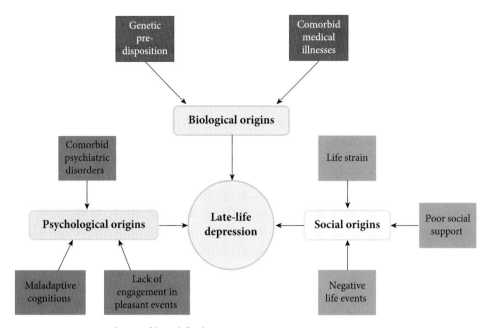

FIGURE 20.1 Aetiology of late-life depression.

Reproduced from *Psychiatric Annals*, 40(1), The Origins of Late-Life Depression, Dan G. Blazer, MD, PhD, pp. 13–18 DOI: 10.3928/00485718–20091229–01 Copyright © 2014, Slack Inc. Reproduced with permission of SLACK Incorporated.

psychological conditions, cognitive activities, stressful or negative events, and social support (see Figure 20.1; Blazer 2010).

Biological origins

There is considerable evidence that biological factors such as genetic predisposition, vascular lesions, and comorbid medical illnesses are associated with late-life depression. For example, an increase with age in the heritability of depression symptoms has been shown in twin studies, which reveal that genes contribute 16–34% of the variability in total depression scores and 55% at ten-year follow-up (Carmelli et al. 2000; Gatz et al. 1992; McGue and Christensen 1997). Zhang et al. (2005) identified a single nucleotide polymorphism (SNP) at the tryptophan hydroxylase-2 (hTPH2) gene (G1463A) as being an important contributor to major depression. Others suggest that cerebrovascular disease may predispose some older adults to depressive disorders (Alexopoulos et al. 1997), which is evidenced by vascular lesions in frontal lobes, as well as decreased volume in the orbitofrontal cortex (Lai et al. 2000; Taylor et al. 2007), subcortical structures (i.e. basal ganglia and hippocampus), and grey and white matter of the anterior cingulate cortex (Artero et al. 2004; Firbank et al. 2004; Hannestad et al. 2006).

Comorbid medical illnesses are one of the most important biological factors contributing to late-life depression. A meta-analysis conducted by Huang and colleagues (2010) found that certain chronic diseases such as stroke, loss of hearing and vision, cardiac disease, and chronic lung disease are risk factors for depression in older adults. Further research has found end-stage renal disease (Balogun et al. 2011) and arthritis (Murphy et al. 2012) to be associated with depression in older adults. For instance, older adults with a stroke are about three times more likely to have depression than those without a stroke (Huang et al. 2010). In addition, depression is prevalent in 42% of older adults with congestive heart disease (Skotzko et al. 2000) and approximately two times more common in older adults with vascular disease (Kivimäki et al. 2012). Mental health conditions are also common among older adults with arthritis, with approximately one-third reporting having either anxiety (31%) or depression (18%; Murphy et al. 2012).

Depression frequently co-exists with chronic health conditions, such that depressive symptoms are detectable in approximately 3.7% of older adults with another non-psychiatric medical condition (Fiest et al. 2011). However, the relationship between depression and chronic disease in older adults is thought to be bidirectional. In other words, chronic health conditions may act as both the 'cause' and the consequence of depression, and vice versa. For instance, chronic health conditions may affect depression directly, as well as indirectly by aggravating strain (e.g. domestic, occupational, and economic) and undermining resources (self-esteem and mastery; Vilhjalmsson 1998). Similarly, depression may both directly and indirectly (e.g. poor adherence to treatment regimens) affect chronic health conditions (Penninx et al. 1999). Therefore, interventions aimed at ameliorating depression are also likely to have beneficial effects on comorbid psychological and physical conditions. For instance, Yon et al. (2009) found that symptoms of insomnia in those with an average (or lower) level of depression can be reduced through psychological treatment for depression.

Psychological origins

Maladaptive information processing and lower pleasurable activities engagement are common psychological factors associated with late-life depression. Maladaptive cognitions can include irrational thoughts, negative self-statements, overgeneralization of adverse events, and catastrophizing of situations. Similarly, depression can emerge in older adults as a function of excess unpleasant events, fewer pleasurable activities, and less positive reinforcement (Lewinsohn et al. 1986).

Late-life depression rarely occurs in isolation (Gum and Cheavens 2008); there is often psychiatric comorbidity. In fact, late-life depression has been associated with, among others, anxiety, insomnia, personality disorders, dementia, and alcohol abuse. Prevalence of comorbid anxiety and depression in older adults has been reported to range from 8.4% to 51.8% (Kvaal et al. 2005). Moreover, researchers have generated estimates of comorbidity between depression and personality disorders in older adults ranging from 24% to 61% (Kunik et al. 1994; Molinari and Marmion 1995). Furthermore, prevalence of depression in patients with dementia ranges from 20% to 54.4% (Tsuno and Homma 2009; Zubenko et al. 2003). In addition, 13.3% of older adults with lifetime major depression also met the criteria for alcohol use disorder (Blow, Serras, and Barry 2007).

Social origins

Many social factors are associated with late-life depression, such as stress or life strain, negative life events, and poor social support. Several studies have established an association between psychological distress and both chronic stressors and daily hassles (Grzywacz et al. 2004; Serido, Almeida, and Wethington 2004). Life strains of older adults include, but are not limited to: financial strain (Ferraro and Su 1999), life-threatening medical disorders or chronic disabling conditions (Couture, Larivière, and Lefraçois 2005; King, Heisel, and Lyness 2005), and care-giving for a demented or disabled relative or spouse (Lavela and Ather 2010). Boey and Chiu (2010) found that life-strain factors were significantly related to mental health status in older women, with financial status and physical health conditions being the most significantly associated with depressive symptoms and life satisfaction. In addition, the diathesis stress model suggests that depressive episodes are catalysed by the combination of biological predisposition and stressful events (Russo, Vitaliano, and Brewer 1995).

There is a positive relationship between depressive symptoms in older adults and negative life events (Fiske, Gatz, and Pedersen 2003). Negative life events that are more commonly faced by older adults include death of significant others, relational stress, the onset of a severe illness in self or spouse, loss of independence in activities of daily living, and decrease in cognitive function (Katsumata et al. 2012; Lövheim et al. 2012). A meta-analysis of twenty-five studies found that almost all negative life events appeared to have a modest but significant relationship to depression (Kraaij, Arensman, and Spinhoven 2002). For example, the total number of negative events and daily hassles was associated with depression, whereas sudden unexpected events were not related to depression scores. Similarly, clinically depressed older adults reported both more frequent and more severe life events than did the control groups (Emmerson et al. 1989).

Social support has also been investigated as a risk factor for development of late-life depression. Results from these studies suggest that poor social support and loneliness have a strong association with late-life depression (Prince et al. 1997). There is a negative correlation between perceived social support and depression in older adults (Alexandrino-Silva et al. 2011). Subjective reports of social support (perceived adequacy) have been found to be more strongly associated with depressive symptoms than objective social support (actual network size) in older participants (George et al. 1989). However, it is unclear if social support independently protects against depression or if it is an important buffer to the stressors of late-life (Blazer 2005).

Protective Factors for
Late-life Depression

Many older adults experience the above risk factors, yet evade late-life depression, suggesting that protective factors exist. Blazer (2010) suggests that the above stressful events and experiences are largely anticipated and 'on time' events for older adults. Therefore, older adults have time to prepare for these events and situations. Fiske, Wetherell, and Gatz (2009) suggest that three themes emerged from their review of the literature on protective factors against late-life depression. The first theme is the importance of resources, such as health, cognitive function, and socio-economic status. Availability of resources provides an explanation for the relation between socio-economic status and depressive symptoms in older adults (Back and Lee 2011). For instance, Rostad, Deeg, and Schei (2009) found that disadvantaged socio-economic status (i.e. lower educational levels and working minimal- to non-paid jobs) was significantly associated with greater self-assessed depression in older women.

The second theme that emerged from Fiske et al. (2009) was that a cohort of older adults gained life experiences that taught them psychological strategies to cope with adversity. For example, the socio-emotional selectivity theory suggests that perception of time causes older adults to have more emotion-focused goals, whereas younger adults have more knowledge-focused goals (Carstensen, Fung, and Charles 2003). In other words, older adults perceive that they have relatively little time left to live and therefore emphasize goals which are emotionally meaningful in the present, instead of planning for the future. For instance, when shown pictures of emotionally charged situations, older adults rated images more positively than younger adults (Mather and Carstensen 2005). In addition, older adults show enhanced emotional control, such that they are able to engage specific emotion regulation processes to compensate for changes in internal and external resources (Urry and Gross 2010). Therefore, there appears to be an age-specific adaptation in late adulthood that confers stability on several aspects of emotion regulation (Orgeta 2009).

Lastly, Fiske et al. (2009) suggest that the role of meaningful engagement is a protective factor against late-life depression. The activity-restriction model is applicable to older adults, who are more likely to be affected by health problems than individuals in other age groups (Areán, Uncapher, and Satre 1998). Activity restriction has been found to mediate the association between medically related stressors and depression, even after controlling for other known causes of depression among older adults (Williamson and Shaffer 2000). In a study of older women with activity restriction due to osteoarthritis, higher perceived control and greater use of active coping strategies were related to lower depressive symptomatology (Rivard 2007). Conversely, increased use of avoidant coping strategies (particularly behavioural disengagement) was related to greater depressive symptomatology. Similarly, Bookwala and Lawson (2011) tested the applicability of the activity restriction model in relation to vision quality in late-life. Poorer self-rated vision in late-life contributes to lower mental health directly by restricting individuals' ability to carry out routine day-to-day physical activities, and indirectly by increasing their feelings of social isolation. These results support the activity-restriction model. Consistent with the above reasoning, Benyamini and Lomranz (2004) found that successfully replacing lost activities was related to lowered depressive symptoms, comparable to those of healthier older adults.

TREATMENT FOR LATE-LIFE DEPRESSION

Pharmacotherapy

Pharmacotherapies (i.e. tricyclic anti-depressants (TCAs), selective serotonin reuptake inhibitors (SSRIs), and monoamine oxidase inhibitors) have been identified as evidence-based interventions for late-life depression (Shanmugham et al. 2005; Wilson et al. 2001). In comparing efficacy of TCAs and SSRIs, Mottram, Wilson, and Strobl (2006) found that both are efficacious, however the total withdrawal rate due to side-effects (i.e.

participants that withdrew from the study) favoured TCAs significantly less. Similarly, SSRIs are thought to produce side-effects that are less threatening to older adults than those associated with TCAs (Shanmugham et al. 2005). The use of anti-depressant medication is more likely to be recommended by medical professionals as a treatment for older adults when depression is severe (Shanmugham et al. 2005). However, depressed older adults tend to have a treatment preference for psychotherapy over pharmacotherapy (Gum et al. 2006; Rokke and Scogin 1995).

Psychotherapies

Cuijpers, Van Straten, and Smit (2006) conducted a meta-analysis which included the comparison of seventeen randomized controlled interventions for late-life depression. They found an overall mean effect size of .72 (95% CI: .57–.87). Similar investigations (e.g. Engels and Verney 1997; Pinquart and Sörensen 2001) provide further evidence that psychological interventions are effective for late-life depression. Furthermore, Scogin and colleagues (2005) have identified specific psychological treatments as evidence-based, using criteria defined by a taskforce of the US-based Society of Clinical Psychology, in the treatment of late-life depression. These treatments include cognitive-behavioural, behavioural, problem-solving, reminiscence, and brief psychodynamic psychotherapies, as well as cognitive bibliotherapy (Scogin et al. 2005). We now provide a review for each of the evidence-based treatments for late-life depression.

Behavioural therapy

Behavioural therapy focuses on the relationship between mood and engagement in pleasant activities (Lewinsohn and Graf 1973; Lewinsohn and Libet 1972). Under this paradigm, late-life depression emerges as a function of excess unpleasant events, fewer pleasurable activities and less positive reinforcement (MacPhillamy and Lewinsohn 1974). Behavioural activation (BA) is designed with the goal of keeping older adults active and engaged in life's activities, rather than leading inactive, withdrawn, and avoidant life styles. Therefore, behavioural therapies for depressed older adults aims to teach them to monitor mood and activity levels, identify behavioural goals within a number of life areas (e.g. hobbies, relationships, etc.), and plan implementation of pleasant events (Hopko et al. 2003). The BA approach encourages the recognition of events that improve or negatively affect mood.

Behavioural therapy in depressed older adults appears to have comparable effectiveness with alternative psychotherapies. The five supported behavioural therapy studies identified by Scogin et al. (2005) were either superior to a control condition or were non-differentially efficacious in comparison to other evidence-based therapies (cognitive-behavioural therapy or brief psychodynamic psychotherapy). Another meta-analysis of four randomized controlled trials (Gallagher and Thompson 1982; Rokke, Tomhave, and Jocic 1999; Scogin, Jamison, and Gochneaur 1989; Thompson, Gallagher, and Breckenridge 1987) determined that behavioural therapy was not significantly more effective than cognitive therapy or brief psychodynamic therapy for post-treatment clinician-rated depression (Samad, Brealey, and Gilbody 2011). However, behavioural therapy was significantly more effective than a wait-list control. In a pilot investigation of the effects of BA in older adults with depression, 71% of participants no longer met criteria for a depressive disorder following a course of individual BA psychotherapy (Yon and Scogin 2008). In addition, a meta-analysis of behavioural therapy for older adults yielded an average effect size of $d = .96$ (Engels and Verney 1997).

Behavioural therapy has been effectively used in various settings, including nursing homes, assisted living, and geriatric psychiatry facilities. For instance, Behavioural Activities Intervention (BE-ACTIV) is a behavioural intervention for depression in nursing homes that emphasizes activation and engagement in pleasant events (Meeks et al. 2008). In a small, randomized pilot study, BE-ACTIV led to increased activity levels and more rapid improvements in depression over treatment as usual for depressed nursing home residents. Similarly, behavioural treatment appears promising for depressed, frail older adults in assisted living facilities. In a small pilot, 37% (four of eleven) of those who initially scored within the depression range scored below it following behavioural treatment (Cernin and Lichtenberg 2009). Lastly, in a sample of older adult patients in a geriatric psychiatry facility, BA treatment improved depression scores compared to treatment as usual (Snarksi et al. 2011).

Cognitive-behavioural therapy (CBT)

The primary goal of CBT is to improve the skills of older adults in examining and modifying maladaptive thoughts and belief systems. Some techniques used in CBT include recognizing and altering irrational thoughts, changing the way in which individuals process information, increasing positive self-statements and experiences, and countering mistaken belief systems. Behavioural techniques are also incorporated into treatment, including behavioural activation, relaxation training, problem-solving and communication skills. The desired outcome of CBT is to assuage depression by developing reinforcing and rewarding experiences and perceptions (Kennedy and Tanenbaum 2000). Derived primarily through the work of Aaron Beck (Beck 1967; Beck et al. 1979), CBT has been modified for use with older adults through the protocols developed by Thompson, Gallagher-Thompson, and colleagues (Thompson et al. 2010).

CBT is an effective treatment for older adults with depressive disorders. Subgroup analyses of a meta-analysis of psychotherapy for older adults showed that CBT (seven studies) was more effective than placebo (Peng et al. 2009). In a sample of low-income older adults, Areán and colleagues (2005) found that clinical case management (CCM) and the combination of CCM with cognitive-behavioural group therapy (CCM + CBGT) led to greater improvements in depressive symptoms than CBGT. Other meta-analyses of cognitive-behavioural therapies for older adults indicate effect sizes ranging from .70 to .85 (Cuijpers et al. 2006; Scogin and McElreath 1994). These effect sizes are comparable to those of younger adults in meta-analyses, using cognitive-behavioural approaches ($d = .72$, Michael and Crowley 2002). Pinquart and Sörensen (2001) conducted a meta-analysis to explore the factors affecting outcomes in older adults. They found that older adults have greater benefits from longer interventions (i.e. more than nine sessions), as well as from interventions that are delivered by therapists with specialized training in working with older adults.

CBT has been used effectively in various settings, including primary care. Laidlaw et al. (2008) found that CBT was non-differentially effective as treatment as usual (TAU) because both produced significant reductions in depressive symptoms both immediately after treatment and six months post-treatment. This study was conducted in the primary care setting and addressed mild to moderate late-life depression. Another study found CBT to be more clinically effective than treatment as usual and talking control (e.g. therapist showed interest and warmth but did not challenge dysfunctional thoughts) for older adults with depression in primary care (Serfaty et al. 2009).

Cognitive bibliotherapy

Cognitive bibliotherapy differs from traditional psychotherapy in that it is self-administered, often at one's own home. Treatment involves reading and written exercises over a four-week period, which is intended to alleviate emotional and psychological problems. Therapist contact during bibliotherapy is minimal, but may include brief (~ 5 minutes) weekly telephone check-ups. Similar to cognitive therapy, the primary aim of the cognitive bibliotherapy for depression is to help participants identify and challenge maladaptive cognitive processes.

Cognitive bibliotherapy has been effective for the treatment of depression in older adults (Floyd et al. 2004; Landreville and Bissonnette 1997; Scogin, Hamblin, and Beutler 1987; Scogin et al. 1989). Some results indicate that the effectiveness of cognitive bibliotherapy is comparable to in-person psychotherapy, with both showing significant improvement compared to control (Scogin et al. 1987; Scogin et al. 1989). Floyd et al. (2004) found that although individual psychotherapy was superior to cognitive bibliotherapy at immediate post-treatment, the bibliotherapy participants continued to improve after treatment, showing no differences from individual psychotherapy at the three-month follow-up evaluation. In another group of studies, treatment gains from cognitive bibliotherapy were maintained through a two- and three-year follow-up period (Floyd et al. 2006; Smith et al. 1997). Finally, a meta-analysis of nine studies of cognitive bibliotherapy for older individuals yielded an average effect size of d = .57 (CI = .37–.77; Gregory et al. 2004). Thus, research has consistently demonstrated that cognitive bibliotherapy is an effective treatment for depression in older adults.

Problem-solving therapy (PST)

In problem-solving therapy (PST), participants learn skills to actively approach problems, select solutions, and make concrete plans for problem resolution. As part of PST, participants are taught to (1) define problems and formulate goals; (2) generate alternative tasks that will alleviate the adverse effects of the problem; (3) apply decision-making to choose a problem-solving strategy; and (4) self-evaluate the outcomes of implementation and verification of solution. The most popular protocol used in PST is based on the work of Nezu and colleagues (Nezu, Nezu, and Perri 1989).

Two relevant studies in depressed older adults found that problem-solving therapy produced significant reduction in depressive symptoms compared with supportive therapy or wait-list control (Alexopoulos, Raue, and Areán 2003; Areán et al. 1993). Williams and colleagues (2000) used problem-solving therapy for primary care older adults and showed more late-course resolution of depressive symptoms than placebo. In a meta-analysis by Cuijpers, van Straten, and Warmerdam (2007), these three studies (Alexopoulos et al. 2003; Areán et al. 1993; Williams et al. 2000) demonstrated an effect size of .27 (CI = .01–.53). Subgroup analyses revealed no efficacy differences between adults and older adults for treating depression, which suggests that problem-solving therapy is suitable for both groups.

Problem-solving therapy has been used effectively in various settings, including in home for medically ill older adults (Ciechanowski et al. 2004; Gellis et al. 2008; Kiosses et al. 2010). For example, Ciechanowski and colleagues (2004) created a home-based problem-solving intervention for the Program to Encourage Active, Rewarding Lives for Seniors (PEARLS). Older adults that received the PEARLS intervention were more likely to have at least 50% reduction in depressive symptoms when compared to the usual care group. To address the needs of older adults with major depression, cognitive impairment, and disability, Kiosses et al. (2010) developed a home-delivered intervention (Problem Adaptation Therapy, PATH) targeting behavioural limitations resulting from depression and disability. In a pre-liminary randomized clinical trial, PATH was more efficacious than home-delivered supportive therapy in reducing depression and disability. Therefore, problem-solving therapy can be successfully adapted to a home-based intervention for homebound older adults, a population that often receives inadequate recognition and treatment.

Treatment for late-life depression in primary care remains challenging. However, problem-solving therapy either as a standalone treatment or as an additive to collaborative care is a viable option for treatment (Areán et al. 2008; Harpole et al. 2005; Hunkeler et al. 2006; Unützer et al. 2002; Williams et al. 2000). As mentioned above, when problem-solving therapy was used in a primary care setting for older adults with minor depression or dysthymia, symptoms improved more rapidly than pill placebo (Williams et al. 2000). In a collaborative treatment programme (IMPACT), older adults had up to twelve months of access to medication support or problem-solving therapy (PST; Unützer et al. 2002). At twelve months, 45% of participants in the IMPACT intervention (PST or anti-depressants) had a 50% or greater reduction in depressive symptoms from baseline compared with only 19% of usual care participants. The IMPACT intervention was also found to be an effective long-term treatment (i.e. eighteen, twenty-four months, and one year after resources were withdrawn) for improving depressive symptoms in older adults (Hunkeler et al. 2006). In older adults with comorbid illness, including arthritis, IMPACT participants experienced significantly lower depression compared with usual care participants (Harpole et al. 2005; Lin et al. 2003). Lastly, older adults receiving problem-solving therapy in IMPACT had fewer depressive symptoms and better functioning than those receiving community-based psychotherapy (Areán et al. 2008).

In addition to being a viable treatment option for primary care and medically frail home-bound older adults, problem-solving therapy has also been found to be an effective inter-vention in older patients with depression and executive dysfunction (Areán et al. 2010; Alexopoulos et al. 2011). At nine and twelve weeks of treatment, PST had a greater reduc-tion in symptom severity, response rate, and remission rate than supportive therapy (ST; Areán et al. 2010). In a post hoc analysis of the same sample, Alexopoulos and colleagues (2011) found that PST reduced disability more than ST. PST's greater effect on disability was thought to contribute to the higher efficacy of PST over ST in improving depressive symptoms.

Brief psychodynamic therapy (BPT)

Brief psychodynamic psychotherapy (BPT) focuses on interpersonal relationships and unconscious processes (i.e. feelings, desires, and thoughts) to treat depressive symptoms. As the name implies, treatment is relatively short in duration (~ 20 sessions). At the start of therapy, the therapist and client agree on a focus, which is often to build awareness of the unconscious affect, cognition, and behaviour that produce depressive symptoms. The role of the therapist is to foster the development of a therapeutic alliance and a positive trans-ference. Like most psychotherapies, the goal of BPT is symptom reduction. However, an additional goal can include personality change, such as decreasing client's vulnerability and increasing long-term resilience. These principles are described in Horowitz and Kaltreider (1979), Mann (1973), and Rose and DelMaestro (1990).

Two studies of brief psychodynamic therapy for depressed community-dwelling older adults (Gallagher and Thompson 1982; Thompson et al. 1987) found BPT to be non-differentially efficacious in relation to other EBTs (cognitive-behavioural therapy and behavioural therapy; Leichsenring 2001). With the addition of a longer form of psy-chodynamic therapy (Steuer et al. 1984), Driessen et al. (2010) found the three studies to have an average effect size of 1.19 (CI = .79–1.60). This indicates that brief psychodynamic therapy can be an effective treatment for depressive symptoms in older adults. In additional subgroup analyses, Driessen et al. (2010) found no efficacy differences from pre- to post-treatment depression change between young and older adults, suggesting brief psy-chodynamic therapy is suited for younger adults as well as older adults.

Reminiscence therapy

In this intervention, older adults are asked to reflect systematically on life and focus on the significant aspects of important positive and negative life events (Haight 1988; Watt and Cappeliez 2000). By reviewing one's life history, it is believed that participants gain self-confidence, socialization, and a better sense of perspective concerning these life events. Goals of reminiscence therapy include resolving conflict from the past and help-ing participants find a balance between successes and failures in their lives (Butler 1963). Reminiscence therapy is one of the few interventions designed specifically for older adults.

Bohlmeijer, Smit, and Cuijpers (2003) conducted a meta-analysis to assess the effective-ness of reminiscence and life review on late-life depression across different target groups and treatment modalities. The mean effect size for twenty studies was .84, indicating a statistically and clinically significant effect of reminiscence and life review on depressive symptomatology in older adults. In addition, participants with greater levels of depressive symptomatology had larger effects ($d = 1.23$) than other subjects ($d = .37$). These effects are comparable to the effects commonly found for other psychological and pharmacotherapy treatments.

Systematic reviews of randomized controlled trials of reminiscence therapy studies have shown significant beneficial effects on depression for older adults (Chin 2007; Peng et al. 2009). Additionally, reminiscence therapy has been found to be non-differentially effica-cious in improving depression than cognitive-behavioural therapy (Peng et al. 2009). Previous studies have found an average reduction in Geriatric Depression Scale-Short Form (GDS-SF) scores ranging from 13.7–6.36 points to 12.3–4.29 points, indicating that reminiscence therapy improves depressive symptoms (as reported in Chiang et al. 2010). Reminiscence therapy was also found to be an effective long-term treatment (i.e. one and three years post-treatment) for improving depressive symptoms in older adults (Haight, Michel, and Hendrix 2000).

Reminiscence therapy is often conducted as an individual modality, but research also supports the use of group reminiscence therapy (Hanaoka and Okamura 2004). Significant differences between group life review activities and discussion control group was found in older adults' depression and hopelessness changes (Hanaoka and Okamura 2004). Similarly, a controlled trial (n = 33) of a community-based intervention, the Life Story Workshop, found a significant improvement for the intervention group compared with the control group (Mastel-Smith et al. 2007).

Reminiscence therapy has also been used to address depressive symptoms in institutionalized older adults. In a quasi-experimental design, both reminiscence and transmissive reminiscence (i.e. telling oral history with a focus on teaching/mentoring) were found to decrease depression scores in geriatric residents of nursing homes (Wilson 2006). There was no significant difference between the two groups. In older adults residing in long-term care facilities, reminiscence therapy produced significant differences between pre- and post-depressive symptoms (Wang 2004; Wang, Hsu, and Cheng 2005). Similarly, Chiang et al. (2010) found that the depression scores of the reminiscence group were significantly lower than control at post-treatment and three-month follow-up on depression, psychological well-being, and loneliness among institutionalized aged.

A multicentre randomized controlled trial found that personal meaning mediated the effects of life review on late-life depressive symptoms (Westerhof et al. 2010). Furthermore, improvement in personal meaning predicted decline in depressive symptoms after the intervention and at follow-up. These results suggest that personal meaning has a critical role in improving depression, as well as sustaining those effects. In addition, Westerhof and colleagues (2010) suggest that improvement in meaning during the intervention may provide older adults with purpose, which in turn results in decreases of depressive symptoms at follow-up.

Implications for Practice

The implications for practice are that depression will continue to be a significant public health concern and that psychological treatments are available to address depressive symptoms experienced by older adults. Moreover, there are a wide range of evidence-based treatments that can be used to match the needs and contexts of the older adults we serve. The findings that older adults often prefer psychological treatments over other forms of depression intervention creates the opportunity for effective service delivery by clinical geropsychologists.

Summary

Even though late-life depression is probably underestimated, potentially because of the age-associated differences in presentation, it is common in older adults. Prevalence rates of late-life depression tend to increase with age, female sex, reduction in severity of symptoms and greater restriction in living arrangements. Given its potential devastating effects (e.g. hospitalization and suicide), it is crucial to expand our understanding of developmental and protective factors in late-life depression. Research suggests that the origin of late-life depression is a combination of biological (e.g. genetic predisposition, vascular lesions, and comorbid medical illnesses), psychological (e.g. maladaptive cognitions, lowered engagement in pleasant events, and comorbid psychiatric disorders) and social factors (e.g. life strain, negative life events, and poor social support). However, many protective factors (resources, psychological strategies, and meaningful engagement) and evidence-based treatments (i.e. pharmacotherapy and psychotherapy) have been identified to ameliorate symptoms of late-life depression. In addition to the evidence-based psychotherapies described above, research has begun to reveal other promising treatments that should be considered, such as acceptance and commitment therapy (Bohlmeijer, Pieterse, and Schreurs 2012), mindfulness-based cognitive therapy (Smith, Graham, and Senthinathan 2007), behavioural bibliotherapy (Moss, Scogin, DiNapoli, and Presnell 2012), and interpersonal therapy (Hinrichsen 2008). To conclude, it is paramount to establish early identification (i.e. self—or physician) of late-life depression so that older adults can have the opportunity to seek effective treatment to alleviate symptoms, which in turn will significantly improve their quality of life.

Key References and Sources for Further Reading

American Psychological Association (2006). *Depression with Older Adults* (DVD). http://www. apa.org/videos/.

American Psychological Association (2008). *Adapting Psychotherapy for Working with Older Adults* (DVD). http://www.apa.org/videos/.

American Psychological Association, Office on Aging (2011). 'Psychology's Role in Addressing the Mental and Behavioral Health Needs of the Geriatric Population'. http://www.apa.org/pi/aging/resources/psychologist-role-geriatric.pdf.

Fiske, A., Wetherell, J. L., and Gatz, M. (2009). Depression in older adults. *Annual Reviews of Clinical Psychology* 5: 363–389.

Karel, M. J., Ogland-hand, S., and Gatz, M. (2002). *Assessing and treating late-life depression: a casebook and resource guide*. New York: Basic Books.

Lavretsky, H., Sajatovic, M., and Reynolds, C. F. III (eds) (2013). *Late-life Mood Disorders*. New York: Oxford University Press.

Scogin, F. and Shah, A. (eds) (2012). *Making Evidence-based Psychological Treatments Work with Older Adults*. Washington, DC: American Psychological Association.

Scogin, F., Welsh, D., Hanson, A., Stump, J., and Coates, A. (2005). 'Evidence-based Psychotherapies for Depression in Older Adults'. *Clinical Psychology: Science and Practice* 12(3): 222–237.

United States Department of Health and Human Services, Substance Abuse and Mental Health Services Administration (2011). *Treatment of Depression in Older Adults Evidence-based Practices (EBP) KIT* (CD-ROM/DVD). http://store.samhsa.gov/home.

References

Akincigil, A., Olfson, M., Walkup, J. T., Siegel, M., Kalay, E., et al. (2011). 'Diagnosis and Treatment of Depression in Older Community-dwelling Adults: 1992–2005'. *Journal of the American Geriatrics Society* 59(6): 1042–1051.

Alexandrino-Silva, C., Alves, T. F., Tófoli, L. F., Wang, Y., and Andrade, L. H. (2011). 'Psychiatry-life Events and Social Support in Late Life Depression'. *Clinics (Sao Paulo)*: 66(2): 233–238.

Alexopoulos, G. S., Meyers, B. S., Young, R. C., Campbell, S., Silbersweig, D., and Charlson, M. (1997). 'Vascular Depression Hypothesis'. *Archives of General Psychiatry* 54(10): 915–922.

Alexopoulos, G. S., Raue, P. and Areán, P. (2003). 'Problem-solving Therapy versus Supportive Therapy in Geriatric Major Depression with Executive Dysfunction'. *American Journal of Geriatric Psychiatry* 11(1): 46–52.

Alexopoulos, G. S., Raue, P. J., Kiosses, D. N., Mackin, R. S., Kanellopoulos, D., et al. (2011). 'Problem-solving Therapy and Supportive Therapy in Older Adults with Major Depression and Executive Dysfunction: Effect on Disability'. *Archives of General Psychiatry* 68(1): 33–41.

American Psychiatric Association (2000). *Diagnostic and Statistical Manual of Mental Disorder* (4th edn; text revised). Washington, DC: American Psychiatric Association.

Aranda, M. P., Lee, P. J., and Wilson, S. (2001). 'Correlates of Depression in Older Latinos'. *Home Health Care Service* 20(1): 1–20.

Areán, P. A., Perri, M. G., Nezu, A. M., Schein, R. L., Christopher, F., et al. (1993). 'Comparative Effectiveness of Social Problem-solving Therapy and Reminiscence Therapy as Treatments for Depression in Older Adults'. *Journal of Consulting and Clinical Psychology* 61(6): 1003–1010.

Areán, P. A., Uncapher, H., and Satre, D. (1998). 'Depression'. In M. Hersen and V. B. van Hasselt (eds), *Handbook of Clinical Geropsychology* (pp. 195–216). New York: Plenum Press.

Areán, P. A., Gum, A., McCulloch, C. E., Bostrom, A., Gallagher-Thompson, D., et al. (2005). 'Treatment of Depression in Low-income Older Adults'. *Psychology and Aging* 20(4): 601–609.

Areán, P., Hegel, M., Vannoy, S., Fan, M., and Unuzter, J. (2008). 'Effectiveness of Problem-solving Therapy for Older, Primary Care Patients with Depression: Results from the IMPACT Project'. *Gerontologist* 48(3): 311–323.

Areán, P. A., Raue, P., Mackin, R. S., Kanellopoulos, D., McCulloch, C., et al. (2010). 'Problem-solving Therapy and Supportive Therapy in Older Adults with Major Depression and Executive Dysfunction'. *American Journal of Psychiatry* 167(11): 1391–1398.

Artero, S., Tiemeier, H., Prins, N. D., Sabatier, R., Breteler, M. M. B., et al. (2004). 'Neuroanatomical Localization and Clinical Correlates of White Matter Lesions in the Elderly'. *Journal of Neurology, Neurosurgery and Psychiatry* 75(9): 1304–1308.

Back, J. H. and Lee, Y. (2011). 'Gender Differences in the Association between Socioeconomic Status (SES) and Depressive Symptoms in Older Adults'. *Archives of Gerontology and Geriatrics* 52(3): 140–144.

Balogun, R. A., Turgut, F., Balogun, S. A., Holroyd, S., and Abdel-Rahman, E. M. (2011). 'Screening for Depression in Elderly Hemodialysis Patients'. *Nephron Clinical Practice* 118(2): 72–77.

Balsis, S. and Cully, J. (2008). 'Comparing Depression Diagnostic Symptoms across Younger and Older Adults'. *Aging & Mental Health* 12(6): 800–806.

Beck, A. T. (1967). *Depression: Causes and Treatment*. Philadelphia, PA: University of Pennsylvania Press.

Beck, A. T., Rush, A. J., Shaw, B. F., and Emery, G. (1979). *Cognitive Therapy of Depression*. New York: Guilford Press.

Benyamini Y. and Lomranz, J. (2004). 'The Relationship of Activity Restriction and Replacement with Depressive Symptoms among Older Adults'. *Psychology and Aging* 19(2): 362–366.

Bergdahl, E., Allard, P., Alex, L., Lundman, B., and Gustafson, Y. (2007). 'Gender Differences in Depression among the Very Old'. *International Psychogeriatrics* 19(6): 1125–1140.

Blazer, D. G. (2003). 'Depression in Late Life: Review and Commentary'. *Journals of Gerontology: Series A* 58(3): 249–265.

Blazer, D. G. (2005). 'Depression and Social Support in Late Life: A Clear but not Obvious Relationship'. *Aging & Mental Health* 9(6): 497–499.

Blazer, D. G. (2010). 'The Origins of Late-life Depression'. *Psychiatric Annals* 40(1): 13–18.

Blow, F. C., Serras, A. M., and Barry, K. L. (2007). 'Late-life Depression and Alcoholism'. *Current Psychiatry Reports* 9(1): 14–19.

Boey, K. W. and Chiu, H. F. (2010). 'Life Strain and Psychological Distress of Older Women and Older Men in Hong Kong'. *Aging & Mental Health* 9(6): 555–562.

Bohlmeijer, E., Smit, F., and Cuijpers, P. (2003). 'Effects of Reminiscence and Life Review on Late-life Depression: A Meta-analysis'. *International Journal of Geriatric Psychiatry* 18(12): 1088–1094.

Bohlmeijer, E. M., Pieterse, M. E., and Schreurs, K. M. G. (2012). 'Acceptance and Commitment Therapy as Guided Self-help for Psychological Distress and Positive Mental Health: A Randomized Controlled Trial'. *Psychological Medicine* 42(3): 485–495.

Bookwala, J. and Lawson, B. (2011). 'Poor Vision, Functioning, and Depressive Symptoms: A Test of the Activity Restriction Model'. *Gerontologist* 51(6): 798–808.

Brodaty, H., Luscombe, G., Parker, G., Wilhelm, K., Hickie, I., et al. (1997). 'Increased Rate of Psychosis and Psychomotor Change in Depression with Age'. *Psychological Medicine* 27(5): 1205–1213.

Butler, R. N. (1963). 'The Life Review: An Interpretation of Reminiscence in the Aged'. *Psychiatry* 26: 65–76.

Carmelli, D., Swan, G. E., Kelly-Hayes, M., Wolf, P. A., Reed, T., et al. (2000). 'Longitudinal Changes in the Contribution of Genetic and Environmental Influences to Symptoms of Depression in Older Male Twins'. *Psychology and Aging* 15(3): 505–510.

Carstensen, L. L., Fung, H. H., and Charles, S. T. (2003). 'Socioemotional Selectivity Theory and the Regulation of Emotion in the Second Half of Life'. *Motivation and Emotion* 27(2): 103–123.

Centers for Disease Control and Prevention (2008). 'Web-Based Injury Statistics Query and Reporting System (WISQARS)'. http://webappa.cdc.gov/sasweb/ncipc/mortrate10_sy.html.

Cernin, P. A., and Lichtenberg, P. A. (2009). 'Behavioral Treatment for Depression Mood: A Pleasant Events Intervention for Seniors Residing in Assisted Living'. *Clinical Gerontologist* 32: 324–331.

Chachamovich, E., Fleck, M., Laidlaw, K., and Power, M. (2008). 'Impact of Major Depression and Subsyndromal Symptoms on Quality of Life and Attitudes toward Aging in an International Sample of Older Adults'. *Gerontologist* 48(5): 593–602.

Chiang, K. J., Chu, H., Chang, H., Chung, M., Chen, C., et al. (2010). 'The Effects of Reminiscence Therapy on Psychological Well-being, Depression, and Loneliness among the Institutionalized Aged'. *International Journal of Geriatric Psychiatry* 25: 380–388.

Chin, A. M. H. (2007). 'Clinical Effects of Reminiscence Therapy in Older Adults: A Meta-analysis of Controlled Trials'. *Hong Kong Journal of Occupational Therapy* 17(1): 10–22.

Ciechanowski, P., Wagner, E., Schmaling, K., Schwartz, S., Williams, B., et al. (2004). 'Community-integrated Home-based Depression Treatment in Older Adults: A Randomized Controlled Trial'. *Journal of the American Medical Association* 291(13): 1569–1577.

Couture, M., Larivière, N., and Lefraçois, R. (2005). 'Psychological Distress in Older Adults with Low Functional Independence: A Multidimensional Perspective'. *Archives of Gerontology and Geriatrics* 41(1): 101–111.

Cuijpers, P., Van Straten, A., and Smit, F. (2006). 'Psychological Treatment of Late-life Depression: A Meta-analysis of Randomized Controlled Trials'. *International Journal of Geriatric Psychiatry* 21(12): 1139–1149.

Cuijpers, P., Van Straten, A., and Warmerdam, L. (2007). 'Problem Solving Therapies for Depression: A Meta-analysis'. *European Psychiatry* 22(1): 9–15.

Driessen, E., Cuijpers, P., De Maat, S. C., Abbass, A. A., De Jonghe, F., et al. (2010). 'The Efficacy of Short-term Psychodynamic Psychotherapy for Depression: A Meta-analysis'. *Clinical Psychology Review* 30(1): 25–36.

Dunlop, D. D., Song, J., Lyons, J. S., Manheim, L. M., and Chang, R. W. (2003). 'Racial/ethnic Differences in Rates of Depression among Preretirement Adults'. *American Journal of Public Health* 93(11): 1945–1952.

Eaton, W., Kramer, M., Anthony, J., Dryman, A., Shapiro, S., et al. (1989). 'The Incidence of Specific DIS/DSM-III Mental Disorders: Data from the NIMH Epidemiological Catchment Area Program'. *Acta Psychiatrica Scandinavica* 79: 109–125.

Edelstein, B. A., Shreve-Neiger, A., and Scheck, S. A. (2004). 'Depression in Late Life'. In C. Spielberger (ed.), *Encyclopedia of Applied Psychology* (vol. 1; pp. 593–599). Oxford, Boston: Elsevier Academic Press.

Emmerson, J. P., Burvill, P. W., Finlay-Jones, R., and Hall, W. (1989). 'Life Events, Life Difficulties and Confiding Relationships in the Depressed Elderly'. *British Journal of Psychiatry* 155: 787–792.

Engels, G. I. and Verney, M. (1997). 'Efficacy of Nonmedical Treatments of Depression in Elders: A Quantitative Analysis'. *Journal of Clinical Geropsychology* 3(1): 17–35.

Ferraro, K. F. and Su, Y. (1999). 'Financial Strain, Social Relations, and Psychological Distress among Older People: A Cross-cultural Analysis'. *Journals of Gerontology: Series B* 54(1): 3–15.

Fiest, K. M., Currie, S. R., Williams, J. V., and Wang, J. (2011). 'Chronic Conditions and Major Depression in Community-dwelling Older Adults'. *Journal of Affective Disorders* 131: 172–178.

Firbank, M. J., Lloyd, A. J., Ferrier, N., and O'Brien, J. T. (2004). 'A Volumetric Study of MRI Signal Hyperintensities in Late-life Depression'. *American Journal of Geriatric Psychiatry* 12(6): 606–612.

Fiske, A., Gatz, M., and Pedersen, N. L. (2003). 'Depressive Symptoms and Aging: The Effects of Illness and Non-health-related Events'. *Journals of Gerontology: Series B* 58(6): 320–328.

Fiske, A., Wetherell, J. L., and Gatz, M. (2009). 'Depression in Older Adults'. *Annual Reviews of Clinical Psychology* 5: 363–389.

Floyd, M., Scogin, F., McKendree-Smith, N. L., Floyd, D. L., and Rokke, P. D. (2004). 'Cognitive Therapy for Depression: A Comparison of Individual Psychotherapy and Bibliotherapy for Depressed Older Adults'. *Behavior Modification* 28(2): 297–318.

Floyd, M., Rohen, N., Shackelford, J. A., Hubbard, K. L., Parnell, M. B., et al. (2006). 'Two-year Follow-up of Bibliotherapy and Individual Cognitive Therapy for Depressed Older Adults'. *Behavior Modification* 30(3): 281–294.

Gallagher, D. E. and Thompson, L. W. (1982). 'Treatment of Major Depressive Disorder in Older Adult Outpatients with Brief Psychotherapies'. *Psychotherapy: Theory, Research and Practice* 19(4): 482–490.

Gallagher, D. E., Mhaolain, A. N., Greene, E., Walsh, C., Denihan, A., et al. (2010). 'Late life Depression: A Comparison of Risk Factors and Symptoms According to Age of Onset in Community Dwelling Older Adults'. *International Journal of Geriatric Psychiatry* 25(10): 981–987.

Gallo, J. J., Cooper-Patrick, L., and Lesikar, S. (1998). 'Depressive Symptoms of Whites and African Americans Aged 60 Years and Older'. *Journal of Gerontology: Series B* 53(5): 277–286.

Gatz, M., Pederson, N. L., Plomin, R., Nesselroade, J. R., and McClearn, G. E. (1992). 'Importance of Shared Genes and Shared Environments for Symptoms of Depression in Older Adults'. *Journal of Abnormal Psychology* 101(4): 701–708.

Gellis, Z. D., McGinty, J., Tierney, L., Jordan, C., Burton, J., et al. (2008). 'Randomized Controlled Trial of Problem-solving Therapy for Minor Depression in Home Care'. *Research on Social Work Practice* 18(6): 596–606.

George, L. K., Blazer, D. G., Hughes, D. C., and Fowler, N. (1989). 'Social Support and the Outcome of Major Depression'. *British Journal of Psychiatry* 154: 478–485.

Gregory, R. J., Canning, S. S., Lee, T. W., and Wise, J. C. (2004). 'Cognitive Bibliotherapy for Depression: A Meta-analysis'. *Professional Psychology: Research and Practice* 35(3): 275–280.

Grzywacz, J. G., Almeida, D. M., Neupert, S. D., and Ettner, S. L. (2004). 'Socioeconomic Status and Health: A Micro-level Analysis of Exposure and Vulnerability to Daily Stressors'. *Journal of Health and Social Behavior* 45: 1–16.

Gum, A. M., Areán, P. A., Hunkeler, E., Tang, L., Katon, W., et al. (2006). 'Depression Treatment Preferences in Older Primary Care Patients'. *Gerontologist* 46(1): 14–22.

Gum, A. M. and Cheavens, J. S. (2008). 'Psychiatric Comorbidity and Depression in Older Adults'. *Current Psychiatry Reports* 10(1): 23–29.

Gureje, O., Oladeji, B., and Abiona, T. (2011). 'Incidence and Risk Factors for Late-life Depression in the Ibadan Study of Ageing'. *Psychological Medicine* 41(9): 1897–1906.

Haight, B. K. (1988). 'The Therapeutic Role of a Structured Life Review Process in Homebound Elderly Subjects'. *Journal of Gerontology* 43(2): 40–44.

Haight, B. K., Michel, Y., and Hendrix, S. (2000). 'The Extended Effects of the Life Review in Nursing Home Residents'. *International Journal of Aging and Human Development* 50(2): 151–168.

Han, B. (2002). 'Depressive Symptoms and Self-rated Health in Community-dwelling Older Adults: A Longitudinal Study'. *Journal of the American Geriatrics Society* 50(9): 1549–1556.

Hanaoka, H. and Okamura, H. (2004). 'Study on Effects of Life Review Activities on the Quality of Life of the Elderly: A Randomized Controlled Trial'. *Psychotherapy and Psychosomatics* 73(5): 302–311.

Hannestad, J., Taylor, W. D., McQuoid, D. R., Payne, M. E., Kirshnan, K. R., et al. (2006). 'White Matter Lesion Volumes and Caudate Volumes in Late-life Depression'. *International Journal of Geriatric Psychiatry* 21(12): 1193–1198.

Harpole, L. H., Williams, J. W., Olsen, M. K., Stechuchak, K. M., Oddone, E., et al. (2005). 'Improving Depression Outcomes in Older Adults with Comorbid Medical Illness'. *General Hospital Psychiatry* 27(1): 4–12.

Harris, Y. (2007). 'Depression as a Risk Factor for Nursing Home Admission among Older Individuals'. *Journal of the American Medical Directors Association* 8(1): 14–20.

Hegeman, J. M., Kok, R. M., Van der Mast, R. C., and Giltay, E. J. (2012). 'Phenomenology of Depression in Older Compared with Younger Adults: Meta-analysis'. *British Journal of Psychiatry* 200: 275–281.

Himelhoch, S., Weller, W., Wu, A. W., Anderson, G. F., and Cooper, L. A. (2004). 'Chronic Medical Illness, Depression, and Use of Acute Medical Services among Medicare Beneficiaries'. *Medical Care* 42(6): 512–521.

Hinrichsen, G. A. (2008). 'Interpersonal Psychotherapy as a Treatment for Depression in Later Life'. *Professional Psychology: Research and Practice* 39(3): 306–312.

Hopko, D. R., Lejuez, C. W., Ruggiero, K. J., and Eifert, G. H. (2003). 'Contemporary Behavioral Activation Treatments for Depression: Procedures, Principles, and Progress'. *Clinical Psychology Review* 23(5): 699–717.

Horowitz, M. J. and Kaltreider. N. B. (1979). 'Brief Therapy of the Stress Response Syndrome'. *Psychiatric Clinics of North America* 2: 365–378.

Huang, C-H., Dong, B. R., Lu, Z. C., Yue, J. R., and Liu, Q. X. (2010). 'Chronic Diseases and Risk for Depression in Old Age: A Meta-analysis of Published Literature'. *Ageing Research Reviews* 9(2): 131–141.

Hunkeler, E. M., Katon, W., Tang, L., Williams, J. W., Kroenke, K., et al. (2006). 'Long Term Outcomes from the IMPACT Randomised Trial for Depressed Elderly Patients in Primary Care'. *British Medical Journal* 332(7536): 259–263.

Husain, M. M., Rush, A. J., Sackeim, H. A., Wisniewski, S. R., McClintock, S. M., et al. (2005). 'Age-related Characteristics of Depression: A Preliminary Star*D report'. *American Journal of Geriatric Psychiatry* 13(10): 852–860.

Katsumata, Y., Arai, A., Ishida, K., Tomimori, M., Lee, R. B., et al. (2012). 'Which Categories of Social and Lifestyle Activities Moderate the Association between Negative Life Events and Depressive Symptoms among Community-dwelling Older Adults in Japan?' *International Psychogeriatrics* 24(2): 307–315.

Kennedy, G. J. and Tanenbaum, S. (2000). 'Psychotherapy with Older Adults'. *American Journal of Psychotherapy* 54: 386–407.

Kessler, R. C., Berglund, P., Demler, O., Jin, R., Koretz, D., et al. (2003). 'The Epidemiology of Major Depressive Disorder: Results from the National Comorbidity Survey Replication (NCS-R)'. *Journal of American Medical Association* 289(23): 3095–3105.

King, D. A., Heisel, M. J., and Lyness, J. M. (2005). 'Assessment and Psychological Treatment of Depression in Older Adults with Terminal or Life-Threatening Illness'. *Clinical Psychology: Science and Practice* 12(3): 339–353.

Kiosses, D. N., Areán, P. A., Teri, L., and Alexopoulos, G. S. (2010). 'Home-delivered Problem Adaptation Therapy (PATH) for Depressed, Cognitively Impaired, Disabled Elders: A Preliminary Study'. *American Journal of Geriatric Psychiatry* 18(11): 988–998.

Kivimäki, M., Shipley, M. J., Allan, C. L., Sexton, C. E., Jokela, M., et al. (2012). 'Vascular Risk Status as a Predictor of Later-Life Depressive Symptoms: A Cohort Study'. *Biologica Psychiatry* 72(4): 324–330.

Koenig, H. G. (1997). 'Differences in Psychosocial and Health Correlates of Major and Minor Depression in Medically Ill Older Adults'. *Journal of the American Geriatrics Society* 45(12): 1487–1495.

Koenig, H. G., Meador, K. G., Shelp, F., Goli, V., Cohen, H. J., et al. (1991). 'Major Depressive Disorder in Hospitalized Medically Ill Patients: An Examination of Young and Elderly Male Veterans'. *Journal of the American Geriatrics Society* 39(9): 881–890.

Kraaij, V., Arensman, E., and Spinhoven, P. (2002). 'Negative Life Events and Depression in Elderly Persons: A Meta-analysis'. *Journals of Gerontology: Series B* 57(1): 87–94.

Kunik, M. E., Mulsant, B. E., Rifai, A. H., Sweet, R. A., Pasternak, R., et al. (1994). 'Diagnostic Rate of Comorbid Personality Disorder in Elderly Psychiatric Inpatients'. *American Journal of Psychiatry* 151(4): 603–605.

Kvaal, K., McDougall, F. A., Brayne, C., Matthews, F. E., and Dewey, M. E. (2008). 'Co-occurrence of Anxiety and Depressive Disorders in a Community Sample of Older People: Result from the MRC CFAS (Medical Research Council Cognitive Function and Ageing Study)'. *International Journal of Geriatric Psychiatry* 23(3): 229–237.

Lai, T., Payne, M. E., Byrum, C. E., Steffens, D. C., and Krishnan, K. R. (2000). 'Reduction of Orbital Frontal Cortex Volume in Geriatric Depression'. *Biological Psychiatry* 48(10): 971–975.

Laidlaw, K., Davidson, K., Toner, H., Jackson, G., Clark, S., et al. (2008). 'A Randomized Controlled Trial of Cognitive Behaviour Therapy vs Treatment as Usual in the Treatment of Mild to Moderate Late Life Depression'. *International Journal of Geriatric Psychiatry* 23(8): 843–850.

Landreville, P. and Bissonnette, L. (1997). 'Effects of Cognitive Bibliotherapy for Depressed Older Adults with a Disability'. *Clinical Gerontologist* 17(4): 35–55.

Lavela, S. L. and Ather, N. (2010). 'Psychological Health in Older Adult Spousal Caregivers of Older Adults'. *Chronic Illness* 6(1): 67–80.

Leichsenring, F. (2001). 'Comparative Effects of Short-term Psychodynamic Psychotherapy and Cognitive-behavioral Therapy in Depression: A Meta-analytic Approach'. *Clinical Psychology Review* 21(3): 401–419.

Lenze, E. J., Rogers, J. C., Martire, L. M., Mulsant, B. H., Rollman, B. L., et al. (2001). 'The Association of Late-life Depression and Anxiety with Physical Disability: A Review of the Literature and Prospectus for Future Research'. *American Journal of Geriatric Psychiatry* 9(2): 113–135.

Lewinsohn, P. M. and Libet, J. (1972). 'Pleasant Activity, Activity Schedules, and Depressions'. *Journal of Abnormal Psychology* 79(3): 291–295.

Lewinsohn, P. M. and Graf, M. (1973). 'Pleasant Activities and Depression'. *Journal of Consulting and Clinical Psychology* 41(2): 261–268.

Lewinsohn, P. M., Munoz, R. F., Youngren, M. A., and Zeiss, A. M. (1986). *Control Your Depression*. New York: Prentice Hall.

Li, C. (2008). 'Racial and Ethnic Disparities among U.S. Elderly: Depression Prevalence, Access and Quality of Healthcare'. Unpublished doctoral dissertation, University of Rochester, New York.

Licht-Strunk, E., Van der Kooij, K. G., Van Schaik, D. J., Van Marwijk, H. W., Van Hout, H. P., et al. (2005). 'Prevalence of Depression in Older Patients Consulting their General Practitioner in the Netherlands'. *International Journal of Geriatric Psychiatry* 20(11): 1013–1019.

Lin, E. H., Katon, W., Von Korff, M., Tang, L., Williams, J. W., et al. (2003). 'Effect of Improving Depression Care on Pain and Functional Outcomes among Older Adults with Arthritis: A Randomized Controlled Trial'. *Journal of the American Medical Association* 290(18): 2428–2429.

Liu, C. P., Leung, D. S., and Chi, I. (2011). 'Social Functioning, Polypharmacy and Depression in Older Chinese Primary Care Patients'. *Aging & Mental Health* 15(6): 732–741.

Lopez, A. D., Mathers, C. D., Ezzati, M., Jamison, D. T., et al. (eds) (2006). 'Global Burden of Disease and Risk Factors'. http://www.dcp2.org/pubs/GBD.

Lövheim, H., Graneheim, U. H., Jonsén, E., Strandberg, G., and Lundman, B. (2012). 'Changes in Sense of Coherence in Old Age: A 5-year Follow-up of the Umeá 85+ Study'. *Scandinavian Journal of Caring Sciences* 27(1): 13–19.

Lue, B., Chen, L., and Wu, S. (2010). 'Health, Financial Stresses, and Life Satisfaction Affecting Late-life Depression among Older Adults: A Nationwide, Longitudinal Survey in Taiwan'. *Archives of Gerontology and Geriatrics* 50(1): 34–38.

Luijendijk, H. J., Van den Berg, J. F., Dekker, M., Van Tuijl, H., Otte, W., et al. (2008). 'Incidence and Recurrence of Late-life Depression'. *Archives of General Psychiatry* 65(12): 1394–1401.

McBride, A. M. and Abeles, N. (2000). 'Depressive Symptoms and Cognitive Performance in Older Adults'. *Clinical Gerontologist* 21(2): 27–47.

McGue, M. and Christensen, K. (1997). 'Genetic and Environmental Contributions to Depression Symptomatology: Evidence from Danish Twins 75 Years of Age and Older'. *Journal of Abnormal Psychology* 106(3): 439–448.

MacPhillamy, D. J. and Lewinsohn, P. M. (1974). 'Depression as a Function of Levels of Desired and Obtained Pleasure'. *Journal of Abnormal Psychology* 83(6): 651–657.

Mann, J. (1973). *Time-limited Psychotherapy*. Cambridge, MA: Harvard University Press.

Mastel-Smith, B. A., McFarlane, J., Sierpina, M., Malecha, A., and Haile, B. (2007). 'Improving Depressive Symptoms in Community-dwelling Older Adults: A Psychosocial Intervention Using Life Review and Writing'. *Journal of Gerontological Nursing* 33(5): 13–19.

Mather, M. and Carstensen, L. L. (2005). 'Aging and Motivated Cognition: The Positivity Effect in Attention and Memory'. *Trends in Cognitive Sciences* 9(10): 496–502.

Meeks, S., Looney, S. W., Van Haitsma, K., and Teri, L. (2008). 'BE-ACTIV: A Staff-assisted Behavioral Intervention for Depression in Nursing Homes'. *Gerontologist* 48(1): 105–114.

Meeks, T. W., Vahia, I. V., Lavretsky, H., Kulkarni, G., and Jest, D. V. (2011). 'A Tune in "A Minor" and "B Major": A Review of Epidemiology, Illness Course, and Public Health Implications of Subthreshold Depression in Older Adults'. *Journal of Affective Disorders* 129: 126–142.

Michael, K. D. and Crowley, S. L. (2002). 'How Effective are Treatments for Child and Adolescent Depression? A Meta-analytic Review'. *Clinical Psychology Review* 22: 247–269.

Mojtabai, R. and Olfson, M. (2004). 'Major Depression in Community-dwelling Middle-aged and Older Adults: Prevalence and 2- and 4-year Follow-up Symptoms'. *Psychological Medicine* 34: 623–634.

Molinari, V. and Marmion, J. (1995). 'Relationship between Affective Disorders and Axis II Diagnoses in Geropsychiatric Patients'. *Journal of Geriatric Psychiatry and Neurology* 8(1): 61–64.

Morrow-Howell, N., Proctor, E., Choi, S., Lawrence, L., Brooks, A., et al. (2008). 'Depression in Public Community Long-term Care: Implications for Intervention Development'. *The Journal of Behavioral Health Services and Research* 35(1): 37–51.

Moss, K., Scogin, F., DiNapoli, E., and Presnell, A. (2012). 'A Self-help Behavioral Activation Treatment for Geriatric Depressive Symptoms'. *Aging & Mental Health* 16(5): 625–635.

Mottram, P. G., Wilson, K., and Strobl, J. J. (2006). 'Antidepressants for Depressed Elderly: Intervention Review'. *Cochrane Database of Systematic Review* 25(1): CD003491.

Murphy, L. B., Sacks, J. J., Brady, T. J., Hootman, J. M., and Chapman, D. P. (2012). 'Anxiety is More Common than Depression among US Adults with Arthritis'. *Arthritis Care and Research* 64(7): 968–976.

Nezu, A. M., Nezu, C. M., and Perri, M. G. (1989). *Problem-solving Therapy for Depression: Theory, Research, and Clinical Guidelines*. New York: Wiley.

Orgeta, V. (2009). 'Specificity of Age Differences in Emotion Regulation'. *Aging & Mental Health* 13(6): 818–826.

Østbye, T., Kristjansson, B., Hill, G., Newman, S. C., Brouwer, R. N., et al. (2005). 'Prevalence and Predictors of Depression in Elderly Canadians: The Canadian Study of Health and Aging'. *Chronic Diseases in Canada* 26(4): 93–99.

Päivärinta, A., Verkkoniemi, A., Niinistö, L., Kivelä, S-L., and Sulkava, R. (1999). 'The Prevalence and Associates of Depressive Disorders in the Oldest-old Finns'. *Social Psychiatry and Psychiatric Epidemiology* 34(7): 352–359.

Parmelee, P. A., Katz, I. R., and Lawton, M. P. (1992). 'Incidence of Depression in Long-term Care Settings'. *Journal of Gerontology* 47(6): 189–196.

Peng, X. D., Huang, C. Q., Chen, L. J., and Lu, Z. C. (2009). 'Cognitive Behavioural Therapy and Reminiscence Techniques for the Treatment of Depression in the Elderly: A Systematic Review'. *Journal of International Medical Research* 37(4): 975–982.

Penninx, B. W., Leveille, S., Ferrucci, L., Van Eijk, J. T., and Guralnik, J. M. (1999). 'Exploring the Effect of Depression on Physical Disability: Longitudinal Evidence from the Established Populations for Epidemiologic Studies of the Elderly'. *American Journal of Public Health* 89(9): 1346–1352.

Pinquart, M. and Sörensen, S. (2001). 'How Effective are Psychotherapeutic and Other Psychosocial Interventions with Older Adults? A Meta-analysis'. *Journal of Mental Health and Aging* 7(2): 207–243.

Prince, M. J., Harwood, R. H., Blizard, R. A., Thomas, A., and Mann, A. H. (1997). 'Social Support Deficits, Loneliness and Life Events as Risk Factors for Depression in Old Age. The Gospel Oak Project VI'. *Psychological Medicine* 27: 323–332.

Rivard, V. (2007). 'Perceived Control and Coping Strategies in Relation to Anxious and Depressive Symptoms in Women with Activity Restriction due to Osteoarthritis'. *Dissertation Abstracts International: Section B* 67: 6075.

Rokke, P. D. and Scogin, F. (1995). 'Depression Treatment Preferences in Younger and Older Adults'. *Journal of Clinical Geropsychology* 1(3): 243–257.

Rokke, P. D., Tomhave, J., and Jocic, Z. (1999). 'The Role of Client Choice and Target Selection in Self-management Therapy for Depression in Older Adults'. *Psychology and Aging* 14(1): 155–169.

Rose, J. and DelMaestro, S. (1990). 'Separation-individuation Conflict as a Model for Understanding Distressed Caregivers: Psychodynamic and Cognitive Case Studies'. *Gerontologist* 20: 693–697.

Rostad, B., Deeg, D. J. H., and Schei, B. (2009). 'Socioeconomic Inequalities in Health in Older Women'. *European Journal of Ageing* 6(1): 39–47.

Roth, M. (1955). 'The Natural History of Mental Disorder in Old Age'. *British Journal of Psychiatry* 10: 281–301.

Rowan, P. J., Davidson, K., Campbell, J. A., Dobrez, D. G., and MacLean, D. R. (2002). 'Depressive Symptoms Predict Medical Care Utilization in a Population-based Sample'. *Psychological Medicine* 32(5): 903–908.

Rumsfeld, J. S., Jones, P. G., Whooley, M. A., Sullivan, M. D., Pitt, B., et al. (2005). 'Depression Predicts Mortality and Hospitalization in Patients with Myocardial Infarction Complicated by Heart Failure'. *American Heart Journal* 150(5): 961–967.

Russo, J., Vitaliano, P. P., and Brewer, D. D. (1995). 'Psychiatric Disorders in Spouse Caregivers of Care Recipients with Alzheimer's Disease and Matched Controls: A Diathesis-stress Model of Psychopathology'. *Journal of Abnormal Psychology* 104: 197–204.

Samad, Z., Brealey, S., and Gilbody, S. (2011). 'The Effectiveness of Behavioural Therapy for the Treatment of Older Adults: A Meta-analysis'. *International Journal of Geriatric Psychiatry* 26(12): 1211–1220.

Scogin, F., Hamblin, D., and Beutler, L. (1987). 'Bibliotherapy for Depressed Older Adults: A Self-help Alternative'. *Gerontologist* 27(3): 383–387.

Scogin, F., Jamison, C., and Gochneaur, K. (1989). 'Comparative Efficacy of Cognitive and Behavioral Bibliotherapy for Mildly and Moderately Depressed Older Adults'. *Journal of Consulting and Clinical Psychology* 57(3): 403–407.

Scogin, F. and McElreath, L. (1994). 'Efficacy of Psychosocial Treatments for Geriatric Depression: A Quantitative Review'. *Journal of Consulting and Clinical Psychology* 62(1): 69–74.

Scogin, F., Welsh, D., Hanson, A., Stump, J., and Coates, A. (2005). 'Evidence-based Psychotherapies for Depression in Older Adults'. *Clinical Psychology: Science and Practice* 12(3): 222–237.

Serfaty, M. A., Haworth, D., Blanchard, M., Buszewicz, M., Murad, S., et al. (2009). 'Clinical Effectiveness of Individual Cognitive Behavioral Therapy for Depressed Older People in Primary Care: A Randomized Controlled Trial'. *Archives of General Psychiatry* 66(12): 1332–1340.

Serido, J., Almedia, D. M., and Wethington, E. (2004). 'Chronic Stressors and Daily Hassles: Unique and Interactive Relationships with Psychological Distress'. *Journal of Health and Social Behavior* 45(1): 17–33.

Shanmugham, B., Karp, J., Drayer, R., Reynolds, C. F. III, and Alexopoulos, G. (2005). 'Evidence-based Pharmacologic Interventions for Geriatric Depression'. *Psychiatric Clinics of North America* 28(4): 821–835.

Simon, G. E. and VonKorff, M. (1995). 'Recognition, Management, and Outcomes of Depression in Primary Care'. *Archives of Family Medicine* 4(2): 99–105.

Skarupski, K. A., Mendes de Leon, C. F., Bienias, J. L., Barnes, L. L., Everson-Rose, S. A., et al. (2005). 'Black-White Differences in Depressive Symptoms among Older Adults over Time'. *Journal of Gerontology: Series B* 60(3): 136–142.

Skotzko, C. E., Krichten, C., Zietowski, G., Alves, L., Freudenberger, R., et al. (2000). 'Depression is Common and Precludes Accurate Assessment of Functional Status in Elderly Patients with Congestive Heart Failure'. *Journal of Cardiac Failure* 6(4): 300–305.

Smith, A., Graham, L., and Senthinathan, S. (2007). 'Mindfulness-based Cognitive Therapy for Recurring Depression in Older People: A Qualitative Study'. *Aging & Mental Health* 11(3): 346–357.

Smith, N. M., Floyd, M. R., Scogin, F., and Jamison, C. S. (1997). 'Three-year Follow-up of Bibliotherapy for Depression'. *Journal of Consulting and Clinical Psychology* 65(2): 324–327.

Snarski, M., Scogin, F., DiNapoli, E., Presnell, A., McAlpine, J., et al. (2011). 'The Effects of Behavioral Activation Therapy with Inpatient Geriatric Psychiatry Patients'. *Behavior Therapy* 42(1): 100–108.

Solhaug, H. I., Romuld, E. B., Romild, U., and Stordal, E. (2012). 'Increased Prevalence of Depression in Cohorts of the Elderly: An 11-year Follow-up in the General Population—the HUNT Study'. *International Psychogeriatrics* 24(1): 151–158.

Steffens, D. C. and McQuoid, D. R. (2005). 'Impact of Symptoms of Generalized Anxiety Disorder on the Course of Late-life Depression'. *American Journal of Geriatric Psychiatry* 13(1): 40–47.

Steuer, J. L., Mintz, J., Hammen, C. L., Hill, M. A., Jarvik, L. F., et al. (1984). 'Cognitive-behavioral and Psychodynamic Group Psychotherapy in Treatment of Geriatric Depression'. *Journal of Consulting and Clinical Psychology* 52(2): 180–189.

St. John, P. D. and Montgomery, P. (2009). 'Does a Single-item Measure of Depression Predict Mortality?' *Canadian Family Physician* 55(6): 1–5.

Taylor, W. D., MacFall, J. R., Payne, M. E., McQuoid, D. R., Steffens, D. C., et al. (2007). Orbitofrontal Cortex Volume in Late Life Depression: Influence of Hyperintense Lesions and Genetic Polymorphisms'. *Psychological Medicine* 37(12): 1763–1773.

Teper, E., and Thomas, A. (2006). 'Is Depression Different in Older Adults?' *Ageing and Health* 2(6): 905–915.

Thompson, L. W., Gallagher, D., and Breckenridge, J. S. (1987). 'Comparative Effectiveness of Psychotherapies for Depressed Elders'. *Journal of Consulting and Clinical Psychology* 55(3): 385–390.

Thompson, L. W., Dick-Siskin, L., Coon, D. W., Powers, D. V., and Gallagher-Thompson, D. (2010). *Treating Late-life depression: A Cognitive Behavioral Therapy Approach-workbook*. Oxford: Oxford University Press.

Tsuno, N. and Homma, A. (2009). 'What is the Association between Depression and Alzheimer's Disease?' *Expert Review of Neurotherapeutics* 9(11): 1667–1676.

Unützer, J., Katon, W., Simon, G., Grembowski, D., Walker, E., et al. (1996). 'Costs of Medical Care in an Elderly Primary Care Population'. Paper presented at the 9th annual meeting of the American Association of Geriatric Psychiatry, Tucson, AZ.

Unützer, J., Katon, W., Callahan, C. M., Williams, J., Hunkeler, E., et al. (2002). 'Collaborative Care Management of Late-life Depression in the Primary Care Setting: A Randomized Controlled Trial'. *Journal of the American Medical Association* 288(22): 2836–2845.

Urry, H. L. and Gross, J. J. (2010). 'Emotion Regulation in Older Age'. *Current Directions in Psychological Science* 19(6): 352–357.

Van Gool, C. H., Kempen, G. I., Penninx, B. W., Deeg, D. J., Beekman, A. T., et al. (2005). 'Impact of Depression on Disablement in Late Middle Aged and Older Persons: Results from the Longitudinal Aging Study Amsterdam'. *Social Science and Medicine* 60(1): 25–36.

Vilhjalmsson, R. (1998). 'Direct and Indirect Effects of Chronic Physical Conditions on Depression: A Preliminary Investigation'. *Social Science and Medicine* 47(5): 603–611.

Wang, J. J. (2004). 'The Comparative Effectiveness among Institutionalized and Non-institutionalized Elderly People in Taiwan of Reminiscence Therapy as a Psychological Measure'. *Journal of Nursing Research* 12(3): 237–245.

Wang, J. J., Hsu, Y. C., and Cheng, S. F. (2005). 'The Effects of Reminiscence in Promoting Mental Health of Taiwanese Elderly'. *International Journal of Nursing Studies* 42(1): 31–36.

Watt, L. M. and Cappeliez, P. (2000). 'Integrative and Instrumental Reminiscence Therapies for Depression in Older Adults: Intervention Strategies and Treatment Effectiveness'. *Aging & Mental Health* 4(2): 166–177.

Westerhof, G. J., Bohlmeijer, E. T., Van Beljouw, I. M. J., and Pot, A. M. (2010). 'Improvement in Personal Meaning Mediates the Effects of a Life Review Intervention on Depressive Symptoms in a Randomized Controlled Trial'. *Gerontologist* 50(4): 541–549.

Williams, J. W., Barrett, J., Oxman, T., Frank, E., Katon, W., et al. (2000). 'Treatment of Dysthymia and Minor Depression in Primary Care: A Randomized Controlled Trial in Older Adults'. *Journal of the American Medical Association* 284(12): 1519–1526.

Williamson, G. M. and Shaffer, D. R. (2000). 'The Activity Restriction Model of Depressed Affect: Antecedents and Consequences of Restricted Normal Activities'. In G. M. Williamson, D. R. Shaffer, and P. A. Parmelee (eds), *Physical Illness and Depression in Older Adults: A Handbook of Theory, Research, and Practice* (pp. 173–200). Dordrecht: Kluwer Academic.

Wilson, K., Mottram, P. G., Sivananthan, A., and Nightingale, A. (2001). 'Antidepressants versus Placebo for the Depressed Elderly'. *Cochrane Database of Systematic Review* 2: CD000561.

Wilson, L. A. (2006). 'A Comparison of the Effects of Reminiscence therapy And Transmissive Reminiscence Therapy on Levels of Depression in Nursing Home Residents'. Unpublished doctoral dissertation, Capella University.

Yon, A. and Scogin, F. (2008). 'Behavioral Activation as a Treatment for Geriatric Depression'. *Clinical Gerontologist* 32(1): 91–103.

Yon, A., Scogin, F., DiNapoli, E. A., McPherron, J., Arean, P. A., et al. 'Do Manualized Treatments for Depression Reduce Insomnia Symptoms?'. Unpublished doctoral dissertation, University of Alabama.

Zhang, X., Gainetdinov, R. R., Beaulieu, J-M., Sotnikova, T. D., Burch, L. H., et al. (2005). 'Loss-of-function Mutation in Tryptophan Hydroxylase-2 Identified in Unipolar Major Depression'. *Neuron* 45(1): 11–16.

Zisook, S. and Downs, N. S. (1998). 'Diagnosis and Treatment of Depression in Late-life'. *Journal of Clinical Psychiatry* 59(4): 80–91.

Zubenko, G. S., Zubenko, W. N., McPherson, S., Spoor, E., Marin, D. B., et al. (2003). 'A Collaborative Study of the Emergence and Clinical Features of the Major Depressive Syndrome of Alzheimer's Disease'. *American Journal of Psychiatry* 160(5): 857–866.

CHAPTER 21

···

PHYSICAL COMORBIDITY WITH MOOD DISORDERS

···

PHILIP E. MOSLEY AND JEFFREY M. LYNESS

INTRODUCTION

The interdependence of psychology and biology

THE historical distinction between medical and mental disorders implies that psychology is irrelevant to the former and biology irrelevant to the latter. Increasingly, however, a contemporary understanding of disease seeks to integrate concepts from both disciplines, rejecting earlier paradigms founded upon Cartesian dualism.

For the clinician, advances in neurology have framed the outmoded nature of mind/body thinking and suggest a more nuanced relationship between the two. For example, neurodegenerative disorders such as Parkinson's disease present a complex array of both motor and psychiatric symptoms tied to the death of neurons in the brain (Weintraub and Burn 2011), notwithstanding the resulting functional and social impairment that may also mediate psychological distress. Patients with conversion disorder display neurological symptoms that are not feigned or malingered but are not explained by existing neurological diagnoses and standard medical investigations. Instead, elaborate psychoanalytic theories of intrapsychic conflict have been advanced to explain their onset (Breuer et al. 1956), suggesting a complex relationship between psyche and soma but often instead used to reinforce the existing dualist dichotomy. Techniques in functional brain imaging, however, have identified unique disruptions to the pattern of neuronal activation in distributed limbic and cortical networks, potentially correlating with the exaggerated self-directed attention, hypersensitivity to stress, and deficits in sense of self-agency seen in these patients (Carson et al. 2012). The emergence of deep brain stimulation for the treatment of both neurological and psychiatric disorders has implications for the role of neuromodulation in the moment-to-moment (Bejjani et al. 1999) or sustained (Mayberg et al. 2005) regulation of mood. Psychological treatment of psychiatric disorders can also induce plastic changes in the brain, on both a functional (Goldapple et al. 2004) and molecular (Karlsson et al. 2010) level.

For the neuroscientist, mind and body also have a close relationship. William James's (1890) contention was that basic feeling states reference the visceral milieu and are tied to somatic events. The neural correlate of this theory exists in the interoceptive system, a collection of afferent neural pathways and brain nuclei that detects and maps the biological processes of the body and triggers innate physiological programmes to restore homeostasis. Many of these are instinctual and stereotyped, occurring without awareness or emotional valence. However, from an evolutionary perspective, the addition of a felt experiential component adds a powerful proxy of biological value and guide of adaptive behaviour (Damasio and Carvalho 2013). The location of these topographically organized internal maps in sub-cortical and brainstem centres also suggests that this is a phylogenetically preserved function. There are significant philosophical objections to this concept, grounded in the rich variety of human emotional experience (Bennett and Hacker 2003). Nonetheless, these hypotheses are reminiscent of a postmodern perspective that considers human perception an active phenomenon embodied in the functioning of a nervous system that brings the world into being (Bracken and Thomas 2005).

If there are meta-representations of the body that form a neural substrate for the experience of emotion, it does not seem excessively reductionistic to propose that any perturbation of the body's functioning would affect the experience of self (including affect) in varied dimensions. Eventually therefore, it may become an anachronism to discuss physical and psychological conditions as if they were separate entities, although currently this convention lingers. This chapter seeks to illuminate some of the ample comorbidity of medical disease with mood disorders appearing in later life, while illustrating a meaningful web of clinically significant reciprocity.

THE SIGNIFICANCE OF COMORBIDITY

Physical comorbidity with mood disorders is clinically meaningful:

- Medical illness burden is a powerful predictor of depression onset and course in older adults (Lyness et al. 2006). Aversive symptoms, disability, and the social implications of chronic illness are demoralizing and may evoke a range of depressive states (Travis et al. 2004).
- Medical conditions and their treatments can directly precipitate an affective disorder, either through damage to the neurological substrate of mood (Alexopoulos et al. 2002) or via metabolic, endocrine, or toxic processes. Affective symptoms may be the earliest manifestation of physical illness, ranging from various cancers (Carney et al. 2003) to neurodegenerative dementias (Green et al. 2003).
- Among older individuals with mood disorder, physical comorbidity is widespread (Scott et al. 2008). Depression is a risk factor for the onset of chronic disease (Patten et al. 2008) and, once established, comorbidity has both indirect behavioural and direct biological sequelae that amplify healthcare costs, worsen symptoms, magnify disability, and increase mortality (Katon and Ciechanowski 2002). Despite this, mood disorder is often under-recognized or undertreated in general medical settings (Rapp,

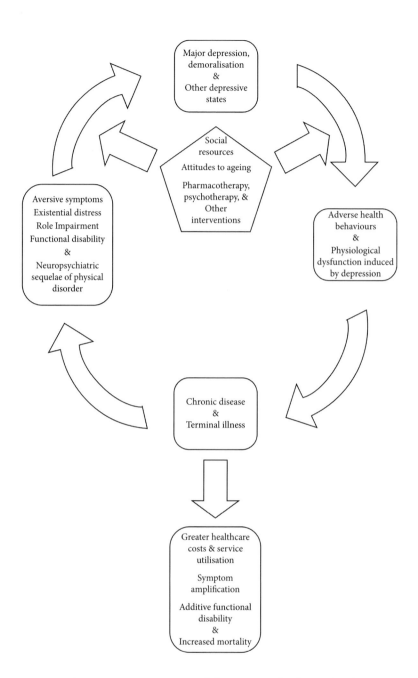

FIGURE 21.1 A schematic representation of the reciprocal relationship between chronic disease and mood disorder in older adults. Those with physical morbidity may suffer a number of injurious phenomena that evoke a range of depressive states, including major depression. In turn, depression augments the damaging effects of medical disorder through inducing physiological dysfunction and affecting health behaviours. Adverse health outcomes may result, but the cycle can be moderated by the influences of attitudes to ageing, social resources, and treatment of the concurrent mood disorder.

Reprinted from *The American Journal of Geriatric Psychiatry*, 19(6), Sergio E. Starkstein, Milan Dragovic, Ricardo Jorge, Simone Brockman, and Robert G. Robinson, Diagnostic Criteria for Depression in Alzheimer Disease: A Study of Symptom Patterns Using Latent Class Analysis, pp. 551–8, figure 2, Copyright (2011), with permission from Elsevier.

Parisi, and Walsh 1988) and psychiatric disorder may limit optimal treatment of medical conditions (DiMatteo, Lepper, and Croghan 2000).

- The extensive comorbidity between mood disorder and physical disease suggests the presence of common antecedent factors, which may include: shared genetic vulnerabilities, pathobiologic mechanisms, personality style, and enduring psychosocial outcomes such as altered role relationships (Lyness 2008). Elucidation of these individual connections may narrow the arbitrary divide between physical and mental health.

Figure 21.1 represents the important interactions between mood disorder and physical disease, serving as a framework for the remainder of the chapter.

DEFINITIONS AND PRINCIPLES

The following are pertinent to the text that follows:

- The terms 'disease', 'illness', and 'sickness' often denote pathobiological, personal and social aspects of human ailments, respectively. Here, these and related synonyms are used interchangeably, noting that evaluative elements pervade all three concepts (Fulford 2001).
- Reflecting the emphasis in the literature, mood disorder is taken to mean those unipolar affective disturbances in the depressed range, unless mania or bipolar disorder is specified. Depending upon the instrument used, some studies predominantly measure depressive symptoms, while others record depressive syndromes. Clearly, states of negative affect and a clinical mood disorder are different classes of emotional response with varying prevalence in a given population, whereas trait depression (a pessimistic cognitive style) may moderate both. Nevertheless, many affective disturbances in older adults can be linked to adverse physical sequelae without necessarily meeting the threshold for major depression (Lyness et al. 2007).
- The standardization of physical comorbidity is methodologically challenging. The attribution of nonspecific symptoms in older adults is difficult; the phenomenology of late-life depression includes more somatic and hypochondriacal symptoms (Hegeman et al. 2012), while older patients are also more likely to attribute symptoms of a mood disorder to a medical condition under the cognitive demands of a screening instrument (Knäuper and Wittchen 1994). Depressed patients are more likely to evaluate their health negatively; therefore studies that rely on self-report risk being confounded unless carefully controlled. The best measures are truly objective (direct visualization of coronary arteries) rather than proxies for health behaviours (number of scripts filled).
- A risk factor is an operationalized entity that increases the probability of a health outcome. Depression can be said to be a risk factor for physical disease and vice versa, but the distinction between correlation and causation must be carefully delineated. Cross-sectional studies generate associations and hypotheses about risk markers but do not establish them as causal factors. Longitudinal studies that use a control group to study the influence of the prospective risk factor are more suitable for this latter

purpose. Other studies may demonstrate that treating the risk factor affects the nature of the outcome variable.

The Epidemiology of Comorbidity

Chronic disease in older adults

Chronic diseases (including malignancy) and conditions that restrict functioning are the principal health concerns of an ageing population. The Global Burden of Disease Study (World Health Organization (WHO) 2008), stratifying cause of death by age and country of origin, showed that for those over the age of 60 living in high-income countries (Western Europe, North America, Australia, and New Zealand), leading causes of mortality were cancer, heart, and cerebrovascular disease, with substantial contributions from respiratory, endocrine and neuropsychiatric disorders. Therefore, in later life deaths are predominantly related to noncommunicable and systemic diseases. In high-income countries most of the total population deaths are from within this aged cohort. Illustrative data from this extensive survey are represented in Table 21.1 and Table 21.2 for men and women, respectively.

The disability-adjusted life year (DALY) extends the concept of mortality to incorporate years of healthy life lost by virtue of being in a state of relative disability, thus more accurately approximating the true burden of a particular disease. Applied to the same population, the DALY confirms that chronic diseases remain significantly linked to morbidity. The very substantial contribution from the dementias, sense organ disorders (problems with vision or hearing), and osteoarthritis also reflects the burdensome influence of functional disability. Illustrative data are again represented in Table 21.3 and Table 21.4 for men and women, respectively.

Globally, as life expectancy increases and risk factors for communicable diseases are addressed, the significance of chronic disease among older adults is likely to expand. Major depression is anticipated to contribute to this morbidity (Murray and Lopez 1997).

Mood disorders in older adults with chronic disease

Surveys of the general population have established an association between chronic medical conditions and depressive disorders (Wells, Golding, and Burnam 1988). As a part of the World Mental Health Survey (Scott et al. 2007), a large household sample from seventeen participating countries completed a checklist for ten chronic physical conditions and the CIDI (Composite International Diagnostic Interview), a structured diagnostic interview for mental disorder. Based on self-report, heart disease and pain disorders (including headache and back pain) were strongly associated with a twelve-month history of *DSM-IV* (*Diagnostic and Statistical Manual of Mental Disorders*, 4th edn) major depressive disorder or dysthymia, as to a lesser extent were ulcers, arthritis, asthma, hypertension, and diabetes.

Using the same data, the rates of medical and psychiatric comorbidity were stratified for age (Scott et al. 2008). Curiously, although the volume of reported physical or pain conditions increased substantially over age 65, the prevalence of twelve-month depressive or

Table 21.1 Selected deaths (thousands) by cause for males over 60 in high-income countries during 2004

Cause	Number of deaths
Malignant neoplasms	985
Ischaemic heart disease	591
Cerebrovascular disease	281
Chronic obstructive pulmonary disease	154
Lower respiratory infections	133
Diabetes mellitus	86
Alzheimer's and other dementias	82
Cirrhosis of the liver	40
Self-inflicted injuries	29
Parkinson's disease	27

Data from: The Global Burden of Disease, 2004 Update (World Health Organisation 2008).

Table 21.2 Selected deaths (thousands) by cause for females over 60 in high-income countries during 2004

Cause	Number of deaths
Malignant neoplasms	779
Ischaemic heart disease	606
Cerebrovascular disease	427
Alzheimer's and other dementias	193
Lower respiratory infections	157
Chronic obstructive pulmonary disease	119
Diabetes mellitus	111
Other endocrine disorders	35
Cirrhosis of the liver	24
Parkinson's disease	24

Data from: The Global Burden of Disease, 2004 Update (World Health Organisation 2008).

anxiety disorders decreased such that the majority of those sampled reported physical problems without psychiatric disorder.

Several points may account for this interesting finding. The most important come from large epidemiological surveys showing that the prevalence of most psychiatric disorders (Kessler et al. 2005) including depression (Hasin et al. 2005; Robins et al. 1984) reduces with age. For many, therefore, older age is a time of relative mental well-being. Age cohort effects may account for this general finding of a reduced prevalence of depression among older adults (Brault, Meuleman, and Bracke 2012). Aged individuals with a common birth era are thought to share protective cultural and social experiences unique to the historical circumstances of their development, while more recent social transformations confer greater vulnerability to depression among younger cohorts. Under these circumstances, future rates of late-life depressive disorder might increase with the succession of each age cohort.

Table 21.3 Selected DALYs (thousands) by cause for males over 60 in high-income countries during 2004

Cause	DALYs
Malignant neoplasms	5611
Ischaemic heart disease	2830
Sense organ disorders	1699
Alzheimer's and other dementias	1354
Cerebrovascular disease	1344
Chronic obstructive pulmonary disease	917
Diabetes mellitus	703
Osteoarthritis	477
Lower respiratory infections	417
Cirrhosis of the liver	305

Data from: The Global Burden of Disease, 2004 Update (World Health Organisation 2008).

Table 21.4 Selected DALYs (thousands) by cause for females over 60 in high-income countries during 2004

Cause	DALYs
Malignant neoplasms	4287
Alzheimer's and other dementias	2694
Ischaemic heart disease	2126
Sense organ disorders	2033
Cerebrovascular disease	1506
Osteoarthritis	934
Diabetes mellitus	876
Chronic obstructive pulmonary disease	693
Unipolar depressive disorders	474
Lower respiratory infections	375

Data from: The Global Burden of Disease, 2004 Update (World Health Organisation 2008).

With regards to sampling of mood disorder in populations with physical comorbidity, however, even structured interviews can be vulnerable to misattribution of somatic symptoms when administered by a layperson. Many studies also exclude the deceased, the institutionalized, and the cognitively impaired, meaning that an incidence-prevalence (Neyman) bias could selectively remove those with substantial physical and mental comorbidity from the sampled cohort. Another methodological issue with cross-sectional surveys is that the relationship between depression and age may not be linear, with data from extremes of age obscured in an inappropriately broad range of sampled age.

Additionally, clinical depressive disorders are not the only affective conditions of significance in older adults. A longitudinal study of ageing has indicated that late-life depressive symptoms increase in the seventh decade of life from an earlier quiescent phase in middle adulthood (Sutin et al. 2013). Proximity to death, physical comorbidity, and functional disability partially but not entirely accounted for these changes in a multivariate analysis. Even if other psychological and social changes occurring in older age mediate this increase in depressive symptoms, they are nonetheless clinically meaningful in individuals with physical comorbidity, associated with a significant downstream increase in functional limitations (Hybels, Pieper, and Blazer 2009) and negative appraisal of disability (Albert, Bear-Lehman, and Burkhardt 2012).

Hospital settings yield a higher prevalence of affective disorder (Rapp et al. 1988), with depression often overlooked by the treating medical team. Predictably, comorbid depression is associated with greater psychological distress and a poorer subjective evaluation of health status.

Without the benefit of temporality it is difficult to assess the correlation between physical morbidity and mood disorder within a cross-sectional study. However, a meta-analysis of twelve longitudinal prospective studies found that the presence of chronic disease (variously defined) or poor self-rated health status at baseline significantly increased the relative risk of developing a depressive disorder in a large pooled cohort of older individuals (Chang-Quan et al. 2010). In these individuals, therefore, it seems possible to conclude that negative health states, either objectively defined or subjectively reported, are a risk factor for the later onset of depressive disorder. Methodological limitations aside, however, the fact remains that at cross-sectional survey many older adults seem to have appreciable levels of physical disorder yet are not currently depressed. Those who do develop a clinical depressive disorder in this context may have specific vulnerability factors linked to their physical morbidity; this is discussed in later sections.

Chronic disease in older adults with mood disorders

In the World Mental Health survey, those community-dwelling older adults who were diagnosed with a mood disorder reported high levels of physical comorbidity (Scott et al. 2008). Medical comorbidity among older psychiatric inpatients with mood disorder is also substantial (Zubenko et al. 1997). A multiplicity of medical problems is the norm, with cardiovascular, respiratory, endocrine, musculoskeletal, and digestive disorders being particularly common. Among older patients with bipolar affective disorder, cross-sectional medical burden is comparable to older patients with unipolar depression (Gildengers et al. 2008).

Longitudinal prospective studies in adult populations have established that depression is a risk factor for the onset of chronic physical disease, including hypertension, heart disease, arthritis, back pain, and chronic respiratory conditions (Patten et al. 2008). Other prospective cohort studies have demonstrated specific links between the presence of antecedent major depressive disorder and the development of clinically diagnosed ischaemic heart disease (Ferketich et al. 2000) and type II diabetes mellitus (Kawakami et al. 1999). Some of these findings have been replicated in exclusively geriatric populations (Atlantis et al. 2010).

Summary: epidemiology

Among older adults, functional disability associated with chronic disease makes a substantial contribution to the overall burden of a health condition. Chronic illness or a negative perception of health status increases the risk for depression onset; this seems to be a general effect rather than linked to a specific organ system. Conversely, depression is also a risk factor for the incidence of chronic disease, and physical comorbidity is the norm among depressed older adults. Both relationships have significant public health implications owing to the additive disability conferred by the co-existence of mood and physical disorders.

The Consequences of Physical Disease

Psychosocial aspects of chronic disease

Chronic disabling disorders, even when not fatal, are a major source of profound long-term suffering and present a significant challenge to existing healthcare systems, in which intervention is often palliative rather than curative in nature. Patients with such disorders must endure distressing symptoms directly related and specific to the character of their condition: the patient with heart disease experiences angina, the patient with emphysema experiences breathlessness, and the patient with arthritis experiences restriction of movement. Pain is a complex cognitive and emotional phenomenon common to many disorders; it can represent an aversive symptom of disease, yet can also be a feature of depressive states, with the link between reported pain and objective tissue damage often indirect. Aside from symptoms, chronic disease may also change physical appearance, restrict independence, and impair social relationships, such that the management of the illness itself comes to dominate the very existence of a sufferer. All of these outcomes may influence mood.

Demoralization

The practical and symbolic consequences of chronic disease are notable. In addition to managing the business of everyday living, patients with chronic illness may struggle to make sense of their illness and reconcile their suffering with existing paradigms of meaning within the universe. The experience of demoralization is an expression of an existential state, including feelings of apprehension, powerlessness, hopelessness, isolation, and purposelessness, occurring as a reaction to overwhelming adversity (Frank 1974). As compared to depression, demoralization syndrome is characterized by a sense of subjective incompetence and indecision rather than by apathy, such that actions are inhibited by uncertainty rather than lack of motivation (De Figueiredo 1993). Moreover, while demoralized patients are denied anticipatory pleasure from a current state of pessimism and entrapment, momentary hedonic capacity is nonetheless retained and cessation of adversity rapidly improves mood. Although existential distress is an almost universal human experience, it has particular relevance to patients whose bodily integrity is threatened by physical illness, particularly if prolonged or accompanied by aversive symptoms and an uncertain prognosis (Clarke and Kissane 2002).

Demoralization is important here because of its ability to threaten the psychological integrity of a patient and thereby magnify suffering. This is a frightening phenomenon related to personhood and the overall illness experience rather than a particular symptom or dysfunction. Demoralization is associated with requests for assisted suicide as it affords some sense of control, mastery, and dignity to patients who otherwise feel powerless.

There may also be a reciprocal relationship with medical illness; demoralization characterized by the attitudes of helplessness and hopelessness, qualitatively different from a depressive syndrome, was first associated with a general vulnerability to somatic disease: 'the giving up–given up complex' (Engel 1967). Demoralized patients also have poor outcomes from their medical disorders, such as an excess mortality from cancer (Watson et al. 1999). The construct of hopelessness seems particularly important to this phenomenon, having been associated with the progression of atherosclerosis (Everson et al. 1997) and mortality from ischaemic heart disease (Anda et al. 1993) as well as requests for a hastened death in terminally ill patients with cancer (Breitbart et al. 2000). It is also an important psychiatric variable, being an established risk factor for completed suicide (Brown et al. 2000; Kuo, Gallo, and Eaton 2004). In older persons, where affects of depression and anxiety are the external manifestations of this internal syndrome, the construct of demoralization may overlap with the concept of subsyndromal depression, a clinically significant and prevalent 'less than major' depressive state associated with considerable medical burden and functional disability (Lyness et al. 2007). The basis of this link between hopelessness, demoralization, depression and physical morbidity may have both biological and behavioural aspects, discussed in the following sections.

Terminal illness

The diagnosis of terminal illness may be associated with a grief reaction that includes depressive symptoms (Kübler-Ross 1970). Modern medical technology facilitates the early detection of chronic degenerative disease; when combined with a curative orientation towards the prolongation of life and the increasing hospitalization of death itself, this means that dying has become a more protracted process with greater opportunity for reflection and anticipatory mourning. It is important not to medicalize transient emotional states that may proceed to adaptive psychological reorganization, yet nonetheless, many terminally ill patients exhibit clinically significant depressive symptoms, which can dramatically impair residual quality of life and justify intervention (Lyness 2004). Depressive symptoms in the dying affect existential deliberation, prevent finances and estates from being settled, impair the quality of remaining relationships, hinder attempts to palliate pain and hasten requests for assisted suicide. Typically, a depressive syndrome can be distinguished by the severity and pervasive nature of the unremitting mood disturbance, with total loss of hedonic capacity and sustained hopelessness. Nevertheless, depression in the terminally ill is often overlooked (Block 2000) as a consequence of the significant overlap between manifestations of depression and of disease, as well as reluctance on the part of clinicians to address psychological difficulties in the dying patient. There is a frequent assumption that distress is a normal feature of the dying process, that frail older patients are unable to tolerate meaningful psychotherapy, and that psychotropic medication is ineffective or unwarranted. However, clinical experience suggests that existing therapies with demonstrated effectiveness in late-life depression can also be applied successfully to this population (King, Heisel, and Lyness 2006). Early identification and recruitment of these depressed patients is key; their progressive attrition may limit the duration of effective treatment.

Functional disability

Overall medical burden, rather than the influence of a particular organ system, is most strongly predictive of depression in an older primary care population (Lyness et al. 2006). Chronic disease burden in a sample of aged secondary care patients with recurrent depressive disorder also increases the risk of relapse (Reynolds et al. 2006). This non-specificity suggests a 'final common pathway', where biological or psychosocial factors shared by many medical disorders lead to depression. Functional disability, typically pertaining to instrumental activities of daily living or self-care, is a measure related to medical burden that could potentially mediate this association. However, while it is intuitive that older individuals may become depressed as a psychological reaction to their disability, in reality both affective and medical illness contribute to low functional status and the temporal relationship between the three cannot be determined within a cross-sectional study (Lyness et al. 1993). Moreover, conditions such as cerebrovascular disease may be more directly connected to mood disorder through the effects of neurological damage. Nevertheless, when disability is present it may be amenable to relatively simple interventions with major consequences for quality of life and well-being. For example, treatment of cataracts can restore sight, improve mobility, and reduce the risk of falls, promoting independence and social interaction. Yet when untreated, immobility, falls, and isolation are risk factors for osteoporosis, fractures, and depression, respectively. Early detection of these problems prevents the insidious development of an irreversible 'iceberg' of mental and physical comorbidity.

Attitudes toward ageing

Growing old may include increased physical morbidity, yet it is nonetheless possible to age without becoming depressed. Indeed, as discussed above, most epidemiological data support the notion of depression becoming less common in old age despite greater self-reported chronic illness (Scott et al. 2008). Internalized, negative stereotypes of ageing as a time of helplessness, decrepitude, and frailty are not only incorrect, but may also be psychologically harmful when expressed by older adults themselves. Here, self-perception and cognitive style mediate the adaptation to functional disability associated with the inevitable biological consequences of increasing age, with positive attitudes to ageing being protective against the development of depression. Accordingly, in a sample of older rural Australians, positive attitudes to ageing were associated with less depression and less psychological disability despite a considerable level of physical morbidity (Bryant et al. 2012). Of course, the relationship between self-perception and mood disorder is likely to be bidirectional as depressed mood will affect the evaluation of ageing, loss, and chronic disease. Longitudinal studies will be instructive in this regard.

Attitudes to ageing are also physically meaningful. A belief that health problems are inevitable in old age reduces the likelihood of older persons engaging in preventative health behaviours such as smoking cessation, medical screening, and exercise, despite evidence of clear benefits in this population. Conversely, individuals with more positive perceptions of their own ageing have more positive health behaviours (Levy and Myers 2004). More positive perceptions are also associated with greater longevity (Levy et al. 2002), although it remains possible, even after taking into account functional limitations and health at base-line, that positive health status itself causes positive perceptions of ageing and an ultimately longer life.

Role function

Related to the influences of functional disability and attitudes to ageing are the effects of chronic disease on role function. Illness inhibits the performance of customary roles, thereby disrupting the collective social system. In contemporary society, such interference is minimized by prescription of a specific social role for the sick, affording its incumbents a legitimate refuge in which to return to a healthy state (Parsons 1951). The older person with chronic disease, however, may suffer with conditions that are unremitting or progressive. Such individuals find it more difficult to exit the sick role, with ensuing ramifications for personal and social functioning.

Physical morbidity can render older adults housebound or prevent attention to personal care. Some chronic illnesses, such as visual defects, are incapacitating but not fatal, while others, such as ischaemic heart disease, may also cause death. Regardless, the older person must increasingly rely on others for care and support. Family roles may alter as the emotional connotations of giving and receiving help become apparent. The person with chronic disease may deny the burdensomeness of their disability and refuse help, placing a strain upon relationships and compounding social isolation.

Cancer is a disease with particular potential to disrupt body image, sexual identity, and the marital relationship. The woman from whom a cancerous breast is removed by mastectomy must reconcile the loss of a highly valued body part with connections to attractiveness and womanhood, with the threat posed by the malignant tissue therein. Similarly, the man with colorectal cancer may regard his colostomy with shame and self-disgust. He must face the taboo of handling his faeces and accept the mutilation of his body. The unpredictable discharge of faeces and flatus can lead to embarrassment and limit intimacy with the marital partner, as well as constraining wider social activities.

The management of symptoms or adherence to complex medical regimens can restrict engagement with more personally gratifying endeavours such as work or leisure pursuits. The patient with joint disease must titrate activity levels to discomfort, with daily life organized so as to prioritize the most valued tasks before pain intercedes and rest is essential. In other conditions, symptoms are controlled through diet, drugs, or the use of advanced technologies such as radiation therapy. In some instances the treatment can be as burdensome as the disease, requiring substantial investment of time and energy.

Stigma can dominate society's perception of the sick older person, with the risk that the sick role becomes the 'master status' for that individual. Here, the older person is seen primarily as a sufferer rather than an individual with unique intellectual and personal strengths. Interactions with care-givers who infantilize or condescend may undermine positive attitudes maintained by the older person and reinforce disability. Through the process of 'secondary deviation', a negative reaction to chronic illness can lead individuals to conform to this stereotype. For example, the institutionalized aged consistently treated as helpless may find it less exacting to concur with this expectation and adopt this role.

Resources

The resources to which individuals have access mitigate the influence of chronic disease. Resources may take the form of money, family support, environmental modifications, or formal care from social services. The fact that personal and social assets must be dedicated to the management of disease is itself part of the handicap related to chronic illness. However, as chronic illnesses progress, available resources may shrink: financial capital may be depleted and family networks may be stressed or eroded. For the older person this may curtail independence and result in premature institutionalization, while informal carers are also affected by loss of their primary paid employment, social life, and holidays. The provision of adequate official assistance is often limited as the needs of an ageing population outstrip the capacity of existing services. Resources are also unevenly distributed in society and certain socio-economic groups may find it more difficult to maintain a satisfactory existence in the face of chronic illness, accentuating earlier inequalities. For example, the high incidence of late-onset depression among older Nigerians has been linked to social instability and attenuated government support (Gureje, Oladeji, and Abiona 2011).

At a cultural level, particular conditions are imbued with meaning that devalues sufferers. For example, the association between chronic obstructive pulmonary disease and heavy smoking leads to the charge that such patients have 'brought the illness upon themselves', with consequential opprobrium and withdrawal of the rights of the sick role. A fear of such enacted stigma may engender a policy of concealment, which may reduce access to appropriate medical and social resources. The importance of perceived isolation in depressive responses to illness is highlighted by the effectiveness of supportive psychotherapy in the treatment of demoralization. Simply 'being with' the patient during their time of distress mobilizes resilient psychological postures and encourages recovery (Griffith and Gaby 2005).

Disorders of the central nervous system

Neurological conditions such as the dementias and cerebrovascular disease are a major cause of mortality and morbidity in later life. Late-onset depressive disorder in older adults is often associated with a high medical burden that includes neurological abnormalities and risk factors for vascular disease with comparatively little family history of mood disorder (Baldwin et al. 2006). In addition to their depressive ideation, such patients are often highly disabled by psychomotor retardation, apathy, and cognitive dysfunction. A poor response to anti-depressant medication is observed in those patients who display features of the dysexecutive syndrome, a disruption of those cognitive processes responsible for abstract reasoning, the shifting of attentional set, and the planning, sequencing, initiation, and inhibition of behaviour (Alexopoulos et al. 2005).

Fronto-limbic and fronto-striatal neurocircuitry play a critical role in the pathogenesis of this 'depression-executive dysfunction syndrome' (Alexopoulos et al. 2002). Functional neuroimaging studies have shown hypoactivity of the caudate nucleus and frontal regions in depressed patients (Drevets et al. 1997), with particular hypometabolism of the rostral anterior cingulate cortex in those with treatment-resistant depression (Mayberg et al. 1997). In addition to their motor symptoms, neurodegenerative disorders of the basal ganglia and its prefrontal projections, such as Huntington's disease, Parkinson's disease, and progressive supranuclear palsy are also complicated by depression and executive dysfunction (Cummings 1993). Thus, in the older patient with medical comorbidity, neurological injury (the aetiology of which may be diverse) seems to confer vulnerability to this characteristic constellation of depressive symptoms.

Cerebrovascular disease

Particular attention has focused on the contribution of vascular disease to the development of late-onset depression in later life (Alexopoulos et al. 1997) and subcortical ischaemic depression has been proposed as a unique diagnostic entity (Alexopoulos 2006). Depression is prevalent in patients with hypertension, coronary heart disease, and vascular dementia, with depression a frequent complication of stroke, particularly stroke affecting the basal ganglia and left frontal regions (Starkstein et al. 1988). White-matter hyperintensities are frequently visualized during structural neuroimaging of depressed older patients; these correspond to atherosclerotic change in perforating arteries supplying blood to the cerebrum and represent end organ damage to the nervous system as a consequence of vascular disease. In asymptomatic individuals, these lesions are associated with reduced cerebral blood flow as well as general cerebrovascular risk factors such as extracranial carotid artery disease, ischaemic heart disease, diabetes mellitus, and hypertension (Fazekas et al. 1988). In depressed patients, particular lesions in the subcortical white matter are most strongly associated with mood disorder and seem to play a key role in the disruption of fronto-striatal neurocircuitry (Krishnan et al. 2006). Of course, depression and vascular disease share a complex reciprocal relationship such that the observed association between white-matter hyperintensities and depression cannot indicate causality in either direction. Depression itself, whether through biological or behavioural mechanisms, may also be a risk factor for the development of cerebrovascular disease. Accordingly, longitudinal studies support a bidirectional relationship: in later life the progression of white matter disease is associated with depression incidence (Firbank et al. 2012), while depressive symptoms predict the progression of white matter disease (Dotson et al. 2012). Important methodological differences exist between these studies, including the population sampled, the ascertainment of mood disorder, and baseline levels of vascular disease and depressive symptoms. Further longitudinal studies would be useful for examining these relationships.

A bidirectional relationship between depression and vascular disease has consequences for the treatment of both conditions. Some geriatric depression might be prevented by addressing risk factors for cerebrovascular disease such as hypertension and hypercholesterolaemia. Similarly, interventions that reduce neurological injury after stroke may lower the risk of subsequent vascular depression by limiting damage to critical subcortical neurocircuitry. Conversely, the treatment of late-onset depression may be neuroprotective in terms of slowing the development of white matter disease and restricting the progression of disability. If evidence of benefit can be demonstrated, the treatment of vascular depression may also include anti-platelet and anti-hypertensive agents that mitigate vascular damage incurred during or contributing to depressive episodes. Regardless of aetiology, behavioural and environmental interventions are necessary to moderate the pronounced functional disability linked to comorbidity in these patients.

Alzheimer's disease

Depression is also commonly comorbid with Alzheimer's disease. Here, reporting of symptoms can be limited by cognitive impairment, and objective assessment can be complicated by misinterpretation of other syndromes such as apathy (Levy et al. 1998). Nevertheless, synthesis of various epidemiological data suggests that 30–50% of patients with Alzheimer's disease suffer with clinically significant depressive symptoms (Lee and Lyketsos 2003). As compared to individuals with late-life depression arising in the absence of cognitive impairment, those with the 'affective syndrome' of Alzheimer's disease are more likely to present with irritability, agitation, neuro-vegetative symptoms and persecutory ideation (Lyketsos and Lee 2004). Lack of interest may be manifest in an inability to sustain basic activities of daily living. Cognitive-emotional symptoms of depression are typically absent and the patient will often deny feeling depressed. Symptoms may also fluctuate throughout the day, highlighting the importance of obtaining a history from an informant and using a validated rating scale such as the Neuropsychiatric Inventory (Cummings 1997) or the Cornell Scale for Depression in Dementia (Alexopoulos et al. 1988). Longitudinal studies indicate that the course of depression in these patients follows a relapsing and remitting course similar to that of idiopathic mood disorder (Brodaty and Luscombe 1996), although high rates of remission in this population might represent the relative insensitivity of existing diagnostic instruments and the subsyndromal nature of concurrent depressive symptoms. The importance of affective disturbance is clear: neuropsychiatric symptoms in Alzheimer's disease (Lyketsos et al. 2006) and depressive symptoms in particular are associated with reduced quality of life (Gonzalez-Salvador et al. 2000), accelerated need for institutionalization (Kopetz et al. 2000), and care-giver burden (Gonzalez-Salvador et al. 1999).

It seems unlikely that the comorbidity of Alzheimer's disease and depression is completely explained by the distressing awareness of progressive cognitive deterioration, as anosognosia (the denial of these deficits) does not confer protection against mood disorder (Migliorelli et al. 1995). In this subgroup of patients, apoptosis of neurons in the brainstem aminergic nuclei proceeds with relative preservation of tissue in cortical areas and in the cholinergic nucleus of Meynert (Zubenko et al. 2003). Comorbidity here thus reflects the selective degeneration of those areas responsible for the synthesis and distribution of the catecholamine neurotransmitters, key regulators of mood, perception, and neuro-vegetative functioning. There may therefore be a specific association between Alzheimer's disease and depression in these patients, who generally present with their first lifetime episode of mood disorder at or shortly after the onset of cognitive impairment. If residual cholinergic integrity is required for the manifestation of depressive symptoms, spontaneous remission might occur with progression of the degenerative disorder and diffuse involvement of cerebral tissue. Accordingly, depression seems more prevalent in those with only mild or moderate cognitive impairment and decreases with duration of follow-up (Holtzer et al. 2005; Li, Meyer, and Thornby 2001), noting, however, that accurate assessment of mood in severely demented patients is challenging.

Depression in Alzheimer's disease may also occur before the onset of cognitive deterioration. In a large retrospective case control study, the strongest association between depressed mood and Alzheimer's disease was seen in those patients whose first depressive episode occurred less than one year prior to the diagnosis of dementia (Green et al. 2003). Clearly, in these patients, late-onset depression heralds the onset of dementia as a prodrome of the dementing illness and a manifestation of the underlying neuropathological degeneration. A more recent study found that depression was associated with the transition from mild cognitive impairment to dementia, but not with the incidence of mild cognitive impairment alone, suggesting that depression accompanies cognitive deterioration rather than precedes it (Richard et al. 2013). Nonetheless, a similar neurodegenerative mechanism is likely to underlie the onset of mood disorder in both groups. Of particular relevance are depressed individuals who present with cognitive deficits that are reversible with treatment of the underlying mood disorder. Such patients with 'pseudo-dementia' (Kiloh 1961) commonly progress to irreversible organic dementia, frequently Alzheimer's disease (Kral 1983). Thus, depression, mild cognitive impairment, and dementia may share a unifying pathophysiology (Panza et al. 2010), although the onset of affective disturbance within this clinical course may be variable.

Depression with first onset well before the start of cognitive deterioration may nevertheless be a true risk factor for the development of Alzheimer's. In the same case-control study noted above (Green et al. 2003), the association between depressive symptoms and Alzheimer's disease remained significant when the first onset of depression was more than twenty-five years prior to the onset of dementia. Severe late-life depression has also been reported to increase the later risk of incident Alzheimer's disease (Gracia-Garcia et al. 2013). However, the mechanism by which a lifetime history of depression confers vulnerability for the later onset of dementia remains unclear. Hippocampal injury has been suggested as a specific neuro-anatomical lesion linking depression and dementia in older adults, with recurrent depression causing prolonged and harmful cortisol release through chronic upregulation of the hypothalamic-pituitary-adrenal axis (Sapolsky 1996). Accordingly, small left hippocampal volumes in patients with late-life depression predict the subsequent onset of dementia (Steffens et al. 2002). Clinically, a synergy of factors is likely to be relevant, including a contribution from vascular disease, potentially significant in the aetiology of both depression and Alzheimer's disease in older adults (Zlokovic 2011).

The relationship between depression and functional impairment in Alzheimer's disease is also bidirectional. Cross-sectionally, the presence of clinically diagnosed (Pearson et al. 1989) or self-reported (Espiritu et al. 2001) depression is associated with additive impairment in instrumental activities of daily living. However, in longitudinal studies both temporal associations are observed: functional deterioration may precede the onset of depression in Alzheimer's dementia (Holtzer et al. 2005), while depression at baseline is also followed by accelerated cognitive and functional decline (Zahodne, Devanand, and Stern 2013). Comorbidity of mood disorder with dementia, therefore, may represent a particularly noxious neuropsychiatric phenotype of dementing illness with worse implications for long-term outcome.

To summarize, depression may be a risk factor for Alzheimer's dementia, a signal of emerging cognitive deterioration and a prognostic marker of long-term cognitive and functional impairment. Once Alzheimer's dementia is established, pharmacological treatment of depressive symptoms does not reverse or ameliorate cognitive deterioration (Munro et al. 2012). Whether treatment of mood disorder might be disease-modifying if administered earlier in the clinical course remains to be established.

Cancer

The prevalence of mood disorder in patients with malignancy is affected by characteristics of the disease itself, including its type, severity, and the nature of treatment. Depression is particularly significant in these individuals, who must often endure disfiguring surgery and long courses of unpleasant chemo- or radiotherapy. Clearly, the diagnosis of cancer is psychologically devastating, but immune activation and the release of pro-inflammatory cytokines may also induce a 'sickness syndrome' that shares many features of a depressive condition (Kent et al. 1992), including fatigue, anhedonia, psychomotor slowing, neuro-vegetative disturbance, and cognitive dysfunction. These symptoms may emerge before the diagnosis of malignancy is made, with depression a particularly common early feature of pancreatic cancer (Carney et al. 2003). Some cytokines such as the interferons are themselves also used in the treatment of certain malignancies and are notorious for inducing affective disturbances, with clear implications for adherence and prognosis. The mechanism of this effect is likely to be related to altered synthesis of monoamine neurotransmitters, overstimulation of the hypothalamic-pituitary-adrenal axis, and inhibition of thyroid hormone metabolism (Raison and Miller 2003). If depression in these patients has a significant biological component, inhibition of pro-inflammatory cytokines or their downstream effects might reduce associated behavioural disturbances. Prophylactic anti-depressant treatment in at-risk patients may reduce the incidence of depression (Musselman et al. 2001).

Drug effects

Many of the drugs commonly used to treat medical disorders can produce neuropsychiatric disturbance through effects upon the central nervous system. Delirium is the most common reaction: an acute organic disturbance of consciousness that in its hypoactive form can present with features of a depressed mood. Older patients are exquisitely vulnerable to such adverse drug reactions, which are typically multifactorial and related to concomitant physical illness, sensory deficits, or incipient dementia. Controlled studies in this area are sparse, but observational data have implicated digoxin, anti-hypertensives, and diuretics (commonly used in the treatment of cardiovascular disease), analgesic and sedative medications such as opiates and benzodiazepines (which may accumulate if excretion is compromised), as well as drugs with anticholinergic properties such as anti-spasmodics, anti-Parkinsonian medications, and tricyclic anti-depressants (Gaudreau et al. 2005). Other medications affect mood in clear consciousness; aside from chemotherapeutic agents, corticosteroids such as prednisolone (often used in the treatment of chronic respiratory, inflammatory, and some malignant conditions) can be problematic (Brown and Suppes 1998).

Neuropsychiatric disturbance may represent an idiosyncratic response to a drug given at normal therapeutic dose, over-administration due to error, excessive self-medication, or drug–drug interactions. The latter are more frequent in older persons, who may have multiple medical problems, multiple prescribers, and multiple medications: 'polypharmacy'. Anti-depressants are often implicated in important pharmacokinetic and pharmacodynamic drug–drug interactions: some inhibit hepatic enzymes responsible for drug metabolism and excretion, while others amplify the tendency of diuretics and oral hypoglycaemics to lower sodium levels (Roxanas, Hibbert, and Field 2007). Both can predispose the older patient to a delirium.

Any psychological assessment of the patient with physical comorbidity must therefore include a careful medication history, with communication between and consolidation of prescribers where necessary. It is not infrequent for physicians to cease psychotropic drugs in the spirit of 'rationalizing' the medication regime of an older patient at risk of adverse reactions. In such cases collaborative input from a psychiatrist may be helpful to clarify the risks and benefits of such an action.

Summary: the consequences of physical disease

Chronic disease is common among older adults and increases the risk of depression. Aversive symptoms, disability, changes in role functioning, and existential crises may lead to grief, demoralization, and a spectrum of other depressive states, moderated by internalized stereotypes of ageing, stigma, and available resources. Other medical conditions and their treatments have more direct neuropsychiatric effects on mood; here depression may herald the onset of varied conditions such dementia, cancer, or endocrine disturbance (Denicoff et al. 1990). Readers are directed to a textbook of neuropsychiatry (e.g. *Lishman's Organic Psychiatry*, David et al. 2012) for a more complete elaboration of these latter associations.

THE CONSEQUENCES OF MOOD DISORDER

Behavioural aspects

Once afflicted with chronic disease, those patients who occupy the sick role are permitted certain privileges contingent upon general social obligations that accompany their position (Parsons 1951). These include the desire to get well as soon as possible and the responsibility of cooperating with medical professionals. The management of many medical disorders involves an organized sequence of consultation with physicians, self-monitoring, medication adherence, and life-style modification. Depressed patients are significantly more likely to be non-adherent to medical treatment recommendations (DiMatteo et al. 2000), leading to adverse health outcomes. In later life, the deleterious effects of depression on memory, energy, motivation, self-efficacy, and interpersonal interactions are particularly relevant.

A collaborative working relationship with the doctor may improve adherence in the patient with chronic disease. Depressed patients, however, are less likely to be satisfied with the quality of care and more likely to be seen as difficult by their medical practitioner (Hahn et al. 1996). Despite higher healthcare utilization and costs, depressed older patients may paradoxically receive a poorer quality of care in terms of preventative screening (Druss et al. 2002) and therapy following myocardial infarction (Druss et al. 2001).

Even prior to the onset of chronic disease, patients with depression may display adverse health behaviours that put them at risk. Depressed patients are more likely to report a high fat diet, a sedentary lifestyle, harmful alcohol use, and smoking (Rosal et al. 2001). Depressed patients are more likely to be obese and suffer from the metabolic syndrome, a constellation of biological markers that confers an increased risk for type II diabetes mellitus and heart disease. Smoking is a negative health behaviour with particularly noxious consequences for future morbidity from cancer, respiratory, and vascular diseases, and which has been consistently associated with depression in previous surveys of comorbidity (Grant 1995). Depression and smoking also share a reciprocal relationship; self-medication with nicotine occurs to regulate a depressed mood while nicotine itself interferes with affective regulation, particularly during withdrawal. There may also be a shared genetic susceptibility to both major depression and nicotine dependence (Kendler et al. 1993).

Biological aspects

Depression is associated with physiological dysfunction that acts systemically and synergistically with behavioural variables to initiate, aggravate, and accelerate pathophysiological changes in the patient with chronic disease.

The neuroendocrine and neurochemical sequelae of depression have been implicated in the development of obesity (Stunkard, Faith, and Allison 2003), osteoporosis (Cizza et al. 2001), and pain disorders (Campbell, Clauw, and Keefer 2003). However, the biological corollaries of depression have been most thoroughly studied in ischaemic heart disease. Here, mood disorder may act through several distinct pathways to promote ischaemic damage to the myocardium as a consequence of atherosclerotic lesions in the coronary blood vessels (Stapelberg et al. 2011). Such pathways include dysregulation of the hypothalamic-pituitary-adrenal axis, excessive sympathetic nervous system tone, release of pro-inflammatory cytokines, platelet activation, and vascular endothelial dysfunction. Atherosclerotic lesions are subsequently fostered through elevations in blood pressure and inflammatory mediators, vasoconstriction, platelet aggregation, and reductions in heart-rate variability. However, behavioural risk factors such as smoking also feed directly into this process by modifying some of the same physiological variables and can confound the interpretation of these findings. Therefore, although heart disease appears to develop by means of a diverse system of connected physiological and behavioural mechanisms, the significance of each 'node' in this complex causal network requires further definition. Indeed, inflammatory mediators and atherosclerosis themselves appear to have a bidirectional link to depression.

Depression has also been implicated in the development of cancer through promotion of immune dysfunction. Proposed mechanisms include reduced production of leucocytes, increased circulating cortisol levels, and defects in cellular DNA repair. Again, however, depression-related behaviours such as smoking, excess alcohol use, and poor nutrition may account for these findings, making the direct effects of depressed mood difficult to quantify (Miller, Cohen, and Herbert 1999). A similar interaction between biological and behavioural variables occurs in type II diabetes mellitus, where insulin resistance is promoted by excess circulating cortisol and adiposity is promoted by binge and comfort eating.

Summary: the consequences of mood disorder

In those older persons with mood disorder, physical comorbidity is considerable. Behaviours associated with depression predispose to the onset of chronic disease and impair effective participation in treatment. Depressed mood may itself exert a directly harmful influence although the interaction with behavioural risk factors is likely to be substantial.

THE IMPLICATIONS OF COMORBIDITY

Thus far, the examination of comorbidity has concentrated upon complex and potentially causal reciprocal relationships. However, comorbidity is also clinically meaningful in an aged population, with consequences for health outcomes, treatment, and the delivery of services.

Healthcare costs and service utilization

Older patients with major depression are over-represented among high users of primary care services, in excess of the expected medical comorbidity associated with mood disorders (Luber et al. 2001). Non-specific symptoms such as fatigue or pain are important determinants of health-service utilization. Similar findings are seen in general hospital inpatients (Mayou, Hawton, and Feldman 1988).

Predictably, depressed community-dwelling older patients amass higher healthcare costs across both the outpatient and inpatient treatment setting (Katon et al. 2003). A trend for increased costs is seen in every component of treatment, from primary care visits to emergency department presentations, even after controlling for the severity of chronic disease. Moreover, this increase is not related to larger mental healthcare costs, which account for only a small fraction of the total healthcare bill.

Symptom amplification

Many individuals can habituate to a certain level of aversive symptoms before becoming distressed. However, possession of a comorbid depressive disorder may interfere with this adaptive process, leading to magnification of disease-specific as well as general somatic symptoms (Katon and Ciechanowski 2002). In patients with coronary artery disease, the presence of depression at one year following cardiac catheterization was significantly associated with pain, disease perception, and fatigue six years later (Sullivan et al. 2000), despite adjustment for the degree of coronary artery occlusion and the nature of medical or surgical intervention. Psychiatric comorbidity may explain why objective measures such as treadmill stress testing and angiography are poor predictors of functioning for patients with ischaemic heart disease. Additional medical consultation and investigation associated with increased symptom reporting may also be one mechanism accounting for the increase in healthcare costs observed in patients with comorbidity.

If depression can intensify the burden of chronic medical illness then it follows that treatment of a comorbid mood disorder could ease the symptoms and improve the functioning of such patients without necessarily making an objective difference to disease markers or pathological processes. Accordingly, patients with tinnitus are not only less depressed, but also less distressed by their symptoms, after treatment with an anti-depressant (Sullivan et al. 1993). Similar results have been reported for patients with chronic obstructive pulmonary disease (COPD) (Borson et al. 1992), with improved respiratory symptoms and physical comfort despite little change in objective measures of lung function.

Additive functional disability

If functional disability can lead to depression then depression can also accentuate disability in those patients with medical comorbidity. Here, mood disorder may not necessarily reflect the severity of concurrent physical illness but it does predict functional impairment and may have greater prognostic value than objective measures of disease alone. Of course, depressed patients may be more likely to perceive themselves as functionally impaired as a consequence of their mood-related cognitive biases, such that to avoid confounding objective measures of disability must be carefully used rather than relying on self-report of functional status.

Among older primary care patients, depression is a leading cause of disability, surpassed only by arthritis and heart disease at a population level (Unutzer et al. 2000). The treatment of depression promises to improve the health-related quality of life in older patients with chronic disease (Von Korff et al. 1992), although experimental support for the effect of depression offset on disability is limited by the absence of appropriate randomized studies.

Increased mortality

Depression confers a risk for developing physical disorders such as diabetes mellitus and ischaemic heart disease that may ultimately increase mortality. However, attempts to synthesize an extensive literature on this topic have been hindered by methodological heterogeneity, publication bias, and failure to control for ill health, alcohol use, smoking, and suicide (Wulsin, Vaillant, and Wells 1999). Moreover, most prospective studies do not assess the chronicity of mood disorder in those patients depressed at baseline and do not account for a history of depression in euthymic individuals. Nevertheless, although the true size and mechanism of the effect remains unclear, it does seem that depression influences mortality in certain populations, particularly males with cardiovascular disease (Ferketich et al. 2000).

Older patients with depression show an excess mortality largely accounted for by cardiovascular or cerebrovascular disease (Bruce and Leaf 1989; Unutzer et al. 2002). Once more, the majority of these patients with clinically significant depressive syndromes are untreated. In the latter study, increased mortality appears related to health behaviours, with risk reduced to non-significant levels after adjustment for alcohol use, smoking, obesity, low levels of exercise, and poor diet. A similar association between depression and mortality is observed in the older persons who are institutionalized, a sample that might permit greater standardization of behavioural factors that affect physical well-being (Parmelee, Katz, and Lawton 1992). However, subsequent analyses of variance demonstrated that the increase in mortality could be largely attributed to the significant association between depression and poor physical health or functional disability, a finding that highlights the inextricable reciprocity of these relationships.

Treatment

Depression in medically ill older adults should be considered a treatable disorder. Pharmacotherapy is effective in depressed patients with ischaemic heart disease, cerebrovascular disease, diabetes mellitus, and cancer (Evans et al. 2005). Even among those patients with late-life depression and high medical burden that respond poorly to first-line treatment, half recover with standard augmentation strategies (Dew et al. 2007). However, anti-depressant use in older people is not a risk-free endeavour (Coupland et al. 2011), and it may be more appropriate to consider a manualized cognitive-behavioural therapy (CBT), as these have also proven effective in similar populations (Cimpean and Drake 2011). Online CBT specifically addressing comorbidity might permit large-scale intervention (Cockayne et al. 2011). Given that treating depression here seems generally effective regardless of the specific medical condition, a large proportion of patients with medical comorbidity stand to benefit.

An effective intervention need not have an explicit mechanism. A relatively non-specific treatment such as the interaction with an attentive clinician may include validation, empowerment, environmental modification, and attention to pain or disability, which may be sufficient to produce sustained changes in mood. In Alzheimer's disease, a condition in which anti-depressant efficacy is more limited and psychological therapies are more difficult to deliver, usual care from an Older Person's Mental Health Service is as effective in reducing depressive symptoms as are active pharmacological treatments (Banerjee et al. 2011). Similarly, in terms of reducing depression scores, education is no less effective than group CBT among individuals with COPD (Kunik et al. 2008) and supportive clinical management is no less effective than interpersonal psychotherapy in patients with coronary heart disease (Lesperance et al. 2007). This is of particular relevance to those patients experiencing 'less than major' depressive states who may not meet the threshold for a trial of anti-depressant medication or a course of psychotherapy. It is also good news for those seeking to address the harmful consequences of comorbidity: many clinicians are capable of effectively intervening to improve depressive symptoms. Of course, this does not preclude the use of targeted pharmacological or psychological treatment among selected patients with severe mood disorders in whom response is likely to be robust (Snowdon 2012).

The repercussions of mood disorder, as a risk factor for incident disease and as a marker of poor prognosis, suggest that intervention will substantially reduce overall morbidity. To date, however, most treatment studies have focused on depressive symptoms, with limited evidence showing that addressing depression improves health behaviours, modifies biological risk factors, or ultimately affects outcomes. Selected exceptions exist for smoking (Trockel et al. 2008), platelet activation (Serebruany et al. 2003), and mortality (Bogner et al. 2007), respectively. Future studies should have the power to identify improvements in these variables. Future research may also consider interventions that promise to have multiple health benefits spanning both medical and psychiatric domains. Exercise on prescription (Sörensen et al. 2011) is one such intervention that can be delivered elegantly in primary care, being mindful that the task of addressing comorbidity will largely fall to the general practitioner.

Service delivery

Comorbidity of mood and medical disorder poses a substantial challenge to existing health-care services, which may be ill-equipped to respond to this relationship in an integrated and efficient manner (Kathol and Clarke 2005). Separation of mental and medical treatment is an almost universal practice, with segregation of financial and operational infra-structures that compete to transfer accountability for services to the opposing stakeholder. This organization reflects a prevailing dualistic assumption that psychiatry is somehow essentially different from the other biomedical specialities. Moreover, such business models, operating under tight fiscal pressures, actively oppose integration of services for complex, high-cost patients with comorbidity. However, future healthcare planning must consider a demographic transition that will result in an increasingly aged population and a potential expansion of comorbidity (Connolly 2012). Addressing comorbidity here will ensure that the increased years of life gained are lived disability-free .

Depressed older adults are high utilizers of healthcare services at all levels of intervention, incurring higher healthcare costs than those with an equivalent level of chronic disease alone (Katon et al. 2003). Significantly, the majority of this additional expenditure is accounted for by an excess of medical rather than psychiatric costs, which may reflect both the power of a mood disorder to augment the morbidity of physical illness and the preponderance of somatic symptoms as a presenting feature of the mood disorder itself. Yet few of these patients with psychiatric illness enter the mental-health sector and few are even recognized as cases at the primary care level. Thus, psychogeriatricians cannot add value to the care of patients with comorbidity because they remain in the general medical setting, with an ensuing cost shift to this sector. Clearly, the interaction of medical and psychiatric illness is not addressed satisfactorily in health systems that handle medical and mental issues separately.

Given that physicians are currently managing the majority of older patients with comorbidity and that the majority of the excess cost is situated within the medical sphere, then early diagnosis and assertive treatment of mood disorder become the business of those who might have traditionally deferred this responsibility to the psychiatric service. This may necessitate a shift in certain existing assumptions about the nature and reversibility of mood disorder in older persons, including that depression is the expected consequence of medical illness. The deleterious effect of untreated depression upon quality of life must be emphasized, including those patients whose lifespan is limited by terminal illness.

Respectively, psychiatric services must be available and accessible in a timely and proximate fashion, reducing the barriers that prevent patients from entering the mental health system, such as additional co-payments to insurance companies or complex referral pathways. Furthermore, those in the mental health sector must remain keenly aware of medical issues among older adults with depression, noting the considerable medical comorbidity in this cohort while actively prioritizing medical issues in their assessment, formulation, and treatment planning. However, such ideological shifts remain challenging in an existing system where administrative, financial, and geographical separation of services precludes communication and collaboration. Moreover, many mental health services themselves prioritize a narrow spectrum of 'severe and enduring mental illnesses' that limit access to public services by diagnosis rather than level of disability. This has disadvantaged those previously supported by a consultation-liaison model of psychiatric care: the somatizers and those with comorbidity (Smith 2003).

General practitioners and their colleagues in the primary care sector are ideally placed at the interface of medical and psychiatric comorbidity. Paradoxically, although it is often in this sector that treatment is most powerful, it is also here that treatment is often overlooked. Nonetheless, there are innovative approaches to improving the care of this cohort. Inter-professional liaison among educational boards and regulatory bodies advocates for a grounding in general psychiatry to be included in the training programmes of all medical practitioners. Treatment models that involve case management by a depression specialist can support general practitioners with the implementation of best practice clinical algorithms that include both pharmacological and psychological therapy, showing evidence of reduced depressive symptoms in patients with comorbidity (Bruce et al. 2004; Williams et al. 2004). In Australia, government funding has increased the availability of specialized psychological services in primary care through the Medicare Better Access Initiative, claiming to meet previously unmet needs for mental health service provision (Pirkis et al. 2011) although the implementation of the scheme and its evaluation have attracted criticism (Hickie, Rosenberry, and Davenport 2011). See also the chapter by Armento and Stanley in this Handbook.

In secondary care, the integration of a psychiatric service within a medical outpatient clinic assists with proactive case finding of complex, resource intensive patients and provides a framework to routinely measure outcomes following psychiatric intervention. Among those patients already managed by a psychiatry service, medically trained nurses can actively coordinate medical treatment and act as 'culture brokers' between the two systems of care (Bartels 2004). Case management here can directly address factors mediating poor outcome, such as medication adherence and self-advocacy within the medical system. Such a model applied to older patients with comorbidity increases access to primary care physicians, the diagnosis of previously unrecognized medical disorders, and the uptake of preventative healthcare (Bartels et al. 2004).

Summary: implications of comorbidity

Older patients with comorbidity carry both the increased burden of chronic physical disease that comes with age, but also the increased morbidity that accompanies mental illness. Combining affective and physical disorder in older adults appears to exert an additive effect in terms of greater healthcare costs, service utilization, symptom burden, functional disability, and mortality. Despite this gloomy prognosis, interventions that address mood disorder in comorbid populations are effective and worthwhile. However, diagnosis and treatment of older adults with depression is often limited by service structure and cultural assumptions about who treats mental illness. Similarly, older persons with depression are liable to receive less than optimal treatment for their physical problems. The serious ramifications of comorbidity necessitate a cultural shift in the organization of care with the incorporation of approaches derived from consultation-liaison psychiatry.

IMPLICATIONS FOR PRACTICE

The following principles summarize the key points of the chapter with respect to clinical practice:

- Maintain a low threshold for depression treatment. Depression is not a necessary consequence of disease or disability, even if mood disorder is felt to be a feature of the pathophysiological process. Quality of life is greatly important, even in terminal illness.
- Mood disorder should not be trivialized with respect to physical disorder. When comorbid with medical illness, depression is robustly associated with a range of poor outcomes and should be assertively addressed. 'Less than major' depressive symptoms are also relevant in the aged population.
- All medically ill older adults should be screened for depression, which is under-recognized in general medical settings. Many such patients with mood disorder do not reach mental health services or access a psychogeriatrician.
- Treatment of depression with pharmacological and psychological therapies is effective in patients with comorbidity. Non-specific interventions may also be successful and can be delivered by any engaged clinician. Early treatment of depression reduces the burden of chronic disease although it remains uncertain whether this crosses over to effects on medical outcomes.
- A large proportion of older adults with mood disorders suffer from chronic medical problems. All clinicians must therefore attend to the physical as well as the psychological and must consider the ramifications of chronic disease. Treatment should not only address aversive symptoms, but also functional disability, the availability of social resources, and the meaning of illness for the patient. A multidisciplinary approach will be most effective, with consideration of the context in which disease arises.
- Early intervention prevents additive disability from untreated medical problems. It may be necessary to encourage patients to consult physicians, address harmful health behaviours, and to advocate on their behalf for the best quality medical care.
- Older patients are at increased risk of adverse outcomes from drug–drug interactions. Some medications directly affect mood and should be reviewed by a physician.
- Positive attitudes to ageing have beneficial effects on health behaviours and adaptation to disability. The cultivation of similar attitudes among clinicians may moderate some of the negative stereotypes that prevent patients with comorbidity from receiving optimal care.
- Holistically treating comorbidity depends upon a collaborative working relationship between providers of 'mental' and 'physical' healthcare. Barriers that restrict access to each speciality should be defined, with increasing cross-disciplinary engagement using innovative models of service delivery.

SUMMARY

In this chapter we have explored the reciprocal and interdependent relationship between physical disease and mood disorder in older adults. Beginning with a conceptual discussion highlighting the clinical and scientific arguments for integration of the two fields, we have ended with a framework for how this might operate in routine practice. We have seen that chronic diseases are the principal health concerns of an older population and that these bring with them aversive physical symptoms, functional impairment, and social changes with the potential to precipitate depressive symptoms in vulnerable individuals. Psychological resilience may be conferred by hopefulness, positive attitudes to ageing, and social resources. However, many medical conditions have specific neuropsychiatric sequelae that can directly precipitate a mood disorder as part of their clinical course, for example through neurodegeneration or neuroendocrine effects. When present, comorbidity of depressive symptoms with medical disorder is almost universally a marker of poorer prognosis, whether this includes functional and cognitive deterioration or higher healthcare costs and utilization. Pathways to these outcomes may be both behavioural and biological with a multitude of potential factors in operation. Effective management of comorbidity must be a target of future healthcare systems in the interests of reducing late-life disability and maintaining efficient service provision. Comorbidity is a complex phenomenon, however, and this is likely to necessitate shifts in both theoretical frameworks as well as business models of healthcare organization.

KEY REFERENCES AND SOURCES FOR FURTHER READING

David, A., Fleminger, S., Kopelman, M., Lovestone, S., and Mellors, J. (2012). *Lishman's Organic Psychiatry: A Textbook of Neuropsychiatry*. Chichester: Wiley-Blackwell.

Raphael, B. (1996). 'The Griefs of Growing Old'. In *The Anatomy of Bereavement* (pp. 283–319). London: Routledge.

Scambler, G. (2008). *Sociology as Applied to Medicine*. Edinburgh: Saunders.

REFERENCES

Albert, S. M., Bear-Lehman, J., and Burkhardt, A. (2012). 'Mild Depressive Symptoms, Self-reported Disability, and Slowing across Multiple Functional Domains'. *International Psychogeriatrics* 24: 253–260.

Alexopoulos, G. S., Abrams, R. C., Young, R. C., and Shamoian, C. A. (1988). 'Cornell Scale for Depression in Dementia'. *Biological Psychiatry* 23: 271–284.

Alexopoulos, G. S., Meyers, B. S., Young, R. C., Campbell, S., Silbersweig, D., et al. (1997). '"Vascular Depression" Hypothesis'. *Archives of General Psychiatry* 54: 915–922.

Alexopoulos, G. S., Kiosses, D. N., Klimstra, S., Kalayam, B., and Bruce, M. L. (2002). 'Clinical Presentation of the "Depression-executive Dysfunction Syndrome" of Late Life'. *American Journal of Geriatric Psychiatry* 10: 98–106.

Alexopoulos, G. S., Kiosses, D. N., Heo, M., Murphy, C. F., Shanmugham, B. (2005). 'Executive Dysfunction and the Course of Geriatric Depression'. *Biological Psychiatry* 58: 204–210.

Alexopoulos, G. S. (2006). 'The Vascular Depression Hypothesis: 10 Years Later'. *Biological Psychiatry* 60: 1304–1305.

Anda, R., Williamson, D., Jones, D., Macera, C., Eaker, E., et al. (1993). 'Depressed Affect, Hopelessness, and the Risk of Ischemic Heart Disease in a Cohort of U.S. Adults'. *Epidemiology* 4: 285–294.

Atlantis, E., Browning, C., Sims, J., and Kendig, H. (2010). 'Diabetes Incidence Associated with Depression and Antidepressants in the Melbourne Longitudinal Studies on Healthy Ageing (MELSHA)'. *International Journal of Geriatric Psychiatry* 25: 688–696.

Baldwin, R. C., Gallagley, A., Gourlay, M., Jackson, A., and Burns, A. (2006). 'Prognosis of Late Life Depression: A Three-year Cohort Study of Outcome and Potential Predictors'. *International Journal of Geriatric Psychiatry* 21: 57–63.

Banerjee, S., Hellier, J., Dewey, M., et al. (2011). 'Sertraline or Mirtazapine for Depression in Dementia (HTA-SADD): A Randomised, Multicentre, Double-blind, Placebo-Controlled Trial'. *Lancet* 378: 403–411.

Bartels, S. J. (2004). 'Caring for the Whole Person: Integrated Health Care for Older Adults with Severe Mental Illness and Medical Comorbidity'. *Journal of the American Geriatrics Society* 52: S249–S257.

Bartels, S. J., Forester, B., Mueser, K. T., Miles, K. M., Dums, A. R., et al. (2004). 'Enhanced Skills Training and Health Care Management for Older Persons with Severe Mental Illness'. *Community Mental Health Journal* 40: 75–90.

Bejjani, B. P., Damier, P., Arnulf, I., Thivard, L., Bonnet, A. M., et al. (1999). 'Transient Acute Depression Induced by High-frequency Deep-brain Stimulation'. *New England Journal of Medicine* 340: 1476–1480.

Bennett, M. R. and Hacker, P. M. S. (2003). *Philosophical Foundations of Neuroscience*. Malden, MA and Oxford: Blackwell.

Block, S. D. (2000). 'Assessing and managing depression in the terminally ill patient. ACP-ASIM End-of-Life Care Consensus Panel. American College of Physicians—American Society of Internal Medicine'. *Annals of Internal Medicine* 132: 209–218.

Bogner, H. R., Morales, K. H., Post, E. P., and Bruce, M. L. (2007). 'Diabetes, Depression, and Death: A Randomized Controlled Trial of a Depression Treatment Program for Older Adults Based in Primary Care (PROSPECT)'. *Diabetes Care* 30: 3005–3010.

Borson, S., McDonald, G. J., Gayle, T., Deffebach, M., Lakshminarayan, S., et al. (1992). 'Improvement in Mood, Physical Symptoms, and Function with Nortriptyline for Depression in Patients with Chronic Obstructive Pulmonary Disease'. *Psychosomatics* 33: 190–201.

Bracken, P. and Thomas, P. (2005). *Postpsychiatry*. Oxford: Oxford University Press.

Brault, M. C., Meuleman, B., and Bracke, P. (2012). 'Depressive Symptoms in the Belgian Population: Disentangling Age and Cohort Effects'. *Social Psychiatry and Psychiatric Epidemiology* 47: 903–915.

Breitbart, W., Rosenfeld, B., Pessin, H., Kaim, M, Funesti-Esch, J., et al. (2000). 'Depression, Hopelessness, and Desire for Hastened Death In Terminally Ill Patients with Cancer'. *Journal of the American Medical Association* 284: 2907–2911.

Breuer, J., Freud, S., Strachey, J., and Strachey, A. (1956). *Studies on Hysteria*. London: Hogarth Press.

Brodaty, H. and Luscombe, G. (1996). 'Depression in Persons with Dementia'. *International Psychogeriatrics* 8: 609–622.

Brown, E. S. and Suppes, T. (1998). 'Mood Symptoms during Corticosteroid Therapy: A Review'. *Harvard Review of Psychiatry* 5: 239–246.

Brown, G. K., Beck, A. T., Steer, R. A., and Grisham, J. R. (2000). 'Risk Factors for Suicide in Psychiatric Outpatients: A 20-year Prospective Study'. *Journal of Consulting and Clinical Psychology* 68: 371–377.

Bruce, M. L. and Leaf, P. J. (1989). Psychiatric Disorders and 15-month Mortality in a Community Sample of Older Adults. *American Journal of Public Health*, 79: 727–730.

Bruce, M. L., Ten Have, T. R., Reynolds, C. F. III, et al. (2004). 'Reducing Suicidal Ideation and Depressive Symptoms in Depressed Older Primary Care Patients: A Randomized Controlled Trial'. *Journal of the American Medical Association* 291: 1081–1091.

Bryant, C., Bei, B., Gilson, K., Komiti, A., Jackson, H., et al. (2012). 'The Relationship between Attitudes to Aging and Physical and Mental Health in Older Adults'. *International Psychogeriatrics* 24(10): 1674–1683.

Campbell, L. C., Clauw, D. J., and Keefe, F. J. (2003). 'Persistent Pain and Depression: A Biopsychosocial Perspective'. *Biological Psychiatry* 54: 399–409.

Carney, C. P., Jones, L., Woolson, R. F., Noyes, R., and Doebbeling, B. N. (2003). 'Relationship between Depression and Pancreatic Cancer in the General Population'. *Psychosomatic Medicine* 65: 884–888.

Carson, A. J., Brown, R., David, A. S., Duncan, R., Edwards, M. J., et al. (2012). 'Functional (Conversion) Neurological Symptoms: Research since the Millennium'. *Journal of Neurology, Neurosurgery and Psychiatry* 83: 842–850.

Chang-Quan, H., Xue-Mei, Z., Bi-Rong, D., Zhen-Chan, L., Ji-Rong, Y., et al. (2010). 'Health Status and Risk for Depression among the Elderly: A Meta-analysis of Published Literature'. *Age and Ageing* 39: 23–30.

Cimpean, D. and Drake, R. E. (2011). 'Treating Co-Morbid Chronic Medical Conditions and Anxiety/Depression'. *Epidemiology and Psychiatric Sciences* 20: 141–150.

Cizza, G., Ravn, P., Chrousos, G. P., and Gold, P. W. (2001). 'Depression: A Major, Unrecognized Risk Factor for Osteoporosis?' *Trends in Endocrinology and Metabolism* 12: 198–203.

Clarke, D. M. and Kissane, D. W. (2002). 'Demoralization: Its Phenomenology and Importance'. *Australian and New Zealand Journal of Psychiatry* 36: 733–742.

Cockayne, N. L., Glozier, N., Naismith, S. L., Christensen, H., Neal, B., et al. (2011). 'Internet-based Treatment for Older Adults with Depression and Co-morbid Cardiovascular Disease: Protocol for a Randomised, Double-blind, Placebo Controlled Trial'. *BMC Psychiatry* 11: 10.

Connolly, M. (2012). 'Futurology and Mental Health Services: Are We Ready for the Demographic Transition?' *Psychiatrist* 36: 161–164.

Coupland, C., Dhiman, P., Morriss, R., Barton, G., Hippisley-Cox, J., et al. (2011). 'Antidepressant Use and Risk of Adverse Outcomes in Older People: Population Based Cohort Study'. *British Medical Journal* 343: d4551.

Cummings, J. L. (1993). 'Frontal-subcortical Circuits and Human Behavior'. *Archives of Neurology* 50: 873–880.

Cummings, J. L. (1997). 'The Neuropsychiatric Inventory: Assessing Psychopathology in Dementia Patients'. *Neurology* 48: S10–S16.

Damasio, A. and Carvalho, G. B. (2013). 'The Nature of Feelings: Evolutionary and Neurobiological Origins'. *Nature Reviews. Neuroscience* 14: 143–152.

De Figueiredo, J. M. (1993). 'Depression and Demoralization: Phenomenologic Differences and Research Perspectives'. *Comprehensive Psychiatry* 34: 308–311.

Denicoff, K. D., Joffe, R. T., Lakshmanan, M. C., Robbins, J., and Rubinow, D. R. (1990). 'Neuropsychiatric Manifestations of Altered Thyroid State'. *American Journal of Psychiatry* 147: 94–99.

Dew, M. A., Whyte, E. M., Lenze, E. J., Houck, P. R., Mulsant, B., et al. (2007). 'Recovery from Major Depression in Older Adults Receiving Augmentation of Antidepressant Pharmacotherapy'. *American Journal of Psychiatry* 164: 892–899.

Dimatteo, M. R., Lepper, H. S., and Croghan, T. W. (2000). 'Depression is A Risk Factor for Noncompliance with Medical Treatment: Meta-analysis of the Effects of Anxiety and Depression on Patient Adherence'. *Archives of Internal Medicine* 160: 2101–2107.

Dotson, V. M., Zonderman, A. B., Kraut, M. A., and Resnick, S. M. (2013). 'Temporal Relationships between Depressive Symptoms and White Matter Hyperintensities in Older Men and Women'. *International Journal of Geriatric Psychiatry* 28(1): 66–74.

Drevets, W. C., Price, J. L., Simpson, J. R., Jr Todd, R. D., Reich, T., et al. (1997). 'Subgenual Prefrontal Cortex Abnormalities in Mood Disorders'. *Nature* 386: 824–827.

Druss, B. G., Bradford, W. D., Rosenheck, R. A., Radford, M. J., and Krumholz, H. M. (2001). 'Quality of Medical Care and Excess Mortality in Older Patients with Mental Disorders'. *Archives of General Psychiatry* 58: 565–572.

Druss, B. G., Rosenheck, R. A., Desai, M. M., and Perlin, J. B. (2002). 'Quality of Preventive Medical Care for Patients with Mental Disorders'. *Medical Care* 40: 129–136.

Engel, G. L. (1967). 'A Psychological Setting of Somatic Disease: The "Giving Up-Given Up" Complex'. *Proceedings of the Royal Society of Medicine* 60: 553–555.

Espiritu, D. A., Rashid, H., Mast, B. T., Fitzgerald, J., Steinberg, J., et al. (2001). 'Depression, Cognitive Impairment and Function in Alzheimer's Disease'. *International Journal of Geriatric Psychiatry* 16: 1098–1103.

Evans, D. L., Charney, D. S., Lewis, L., Golden, R. N., Gorman, J. M., et al. (2005). 'Mood Disorders in the Medically Ill: Scientific Review and Recommendations'. *Biological Psychiatry* 58: 175–189.

Everson, S. A., Kaplan, G. A., Goldberg, D. E., Salonen, R., and Salonen, J. T. (1997). 'Hopelessness and 4-year Progression of Carotid Atherosclerosis. The Kuopio Ischemic Heart Disease Risk Factor Study'. *Arteriosclerosis, Thrombosis, and Vascular Biology* 17: 1490–1495.

Fazekas, F., Niederkorn, K., Schmidt, R., et al. (1988). 'White Matter Signal Abnormalities in Normal Individuals: Correlation with Carotid Ultrasonography, Cerebral Blood Flow Measurements, and Cerebrovascular Risk Factors'. *Stroke* 19: 1285–1288.

Ferketich, A. K., Schwartzbaum, J. A., Frid, D. J., and Moeschberger, M. L. (2000). 'Depression as an Antecedent to Heart Disease among Women and Men in the NHANES I study. National Health and Nutrition Examination Survey'. *Archives of Internal Medicine* 160: 1261–1268.

Firbank, M. J., Teodorczuk, A., Van Der Flier, W. M., et al. (2012). 'Relationship between Progression of Brain White Matter Changes and Late-life Depression: 3-year Results from the LADIS Study'. *British Journal of Psychiatry* 201: 40–45.

Frank, J. D. (1974). 'Psychotherapy: The Restoration of Morale'. *American Journal of Psychiatry* 131: 271–274.

Fulford, K. W. (2001). '"What is (Mental) Disease?": An Open Letter to Christopher Boorse'. *Journal of Medical Ethics* 27: 80–85.

Gaudreau, J. D., Gagnon, P., Roy, M. A., Harel, F., and Tremblay, A. (2005). 'Association between Psychoactive Medications and Delirium in Hospitalized Patients: A Critical Review'. *Psychosomatics* 46: 302–316.

Gildengers, A. G., Whyte, E. M., Drayer, R. A., et al. (2008). 'Medical Burden in Late-life Bipolar and Major Depressive Disorders'. *American Journal of Geriatric Psychiatry* 16: 194–200.

Goldapple, K., Segal, Z., Garson, C., Soreca, I., Fagiolini, A., et al. (2004). 'Modulation of Cortical-limbic Pathways in Major Depression: Treatment-specific Effects of Cognitive Behavior Therapy'. *Archives of General Psychiatry* 61: 34–41.

Gonzalez-Salvador, M. T., Arango, C., Lyketsos, C. G., and Barba, A. C. (1999). 'The Stress and Psychological Morbidity of the Alzheimer Patient Caregiver'. *International Journal of Geriatric Psychiatry* 14: 701–710.

Gonzalez-Salvador, T., Lyketsos, C. G., Baker, A., Hovanec, L., Roques, C., et al.(2000). 'Quality of Life in Dementia Patients in Long-term Care'. *International Journal of Geriatric Psychiatry* 15: 181–189.

Gracia-Garcia, P., De-La-Camara, C., Santabarbara, J., Lopez-Anton, R., Quintanilla, M. A., et al. (2013). 'Depression and Incident Alzheimer Disease: The Impact of Disease Severity'. *American Journal of Geriatric Psychiatry* (epub ahead of print).

Grant, B. F. (1995). 'Comorbidity between DSM-IV Drug Use Disorders and Major Depression: Results of a National Survey of Adults'. *Journal of Substance Abuse* 7: 481–497.

Green, R. C., Cupples, L. A., Kurz, A., Auerbach, S., Go, R., et al.(2003). 'Depression as a Risk Factor for Alzheimer Disease: The MIRAGE Study'. *Archives of Neurology* 60: 753–759.

Griffith, J. L. and Gaby, L. (2005). 'Brief Psychotherapy at the Bedside: Countering Demoralization from Medical Illness'. *Psychosomatics* 46: 109–116.

Gureje, O., Oladeji, B., and Abiona, T. (2011). 'Incidence and Risk Factors for Late-life Depression in the Ibadan Study of Ageing'. *Psychological Medicine* 41: 1897–1906.

Hahn, S. R., Kroenke, K., Spitzer, R. L., Brody, D., Williams, J. B., et al. (1996). 'The Difficult Patient: Prevalence, Psychopathology, and Functional Impairment'. *Journal of General Internal Medicine* 11: 1–8.

Hasin, D. S., Goodwin, R. D., Stinson, F. S., and Grant, B. F. (2005). 'Epidemiology of Major Depressive Disorder: Results from the National Epidemiologic Survey on Alcoholism and Related Conditions'. *Archives of General Psychiatry* 62: 1097–1106.

Hegeman, J. M., Kok, R. M., Van Der Mast, R. C., and Giltay, E. J. (2012). 'Phenomenology of Depression In Older Compared with Younger Adults: Meta-analysis'. *British Journal of Psychiatry* 200: 275–281.

Hickie, I. B., Rosenberg, S., and Davenport, T. A. (2011). 'Australia's Better Access Initiative: Still Awaiting Serious Evaluation?' *Australian and New Zealand Journal of Psychiatry* 45: 814–823.

Holtzer, R., Scarmeas, N., Wegesin, D. J., et al. (2005). 'Depressive Symptoms in Alzheimer's Disease: Natural Course and Temporal Relation to Function and Cognitive Status'. *Journal of the American Geriatrics Society* 53: 2083–2089.

Hybels, C. F., Pieper, C. F., and Blazer, D. G. (2009). 'The Complex Relationship between Depressive Symptoms and Functional Limitations in Community-dwelling Older Adults: The Impact of Subthreshold Depression'. *Psychological Medicine* 39: 1677–1688.

James, W. (1890). *The Principles of Psychology*. New York, Henry Holt.

Karlsson, H., Hirvonen, J., Kajander, J., Markula J., Rasi-Hakal, H., et al. (2010). 'Research Letter: Psychotherapy Increases Brain Serotonin 5-HT1A Receptors in Patients with Major Depressive Disorder'. *Psychological Medicine* 40: 523–528.

Kathol, R. G. and Clarke, D. (2005). 'Rethinking the Place of the Psyche in Health: Toward the Integration of Health Care Systems'. *Australian and New Zealand Journal of Psychiatry* 39: 816–825.

Katon, W. and Ciechanowski, P. (2002). 'Impact of Major Depression on Chronic Medical Illness'. *Journal of Psychosomatic Research*, 53: 859–863.

Katon, W. J., Lin, E., Russo, J., and Unutzer, J. (2003). 'Increased Medical Costs of a Population-based Sample of Depressed Elderly Patients'. *Archives of General Psychiatry* 60: 897–903.

Kawakami, N., Takatsuka, N., Shimizu, H., and Ishibashi, H. (1999). 'Depressive Symptoms and Occurrence of Type 2 Diabetes among Japanese Men'. *Diabetes Care* 22: 1071–1076.

Kendler, K. S., Neale, M. C., Maclean, C. J., Heath, A. C., Eaves, L. J., et al. (1993). 'Smoking and Major Depression. A Causal Analysis'. *Archives of General Psychiatry* 50: 36–43.

Kent, S., Bluthe, R. M., Kelley, K. W., and Dantzer, R. (1992). 'Sickness Behavior as a New Target for Drug Development'. *Trends in Pharmacological Sciences* 13: 24–28.

Kessler, R. C., Berglund, P., Demler, O., Jin, R., Merikangas, K., et al. (2005). 'Lifetime Prevalence and Age-of-Onset Distributions of DSM-IV Disorders in the National Comorbidity Survey Replication'. *Archives of General Psychiatry* 62: 593–602.

Kiloh, L. G. (1961). 'Pseudo-dementia'. *Acta Psychiatrica Scandinavica* 37: 336–351.

King, D. A., Heisel, M. J., and Lyness, J. M. (2006). 'Assessment and Psychological Treatment of Depression in Older Adults with Terminal or Life-Threatening Illness'. *Clinical Psychology* 12: 339–353.

Knäuper, B. and Wittchen, H.-U.(1994). 'Diagnosing Major Depression in the Elderly: Evidence for Response Bias in Standardized Diagnostic Interviews?' *Journal of Psychiatric Research* 2: 147–164.

Kopetz, S., Steele, C. D., Brandt, J., Baker, A., Kronberg, M., et al. (2000). 'Characteristics and Outcomes of Dementia Residents in an Assisted Living Facility'. *International Journal of Geriatric Psychiatry* 15: 586–593.

Kral, V. A. (1983). 'The Relationship between Senile Dementia (Alzheimer Type) and Depression'. *Canadian Journal of Psychiatry* 28: 304–306.

Krishnan, M. S., O'Brien, J. T., Firbank, M. J., et al. (2006). 'Relationship between Periventricular and Deep White Matter Lesions and Depressive Symptoms in Older People. The LADIS Study'. *International Journal of Geriatric Psychiatry* 21: 983–989.

Kübler-Ross, E. (1970). *On Death and Dying*. London: Tavistock Publications.

Kunik, M. E., Veazey, C., Cully, J. A., Souchek, J., Graham, D. P., et al. (2008). 'COPD Education and Cognitive Behavioral Therapy Group Treatment for Clinically Significant Symptoms of Depression and Anxiety in COPD Patients: A Randomized Controlled Trial'. *Psychological Medicine* 38: 385–396.

Kuo, W. H., Gallo, J. J., and Eaton, W. W. (2004). 'Hopelessness, Depression, Substance Disorder, and Suicidality: A 13-year Community-based Study'. *Social Psychiatry and Psychiatric Epidemiology* 39: 497–501.

Lee, H. B. and Lyketsos, C. G. (2003). 'Depression in Alzheimer's Disease: Heterogeneity and Related Issues'. *Biological Psychiatry* 54: 353–362.

Lesperance, F., Frasure-Smith, N., Koszycki, D., Laliberté, M. A., Van Zyl, L. T., et al. (2007). 'Effects of Citalopram and Interpersonal Psychotherapy on Depression in Patients with Coronary Artery Disease: The Canadian Cardiac Randomized Evaluation of Antidepressant and Psychotherapy Efficacy (CREATE) Trial'. *Journal of the American Medical Association* 297: 367–379.

Levy, B. R., Slade, M. D., Kunkel, S. R., and Kasl, S. V. (2002). 'Longevity Increased by Positive Self-perceptions of Aging'. *Journal of Personality and Social Psychology* 83: 261–270.

Levy, B. R. and Myers, L. M. (2004). 'Preventive Health Behaviors Influenced by Self-perceptions of Aging'. *Preventive Medicine* 39: 625–629.

Levy, M. L., Cummings, J. L., Fairbanks, L. A., Masterman, D., Miller, B. L., et al. (1998). 'Apathy Is Not Depression'. *Journal of Neuropsychiatry and Clinical Neurosciences* 10: 314–319.

Li, Y. S., Meyer, J. S., and Thornby, J. (2001). 'Longitudinal Follow-up of Depressive Symptoms among Normal versus Cognitively Impaired Elderly'. *International Journal of Geriatric Psychiatry* 16: 718–727.

Luber, M. P., Meyers, B. S., Williams-Russo, P. G., et al. (2001). 'Depression and Service Utilization in Elderly Primary Care Patients'. *American Journal of Geriatric Psychiatry* 9: 169–176.

Lyketsos, C. G. and Lee, H. B. (2004). 'Diagnosis and Treatment of Depression in Alzheimer's Disease. A Practical Update for the Clinician'. *Dementia And Geriatric Cognitive Disorders* 17: 55–64.

Lyketsos, C. G., Colenda, C. C., Beck, C., Blank, K., Doraiswamy, M. P., et al. (2006). 'Position Statement of the American Association for Geriatric Psychiatry Regarding Principles of Care for Patients with Dementia Resulting from Alzheimer Disease'. *American Journal of Geriatric Psychiatry* 14: 561–572.

Lyness, J. M., Caine, E. D., Conwell, Y., King, D. A., and Cox, C. (1993). 'Depressive Symptoms, Medical Illness, and Functional Status in Depressed Psychiatric Inpatients'. *American Journal of Psychiatry* 150: 910–915.

Lyness, J. M. (2004). 'End-of-Life Care: Issues Relevant to the Geriatric Psychiatrist'. *American Journal of Geriatric Psychiatry* 12: 457–472.

Lyness, J. M., Niculescu, A., Tu, X., Reynolds, C. F. III, and Caine, E. D. (2006). 'The Relationship of Medical Comorbidity and Depression in Older, Primary Care Patients'. *Psychosomatics* 47: 435–439.

Lyness, J. M., Kim, J., Tang, W., et al. (2007). 'The Clinical Significance of Subsyndromal Depression in Older Primary Care Patients'. *American Journal of Geriatric Psychiatry* 15: 214–223.

Lyness, J. M. (2008). 'Depression and Comorbidity: Objects in the Mirror Are More Complex than they Appear'. *American Journal of Geriatric Psychiatry* 16: 181–15.

Mayberg, H. S., Brannan, S. K., Mahurin, R. K., Jerabek, P. A., Brickman, J., et al. (1997). 'Cingulate Function in Depression: A Potential Predictor of Treatment Response'. *Neuroreport* 8: 1057–1061.

Mayberg, H. S., Lozano, A. M., Voon, V., McNeely, H. E., Seminowicz, D., et al (2005). 'Deep Brain Stimulation for Treatment-resistant Depression'. *Neuron* 45: 651–660.

Mayou, R., Hawton, K., and Feldman, E. (1988). 'What Happens to Medical Patients with Psychiatric Disorder?' *Journal of Psychosomatic Research* 32: 541–549.

Migliorelli, R., Teson, A., Sabe, L., Petracchi, M., Leiguardia, R., et al. (1995). 'Prevalence and Correlates of Dysthymia and Major Depression among Patients with Alzheimer's Disease'. *American Journal of Psychiatry* 152: 37–44.

Miller, G. E., Cohen, S., and Herbert, T. B. (1999). 'Pathways Linking Major Depression and Immunity in Ambulatory Female Patients'. *Psychosomatic Medicine* 61: 850–860.

Munro, C. A., Longmire, C. F., Drye, L. T., et al. (2012). 'Cognitive Outcomes after Sertaline Treatment in Patients with Depression of Alzheimer Disease'. *American Journal of Geriatric Psychiatry* 20: 1036–1044.

Murray, C. J. and Lopez, A. D. (1997). 'Alternative Projections of Mortality and Disability by Cause 1990–2020: Global Burden of Disease Study'. *Lancet* 349: 1498–1504.

Musselman, D. L., Lawson, D. H., Gumnick, J. F., Manatunga, A. K., Penna, S., et al. (2001). 'Paroxetine for the Prevention of Depression Induced by High-dose Interferon Alfa'. *New England Journal of Medicine* 344: 961–966.

Panza, F., Frisardi, V., Capurso, C., D'Introno, A., Colacicco, A. M., et al.(2010). 'Late-life Depression, Mild Cognitive Impairment, and Dementia: Possible Continuum?' *American Journal of Geriatric Psychiatry* 18: 98–116.

Parmelee, P. A., Katz, I. R., and Lawton, M. P. (1992). 'Depression and Mortality among Institutionalized Aged'. *Journal of Gerontology* 47: P3–P10.

Parsons, T. (1951). 'Illness and the Role of the Physician: A Sociological Perspective'. *American Journal of Orthopsychiatry* 21: 452–460.

Patten, S. B., Williams, J. V., Lavorato, D. H., Modgill, G., Jetté, N. et al. (2008). 'Major Depression as a Risk Factor for Chronic Disease Incidence: Longitudinal Analyses in a General Population Cohort'. *General Hospital Psychiatry* 30: 407–413.

Pearson, J. L., Teri, L., Reifler, B. V., and Raskind, M. A. (1989). 'Functional Status and Cognitive Impairment in Alzheimer's Patients With and Without Depression'. *Journal of the American Geriatrics Society* 37: 1117–1121.

Pirkis, J., Ftanou, M., Williamson, M., Machlin A., Spittal, M. J., et al. (2011). 'Australia's Better Access Initiative: An Evaluation'. *Australian and New Zealand Journal of Psychiatry* 45: 726–739.

Raison, C. L. and Miller, A. H. (2003).' Depression in Cancer: New Developments Regarding Diagnosis and Treatment'. *Biological Psychiatry* 54: 283–294.

Rapp, S. R., Parisi, S. A., and Walsh, D. A. (1988). 'Psychological Dysfunction and Physical Health among Elderly Medical Inpatients'. *Journal of Consulting and Clinical Psychology* 56: 851–855.

Reynolds, C. F. III, Dew, M. A., Pollock, B. G., Mulsant, B. H., Frank, E., et al. (2006). 'Maintenance Treatment of Major Depression in Old Age'. *New England Journal of Medicine* 354: 1130–1138.

Richard, E., Reitz, C., Honig, L. H., Schupf, N., Tang, M. X., et al. (2013). 'Late-life Depression, Mild Cognitive Impairment, and Dementia'. *JAMA Neurology* 70: 374–382.

Robins, L. N., Helzer, J. E., Weissman, M. M., Orvaschel, H., Gruenberg, E., et al. (1984). 'Lifetime Prevalence of Specific Psychiatric Disorders in Three Sites'. *Archives of General Psychiatry* 41: 949–958.

Rosal, M. C., Ockene, J. K., Ma, Y., Herbert, J. R., Merriam, P. A., et al. (2001). 'Behavioral Risk Factors among Members of a Health Maintenance Organization'. *Preventive Medicine* 33: 586–594.

Roxanas, M., Hibbert, E., and Field, M. (2007). 'Venlafaxine Hyponatraemia: Incidence, Mechanism and Management'. *Australian and New Zealand Journal of Psychiatry* 41: 411–418.

Sapolsky, R. M. (1996). 'Why Stress is Bad for your Brain'. *Science* 273: 749–750.

Scott, K. M., Bruffaerts, R., Tsang, A., Ormel, A., Alonso, J., et al. (2007). 'Depression–Anxiety Relationships with Chronic Physical Conditions: Results from the World Mental Health Surveys'. *Journal of Affective Disorders* 103: 113–120.

Scott, K. M., Von Korff, M., Alonso, J., Angermeyer, M., Bromet, E. J., et al. (2008). 'Age Patterns in the Prevalence of DSM-IV Depressive/Anxiety Disorders with and without Physical Co-morbidity'. *Psychological Medicine* 38: 1659–1669.

Serebruany, V. L., Glassman, A. H., Malinin, A. I., Nemeroff, C. B., Musselman, D. L., et al. (2003). 'Platelet/Endothelial Biomarkers in Depressed Patients Treated with the Selective Serotonin Reuptake Inhibitor Sertraline after Acute Coronary Events: The Sertraline AntiDepressant Heart Attack Randomized Trial (SADHART) Platelet Substudy'. *Circulation* 108: 939–944.

Smith, G. C. (2003). 'The Future of Consultation-liaison Psychiatry'. *Australian and New Zealand Journal of Psychiatry* 37: 150–159.

Snowdon, J. (2012). 'Tailored Treatment for Depression with Co-morbid Dementia'. *Australian and New Zealand Journal of Psychiatry* 46: 678–679.

Sörensen, J., Sörensen, J. B., Skovgaard, T., Bredahl, T., and Puggaard, L. (2011). 'Exercise on Prescription: Changes in Physical Activity and Health-related Quality of Life in Five Danish Programmes'. *European Journal of Public Health* 21: 56–62.

Stapelberg, N. J., Neumann, D. L., Shum, D. H., Mcconnell, H., and Hamilton-Craig, I. (2011). 'A Topographical Map of the Causal Network of Mechanisms Underlying the Relationship between Major Depressive Disorder and Coronary Heart Disease'. *Australian and New Zealand Journal of Psychiatry* 45: 351–369.

Starkstein, S. E., Robinson, R. G., Berthier, M. L., Parikh, R. M., and Price, T. R. (1988). 'Differential Mood Changes Following Basal Ganglia vs Thalamic Lesions'. *Archives of Neurology* 45: 725–730.

Steffens, D. C., Payne, M. E., Greenberg, D. L., Byrum, C. E., Welsh-Bohmer, K. A., et al. (2002). 'Hippocampal Volume and Incident Dementia in Geriatric Depression'. *American Journal of Geriatric Psychiatry* 10: 62–71.

Stunkard, A. J., Faith, M. S., and Allison, K. C. (2003). 'Depression and Obesity'. *Biological Psychiatry* 54: 330–337.

Sullivan, M., Katon, W., Russo, J., Dobie, R., and Sakai, C. (1993). 'A Randomized Trial of Nortriptyline for Severe Chronic Tinnitus. Effects on Depression, Disability, and Tinnitus Symptoms'. *Archives of Internal Medicine* 153: 2251–2259.

Sullivan, M. D., Lacroix, A. Z., Spertus, J. A., and Hecht, J. (2000). 'Five-year Prospective Study of the Effects of Anxiety and Depression in Patients with Coronary Artery Disease'. *American Journal of Cardiology* 86: 1135–1138, A6, A9.

Sutin, A. R., Terracciano, A., Milaneschi, Y., An, Y., Ferrucci, L., et al. (2013). 'The Trajectory of Depressive Symptoms across the Adult Life Span'. *JAMA Psychiatry* 70: 803–811.

Travis, L. A., Lyness, J. M., Shields, C. G., King, D. A., and Cox, C. (2004). 'Social Support, Depression, and Functional Disability in Older Adult Primary-care Patients'. *American Journal of Geriatric Psychiatry* 12: 265–271.

Trockel, M., Burg, M., Jaffe, A., Barbour, K., and Taylor, C. B. (2008). 'Smoking Behavior Postmyocardial Infarction among ENRICHD Trial Participants: Cognitive Behavior Therapy Intervention for Depression and Low Perceived Social Support Compared with Care as Usual'. *Psychosomatic Medicine* 70: 875–882.

Unutzer, J., Patrick, D. L., Diehr, P., Simon, G., Grembowski, D., et al. (2000). 'Quality Adjusted Life Years in Older Adults with Depressive Symptoms and Chronic Medical Disorders'. *International Psychogeriatrics* 12: 15–33.

Unutzer, J., Patrick, D. L., Marmon, T., Simon, G. E., and Katon, W. J. (2002). 'Depressive Symptoms and Mortality in a Prospective Study of 2,558 Older Adults'. *American Journal of Geriatric Psychiatry* 10: 521–530.

Von Korff, M., Ormel, J., Katon, W., and Lin, E. H. (1992). 'Disability and Depression among High Utilizers of Health Care. A Longitudinal Analysis'. *Archives of General Psychiatry* 49: 91–100.

Watson, M., Haviland, J. S., Greer, S., Davidson, J., and Bliss, J. M. (1999). 'Influence of Psychological Response on Survival in Breast Cancer: A Population-based Cohort Study'. *Lancet* 354: 1331–1336.

Weintraub, D. and Burn, D. J. (2011). 'Parkinson's Disease: The Quintessential Neuropsychiatric Disorder'. *Movement Disorders* 26: 1022–1031.

Wells, K. B., Golding, J. M., and Burnam, M. A. (1988). 'Psychiatric Disorder in a Sample of the General Population With and Without Chronic Medical Conditions'. *American Journal of Psychiatry* 145: 976–981.

Williams, J. W., Jr, Katon, W., Lin, E. H., Noël, P. H., Worchel, J., et al. (2004). 'The Effectiveness of Depression Care Management on Diabetes-related Outcomes in Older Patients'. *Annals of Internal Medicine* 140: 1015–1024.

World Health Organization (2008). *The Global Burden of Disease: 2004 Update*. Geneva: WHO.

Wulsin, L. R., Vaillant, G. E., and Wells, V. E. (1999). 'A Systematic Review of the Mortality of Depression'. *Psychosomatic Medicine* 61: 6–17.

Zahodne, L. B., Devanand, D. P., and Stern, Y. (2013). 'Coupled Cognitive and Functional Change in Alzheimer's Disease and the Influence of Depressive Symptoms'. *Journal of Alzheimer's Disease* 34: 851–860.

Zlokovic, B. V. (2011). 'Neurovascular Pathways to Neurodegeneration in Alzheimer's Disease and Other Disorders'. *Nature Reviews. Neuroscience* 12: 723–738.

Zubenko, G. S., Marino, L. J., Jr, Sweet, R. A., Rifai, A. H., Mulsant, B. H., et al. (1997). 'Medical Comorbidity in Elderly Psychiatric Inpatients'. *Biological Psychiatry* 41: 724–736.

Zubenko, G. S., Zubenko, W. N., Mcpherson, S., Spoor, E., Marin, D. B., et al. (2003). 'A Collaborative Study of the Emergence and Clinical Features of the Major Depressive Syndrome of Alzheimer's Disease'. *American Journal of Psychiatry* 160: 857–866.

CHAPTER 22

....

LATE-LIFE ANXIETY

....

BEYON MILOYAN, GERARD J. BYRNE, AND NANCY A. PACHANA

Introduction

ANXIETY ranks among the most pressing public health issues today. Anxiety disorders are associated with high levels of service use in the general population, and studies across the globe suggest that anxiety disorders cause considerable economic burden (Andlin-Sobocki and Wittchen 2005; Brenes et al. 2005, 2008; De Beurs et al. 1999; Greenberg et al. 1999; Oliva-Moreno, Lopez-Bastida, and Y Montejo 2006; Porensky et al. 2009; Smit et al. 2006; Teeson et al. 2011; Vasiliadis et al. 2013; Wang et al. 2005; Wetherell et al. 2004). Untreated anxiety disorders may also impose great societal burden due to reduced levels of individual productivity and increased levels of care required by others (Candilis and Pollack 1997; Hoffman, Dukes, and Wittchen 2008). In addition to chronicity and persistence, clinical anxiety is associated with a number of cognitive and somatic symptoms, distress, and disability. Due to age-related changes in anxiety, with respect to aetiology and prevalence, there are significant challenges in the management of anxiety disorders among older adults. This chapter will begin by reviewing age-related changes in the prevalence, phenomenology, and clinical significance of anxiety, consider biological factors (neuroanatomical and genetic correlates) associated with anxiety, and deal with the various contexts and settings in and around which late-life anxiety most frequently occurs. Finally, treatment approaches for anxiety in later life, and their efficacy, will be reviewed.

Prevalence

Baxter et al. (2013) recently performed a systematic review and meta-regression of eighty-seven studies across forty-four countries in order to estimate global trends in the prevalence of anxiety disorders. The results of the analysis revealed that the current global prevalence of anxiety disorders is 7.3%, and higher (10.4%) among developed (i.e. Anglo/European) compared to developing (i.e. African) nations (5.3%). The authors of this study used the term 'current' to refer to any estimate between point prevalence and three-month prevalence on grounds that such estimates were statistically similar. Given the chronicity of anxiety disorder, we will adopt the term 'current' to refer to any estimate between point-prevalence and twelve-month prevalence in this chapter.

In terms of age, epidemiological studies have found that there is a decrease in the lifetime prevalence of mental health disorders in general, and particularly anxiety disorders, after middle age and into older adulthood (Kessler et al. 2005). Nonetheless, anxiety disorders are among the most highly prevalent mental health disorders in older adults (Bryant, Jackson, and Ames 2008; Byers et al. 2010; Kessler et al. 2005), with a range of current prevalence estimates reported across the globe: 5.4%, Australia; 7%, US; 10.2%, Netherlands; and 14.2%, France (Australian Bureau of Statistics 2007; Beekman et al. 1998; Gum, King-Kallimanis, and Kohn 2009; Ritchie et al. 2004). Although age-related decreases in prevalence have evaded a straightforward explanation, it appears that there are a number of age-related changes which pose challenges to the detection and diagnosis of late-life anxiety disorders.

Phenomenology

One such challenge in the identification of anxiety disorders pertains to age-related changes in the phenomenology of anxiety-related processes. First, older adults tend to worry less frequently than younger adults do (Basevitz et al. 2008; Gonçalves and Byrne 2013; Gould and Edelstein 2010; Hunt, Wisocki, and Yanko 2003). Older adults also ascribe less functional value to worrying and utilize fewer coping strategies to attempt to control their worries (Basevitz et al. 2008; Hunt et al. 2003). Second, older adults tend to worry more about the health and welfare of loved ones, whereas younger adults tend to worry more about work, finances, and interpersonal relations (Gonçalves and Byrne 2013; Lindesay et al. 2006; Powers, Wisocki, and Whitbourne 1992).

A qualitatively distinct set of symptoms has been found to distinguish older adults with and without a GAD diagnosis compared to young and middle-aged adults, and numerically fewer symptoms have also been found to distinguish older adults with and without GAD compared to younger age groups (Miloyan, Byrne, and Pachana 2014). Similar age-related changes have been observed in other types of anxiety as well. For instance, older adults with post-traumatic stress disorder (PTSD) report lower symptom severity relative to younger adults (Bottche, Kuwert, and Knaevelsrud 2012; Frueh et al. 2004). Older adults experience fewer symptoms of panic, and panic attacks are reported to be less intense and shorter in duration compared to those in younger adults; and older adults with late-onset panic attacks report fewer panic symptoms than both younger and older adults with early-onset panic attacks (Deer and Calamari 1998). Considered together, these findings suggest that older adulthood is associated with quantitative and qualitative changes in anxiety, such that older adults endorse numerically fewer and distinctive types of anxiety symptoms.

Clinical Significance

The term 'clinical significance' typically refers to the extent to which psychiatric symptoms cause impairment. In order to constitute a disorder, anxiety symptoms should be associated with significant levels of disability and/or distress. As such, late-life anxiety is associated with diminished well-being, impaired social functioning, reduced life satisfaction, poor general and health-related quality of life (QOL), and increased risk of physical and functional disability (Brenes et al. 2005; Bryant, Jackson, and Ames 2009; Mendlowicz and Stein 2000; Henning et al. 2007; Porensky et al. 2009; Wetherell et al. 2004). Anxiety is also associated with suicidal feelings, suicide attempts, and excess risk of mortality (Brenes et al. 2007; Jonson et al. 2012; Nepon Belik, Bolton, and Sareen 2010; Tully, Baker, and Knight 2008; Van Hout et al. 2004).

At the moment, however, age-related changes in the contribution of anxiety symptoms to disability and distress remain unclear. As noted in the previous section, older adults typically endorse fewer and less severe symptoms compared with younger adults. At the same time, however, older adults represent the highest proportion of the population with a physical disability (Brault 2012; Lenze et al. 2001). Moreover, older adults with anxiety have been found to report higher levels of disability than younger adults with anxiety, even after controlling for socio-demographic variables and medical conditions (Brenes et al. 2008). Consistent with these findings, the results of a recent study indicated that subthreshold anxiety was highly prevalent among older adults, and associated with similar health characteristics when compared with an age-matched threshold group (Grenier et al. 2011). These findings suggest that the fewer number of symptoms endorsed by older adults may suffice to account for significant levels of physical/functional disability. Due to higher rates of disability among older adults, the threshold for clinical impairment might be lower in older adults (See Figure 22.1). More work is needed to investigate age-related changes in anxiety symptoms and disability.

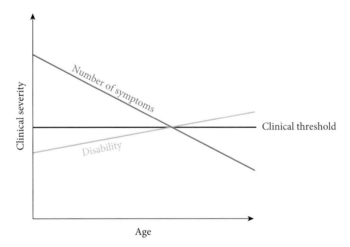

FIGURE 22.1 Age-related decreases in the number/severity of anxiety symptoms might account for decreased prevalence of anxiety disorders in older adults. However, older adults with subclinical anxiety symptoms are similar to clinical groups in terms of health characteristics (Grenier et al. 2011). Moreover, disability is more highly prevalent among older adults compared to younger adults (Brault 2012; Lenze et al. 2001). Therefore, due to higher susceptibility to disability, fewer symptoms might suffice to account for clinically significant anxiety among older adults.

Biological Factors

Genetic correlates

Genetic studies have found that 30–40% of the variance contributing to anxiety disorders is heritable (Norrholm and Ressler 2009). In a study of 10 566 individuals (M_{age} = 62, R = 55–74) from the Swedish Twin Registry, one-third of the genetic influence on GAD was shared with neuroticism, suggesting that anxiety might be at least partly accounted for by genetic predisposition to certain personality traits (Mackintosh et al. 2006).

Mutations in the glucocorticoid receptor gene, which impair regulation of the hypothalamus-pituitary-adrenal (HPA) axis, have been found to reduce anxiety and create an impaired response pattern toward stress in mice (Tronche et al. 1999). The role of the HPA axis in generating emotional behaviours, and specifically anxiety-related behaviours, might partially explain these findings. Polymorphisms in the human serotonin transporter gene (5-HTTLPR) have also been implicated in anxiety symptoms and disorders (Lesch et al. 1996). The same gene has been found to be associated with hyperactive amygdala responses toward fearful stimuli as measured by functional magnetic resonance imaging (fMRI), and to play an important role in modulating amygdala reactivity toward environmental threat (Hariri et al. 2002, 2005).

Neuroanatomical correlates

An emerging body of research is beginning to reveal the key neural substrates underlying fear and anxiety in humans. Largely implicated is a network of emotional brain sectors including, most notably, the amygdala and portions of the prefrontal cortex (PFC). The amygdala is involved in the acquisition and expression of conditioned fear responses across species (LeDoux 1995, 2000), and, more specifically, in the development of phobic fear and anxiety in humans (Bishop 2008; Indovina et al. 2010). Patients with bilateral damage to the amygdala fail to trigger a fear response to threatening stimuli in the external environment (Feinstein et al. 2011). In fact, damage to the amygdala has been found to protect against PTSD in a sample of combat veterans (Koenigs et al. 2008b). The amygdala shares strong reciprocal connections with the ventromedial prefrontal cortex (vmPFC) (Ongur and Price 2000), which has also been found to play a critical role in anxiety. It has been suggested that the ventral PFC (vPFC) biases attention to threat-related responses based on relevant input from the amygdala (Bishop 2007; Indovina et al. 2010). In line with this interpretation, which favours a role for the vPFC in the maintenance of anxiety, early case reports of psychiatric patients indicated marked reductions in anxiety and associated somatic symptoms following prefrontal leucotomy (Moniz 1936; Steele 1951). More recently, human lesion studies have demonstrated that damage to the vmPFC—a heterogeneous brain sector comprised of medial portions of orbitofrontal cortex (OFC) and ventral portions of medial prefrontal cortex—confers resistance to PTSD and depression in humans (Koenigs et al. 2008a, 2008b).

Contexts and Settings

Primary care and nursing homes

Primary care

Primary care is emerging as a key context for diagnosis and intervention with older adults with elevated anxiety levels. A US-based study randomly sampled 965 patients (M_{age} = 47, R = 18–87) across fifteen primary care clinics, and employed two mental health professionals to make diagnoses based on the Structured Clinical Interview for DSM-IV (SCID) (Kroenke et al. 2007). The study estimated current prevalence of anxiety disorders among primary care patients to be 19.5%, with PTSD (8.6%), GAD (7.6%), panic disorder (6.8%), and social anxiety disorder (6.2%) the most prevalent subtypes. Anxiety frequently co-occurred with depressive and somatic symptoms, and was associated with a comorbid depressive disorder. Of patients with an anxiety disorder, 41% reported that they were not currently receiving treatment, consistent with the results of a study conducted in the Netherlands, which indicated that a large number of primary care patients expressed a need for counselling and information regarding their anxiety and/or depression (Prins et al. 2009).

Two European studies have found comparable estimates. In the first study, 2316 patients (approximately 30% of whom were older adults) were randomly sampled across eighty-six primary care settings in Belgium. Diagnoses were made using the Primary Care Evaluation of Mental Disorders (PRIME-MD), which consists of a patient questionnaire and a structured interview administered by the primary care physician. The estimated prevalence of anxiety disorders was, as in the previous study, 19%. In the second study, 13 677 patients (M_{age} = 50; SD = 17.3) aged 18 years and older were randomly sampled across 300 primary care clinics (Ansseau et al. 2005). Diagnoses were made by the primary care physician using the Mini Neuropsychiatric Interview (MINI). The estimated prevalence of GAD was 8.3%, similar to the aforementioned US study. Living alone, being unemployed, and having a low level of education have also been found to be associated with anxiety among patients in primary care (Ansseau et al. 2008). However, it is important to note that all of these studies evaluated participants of a wide age range. Thus, a better understanding of the prevalence and correlates of anxiety disorders among older adults in primary care settings is still needed.

Regarding efficacy of treatments for anxious older adults in primary care, cognitive-behavioural therapy (CBT) has demonstrated improvements in worry severity, depressive symptoms, and overall mental health relative to enhanced usual care (Richards et al. 2003; Stanley et al. 2009). Participants who felt that they understood the treatment reported higher levels of satisfaction with their treatment (Hundt et al. 2013). Computer-based CBT treatments and self-help treatments appear promising; however, more rigorous investigation is required before determining whether such programmes could be routinely implemented (Bower, Richards, and Lovell 2001; Craske et al. 2009; Hoifodt et al. 2011). These studies were not without limitation. In one study, participants were self-referred from an insurance-based care provider, and therapy was administered in person for approximately one hour per week, which is typically not the case for primary care patients (Stanley et al. 2009). In the other study, patients were included based on distress ratings, and attrition rates were markedly high (Richards et al. 2003).

Nursing homes

Anxiety in long-term care settings has only recently been the subject of systematic investigations. Two European studies by Smalbrugge et al. (2005a, 2005b) assessed occurrence and risk factors associated with anxiety among 333 nursing home patients (M_{age} = 79 years, R = 55–99) in the Netherlands. Diagnoses were made using the Schedules for Clinical Assessment in Neuropsychiatry (SCAN). Current prevalence for anxiety disorders (5.7%), comorbid anxiety and depression (5.1%), subthreshold anxiety (4.2%), and anxiety symptoms (29.7%) were estimated. Anxiety disorders were correlated with history of stroke, cognitive impairment, depression, and perceived lack of adequate care; comorbid anxiety and depression were correlated with advancing age and lack of social support; and anxiety symptoms were associated with education, health-related characteristics, and a negative life event within the past year.

Neurologic comorbidities

Anxiety is highly prevalent among older adults with neurological conditions; however, formal diagnosis of anxiety in some neurologic populations (e.g. Parkinson's disease [PD]) is challenging due to considerable overlap of symptoms. This portion of the review will focus on anxiety in two neurologic populations (Alzheimer's disease [AD] and PD) where anxiety has been studied in some depth. See also chapter on 'Neuropsychiatric Approaches to Working with Older People' in this Handbook.

Cognitive impairment, Alzheimer's disease, and dementia

Symptoms of anxiety frequently co-occur with mild cognitive impairment (MCI) and AD, and have been reported to range in prevalence from 47% to 50% in MCI, and 48–70% in AD (Ferretti et al. 2001; Gallagher et al. 2011; Geda et al. 2008; Mega et al. 1996; Palmer et al. 2007; Teri et al. 1999). Symptoms and disorders of anxiety are also associated with poorer cognitive and functional performance in these groups (Beaudreau and O'Hara 2008; Butters et al. 2011; Teri et al. 1999). Self-report measures have been found to be suboptimal for use with persons with significant cognitive impairment, in which case informant reports are preferable, particularly for visibly observable symptoms (McDade-Montez et al. 2008). The impact of anxiety symptoms as a risk factor for AD incidence and cognitive decline has also been examined, with conflicting results. Current anxiety has been found to be associated with an increased risk of incident cognitive impairment, cognitive decline, and incident AD, and a lifetime diagnosis of anxiety disorder has been found to predict incident dementia (Burton et al. 2012; Palmer et al. 2007; Potvin et al. 2011; Sinoff and Werner 2003). Moreover, persistent worrying has been found to be associated with a five-fold increase in the risk of incident AD among patients with MCI (Palmer et al. 2007). In contrast to these findings, however, one study found that trait anxiety is associated with a lower risk of conversion from MCI to AD (Devier et al. 2009). The discrepancy between the two sets of findings might be explained by the observation that MCI in the latter study was identified retrospectively, such that participants were recruited from a memory clinic prior to the publication of MCI criteria.

Parkinson's disease

Current prevalence of anxiety disorders in PD ranges from 25% to 43%, and one study has esti-mated lifetime prevalence at 49% (Dissanayaka et al. 2010; Leentjens et al. 2011; Pontone et al. 2009). Both anxiety disorders and symptoms are common, with one study indicating current prevalence estimates of 34% and 11.4%, respectively (Leentjens et al. 2011). Anxiety is posi-tively correlated with PD severity and motor impairments, and is especially prevalent among patients with postural and gait dysfunction (Dissanayaka et al. 2010; Leentjens et al. 2011; Pontone et al. 2009). A twelve-year prospective longitudinal study of 35 815 male health profes-sionals reported that those with higher levels of anxiety were found to have a 1.5 times greater relative risk of incident PD (Weisskopf et al. 2003). Comorbid anxiety and depression are also common in PD, and motor impairments may contribute to challenges in the identification and treatment of anxiety and depression (Aarsland, Marsh, and Schrag 2009; Dissanayaka et al. 2010; Menza, Robertson-Hoffman, and Bonapace 1993). It has been suggested that CBT is an effective treatment approach for anxiety and depression in PD (Pachana et al. 2013).

Psychiatric comorbidity

Late-life anxiety disorders have been reported to be more highly prevalent in outpatient care settings (e.g. primary care, private practice) as compared with inpatient psychiatric settings and in community-based samples (Ansseau et al. 2005; Australian Bureau of Statistics 2007; Beekman et al. 1998; Gum, King-Kallimanis, and Kohn 2009; Kroenke et al. 2007; Ritchie et al. 2004; Smalbrugge et al. 2005a, 2005b). However, anxiety symptoms are highly preva-lent in inpatient settings, and frequently co-occur with other psychiatric and medical condi-tions (Smalbrugge et al. 2005a, 2005b).

Depression

Anxiety and depression are highly comorbid in late-life, and are associated with poor detection and treatment outcomes, and poor quality of life (Almeida et al. 2012). Consistently high rates of comorbid anxiety and depression among older adults raise ques-tions about the degree of convergence between aspects of anxiety and depression in late-life. A recent study utilized structural equation modelling to examine the factor structure of neuroticism, anxiety, and depressive symptoms in 335 participants ranging across the adult lifespan (18–93 years; Teachman, Siedlecki, and Magee 2007). A three-factor model com-prised of negative affect, low positive affect, and arousal was found to be (1) the best fit for all age groups and (2) age invariant (the factor structure reflected the same underlying traits in the sample regardless of age), indicating that anxiety and depression remain largely consist-ent throughout the lifespan and represent distinct clinical entities that withstand age-related changes in presentation and symptomatology (See Figure 22.2).

Nonetheless, the high rate of comorbidity between anxiety and depression in late-life continues to raise important questions about the high degree of convergence between these disorders. For instance, a large-scale community-based study in the Netherlands investigated risk factors for anxiety–depression comorbidity in a sample of 3056 older adults (M_{age} = 71 years, 58% female) (Beekman et al. 2000). Of participants with anxiety

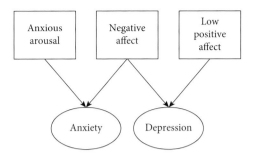

FIGURE 22.2 The factor structure of Clark and Watson's (1991) tripartite model of anxiety and depression has been found to be age invariant (Teachman, Siedlecki, and Magee 2007), which suggests that it represents a good conceptual model of anxiety and depression across the lifespan.

disorders, 26.1% met criteria for a comorbid major depressive disorder, and of those with major depressive disorder 47.5% met criteria for a comorbid anxiety disorder. Despite this high level of comorbidity, the constellations of risk factors for each disorder were markedly different. Significant risk factors associated with anxiety disorders included a host of stress and vulnerability factors, whereas major depression was associated with younger age and external locus of control. Importantly, past depressive episodes may also contribute to onset of late-life anxiety disorders (Huk et al. 2011).

General Medical Comorbidity

Chronic obstructive pulmonary disease (COPD)

Wilgoss and Yohannes (2013) recently conducted a systematic review of anxiety disorders in COPD. They reported that the prevalence of clinical anxiety ranged from 10% to 55% among COPD patients. Though it is important to note that the review article was not selectively concerned with older adults, all but one of the studies included in the review reported a mean age greater than 60. Moreover, these findings coincide with the results of a previous systematic review by the same authors assessing mood and anxiety symptoms among older adults with COPD (Yohannes, Baldwin, and Connolly 2000). This review article reported that the prevalence of anxiety symptoms ranged from 13% to 55%, with the exception of one study, which estimated prevalence to be 2% using the STAI. Overall, these findings suggest that anxiety is highly prevalent among older adults with COPD.

Cardiovascular diseases

Anxiety disorders are common among older adults with cardiovascular diseases (Grenier et al. 2012). In a Canadian sample of 2811 community-dwelling older adults with cardiovascular diseases, the twelve-month prevalence of anxiety disorders (5.1%) and subthreshold anxiety (14.8%) were estimated. Obsessive compulsive disorder (35%), GAD (29%), and specific phobias (29%) were the most common anxiety disorders. The most common sub-threshold anxiety disorders were specific phobias (53.8%), agoraphobia (50.5%), and panic disorder (20.9%). Sex (female), high blood pressure, and depressive disorders were sig-nificant predictors of anxiety in this sample of older adults with cardiovascular diseases. A ten-year longitudinal study assessed GAD-related risk of adverse outcomes among 438 participants with myocardial infarctions, 414 without GAD (M_{age} = 61), and 24 with GAD (M_{age} = 58) (Roest, Zuidersma, and De Jonge 2012). GAD was associated with an almost two-fold risk of mortality and cardiovascular-related hospital readmission. In terms of mental health, physical activity has been found to be negatively associated with mental health disorders and positively associated with survival and well-being among older adults (Goodwin 2003; Scarmeas et al. 2011). In terms of cardiovascular health, aerobic physical activity has been found to reduce the risk of myocardial infarctions (Chomistek et al. 2011; Fransson et al. 2004; Lakka 1994). Physical activity may thus serve as a preventative factor against the detrimental effects of anxiety and some frequently co-occurring general medical conditions.

Care-giving

Cross-sectional studies in the US and Europe demonstrate that older adult female care-givers of patients with AD and dementia score significantly above normative levels for their age group on a host of psychiatric symptoms, including anxiety and obsessive-compulsive symptoms (Anthony-Bergstone, Zarit, and Gatz 1988; Cooper, Balamurali, and Livingston 2007; Sansoni, Vellone, and Piras 2004). High anxiety and depression are positively cor-related with hours of care and care-giver physical and psychological illness, and negatively correlated with level of education and time for leisure activities (Anthony-Bergstone et al. 1988; Sansoni et al. 2004). Longitudinal studies of spousal care-givers of AD patients indi-cate marked increases in the portion of care-givers who report significant anxiety symptoms between baseline and follow-up (one and a half years), and these symptoms are correlated with physical illness and frequency of recent doctor visits among care-givers (Vitaliano et al. 1991). Interestingly, anxiety levels and subjective burden among care-givers of individuals with MCI are lower than those normally reported in care-givers of AD patients, consistent with the blunted severity of MCI relative to AD (Garand et al. 2005, 2012). Thus, care-giver burden and anxiety may increase in proportion to care recipients' degree of impairment.

A recent systematic review indicated an overall increase in levels of psychological distress, symptoms of anxiety and depression, and physical health problems among care-givers of cancer patients (Stenberg, Ruland, and Miaskowski 2010). Further analysis of the frequency of subjectively reported emotional problems by care-givers included: persistent anxiety, anxiety for own health, worry, fear, and uncertainty, as well as helping care recipients deal with anxiety and depression regarding their condition. Overall, anxiety symptoms appear to be significantly greater among older adult care-givers than among non-care-givers (Russo et al. 1995). Additionally, care-givers who live with care recipients appear more likely to be anxious, whereas care-givers who do not live with care recipients appear more likely to be depressed. Notably, care-givers reporting greater burden and distress are more likely to place their care recipient in long-term care (Schulz et al. 2004). However, those care-givers who place their care recipient in long-term care report comparably high depression and anxiety scores at baseline and follow-up. Thus, care-giver anxiety seems unlikely to subside by placing a care recipient in long-term care. Taken together, these studies indicate that psychiatric symptoms in general, and specifically anxiety, are highly prevalent among care-givers. Moreover, these results suggest that care-giving responsibilities in old age lead to notable increases in anxiety symptoms and reductions in self-rated health. For more on care-giving, see the chapter on that topic in this Handbook.

TREATMENT APPROACHES

Pharmacotherapy has been found to be efficacious for treating late-life anxiety disorders. A recent meta-analytic study of nine pharmacotherapy trials found that these studies had a moderate pooled effect for treating late-life GAD (Gonçalves and Byrne 2012). Clinicians have been cautioned against using benzodiazepines due to the observation that they are associated with potentially costly risks (e.g. falls and increased confusion, Allain et al. 2005; Ray, Thapa, and Gideon 2000). Therefore, selective serotonin reuptake inhibitor (SSRI) and serotonin-norepinephrine reuptake inhibitor (SNRI) anti-depressants, which appear to be associated with fewer adverse risks, are preferred. A series of five RCTs in the US and Europe explored the efficacy of an SNRI anti-depressant (Venlafaxine ER) for treating GAD in younger ($\leq$ 60 years) and older ($\geq$ 60 years) adults (Katz et al. 2002). There were no age effects on treatment and no age-by-treatment interactions, such that similar proportions of younger and older adults showed comparable treatment effects. These findings suggest that pharmacotherapy, and more specifically SNRIs, can be an effective and relatively safe option for treating late-life anxiety disorders. However, it is important to note that SNRIs might not be a feasible option for all older adults due to possible adverse interactions with other medications.

Although the first randomized controlled trial (RCT) that compared the efficacy of SSRI, CBT, and a waitlist control condition found that CBT was significantly more efficacious than both other conditions for treating late-life anxiety disorders (GAD, panic disorder, agoraphobia, or social phobia) (Schuurmans et al. 2006), the results of more recent meta-analyses suggest that CBT and pharmacotherapy share similar effect sizes for treating late-life anxiety disorders (Gonçalves and Byrne 2012; Thorp et al. 2009).

A review of seventeen evidence-based psychological treatment studies for late-life anxiety recently concluded that CBT was more efficacious than relaxation therapy, supportive therapy, and cognitive therapy (Ayers et al. 2007). However, it is important to note that there was only limited support for the efficacy of CBT for improving subjective anxiety symptoms. The study also concluded that relaxation training might represent an effective and low-cost option. More recently, the authors of two meta-analyses and a review article all concluded that CBT is moderately and significantly more effective than waitlist or usual care control conditions in treating anxiety (Gonçalves and Byrne 2012; Hendricks et al. 2008; Nordhus and Pallesen 2003). However, when compared with other active treatments the effectiveness of CBT is negligible. Taken together, these findings suggest that pharmacotherapy and active forms of psychological treatment in general are equally effective in treating late-life anxiety disorders.

There is an important need for more research in determining appropriate treatment approaches for anxiety in later life. Some authors have recommended that existing CBT treatments be modified for use in older adults due to cohort effects, changes in life circumstances, and co-occurrence of physical and general medical conditions (Laidlaw, Thompson, and Gallagher-Thompson 2004; Laidlaw and McAlpine 2008). The proposed modifications include greater emphasis on treatment rationale, clarifying differences between typically passive medical treatment and collaborative CBT treatment, correcting misconceptions about psychotherapy, carrying out the intervention at a slower pace, and increased use of reminders due to memory impairments (Ladouceur et al. 2004; Pachana, Woodward, and Byrne 2007). Additionally, given the varied circumstances surrounding late-life anxiety, interventions that can be flexibly administered would most likely have the greatest utility (e.g. McMurchie et al. 2013). More research is needed to evaluate the efficacy of combined psychological and pharmacological interventions for treating late-life anxiety.

Research assessing the effect of lifestyle factors on late-life anxiety is also wanting. One study using nationally representative data found that individuals aged 15–54 in the US who reported regular physical activity had a lower prevalence of mental disorders (Goodwin 2003). Physical exercise has also been found to be mildly efficacious for reducing anxiety symptoms (Herring, O'Connor, and Dishman 2010). However, the first study excluded older adults and the second study assessed adults across the entire lifespan. Therefore, the extent to which physical activity might confer mental health benefits for older adults remains unclear.

IMPLICATIONS FOR PRACTICE

Due to high rates of anxiety in numerous medical contexts, active screening of older adults across a range of medical settings (e.g. older adults visiting primary care settings, spouses and care-givers of older adults with cognitive impairment and/or other medical conditions) is highly recommended. Older care-givers of family members in medical settings also represent a particularly vulnerable group, and the development and implementation of appropriate interventions for this group represents a major priority. In assessing older adults, clinicians are likely to benefit from utilization of self- and informant-report measures to assess non-visible (i.e. mental and phenomenal) and visible (i.e. somatic and behavioural) symptoms, respectively, when screening for late-life anxiety (McDade-Montez et al. 2008). Interventions that can be flexibly administered, and which are tailored specifically to older adults, are likely to be most effective.

SUMMARY

This chapter reviewed age-related changes in the prevalence, phenomenology, and clinical significance of late-life anxiety. Anxiety disorders become less prevalent after middle age and into older adulthood, but it remains unclear whether this is accurate, or whether this decrease in prevalence can be explained by the fact that age-related changes in phenomenology and clinical significance are not accounted for in the diagnostic criteria. In terms of phenomenology, older adults tend to endorse fewer symptoms of anxiety. These symptoms are reported to be less severe in nature than those reported by younger adults, and there are also qualitative differences in the symptoms endorsed by young and older adults. In terms of clinical significance, older adults appear to be more vulnerable to disability and less vulnerable to distress. Therefore, even though older adults report numerically fewer and less severe symptoms, these might suffice to contribute to clinically significant levels of disability. High levels of distress among older adults, on the other hand, might represent more severe forms of anxiety. This chapter also reviewed the prevalence and correlates of late-life anxiety in a number of medical and social contexts. Late-life anxiety frequently co-occurs with depression, cognitive impairment, dementia, general medical conditions, and care-giving responsibilities, and is markedly prevalent among older adults in medical settings such as primary care and nursing homes. Finally, more research is needed to refine psychological approaches, and to evaluate the efficacy of combined psychological and pharmacological interventions, for treating anxiety disorders in later life.

KEY REFERENCES AND SOURCES FOR FURTHER READING

Ayers, C. R., Sorrell, J. T., Thorp, S. R., and Wetherell, J. L. (2007). 'Evidence-based Psychological Treatments for Late-life Anxiety'. *Psychology and Aging* 22: 8–17.

Beck, J. G. (2005). 'Cognitive Aspects of Anxiety and Depression in the Elderly'. *Current Psychiatry Reports* 7: 27–31.

Bishop, S. J. (2007). 'Neurocognitive Mechanisms of Anxiety: An Integrative Account'. *Trends in Cognitive Sciences* 11: 307–316.

Hendricks, G. J., Oude Voshaar, R. C., Keijsers, G. P., Hoogduin, C. A., and Van Balkom, A. J. (2008). 'Cognitive-behavioural Therapy for Late-life Anxiety Disorders: A Systematic Review and Meta-analysis'. *Acta Psychiatrica Scandinavica* 117: 403–411.

Lenze, E. J. and Wetherell, J. L. (2009). 'Bringing the Bedside to the Bench, and then to the Community: A Prospectus for Intervention Research in Late-life Anxiety Disorders'. *International Journal of Geriatric Psychiatry* 24: 1–14.

Mohlman, J., Bryant, C., Lenze, E. J., Stanley, M. A., Gum, A., et al. (2011). 'Improving Recognition of Late Life Anxiety Disorders in Diagnostic and Statistical Manual of Mental Disorders, Fifth Edition: Observations and Recommendations of the Advisory Committee to the Lifespan Disorders Work Group'. *International Journal of Geriatric Psychiatry* 27: 549–556.

Wolitzky-Taylor, K. B., Castriotta, N., Lenze, E. J., Stanley, M. A., and Craske, M. G. (2010). 'Anxiety Disorders in Older Adults: A Comprehensive Review'. *Depression & Anxiety* 27: 190–211.

REFERENCES

Aarsland, D., Marsh, L., and Schrag, A. (2009). 'Neuropsychiatric Symptoms in Parkinson's Disease'. *Movement Disorders* 24: 2175–2186.

Allain, H., Bentue-Ferrer, D., Polard, E., Akwa, Y., and Patat, A. (2005). 'Postural Instability and Consequent Falls and Hip Fractures Associate with Use of Hypnotics in the Elderly: A Comparative Review'. *Drugs and Aging* 22: 749–765.

Almeida, O. P., Draper, B., Pirkis, J., Snowdon, J., Lautenschlager, N. T., et al. (2012). 'Anxiety, Depression, and Comorbid Anxiety and Depression: Risk Factors and Outcome over Two Years'. *International Psychogeriatrics* 24: 1622–1632.

Andlin-Sobocki, P. and Wittchen, H. U. (2005). 'Cost of Anxiety Disorders in Europe'. *European Journal of Neurology* 12 (suppl. 1): 39–44.

Ansseau, M., Fischler, B., Dierick, M., Mignon, A., and Leyman, S. (2005). 'Prevalence and Impact of Generalized Anxiety Disorder and Major Depression in Primary Care in Belgium and Luxemburg: The GADIS Study'. *European Psychiatry* 20: 229–235.

Ansseau, M., Fischler, B., Dierick, M., Albert, A., Leyman, S., and Mignon, A. (2008). 'Socioeconomic Correlates of Generalized Anxiety Disorder and Major Depression in Primary Care: The GADIS II Study (Generalized Anxiety and Depression Impact Survey II)'. *Depression & Anxiety* 25: 506–513.

Anthony-Bergstone, C. R., Zarit, S. H., and Gatz, M. (1988). 'Symptoms of Psychological Distress among Caregivers of Dementia Patients'. *Psychology and Aging* 3: 245–248.

Australian Bureau of Statistics (2007). National Survey of Mental Health and Wellbeing. ABS Cat. No. 4326.0

Ayers, C. R., Sorrell, J. T., Thorp, S. R., and Wetherell, J. L. (2007). 'Evidence-based Psychological Treatments for Late-life Anxiety Disorders: A Systematic Review and Meta-analysis'. *Psychology and Aging* 22: 8–17.

Basevitz, P., Pushkar, D., Chaikelson, J., Conway, M., and Dalton, C. (2008). 'Age-related Differences in Worry and Related Processes'. *International Journal of Aging & Human Development* 66: 283–305.

Baxter, A. J., Scott, K. M., Vos, T., and Whiteford, H. A. (2013). 'Global Prevalence of Anxiety Disorders: A Systematic Review and Meta-regression'. *Psychological Medicine* 43: 897–910.

Beaudreau, S. A. and O'Hara, R. (2008). 'Late-life Anxiety and Cognitive Impairment: A Review'. *American Journal of Geriatric Psychiatry* 16: 790–803.

Beekman, A. T., Bremmer, M. A., Deeg, D. J., Van Balkom, A. J., Smit, J. H., et al. (1998). 'Anxiety Disorders in Later Life: A Report from the Longitudinal Aging Study Amsterdam'. *International Journal of Geriatric Psychiatry* 13: 717–726.

Beekman, A. T., de Beurs, E., Van Balkom, A. J., Deeg, D. J., Van Dyck, R., et al. (2000). 'Anxiety and Depression in Later Life: Co-occurrence and Communality of Risk Factors'. *American Journal of Psychiatry* 157: 89–95.

Bishop, S. J. (2007). 'Neurocognitive Mechanisms of Anxiety: An Integrative Account'. *Trends in Cognitive Sciences* 11: 307–316.

Bishop, S. J. (2008). 'Neural Mechanisms Underlying Selective Attention to Threat'. *Annals of the New York Academy of Sciences* 1129: 141–152.

Bottche, M., Kuwert, P., and Knaevelsrud, C. (2012). 'Posttraumatic Stress Disorder in Older Adults: An Overview of Characteristics and Treatment Approaches'. *International Journal of Geriatric Psychiatry* 27: 230–239.

Bower, P., Richards, D., and Lovell, K. (2001). 'The Clinical and Cost-effectiveness of Self-help Treatments for Anxiety and Depressive Disorders in Primary Care: A Systematic Review'. *British Journal of General Practice* 51: 838–845.

Brault, M. W. (2012). *Americans with Disabilities: 2010. Household Economic Studies. Current Population Reports.* Washington, DC: US Census Bureau.

Brenes, G. A., Guralnik, J. M., Williamson, J. D., Fried, L. P., Simpson, C., et al. (2005). 'The Influence of Anxiety on the Progression of Disability'. *Journal of the American Geriatrics Society* 53: 34–39.

Brenes, G. A., Kritchevsky, S. B., Mehta, K. M., Yaffe, K., Simonsick, E. M., et al. (2007). 'Scared to Death: Results from the Health, Aging, and Body Composition Study'. *American Journal of Geriatric Psychiatry* 15: 262–265.

Brenes, G. A., Penninx, B. W., Judd, P. H., Rockwell, E., Sewell, D. D., et al. (2008). 'Anxiety, Depression and Disability across the Lifespan'. *Aging & Mental Health* 12: 158–163.

Bryant, C., Jackson, H., and Ames, D. (2008). 'The Prevalence of Anxiety in Older Adults: Methodological Issues and a Review of the Literature'. *Journal of Affective Disorders* 109: 233–250.

Bryant, C., Jackson, H., and Ames, D. (2009). 'Depression and Anxiety in Medically Unwell Older Adults: Prevalence and Short-term Course'. *International Psychogeriatrics* 21: 754–763.

Burton, C., Campbell, P., Jordan, K., Strauss, V., and Mallen, C. (2012). 'The Association of Anxiety and Depression with Future Dementia Diagnosis: A Case-control Study in Primary Care'. *Family Practice* 30: 25–30.

Butters, M. A., Bhalla, R. K., Andreescu, C., Wetherell, J. L., Mantella, R., et al. (2011). 'Changes in Neuropsychological Functioning following Treatment for Late-life Generalised Anxiety Disorder'. *British Journal of Psychiatry* 199: 211–218.

Byers, A. L., Yaffe, K., Covinsky, K. E., Friedman, M. B., and Bruce, M. L. (2010). 'High Occurrence of Mood and Anxiety Disorders among Older Adults: The National Comorbidity Survey Replication'. *Archives of General Psychiatry* 67: 489–496.

Candilis, P. J. and Pollack, M. H. (1997). 'The Hidden Costs of Untreated Anxiety Disorders'. *Harvard Review of Psychiatry* 5: 40–42.

Chomistek, A. K., Chiuve, S. E., Jensen, M. K., Cook, N. R., and Rimm, E. B. (2011). 'Vigorous Physical Activity, Mediating Biomarkers, and Risk of Myocardial Infarction'. *Medicine and Science in Sports Exercise* 43: 1884–1890.

Clark, L. A. and Watson, D. (1991). 'Tripartite Model of Anxiety and Depression: Psychometric Evidence and Taxonomic Implications'. *Journal of Abnormal Psychology* 100: 316–336.

Cooper, C., Balamurali, T. B. S., and Livingston, G. (2007). 'A Systematic Review of the Prevalence and Covariates of Anxiety in Caregivers of People with Dementia'. *International Psychogeriatrics* 19: 175–195.

Craske, M. G., Rose, R. D., Lang, A., Welch, S. S., Campbell-Sills, L., et al. (2009). 'Computer-assisted Delivery of Cognitive Behavioural Therapy for Anxiety Disorders in Primary-care Settings'. *Depression & Anxiety* 26: 235–242.

De Beurs, E., Beekman, A. T. F., Van Balkom, A. J., Deeg, D. J., Van Dyck, R., et al. (1999). 'Consequences of Anxiety in Older Persons: Its Effect on Disability, Well-being and Use of Health Services'. *Psychological Medicine* 29: 583–593.

Deer, T. M. and Calamari, J. E. (1998). 'Panic Symptomatology and Anxiety Sensitivity in Older Adults'. *Journal of Behavior Therapy & Experimental Psychiatry* 29: 303–316.

Devier, D., Pelton, G. H., Tabert, M. H., Liu, X., Cuasay, K., et al. (2009). 'The Impact of Anxiety on Conversion from Mild Cognitive Impairment to Alzheimer's Disease'. *International Journal of Geriatric Psychiatry* 24: 1335–1342.

Dissanayaka, N. N., Sellbach, A., Matheson, S., O'Sullivan, J. D., Silburn, P. A., et al. (2010). 'Anxiety Disorders in Parkinson's Disease: Prevalence and Risk Factors'. *Movement Disorders* 25: 838–845.

Feinstein, J. S., Adolphs, R., Damasio, A., and Tranel, D. (2011). 'The Human Amygdala and the Induction and Experience of Fear'. *Current Biology* 21: 34–38.

Ferretti, L., McCurry, S. M., Logsdon, R., Gibbons, L., and Teri, L. (2001). 'Anxiety and Alzheimer's Disease'. *Journal of Geriatric Psychiatry and Neurology* 14: 52–58.

Fransson, E., De Faire, U., Ahlbom, A., Reuterwall, C., Hallqvist, J., et al. (2004). 'The Risk of Acute Myocardial Infarction: Interactions of Types of Physical Activity'. *Epidemiology* 15: 573–582.

Frueh, B. C., Elhai, J. D., Hamner, M. B., Magruder, K. M., Sauvageot, J. A., et al. (2004). 'Elderly Veterans with Combat-related Posttraumatic Stress Disorder in Speciality Care'. *Journal of Nervous and Mental Disease* 192: 75–79.

Gallagher, D., Coen, R., Kilroy, D., Belinski, K., Bruce, L., et al. (2011). 'Anxiety and Behavioural Disturbance as Markers of Prodromal Alzheimer's Disease in Patients with Mild Cognitive Impairment'. *International Journal of Geriatric Psychiatry* 26: 166–172.

Garand, L., Dew, M. A., Eazor, L. R., DeKosky, S. T., and Reynolds, C. F. (2005). 'Caregiving Burden and Psychiatric Morbidity in Spouses of Persons with Mild Cognitive Impairment'. *International Journal of Geriatric Psychiatry* 20: 512–522.

Garand, L., Lingler, J. H., Deardorf, K. E., DeKosky, S. T., Schulz, R., et al. (2012). 'Anticipatory Grief in New Family Caregivers of Persons with Mild Cognitive Impairment and Dementia'. *Alzheimer Disease & Associated Disorders* 26: 159–165.

Geda, Y. E., Roberts, R. O., Knopman, D. S., Petersen, R. C., Christianson, T. J., et al. (2008). 'Prevalence of Neuropsychiatric Symptoms in Mild Cognitive Impairment and Normal Cognitive Aging: A Population-based Study'. *Archives of General Psychiatry* 65: 1193–1198.

Gonçalves, D. C. and Byrne, G. J. (2012). 'Interventions for Generalized Anxiety Disorder in Older Adults: Systematic Review and Meta-analysis'. *Journal of Anxiety Disorders* 26: 1–11.

Gonçalves, D. C. and Byrne, G. J. (2013). 'Who Worries Most? Worry Prevalence and Patterns across the Lifespan'. *International Journal of Geriatric Psychiatry* 28: 41–49.

Goodwin, R. D. (2003). 'Association between Physical Activity and Mental Disorders among Adults in the United States'. *Preventive Medicine* 36: 698–703.

Gould, C. E. and Edelstein, B. A. (2010). 'Worry, Emotion Control, and Anxiety Control in Older and Younger Adults'. *Journal of Anxiety Disorders* 24: 759–766.

Greenberg, P. E., Sisitsky, T., Kessler, R. C., Finkelstein, S. N., Berndt, E. R., et al. (1999). 'The Economic Burden of Anxiety Disorders in the 1990s'. *Journal of Clinical Psychiatry* 60: 427–435.

Grenier, S., Préville, M., Boyer, R., O'Connor, K., Béland, S.-G., et al. (2011). 'The Impact of DSM-IV Symptom and Clinical Significance Criteria on the Prevalence Estimates of Subthreshold and Threshold Anxiety in the Older Adult Population'. *American Journal of Geriatric Psychiatry* 19: 316–326.

Grenier, S., Potvin, O., Hudon, C., Boyer, R., Preville, M., et al. (2012). 'Twelve-month Prevalence and Correlates of Subthreshold and Threshold Anxiety in Community-dwelling Older Adults with Cardiovascular Diseases'. *Journal of Affective Disorders* 136: 724–732.

Gum, A. M., King-Kallimanis, B., and Kohn, R. (2009). 'Prevalence of Mood, Anxiety, Substance-abuse Disorders for Americans in the National Comorbidity Survey-Replication'. *American Journal of Geriatric Psychiatry* 17: 782–792.

Hariri, A. R., Mattay, V. S., Tessitore, A., Kolachana, B., Fera, F., et al. (2002). 'Serotonin Transporter Genetic Variation and the Response of the Human Amygdala'. *Science* 297: 400–403.

Hariri, A. R., Drabant, E. M., Munoz, K. E., Kolachana, B. S., Mattay, V. S., et al. (2005). 'A Susceptibility Gene for Affective Disorders and the Response of the Human Amygdala'. *Archives of General Psychiatry* 62: 146–152.

Hendricks, G. J., Oude Voshaar, R. C., Keijsers, G. P. J., Hoogduin, C. A. L., and Van Balkom, A. J. L. M. (2008). 'Cognitive-behavioural Therapy for Late-life Anxiety Disorders: A Systematic Review and Meta-analysis'. *Acta Psychiatrica Scandinavica* 117: 403–411.

Henning, E. R., Turk, C. L., Mennin, D. S., Fresco, D. M., and Heimberg, R. G. (2007). 'Impairment and Quality of Life in Individuals with Generalized Anxiety Disorder'. *Depression & Anxiety* 24: 342–349.

Herring, M. P., O'Connor, P. J., and Dishman, R. K. (2010). 'The Effect of Exercise Training on Anxiety Symptoms among Patients: A Systematic Review'. *Archives of Internal Medicine.* 170(4): 321–333.

Hoffman, D. L., Dukes, E. M., and Wittchen, H. U. (2008). 'Human and Economic Burden of Generalized Anxiety Disorder'. *Depression & Anxiety* 25: 72–90.

Hoifodt, R. S., Strom, C., Kolstrup, N., Eisemann, M., and Waterloo, K. (2011). 'Effectiveness of Cognitive Behavioural Therapy in Primary Health Care: A Review'. *Family Practice* 28: 489–504.

Huk, K., Tiemeier, H., Newson, R. S., Luijendijk, H. J., Hofman, A., et al. (2011). 'Anxiety Disorders and Comorbid Depression in Community Dwelling Older Adults'. *International Journal of Methods in Psychiatric Research* 20: 157–168.

Hundt, N. E., Armento, M. E. A., Porter, B., Cully, J. A., Kunik, M. E., et al. (2013). 'Predictors of Treatment Satisfaction among Older Adults with Anxiety in a Primary Care Psychology Program'. *Evaluation & Program Planning* 37: 58–63.

Hunt, S., Wisocki, P., and Yanko, J. (2003). 'Worry and Use of Coping Strategies among Older and Younger Adults'. *Journal of Anxiety Disorders* 17: 547–560.

Indovina, I., Robbins. T. W., Nunez-Elizalde, A. O., Dunn, B. D., and Bishop, S. J. (2010). 'Fear-conditioning Mechanisms Associated with Trait Vulnerability to Anxiety in Humans'. *Neuron* 69: 563–571.

Jonson, M., Skoog, I., Marlow, T., Fässberg, M. M., and Waern, M. (2012). 'Anxiety Symptoms and Suicidal Feelings in a Population Sample of 70-year-olds without Dementia'. *International Psychogeriatrics* 24: 1865–1871.

Katz, I. R., Reynolds, C. F., Alexpoulos, G. S., and Hackett, D. (2002). 'Venlafaxine ER as a Treatment for Generalized Anxiety Disorder in Older Adults: Pooled Analysis of Five Randomized Placebo-controlled Clinical Trials'. *Journal of the American Geriatrics Society* 50: 18–25.

Kessler, R. C., Berglund, P., Demler, O., Jin, R., Merikangas, K. R., et al. (2005). 'Lifetime Prevalence and Age-of-onset Distributions of DSM-IV Disorders in the National Comorbidity Survey Replication'. *Archives of General Psychiatry* 62: 593–602.

Koenigs, M., Huey, E. D., Calamia, M., Raymont, V., Tranel, D., et al. (2008a). 'Distinct Regions of Prefrontal Cortex Mediate Resistance and Vulnerability to Depression'. *Journal of Neuroscience* 28: 12341–12348.

Koenigs, M., Huey, E. D., Raymont, V., Cheon, B., Solomon, J., et al. (2008b). 'Focal Brain Damage Protects against Post-traumatic Stress Disorder in Combat Veterans'. *Nature Neuroscience* 11: 232–237.

Kroenke, K., Spitzer, R. L., Williams, J. B., Monahan, P. O., et al. (2007). 'Anxiety Disorders in Primary Care: Prevalence, Impairment, Comorbidity, and Detection'. *Annals of Internal Medicine* 146: 317–325.

Ladouceur, R., Léger, E., Dugas, M., and Freeston, M. H. (2004). 'Cognitive-behavioral Treatment of Generalized Anxiety Disorder (GAD) for Older Adults'. *International Psychogeriatrics* 16: 195–207.

Laidlaw, K., Thompson, L. W., and Gallagher-Thompson, D. (2004). 'Comprehensive Conceptualization of Cognitive Behaviour Therapy for Late Life Depression'. *Behavioural and Cognitive Psychotherapy* 32: 389–399.

Laidlaw, K. and McAlpine, S. (2008). 'Cognitive Behaviour Therapy: How Is It Different with Older People?' *Journal of Rational-Emotional Cognitive-Behavioural Therapy* 26: 250–262.

Lakka, T. A., Venalainen, J. M., Rauramaa, R., Salonen, R., Tuomilehto, J., et al. (1994). 'Relation of Leisure-time Physical Activity and Cardiorespiratory Fitness to the Risk of Acute Myocardial Infarction in Men'. *New England Journal of Medicine* 330: 1549–1554.

LeDoux, J. E. (1995). 'Emotion: Clues from the Brain'. *Annual Review of Psychology* 46: 209–235.

LeDoux, J. E. (2000). 'Emotion Circuits in the Brain'. *Annual Review of Neuroscience* 23: 155–184.

Leentjens, A. F., Dujardin, K., Marsh, L., Martinez-Martin, P., Richard, I. H., et al. (2011). 'Symptomatology and Markers of Anxiety Disorders in Parkinson's Disease: A Cross-sectional Study'. *Movement Disorders* 26: 484–492.

Lenze, E. J., Rogers, J. C., Martire, L. M., Mulsant, B. H., Rollman, B. L., et al. (2001). 'The Association of Late-life Depression and Anxiety with Physical Disability'. *American Journal of Geriatric Psychiatry* 9: 113–135.

Lesch, K.-P., Bengel, D., Heils, A., Sabol, S. Z., Greenberg, B. D., et al. (1996). 'Association of Anxiety-related Traits with a Polymorphism in the Serotonin Transporter Gene Regulatory Region'. *Science* 274: 1527–1531.

Lindesay, J., Baillon, S., Brugha, T., Dennis, M., Stewart, R., et al. (2006). 'Worry Content across the Lifespan: An Analysis of 16- to 74-year old Participants in the British National Survey of Psychiatric Morbidity 2000'. *Psychological Medicine* 36: 1625–1633.

McDade-Montez, E. A., Watson, D., O'Hara, M. W., and Denburg, N. L. (2008). 'The Effect of Symptom Visibility on Informant Reporting'. *Psychology and Aging* 23: 940–946.

Mackintosh, M. A., Gatz, M., Wetherell, J. L., and Pedersen, N. L. (2006). 'A Twin Study of Lifetime Generalized Anxiety Disorder (GAD) in Older Adults: Genetic and Environmental Influences Shared by Neuroticism and GAD'. *Twin Research & Human Genetics* 9: 30–37.

McMurchie, W., Macleod, F., Power, K., Laidlaw, K., and Prentice, N. (2013). 'Computerised Cognitive Behavioural Therapy for Depression and Anxiety with Older People: A Pilot Study to Examine Patient Acceptability and Treatment Outcome'. *International Journal of Geriatric Psychiatry* 28(11): 1147–1156.

Mega, M. S., Cummings, J. L., Fiorello, T., and Gornbein, J. (1996). 'The Spectrum of Behavioral Changes in Alzheimer's Disease'. *Neurology* 46: 130–135.

Mendlowicz, M. V. and Stein, M. B. (2000). 'Quality of Life in Individuals with Anxiety Disorders'. *American Journal of Psychiatry* 157: 669–682.

Menza, M. A., Robertson-Hoffman, D. E., and Bonapace, A. S. (1993). 'Parkinson's Disease and Anxiety: Comorbidity with Depression'. *Biological Psychiatry* 34: 465–470.

Miloyan, B., Byrne, G. J., and Pachana, N. A. (2014). 'Age-related Changes in GAD Symptoms'. *International Psychogeriatrics* 26: 565–572.

Moniz, E. (1936). *Tentatives operatoires dans le traitment de certaines psychoses.* Paris: Masson.

Nepon, J., Belik, S-L., Bolton, J., and Sareen, J. (2010). 'The Relationship Between Anxiety Disorders and Suicide Attempts: Findings from the National Epidemiological Survey on Alcohol and Related Conditions'. *Depression and Anxiety* 27: 791–798.

Nordhus, I. H. and Pallesen, S. (2003). 'Psychological Treatment of Late-life Anxiety: An Empirical Review'. *Journal of Consulting and Clinical Psychology* 71: 643–651.

Norrholm, S. D. and Ressler, K. J. (2009). 'Genetics of Anxiety and Trauma-related Disorders'. *Neuroscience* 164: 272–287.

Oliva-Moreno, J., Lopez-Bastida, J., and Y Montejo, A. L. (2006). 'The Economic Costs of Anxiety in Spain'. *Estudios De Economia Aplicada* 24: 821–836.

Ongur, D. and Price, J. L. (2000). 'The Organization of Networks within the Orbital and Medial Prefrontal Cortex of Rats, Monkeys and Humans'. *Cerebral Cortex* 10: 206–219.

Pachana, N. A., Woodward, R. M., and Byrne, G. J. A. (2007). 'Treatment of Specific Phobia in Older Adults'. *Clinical Interventions in Aging* 2: 469–476.

Pachana, N. A., Egan, S. J., Laidlaw, K., Dissanayaka, N., Byrne, G. J., et al. (2013). 'Clinical Issues in the Treatment of Anxiety in Parkinson's Disease from a Cognitive Behavior Therapy Perspective'. *Movement Disorders* 28: 1930–1934.

Palmer, K., Berger, A. K., Monastero, R., Winblad, B., Bäckman, L., et al. (2007). 'Predictors of Progression from Mild Cognitive Impairment to Alzheimer Disease'. *Neurology* 68: 1596–1602.

Pontone, G. M., Williams, J. R., Anderson, K. E., Chase, G., Goldstein, S. A., et al. (2009). 'Prevalence of Anxiety Disorders and Anxiety Subtypes in Patients with Parkinson's Disease'. *Movement Disorders* 24: 1333–1338.

Porensky, E. K., Dew, M. A., Karp, J. F., Skidmore, E., Rollman, B. L., et al. (2009). 'The Burden of Late-life Generalized Anxiety Disorder: Effects on Disability, Health-related Quality of Life, and Healthcare Utilization'. *American Journal of Geriatric Psychiatry* 17: 473–482.

Potvin, O., Forget, H., Grenier, S., Preville, M., and Hudon, C. (2011). 'Anxiety, Depression, and 1-year Incident Cognitive Impairment in Community-dwelling Older Adults'. *Journal of the American Geriatrics Society* 59: 1421–1428.

Powers, C. B., Wisocki, P. A., and Whitbourne, S. K. (1992). 'Age Differences and Correlates of Worrying in Young and Elderly Adults'. *Gerontologist* 32: 82–88.

Prins, M. A., Verhaak, P. F., Van Der Meer, K., Penninx, B. W., and Bensing, J. M. (2009). 'Primary Care Patients with Anxiety and Depression: Need for Care from the Patient's Perspective'. *Journal of Affective Disorders* 119: 163–171.

Ray, W. A., Thapa, P. B., and Gideon, P. (2000). 'Benzodiazepines and the Risk of Falls in Nursing Home Residents'. *Journal of the American Geriatrics Society* 48: 682–685.

Richards, A., Barkham, M., Cahill, J., Richards, D., Williams, C., et al. (2003). 'PHASE: A Randomized, Controlled Trial of Supervised Self-help Cognitive Behavioural Therapy in Primary Care'. *British Journal of General Practice* 53: 764–770.

Ritchie, K., Artero, S., Beluche, I., Ancelin, M. L., Mann, A., et al. (2004). 'Prevalence of DSM-IV Psychiatric Disorder in the French Elderly Population'. *British Journal of Psychiatry* 184: 147–152.

Roest, A. M., Zuidersma, M., and De Jonge, P. (2012). 'Myocardial Infarction and Generalised Anxiety Disorder: 10-year Follow-up'. *British Journal of Psychiatry* 200: 324–329.

Russo, J., Vitaliano, P. P., Brewer, D. D., Katon, W., and Becker, J. (1995). 'Psychiatric Disorders in Spouse Caregivers of Care Recipients with Alzheimer's Disease and Matched Controls: A diathesis-stress Model for Psychopathology'. *Journal of Abnormal Psychology* 104: 197–204.

Sansoni, J., Vellone, E., and Piras, G. (2004). 'Anxiety and Depression in Community-dwelling, Italian Alzheimer's Disease Caregivers'. *International Journal of Nursing Practice* 10: 93–100.

Scarmeas, N., Luchsinger, J. A., Brickman, A. M., Cosentino, S., Schupf, N., et al. (2011). 'Physical Activity and Alzheimer's Disease Course'. *American Journal of Geriatric Psychiatry* 19: 471–481.

Schulz, R., Belle, S. H., Czaja, S. J., McGinnis, K. A., Stevens, A., et al. (2004). 'Long-term Care Placement of Dementia Patients and Caregiver Health and Well-being'. *Journal of the American Medical Association* 292: 961–967.

Schuurmans, J., Comijs, H., Emmelkamp, P. M. G., Gundy, C. M. M., Weijnen, I., et al. (2006). 'A Randomized, Controlled Trial of the Effectiveness of Cognitive-behavioral Therapy and Sertraline versus a Waitlist Control Group for Anxiety Disorders in Older Adults'. *American Journal of Geriatric Psychiatry* 14: 255–263.

Sinoff, G. and Werner, P. (2003). 'Anxiety Disorder and Accompanying Subjective Memory Loss in the Elderly as a Predictor of Future Cognitive Decline'. *International Journal of Geriatric Psychiatry* 18: 951–959.

Smalbrugge, M., Jongenelis, L., Pot, A. M., Beekman, A. T., and Eefsting, J. A. (2005a). 'Comorbidity of Depression and Anxiety in Nursing Home Patients'. *International Journal of Geriatric Psychiatry* 20: 218–226.

Smalbrugge, M., Pot, A. M., Jongenelis, K., Beekman, A. T. F., and Eefsting, J. A. (2005b). 'Prevalence and Correlates of Anxiety among Nursing Home Patients'. *Journal of Affective Disorders* 88: 145–153.

Smit, F., Cuijpers, P., Oostenbrink, J., Batelaan, N., De Graaf, R., et al. (2006). 'Costs of Nine Common Mental Disorders: Implications for Curative and Preventive Psychiatry'. *Journal of Mental Health Policy and Economics* 9: 193–200.

Stanley, M. A., Wilson, N. L., Novy, D. M., Rhoades, H. M., Wagener, P. D., et al. (2009). 'Cognitive Behavior Therapy for Generalized Anxiety Disorder among Older Adults in Primary Care'. *Journal of the American Medical Association* 301: 1460–1467.

Steele, G. D. F. (1951). 'Persistent Anxiety and Tachycardia Successfully Treated by Prefrontal Leucotomy'. *British Medical Journal* 2: 84–86.

Stenberg, U., Ruland, C. M., and Miaskowski, C. (2010). 'Review of the Literature on the Effects of Caring for a Patient with Cancer'. *Psycho-Oncology* 19: 1013–1025.

Teachman, B. A., Siedlecki, K. L., and Magee, J. C. (2007). 'Aging and Symptoms of Anxiety and Depression: Structural Invariance of the Tripartite Model'. *Psychology and Aging* 22: 160–170.

Teeson, M., Mitchell, P. B., Deady, M., Memedovic, S., Slade, T., et al. (2011). 'Affective and Anxiety Disorders and their Relationship with Chronic Physical Conditions in Australia: Findings of the 2007 National Survey of Mental Health and Wellbeing'. *Australian and New Zealand Journal of Psychiatry* 45: 939–946.

Teri, L., Ferretti, L. E., Gibbons, L. E., Logsdon, R. G., McCurry, S. M., et al. (1999). 'Anxiety in Alzheimer's Disease: Prevalence and Correlates'. *Journal of Gerontology: Medical Sciences* 54A: 348–352.

Thorp, S. R., Ayers, C. R., Nuevo, R., Stoddard, J. A., Sorrell, J. T., et al. (2009). 'Meta-analysis Comparing Different Behavioural Treatments for Late-life Anxiety'. *American Journal of Geriatric Psychiatry* 17: 105–115.

Tronche, F., Kellendonk, C., Kretz, O., Gass, P., Anlag, K., et al. (1999). 'Disruption of the Glucocorticoid Receptor Gene in the Nervous System Results in Reduced Anxiety'. *Nature Genetics* 23: 99–103.

Tully, P. J., Baker, R. A., and Knight, J. L. (2008). 'Anxiety and Depression as Risk Factors for Mortality after Coronary Artery Bypass Surgery'. *Journal of Psychosomatic Research* 64: 285–290.

Van Hout, H. P., Beekman, A. T., De Beurs, E., Comijs, H., Van Marwijk, H., et al. (2004). 'Anxiety and the Risk of Death in Older Men and Women'. *British Journal of Psychiatry* 185: 399–404.

Vasiliadis, H.-M., Dionne, P.-A., Preville, M., Gentil, L., Berbiche, D., et al. (2013). 'The Excess Healthcare Costs Associated with Depression and Anxiety in Elderly Living in the Community'. *American Journal of Geriatric Psychiatry*, 21: 536-548.

Vitaliano, P. P., Russo, J., Young, H. M., Teri, L., and Maiuro, R. D. (1991). 'Predictors of Burden in Spouse Caregivers of Individuals with Alzheimer's Disease'. *Psychology and Aging* 6: 392–402.

Wang, P. S., Lane, M., Olfson, M., Pincus, H. A., Wells, K. B., et al. (2005). 'Twelve-month Use of Mental Health Services in the United States: Results from the National Comorbidity Survey Replication'. *Archives of General Psychiatry* 62: 629–640.

Weisskopf, M. G., Chen, H., Schwarzschild, M. A., Kawachi, I., and Ascherio, A. (2003). 'Prospective Study of Phobic Anxiety and Risk of Parkinson's Disease'. *Movement Disorders* 18: 646–651.

Wetherell, J. L., Thorp, S. R., Patterson, T. L., Golshan, S., Jeste, D. V., et al. (2004). 'Quality of Life in Geriatric Generalized Anxiety Disorder: A Preliminary Investigation'. *Journal of Psychiatric Research* 38: 305–312.

Wilgoss, T. G. and Yohannes, A. M. (2013). 'Anxiety Disorders in Patients with COPD: A Systematic Review'. *Respiratory Care* 58: 858–866.

Yohannes, A., Baldwin, R. C., and Connolly, M. J. (2000). 'Mood Disorders in Elderly Patients with Chronic Obstructive Pulmonary Disease'. *Reviews in Clinical Gerontology* 10: 193–202.

CHAPTER 23

....

PSYCHOSIS IN OLDER ADULTS

....

JENNIFER CEGLOWSKI, LAURA VERGEL DE DIOS, AND COLIN DEPP

INTRODUCTION

PSYCHOSIS is relatively common among older adults. Compared to younger adults, psychosis in older people stems from a wide array of causes, which can complicate diagnosis and treatment planning. Regardless of how psychotic symptoms manifest, the symptoms are frequently highly distressing to care-givers. Moreover, psychosis is a risk factor for increased risk of mortality, institutionalization, functional decline, and increased healthcare costs (Okura et al. 2010). Risk of suicide also increases in older adults who experience psychosis in certain conditions (Kreyenbuhl, Kelly, and Conley 2002; Schaffer et al. 2008). In this chapter, we describe psychosis in older adults, focusing on late-life schizophrenia, affective disorders, and dementia, including the prevalence, course and associated symptoms, and current treatment approaches.

Broadly speaking, psychosis is defined as a loss of contact with reality, characterized by disturbances in thought process manifested in delusions and hallucinations. Psychosis can sometimes be accompanied by disruptive behavioural changes or aggressiveness as well as disorganized thought processes and speech. Hallucinations are false sensory perceptions that present as auditory, visual, olfactory, tactile, gustatory or other somatic sensations (body being invaded, twisted, or torn). Among hallucinations, some are command hallucinations in which patients are instructed to perform actions. Hallucinations must be differentiated from illusions, which are transient perceptual disturbances that are more frequent in dementia or delirium. Delusions are persistent false beliefs that persevere despite strong contradictory evidence. Delusions can be categorized as bizarre, non-bizarre, mood-congruent or mood-neutral. The delusional content might include delusions of reference, control, persecutory, paranoia, grandiosity, somatic, or jealousy/guilt. Some specific delusions are particularly common in older people with dementia, which include Capgras delusion, believing that an unfamiliar person has replaced a care-giver or family member, and Phantom Boarder Syndrome, imagining that there are people in the home.

The phenomenology of psychotic symptoms, both in terms of the kinds of symptoms expressed and their course, can offer clues as to the likely source. Further assessment of the type of delusion and hallucination can help determine in what context the psychosis may be present. For instance, visual, tactile, and olfactory hallucinations are more often related to psychosis caused by a medical condition or medication, while auditory hallucinations would be more indicative of a psychiatric disorder such as schizophrenia. Additionally, psychosis in the presence of sudden changes in cognition or disorientation might suggest delirium. Delusions that are intricate and persistent would most likely suggest psychosis in schizophrenia.

Combining all causes, psychosis is actually quite common in older people with prevalence rates ranging from 4% to 10% in community-dwelling older adults (Henderson et al. 1998; Ostling and Skoog 2002). The prevalence is even higher among those who are over the age of 95 and among those residing in institutional settings (Ostling et al. 2007). Factors that increase the risk of psychosis in the general population of older adults are social isolation, sensory deficits, physical illness, changes in cognition, and polypharmacy. As opposed to younger adults, among whom the most likely causes of psychosis are psychotic disorders, the most common cause of psychosis in older people is dementia.

GENERAL ASSESSMENT APPROACH

In order to properly assess for psychosis in older adults, a first step is to rule out possible medical conditions and medications that might cause these symptoms, including head trauma, infection, deliberate or accidental medication overdoses, and use of illicit substances. Of note, certain medical conditions can produce psychosis among individuals with a history of psychiatric disorder. Therefore, a thorough medical history should be taken when psychotic symptoms are present or if previous symptoms have gotten worse, even among patients who have a remote history of psychosis. Information should be gathered from the individual's medical records and from informants such as family members and primary care providers. Blood work, neuroimaging, and assessment of sensory and motor function, coordination, and gait can aid in determining if there are any medical causes of the current psychosis.

Faison and Armstrong (2003) stressed the importance of understanding the important role of culture in assessing for psychosis in older adults. Culture can influence the way in which people explain or define their symptoms, who they approach for help and how likely they are to access mental health services. Certain cultural or religious behaviours could be interpreted as symptoms of paranoia, delusion, or hallucination (e.g. seeing spirits) and yet these are normative and not considered to be psychosis. In the next sections, we provide an overview of selected common causes of psychosis in older adults.

Paraphrenia, which is no longer found in the *DSM* or International Classification of Diseases (ICD), is a term that was first used by Kraeplin to describe a group between paranoia and dementia praecox. Marked by persistent delusions and hallucinations, it was believed to be closely related to schizophrenia with less deterioration and without the full characteristics of delusional disorder. A diagnosis of paraphrenia included semi-systematized delusions and auditory hallucinations without severe personality or thought disturbances and relatively appropriate affect and behaviours. Paraphrenia has been suggested to be an illness related to older age; however, there is not substantial information to support this. Since paraphrenia is absent from the *DSM* and ICD people who might otherwise meet criteria for this diagnosis were instead diagnosed with delusional disorder, paranoid schizophrenia, and depression/dysthymia (Ravindran, Yatham, and Munro 1999).

We will examine psychotic symptoms, such as those that accompany dementia, in older adults as well as psychotic disorders in later life, focusing on schizophrenia and bipolar disorder. We will discuss prevalence, course, assessment, and management of psychosis in older age. We will then provide various treatment options to manage symptoms and implications for practice.

Schizophrenia

Prevalence

Schizophrenia affects about .1% to .5% of adults over the age of 65 (Howard et al. 2000). Approximately 85% of patients reside in the community and the remainder live in long-term care settings/supported living. Admission data suggests that as people over the age of 60 get older the risk for onset of schizophrenia-like psychosis increases by 11% with each five-year age increase (Van Os et al. 1995).

Although early-onset schizophrenia (below age 40) presents more commonly in men than women, women outnumber men with late-onset schizophrenia (40–65) and very late onset schizophrenia (65+) (Palmer, McClure, and Jeste 2001). Among people with schizophrenia, symptoms tend to be similar across ethnicities and cultures. However, there is a recognized tendency for African Americans to be diagnosed more often as having schizophrenia than mood disorders across the lifespan (Minsky et al. 2003). Also worth noting is the influence of culture among Latinos with schizophrenia. For example, Latinos with schizophrenia tend to live with family members instead of in supportive housing, which might lead to improved prognosis. On the other hand, Latinos with schizophrenia may access services at a lower rate than non-Latinos (Vega and Lopez 2001), and thus a greater proportion of Latinos with schizophrenia do not receive adequate treatment or therapy.

In relation to schizophrenia, symptoms are generally divided into negative and positive symptoms. A positive symptom is thought of as an excess or distorted version of normal functions, such as psychosis, including delusions and hallucinations, disorganized speech, or disorganized catatonic behaviour (*DSM-IV*). A negative symptom is thought of as a loss of normal functions such as flat affect, avolition, or anhedonia. While psychosis in the form of hallucinations or delusions seems to be more widely connected to schizophrenia, it is not required to meet criteria for the disorder as long as the patient exhibits prominent disorganized behaviour and negative symptoms (*DSM-IV*).

Course

A majority of the cases of schizophrenia experience onset in late teens and mid twenties. However, a late onset (after 40 years) and very late onset (after 60 years) of schizophrenia is also possible, with onset after 40 occurring in fewer than 10% of patients and onset after age 60 in fewer than 1%. In general, there are more similarities than differences in comparing early-and late-onset subtypes of schizophrenia. However, more typically among late-onset schizophrenia in comparison with earlier-onset schizophrenia, clinical symptoms include persecutory delusions and auditory hallucinations (Jeste et al. 1988). Additionally, in late-onset schizophrenia, executive functioning and learning impairments are less severe than in early-onset schizophrenia. In the very late-onset schizophrenia subgroup, sensory deficits such as hearing loss tend to occur more commonly. As with many psychiatric illnesses, early onset tends to indicate a worse outcome than later onset, in part because late-onset patients have more years of life asymptotic in which they may have been able to attain functional milestones such as marriage and education. Longer duration of illness is associated with worse prognosis among long-term institutionalized patients (Harvey et al. 1998). Social isolation and sensory impairment may contribute to very-late-onset schizophrenia (Howard et al. 2000). Regardless of age of onset, the course of schizophrenia (including clinical features, psychopathology, cognitive impairments, quality of well-being, and everyday functioning) tends to stabilize in late life (Jeste et al. 2003). Heaton et al. (2001) found that ambulatory patients with schizophrenia illustrated comparable test-retest reliability and cognitive stability with normal control subjects over a period up to five years on neuropsychological examination. Another important aspect of clinical course is duration of time until initiation of treatment. In a study by Haan et al. (2003), the duration of untreated psychosis with anti-psychotics as well as the delay in psychosocial treatment were associated with negative symptoms at outcome (six years after onset). However, when controlling for age at onset, gender, and length of time between onset and first treatment, the delay in psychosocial treatment seemed to be a stronger predictor of negative symptoms at outcome than the delay in anti-psychotic treatment.

Associated symptoms and disability

Even though cognitive impairments do not worsen any faster than those associated with normal ageing, the impact of cognitive impairment on the functioning of older adults with schizophrenia is substantial. Subjects with schizophrenia between the ages of 40 and 49 performed worse than older (70+) healthy controls in domains such as episodic memory, executive functioning and high-processing working memory, but both populations performed similarly in processing speed and simple working memory tests. Age-related effects were significantly larger for cognitive performance variables among patients with schizophrenia (largest age-related differences in those aged 70 and above) than for healthy controls (Loewenstein et al. 2011).

Social skills impairments in patients with schizophrenia also impact daily lives. While those diagnosed with late and very-late-life schizophrenia tend to have better developed social skills than those diagnosed with earlier onset, many older adults with schizophrenia still struggle with the daily social skills necessary to lead an independent life style. As measured with the Social Skills Performance Assessment (SSPA), performance-based assessed social skills are lower than those for older adults with bipolar disorder or major depression (Muesser et al. 2010).

Treatment

The cornerstone of treatment for schizophrenia is anti-psychotic medication. Anti-psychotic medications are more effective in treating positive symptoms than negative symptoms and cognitive impairments (Tandon, Nasrallah, and Keshavan 2010). Notably, the risks of side-effects increase with age; conventional anti-psychotics are associated with risks of extra-pyramidal symptoms such as tardive dyskinesia. Second-generation anti-psychotics (e.g. clozapine, olanzapine) are typically more tolerable in terms of extra-pyramidal side-effects, as well as more effective in treating some symptoms (depression, negative symptoms, cognition) than conventional anti-psychotic medications (Geddes 2000). Atypicals also have a higher risk of metabolic symptoms. Metabolic syndrome is characterized by increased cardiac risk factors such as diabetes, abdominal obesity, high cholesterol, and high blood pressure and is prevalent (42.7%) among patients with schizophrenia (Brunero, Lamont, and Fairbrother 2009). Other patterns observed between metabolic syndrome and patients with anti-psychotic treatment include a higher metabolic risk in those with longer illness duration and older age. Responsiveness to anti-psychotics varies with stage of illness: those treated in their first episode generally respond faster and at higher rates to treatment than those treated at a later stage (Tandon et al. 2010). Given the risk of side-effects, the general recommendation is to 'start low and go slow'.

When considering treatments for patients with schizophrenia, one must keep in mind that there are other issues not addressed by pharmacotherapy (i.e. medical adherence and general quality of life) which psychosocial interventions aim to improve. Medication adherence is an important issue to address because of its link to patient relapse and hospitalization (Patterson and Leeuwenkamp 2008). While pharmacotherapy, specifically anti-psychotics, has been deemed the standard care for schizophrenia, there is evidence that a combination of pharmacotherapy and psychosocial interventions can reduce the average cost and need of treatment per individual (Patterson and Leeuwenkamp 2008). There are four main categories of psychosocial interventions: cognitive-behavioural therapy (CBT), family intervention therapy (FIT), social skills therapy (SST), and cognitive remediation therapy (CRT). There are a few integrated therapies that combine aspects from each of these categories, such as functional adaption skills training (FAST) and integrated psychological therapy (IPT). These integrated therapies help to minimize the weaknesses and enhance the strengths of the different approaches. CBT attempts to reduce symptoms and relapse, and enhance functioning by having patients provide rational perspectives on their experiences. Studies have found that CBT provided lasting effects and improved mental state, especially in the early stages of schizophrenia. Despite some of these benefits, there is little evidence that CBT reduces relapse or re-hospitalization, and this modality can be difficult to implement. Each of these approaches effectively targets specific areas. For CBT, these areas are psychopathology and symptoms, whereas for FIT the outcome is adherence, relapse, and re-hospitalization. SST is effective in improving social skills and employment, and CRT can help with neurocognitive function. Table 23.1 illustrates the different outcomes across the four interventions: CBT, SST, FIT, and CRT. IPT is a group-based CBT programme combined with neurocognitive and social cognitive components and psychosocial rehabilitation that has been found significantly to improve neurocognition, negative and positive symptoms, and psychosocial functioning. Additionally FAST, a combination of CBT and SST, improves social function and negative symptoms for up to six months (Patterson and Leeuwenkamp 2008).

Table 23.1 Psychosocial treatments in schizophrenia

Intervention	Domains most consistently improved	Domains less consistently improved
Cognitive-behavioural therapy (CBT)	Psychopathology, residual symptoms	Adherence, social function
Family intervention therapy (FIT)	Adherence, relapse, hospitalization, disease burden	Residual symptoms, social function
Social skills therapy (SST)	Social function, activities of daily life	Adherence, residual symptoms
Cognitive remediation therapy (CRT)	Cognitive function	Residual symptoms, social function

PSYCHOSIS AND BIPOLAR DISORDER

Bipolar disorder is a mood disorder characterized by alternating periods of depression, hypomania/mania, and euthymia. As with schizophrenia, the next several decades will be accompanied by an increase in the absolute number of older adults diagnosed with bipolar disorder. Compared to schizophrenia, far less empirical research has been conducted on late-life bipolar disorder and most of the knowledge base about late-life bipolar disorder is derived from mixed-age studies.

Prevalence

Based on an international review of Bipolar I and II, the aggregate lifetime prevalence in population studies was 1.2% (Merikangas et al. 2011). Morgan, Mitchell, and Jablensky (2005) estimated that the prevalence rate of psychosis in bipolar disorder was 70–85%. Bipolar disorder can start in early childhood or later in life but the median age of onset is 25 years. Patients with late-onset bipolar disorder (>49 years) are at a greater risk for psychotic features and cerebrovascular problems (Wylie et al. 1999). While prevalence rates for bipolar disorder are difficult to determine and typically underreported, Blow (2005) estimated that bipolar disorder accounts for 5–19% of mood disorders in older adults. In a comprehensive review by Depp and Jeste (2004), 60% of older adults with bipolar disorder had psychotic symptoms.

Course

It is not uncommon for bipolar disorder to present alongside other psychiatric disorders, such as substance abuse, anxiety disorder, and personality disorder. Substance abuse comorbidity affects fewer older adults compared to the younger population; cognitive impairment and medical comorbidity are more common among the older adult population (Depp and Jeste 2004).

Little is known about the course of psychosis in bipolar older adults. However, based on some long-term studies, it seems that bipolar disorder is a chronic illness with periods of symptomatic recovery but few instances of fully functional recovery. Negative life events seem to be a causative factor for affective episodes. Anecdotal evidence suggests that older adults have longer and more frequent episodes; however, there is little data that actually supports this.

Psychotic symptoms generally predict a worse prognosis in bipolar disorder. Cognitive impairment in older adults is consistently found in bipolar disorder and can cause substantial disability. Additionally, mixed-age studies have revealed that psychotic features can put patients at a greater risk for cognitive impairment and death (Keller et al. 2006; Kisely et al. 2005). Psychotic symptoms such as hallucinations and paranoia predict lower global functioning, lower health-related quality of life, re-hospitalization, manic recurrence, and number of psychotic episodes (Carlson et al. 2012; Depp et al. 2006).

Associated symptoms and disability

In bipolar disorder, delusions tend to be more common than hallucinations (Meyers 1995). Psychosis associated with bipolar disorder is most commonly mood congruent, meaning the hallucinations or delusions represent the extreme mood state that the individual is currently experiencing. In manic episodes the content of delusions might be grandiose while delusions experienced during a depressive episode might include themes of persecution, jealousy, or guilt.

Treatment

Medication is the first-line approach to treating psychosis in bipolar disorder. Older adults with bipolar disorder often take several different medications including anti-psychotic drugs, mood stabilizers, and anti-depressants (Sajatovic 2002). Polypharmacy puts patients at greater risk for adverse drug reactions and death (Onder et al. 2003).

There is a lack of randomized controlled trials (RCT) for bipolar disorder in older adults, which makes it difficult to draw conclusions about the most effective treatment. The GERI-BD study is the first RCT of any medication in late-life bipolar disorder, comparing lithium and valproate for acute mania in bipolar adults aged 60 years and older (Young et al. 2010). Results from the study could provide additional information about the best pharmacological treatment for older adult bipolar patients.

The use of atypical anti-psychotics as a treatment for bipolar disorder has increased over the past several years. Unfortunately, most of the studies regarding the use of these agents are derived from anecdotal evidence from mixed-aged studies and case reports. Therefore, little is known about the relationship of adverse effects and ageing in bipolar disorder.

Psychosocial interventions can be used to complement medication treatment and increase medication adherence. Education, motivational interviewing, and skills training are all used to increase the likelihood that individuals adhere to medication. For these interventions to be effective with older adults they should be structured as brief, in-person practice sessions in which content is broken down into smaller steps. Training should be accompanied by manual and weekly homework assignments (Depp and Lebowitz 2007). One example of an intervention used to increase medication adherence is the Medication Adherence Skills Training for Bipolar Disorder (MAST-BD) (Depp et al. 2007). This twelve-week group intervention focuses on four components—education, motivational training, medication management, and symptom management—and teaches older adults the importance of medication adherence and how to properly manage medications and their symptoms.

Psychosis in Dementia

Alzheimer's disease (AD) and other dementias are the most common causes of psychosis in older adults. Psychotic features are not recognized as a specific symptom of dementia but rather are categorized under the behavioural disturbances modifier. Psychosis in older adults with dementia is associated with negative outcomes, including increased hostility, decreased ability to perform ADLs independently, increased care-giver distress, and premature institutionalization. In particular, two common behavioural problems for people with dementia that can be related to psychotic symptoms are wandering and aggression. These behaviours might increase in individuals who experience persistent delusions or misidentify their familiar surroundings.

Neurobiological studies have shown that psychosis in dementia is biologically different from psychosis due to schizophrenia. Table 23.2 illustrates the distinction between psychosis in schizophrenia and AD and what criteria must be met for both disorders (Jeste and Finkel 2000).

Prevalence

Alzheimer's disease is the most common cause of dementia and accounts for the highest proportion of psychosis in dementias. While the range in prevalence varies greatly, Ropacki and Jeste (2005) reported that 40% of people with dementia show signs of symptoms of psychosis. In Ropacki and Jeste's (2005) extensive review they found that delusions tend to

Table 23.2 Psychosis of Alzheimer's disease vs late-life schizophrenia

	Alzheimer's disease	Schizophrenia
Bizarre delusions	Rare	Frequent
Misidentifications	Common	Rare
Hallucinations	Mostly visual	Mostly auditory
Suicidality	Rare	Frequent
Past history	Rare	Common
Anti-psychotic doses	Low	Moderate

be more common than hallucinations in AD, with 36% of patients showing symptoms of delusion and 18% exhibiting hallucinations. A recent study on psychosis and dementia in adults over 85 years old produced similar results: prevalence of psychosis was 44%, where approximately 27% experienced hallucinations and 32% experienced delusions (Ostling et al. 2011). Patients with more severe cognitive impairment (MMSE scores <21) were more likely to present with psychotic features (Ostling et al. 2011). AD is not the only type of dementia that presents with psychosis, however. Lewy body dementia, Parkinson's disease, and fronto-temporal dementia also frequently co-occur with psychotic features (Werner 2003).

Course

The course of psychotic symptoms in AD is a gradual one in which symptoms may emerge slowly, last for several months to several years, then might decrease in occurrence or even disappear, and then reappear months later. The incidence of psychosis increases as AD progresses. One study found that psychosis was present in 20% of patients at year 1 and progressively increased to 51% by year 4 (Paulsen et al. 2000). Overall, psychosis is most often present during the middle stage of AD. This does not mean that patients in the later stages do not experience psychotic symptoms; however, they may not be able to explain their delusions or hallucinations verbally and their reactions may manifest instead in agitation. Psychosis in earlier stages is less common as this stage is normally associated with depression and anxiety (Devanand 1999).

Associated symptoms and disability

Psychosis in AD can have a negative impact on the quality of life of both the patient and the care-giver. There is a strong association between the presence of psychosis and care-giver distress. Often, psychosis hastens placement of patients in nursing homes (Balestreri, Grossberg, and Grossberg 2000). Research has shown that individuals with AD with psychotic features experience greater cognitive impairment and a more rapid cognitive decline and this might put the patient at an increased risk of death (Mizrahi et al. 2006).

There are a number of delusions that are common in dementia. These include delusions of infidelity, delusions of misidentification, delusions of theft, delusions of abandonment, delusions of danger, and delusions that their house is not their own house or that there is someone else living there (Fischer, Bozanovic-Sosic, and Norris 2004). There has been some debate about whether misidentification should be considered a delusion, as it may be more closely related to confusion rather than a loss of contact with reality. According to Cohen-Mansfield et al. (2011), delusions fall into different themes including disorientation, re-experiencing of past events, and loneliness and insecurity. A person might also experience delusions of boredom—taking on other roles when they experience inactivity and trigger/environmental stimuli like shift-changes, or as a result of listening to the conversations of others or even the television.

Treatment

The first-line treatment of choice for psychosis in AD is redirection and reassurance; however, if symptoms place the patient or care-giver at risk then pharmacological treatment may be necessary (American Psychiatric Association 2007). Anxiolytic medications can be used to help manage agitation that might accompany psychosis in patients with dementia; however, the side-effects associated with these medications may produce negative effects on balance and orientation that may outweigh the benefits. Additionally, neuroleptic medications have often been used to target psychotic symptoms in patients with AD, though these can produce adverse effects in older adults with dementia who may require lower doses. In the past, haloperidol has been the initial drug of choice but more recently drugs such as risperidone and olanzapine have been used as the initial choice due to their safer side-effect profile. Adverse side-effects related to the use of anti-psychotic drugs can include increased sedation and cognitive impairment, metabolic disturbances, and higher risk for cerebrovascular events and stroke. Additionally, in the US the Federal Drug Administration has issued a black box warning regarding the association between atypical anti-psychotic use and increased risk for mortality. This risk may be especially high with conventional anti-psychotics compared to the atypical anti-psychotics.

IMPLICATIONS FOR PRACTICE

Not much is known about psychosis and older adults, but clinicians should be aware that this is a common issue in late life. Psychotic symptoms can be from a variety of causes including the ones we mentioned, schizophrenia, bipolar disorder, and dementia. Proper assessment is crucial in order to differentiate between the causes of psychosis and time of onset. Schizophrenia and bipolar disorder are frequently associated with psychotic symptoms in late life. Effective treatment for this is a combination of psychopharmacotherapy and behavioural interventions. Psychosis in dementia is very common, especially in the middle stages of the illness and should be identified by a proper medical workup. Less is known about the treatment of psychosis in dementia and there is much controversy on the use of pharmacotherapy in this population. It is clear that we need more research in order to better understand psychosis in late life.

SUMMARY

As described in this chapter, psychotic symptoms are common among older people, cause substantial distress to care-givers and are associated with many negative outcomes. Identifying the cause of psychosis can often present a challenge in older people, given that many more illnesses can produce psychosis in older age as compared to younger people. As such, a multimodal assessment is often needed, and close monitoring as symptoms are managed. The current armamentarium of medication treatment options are often associated with significant side-effects, and thus require careful weighing of benefits to potential harms. Practitioners working with older adults can have a major positive impact by educating and reassuring care-givers about the causes and behavioural management of psychotic symptoms.

KEY REFERENCES AND SOURCES FOR FURTHER READING

Depp, C. A. and Jeste, D. V. (2004). 'Bipolar Disorder in Older Adults: A Critical Review'. *Bipolar Disorders* 6: 343–367.

Harvey, P. D. (2005). *Schizophrenia in Late Life: Aging Effects on Symptoms and Course of Illness*. Washington, DC: American Psychological Association.

Howard, R., Rabins, P. V., Seeman, M. V., Jeste, D. V., and the International Late-onset Schizophrenia Group (2000). 'Late-onset Schizophrenia and Very-late-onset Schizophrenia-like Psychosis: An International Consensus'. *American Journal of Psychiatry* 157: 172–178.

Ropacki, S. A. and Jeste, D. V. (2005). 'Epidemiology of and Risk Factors for Psychosis of Alzheimer Disease: A Review of 55 Studies Published from 1990 to 2003'. *American Journal of Psychiatry* 162: 2022–2030.

Tandon, R., Nasrallah, H. A., and Keshavan, M. S. (2010). 'Schizophrenia, "Just the Facts" 5. Treatment and Prevention Past, Present and Future'. *Schizophrenia Research* 122: 1–23.

REFERENCES

American Psychiatric Association (2007). *Practice Guidelines for the Treatment of Patients with Alzheimer's Disease and Other Dementias*. Washington, DC: American Psychiatric Association.

Balestreri, L., Grossberg, A., and Grossberg G. T. (2000). 'Behavioral and Psychological Symptoms of Dementia as a Risk Factor for Nursing Home Placement'. *International Psychogeriatrics* 12: 59–62.

Blow, F. C. (2005). 'Epidemiology and Health Services Utilization of Late-life Bipolar Disorder'. Program and Abstracts of the 18th Annual Meeting of the American Association for Geriatric Psychiatry, 3–6 March, San Diego, CA.

Brunero, S., Lamont, S., and Fairbrother, G. (2009). 'Prevalence and Predictors of Metabolic Syndrome Among Patients Attending an Outpatient Clozapine Clinic in Australia'. *Archives of Psychiatric Nursing* 23: 261–268.

Carlson, G. A., Kotov, R., Chang, S., Ruggero, C., and Bromet, E. (2012). 'Early Determinants of Four-year Clinical Outcomes in Bipolar Disorder with Psychosis'. *Bipolar Disorders* 14: 19–30.

Cohen-Mansfield, J., Golander, H., Ben-Israel, J., and Garfinkel, D. (2011). 'The Meanings of Delusions in Dementia: A Preliminary Study'. *Psychiatry Research* 189: 97–104.

Depp, C. A., Davis, C. E., Mittal, D., Patterson, T. L., and Jeste, D. V. (2006). 'Health-related Quality of Life and Functioning of Middle-aged and Elderly Adults with Bipolar Disorder'. *Journal of Clinical Psychiatry* 67: 215–221.

Depp, C. A. and Lebowitz, B. D. (2007). 'Enhancing Medication Adherence: In Older Adults with Bipolar Disorder'. *Psychiatry* 4: 22–32.

Depp, C. A., Lebowitz, B. D., Patterson, T. L., Lacro, J. P., and Jeste, D. V. (2007). 'Medication Adherence Skills Training for Middle-aged and Elderly Adults with Bipolar Disorder: Development and Pilot Study'. *Bipolar Disorder* 9: 636–645.

Devanand, D. P. (1999). 'The Interrelations between Psychosis, Behavioral Disturbance, and Depression in Alzheimer Disease'. *Alzheimer Disease and Associated Disorders* 13: 53–58.

Faison, W. E. and Armstrong, D. (2003). 'Cultural Aspects of Psychosis in the Elderly'. *Journal of Geriatric Psychiatry and Neurolology* 16: 225–231.

Fischer, C., Bozanovic-Sosic, R., and Norris, M. (2004). 'Review of Delusions in Dementia'. *American Journal of Alzheimer's Disease and Other Dementias* 19: 19–23.

Geddes, J., Freemantle, N., Harrison, P., and Bebbington, P. (2000). 'Atypical Antipsychotics in the Treatment of Schizophrenia: Systematic Overview and Meta-regression Analysis'. *British Medical Journal* 321: 1371–1376.

Haan, L., Linszen, D. H., Lenior, M. E., De Win, E. D., and Gorsira, R. (2003). 'Duration of Untreated Psychosis and Outcome of Schizophrenia: Delay in Intensive Psychosocial Treatment versus Delay in Treatment with Antipsychotic Medication'. *Schizophrenia Bulletin* 29: 341–348.

Harvey, P. D., Howanitz, E., Parrella, M., White, L., Davidson, M., et al. (1998). 'Symptoms, Cognitive Functioning and Adaptive Skills in Geriatric Patients with Lifelong Schizophrenia: A Comparison Across Treatment Sites'. *American Journal of Psychiatry* 155: 1080–1086.

Heaton, R. K., Gladsjo, J. A., Palmer, B. W., Kuck, J., Marcotte, T. D., et al. (2001). 'Stability and Course of Neuropsychological Deficits in Schizophrenia'. *Archives of General Psychiatry* 58: 24–32.

Henderson, A.S., Korten, A.E., Levings, C., Jorm, A.F., Christensen, H., et al. (1998) 'Psychotic Symptoms in the Elderly: A Prospective Study in a Population Sample'. *International Journal of Geriatric Psychiatry* 13: 484–492.

Howard, R., Rabins, P. V., Seeman, M. V., Jeste, D. V., and the International Late-onset Schizophrenia Group (2000). 'Late-onset Schizophrenia and Very-late-onset Schizophrenia-like Psychosis: An International Consensus'. *American Journal of Psychiatry* 157: 172–178.

Jeste, D.V. and Finkel, S.I. (2000). Psychosis of Alzheimer's Disease and Related Dementias: Diagnostic Criteria for a Distinct Syndrome. *American Journal of Geriatric Psychiatry* 8: 29–34.

Jeste, D. V., Harris, M. J., Pearlson, G. D., Rabins, P., Lesser, I., et al. (1988). 'Late-onset Schizophrenia: Studying Clinical Validity'. *Psychiatric Clinics of North America* 11: 1–14.

Jeste, D. V., Twamley, E. W., Eyler Zorrilla, L. T., Golshan, S., Patterson, T. L., et al. (2003). 'Aging and Outcome in Schizophrenia'. *Acta Psychiatrica Scandinavica* 107: 336–343.

Keller, J., Gomez, R.G., Kenna, H.A., Poesner, J., DeBattista, C., et al. (2006). 'Detecting Psychotic Major Depression Using Psychiatric Rating Scales'. *Journal of Psychiatric Research* 40: 22–29.

Kisely, S., Smith, M., Lawrence, D., and Maaten, S. (2005). 'Mortality in Individuals who Have Had Psychiatric Treatment: Population-based Study in Nova Scotia'. *British Journal of Psychiatry* 187: 552–558.

Kreyenbuhl, J. A., Kelly, D. L., and Conley, R. R. (2002). 'Circumstances of Suicide among Individuals with Schizophrenia'. *Schizophrenia Research* 58: 253–261.

Loewenstein, D. A., Czaja, S. J., Bowie, C. R., and Harvey, P. D. (2011). 'Age Associated Difference in Cognitive Performance in Older Patients with Schizophrenia: A Comparison with Healthy Older Adults'. *American Journal of Geriatric Psychiatry* 20: 29–40.

Merikangas, K. R., Jin, R., He, J., Kessler, R. C., Lee, S., et al. (2011). 'Prevalence and Correlates of Bipolar Spectrum Disorder in the World Mental Health Survey Initiative'. *Archives of General Psychiatry* 68: 241–251.

Meyers, B. (1995). 'Late-life Delusional Depression: Acute and Long-term Treatment'. *International Psychogeriatrics* 7: 113–124.

Minsky, S, Vega, W., Miskimen, T., Gara, M., and Escobar, J. (2003). 'Diagnostic Patterns in Latino, African American, and European American Psychiatric Patients'. *Archives of General Psychiatry* 60: 637–644.

Mizrahi, R., Starkstein, S. E., Jorge, R., and Robinson, R. G. (2006). Phenomenology and Clinical Correlates of Delusions in Alzheimer Disease. *The American Journal of Geriatric Psychiatry* 14: 573–581.

Morgan, V. A., Mitchell, P. B., and Jablensky, A. V. (2005). 'The Epidemiology of Bipolar Disorder: Sociodemographic, Disability and Service Utilization Data from the Australian National Study of Low Prevalence (Psychotic) Disorders'. *Bipolar Disorder* 7: 326–337.

Muesser, K. T., Pratt, S. I., Bartels, S. J., Forester, B., Wolfe, R., et al. (2010). 'Neurocognition and Social Skill in Older Persons with Schizophrenia and Major Mood Disorders: An Analysis of Gender and Diagnosis Effects'. *Journal of Neurolinguistics* 23: 297–317.

Okura, T., Plassman, B. L., Steffens, D. C., Llewellyn, D. J., Potter, G. G., et al. (2010). 'Prevalence of Neuropsychiatric Symptoms and their Association with Functional Limitations in Older Adults in the United States: The Aging, Demographics, and Memory Study'. *Journal of the American Geriatrics Society* 58: 330–337.

Onder, G., Landi, F., Cesari, M., Gambassi, G., Carbonin, P., et al. (2003). 'Inappropriate Medication Use among Hospitalized Older Adults in Italy: Results from the Italian Group of Pharmacoepidemiology in the Elderly'. *European Journal of Clinical Pharmacology* 59: 157–162.

Ostling, S., Börjesson-Hanson, A., and Skoog, I. (2007). 'Psychotic Symptoms and Paranoid Ideation in a Population-based Sample of 95-year-olds'. *American Journal of Geriatric Psychiatry* 15: 999–1004.

Ostling, S., Gustafson, D., Blennow, K., Börjesson-Hanson, A., and Waern, M. (2011). 'Psychotic Symptoms in a Population-based Sample of 85-year-old Individuals with Dementia'. *Journal of Geriatric Psychiatry Neurology* 24: 3–8.

Ostling, S., and Skoog, I. (2002). 'Psychotic Symptoms and Paranoid Ideation in a Nondemented Population-based Sample of the Very Old'. *Archives of General Psychiatry* 59: 53–59.

Palmer, B. W., McClure, F. S., and Jeste, D. V. (2001). 'Schizophrenia in Late Life: Findings Challenge Traditional Concepts'. *Harvard Review of Psychiatry* 9: 51–58.

Patterson, T. L. and Leeuwenkamp, O. R. (2008). 'Adjunctive Psychosocial Therapies for the Treatment of Schizophrenia'. *Schizophrenia Research* 100: 108–119.

Paulsen, J. S., Salmon, D. P., Thal, L. J., Romero, R., Weisstein-Jenkins, C., et al. (2000). 'Incidence of and Risk Factors for Hallucinations and Delusions in Patients with Probable Alzheimer's Disease'. *Neurology* 54: 1965–1971.

Ravindran, A. V., Yatham, L. N., and Munro, A. (1999). 'Paraphrenia Redefined'. *Canadian Journal of Psychiatry* 44: 133–137.

Sajatovic, M. (2002). 'Treatment of Bipolar Disorder in Older Adults'. *International Journal of Geriatric Psychiatry* 17: 865–873.

Schaffer, A., Flint, A. J., Smith, E., Rothschild, A. J., Mulsant, B. H., et al. (2008). 'Correlates of Suicidality among Patients with Psychotic Depression'. *Suicide and Life-threatening Behavior* 38: 403–414.

Tandon, R., Nasrallah, H. A., and Keshavan, M. S. (2010). 'Schizophrenia, "Just the Facts" 5. Treatment and Prevention Past, Present and Future'. *Schizophrenia Research* 122: 1–23.

Van Os, J., Howard, R., Takei, N., and Murray, R. M. (1995). 'Increasing Age is a Risk Factor for Psychosis in the Elderly'. *Social Psychiatry and Psychiatric Epidemiology* 30: 161–164.

Vega, W. A. and Lopez, S. R. (2001). 'Priority Issues in Latino Mental Health Services Research'. *Mental Health Services Research* 3: 189–200.

Werner, P. (2003). 'Psychosis in Parkinson's Disease'. *Movement Disorders* 18: 80–87.

Wylie, M. E., Mulsant, B. H., Pollock, B. G., Sweet, R. A., Zubenko, G. S., et al. (1999). 'Age at Onset in Geriatric Bipolar Disorder: Effects on Clinical Presentation and Treatment Outcomes in an Inpatient Sample'. *American Journal of Geriatric Psychiatry* 7: 77–83.

Young, R.C., Schulberg, H.C., Gildengers, A.G., Sajatovic, M., Mulsant, B.H., et al. (2010). 'Conceptual and Methodological Issues in Designing a Randomized, Controlled Treatment Trial for Geriatric Bipolar Disorder: GERI-BD'. *Bipolar Disorder* 12: 56–67.

CHAPTER 24

DISORDERS OF PERSONALITY IN LATE-LIFE

JOEL SADAVOY

INTRODUCTION

So often, the categorical diagnosis of personality disorder (PD) is avoided or 'deferred' by clinicians. In geriatric work, part of the clinical diagnostic challenge of determining the presence of personality disorder lies in trying to disentangle the habitual lifelong reactions of an older patient, i.e. their personality traits, from categorically defined psychopathology of other sorts such as depression or anxiety disorders, the symptoms of which can overlap with the phenomenology of PD. This challenge is more pronounced when trying to apply categorical diagnostic criteria designed for younger adults to older adults whose life circumstances, such as losses, or physical condition, such as frailty or immobility, introduce emotional and behavioural reactions to stressors which may be enduring and hence hard to distinguish from personality-based disturbances.

Since their introduction, the utility and accuracy of Diagnostic and Statistical Manual (DSM) categorical phenomenological threshold criteria for diagnosis have been the subject of an ongoing debate. The *DSM-5* (American Psychiatric Association 2013) has essentially retained the *DSM-IV* criteria for personality disorders adding a more sophisticated and refined theoretical model in section 3 of the manual (Emerging Measures and Models) as a stimulus to further research and possible change in future editions of the *DSM-5*. This model recognizes the inherent dimensionality of personality expression in a given individual and the need to incorporate both observable trait-based behaviours with underlying, less overtly observable impairments in self- and interpersonal functioning. In other words, in this alternative model, while categorical diagnosis might be retained, it would be integrated with a dimensional approach to diagnosis including making room for dimensional descriptors of trait-modifiers in the diagnosis. Unfortunately, however, the *DSM-5* has still ignored the issue of diagnostic variations in older adults. As will become evident later in this chapter, this is a major problem that should be addressed.

One may ask why it is necessary to be specifically concerned about personality and its disorders in old age. There are several important diagnostic and clinical reasons. Personality disturbances and disorders may impair capacity to adapt to old age; PD is well known to distort psychiatric and psychological assessment and diagnosis; PD increases the complexity of treatment and leads to poorer prognosis; PD negatively impacts the relationships of the older person especially in the care-giving context; PD increases the risks inherent in management of older adults in institutions because of the suicidality sometimes associated with older patients with PD; the interpersonal problems associated with PD may predispose to earlier institutionalization because of breakdown in care-giving relationships; and finally PD negatively affects the morale and function of healthcare providers because of the impaired capacity of older adults with PD to trust and rely on others without conflict.

What Happens to Personality with Ageing?

For clinical reasons it is increasingly necessary for clinicians to understand the normal evolution of personality traits across the lifespan. While the final answers to whether personality changes or remains unchanged with ageing are not in yet, the best data we have at the moment comes down on the side of stability of personality and personality traits over time. Tackett et al. (2009) recently reviewed data from longitudinal studies in normal populations and, overall, concluded that traits remain relatively stable. When traits do show changes, as shown in the review of Roberts, Walton, and Viechtbauer (2006), careful examination of data reveals that the extent of change is probably small. Hence there is evidence that traits of neuroticism, extraversion, and openness decrease slightly while agreeableness and conscientiousness increase slightly. Whether these changes reach observable significance in large populations or have clinical significance is not yet determined; however, clinical experience does show that interaction of personality with life stressors can exacerbate some traits that may not have been as evident when the individual was younger.

Epidemiology

Determining accurately the epidemiology of PD is not easy for any age cohort. But the task is confounded further for older persons by the absence of adequate epidemiological tools. The rates of PD among older persons have not been accurately determined because of the limitations of the existing diagnostic criteria and assessment tools when used for older adults.

Balsis et al. (2007a), using cross-sectional design in 18–98-year-olds, found that 29% of the *DSM* criteria for PD led to measurement errors in older people (Balsis et al. 2007b). In a small Dutch study, only three of the seven *DSM-IV* criteria for antisocial PD were viewed by forensic psychiatrists and psychologists as useful for diagnosis in older people (Van Alphen, Nijhuis, and Oei 2007).

There are few validated instruments to detect PD in older adults (Oltmanns and Balsis 2011) as well as many practical challenges in the valid administration of the tests (Van

Alphen et al. 2006a). One published measurement instrument, the Gerontological Personality Disorders Scale (GPS; Van Alphen et al. 2006b; Tummers et al. 2011), specifically developed and validated for older people is available, but not yet in wide use.

Diagnosis in older persons is often aided by collateral information. However, in the area of PD, using collateral information of informants poses significant risk of bias and inaccuracy, particularly for factors related to less clearly observable phenomena such as mood and self-perception (Van Alphen et al. 2005; Vine and Steingart 1994).

In light of research limitations, epidemiological findings about PD in later life must be approached with caution. Best estimates at this point suggest that the lifetime prevalence of PD among older adults in nonclinical populations, using tools designed for general adults, ranges widely. Some studies estimate a range of 2.8% to 13% (Ames and Molinari 1994; Weissman 1993). Abrams and Horowitz (1996), in a meta-analysis of eleven studies, reported a PD rate of 10% (range of 6% to 33%) similar to the community sample reported by Segal, Coolidge, and Rosowsky (2006) of 11%. In another analysis of sixteen studies of the same age group, Abrams and Horowitz (1999) found a higher mean prevalence of 20%.

The prevalence of specific types of PD in later life remains unclear. Antisocial and histrionic PD are probably under-represented in the older population (Cohen et al. 1994). Abrams and Horowitz (1999) found that paranoid PD was the most common form of PD in those over 50. As noted by Van Alphen et al. (2012a), the wide prevalence spread in studies of PD in clinical older adult populations reflects the different research methods, diagnostic criteria and instruments used in the studies as well as the variation in the size of the samples ranging from 30 subjects (Silberman et al. 1997) to 547 subjects (Kunik et al. 1994).

Data on older clinical populations generally show higher rates of PD. For example, in ambulatory settings, prevalence ranges from 5% to 33% (Mezzich et al. 1987; Molinari and Marmion 1995); among depressed older adults, Molinari and Marmion (1995) reported a prevalence rate of 63%; and in older inpatients receiving mental health treatment prevalence has been reported as between 7% and 80% (Casey and Schrodt 1989; Silberman et al. 1997).

The comorbidity of PD with axis 1 disorders, particularly depression, its interaction with psychodynamically determined developmental factors, and the negative effect of PD on prognosis for treatment of depression have been reviewed elsewhere (Sadavoy 1999, Segal et al. 2006). Of special note, however, is the necessary caution when evaluating patients including older adults who have both an axis 1 disorder and apparent PD. While it is probably true that personality-based vulnerabilities, such as narcissism or impairments in trust and security, can predispose to axis 1 disorders such as depression, anxiety, or somatoform disorders (see Sadavoy 1999, Segal et al. 2006), it is also evident that depression as well as other life events and circumstances such as severe illness can produce symptoms that resemble those of PD which melt away once treatment has been successful or the stressor has been removed (Thompson, Gallagher, and Czirr 1988). Hence diagnostic caution is warranted when determining whether comorbid PD is present with an active comorbid axis 1 or serious medical disorder in a given patient (Fogel and Stoudemire 2000).

Cross-sectional prevalence studies on specific PDs in different venues indicate that personality disorders from the A and C clusters remain relatively stable over time, while those from the B cluster tend to diminish during mid-life and older age (Coolidge et al. 1992; Engels et al. 2003; Molinari, Ames, and Essa 1994; Stevenson, Meares, and Comerford 2003; Ullrich and Coid 2009; Watson and Sinha 1996).

Borderline PD (BPD) is among the most researched of the personality disorder constructs. One question for geriatrics is whether this diagnostic construct remains relevant in old age. Certainly there seems to be a general consensus that the most dramatic and often challenging behaviours of BPD such as impulsivity, aggression, self-destructiveness, and fluctuating mood states seem to calm down in mid-life and become less relevant to diagnosis in old age (Rosowsky and Gurian 1992; Sadavoy 1996; Van Alphen et al. 2006a). In contrast, symptoms of paranoid, schizoid, schizotypal, or obsessive-compulsive PD seem to change less although elements such as rigid behaviour or suspicion may increase (Agronin and Maletta 2000; Solomon 1981).

Overall, BPD in younger adults seems to arise from dysfunction in emotional stability, interpersonal relations, and constraint or self-control (Trull et al. 2010). For example, Trull et al. 2011 note that in BPD the dimensions that are most consistently identified are affective dysregulation or affective instability, impulsivity or behavioural dysregulation, and interpersonal hypersensitivity. From a diagnostic perspective therapists dealing with older adults must reframe their clinical lens to look less for dramatic acting-out behaviours which decline with age and focus on more subtle core elements of PD (Sadavoy 1996).

Stevenson et al. (2003) investigated the common wisdom that borderline personalities 'burn out ' with age (McGlashan 1986; Stone 1990) and asked whether all the key *DSM-IV* diagnostic features of BPD, i.e. impulsivity, interpersonal disturbances, cognitive self-perceptions, and affective disruptions, burn out or whether it is only specific elements that become less evident with ageing. To answer this question they used a vertical design and examined only outpatients. They screened 154 outpatients and ended up with 123 subjects (24 males, 99 females). The instruments they used for inclusion were the Westmead Severity Scale and the DIB-R (*DSM-IV* criteria for borderline). Mean age was 31.56 (range 18–52). They found that only impulsivity declined with age but that identity disturbances remained strong. While not a 'geriatric study' per se, the implication of this study is that while certain forms of impulsivity such as self-harm and other dramatic acting out decline, the core dynamics of BPD remain, including impaired self- and relational perceptions of trust and abandonment, which remain stable. Similarly, Silver (personal communication) conducted a long-term twenty-year clinical follow-up of his borderline patients in 1995 and concluded that while they had become more behaviourally and interpersonally stable, their underlying psychological conflicts, disturbances in their sense of self, and their ability to trust others remained unchanged. These findings correspond with much older clinical and theoretical positions on the effect of ageing on the inner developmental world of the individual. Forty years ago Berezin (1972) restated a long-held psychoanalytic principle that the unconscious is 'timeless' and does not change with ageing.

THE IMPACT OF PERSONALITY DISTURBANCE ON ADAPTATION IN LATE-LIFE

At a time in life when many individuals begin to struggle with decline in various capacities and abilities, older adults are often confronted with the most difficult adaptational challenges. Having said that we must ask why most older adults do not simply succumb to the daunting emotional stressors that they have to face, such as loss of lifelong partners, decline in status and prestige, relocation to a long-term care environment, or chronic physical disability and illness. The answer of course is that there are varying levels of adaptive capacity among older people, many of which derive from personality development.

It may be said with some confidence that many life challenges are only experienced as overwhelming stressors when they are perceived as such by the individual (Devanand et al. 2002). In turn the individual's perception is a direct outcome of their personality structure.

Every challenge can become a stress if it hits the ageing individual at a point of psychological vulnerability (diathesis–stress theory of Holmes and Rahe; Aaron Beck). The more mature the older person is, the fewer the points of psychological vulnerability. The more vulnerable (fragile, immature, primitive) the older person is, the greater the risk of life events and other challenges becoming stress that overwhelms their capacity to adapt to the challenges of ageing.

A promising line of investigation that has the potential to link personality factors, physiology, and psychopathology is the association of depression with elevated serum cytokine levels (especially interleukin 6 and 1 and tumour necrosis factor) (Brebner 2000).

Alterations of cytokines may be especially relevant in old age. Cytokines are increased in depression although the cause and effect relationship with depression is not yet clear. (Capuron et al. 2001). Cytokines are stimulated by inflammatory disorders and diseases especially common in older adults including cardiovascular disease, osteoporosis, arthritis, type 2 diabetes, various cancers, lymphoproliferative diseases, Alzheimer's disease. and some treatments such as interferon in cancer (Dantzer 2001; Konsman et al. 2002). Depression is associated with increased cardiovascular disease, but the underlying mechanisms are not well understood. In one study Kop et al. (2002) found that depression and exhaustion are associated with low-grade inflammation and elevated coagulation factors in persons aged over 65 years. Inflammatory markers such as interleukin 6 and C-reactive protein are associated with age and predict functional decline, mortality, decreased functional status, and disability (Ferrucci et al. 1999; Hamerman et al. 1999; Pieper et al. 2000).

There is reason to be particularly concerned about the vulnerability of older adults to cytokine activity and immunological factors. Distress or depression seems to be associated with greater immunological impairments in older adults (Kiecolt-Glaser et al. 2003). IL-6 may be a marker for impending deterioration in health status in older adults and IL-6 levels increase with age (Ferrucci et al. 1999). Care-givers of spouses with Alzheimer's disease are at greater risk of impaired immunological function particularly if they have poor levels of social support (Bauer et al. 2000; Kiecolt-Glaser et al. 1991).

Why be concerned about immunology and depression when discussing personality and its disorders? The mechanism of how a personality-emotion-immune interaction works is not entirely clear yet, but some data support the hypothesis that personality structure may predispose an individual to greater relative positive or negative emotions which in turn influence immune function such as immune cell counts in peripheral blood (Segerstrom 2000). Importantly, for example, there is an association between elevated cytokine levels and personality traits which predispose individuals to negative emotional states such as pessimism, sense of meaninglessness, and negative self perceptions, which in turn further contribute to a possible depressogenic cascade in older adults (Kiecolt-Glaser et al. 2002; Maruta et al. 2000).

Data from other studies help us to specify the nature of these positive and negative emotional states. Positive emotions that may be an indicator of resilience in the face of stress and adversity include the following: the ability to make a positive reappraisal of stressful life experience and to find meaning in life and events, and developing positive illusions about the self and situational optimism (Maruta et al. 2000.). Some have hypothesized that these characteristics can have a positive effect on health outcomes possibly mediated through endocrine and immune mechanisms (Kiecolt-Glaser et al. 2002). Data support the contention that personality and coping characteristics of optimism vs pessimism may predict physical illness and mortality in initially healthy adults (Maruta et al. 2000). Moreover, personality traits such as conscientiousness, activity, and emotional stability appear to have a direct impact not only on the capacity to adapt to ageing but to longevity itself (Terracciano 2008).

One personality factor that is associated with negative emotional states and that may be particularly important in predicting late-onset depression is sociotropy, defined as an unusual need for approval and reassurance in interpersonal relationships. This trait, combined with negative interpersonal events, poorer physical functioning, and medical illness were the primary predictive factors of late-life depression in a study by Mazure et al. (2002). This line of research becomes particularly relevant when taken together with the data that shows that internal states of self-image and views of self and others remain stable over the lifespan. A trait like sociotropy, which has its origins in earlier life development, is not only likely to remain stable into old age but to be particularly vulnerable to the nature of late-life assaults and adaptive challenges. Old age is notoriously hard on self-esteem because of the frequent devaluation or ignoring of older persons by those who are younger, as well as by society as a whole.

This research demonstrates the remarkable complexity of a feedback system in which the experiences of old age induce negative emotional states in those with pre-existing vulnerable personality structures which leads to physiological (immunological) changes that in turn further exacerbate the negative emotional states. A complex cascade can now be hypothesized for late-life depression as follows: older adults are at risk of depressive symptoms when stress, i.e. their environment, illness, or life events, interacts with personality-based vulnerabilities to induce negative emotions causing demoralization and fear. In turn, these emotional states alter immune responses to produce pro-inflammatory changes that raise cytokine levels and induce depressive symptoms. Alternatively or concurrently, certain illnesses like cancer, heart disease, or arthritis themselves may be pro-inflammatory, which both raises cytokines and induces negative emotional states which then go on to autoinduce further depression.

IMPLICATIONS FOR TREATMENT OF PERSONALITY AND ITS DISORDERS IN LATE-LIFE

The therapist of the older patient with PD has a basic decision to make initially: what is the primary target of therapy? Most patients come with a symptomatic concern such as mood change or anxiety often precipitated by alterations in life circumstances. Inevitably, as the therapist uncovers the factors that affect the decision of which therapy to use and for how long, it becomes evident that the patient's personality is a key context within which the symptoms and response to life events are taking place. The personality structure of the patient will determine the adaptive capacity of the patient, the nature of the therapeutic relationship that develops, i.e. the transference, and the way in which the patient's family or other relations need to be taken into account in the process.

For all of these reasons the prudent therapist will assess personality structure with particular reference to the defensive style of the patient and the interpersonal relationships they have had in the past and currently. Key to this evaluation in older adults is evaluating their adaptive capacities throughout their life. This evaluation provides the raw data for understanding the personality-based factors that affect the older patient's reactions to life circumstances and equally important their likely reactions within the therapeutic relationship.

It is beyond the scope of this chapter to attempt a detailed discussion of the origins of personality vulnerability and disorder. However, since internal psychological organization remains relatively stable throughout the lifespan, the therapist of the geriatric patient will need to evaluate developmental factors similar to those that are relevant to younger adults, but place them into the context of the special stressors associated with adaptation to ageing.

Adaptation to ageing places great strain on both the cognitive and psychodynamically determined defences of the individual. While little formal research has addressed these issues in clinical practice, clinical experience strongly suggests that individuals with PD or personality-based vulnerabilities will have greater difficulty adapting. In other words, life events only become stressful when they are interpreted as such and those with vulnerable personality structures are more prone to negative interpretations of life events. Hence, rather than looking only at the events in an individual's life it is important to evaluate the subjective impact of adverse life events...and consider them in clinical management (Devanand et al. 2002). To understand the interaction between personality and environment, the clinician might consider answering these three interrelated questions:

1 What are the environmental factors that are creating *psychological stress* in this older individual?
2 What are the *core vulnerabilities* in this patient (i.e. vulnerable aspects of this particular older self) that may react characteristically and adversely to challenge, and cause the person to interpret the events as overwhelming stress?
3 What are the *behaviours or symptoms* that this person is manifesting that seem to result from the interaction of the stressors on the vulnerable aspect of their personality structure?

Stress factors in old age

Anyone can be overwhelmed by life if the pressures are great enough—for example severe illness associated with recent bereavement and economic uncertainty in the context of psychological vulnerability. Intuitively, it seems probable that perfect storms of stress are more likely in old age when as Shakespeare's Claudius said 'When sorrows come they come not single spies but in battalions'. Table 24.1 is a partial list of these stressors. When we

Table 24.1 Common age-related stressors

Physical change, chronic illness	Loss of control, influence, vitality, leadership,
Loss/grief/bereavement—actual, anticipated	and authority
Cognitive decline	Economic losses
Roles—e.g. retirement, parenting, spousal	Displacement by youth
Productivity/creativity	Sexual decline/attractiveness
Abandonment—institutionalization	Facing regrets
Forced dependency	Relinquishing fantasies
Societal devaluation—shame, humiliation	Facing foreshortened future
	Death

examine the common stresses of old age it becomes possible to group them according to key personality-based vulnerabilities.

Core vulnerabilities and therapy

Various schools of thought have vied for primacy in developing '*the* model' to explain psychological vulnerability but no one has achieved universality. Some models seem more appropriate than others depending on the individual. Hence it is clinically prudent to keep an open mind clinically and tailor the model of understanding to the patient rather than the other way around.

In this spirit the following is proposed as an organizing structure to help formulate personality-based vulnerability in older patients. Five key determinants of vulnerability seem most relevant to old age:

- oversensitivity to narcissistic assault,
- excessive fear of abandonment,
- impaired capacity for intimacy and trust,
- attachment pathology such as intense and insecure attachment/dependency needs (impaired individuation, separation, and autonomy), and
- overly intense emotional reactivity (impaired affect regulation).

While important at any age, the struggles and challenges of old age are perhaps more assaultive to these underlying dynamic vulnerabilities. If we examine the common challenges of ageing, the relevance of these five factors becomes more evident. Table 24.2 lists common adaptive challenges of old age, the particular personality vulnerability they are likely to assault, and examples of behaviours that may result.

Table 24.2 provides a concise illustration of the task of the clinician when encountering the older patient with behavioural or emotional disturbances. Naturally, the first question to ask (beyond a diagnostic categorization) is whether the behaviours or reactions have psychological meaning and if so how they should be understood. From the point of view of integrating personality-based pathology or vulnerability into the practical treatment of older adults, it is helpful to try to tie the behaviour to the precipitant (e.g. institutionalization),

Table 24.2

Adaptive challenges	Personality vulnerability	Behavioural expression
Physical change, chronic illness; forced dependency	Narcissistic assault; impaired ability to trust others	Desperately seeking help; mistrust and rejection of help; pseudo-independence; devaluation of others; anxiety; "depression"; withdrawal
Loss/grief/ bereavement— actual, anticipated	Mobilization of abandonment fears	Pathological grief; searching for a saviour; clinging and demanding; anxiety; rage
Role changes—e.g. retirement, parenting, spousal	Abandonment; trust	Identity challenges; loss of purpose; inner emptiness; resentment; withdrawal; demanding
Productivity/ creativity; loss of control, influence, vitality, leadership and authority; displacement by youth; societal devaluation— shame, humiliation	Narcissistic assault	Worthlessness; clinging to the past; resentment/devaluation of others
Institutionalization	Abandonment anxiety; impaired capacity for trust	Acting out, complaintive, demanding, depressive withdrawal
Economic losses	Dependency fears	Clinging; denial; pseudo-independence;
Sexual decline/ attractiveness	Narcissistic assault; loss of the other	Denial of ageing; haughty devaluation of others; forming idealized relationships
Facing regrets; relinquishing fantasies	Abandonment	Inability to grieve losses; 'depression'
Death; facing foreshortened future	Affective instability	Primitive fantasies; difficulty modulating anxiety

and the precipitant to the underlying, often hidden personality vulnerabilities (e.g. lifelong fears of abandonment).

Once the underlying personality-based vulnerabilities are 'diagnosed', interventions can be tailored to the older person's powerful but often unspoken internal needs. There is little to no research on interventions specific to PD in later life. However, while pharmacotherapy and social/environmental techniques are sometimes useful, the core of any successful intervention for PD is psychotherapy. The method of intervention will be derived from the standard clinical toolbox and may include dialectical behavioural therapy (DBT), cognitive-behavioural therapy (CBT), problem-solving or solution-focused approaches (PST, SFT), interpersonal therapeutic approaches (IPT), or brief or longer-term psychodynamically informed therapy delivered in individual or group formats. Very preliminary indications of the suitability of DBT for geriatric patients has emerged (although the data is confounded by diagnostic uncertainties in the sample) (Lynch et al. 2007). Other data suggest that brief dynamic and CBT therapies have been found useful for older adults with anxiety and depressive disorders, and so, by implication, that they may be suitable for the older patient with personality disturbances (Bizzini 1998; Dick and Gallagher-Thompson 1995; Hendriks et al. 2008; Laidlaw 2001; Pinquart, Duberstein, and Lyness 2007; Van Alphen 2010; Wilson, Mottram, and Vassilas 2008). Whatever the technique being used, therapy of the patient with PD must take into account the therapeutic relationship since it is the management of this element of therapy with the person with PD that will determine success or failure.

Goldfried and Davila (2005) state that the relationship is the active ingredient in all psychotherapy regardless of technique:

> It is then proposed that there are general principles of therapeutic change that are facilitated by both the relationship and technique. It is suggested that these principles of change should be seen as the active ingredients of therapy, thereby moving the field away from a debate about whether technique or the relationship is more important. Instead, an emphasis on studying general principles of change and the processes by which technique and relationship facilitate these principles is encouraged.

There is considerable empirical support for the importance of the therapy relationship across different forms of psychotherapy (Castonguay et al. 2004; Constantino et al. 2008; Crits-Christoph and Barber 1991; Kanter, Schildcrout, and Kohlenberg 2005; Kohlenberg et al. 2002; Lambert and Barley 2001; Safran and Muran 2000; Vocisano et al 2004).

Whatever the chosen form of intervention used for the older patient with PD, therefore, it is unlikely to be effective unless a therapeutic alliance can be established. This requires management of one of the most challenging aspects of therapy of the person with personality disturbance: the transferential relationship.

PD and Relationships in Old Age

It is well recognized that one of the most important outcomes of personality disorder is its destructive effect on close or care-giving relationships. Impairment in relationships arise because of the distorted perceptions of the personality disordered individual regarding the motivations, intent, reliability, or caring of the other. In other words, the person with personality disturbance develops impaired perceptions of themselves in relationship to others. Table 24.3 illustrates some common self–other paradigms often associated with PD in older adults. If the therapist can identify these paradigms accurately when dealing with the older patient with PD, it then becomes possible to understand the reasons behind the patient's reactions during therapy. Similarly, such understanding can help the therapist understand the reasons behind behavioural interactions of the patient with others such as care-givers, family members, or friends. This puts the therapist in a much stronger position to defuse problematic behaviours as well as coach others to understand and deal appropriately with the person. Effective coaching is of particular relevance and value in intense care-giving

Table 24.3 Self/other model

Experience of self (trait)	Experience of other	Observed emotional state
Humiliated (narcissistic)	Demeaning	Anger, demoralized
Abandoned (abandonment fears)	Uncaring, rejecting	Depressed, hopeless, panic
Vulnerable, endangered (impaired trust)	Powerful, dangerous	Submissive, avoidant, anxious

situations where family or professional care-givers must interact closely with someone with PD over long periods of time. This is often very challenging for care-givers, who might prefer to withdraw from their role but cannot because of feeling trapped by the frailty and needs of the older person. Indeed, the children of a parent with PD often cope by creating distance from their parent. The problems of old age, however, often require that the parent be cared for much more intensively. The 'whirlpool' of ageing draws children back into the vortex of the relationship.

The Therapeutic Alliance

PD is selectively challenging to the development and maintenance of the therapeutic alliance, an essential part of any psychotherapy. The work of Bordin (1979) has specified the components of the alliance, each of which can be measured and adapted to facilitate the change process in older patients. According to Bordin, the therapeutic alliance is composed of three factors: (1) The presence of a personal *bond* between therapist and client, where the client views the therapist as caring, understanding, and knowledgeable; (2) an agreement between client and therapist regarding the *goals* of treatment (e.g., reducing symptoms, improving relationships with others); and (3) an agreement as to the *means* by which these goals may be achieved (i.e. therapeutic method). Anyone who has worked with individuals with PD will readily recognize that forming a bond or agreeing on goals and methods is often very difficult and at times impossible.

Closely allied to concepts of the therapeutic alliance are aspects of therapeutic relationship that emerge moment by moment during therapy and which the therapist has to handle in a way that both maintains the alliance and advances the goals of therapy. The skilful handling of the 'present moment' in therapy has long been a core tool of the best psychotherapists and is highly relevant to work with patients at any age. The ability to understand and manage patients' reactions as they arise in therapy will be a crucial determinant of outcome in patients with personality disorder.

Working in the present moment requires the therapist to be empathically tuned in to the patient's emotional and behavioural states and to respond accurately and skilfully. The emergence of feelings and reactions in patients is determined both by what is happening in the moment and by the longstanding deeper emotions, psychological conflicts, and ability to engage in an intimate trusting relationship. In other words, the transference. Transference may be viewed as the intermingling of the unconscious inner feelings of any two individuals who become involved in a relationship with each other. "Essentially a person in the present is reacted to as though he were a person in the past" (Greenson 1972, p152). Is the transference a practical and valuable focus of therapy in PD? Limited research, which admittedly needs to be interpreted with caution, suggests it is an important focus and predictor of outcome. For example, Høglend et al. (2008) demonstrated that outcome in brief dynamic psychotherapy is particularly improved by transference-based interpretations in the subset of patients with personality disorders.

In psychodynamic psychoanalytically informed therapy, the transference is a key therapeutic focus both to understand the patient's behaviours and reactions and as the basis of interpretive intervention. Other present-moment therapies have emerged more recently which recognize the centrality of the relationship and transference, and address it as a primary therapeutic target during various forms of therapy. This integrated perspective is nowhere more important than in geriatric psychotherapy, where multiple techniques are often used with a given patient. What grounds the therapy however, is understanding and management of the way the patient relates to the therapist and vice versa (Goldfried and Davila 2005).

WORKING IN THE PRESENT MOMENT

Kanter et al. (2009) has reviewed cognitive and interpersonal therapies that actively address the relationship as a key focus of therapy and emphasize the central role of empathy. He points out that in traditional CBT the primary focus is on changing thoughts and behaviour related to the world outside of therapy, but not in relation to the here-and-now therapy moment, the therapy relationship, or the therapy process. However, more recently the role of the present moment in therapy has begun to emerge as a primary concern in a variety of therapeutic techniques, some particularly relevant to personality disorder such as Beck's (2005) approach to cognitive therapy (CT) for challenging problems, and Leahy's (2001) guidelines for overcoming resistance in cognitive therapy and cognitive therapy for personality disorders (CT-PD) (Beck et al. 1990). Many other therapeutic variants of various theoretical perspectives that integrate developmental and present-moment with cognitive approaches have emerged, some of which have gained wider acceptance than others. These include cognitive-behavioural analysis system of psychotherapy (CBASP; McCullough 2000), schema-focused therapy (SFT; Young 1999), short-term cognitive therapy (STCT; Newman 1998), and integrated CT (ICT; Castonguay et al. 2004) among others.

Managing and enhancing the therapeutic alliance is at the core of some of the present-moment therapies. For example, integrated cognitive therapy (ICT) employs techniques empathically to reveal and heal alliance ruptures as they arise (Safran and Segal 1990; Safran and Muran 2000), and encourages exploring and understanding with the patient their feelings and reactions toward the therapist (Castonguay et al. 2004). Other approaches emphasize the therapeutic relationship more broadly (Gelso and Samstag 2008; Lejuez, et al. 2005).

In varying ways these newer versions of integrated therapy highlight and systematize well-known aspects of the therapeutic encounter and provide techniques for managing such things as the therapist's feelings of frustration and incompetence, patient resistances, hostility and anger, passivity, as in the cognitive-behavioural analysis system of psychotherapy (CBASP, McCullough 2000), mistrust and sensitivity to abandonment (Newman 1998), and non-collaboration in the therapeutic process. Present-moment techniques emphasize several approaches, including SFT (Young 1999), CT-PD (Beck et al. 1990), STCT (Newman 1998), and functional analytic enhanced cognitive therapy (FECT; Kohlenberg et al. 2002), and applying cognitive restructuring strategies as emotional reactions to the relationship emerge in therapy.

In psychotherapy, both the older patient and the therapist can doubt the enduring presence and power of early life relationships and fail to recognize their effect on the transference and, in turn, interactions which emerge between therapist and patient during the course of therapy. What is the value of addressing this matter? There are two reasons. The first is that a transference model gives the therapist a tool to understand the sometimes puzzling or difficult behaviours seen in patients with immature personality development. The second reason is that in some therapies transference interpretations may be very helpful to the patient.

The following clinical vignette illustrates the continuing effect of primitive psychodynamics, the 'timelessness of the unconscious', and the complicated therapy that can result. This case demonstrates a therapeutic rupture associated with a rapid breakdown of trust stemming from unconscious conflicts and the intense therapeutic fallout that is characteristic of some forms of PD. As in this case, the precipitant for the rupture in the therapeutic relationship does not have to be obvious or dramatic. It can be a misinterpreted look, tone of voice, or minor therapeutic failure that is the trigger. While one never intentionally provokes such negative transference feelings in therapy, they are inevitable because no therapist can avoid being disappointing at times. Sometimes, because of deeply ingrained mistrust and insecurity, the patient expects that the therapist will be depriving, re-enacting the self– other paradigm of the hurt abandoned child and the domineering, dangerous, or uncaring parent. These moments in therapy can be extremely uncomfortable for the therapist and the patient alike, causing the therapist to feel guilty at their failure or angry at the implicit accusations; but when these moments arise it is an opportunity to address the deepest level of feeling of the patient and to enable them to work through inner conflicts which otherwise would never be addressed.

Vignette

The patient Barbara was 76 years old. She had had recent disfiguring surgery complicated by severe and life-threatening post-operative complications. While these complications gradually remitted she continued to be deeply troubled by a casual comment by a psychiatrist who had seen her once while she was in hospital to consult around her peri-operative anxiety. The psychiatrist deeply affected her when she made an apparently innocent comment that she was 'in the later stages of her life'. When she left hospital, this previously self-reliant woman became preoccupied with the comment. She described going to an old-age facility in a panic to inquire about admission despite the fact that there was no indication at all that she needed any kind of supportive care. She could not sleep, was preoccupied with fears of old age, recurrence of cancer, and dying. She felt old, deformed, and that a man would never be interested in her again. She withdrew from her prior creative pleasures and activities. She came to therapy on her own initiative for help dealing with symptoms of depression and panic.

In earlier years she was a beautiful woman pursued by many proposals of marriage which she always rejected because of her exquisite fears of being hurt and her overly developed watchfulness for any perceived slight, disrespect, or feeling of being betrayed. Consequently, her younger adult history was punctuated by a series of intense relationships with men that she always broke off, blaming the inattention or failures of the man. While she was unsuccessful in relationships, other aspects of her life were characterized by creativity and business success. She was an avid amateur painter and pianist, financially secure from her own efforts and had an active, albeit superficial, social life. Her therapist diagnosed her with borderline personality disorder. She demonstrated impaired trust and unstable relationships, a poorly developed sense of identity, emotional instability, impulsivity, and acting out. While her more dramatic elements of sexual impulsivity and relational storms had quieted with ageing, her sense of self and her impaired relational capacities remained.

Her childhood had been very difficult and had distorted her emotional and psychological development. Her mother had schizophrenia and was hospitalized many times. At home she felt very insecure and that her many talents were devalued. Her father was cold and unresponsive, unable to protect her against the bizarre and frightening behaviour of her mother. She had two older sisters whom she also feared.

While never diagnosed with a formal psychiatric disorder, she had sought psychotherapy many years earlier as a young woman in her 20s. This therapy, while supportive, did not help her work through her conflicts. Only now in her 70s did she seek out therapy once again to cope with this new emotional crisis.

Perhaps not surprisingly, her therapy was often stormy. The sensitivity, suspicion, and mistrust that she described in her earlier relationships emerged during therapy. She often cross-examined the therapist about his motivations, and frequently focused on small perceived failures or what she experienced as unempathic comments by asking in the finest detail what the therapist was thinking when he said 'such and such'. Despite her challenging qualities she was not unpleasant to deal with most of the time. She had a sense of humour, was bright and between sessions often tried to reflect on herself and the therapy. She rarely acted out but therapy was challenging for her.

About a year and a half into therapy an administrative error led to Barbara being double booked with another patient. Because the new patient had travelled many hours from out of town, the therapist reluctantly elected to tell Barbara that her appointment that day had to be cancelled but that she could return in two days. She was initially quietly compliant. The therapist did not suspect that this error would evoke profound and very longlasting hurt and anger that was to plunge the therapeutic relationship into the depths of distrust and withdrawal. In ensuing sessions she repeatedly asked why the therapist had done this to her and described intense ruminations about what it had meant that the therapist had chosen the other patient over her. Logical explanations and apology were temporarily calming for her but had no lasting effect. To compound the difficulties the therapist then went on a long-planned three-week vacation.

When the therapist returned to his first session with her after his vacation, Barbara began the session abruptly by saying there was unfinished business, i.e. how confused she still felt about everything since the day of the double-booked appointment. Once again she said it was deeply disrespectful and had tormented her for weeks ever since. She thought about it while the therapist was away and wondered if this was his way of telling her he did not want to work with her and make her quit. She coldly said she felt very betrayed and now felt unsafe with him. While she recalled that the therapist had apologized and explained the unfortunate conflict in timing at the time, she did not accept his explanation and said she wondered if he had 'unconsciously' done this and not even realized what he had done to her.

Naturally the therapist felt tense, accused and under attack, although the feelings were not unfamiliar. In less intense forms the patient had expressed similar briefer reactions each time the therapist had inadvertently failed accurately to tune in to her emotions, was a few minutes late, or otherwise let her down.

This time, however, when the moment seemed right, the therapist decided on a different approach. He pointed out that her mistrust seemed to be a familiar feeling that she had described before. He went on to relate her current feelings to her earliest childhood experiences with her unpredictably rejecting and sometimes violent mother.

Interestingly, this transference and relational intervention calmed her. She said she actually had been surprised at the intensity of her feelings and acknowledged that it was no wonder she felt this way about him considering how she was always treated this way by her parents. She said 'no wonder I don't feel safe in relationships' but also reflected that it frightened her that if this is how she reacts it is understandable why she cannot have a close relationship in her life. The therapist reflected that he could understand what she was saying but added that all important relationships have elements of emotional risk. He went on to add that there are inevitably unpredictable and sometimes disappointing elements in close relationships but that a strong relationship can tolerate and survive anger or disappointment.

This opened other deeper thoughts in Barbara. She said she still wanted a hero as she always had; a hero, 'someone safe like Santa Claus or God', who would not let her down she said. The therapist pointed out that even heroes are flawed. She acknowledged that she wanted perfection and said that if there are flaws in the other she gets overwhelmed with fear and disappointment.

This vignette highlights so clearly the importance of recognizing how vibrant transference-based interactions can continue to be in a 76-year-old woman and how crucial it is that the therapist be aware of what is happening so that he can respond accurately. The idea that the past is so distant that it has lost its relevance for the older patient is clearly untrue. For this reason, the therapeutic work with older patients like Barbara needs to be in the here and now of the therapeutic process as it is with younger patients. Patients with immature personality structures such as Barbara are especially sensitive to empathic failures and can become angry, hurt, or withdrawn in response. Older adults easily feel alienated from younger therapists and can be very sensitive to failures of empathy in the therapeutic context, although often they may not acknowledge it.

While they are important in individual therapy, it is also crucial to keep these interpersonal dynamics in mind when understanding the reaction of older patients with PD to other situations such as relating to a new personal care-giver, dealing with acute illness in a hospital setting, or finding a way to adapt to the intense closeness of the long-term care environment.

SUMMARY

The clinician is challenged by the complexity of diagnosing PD; reliance on external observable behaviour, i.e. phenomenology, is insufficient. It is essential that clinical skills include tools to conduct a more refined evaluation of internal states, of concepts of self and others, intimacy, empathy, and identity, and self direction among others. This may be challenging in older adults where lifelong patterns may be overlaid by daily challenges that may distort perceptions of self and others.

It is unwise at this point to rely too heavily on epidemiological data regarding PDs because instruments designed for use in older adults have not been developed. While diagnosis is clinically challenging in some geriatric patients precision is important. The presence of PD will alter both treatment planning as well as expectations of outcome.

Important to understanding PD in late-life is the interplay of late-life stressors and the specific vulnerability of the ageing person, similar to the diathesis stress approach to understanding mental health. History taking and evaluation of older persons therefore not only must catalogue potential stressors but seek to link these stresses to the defensive structure of the individual and determine where and how they may be producing specific challenges that are leading to impaired function and symptomatic behaviours, especially depression and anxiety.

Five key factors are hypothesized as diatheses of vulnerability in later life: oversensitivity to narcissistic assault; excessive fear of abandonment; impaired capacity for intimacy and trust; attachment pathology such as intense and insecure attachment/dependency needs (impaired individuation, separation, and autonomy); and overly intense emotional reactivity (impaired affect regulation). The evaluation of concepts of self and other can be enhanced by employing a self–other paradigm and linking its effects to the observable behaviours of the patient.

Therapy is heavily impacted by the presence of PD or significant PD traits. A key challenge is managing the crucial therapeutic alliance without which therapy will fail. Various techniques have evolved recently that incorporate CBT principles with essential processes of working on the relationship as it emerges in the day-to-day therapy: so-called present-moment therapeutic techniques. Finally, the patient's behaviours and responses in therapy can provide important data on conflicts and reactions that may be emerging in other settings, such as with family or associated with home and institutional care.

KEY REFERENCES AND SOURCES FOR FURTHER READING

Balsis, S., Woods, C. M., Gleason, M. E., and Oltmanns, T. F. (2007). 'Over and Underdiagnosis of Personality Disorders in Older Adults'. *American Journal of Geriatric Psychiatry* 15(9): 742–753.

Kanter, J. W., Rusch, L. C., Lands, S. J., Holman, G. I., Whiteside, U., and Sedivy, S. K. (2009). 'The Use and Nature of Present-focused Interventions in Cognitive and Behavioral Therapies for Depression'. *Psychotherapy: Theory, Research, Practice* 46(2): 220–232.

Sadavoy, J. (1987). 'Character Disorders in the Elderly: An Overview'. In J. Sadavoy and M. Leszcz (eds), *Treating the Elderly with Psychotherapy: The Scope for Change in Later Life* (pp. 175–229). Madison, CT: International Universities Press.

Sadavoy, J. (1999). 'The Effect of Personality Disorder on Axis 1 Disorders in the Elderly'. In Michael Duffy (ed.), *Handbook of Counselling and Psychotherapy with Older Adults* (pp. 397–413). New York: Wiley.

Segal, D. L., Coolidge, F. L., and Rosowsky, E. (2006). *Personality Disorders and Older Adults: Diagnosis, Assessment and Treatment*. Hoboken, NJ: Wiley.

Tackett, J. L., Balsis, S., Oltmanns, T. F., and Krueger, R. F. (2009). 'A Unifying Perspective on Personality Pathology across the Life Span: Developmental Considerations for the Fifth Edition of the Diagnostic and Statistical Manual of Mental Disorders'. *Development and Psychopathology* 21: 687–713.

References

Abrams, R. C. and Horowitz, S. V. (1996). 'Personality Disorders after Age 50: A Meta-analysis'. *Journal of Personality Disorders* 35: 383–386.

Abrams, R. C. and Horowitz, S. V. (1999). 'Personality Disorders after Age 50: A Meta-analytic Review of the Literature'. In E. Rosowsky, R. C. Abrams, and R. A. Zweig (eds), *Personality Disorders in Older Adults* (pp. 55–68). Mahwah, NJ: Lawrence Erlbaum Associates.

Agronin, M. E. and Maletta, G. (2000). 'Personality Disorders in Late Life. Understanding and Overcoming the Gap in Research'. *American Journal of Geriatric Psychiatry* 8(1): 4–18.

American Psychiatric Association (2013). *Diagnostic and Statistical Manual of Mental Disorders* (5th edn). Arlington, VA: American Psychiatric Association.

Ames, A. and Molinari, V. (1994). 'Prevalence of Personality Disorders in Community Living Elderly'. *Journal of Geriatric Psychiatry and Neurology* 7: 189–194.

Balsis, S., Gleason, M. E., Woods, C. M., and Oltmanns, T. F. (2007a). 'An Item Response Theory Analysis of DSM-IV Personality Disorder Criteria across Younger and Older Age Groups'. *Psychological Aging* 22(1): 171–185.

Balsis, S., Woods, C. M., Gleason, M. E., and Oltmanns, T. F. (2007b). 'Overdiagnosis and Underdiagnosis of Personality Disorders in Older Adults'. *American Journal of Geriatric Psychiatry* 15(9): 742–753.

Bauer, M. E., Vedhara, K., Perks, P., Wilcock, G. K., Lightman, S. L., and Shanks, N. (2000). 'Chronic Stress in Caregivers of Dementia Patients is Associated with Reduced Lymphocyte Sensitivity to Glucocorticoids'. *Journal of Neuroimmunology* 103: 84–92.

Beck, A. T., Freeman, A., Davis, D. D., and Associates (1990). *Cognitive Therapy of Personality Disorders*. New York: Guilford Press.

Beck, J. S. (2005). *Cognitive Therapy for Challenging Problems: What to Do When the Basics Don't Work*. New York: Guilford Press.

Berezin, M. A. (1972). 'Psychodynamic Considerations of Aging and the Aged: An Overview'. *American Journal of Psychiatry* 128(12): 1483–1491.

Bizzini, L. (1998). 'Cognitive Psychotherapy in the Treatment of Personality Disorders in the Elderly'. In C. Perris and P. D. McGorry (eds), *Cognitive Psychotherapy of Psychotic and Personality Disorders: Handbook of Theory and Practice*. Chicester: Wiley.

Bordin, E. S. (1979). 'The Generalizability of the Psychoanalytic Concept of the Working Alliance'. *Psychotherapy: Theory, Research, and Practice* 16: 252–260.

Brebner, K., Hayley, S., Zacharko, R., Merali, Z., and Anisman, H. (2000). 'Synergistic Effects of Interleukin-1beta, Interleukin-6, and Tumor Necrosis Factor-Alpha: Central Monoamine, Corticosterone, and Behavioral Variations'. *Neuropsychopharmacology* 22: 566–580.

Capuron, L., Bluthé, R. M., and Dantzer, R. (2001). 'Cytokines in Clinical Psychiatry'. *American Journal of Psychiatry* 158: 1163–1164.

Casey, D. A. and Schrodt, C. J. (1989). 'Axis II Diagnoses in Geriatric Inpatients'. *Journal of Geriatric Psychiatry and Neurology* 2: 87–88.

Castonguay, L. G., Schut, A. J., Aikins, D. E., Constantino, M. J., Laurenceau, J., Bologh, L., et al. (2004). 'Integrative Cognitive Therapy for Depression: A Preliminary Investigation'. *Journal of Psychotherapy Integration* 14: 4–20.

Cohen, B. J., Nestadt, G., Samuels, J. F., Romanski, A. J., McHuch, P. R., and Rabins P. V. (1994). 'Personality Disorder in Later Life: A Community Study'. *British Journal of Psychiatry* 165: 493–499.

Constantino, M., Marnell, M., Haile, A., Kanthersista, S., Wolman, K., Zappert, L., et al. (2008). 'Integrative Cognitive Therapy for Depression: A Randomized Pilot Comparison'. *Psychotherapy: Theory, Research, Practice, Training* 45: 122–134.

Coolidge, F. L., Burns, E. M., Nathan, J. H., and Mull, C. E. (1992). 'Personality Disorders in the Elderly'. *Clinical Gerontologist* 12: 41–55.

Crits-Christoph, P. and Barber, J. (1991). *Handbook of Short-term Dynamic Psychotherapy.* New York: Basic Books.

Dantzer, R. (2001). 'Cytokine-Induced Sickness Behavior: Mechanisms and Implications'. *Annals of the New York Academy of Sciences* 933: 222–234.

Devanand, D. P., Kim, M. K., Paykina, N., and Sackeim, H. A. (2002). 'Adverse Life Events in Elderly Patients with Major Depression or Dysthymic Disorder and in Healthy-Control Subjects'. *American Journal of Geriatric Psychiatry* 10: 265–274.

Dick, L. P. and Gallagher-Thompson, D. (1995). 'Cognitive Therapy with the Core Beliefs of a Distressed Lonely Caregiver'. *Journal of Cognitive Psychotherapy* 9(4): 215–227.

Dobson, K. S. (1989). 'A Meta-analysis of the Efficacy of Cognitive Therapy for Depression'. *Journal of Consulting and Clinical Psychology* 57: 414–419.

Ekers, D., Richards, D., and Gilbody, S. (2008). 'A Meta-analysis of Randomized Trials of Behavioural Treatment of Depression'. *Psychological Medicine* 38: 611–623.

Engels, G. I., Duijsens, I. J., Haringsma, R., and van Putten, C. M. (2003). 'Personality Disorders in the Elderly Compared to Four Younger Age Groups: A Cross-sectional Study of Community Residents and Mental Health Patients'. *Journal of Personality Disorders* 17: 447–459.

Ferrucci, L., Harris, T. B., Guralnik, J. M., Tracy, R. P., Corti, M. C., Cohen, H. J., Penninx, B., Pahor, M., Wallace, R., and Havlik, R. J. (1999). 'Serum IL-6 Level and the Development of Disability in Older Persons'. *Journal of the American Geriatrics Society* 47: 639–646.

Fogel, B. S. and Stoudemire, A. (2000). 'Personality Disorders in the Medical Setting'. In A. Stoudemire, B. S. Fogel, and D. Greenberg (eds), *Psychiatric Care of the Medical Patient* (pp. 443–457). New York: Oxford University Press.

Gelso, C. and Samstag, L. (2008). 'A Tripartite Model of the Therapeutic Relationship'. In S. Brown and R. Lent (eds), *Handbook of Counseling Psychology* (4th edn; pp. 267–283). New York: Wiley.

Goldfried, M., Raue, P., and Castonguay, L. (1998). 'The Therapeutic Focus in Significant Sessions of Master Therapists: A Comparison of Cognitive-behavioral and Psychodynamic-Interpersonal Interventions'. *Journal of Consulting and Clinical Psychology* 66: 803–810.

Goldfried, M. and Davila, J. (2005). 'The Role of Relationship and Technique in Therapeutic Change'. *Psychotherapy: Theory, Research, Practice, Training* 42: 421–430.

Gortner, E. T., Gollan, J. K., Dobson, K. S., and Jacobson, N. S. (1998). 'Cognitive-behavioral Treatment for Depression: Relapse Prevention'. *Journal of Consulting and Clinical Psychology* 66: 377–384.

Greenson, R. (1972). *The Technique and Practice of Psychoanalysis* (p. 152). New York: International Universities Press.

Hamilton, M. (1967). 'Development of a Rating Scale for Primary Depressive Illness'. *British Journal of Social and Clinical Psychology* 6: 278–296.

Hamerman, D., Berman, J. W., Albers, G. W., Brown, D. L., and Silver, D. (1999). 'Emerging Evidence for Inflammation in Conditions Frequently Affecting Older Adults: Report of a Symposium'. *Journal of the American Geriatrics Society* 47: 1016–1025.

Hendriks, G. J., Oude Voshaar, R. C., Keijsers, G. P., Hoogduin, C. A., and van Balkom, A. J. (2008). 'Cognitive-behavioural Therapy for Late-life Anxiety Disorders: A Systematic Review and Meta-analysis'. *Acta Psychiatrica Scandinavica* 117: 403–411.

Høglend, P., Bøgwald, K.-P., Amlo, S., Marble, A., Ulberg, R., Sjaastad, M. C., et al. (2008). 'Transference Interpretations in Dynamic Psychotherapy: Do they Really Yield Sustained Results'. *American Journal of Psychiatry* 165: 763–771.

Jacobson, N. S., Dobson, K. S., Truax, P. A., Addis, M. E., Koerner, K., Gollan, J. K., et al. (1996). 'A Component Analysis of Cognitive Behavioral Treatment for Depression'. *Journal of Consulting and Clinical Psychology* 64: 295–304.

James, I. A. (2008). 'Schemas and Schema-focused Approaches in Older People'. In K. Laidlaw and B. Knight (eds), *Handbook of Emotional Disorders in Later Life: Assessment and Treatment* (pp. 111–140). Oxford: Oxford University Press.

Kanter, J. W., Schildcrout, J. S., and Kohlenberg, R. J. (2005). 'In Vivo Processes in Cognitive Therapy for Depression: Frequency and Benefits'. *Psychotherapy Research* 15: 366–373.

Kanter, J. W., Manos, R. C., Busch, A. M., and Rusch, L. C. (2008). 'Making Behavioral Activation More Behavioral'. *Behavioral Modification* 32: 780–803.

Kanter, J. W., Rusch, L. C., Lands, S. J., Holman, G. I., Whiteside, U., and Sedivy, S. K. (2009). 'The Use and Nature of Present-focused Interventions in Cognitive and Behavioral Therapies for Depression'. *Psychotherapy: Theory, Research, Practice* 46(2): 220–232.

Keller, M. B., Mccullough, J. P., Klein, D. N., Arnow, B. A., Rush, A. J., Nemeroff, C. B., et al. (2000). 'A Comparison of Nefazadone, the Cognitive Behavioral Analysis System of Psychotherapy and their Combination for the Treatment of Chronic Depression'. *New England Journal of Medicine* 322: 1462–1470.

Kiecolt-Glaser, J. K., Dura, J. R., Speicher, C. E., Trask, O. J., and Glaser, R. (1991). 'Spousal Caregivers of Dementia Victims: Longitudinal Changes in Immunity and Health'. *Psychosomatic Medicine* Jul–Aug; 53(4): 345–362.

Kiecolt-Glaser, J. K. and Glaser, R. (2002). 'Depression and Immune Function: Central Pathways to Morbidity and Mortality'. *Journal of Psychosomatic Research* 53: 873–876.

Kiecolt-Glaser, J. K., Preacher, K. J., MacCallum, R. C., Atkinson, C., Malarkey, W. B., and Glaser, R. (2003). 'Chronic Stress and Age-Related Increases in the Proinflammatory Cytokine IL-6'. *Proceedings of the National Academy of Sciences of the United States of America* 100: 9090–9095.

Klein, D. N., Santiago, N. J., Vivian, D., Arnow, B. A., Blalock, J. A., Dunner, D. L., et al. (2004). 'Cognitive-behavioral Analysis System of Psychotherapy as a Maintenance Treatment for Chronic Depression'. *Journal of Consulting and Clinical Psychology* 72: 681–688.

Kohlenberg, R. J. and Tsai, M. (1991). *Functional Analytic Psychotherapy: A Guide for Creating Intense and Curative Therapeutic Relationships*. New York: Plenum Press.

Kohlenberg, R. J., Kanter, J. W., Bolling, M. Y., Parker, C. R., and Tsai, M. (2002). 'Enhancing Cognitive Therapy for Depression with Functional Analytic Psychotherapy: Treatment Guidelines and Empirical Findings'. *Cognitive and Behavioral Practice* 9: 213–229.

Konsman, J. P., Parnet, P., and Dantzer, R. (2002). 'Cytokine-Induced Sickness Behaviour: Mechanisms and Implications'. *Trends in Neuroscience* 25: 154–9.

Kop, W. J., Gottdiener, J. S., Tangen, C. M., Fried, L. P., McBurnie, M. A., Walston, J., Newman, A., Hirsch, C., and Tracy, R. P. (2002). 'Inflammation and Coagulation Factors in Persons >65 Years of Age with Symptoms of Depression but without Evidence of Myocardial Ischemia'. *American Journal of Cardiology* 89: 419–24.

Kunik, M. E., Mulsant, B. H., Rifai, A. H., Sweet, R. A., Pasternak, R., and Zubenko, G. S. (1994). 'Diagnostic Rate of Comorbid Personality Disorder in Elderly Psychiatric Inpatients'. *American Journal of Psychiatry* 154: 603–605.

Laidlaw K. (2001). 'An Empirical Review of Cognitive Therapy for Late Life Depression: Does Research Evidence Suggest Adaptations are Necessary for Cognitive Therapy with Older Adults?' *Clinical Psychology & Psychotherapy* 8: 1–14.

Laidlaw, K., Thompson, L. W., Dick-Siskin, L., and Gallagher-Thompson, D. (2003). *Cognitive Behaviour Therapy with Older People*. Chichester: Wiley.

Laidlaw, K. and Thompson, L. W. (2008). 'Cognitive Behaviour Therapy with Depressed Older People'. In K. Laidlaw and B. Knight (eds), *Handbook of Emotional Disorders in Later Life: Assessment and Treatment* (pp. 91–116). Oxford: Oxford University Press.

Lambert, M. and Barley, D. (2001). 'Research Summary on the Therapeutic Relationship and Psychotherapy Outcome'. *Psychotherapy: Theory, Research, Practice, Training* 38: 357–361.

Lazarus, A. (2003). 'Some Reactions to Robert Kohlenberg's Article'. *Behavior Therapist* 26: 380.

Leahy, R. (2001). '*Overcoming Resistance in Cognitive Therapy*'. New York: Guilford Press.

Lejuez, C. W., Hopko, D. R., Levine, S., Gholkar, R., and Collins, L. M. (2005). 'The Therapeutic Alliance in Behavior Therapy'. *Psychotherapy: Theory, Research, Practice, Training* 42: 456–468.

Lynch, T. R., Cheavens, J. S., Cukrowitz, K. C., Thorp, S. R., Bronner, L., and Beyer, J. (2007). 'Treatment of Adults with Co-morbid Personality Disorder and Depression: A Dialectical Behaviour Therapy Approach'. *International Journal of Geriatric Psychiatry* 22: 131–143.

Maruta, T., Colligan, R. C., Malinchoc, M., and Offord, K. P. (2000). 'Optimists vs Pessimists: Survival Rate Among Medical Patients Over a 30-Year Period'. *Mayo Clinic Proceedings* 75: 140–3.

Mazure, C. M., Maciejewski, P. K., Jacobs, S. C., and Bruce, M. L. (2002). 'Stressful Life Events Interacting with Cognitive/Personality Styles to Predict Late-Onset Major Depression'. *American Journal of Geriatric Psychiatry* 10: 297–304.

McCullough, J. P. (2000). *Treatment for Chronic Depression: Cognitive Behavioral Analysis System of Psychotherapy (CBASP)*. New York: Guilford Press.

McGlashan, T. H. (1986). 'The Chestnut Lodge Follow-up Study III: Long Term Outcome of Borderline Personalities'. *Archives of General Psychiatry* 43: 20–30.

Martell, C. R., Addis, M. E., and Jacobson, N. S. (2001). *Depression in Context: Strategies for Guided Action*. New York: Norton.

Marvin, R., Goldfried, M., and J. Davila (2005). 'The Role of Relationship and Technique in Therapeutic Change'. *Psychotherapy: Theory, Research, Practice, Training* 42: 421–430.

Mergenthaler, E. and Stinson, C. H. (1992). 'Psychotherapy Transcription Standards'. *Psychotherapy Research* 2: 125–142.

Mezzich, T. E., Fabrega, H., Coffman, G. A., and Glavin, Y. F. (1987). 'Comprehensively Diagnosing Geriatric Patients'. *Comprehensive Psychiatry* 28: 68–76.

Molinari, V. and Marmion, J. (1993). 'Personality Disorders in Geropsychiatric Outpatients'. *Psychological Reports* 73: 256–258.

Molinari, V., Ames, A., and Essa, M. (1994). 'Prevalence of Personality Disorders in Two Psychiatric Inpatients Units'. *Journal of Geriatric Psychiatry and Neurology* 7: 209–215.

Molinari, V. and Marmion, J. (1995). 'Relationship between Affective Disorders and Axis II Diagnoses in Geropsychiatric Patients'. *Journal of Geriatric Psychiatry and Neurology* 8: 61–64.

Muran, J., Safran, J., Samstag, L., and Winston, A. (2005). 'Evaluating an Alliance-focused Treatment for Personality Disorders'. *Psychotherapy: Theory, Research, Practice, Training* 42: 532–545.

Newman, C. F. (1998). 'The Therapeutic Relationship and Alliance in Short-term Cognitive Therapy'. In J. D. Safran and J. C. Muran (eds), *The Therapeutic Alliance in Brief Psychotherapy* (pp. 95–122). Washington, DC: American Psychological Association.

Oltmanns, T. F. and Balsis, S. (2011). 'Personality Disorders in Later Life: Questions about the Measurement, Course and Impact of Disorders'. *Annual Review of Clinical Psychology* 27(7): 321–349.

Pieper, C. F., Rao, K. M., Currie, M. S., Harris, T. B., and Cohen, H. J. (2000). 'Age, Functional Status, and Racial Differences in Plasma D-dimer Levels in Community-Dwelling Elderly Persons'. *Journals of Gerontology Series A: Biological Sciences and Medical Sciences* 55: M649–57.

Pinquart, M., Duberstein, P. R., and Lyness, J. M. (2007). 'Effects of Psychotherapy and Other Behavioral Interventions on Clinically Depressed Older Adults: A Meta-analysis'. *Aging & Mental Health* 11: 645–657.

Piper, W. E., Joyce, A. S., McCallum, M., and Azim, H. F. A. (1993). 'Concentration and Correspondence of Transference Interpretations in Short-term Psychotherapy'. *Journal of Consulting and Clinical Psychology* 61: 586–595.

Raudenbush, S. W. and Bryk, A. S. (2002). *Hierarchical Linear Models: Applications and Data Analysis Methods* (2nd edn). Newbury Park, CA: Sage.

Raudenbush, S. W., Bryk, A. S., Cheong, Y. F., Congdon, R., and Du Toit, M. (2004). *HLM6: Hierarchical Linear and Nonlinear Modeling*. Lincolnwood, IL: Scientific Software International.

Roberts, B. W., Walton, K. E., and Viechtbauer, W. (2006). 'Patterns of Mean-level Change in Personality Traits across the Life Course: A Metaanalysis of Longitudinal Studies'. *Psychological Bulletin* 132: 1–25.

Rosowsky, E. and Gurian, B. (1992). 'Impact of Borderline Personality Disorder in Late Life on Systems of Care'. *Hospital and Community Psychiatry* 43: 386–389.

Sadavoy, J. (1987). 'Character Disorders in the Elderly: An Overview'. In J. Sadavoy and M. Leszcz (eds), *Treating the Elderly with Psychotherapy: The Scope for Change in Later Life* (pp. 175–229). Madison, CT: International Universities Press.

Sadavoy, J. (1996). 'The Symptom Expression of Personality Disorder in Old Age'. *Clinical Gerontologist* 16(3): 19–36.

Sadavoy, J. (1999). 'The Effect of Personality Disorder on Axis 1 Disorders in the Elderly'. In M. Duffy (ed.), *Handbook of Counselling and Psychotherapy with Older Adults* (pp. 397–413). New York: Wiley.

Safran, J. D. and Segal, Z. V. (1990). *Interpersonal Process in Cognitive Therapy*. New York: Basic Books.

Safran, J. D. and Muran, J. C. (2000). *Negotiating the Therapeutic Alliance: A Relational Treatment Guide*. New York: Guilford Press.

Segal, D. L., Coolidge, F. L., and Rosowsky, E. (2006). 'Personality Disorders and Older Adults'. *Annals of Behavioral Medicine*. 2000 Summer; 22(3): 180–90.

Segerstrom, S. C. (2000). *Personality and the immune system: models, methods, and mechanisms. Diagnosis, Assessment and Treatment*. Hoboken, NJ: Wiley.

Shakespeare W. *The Tragedy of Hamlet, Prince of Denmark* Act 4 Scene 5.

Shrout, P. and Fleiss, J. (1979). 'Intraclass Correlations: Uses in Assessing Rater Reliability'. *Psychological Bulletin* 86: 420–428.

Silberman, C. S., Roth, L., Degal., D. L., and Burns, W. (1997). 'Relationship between the Millon Clinical Multiaxial Inventory-II and Coolidge Axis II Inventory in Chronically Mentally Ill Older Adults: A Pilot Study'. *Journal of Clinical Psychology* 53: 559–566.

Solomon, K. (1981). 'Personality Disorders in the Elderly'. In J. R. Lion (ed.), *Personality Disorders, Diagnosis, and Management* (pp. 310–338). Baltimore: Williams and Wilkins.

Spitzer, R. L. (1983). 'Psychiatric Diagnosis: Are Clinicians Still Necessary?' *Comprehensive Psychiatry* 24: 399–411.

Stevenson, J., Meares, R., and Comerford, A. (2003). 'Diminished Impulsivity in Older Patients with Borderline Personality Disorder'. *American Journal of Psychiatry* 160: 165–166.

Stone, M. H. (1990). *The Fate of Borderline Patients*. New York: Guilford Press.

Stone, M. H. (1993). 'Long-term Outcome in Personality Disorders'. *British Journal of Psychiatry* 162: 299–313.

Tackett, J. L., Balsis, S., Oltmanns, T. F., and Krueger, R. F. (2009). 'A Unifying Perspective on Personality Pathology across the Life Span: Developmental Considerations for the Fifth Edition of the Diagnostic and Statistical Manual of Mental Disorders'. *Development and Psychopathology* 21: 687–713.

Terracciano, A., Löckenhoff, C., Zonderman, A., Ferrucci, L., and Costa, P. (2008). 'Personality Predictors of Longevity: Activity, Emotional Stability, and Conscientiousness'. *Psychosomatic Medicine* 70: 621–627.

Thompson, L. W., Gallagher, D., and Czirr, R. (1988). 'Personality Disorders and Outcome in the Treatment of Late-life Depression'. *Journal of Geriatric Psychiatry* 21: 133–146.

Trull, T. J., Tomko, R. L., Brown, W. C., and Scheiderer, E. M. (2010). 'Borderline Personality Disorder in 3-D: Dimensions, Symptoms, and Measurement Challenges'. *Social and Personality Psychology Compass* 11: 1057–1069.

Trull, T. J., Distel, M. A., and Carpenter, R. W. (2011). 'DSM-5 Borderline Personality Disorder: At the Border Between a Dimensional and a Categorical View'. *Current Psychiatry Reports* 13: 43–49.

Tsai, M., Kohlenberg, R. J., Kanter, J. W., Kohlenberg, B., Follette, W. C., and Callaghan, G. M. (eds) (2008). *A Guide to Functional Analytic Psychotherapy: Awareness, Courage, Love, and Behaviorism in the Therapeutic Relationship*. New York: Springer.

Tummers, J. A., Hoijtink, J. A., Penders, K. P., Derksen, J. L., and van Alphen, S. J. (2011). 'Screening Items for Personality Disorders in Older Adults: A Multi-center Study of Psychiatric Inpatients and Outpatients in the Netherlands'. *Clinical Gerontologist* 34(1): 34–44.

Ullrich, S. and Coid, J. (2009). 'The Age Distribution of Self-reported Personality Disorder Traits in a Household Population'. *Journal of Personality Disorders* 23: 187–200.

Van Alphen, S. P. J., Rettig, A. M., Engelen, G. J. J. A., Kuin, Y., and Derksen, J. J. L. (2005). 'Patiënt-informant overeenkomst op de Gerontologische Personality disorders Schaal (GPS)' [Patient-informant concordance of the Gerontological Personality Disorder Scale]. *Tijdschrift voor Psychiatrie* 47: 613–617.

Van Alphen, S. P. J., Engelen, G. J. J. A., Kuin, Y., and Derksen, J. J. L. (2006a). 'Editorial: The Relevance of a Geriatric Sub-classification of Personality Disorders in the DSM-V'. *International Journal of Geriatric Psychiatry* 21: 205–209.

Van Alphen, S. P. J., Engelen, G. J. J. A., Kuin, Y., Hoijtink, H. J. A., and Derksen, J. J. L. (2006b). 'A Preliminary Study of the Diagnostic Accuracy of the Gerontological Personality Disorders Scale (GPS)'. *International Journal of Geriatric Psychiatry* 21: 862–868.

Van Alphen, S. P. J., Nijhuis, P. E. P., and Oei, T. I. (2007). 'Antisocial Personality Disorder in Older Adults: A Qualitative Study of Dutch Forensic Psychiatrists and Forensic Psychologists'. *International Journal of Geriatric Psychiatry* 22: 813–815.

Van Alphen, S. P. J. (2010). 'Treatment of Avoidant Personality Pathology in Late Life'. *International Psychogeriatrics* 30: 1–4.

Van Alphen, S. P. J., Derksen, J. J. L., Sadavoy, J., Rosowsky, E. (2012a). 'Features and Challenges of Personality Disorders in Late Life'. *Aging & Mental Health* 16(7): 805–810.

Van Alphen, S. P. J., Bolwerk, N., Videler, A. C., Tummers, J. H. A., Van Royen, R. J. J., Barendse, H. P. J., et al. (2012b). 'Age Related Aspects and Clinical Implications of Diagnosis and Treatment of Personality Disorders in Older Adults'. *Clinical Gerontologist* 35(1): 27–41.

Vine, R., and Steingart, A. (1994). 'Personality Disorder in the Elderly Depressed'. *Canadian Journal of Psychiatry* 39: 392–398.

Vocisano, C., Klein, D. N., Arnow, B., Rivera, C. Blalock, J. A., Rothbaum, R., et al. (2004). 'Therapist Variables that Predict Symptom Change in Psychotherapy with Chronically Depressed Outpatients'. *Psychotherapy: Theory, Research, Practice, Training* 41: 255–265.

Waddington, L. (2002). 'The Therapy Relationship in Cognitive Therapy: A Review'. *Behavioural and Cognitive Psychotherapy* 30: 179–192.

Watson, D. C. and Sinha, K. B. (1996). 'A Normative Study of the Coolidge Axis II Inventory'. *Journal of Clinical Psychology* 52: 631–637.

Weissman, M. M. (1993). 'The Epidemiology of Personality Disorders: A 1990 Update'. *Journal of Personality Disorders* 7: 44–62.

Williams, J. B. W. (1988). 'A Structured Interview Guide for the Hamilton Depression Rating Scale'. *Archives of General Psychiatry* 45: 742–747.

Wilson, K. C., Mottram, P. G., and Vassilas, C. A. (2008). 'Psychotherapeutic Treatments for Older Depressed People'. *Cochrane Database of Systematic Reviews* 1: CD004853. doi:10.1002/14651858.CD004853.pub2.

Young, J. E. (1999). *Cognitive Therapy for Personality Disorders: A Schema-focused Approach.* Sarasota, FL: Professional Resource Press.

Zimmerman, M. (1994). 'Diagnosing Personality Disorders: A Review of Issues and Research Methods'. *Archives of General Psychiatry* 51: 225–245.

....

CHAPTER 25

LATE-LIFE INSOMNIA

....

MEGAN E. RUITER PETROV,
GREGORY S.VANDER WAL, AND
KENNETH L.LICHSTEIN

LATE-LIFE INSOMNIA

OLDER adults are a burgeoning segment of the global population. Adults aged 60 or older are projected to represent 21.4% of the population in 2050 compared to 10% in 2000 (Cohen 2003). Common health-related changes that occur in older adulthood are the lightening (i.e. increased time spent in the stages of sleep that are easiest to wake from) and greater fragility of sleep. These changes are a natural part of the ageing process, yet sleep complaints such as difficulty maintaining sleep and early-morning awakenings are commonly reported in older adulthood (Foley et al. 1995, 1999). These complaints are not wholly accounted for by normal age-related changes in sleep. Instead, the greater fragility of the sleep-wake cycle, concomitant with an accumulation of other age-related changes such as illness, polypharmacy, institutionalization, and social role transitions, are considered collectively to increase the likelihood of incident sleep complaints and chronic insomnia (Lichstein et al. 2004). Recent reviews have been conducted on age-related sleep changes and late-life insomnia (Ancoli-Israel, Ayalon, and Salzman 2008; Krishnan and Hawranik 2008; Neikrug and Ancoli-Israel 2010; Ruiter et al. 2010b). This chapter summarizes these reviews and merges them with up-to-date evidence describing the prevalence and clinical presentation of insomnia symptoms and chronic insomnia among older adults. It will also outline guidelines for the assessment, diagnosis, and treatment of late-life insomnia. Non-pathological age-related changes in sleep will be briefly reviewed first in order to assist the clinician and researcher alike in distinguishing these sleep patterns from chronic late-life insomnia.

Normal Changes in Sleep Patterns
with Age

Sleep structure and continuity

The structure of sleep has been described previously (Iber 2007; Rechtschaffen and Kales 1968) and is beyond the scope of the current chapter. In brief, sleep is divided into four stages of sleep as defined by electroencephalography, electrooculography, and electromyography. Stages 1, 2, and 3 comprise non-rapid eye movement (NREM) sleep, and these stages cyclically occur along with rapid eye movement (REM) sleep every 90–120 minutes during the sleep state. Stages 1 and 2 are described as 'lighter' stages of sleep that are easier to arouse from, whereas Stage 3 sleep, also known as slow wave sleep, is known for being more restorative and more difficult from which to awaken. REM sleep is characterized by rapid eye movements, muscle atonia, and vivid dreams.

As we age, the structure of sleep alters, generally resulting in lighter sleep that is more easily disrupted. Compared to younger adults, older adults' percentage of time slept in stage 3 and REM sleep is less. Consequently their percentage time slept in lighter stages of sleep, stages 1 and 2, is greater (Gillin and Ancoli-Israel 2005). These findings were confirmed within a meta-analysis of objectively assessed sleep on 3577 participants across the lifespan (Ohayon et al. 2004). The participants in their latter years were selected for their optimal health; thus these results represent healthy ageing of sleep. The meta-analysis demonstrated that most of these age-related changes occur between young adulthood and 60 years of age, and from thereon alter only minimally (Ohayon et al. 2004). In particular, slow wave sleep declines by 2% per decade until age 60. Thereafter, the decline appears to plateau; however, further studies that screen comprehensively for psychiatric and medical disorders need to be conducted in older adults to verify this plateau.

With lightening of sleep comes a greater risk of spontaneous, biological, and environmental disruption that can alter the quality and quantity of sleep. Sleep continuity continues to decrease modestly in healthy older adults by 3% per decade (Ohayon et al. 2004). It is likely that the decrease is modest because healthy older adults have the ability to fall back asleep just as easily as young adults even though they awaken more often (Klerman et al. 2004). With ill health and other stressors, however, this increase in sleep fragmentation can be exaggerated and characterized by frequent sleep stage shifts (Morgan 2000). This deterioration of sleep continuity may have contributed to the common adage that older adults sleep less, and do not need as much sleep as younger adults. Although total sleep time decreases as we age (Ohayon et al. 2004) and the sleep duration of older adults is on average shorter (Campbell and Murphy 2007), the amount is still comparable to younger adults (Foley et al. 2004). Rather, multiple health, social, and environmental risk factors capitalize on already present age-related sleep continuity changes to explain reductions in older adults' sleep quantity and quality. Therefore, the sleep need of older adults is *not altered* (Foley et al. 2004), but the ability to achieve that need is frequently more challenging.

Circadian rhythm changes

The sleep-wake cycle follows a 24-hour circadian rhythm moderated by the hypothalamic suprachiasmatic nucleus. With age, the nucleus and other brain areas experience neuronal degeneration, which disrupts the rhythmicity of sleep-wake patterns. A common change in rhythmicity among older adults is an advanced phase shift that causes sleepiness to occur in the early evening hours and awaking in the early-morning hours (Monk 2005). These changes are not pathological. However, insomnia symptoms and sleep loss can result if older adults resist these changes by attempting sleep outside of their natural sleep phase.

Daytime Sleep

The degradation in sleep continuity, depth, duration, and circadian rhythmicity has been hypothesized to explain increasing amounts of daytime sleep in older adults (McCrae et al. 2006). A current debate in the field concerns whether daytime sleep is beneficial by contributing to the overall 24-hour sleep duration (Campbell, Murphy, and Stauble 2005), or if it is deleterious, leading to insomnia symptoms (Boden-Albala et al. 2008). A study comparing community-dwelling older adult 'nappers' to 'non-nappers' revealed that self-reported sleep duration and quality were not significantly different between groups (Picarsic et al. 2008). However, a study using objectively assessed sleep indicated that greater sleep fragmentation increased the odds of napping (Goldman et al. 2008). Further research is necessary to determine if and what aspects of daytime sleep in older adults are pathological.

In review, the sleep of healthy older adults is lighter, more fragmented, and more likely to be phase advanced and occur during the day compared to younger adults. These changes represent risk factors rather than causes of chronic insomnia. There are numerous causes of insomnia that older adults have a greater probability of encountering than their younger counterparts. Poor physical health status is usually the primary culprit (Ohayon et al. 2001), though polypharmacy, other primary sleep disorders, and mental health, behavioural, and psychosocial dynamics are also major factors (Ohayon 2004). Thus, chronic insomnia is more prevalent in older adults (discussed later in this chapter), and is associated with objective impairments in sleep (Gooneratne et al. 2011) more than in younger adults (Edinger et al. 2000).

DIAGNOSIS

Multiple nosological systems, such as the *Diagnostic and Statistical Manual of Mental Disorders* (*DSM-IV-TR*; American Psychiatric Association (APA) 2000), the International Classification of Disease (ICD-10;World Health Organization 1993), and the International Classification of Sleep Disorders (ICSD-II; American Academy of Sleep Medicine 2005), provide diagnostic criteria for insomnia. Despite differences in the subtypes of insomnia, there are essentially three components of an insomnia diagnosis: (1) complaint of a sleep difficulty; (2) adequate opportunity to attain sufficient sleep; and (3) complaint of daytime functioning impairment. The presence of distress about sleep is especially important in older adults as many who exhibit poor sleep are not distressed by it (McCrae et al. 2005). Night-time insomnia symptoms include difficulty falling asleep, difficulty staying asleep, and early-morning awakenings. Common daytime functioning impairment complaints include fatigue, poor concentration, excessive sleepiness, worries about sleep, depressed mood, and impaired cognitive functioning (Riedel and Lichstein 2000). For diagnosis, these functioning deficits must have a negative impact on social, occupational, or physical functioning (APA 2000).

None of the current classification systems provide specific quantitative criteria for measuring insomnia symptoms. General recommendations for quantitative sleep distur-bance criteria have been established, which include $\geq$ 31 minutes of sleep onset latency (SOL) or wake time after sleep onset (WASO), and experiencing these symptoms three nights a week, for six months or longer (Buysse et al. 2006). These criteria appear to best differentiate older adults with insomnia (OAWI) from normal sleepers. Quantification of early-morning awakenings have received attention in the literature on OAWI (Bonanni et al. 2010; Jaussent et al. 2011a), but not to the extent of onset and maintenance sleep disturbance.

Epidemiology

The prevalence of insomnia symptoms has been investigated in numerous samples of older adults across multiple countries and cultures. The estimated global prevalence of insomnia symptoms among older adults shows great diversity, falling between 23% and 70% across studies (Bonanni et al. 2010; Foley et al. 1995; Gureje et al. 2009; Jaussent et al. 2011b; Kim et al. 2009; Liu and Liu 2005). The prevalence of chronic insomnia variously defined among older people/adults also shows a wide range, from 11.6% to 40% (Foley et al. 1995; Ford and Kamerow 1989; Ohayon 1996; Sateia et al. 2000), compared to a point prevalence of 15.9% in the general population (Lichstein et al. 2004). Epidemiological studies show that the prev-alence of insomnia increases with advancing age (Bonanni et al. 2010; Gureje et al. 2009; Ohayon 2002). Using empirically based, quantitative criteria for insomnia, our research group has examined prevalence changes across the adult lifespan (Lichstein et al. 2004). We found that prevalence is fairly constant until decades 70–79 and 80–89, during which insomnia prevalence doubled in mean rate.

Incidence rates of insomnia also increase with age. One- to four-year incidence rates have been shown to range between 2.8% and 7.3% (Foley et al. 1999; Ford and Kamerow 1989; Morgan and Clark 1997). One study examined the cumulative four- to eight-year insomnia incidence and concluded that, on average, there is a 3.6% per year increase in individuals 65 years and older (Morgan 2003). Furthermore, the probability of reporting sleep distur-bance almost doubled in individuals 75 and older. Predictors of incident insomnia in older age include depression, an increased number of physical disorders, previous manual occu-pation, and physical inactivity (Kim et al. 2009).

Another study demonstrated that increased insomnia persistence was associated with older age (Morphy et al. 2007). This led them to suggest that the rate of new cases may not increase with age but that remission rates may decline with age. They ascertained that each decade increase in age is associated with a 1.1 increase in risk of persistent insomnia. A study of sleep in an African community showed that the mean duration of insomnia symptoms is lower for individuals aged 65–74 (16.4 weeks) compared to those aged 75 or older (19.6 weeks; Gureje et al. 2009). Women appear to experience more prominent amplifications of insomnia symptoms than men in their later years (Foley et al. 1995; Gureje et al. 2009; Liu and Liu 2005; Morgan 2003; Ohayon 1996). A meta-analysis of gender differences in insomnia found an overall greater risk for women to develop insomnia compared to men across all ages (Zhang and Wing 2006). Data from our research group show that insomnia prevalence peaks at 41% in women between the ages of 80 and 89 while in men it culminates at 23% (Lichstein et al. 2004). Menopause, oestrogen deficiency, and other hormonal changes that occur as women age may augment the susceptibility of women to developing insomnia (Manber and Armitage 1999; Moe 1999).

There is also a growing pool of evidence indicating ethnic differences in the epidemiology of insomnia. The wide range of global prevalence of insomnia symptoms discussed previously may suggest the presence of ethnic differences in OAWI. Ethnicity has been shown to be a significant predictor of sleep onset, maintenance, and early-morning awakenings (Jean-Louis et al. 2001). Our research group completed meta-analyses comparing Caucasian-American and African-American sleep in individuals with insomnia symptoms (Ruiter et al. 2010a). Results showed that Caucasian-Americans report significantly higher prevalence of sleep complaints, difficulty maintaining sleep, and early-morning awakenings. Epidemiological data on older African Americans also suggest they report fewer sleep complaints than Caucasian Americans and the pointed rise in insomnia prevalence in older adults described earlier is less robust among African Americans (Durrence and Lichstein 2006).

There has been recent interest as to whether certain types of insomnia symptoms are more common at different ages. It is widely held that sleep maintenance insomnia is more common in older adults (Morgan 2000). There is some evidence to support this opinion (Gureje et al. 2009; Jaussent et al. 2011b), though it may not hold true for insomnia symptoms in the presence of other clinical conditions, such as depression (Yokoyama et al. 2010). The high prevalence of maintenance problems might be accounted for by the greater variability in the night-to-night ability to maintain sleep among OAWI (Buysse et al. 2010). Greater unpredictability of sleep patterns may breed more complaints. Our research group found a trend for type of insomnia to correlate with age as suggested above, but that all types of insomnia were common in all age groups (Lichstein et al. 2004). Similarly, Ohayon and his colleagues (2001), in a survey of over 13 000 people between the ages of 15 and 100, reported that type of insomnia was not associated with age. Overall, the data appear to be unclear on this matter.

CLINICAL RISK FACTORS OF INSOMNIA

Multiple life factors can precipitate, perpetuate, and exaggerate insomnia. We will address the most common biopsychosocial events that increase risk for insomnia in older adults (see Table 25.1). Detailed discussion will be focused on insomnia comorbid with depression and chronic pain.

Table 25.1 Risk factors for insomnia in later life

Risk Factors for Insomnia in Older Adulthood		
Physiological/Biological	Psychological	Social/Behavioural
Medical Disorders	Depression	Retirement
Cardiovascular (e.g. CHF)	Anxiety disorders	Nursing home placement
Pulmonary (e.g. COPD)	Psychosis	Hospitalization
Gastrointestinal (e.g. GERD)	Schizophrenia	Bereavement
Chronic pain (e.g. arthritis)	Dementia	↓ Physical activity
Medications		Napping
Anti-depressants		Financial strain
Opiates		Low social support
Antihistamines		Worry
B-Blockers		Poor sleep habits
Corticosteroids		Unrealistic sleep beliefs
Alcohol, nicotine, caffeine		
Sleep disorders		
Sleep-disordered breathing		
Restless legs syndrome		
PLMD		
REM behaviour disorder		

Note: CHF = congestive heart failure; COPD = chronic obstructive pulmonary disease; GERD = gastroesophageal reflux disease; PLMD = periodic limb movement disorder.

Medical and psychiatric illnesses

Medical and psychiatric conditions can disrupt sleep and lead to comorbid insomnia through various mechanisms. The prevalence of insomnia in older adults is compounded the more conditions that are present (Foley et al. 2004). Medical conditions are the strongest predictors of the incidence and persistence of insomnia in older adults (Gureje et al. 2011). Insomnia among older adults has been associated with stroke, cardiovascular disease, pulmonary diseases, depression, and incidence of Alzheimer's disease (Foley et al. 2004; Lobo et al. 2008; Osorio et al. 2011). Other medical and psychiatric illnesses that are known for their sleep-disruptive properties are as follows: pain conditions such as cancer and arthritis; gastrointestinal diseases; neurological disorders; genitourinary disorders; endocrine disorders; anxiety disorders; psychosis; dementia; schizophrenia; and primary sleep disorders, notably obstructive sleep apnoea, restless leg syndrome, periodic limb movement disorder, and REM behaviour disorder (Ancoli-Israel et al. 2008; Krishnan and Hawranik 2008; Neikrug and Ancoli-Israel 2010). The medications intended to treat these disorders, and the interactions between them, can also prelude insomnia. For more information on how medications affect sleep and alertness, see the review by Roux and Kryger (2010).

LATE-LIFE INSOMNIA AND DEPRESSION

Insomnia comorbid with depression is common across the lifespan. There is ongoing inquiry regarding whether untreated insomnia predicts incident depression in older people. Evidence from small studies suggests insomnia is a risk factor for depression in older adulthood (Perlis et al. 2006) and vice versa (Cole and Dendukuri 2003). Two large longitudinal studies demonstrated that chronic insomnia and insomnia symptoms predict greater odds of incident depression and depressive symptoms in older adults (Jaussent et al. 2011a; Kim et al. 2009). Furthermore, frequent difficulty initiating and maintaining sleep, but not early-morning awakenings, predicted greater risk for depressive symptoms (Jaussent et al. 2011a). A three-year longitudinal study in community-dwelling older adults found corroborating evidence for difficulty initiating sleep, but not difficulty maintaining sleep (Yokoyama et al. 2010). Chronic insomnia also appears to increase the risk of persistent major depression despite treatment by 1.8 to 3.5 times that of older adult patients with no insomnia (Pigeon et al. 2008).

LATE-LIFE INSOMNIA AND CHRONIC PAIN

Poor sleep often accompanies chronic pain (Smith et al. 2000). Evidence suggests the relationship between chronic pain and sleep disturbance is bidirectional (Smith and Haythornthwaite 2004). Chronic, widespread pain and moderate-to-severe pain were both associated with greater odds of difficulty falling asleep and experiencing restless sleep among older adults (Chen et al. 2011). When examining objectively assessed sleep and self-reported pain in OAWI, one study found night-to-night variability in sleep is associated with day-to-day variability in pain reports (Dzierzewski et al. 2010). This study provides evidence that the experiences of insomnia and pain are sensitive to changes in the other.

SOCIAL AND BEHAVIOURAL CHANGES

Psychosocial, cultural, behavioural, and environmental factors that occur more frequently in our latter years contribute to the development and maintenance of chronic insomnia. Common risk factors are retirement, nursing home placement, hospitalization, loss and bereavement, decreased activity, and chronic stressors and cultural influences specific to nations and regions (Wolkove et al. 2007). These events produce stress that may alter sleep-related behaviours, thus increasing risk for chronic insomnia. For example, one study found self-reported sleep disturbance of older adults who recently lost a spouse was more severe than experienced by good sleepers but less severe than experienced by OAWI (Monk, Germain, and Buysse 2009). An exception was that the reported SOL of bereaved people was comparable to patients with insomnia. Institutional settings such as nursing homes and hospitals are also ripe environments for sleep disruption. Patients of these institutions have limited exposure to bright light to entrain their circadian rhythms, experience more noise in their environment, and spend more time at bed rest, all of which negatively affects their sleep quality (Middelkoop et al. 1994; Schnelle et al. 1998). Lastly, regular physical activity levels may decrease as health and consistent daily schedules deteriorate due to retirement and other factors. Being sedentary has been found to be predictive of acute and persistent insomnia (Morgan 2003), and physical activity may be a buffer against poor sleep (de Castro Toledo Guimaraes et al. 2008).

Other psychosocial stressors that negatively impact on the sleep of older adults are economic factors and social status. Beyond common confounders, ongoing financial strain, as a proxy for chronic stress, is independently associated with objectively assessed poor sleep efficiency (Hall et al. 2008). Low social support may also be a risk factor. A study comparing OAWI to age-matched participants found high levels of social support were a protective buffer against WASO for both groups, and specifically decreased SOL among the insomnia group (Troxel et al. 2010).

BELIEFS AND PERSONALITY

Personality traits and personal beliefs about sleep are also predisposing and perpetuating factors for insomnia in older adults. It is likely that these traits and beliefs were present during earlier years, but with age-related sleep changes they may increase the risk of activating an insomnia state. For example, subclinical levels of trait anxiety are associated with greater self-reported WASO in older adults (Spira et al. 2008). A greater tendency to worry excessively, feel distressed about bodily dysfunction, and frequently experience cognitive intrusions are other traits found at higher levels among OAWI compared to older adults without insomnia (Pallesen et al. 2002). Several unrealistic beliefs have been identified that differentiate OAWI from good sleepers. These beliefs include attributing lack of energy, mood disturbances, and poor performance on daily tasks to poor sleep, predicting poor sleep will ruin future sleep and foster poor health, and worrying about losing control of mind-racing cognitions and sleep in general (Ellis, Hampson, and Coley 2007).

NEGATIVE CONSEQUENCES OF INSOMNIA

Schutte-Rodin and colleagues (2008) emphasize five major categories of negative consequences of insomnia: poor quality of life; exacerbation of illness; mood disturbances; subjective sleepiness and fatigue; and cognitive impairments. Poor quality of life is highly prevalent in patients with insomnia (Roth and Ancoli-Israel 1999). Insomnia symptoms and daytime sleepiness increase the odds of poor quality of life in older adults (Yokoyama et al. 2008). Disturbances in family, social, and professional roles due to insomnia (Leger et al. 2002) and ill health likely contribute to mood disturbances and poor quality of life.

Excessive daytime sleepiness is a common complaint for OAWI. Difficulty initiating sleep, early-morning awakenings, and difficulty maintaining sleep are also associated with excessive daytime sleepiness in older adults with the latter being most strongly correlated (Hara et al. 2011). Sleepiness also appears to be more prevalent in OAWI than middle-aged patients (Stone et al. 2006). Increased sleepiness as demonstrated by frequent napping has been found to be a risk factor for falls and hip fractures (Stone et al. 2008). Actigraphy-measured poor sleep continuity and short sleep duration were also found to be risk factors for falls (Riedel and Lichstein 2000).

Decrements in daytime performance of cognitive tasks are often reported by patients with insomnia. Several investigations in patients across the lifespan have been undertaken to determine if these reported neurocognitive impairments have an objective basis. These studies generally found no major differences in objective cognitive abilities between patients with insomnia and age-matched controls (Schutte et al. 2006). The recent literature has re-examined this discrepancy among older adults. These studies in OAWI have revealed that while performance on simple cognitive tasks is comparable to patients without insomnia, performance on more cognitively demanding tasks is reduced (Altena et al. 2008). Objective impairments have been observed in attention, memory span, time estimation, integration of cognitive dimensions, executive-order functioning (Haimov, Hanuka, and Horowitz 2008), and visual-perceptual processing (Haimov, Hadad, and Shurkin 2007). OAWI also have a reduced ability to detect impaired cognitive performance (Bonnefond 2006). However, these impairments may be reversed with multicomponent cognitive-behavioural interventions for insomnia, as evidenced by improvements in vigilance in a treatment study by Altena and colleagues (2008).

ASSESSMENT

Clinical guidelines for the evaluation of chronic insomnia in all adults are outlined by Schutte-Rodin and colleagues (2008). A standard clinical assessment includes a comprehensive sleep, physical, substance, and mental health history accompanied by a physical and mental status examination. It is highly preferable to obtain a collateral report from a bed partner. Self-reported retrospective and prospective measures of sleep patterns are standard tools of assessment. These measures may include sleep-wake diaries (Carney et al. 2012; Figure 25.1), questionnaires, screening tools, and symptom checklists. Objective measures of sleep and daytime sleepiness, such as polysomnography, actigraphy, and the multiple sleep latency test, are generally not recommended, though they may be more indicated for older adults since higher rates of sleep disorders are experienced with advancing age (Littner et al. 2003). Approximately 29% of older adults with insomnia have undiagnosed sleep apnoea (Gooneratne et al. 2006; Lichstein et al. 1999). For certain older adults, wrist actigraphy may be a valuable tool to ascertain sleep disruption. The following groups may have greater difficulty using traditional sleep logs and questionnaires: nursing home residents, depressed patients, patients with circadian rhythm disturbances, and patients whose activity patterns are suspected to be influencing their sleep (Buysse et al. 2006; Morgenthaler et al. 2007). If you do chose to use actigraphy, then seven days of data are usually sufficient to examine meaningful sleep patterns, especially if the presentation is variable (Rowe et al. 2008).

What differs in an evaluation of chronic insomnia in older adults is oftentimes that the clinical presentation can be more complex due to a higher propensity for medical comorbidities and polypharmacy. The first major determination is if the insomnia complaint is in excess of normal age-related changes in sleep and not better accounted for by other primary sleep disorders. Useful ways to help rule out these conditions are in the following: assessing movement and restlessness while asleep or relaxed; measuring neck size; assess snoring and daytime sleepiness through clinical interview; calculating body-mass index (Buysse et al. 2006); and obtaining corroborating reports from bed partners. Then you must examine the older adult with insomnia within their personal and situational contexts accurately to identify all treatable precipitating and perpetuating factors contributing to the insomnia complaint whether they are medical, substance-based, psychiatric, environmental, or behavioural (see Figure 25.2). For example, assessment of alcohol consumption among OAWI is important because alcohol may be used as an aide to fall asleep, though physiologically it worsens sleep due to withdrawal effects that promote wakefulness later in the night. It is also important to ask if OAWI are taking medications or substances not prescribed for them, who organizes their medications, and how medications are organized since negative interactions among medications are a risk factor for insomnia.

Schutte-Rodin and colleagues provide six standard categories for assessment (Schutte-Rodin 2008). (1) You must determine the primary sleep complaint(s) such as difficulty initiating sleep, difficulty maintaining sleep, early-morning awakenings, and non-restorative sleep. The following characteristics of the primary complaint(s) should be determined: duration; frequency; course; distress, and daytime impairment severity; agonists and antagonists of the complaint; history of precipitating, perpetuating factors; previous treatments, and treatment responses. (2) Mental and environmental conditions prior to sleep need to be evaluated for the presence of behaviours and attitudes that are counteractive to sleep. Such behaviours and attitudes include using the bed or bedroom as a place for mental stimulation and entertainment (e.g. using electronic devices, exercising, negative interactions with bed partner), and adopting an anxious or anticipatory mindset toward sleep (e.g. hypervigilance, problem-solving/rehearsing in bed, predicting a poor night of sleep). (3) The measurement of the variability in the patient's sleep complaint and sleep-wake schedule allows for the estimation of sleep-wake patterns within the context of their daily life. Sleep-wake diaries are standard tools to quantify parameters of bedtime, wake time, SOL, frequency of awakenings, WASO, time in bed, total sleep time, nap times, and sleep efficiency. For the calculation of sleep efficiency, see below:

$$\frac{Total\ Sleep\ Time}{Total\ Sleep\ in\ Bed} \times 100\%$$

(4) Somatic and emotional symptoms occurring during the night also harbour valuable information regarding differential diagnosis from other sleep disorders, medical conditions, and psychiatric illnesses (e.g. snoring, kicking, reflux, sadness). (5) The five major categories of negative daytime consequences mentioned earlier also should be examined to determine treatable causes of the complaint and outcomes important to the patient. (6) Lastly, the current and personal history of medical and psychiatric conditions, and medication/substance usage must be identified. Physical and mental status examinations and a family sleep history review are also highly recommended.

Figure 25.1 Consensus Sleep Diary. This tool is distributed under the terms of an Attribution Non-Commercial license (http://creativecommons.org/licenses/by-nc-nd/3.0/legalcode). Unrestricted use is granted to individual practising clinicians. Industry, organizations, or researchers wishing to use this questionnaire should contact Dr Colleen Carney (ccarney@psych.ryerson.ca) for permission.

Consensus Sleep Diary-Core

	Sample	ID/Name:__________						
Today's date	4/5/11							
1. What time did you get into bed?	10:15 p.m.							
2. What time did you try to go to sleep?	11:30 p.m.							
3. How long did it take you to fall asleep?	55 min.							
4. How many times did you wake up, not counting your final awakening?	3 times							
5. In total, how long did these awakenings last?	1 hour 10 min.							
6. What time was your final awakening?	6:35 a.m.							
7. What time did you get out of bed for the day?	7:20 a.m.							
8. How would you rate the quality of your sleep?	☐ Very poor ☐ Poor ☐ Fair ☐ Good ☐ Very good	☐ Very poor ☐ Poor ☐ Fair ☐ Good ☐ Very good	☐ Very poor ☐ Poor ☐ Fair ☐ Good ☐ Very good	☐ Very poor ☐ Poor ☐ Fair ☐ Good ☐ Very good	☐ Very poor ☐ Poor ☐ Fair ☐ Good ☐ Very good	☐ Very poor ☐ Poor ☐ Fair ☐ Good ☐ Very good	☐ Very poor ☐ Poor ☐ Fair ☐ Good ☐ Very good	☐ Very poor ☐ Poor ☐ Fair ☐ Good ☐ Very good
9. Comments (if applicable)	I have a cold							

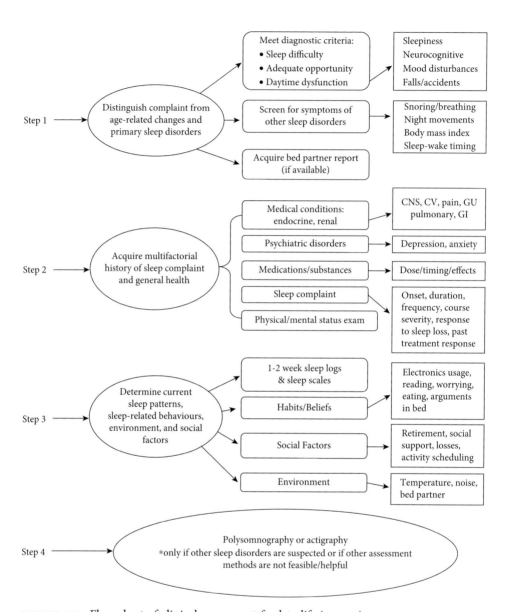

FIGURE 25.2 Flow chart of clinical assessment for late-life insomnia.

Data from Ancoli-Israel, S, Ayalon, L & Salzman, C, Sleep in the elderly: normal variations and common sleep disorders, *Harvard Review of Psychiatry*, 16(5), pp. 279–286, 2008, Lippincott, Williams, and Wilkins, Krishnan, P & Hawranik, P., Diagnosis and management of geriatric insomnia: a guide for nurse practitioners, *Journal of the American Academy of Nurse Practitioners*, 20(12), pp. 590–599, 2008, American Academy of Nurse Practitioners, Ruiter, ME, DeCoster, J, Jacobs, L & Lichstein, KL, Sleep disorders in african americans and caucasian americans: a meta-analysis, *Behavioral Sleep Medicine*, 8(4), pp. 246–259, 2010, Taylor and Francis, and Schutte-Rodin, S, Broch, L, Buysse, D, Dorsey, C and Sateia, M., Clinical guideline for the evaluation and management of chronic insomnia in adults, *Journal of Clinical Sleep Medicine*, 4(5), pp. 487–504, 2008, American Academy of Sleep Medicine.

Note: CNS refers to central nervous system; CV refers to cardiovascular; GU refers to genitourinary; GI refers to gastrointestinal.

EVIDENCE-BASED INTERVENTIONS

There are many evidence-based treatments for insomnia, both pharmacological and cognitive-behavioural, that have been implemented with OAWI. These treatments and their empirical support have been laid out extensively in other sources (Lichstein 2000; McCrae, Ozierzewski, and Kay 2009). We will provide a brief overview of the most common approaches to treating late-life insomnia. Table 25.2 highlights specific treatment recommendations for OAWI.

Cognitive-behavioural therapy

Cognitive-behavioural therapy (CBT) interventions for insomnia are sometimes implemented in isolation but are more commonly and efficaciously implemented in various packaged multicomponent treatments (McCurry et al. 2007). Their efficacy has been well established in other reviews and meta-analyses (Bain 2006; Irwin, Cole, and Nicassio 2006). There is evidence that older adults benefit as much from these interventions as their younger counterparts (Lichstein et al. 2001; Sivertsen et al. 2006).

Stimulus control was originally developed by Dr Richard Bootzin and is based on learning principles that suggest the bed and bedroom have become a learned stimulus for arousal and wakeful behaviours through misuse of the bedroom space (see Bootzin and Epstein 2000). The goal is to restore the bed and bedroom as a cue for sleep by confining all sleep behaviours to the bed and removing wakeful behaviours from the bedroom (except sex). This is accomplished through a series of instructions, described in Table 25.2.

Sleep-restriction therapy is an intervention aimed at maximizing sleep efficiency by eliminating time awake in bed through restricting the amount of time allowed for sleep each night (Wohlgemuth and Edinger 2000). It works by both breaking the associations of the bed with wakefulness and by helping the patient build sufficient sleep debt to experience an uninterrupted block of sleep (McCrae et al. 2009). Sleep restriction has been shown to be efficacious in older adults as a standalone treatment (McCurry et al. 2007).

Cognitive therapy is aimed at reducing cognitive arousal that results from worry about sleep at night, dysfunctional beliefs about sleep, and daytime anxiety about poor sleep (Harvey 2002; Morin, Savard, and Blais 2000). This is typically accomplished through cognitive restructuring, identifying and challenging maladaptive beliefs and thoughts, and helping patients develop realistic alternative thoughts and beliefs (Morin et al. 2000). Unlike behavioural interventions for insomnia, more training is necessary successfully to implement cognitive strategies.

Other treatment package components include relaxation strategies and sleep hygiene education. Relaxation techniques help combat mental and physical arousal that may interfere with sleep. Common techniques include progressive muscle relaxation, passive relaxation, breathing strategies, guided imagery, and meditation (Lichstein 2000). For older adults with acute and chronic pain, passive relaxation is recommended as a less intensive strategy (see Lichstein 2000 for detailed instructions). Education about sleep-promoting and inhibiting behaviours can also be an effective intervention (McCurry et al. 2007).

Table 25.2 CBT interventions and special considerations for older adult populations.

Intervention	Considerations for elderly populations*
Stimulus control: 1 Go to bed only when sleepy. 2 Set a fixed morning wake time. 3 Eliminate napping. 4 Remove all non-sleep behaviours from the bedroom (i.e. reading, watching television, worrying). 5 Leave the bedroom if not asleep within 15–20 minutes and engage in a non-stimulating activity. 6 Return to bed only when sleepy again (this applies to the beginning of the night and to awakenings during the middle of the night). 7 Repeat steps 5 and 6 as often as necessary.	• Sleep may initially get worse before it gets better. • Telling people to get out of bed to help improve sleep is counter-intuitive for some. Provide adequate rationale to increase buy-in. • Problem solve ahead of time (i.e. anticipate physical discomfort or difficulty getting out of bed and plan to have measures in place to help alleviate barriers, such as having the patient sit up in bed instead of leaving bed). • If stopping naps is a problem, try slowly reducing duration and moving them earlier in the day. Naps should be taken in bed.
Relaxation: Progressive muscle relaxation Passive muscle relaxation Deep breathing Meditation Autogenic phrases Guided imagery	• Use passive methods instead of progressive muscle relaxation if pain is a concern. • Allow the patient to choose what best works for them and encourage them to go at their own pace. • Be aware of the potential for hearing loss when administering relaxation. • Encourage home practice.
Sleep hygiene: Avoid napping Avoid caffeine after noon Avoid nicotine Avoid alcohol within 2 hours of bedtime Avoid heavy meals within 2 hours of bedtime Increase daily exercise, though avoid within 2 hours of bedtime Create an adequate sleep environment (i.e. cool, dark, free of outside noise)	• Gradual withdrawal from caffeine, nicotine, or napping, and gradual increases in exercise will help the patient find success and build efficacy. • Developing a baseline for disruptive behaviours can help the patient see how they affect their sleep.
Sleep Restriction: 1 Gather baseline data on time in bed and total sleep time. 2 Prescribe time in bed at the patient's average baseline total sleep time plus 30 min. 3 Set bedtime and wake time to meet time in bed prescription. 4 If average sleep efficiency is >90%, increase time in bed by 15–30 min. 5 If average sleep efficiency is <85%, decrease time in bed by 15–30 min.	• Help patient identify additional activities to engage in during their newly increased time awake to combat boredom and help improve treatment compliance. • Emphasize positive changes during treatment to help improve sleep self-efficacy.

(Continued)

Table 25.2 (Continued)

Intervention	Considerations for elderly populations*
Cognitive therapy: Cognitive restructuring Correct misconceptions about insomnia and its daytime consequences	• Older adults may have more established beliefs about their sleep and may be less flexible when attempting to change them. • Be concrete when describing principles and provide many practical examples to illustrate concepts.

* Many tips for older adults derived from chapters out of Lichstein and Morin (2000).

Pharmacological

Numerous pharmacological drugs are used to treat insomnia symptoms in OAWI including antihistamines, anti-depressants, atypical anti-psychotics, sedatives, and sedative-hypnotics (Taylor and Weiss 2009). Only sedative-hypnotics, which include benzodiazepines (e.g. estazolam, temazepam), non-benzodiazepines (e. g. eszopiclone, zolpidem), melatonin receptor agonists (e.g. ramelteon), and low doses of anti-depressants (doxepin) are approved for treatment of insomnia by the US Food and Drug Administration (Patel and Goldman-Levine 2011; Taylor and Weiss 2009). Outside the US, specific drugs approved for use differ, but the classifications generally do not. For example, the European Medicines Agency lists zaleplon and Circadin (extended-release melatonin) as approved medications for the treatment of sleep initiation and maintenance disorders.

There is some evidence that insomnia medications can safely treat OAWI (Cotroneo et al. 2007), but there remains a vast dearth of knowledge as to the effectiveness of these medications in OAWI (McCrae et al. 2009). Sedative hypnotics carry with them the possibility of negative side-effects, such as dizziness, increased risk of falls, headaches, fatigue, and excessive sleepiness (Bain 2006; Glass et al. 2005). There is also a risk that they will have negative interactions with other medications (Dolder, Nelson, and McKinsey 2007), a risk that is potentially higher in older adults. Recently, some sedative hypnotics, such as benzodiazepines, have been deemed potentially inappropriate for use in older adults (American Geriatrics Society Beers Criteria Update Expert Panel 2012). In general, CBT has been shown to be more effective than pharmacotherapy (Smith et al. 2002) for the treatment of late-life insomnia and to have better maintenance of gains in the general population (Morin et al. 1999).

IMPLICATIONS FOR PRACTICE

Insomnia is a highly prevalent problem in older adults that warrants appropriate attention, assessment, and intervention. We recommend the use of CBT interventions as the primary treatment option for OAWI. Table 25.2 provides a list of special considerations for using CBT for insomnia in older adults. Pharmacological approaches can be beneficial, but caution should be used in prescribing them given the potential for negative side-effects. Further consideration should be given to what medications are prescribed given that some sedative hypnotics, such as benzodiazepines, have been deemed potentially inappropriate for use in older adults.

SUMMARY

As we age, our sleep naturally lightens, increases during the daytime, becomes more fragmented, and tends to phase advance. Late-life insomnia can be defined as a complaint of difficulty sleeping, with associated daytime impairment, despite adequate circumstances to obtain sleep, and is in excess of normal age-related sleep and circadian rhythm changes. Late-life insomnia is often comorbid with or related to medical conditions, psychiatric disorders, primary sleep disorders, polypharmacy, social role shifts, poor behavioural habits, and environmental changes (i.e. chronic pain, depression, institutionalization, bereavement, etc.). Because of an increase in these risk factors with older age, insomnia is more prevalent, severe, persistent, and associated with greater objective daytime impairments such as excessive sleepiness and neurocognitive deficits. Given that the presentation of late-life insomnia is multifactorial, it is highly recommended that the assessment of the sleep complaint and health status be comprehensive, and the current sleep pattern, reported by the patient and bed partner, to be well documented. Objective assessment of insomnia may be more indicated for older adults as other sleep disorders increase with age, and other health conditions can make assessment more challenging. Despite a more complicated clinical presentation of insomnia, cognitive-behavioural and pharmacological interventions benefit OAWI as well as younger adults. However, cognitive-behavioural interventions are more recommended as the side-effect profile is minimal, and the persistence of successful treatment outcomes is greater.

KEY REFERENCES AND SOURCES FOR FURTHER READING

Irwin, M. R., Cole, J. C., and Nicassio, P. M. (2006). 'Comparative Meta-analysis of Behavioral Interventions for Insomnia and their Efficacy in Middle-aged Adults and in Older Adults 55+ Years of Age'. *Health Psychology* 25: 3–14.

Glass, J., Lanctot, K. L., Herrmann, N., Sproule, B. A., and Busto, U. E. (2005). 'Sedative Hypnotics in Older People with Insomnia: Meta-analysis of Risks and Benefits'. *British Medical Journal* 331: 1169. doi:10.1136/bmj.38623.768588.47.

Lichstein, K. L. and Morin, C. M. (eds) (2000). *Treatment of Late-life Insomnia*. Thousand Oaks, CA: Sage.

Lichstein, K. L., Durrence, H. H., Riedel, B. W., Taylor, D. J. and Bush, A. J. (2004). *Epidemiology of Sleep: Age, Gender, and Ethnicity*. Mahwah, NJ: Erlbaum.

REFERENCES

Altena, E., van der Werf, Y., Strijers, R. L. M., and Van Someren, E. J. W. (2008). 'Sleep Loss Affects Vigilance: Effects of Chronic Insomnia and Sleep Therapy'. *Journal of Sleep Research* 17(3): 335–343.

American Academy of Sleep Medicine (2005). *International Classification of Sleep Disorders* (2nd edn). Westchester, IL: American Academy of Sleep Medicine.

American Geriatrics Society Beers Criteria Update Expert Panel (2012). 'American Geriatrics Society Updated Beers Criteria for Potentially Inappropriate Medication Use in Older Adults'. *Journal of the American Geriatrics Society* 60: 616–631.

American Psychiatric Association (2000). *Diagnostic and Statistical Manual of Mental Disorders* (4th edn). Washington, DC: American Psychiatric Association.

Ancoli-Israel, S., Ayalon, L., and Salzman, C. (2008). 'Sleep in the Elderly: Normal Variations and Common Sleep Disorders'. *Harvard Review of Psychiatry* 16(5): 279–286.

Bain, K. T. (2006). 'Management of Chronic Insomnia in Elderly Persons'. *American Journal of Geriatric Pharmacotherapy* 4(2): 168–192.

Boden-Albala, B., Bazil, C., Moon, Y., De Rosa, J., Elkind, M. S, Paik, M. C., et al. (2008). 'Unplanned Napping Causes Seniors Vascular Events', Paper presented at the International Stroke Conference, American Stroke Association, February, New Orleans.

Bonanni, E., Tognoni, G., Maestri, M., Salvati, N., Fabbrini, M., Borghetti, D., et al. (2010). 'Sleep Disturbances in Elderly Subjects: An Epidemiological Survey in an Italian District'. *Acta Neurologica Scandinavica* 122(6): 389–397.

Bonnefond, A. (2006). 'Interaction of Age with Shift-related Sleep-wakefulness, Sleepiness, Performance, and Social Life' *Experimental Aging Research* 32(2): 185–208.

Bootzin, R. R. and Epstein, D. R. (2000). 'Stimulus Control'. In K. L.Lichstein and C. M.Morin (eds), *Treatment of Late-life Insomnia* (pp. 167–184). Thousand Oaks, CA: Sage.

Buysse, D. J., Ancoli-Israel, S., Edinger, J. D., Lichstein, K. L., and Morin, C. M. (2006). 'Recommendations for a Standard Research Assessment of Insomnia'. *Sleep* 29(9): 1155–1173.

Buysse, D. J., Cheng, Y., Germain, A., Moul, D., Franzen, P. L., Fletcher, M., et al. (2010). 'Night-to-night Sleep Variability in Older Adults with and without Chronic Insomnia'. *Sleep Medicine* 11(1): 56–64.

Campbell, S. S., Murphy, P. J., and Stauble, T. N. (2005). 'Effects of a Nap on Nighttime Sleep and Waking Function in Older Subjects'. *Journal of the American Geriatrics Society* 53(1): 48–53.

Campbell, S. S. and Murphy, P. J. (2007). 'The Nature of Spontaneous Sleep across Adulthood'. *Journal of Sleep Research* 16(1): 24–32.

Carney, C. E., Buysse, D. J., Ancoli-Israel, S., Edinger, J. D., Krystal, A. D., Lichstein, K. L., et al. (2012). 'The Consensus Sleep Diary: Standardizing Prospective Sleep Self-monitoring'. *Sleep* 35: 287–302.

de Castro Toledo Guimaraes, L. H., de Carvalho, L. B., Yanaguibashi, G., and do Prado, G. F. (2008). 'Physically Active Elderly Women Sleep More and Better than Sedentary Women'. *Sleep Medicine* 9(5): 488–493.

Chen, Q., Hayman, L. L., Shmerling, R. H., Bean, J. F., and Leveille, S. G. (2011). 'Characteristics of Chronic Pain Associated with Sleep Difficulty in Older Adults: The Maintenance of Balance, Independent Living, Intellect, and Zest in the Elderly (MOBILIZE) Boston Study'. *Journal of the American Geriatrics Society* 59(8): 1385–1392.

Cohen, J. (2003). 'Human Population: The Next Half Century'. *Science* 302(5648): 1172–1175.

Cole, M. G. and Dendukuri, N. (2003). 'Risk Factors for Depression among Elderly Community Subjects: A Systematic Review and Meta-analysis'. *American Journal of Psychiatry* 160(6): 1147–1156.

Cotroneo, A., Gareri, P., Nicoletti, N., Lacava, R., Grassone, D., Maina, E., et al. (2007). 'Effectiveness and Safety of Hypnotic Drugs in the Treatment of Insomnia in over 70-year Old People'. *Archives of Gerontology and Geriatrics* 44(suppl.): 121–124.

Dolder, C., Nelson, M., and McKinsey, J, (2007). 'Use of Non-benzodiazepine Hypnotics in the Elderly: Are All Agents the Same?' *CNS Drugs* 21(5): 389–405.

Durrence, H. H. and Lichstein, K. L. (2006). 'The Sleep of African Americans: A Comparative Review'. *Behavioral Sleep Medicine* 4(1): 29–44.

Dzierzewski, J., Williams, J. M., Roditi, D., Marsiske, M., McCoy, K., McNamara, J., et al. (2010). 'Daily Variations in Objective Nighttime Sleep and Subjective Morning Pain in Older Adults with Insomnia: Evidence of Covariation over Time'. *Journal of the American Geriatrics Society* 58(5): 925–930.

Edinger, J. D., Fins, A. I., Glenn, D. M., Sullivan, R. J., Bastian, L. A., Marsh, G. R., et al. (2000), 'Insomnia and the Eye of the Beholder: Are There Clinical Markers of Objective Sleep Disturbances among Adults with and without Insomnia Complaints?' *Journal of Consulting and Clinical Psychology* 68(4): 586–593.

Ellis, J., Hampson, S. E., and Cropley, M. (2007). 'The Role of Dysfunctional Beliefs and Attitudes in Late-life Insomnia'. *Journal of Psychosomatic Research* 62(1): 81–84.

Foley, D. J., Monjan, A. A., Brown, S. L., Simonsick, E. M., Wallace, R. B., and Blazer, D. G. (1995). 'Sleep Complaints among Elderly Persons: An Epidemiologic Study of Three Communities'. *Sleep* 18(6): 425–432.

Foley, D. J., Ancoli-Israel, S., Britz, P., and Walsh, J. (2004). 'Sleep Disturbances and Chronic Disease in Older Adults: Results of the 2003 National Sleep Foundation Sleep in America Survey'. *Journal of Psychosomatic Research* 56(5): 497–502.

Foley, D. J., Monjan, A., Simonsick, E. M., Wallace, R. B., and Blazer, D. G. (1999). 'Incidence and Remission of Insomnia among Elderly Adults: An Epidemiologic Study of 6,800 Persons over Three Years'. *Sleep* 22(suppl. 2): S366–S372.

Ford, D. E. and Kamerow, D. B. (1989). 'Epidemiologic Study of Sleep Disturbances and Psychiatric Disorders'. *Journal of the American Medical Association* 262(11): 1479–1484.

Gillin, J. C. and Ancoli-Israel, S. (2005). 'The Impact of Age on Sleep and Sleep Disorders'. In C. Salzman (ed.), *Clinical Geriatric Psychopharmacology* (4th edn; 483–512). Philadelphia, PA: Lippincott Williams and Wilkins.

Glass, J., Lanctot, K. L., Herrmann, N., Sproule, B. A., and Busto, U. E. (2005). 'Sedative Hypnotics in Older People with Insomnia: Meta-analysis of Risks and Benefits'. *British Medical Journal* 331. doi:10.1136/bmj.38623.768588.47.

Goldman, S. E., Hall, M., Boudreau, R., Matthews, K. A., Cauley, J. A., Ancoli-Israel, S., et al. (2008). 'Association between Nighttime Sleep and Napping in Older Adults'. *Sleep* 31(5): 733–740.

Gooneratne, N. S., Gehrman, P. R., Nkwuo, J. E., Bellamy, S. L., Schutte-Rodin, S., Dinges, D. F., et al. (2006). 'Consequences of Comorbid Insomnia Symptoms and Sleep-related Breathing Disorder in Elderly Subjects'. *Archives of Internal Medicine* 166(16): 1732–1738.

Gooneratne, N. S., Bellamy, S. L., Pack, F., Staley, B., Schutte-Rodin, S., Dinges, D. F., et al. (2011). 'Case-control Study of Subjective and Objective Differences in Sleep Patterns in Older Adults with Insomnia Symptoms'. *Journal of Sleep Research* 20(3): 434–444.

Gureje, O., Kola, L., Ademola, A., and Olley, B. O. (2009). 'Profile, Comorbidity and Impact of Insomnia in the Ibadan Study of Ageing'. *International Journal of Geriatric Psychiatry* 24(7): 686–693.

Gureje, O., Loadeji, B. D., Abiona, T., Makanjuola, V., and Esan, O. (2011). 'The Natural History of Insomnia in the Ibadan Study of Ageing'. *Sleep* 34(7): 965–973.

Haimov, I., Hadad, B. S., and Shurkin, D. (2007). 'Visual Cognitive Function: Changes Associated with Chronic Insomnia in Older Adults'. *Journal of Gerontological Nursing* 33(10): 32–41.

Haimov, I., Hanuka, E., and Horowitz, Y. (2008). 'Chronic Insomnia and Cognitive Functioning among Older Adults'. *Behavioral Sleep Medicine* 6(1): 32–54.

Hall, M., Buysee, D. J., Nofzinger, E. A., Reynolds, C. F.,III, Thompson, W., Mazumdar, S., et al. (2008). 'Financial Strain is a Significant Correlate of Sleep Continuity Disturbances in Late-life'. *Biological Psychology* 77(2): 217–222.

Hara, C., Stewart, R., Lima-Costa, M. F., Rocha, F. L., Fuzikawa, C., Uchoa, E., et al. (2011). 'Insomnia Subtypes and their Relationship to Excessive Daytime Sleepiness in Brazilian Community-dwelling Older Adults'. *Sleep* 34(8): 1111–1117.

Harvey, A. G. (2002). 'A Cognitive Model of Insomnia'. *Behaviour Research and Therapy* 40(8): 869–893.

Iber, C. (2007). *The AASM Manual for the Scoring of Sleep and Associated Events: Rules, Terminology and Technical Specification*. Westchester, IL: American Academy of Sleep Medicine.

Irwin, M. R., Cole, J. C., and Nicassio, P. M. (2006). 'Comparative Meta-analysis of Behavioral Interventions for Insomnia and their Efficacy in Middle-aged Adults and in Older Adults 55+ Years of Age'. *Health Psychology* 25(1): 3–14.

Jaussent, I., Bouyer, J., Ancelin, M. L., Akbaraly, T., Pérès, K., Ritchie, K., et al. (2011a). 'Insomnia and Daytime Sleepiness are Risk Factors for Depressive Symptoms in the Elderly'. *Sleep* 34(8): 1103–1110.

Jaussent, I., Dauvilliers, Y., Ancelin, M., Darigues, J., Tavernier, B., Touchon, J., et al. (2011b). 'Insomnia Symptoms in Older Adults: Associated Factors and Gender Differences'. *American Journal of Geriatric Medicine* 19(1): 88–97.

Jean-Louis, G., Magai, C. M., Cohen, C. I., Zizi, F., von Gizycki, H., DiPalma, J., et al. (2001). 'Ethnic Differences in Self-reported Sleep Problems in Older Adults'. *Sleep* 24(8): 926–933.

Kim, J., Stewart, R., Kim, S., Yang, S., Shin, I., and Yoon, J. (2009). 'Insomnia, Depression, and Physical Disorders in Late Life: A 2-year Longitudinal Community Study in Koreans'. *Sleep* 39(9): 1221–1228.

Klerman, E. B., Davis, J. B., Duffy, J. F., Dijk, D. J., and Kronauer, R. E. (2004). 'Older People Awaken More Frequently but Fall Back Asleep at the Same Rate as Younger People'. *Sleep* 27(4): 793–798.

Krishnan, P. and Hawranik, P. (2008). 'Diagnosis and Management of Geriatric Insomnia: A Guide for Nurse Practitioners'. *Journal of the American Academy of Nurse Practitioners* 20(12): 590–599.

Leger, D., Guilleminault, C., Bader, G., Levy, E., and Paillard, M. (2002). 'Medical and Socio-professional Impact of Insomnia'. *Sleep* 25(6): 625–629.

Lichstein, K. L., Riedel, B. W., Lester, K. W., and Aguillard, R. N. (1999). 'Occult Sleep Apnea in a Recruited Sample of Older Adults with Insomnia'. *Journal of Consulting and Clinical Psychology* 67(3): 405–410.

Lichstein, K. L. (2000). 'Relaxation'. In K. L. Lichstein and C. M. Morin (eds), *Treatment of Late-life Insomnia* (pp. 185–206). Thousand Oaks, CA: Sage.

Lichstein, K. L., Riedel, B. W., Wilson, N. M., Lester, K. W., and Aguillard, R. N. (2001). 'Relaxation and Sleep Compression for Late-life Insomnia: A Placebo Controlled Trial'. *Journal of Consulting and Clinical Psychology* 69(2): 227–239.

Lichstein, K. L., Durrence, H. H., Riedel, B. W., Taylor, D. J., and Bush, A. J. (2004). *Epidemiology of Sleep: Age, Gender, and Ethnicity*. Mahwah, NJ: Erlbaum.

Littner, M., Hirshkowitz, M., Kramer, M., Kapen, S., Anderson, W. M., Bailey, D., et al. (2003). 'Practice Parameters for Using Polysomnography to Evaluate Insomnia: an Update'. *Sleep* 26(6): 754–760.

Liu, X. and Liu, L. (2005). 'Sleep Habits and Insomnia in a Sample of Elderly Persons in China'. *Sleep* 28(12): 1579–1587.

Lobo, A., Lopez-Anton, R., de-la-Camara, C., Quintanilla, M. A., Campayo, A., and Saz, P. (2008). 'Non-cognitive Psychopathological Symptoms Associated with Incident Mild Cognitive Impairment and Dementia, Alzheimer's Type'. *Neurotoxicity Research* 14(2–3): 263–272.

McCrae, C. S., Rowe, M. A., Tierney, C. G., Dautovich, N. D., DeFinis, A. L.. and McNamara, J. P. H. (2005). 'Sleep Complaints, Subjective and Objective Sleep Patterns, Health, Psychological Adjustment, and Daytime Functioning in Community-dwelling Older Adults'. *Journal of Gerontology: Psychological Sciences* 60(4): 182–189.

McCrae, C. S., Rowe, M. A., Dautovich, N. D., Lichstein, K. L., Durrence, H. H., Riedel, B. W., et al. (2006). 'Sleep Hygiene Practices in Two Community Dwelling Samples of Older Adults'. *Sleep* 29(12): 1551–1560.

McCrae, C. S., Dzierzewski, J. M., and Kay, D. B. (2009). 'Treatment of Late-life Insomnia'. *Sleep Medicine Clinics* 4(4): 593–604.

McCurry, S. M., Logsdon, R. G., Teri, L., and Vitiello, M. V. (2007). 'Evidence-based Psychological Treatments for Insomnia in Older Adults'. *Psychology and Aging* 22(1): 18–27.

Manber, R. and Armitage, R. (1999). 'Sex, Steroids, and Sleep: A Review'. *Sleep* 22(5): 540–555.

Middelkoop, H. A., Kerkhof, G. A., Smilde-van den Doel, D. A., Ligthart, G. J., and Kamphuisen, H. A. (1994). 'Sleep and Ageing: The Effect of Institutionalization on Subjective and Objective Characteristics of Sleep'. *Age and Ageing* 23(5): 411–417.

Moe, K. E. (1999). 'Reproductive Hormones, Aging, and Sleep'. *Seminars in Reproductive Endocrinology* 17(4): 339–348.

Monk, T. H. (2005). 'Aging Human Circadian Rhythms: Conventional Wisdom May Not Always Be Right'. *Journal of Biological Rhythms* 20(4): 366–374.

Monk, T. H., Germain, A., and Buysse, D. J. (2009). 'The Sleep of the Bereaved'. *Sleep and Hypnosis* 11(1): 219–229.

Morgan, K. and Clark, D. (1997). 'Longitudinal Trends in Late-life Insomnia: Implications for Prescribing'. *Age and Aging* 26(3): 179–184.

Morgan, K. (2000). 'Sleep and Aging'. In K. L. Lichstein and C. M. Morin (eds), *Treatment of Late-life Insomnia* (pp. 3–36). Thousand Oaks, CA: Sage.

Morgan, K. (2003). 'Daytime Activity and Risk Factors for Late-life Insomnia'. *Journal of Sleep Research* 12(3): 231–238.

Morgenthaler, T., Alessi, C., Friedman, L., Owens, J., Kapur, V., Boehlecke, B., et al. (2007). 'Practice Parameters for the Use of Actigraphy in the Assessment of Sleep and Sleep Disorders: An Update for 2007'. *Sleep* 30(4): 519–529.

Morin, C. M., Colecchi, C., Stone, J., Sood, R., and Brink, D. (1999). 'Behavioral and Pharmacological Therapies for Late Life Insomnia: A Randomized Controlled Trial'. *Journal of the American Medical Association* 281(11): 991–999.

Morin, C. M., Savard, J., and Blais, F. C. (2000). 'Cognitive Therapy'. In K. L. Lichstein and C. M. Morin (eds), *Treatment of Late-life Insomnia* (pp. 207–230). Thousand Oaks, CA: Sage.

Morphy, H., Dunn, K. M., Lewis, M., Boardman, H. F., and Croft, P. R. (2007). 'Epidemiology of Insomnia: A Longitudinal Study in a UK Population'. *Sleep* 30(3): 274–280.

Neikrug, A. B. and Ancoli-Israel, S. (2010). 'Sleep Disorders in the Older Adult: A Mini Review'. *Gerontology* 56(2): 181–189.

Ohayon, M. M. (1996). 'Epidemiologic Study on Insomnia in the General Population'. *Sleep* 19(suppl. 1): S7–S15.

Ohayon, M. M., Zulley, J., Guilleminault, C., Smirne, S., and Priest, R. G. (2001). 'How Age and Daytime Activities are Related to Insomnia in the General Population: Consequences for Older People'. *Journal of the American Geriatrics Society* 49(4): 360–366.

Ohayon, M. M. (2002). 'Epidemiology of Insomnia: What We Know and What We Still Need to Learn'. *Sleep Medicine Reviews* 6(2): 97–111.

Ohayon, M. M. (2004). 'Interactions between Sleep Normative Data and Sociocultural Characteristics in the Elderly'. *Journal of Psychosomatic Research* 56(5): 479–486.

Ohayon, M. M., Carskadon, M. A., Guilleminault, C., and Vitiello, M. V. (2004). 'Meta-analysis of Quantitative Sleep Parameters from Childhood to Old Age in Healthy Individuals: Developing Normative Sleep Values across the Human Lifespan'. *Sleep* 27(7): 1255–1273.

Osorio, R., Pirraglia, E., Aguera-Ortiz, L. F., During, E. H., Sacks, H., Ayappa, I., et al. (2011). 'Greater Risk of Alzheimer's Disease in Older Adults with Insomnia'. *Journal of the American Geriatrics Society* 59(3): 559–561.

Pallesen, S., Nordhus, I. H., Kvale, G., Havik, O. E., Nielsen, G. H., Johnsen, B. H., et al. (2002). 'Psychological Characteristics of Elderly Insomniacs'. *Scandinavian Journal of Psychology* 43(5): 425–432.

Patel, D. and Goldman-Levine, J. D. (2011). 'Doxepin (Silenor) for Insomnia'. *American Family Physician* 84: 453–454.

Perlis, M. L., Smith, L. J., Lyness, J. M., Matteson, S. R., Pigeon, W. R., Jungquist, C. R., et al. (2006). 'Insomnia as a Risk Factor for Onset of Depression in the Elderly'. *Behavioral Sleep Medicine* 4(2): 104–113.

Picarsic, J. L., Glynn, N. W., Taylor, C. A., Katula, J. A., Goldman, S. E., Studenski, S. A., et al. (2008). 'Self-reported Napping and Duration and Quality of Sleep in the Interventions and Independence for Elders Pilot Study'. *Journal of the American Geriatrics Society* 56(9): 1674–1680.

Pigeon, W. R., Hegel, M., Unützer, J., Fan, M. Y., Sateia, M. J., Lyness, J. M., et al. (2008). 'Is Insomnia a Perpetuating Factor for Late-life Depression in the IMPACT Cohort?'. *Sleep* 31(4): 481–488.

Rechtschaffen, A. and Kales, A. A. (1968). *A Manual of Standardized Terminology, Techniques and Scoring System for Sleep Stages of Human Subjects*. Los Angeles, CA: Brain Information Service, UCLA.

Riedel, B. W. and Lichstein, K. L. (2000). 'Insomnia and Daytime Functioning'. *Sleep Medicine Reviews* 4(3): 277–298.

Roth, T. and Ancoli-Israel, S. (1999). 'Daytime Consequences and Correlates of Insomnia in the United States: Results of the 1991 National Sleep Foundation Survey. II'. *Sleep* 22(suppl. 2): S354–S358.

Roux, F. J. and Kryger, M. H. (2010). 'Medication Effects on Sleep'. *Clinics in Chest Medicine* 31(2): 397–405.

Rowe, M., McCrae, C., Campbell, J., Horne, C., Tiegs, T., Lehman, B., et al. (2008). 'Actigraphy in Older Adults: Comparison of Means and Variability of Three Different Aggregates of Measurement'. *Behavioral Sleep Medicine* 6(2): 127–145.

Ruiter, M. E., DeCoster, J., Jacobs, L., and Lichstein, K. L. (2010a). 'Sleep Disorders in African Americans and Caucasian Americans: A Meta-analysis'. *Behavioral Sleep Medicine* 8(4): 246–259.

Ruiter, M. E., Vander Wal, G. V., and Lichstein, K. L. (2010b). 'Insomnia in the Elderly'. In J. M. Monti, A. Monjan, and S. R. Pandi-Perumal (eds), *Principles and Practice of Geriatric Sleep Medicine* (pp. 271–279). Cambridge: Cambridge University Press.

Sateia, M. J., Doghramji, K., Hauri, P. J., and Morin, C. M. (2000). 'Evaluation of Chronic Insomnia: An American Academy of Sleep Medicine Review'. *Sleep* 23(2): 237–241.

Schnelle, J. F., Cruise, P. A., Alessi, C. A., Al-Samarrai, N., and Ouslander, J. G. (1998). 'Sleep Hygiene in Physically Dependent Nursing Home Residents'. *Sleep* 21(5): 515–523.

Schutte, R., Altena, E., Van der Werf, Y., Sans-Arigita, E., and Van Someren, E. (2006). 'Task-switching in Elderly Patients Suffering from Psychophysiological Insomnia: A Functional MRI Study'. *Journal of Sleep Research* 15(suppl. 1): 155.

Schutte-Rodin, S., Broch, L., Buysse, D., Dorsey, C., and Sateia, M. (2008). 'Clinical Guideline for the Evaluation and Management of Chronic Insomnia in Adults'. *Journal of Clinical Sleep Medicine* 4(5): 487–504.

Sivertsen, B., Omvik, S., Pallesen, S., Bjorvatn, B., Havik, O. E., Kvale, G. et al. (2006). 'Cognitive Behavioral Therapy vs Zopiclone for Treatment of Chronic Primary Insomnia in Older Adults'. *Journal of the American Medical Association* 295(24): 2851–2858.

Smith, M. T., Perlis, M. L., Smith, M. S., Giles, D. E., and Carmody, T. P. (2000). 'Sleep Quality and Presleep Arousal in Chronic Pain'. *Journal of Behavioral Medicine* 23(1): 1–13.

Smith, M. T., Perlis, M. L., Park, A., Smith, M. A., Pennington, J., Giles, D. E. et al. (2002). 'Comparative Meta-analysis of Pharmacotherapy and Behavior Therapy for Persistent Insomnia'. *American Journal of Psychiatry* 159(1): 5–11.

Smith, M. T. and Haythornthwaite, J. A. (2004). 'How Do Sleep Disturbance and Chronic Pain Inter-relate? Insights from the Longitudinal and Cognitive-behavioral Clinical Trials Literature'. *Sleep Medicine Reviews* 8(2): 119–132.

Spira, A. P., Friedman, L., Aulakh, J. S., Lee, T., Sheikh, J. I., and Yesavage, J. A. (2008). 'Sublinical Anxiety Symptoms, Sleep, and Daytime Dysfunction in Older Adults with Primary Insomnia'. *Journal of Geriatric Psychiatry and Neurology* 21(2): 149–153.

Stone, K. L., Ewing, S. K., Lui, L. Y., Ensurd, K. E., Ancoli-Israel, S., Bauer, D. C., et al. (2006). 'Self-reported Sleep and Nap Habits and Risk of Falls and Fractures in Older Women: The Study of Osteoporotic Fractures'. *Journal of the American Geriatrics Society* 54(8): 1177–1183.

Stone, K. L., Ancoli-Israel, S., Blackwell, T., Ensrud, K. E., Cauley, J. A., Redline, S., et al. (2008). 'Actigraphy-measured Sleep Characteristics and Risk of Falls in Older Women'. *Archives of Internal Medicine* 168(16): 1768–1775.

Taylor, S. R. and Weiss, J. S. (2009). 'Review of Insomnia Pharmacotherapy Options for the Elderly: Implications for Managed Care'. *Population Health Management* 12(6): 317–323.

Troxel, W. M., Buysse, D. J., Monk, T. H., Begley, A., and Hall, M. (2010). 'Does Social Support Differentially Affect Sleep in Older Adults with versus without Insomnia?' *Journal of Psychosomatic Research* 69: 459–466.

Wohlgemuth, W. K. and Edinger, J. D. (2000). 'Sleep Restriction Therapy'. In K. L. Lichstein and C. M. Morin (eds), *Treatment of Late-life Insomnia* (pp. 147–166). Thousand Oaks, CA: Sage.

Wolkove, N., Elkholy, O., Baltzan, M., and Palayew, M. (2007). 'Sleep and Aging: 1. Sleep Disorders Commonly Found in Older People'. *Canadian Medical Association Journal* 176(9): 1299–1304.

World Health Organization (1993). *The ICD-10 Classification of Mental and Behavioral Disorders*. Geneva: WHO.

Yokoyama, E., Saito, Y., Kaneita, Y., Ohida, T., Harano, S., Tamaki, T., et al. (2008). 'Association between Subjective Well-being and Sleep among the Elderly in Japan'. *Sleep Medicine* 9(2): 157–164.

Yokoyama, E., Kaneita, Y., Saito, Y., Uchiyama, M., Matsuzaki, Y., Tamaki, T., et al. (2010). 'Association between Depression and Insomnia Subtypes: A Longitudinal Study on the Elderly in Japan'. *Sleep* 33(12): 1693–1702.

Zhang, B. and Wing, Y. (2006). 'Sex Differences in Insomnia: A Meta-analysis'. *Sleep* 29(1): 85–93.

CHAPTER 26

SUBSTANCE USE, MISUSE, AND ABUSE

Special Issues for Older Adults

KRISTEN L. BARRY AND FREDERIC C. BLOW

INTRODUCTION

WE are well into a new millennium that is bringing new challenges in caring for the growing population of older adults. According to the *2010 Revision of World Population Prospects*, life expectancy at birth for the world as a whole rose from 46.6 years in 1950–1955 to 69.3 years in 2010–2015. The proportion of the world's population living in countries where life expectancy was below 60 years fell from 68% in the early 1950s to 12% in 2010–2015, while the share living in countries with life expectancy of 70 years or higher rose from 1% to 57% (United Nations Department of Economic and Social Affairs 2011). Over the same period, the probability of dying in early childhood—that is, the number of deaths under age 5 per 1000 live births—fell from 203 per 1000 to 60 per 1000. For the first time, there are more people over age 60 than children below the age of 5 (UNFPA 2012). The number and proportion of older persons is growing faster than any other age group, and will surpass one billion people worldwide in less than ten years. The US Census Bureau also estimates that the older adult population is growing rapidly, beginning in 2010 and extending through 2030, as the 'Baby Boom' cohort reaches the age of 65. By 2030, there will be about 72.1 million older persons in the US (19.3% of the total population), almost twice the number reported in 2008 (Administration on Aging 2010; US Census Bureau 2008).

As this current cohort of ageing adults transitions from mid- to later life, the emerging research indicates that they are continuing to use alcohol and psychoactive prescription medications at a higher rate than previous generations and they are beginning to present larger issues for the healthcare system and the intervention and treatment communities (Blow, Oslin, and Barry 2002; Korper and Council 2002). Accompanying the demographic and substance use changes that are underway, we are beginning to see the documented increases in problems related to substance use that result in costly negative health outcomes (Agency for Healthcare Research and Quality 2010). Having evidence-based practices to address these problems and provide prevention and early intervention services will be crucial to meeting the needs of this growing population.

The purpose of this chapter is to provide:

1 Background on the extent of the issue related to alcohol misuse/abuse and psychoactive prescription medication misuse.
2 Guidelines for alcohol and psychoactive medication use/misuse.
3 The evidence base for screening and early intervention for alcohol and psychoactive prescription medication misuse.
4 Potential screening questions and techniques appropriate for use with older adults.
5 A short guide to the steps in a brief intervention.

Extent of the Problem

There are two main categories of substances that generate the most concerns when working with older adults—(1) alcohol, and (2) psychoactive prescription medications (e.g. medications for anxiety (e.g. benzodiazepines), medications for sleep, and pain medications). Although illicit drug use is a growing concern and it is anticipated that it could be a larger problem with the ageing of the Baby Boomer cohort, illicit drug use is low in the current cohort of older adults.

The misuse and abuse of alcohol and medications in older adults pose challenges in terms of recognition, interventions, and treatment options. Problems related to use of substance in this age group are often not recognized and, if recognized, are generally undertreated. The standard diagnostic criteria for abuse/dependence have been difficult to apply to older adults (Blow, Center for Substance Abuse Treatment 1998), compounding the tendency to under-identify more serious problems. From a positive standpoint, however, older adults are more likely than younger adults to seek care from their primary and specialty care providers which affords opportunities for recognizing and intervening with the older adults who drink/use psychoactive medications at hazardous levels.

Prevalence of alcohol and drug misuse/abuse

Over a number of years, community surveys have estimated the prevalence of problem drinking among older adults to range from 1% to 16% (Adams, Barry, and Fleming 1996; Barry 1997; Fleming et al. 1999; Menninger 2002; Moore et al. 1999; Office of Applied Studies 2004, 2005). The rates vary widely depending on the definitions of older adults, at-risk and problem drinking, and alcohol abuse/dependence. The 2002–2003 National Survey on Drug Use and Health (NSDUH) found that, for individuals aged 50+ in the US, 12.2% were heavy drinkers, 3.2% were binge drinkers, and 1.8% used illicit drugs (Huang et al. 2006; Office of Applied Studies 2005). A later NSDUH (2005–2006) found a significant level of binge drinking among individuals age 50–64 (Blazer and Wu 2009). This group is included in the 'Baby Boomer' cohort. They also found that 19% of men and 13% of women had two or more drinks a day. The survey also showed a relatively high level of binge drinking in those over 65, with 14% of men and 3% of women engaging in binge drinking.

Mental and physical health risks associated with use/misuse/abuse

There are a number of mental and physical health problems that have been associated with alcohol use/misuse/abuse. Drinking at hazardous levels increases the risk of hypertension (Chermack, Blow, and Hill 1996; National Institute on Alcohol Abuse and Alcoholism 1995) and diabetes (Vestal et al. 1977), among other medical conditions in this population. Hazardous drinking can significantly affect a number of other conditions in this age group, including mood disorders and sleep, as well as general health functioning (Blow et al. 2000). Depression has been linked to relapse in drinking and increased alcohol intake. Blow and colleagues (2000) found negative effects of drinking status on general health, physical functioning, pain, mental health, and emotional functioning, with low-risk drinkers scoring better than abstainers and better than hazardous drinkers.

GUIDELINES FOR ALCOHOL USE

Among other factors, WHO advocates moderation in alcohol use as essential to healthy ageing (Stein and Moritz 1999). In the US, the National Institute of Alcohol Abuse and Alcoholism (NIAAA) set the following limits: 'Under age 65: more than 7 standard drinks/week for women, and more than 14 standard drinks/week for men are considered at-risk drinking. The guidelines recommend no more than one drink a day for both men and women over 65' (National Institute of Alcholism and Alcohol Abuse 1995). In the US, a 'standard drink' contains 12 grammes of alcohol. Therefore, a 12 oz beer = 5 oz of wine = 1½ oz of liquor = 4 oz of a liqueur (see Figure 26.1).

However, the guidelines differ across countries. For example, in England and Australia in particular, a standard drink contains 10 grammes of alcohol. This has implications for determining the prevalence of risk drinking and setting guidelines for use. Even within countries, the guidelines for alcohol usage by age may be a topic of discussion (e.g. McLaughlin et al. 2011).

Across countries, recommendations include the use of lower quantities of alcohol with ageing (Chermack et al. 1996). Because patients with a previous history of problems with alcohol or other drugs are at risk for relapse, establishing a history of use can provide important clues for future problems. Although alcohol and drug/medication dependence are less common in older adults when compared to younger adults, the mental and physical health consequences of use at this level are serious (Barry and Blow 2009). For example, the combined use of alcohol with psychoactive medications (e.g. benzodiazepines) can lead to negative central nervous system (CNS) effects. Older adults have a comparatively high rate of completed suicides. The causes of suicide in later life are multifaceted. Although no predominant factor precipitates or explains geriatric suicide, both depression and alcohol are strongly linked to suicide attempts and completions (Blow, Brockmann, and Barry 2004). In

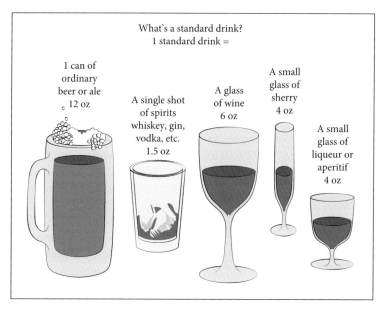

FIGURE 26.1 Standard Drink Equivalents.

Note: In the US, a standard drink contains 12 grammes of alcohol. In the UK and Australia, a standard drink contains 10 grammes of alcohol. Reproduced from Barry KL. Center for Substance Abuse Treatment Brief Interventions and Brief Therapies for Substance Abuse. Treatment Improvement Protocol (TIP) Series 34. DHHS Publication No. (SMA) pp. 99–3353. Rockville, MD: Substance Abuse and Mental Health Services Administration © 1999, The Authors.

addition, with changes in liver functioning with ageing and decreases in lean muscle mass, older adults metabolize alcohol differently than younger individuals. What might be considered light or moderate drinking for individuals in their thirties may have multiple negative health effects in an older person. Therefore, there is a need for further training for clinicians who treat older patients so that the clinicians understand alcohol use levels and are aware of health implications of the older adult's alcohol and psychoactive medication use.

Psychoactive prescription medication misuse

Misuse of psychoactive medications by older adults can be an even more challenging issue to identify than alcohol misuse. Despite high rates of medication use among older adults, few studies have specifically examined the prevalence and nature of psychoactive medication misuse and abuse in this population. The small amount of existing literature on this topic indicates that psychoactive medication misuse affects a small but significant minority of the older adult population (Simoni-Wastila et al. 2005). Older adults are at higher risk for inappropriate use of medications than younger individuals. A relatively recent study found that 25% of older adults use prescription psychoactive medications that have abuse potential (Simoni-Wastila and Yang 2006).

Psychoactive prescription misuse and abuse among older adults is quantitatively and qualitatively different than misuse/abuse in younger age groups. Prescription drugs misuse and abuse by older adults is usually unintentional (Simoni-Wastila and Yang 2006). Most of these drugs are obtained legally and they are not typically used to 'get high' (Blow et al. 2006b).

The psychoactive medications of most concern in this population are: (1) opioid medications for the treatment of pain, and (2) benzodiazepines used to treat anxiety and insomnia because these are the medications that cause some of the most serious problems for seniors who use them. These two classes of medication are often prescribed for older adults and have a high dependence and abuse potential.

Being female (Finlayson and Davis 1994; Jinks and Raschko 1990; Simoni-Wastila and Yang 2006), being socially isolated (Jinks and Raschko 1990; Simoni-Wastila and Yang 2006), and having a history of substance abuse or a mental health disorder (Jinks and Raschko 1990; Simoni-Wastila and Strickler 2004; Simoni-Wastila and Yang 2006; Solomon et al. 1993) are all associated with an increased risk of problems related to psychoactive medications. Longer-term use of psychotropic medications, especially benzodiazepines, has been associated with depression and cognitive losses (Dealberto et al. 1997; Hanlon et al. 1998; Hogan et al. 2003). Benzodiazepine use can also increase confusion and has the potential to increase falls and hip fractures in older adults (Leipzig, Cumming, and Tinetti 1999).

The misuse of psychoactive prescription medications (use in greater quantities or more often than prescribed) with or without the additional use of alcohol is now seen as a growing problem (Agency for Healthcare Research and Quality 2010). In fact, in the US admission to hospitals for all drug-related conditions grew by 117% for individuals age 45–64 (the Baby Boom cohort) over a recent ten-year period. The rates of hospital admission for all drug-related conditions among those aged 65–84 followed closely, growing by 96%. Studies have also found that higher scores on measures of psychoactive prescription misuse have been associated with a history of substance abuse, higher levels of psychosocial distress, and poorer functioning (Adams 2002; Holmes et al. 2006). Although the real scale of the problem is unknown, the United Nations Office on Drugs and Crime (UNODC) (2011) cautioned that the non-medical use of prescription drugs is a global health concern. The World Drug Report (UNODC 2010) stated that 'the misuse of prescription drugs, including opioids, benzodiazepines, and synthetic prescription stimulants, is a growing health problem in a number of developed and developing countries'. Compton and Volkow (2006) stated that older adults are one of the most vulnerable groups, particularly in term of the use of benzodiazipines and pain medications.

COMBINING ALCOHOL AND PSYCHOACTIVE MEDICATIONS

In addition to the concerns about the misuse of psychoactive medications alone, combined alcohol and medication misuse is a growing concern in the field. Substance abuse problems among older individuals often occur from misuse of over-the-counter and psychoactive prescription drugs. Misuse can fairly easily move to abuse, particularly if the older individual is experiencing pain, anxiety, and/or sleep disturbance (Blow, Oslin, and Barry 2002; Patterson and Jeste 1999; Schonfeld et al. 2010).

USE OF ILLICIT DRUGS

The use of illicit drugs is relatively rare in the current cohort of older adults. For example, in the US, the NSDUH (2002–2003) found that, for individuals age 50+, 1.8% used illicit drugs (Huang et al. 2006; Office of Applied Studies 2005). It is anticipated that the number of illicit drug users (as well as those with problems related to alcohol) in older adulthood will increase due to the ageing of the Baby Boom generation. Blow, Barry and colleagues (2002) analysed the National Health and Nutrition Examination Survey (NHANES) data, which suggested that the Baby Boom cohort, as it continues to age, could maintain a higher level of alcohol consumption than in previous older adult cohorts. It is anticipated that this cohort, unlike the current older adult population, will also be more likely to use illicit drugs. Consequently, a larger percentage of future older adults may have use patterns that place their health at risk.

DEFINITIONS

Many older adults have problems related to their alcohol use without meeting any standardized criteria for abuse and/or dependence. This same statement can be made for problems in this age group related to psychoactive prescription medication misuse. In order to address the range of problems, particularly in terms of alcohol and older adults, screening and assessment procedures need to focus on levels of use. In this age group, decisions regarding interventions and treatment may need to be made partly based on level of alcohol/medication use and misuse and partly based on problems manifested, regardless of amount used.

To diagnose alcohol use disorders clinicians generally look for behavioural factors such as the inability to cut down or stop, social and emotional consequences such as family problems, and physiological symptoms such as insomnia, gastrointestinal pain, liver toxicity, tolerance (it takes more of the substance to feel an effect over time), and withdrawal. There is generally a positive relationship between level of drinking (consumption) and severity of alcohol-related problems. This relationship is often true for younger adults but is not as applicable for older adults. In older adults, problems with alcohol can occur with relatively low levels of use. Screening and intervention efforts should include both an evaluation of: (1) psychosocial and medical problems that can be related to alcohol; and (2) a determination of consumption levels.

Because of the potential for interactions between alcohol and medications in this age group, the definitions of low-risk, at-risk, problem use, and abuse/dependence should always include an evaluation of medication use (including over-the-counter and a broad range of prescription medications) along with the use of alcohol. Additionally, it is important to understand the broad range of problematic use of prescription medications that can be found in this population. The following definitions based on level of risk can provide a guide for determining prevention/intervention strategies for assisting older adults.

Low-risk use

Alcohol use that does not lead to problems is called *low-risk use* (adapted from Barry and Blow 2010). People in this category can set reasonable limits on alcohol consumption, do not drink when driving a car or boat, operating machinery, and/or do not use contraindicated medications. They also do not engage in binge drinking. Low-risk use of medications could include short-term use of an anti-anxiety medication for an acute anxiety state during which the physician's prescription is followed and no alcohol is used; or drinking one drink three times/week without the use of any contraindicated medications.

At-risk use

At-risk use is use that increases the chances of developing problems and complications. In the US, these individuals consume more than seven drinks/week, binge drink (women age 60+: three or more drinks on a drinking occasion; men age 60+: four or more drinks on a drinking occasion), or drink in risky situations (e.g. driving, operating machinery). They do not currently have major health problems caused by alcohol, but if their drinking pattern continues, problems could result. In Australia and England, the cut-offs are slightly higher because a standard drink is 10 grammes of alcohol compared to 12 grammes in the US.

There are two types of medication misuse that may fit into at-risk use or problem use depending on severity. The types are misuse by the patient and misuse by the practitioner. Misuse by the patient includes taking more or less medication than prescribed; hoarding or skipping doses of a medication; use of medication for purposes other than those prescribed; and use of the medication in conjunction with alcohol or other contraindicated medications. Misuse by the practitioner includes prescribing medication for an inappropriate indication; prescribing a dosage that is unnecessarily high; or failure to monitor or fully explain the appropriate use of a medication (Culberson and Ziska 2008).

Problematic use

Problematic use refers to a level of use that has already resulted in adverse medical, psychological, or social consequences. Although most problem drinkers consume more than the low-risk limits, some older adults who drink smaller amounts may experience alcohol-related problems. As mentioned above, medication misuse can also fit into the problem-use category. Individuals in this category would benefit from a more extensive assessment to determine the severity of the problems and offer appropriate interventions/treatments.

ALCOHOL AND OTHER DRUG DEPENDENCE

Those who use at the level of *dependence* have a medical disorder that is characterized by loss of control, preoccupation with alcohol/psychoactive medications, continued use despite adverse consequences, and physiological symptoms such as tolerance. Although not always present, it is important to assess for withdrawal. A wide range of legal and illegal substances can be addictive.

Medication abuse involves medication use that results in diminished physical or social functioning; medication use in risky situations; and continued medication use despite adverse social or personal consequences (Culberson and Ziska 2008). Dependence includes medication use that results in tolerance or withdrawal symptoms, unsuccessful attempts to stop or control medication use, and preoccupation with attaining or using a medication.

Note: It is clear that some older individuals should not consume alcohol at all, and it is critical that this is part of the recommended drinking limit for those individuals. Older adults taking certain prescription medications, especially psychoactive prescription medications (e.g. opioid analgesics and benzodiazepines), certain over-the-counter medications (e.g. sleep aids), those with medical conditions that can be made worse by alcohol (e.g. diabetes, heart disease), individuals planning to drive a car or engage in other activities requiring alertness and skill, and those who are recovering from alcohol dependence, should not drink alcohol.

Screening

Pre-screening and screening

Because of the relationship between alcohol consumption and health problems, questions about consumption (quantity and frequency of use) provide a method to categorize patients into levels of risk for alcohol use. The traditional assumption that all patients who drink have a tendency to under-report their alcohol use is not supported by research over many years. People who are not alcohol dependent often give accurate answers.

Clinicians can get more accurate histories by asking questions about the recent past; embedding the alcohol use questions in the context of other health behaviours (i.e. exercise, weight, smoking, alcohol use); and paying attention to nonverbal cues that suggest the patient is minimizing use (i.e. blushing, turning away, fidgeting, looking at the floor, change in breathing pattern). Screening questions can be asked by verbal interview, by paper-and-pencil questionnaire, or by computerized questionnaire. All three methods have equivalent reliability and validity (Barry and Fleming 1990). However, patients are often more comfortable answering questions on either paper-and-pencil or computerized screeners. Any positive responses can lead to further questions about consequences. *To successfully incorporate alcohol (and other drug) screening into clinical practice, it should be simple and consistent with other screening procedures already in place.*

Before asking any screening questions the following conditions are needed: (1) the interviewer needs to be friendly and non-threatening; (2) the purpose of the questions should be clearly related to their health status; (3) the patient should be alcohol-free at the time of the screening; if the patient is intoxicated at the time of screening, either waiting until their blood alcohol levels decrease (e.g. in the Emergency Department) or screening at another time (e.g. primary care settings) would be appropriate; (4) the information should be confidential; and (5) the questions should be easy to understand. Screening questions can be used with the older adult who may have alcohol-related problems as well as to guide an interview with a concerned friend, spouse, or family member. In some settings (such as waiting rooms), screening instruments are given as self-report questionnaires, with instructions for the patient to discuss the meaning of the results with their healthcare provider.

Table 26.1 Audit

1. How often do you have a drink containing alcohol?
   - ☐ 0 Never
   - ☐ 1 Monthly or less
   - ☐ 2 2 to 4 times a month
   - ☐ 3 2 to 3 times a month
   - ☐ 4 4 or more times a week

2. How many drinks containing alcohol do you have on a typical day when you are drinking?
   - ☐ 0 1 or 2
   - ☐ 1 3 or 4
   - ☐ 2 5 or 6
   - ☐ 3 7 or 9
   - ☐ 4 10 or more

3. How often do you have 6 or more drinks on one occasion?
   - ☐ 0 Never
   - ☐ 1 Less than monthly
   - ☐ 2 Monthly
   - ☐ 3 Weekly
   - ☐ 4 Daily or almost daily

4. How often during the last year have you found that you were not able to stop drinking once you had started?
   - ☐ 0 Never
   - ☐ 1 Less than monthly
   - ☐ 2 Monthly
   - ☐ 3 Weekly
   - ☐ 4 Daily or almost daily

5. How often during the last year have you failed to do what was normally expected from you because of drinking?
   - ☐ 0 Never
   - ☐ 1 Less than monthly
   - ☐ 2 Monthly
   - ☐ 3 Weekly
   - ☐ 4 Daily or almost daily

6. How often during the last year have you needed a first drink in the morning to get yourself going after a heavy drinking session?
   - ☐ 0 Never
   - ☐ 1 Less than monthly
   - ☐ 2 Monthly
   - ☐ 3 Weekly
   - ☐ 4 Daily or almost daily

7. How often during the last year have you had a feeling of guilt or remorse after drinking?
   - ☐ 0 Never
   - ☐ 1 Less than monthly
   - ☐ 2 Monthly
   - ☐ 3 Weekly
   - ☐ 4 Daily or almost daily

(Continued)

Table 26.1 (Continued)

8. How often during the last year have you been unable to remember what happened the night before because of your drinking?

    ☐ 0 Never

    ☐ 1 Less than monthly

    ☐ 2 Monthly

    ☐ 3 Weekly

    ☐ 4 Daily or almost daily

9. Have you or someone else been injured as a result of your drinking?

    ☐ 0 No

    ☐ 2 Yes, but not in the last year

    ☐ 4 Yes, during the last year

10. Has a relative, friend, doctor or other health worker been concerned about your drinking or suggested you cut down?

    ☐ 0 No

    ☐ 2 Yes, but not in the last year

    ☐ 4 Yes, during the last year

Record sum of individual item scores here:

SCORING: The following are guidelines for scoring the AUDIT. However, some older adults who use contraindicated medications or are experiencing cognitive or health problems should not use alcohol at all.

0–4: Lower risk use; 5–8: At-risk use; 8–10: Alcohol abuse; 11-up: Alcohol dependence

The AUDIT is in public domain. Readers can find out more about it at the following websites:

Australia: http://www.health.nt.gov.au/library/scripts/objectifyMedia.aspx?file=pdf/63/68.pdf

US: http://pubs.niaaa.nih.gov/publications/aa65/aa65.htm

UK: http://www.patient.co.uk/doctor/alcohol-use-disorders-identification-test-audit

Brief pre-screening for substance use is a critical first step in identifying older adults who may need further in-depth screening/assessments and those who may be suitable candidates for brief interventions. The screening process should help determine if an individual's alcohol/psychoactive medication use is appropriate for brief intervention or warrants a different approach (e.g. brief treatment; referral to specialized treatments).

Adapted from *The NIAAA Clinician's Guide to Helping Patients who Drink too Much* (US National Institute for Alcohol Abuse and Alcoholism 2005), simple questions about heavy substance use days can be used during a clinical interview or before an older adult is seen, followed up with further questions as indicated. The UK (National Institute for Health and Clinical Excellence 2010) recommends using the Alcohol Use Disorders Identification Test (AUDIT) and revising the scores downward for older adults (Babor, Higgins-Biddle, and Saunders 2001). Note: In addition to individual screening and interventions, countries have adopted policies regarding taxation of alcohol, etc. to address alcohol problems from a societal level. For example, the Scottish Health Action on Alcohol Problems (SHAAP) was established by the Scottish Medical Royal Colleges and Faculties to raise awareness about alcohol-related harm and to promote solutions based on the best available evidence and has addressed both screening and interventions for individuals as well as societal measures to reduce alcohol misuse/abuse (SHAAP 2007).

The following are pre-screening questions that can be asked in a clinical setting to determine which patients should complete more complete screening assessments:

Pre-screening question: Do you drink beer, wine, or other alcoholic beverages?

Follow-up: If yes, how many times in the [past year; past three months; past six months] have you had five or more drinks in a day (for men)/four or more drinks in a day (for women)?

On average, how many days/week do you drink alcoholic beverages? *If weekly or more:* On a day when you drink alcohol, how many drinks do you have?

Pre-screening questions: Do you use prescription medicines for pain? anxiety? sleep? Do you use any of these prescription drugs in a way that is different from how they were prescribed?

Follow-up: If yes, follow up with additional questions regarding which substances, frequency, and quantity of use.

When using standardized alcohol screening questionnaires in an interview format, it is important to read the questions as written and in the order indicated. By following the exact wording, better comparability will be obtained between your results and those obtained by other interviewers. This section of the chapter focuses primarily on two widely used alcohol screening instruments: the Alcohol Use Disorders Identification Test (AUDIT) developed by the WHO, and the Short Michigan Alcoholism Screening Test-Geriatric Version (SMAST-G), as well as a drug use questionnaire developed by the National Institute on Drug Abuse (NIDA), the ASSIST which was modified to address psychoactive prescription medication misuse and tested with older adults (Schonfeld et al. 2010). These three instruments are included here because they have been tested across age groups including older adults. There are additional alcohol screening instruments that are widely used internationally such as the Fast Alcohol Screening Test (FAST) developed by the Health Development Agency (HDA), part of the NHS in the UK (HDA and University of Wales College of Medicine 2002). The FAST includes four questions (binge drinking, blackouts, failure to do what is normally expected, and concern from a healthcare provider).

The Alcohol Use Disorders Identification Test (AUDIT) (Table 26.1), which was developed by the World Health Organization (WHO) as a brief screening tool for excessive drinking (Babor et al. 1989; Barry and Fleming 1993; Fiellin et al. 2000; Fleming, Barry, and MacDonald 1991; Schmidt, Barry, and Fleming 1995), is a well-validated screener. The AUDIT can also be helpful in developing a framework for brief interventions for individuals drinking at hazardous or harmful levels. The AUDIT has been used in age groups across the lifespan. The AUDIT is a ten-item questionnaire introduced by a section explaining to the respondent that questions about alcohol use in the *previous year only* are included. The questionnaire is often used as a screener without the clinical examination. The recommended cut-off score for the AUDIT has been 8. A copy of this tool can be found at: http://www.niaaa.nih.gov/Publications/EducationTrainingMaterials/Documents/Audit.pdf.

The Short Michigan Alcoholism Screening Test-Geriatric Version (SMAST-G) (see Table 26.2) is the short form of the MAST-G and was developed for use in busy clinical settings and in research settings where brevity is an issue (Blow et al. 1998). Major barriers to using the longer scale in busy clinical settings are length and administration time. To address these issues, a short version of the MAST-G was developed. The ten items on the short version of the MAST-G (SMAST-G) were selected by factor analysis. The initial sensitivity and specificity of the SMAST-G were tested in a sample of fifty older adult subjects (age range 55–81). The testing criteria were *DSM-III-R* diagnoses of alcohol abuse and/or dependence as measured by the Diagnostic Interview Schedule-Revised. Of the sample 26% were diagnosed with alcohol abuse and/or dependence. Based on an ROC analysis, an SMAST-G cut-off point between 3 and 4 yielded a sensitivity of .85 and specificity of .97. The SMAST-G fared as well as the AUDIT, and may be more acceptable to older individuals. In this sample, SMAST-G is also an acceptable alternative to the MAST-G for elder-specific brief alcohol screening and is superior to other screening instruments developed in younger populations. A score of 2 or more (e.g. two 'yes' responses) indicates probable alcohol problems. The SMAST-G questions ask about participants' experiences within the last year.

The National Institute on Drug Abuse (NIDA) Modified ASSIST instrument, developed originally to measure illicit drug use/abuse, has been adapted in the field and is now more widely used to measure psychoactive prescription medication problems (e.g. Schonfeld et al. 2010).

Screening opportunities include during routine appointments, when filling out intake forms, before prescribing medications (particularly those that interact with alcohol or other drugs), in emergency departments/urgent care centres, and for older individuals with

---

Table 26.2 Short Michigan Alcoholism Screening Test–Geriatric Version (SMAST–G)

YES (1) NO (0)

1. When talking with others, do you ever underestimate how much you actually drink?   _____ _____

2. After a few drinks, have you sometimes not eaten or been able to skip a meal because you didn't feel hungry?   _____ _____

3. Does having a few drinks help decrease your shakiness or tremors?   _____ _____

4. Does alcohol sometimes make it hard for you to remember parts of the day or night?   _____ _____

5. Do you usually take a drink to relax or calm your nerves?   _____ _____

6. Do you drink to take your mind off your problems?   _____ _____

7. Have you ever increased your drinking after experiencing a loss in your life?   _____ _____

8. Has a doctor or nurse ever said they were worried or concerned about your drinking?   _____ _____

9. Have you ever made rules to manage your drinking?   _____ _____

10. When you feel lonely, does having a drink help?   _____ _____

Total SMAST-G Score (0-10) _____
© The Regents of the University of Michigan, Frederic C. Blow, Ph.D., 1991.

health conditions that may be alcohol related, and those with illnesses that are not responding to treatment as expected.

In the US, the Substance Abuse and Mental Health Services Administration (SAMHSA), Center for Substance Abuse Treatment (CSAT) developed a series of Treatment Improvement Protocols (TIPs) including TIP #26, 'Substance Abuse in Older Adults' (Blow, Center for Substance Abuse Treatment 1998). The expert panel convened to develop these guidelines recommended that all adults age 60+ should be screened on a yearly basis (generally, embedded with other health-screening questions) and rescreened if there are major life changes that could precipitate increased use and problems (e.g. retirement, death of a partner/spouse, etc).

BRIEF INTERVENTIONS

There is a large body of evidence that motivational brief interventions, delivered in a variety of healthcare and social service settings, can effectively reduce drinking, particularly for at-risk and problem users. Over the last 30+ years, preventive interventions in a variety of medical and social service care settings have proven to be efficacious in reducing alcohol misuse among younger adults (e.g. Babor and Grant 1992; Blow et al. 2006b; Chick, Lloyd, and Crombie 1985; Fleming et al. 1997, 1999; Harris and Miller 1990; Wallace, Cutler, and Haines 1988). See meta-analytic reviews including: Whitlock et al. (2004) and Havard, Shakeshaft, and Sanson-Fisher (2008).

The general form of the interventions in these studies has included personalized feedback based on the patients' responses to screening questions and untailored (generic) messages to cut down or stop drinking. Meta-analyses of randomized controlled studies have found that these techniques generally reduce drinking in the intervention vs control conditions. Results indicate that, across studies, participants reduced their average number of drinks/week by 13% to 34% compared to controls. The reduction in drinking due to these very brief interventions generally lasted at least one year. The proportion of participants in intervention condition drinking at moderate or safe levels was 10–19% greater than controls over twelve months.

The randomized controlled brief intervention trials with older adults (Blow and Barry 1999; Fleming et al. 1999; Lin et al. 2010; Moore et al. 2011) have exhibited the same positive results. In addition to the randomized controlled trials, two notable large-scale effectiveness studies have been conducted to study the implementation of these models in practice: the Primary Care Research in Substance Abuse and Mental Health for the Elderly study (PRISM-E) (Oslin et al. 2006) and the Florida BRITE (Brief Intervention and Treatment for Elders) project (Schonfeld et al. 2010). These two effectiveness studies demonstrated that, despite the strong evidence of the efficacy of screening and brief intervention approaches, and deliberate attempts at implementing these evidence-based interventions in practice, enormous barriers in implementation continue to exist for the implementation of preventive interventions that work with older adults in real-world settings. These barriers include stigma from the perspective of older adults, difficulty in outreach to older adults, lack of healthcare and other professionals trained in screening and brief interventions, chronic medical conditions that may make it more difficult for providers to recognize the role of alcohol and psychoactive medication misuse in decreases in functioning and quality of life, and few or low reimbursement/funding sources for SBI. These and other barriers and possible solutions are discussed in the second section of this chapter.

Although the efficacy and effectiveness of screening and brief interventions, particularly for alcohol misuse/abuse is well-documented, there is a science-to-service gap in providing these evidence-based practices for the growing population of older adults worldwide. This need is becoming more acute as the evidence grows regarding the widespread use and misuse of alcohol and psychoactive prescription medications, such as opioid analgesics and benzodiazepines, in this ageing population, particularly the Baby Boom cohort.

Screening, Brief Intervention, and Referral to Treatment (SBIRT) Model (see Figure 26.2)

A comprehensive model for addressing alcohol and psychoactive prescription misuse in a variety of health-related settings is called SBIRT. SBIRT consists of **S**creening, **B**rief **I**ntervention, and **R**eferral to **T**reatment. The SBIRT model was based on all of the research conducted to establish the efficacy and effectiveness of screening and brief intervention techniques.

Screening quickly assesses the severity of substance use and identifies the appropriate level of intervention. *Brief Intervention* focuses on increasing insight and awareness regarding substance use and motivation for behavioural change. *Referral to Treatment* provides access to specialty substance abuse assessment and care, if needed. Most trials have tested the brief intervention portion of SBIRT, particularly those with older adults. However, Schonfeld et al. (2010) studied the entire SBIRT model with older adults.

Practical Steps in a Brief Intervention

Effective brief interventions generally follow the FRAMES model (Barry, Center for Substance Abuse Treatment 1999; Barry, Oslin, and Blow 2001). In this model:

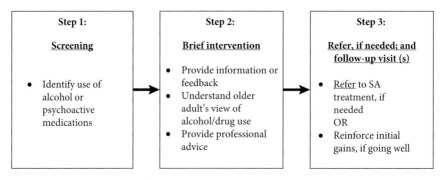

FIGURE 26.2 Screening, Brief Intervention and Referral to Treatment (SBIRT) steps.

SAMHSA, Committee on Trauma Quick Guide (http://www.aoa.gov/AoARoot/AoA_Programs/HPW/Behavioral/docs2/Issue%20Brief%203%20Screening%20Brief%20Interventions.pdf).

Feedback is given to the individual about risk.
Responsibility for change is placed with the individual receiving the intervention.
Advice for changing behaviour is given by the clinician.
Menu of alternative options for change is offered.
Empathic and motivational style is used by the intervener.
Self-efficacy or empowerment is promoted.

Brief intervention protocols often use a workbook containing the steps listed below. Using a workbook can make it easier for both the client and the clinician to discuss cues to use, reasons for the level of use, reasons to cut down or quit, to negotiate an agreement for next steps, and to introduce using daily diary cards for self-monitoring. Brief interventions take ~20–30 minutes to conduct (Barry, Center for Substance Abuse Treatment TIP—Treatment Improvement Protocol 1999). A brief intervention workbook is included in the TIP (Barry, Center for Substance Abuse Treatment 1999) and in Barry, Oslin, and Blow (2001). Providers can be trained to use the intervention protocol through role-playing and general skills training techniques in educational programmes. Following motivational interviewing principles, the interventions using a workbook have been tested in a variety of clinical settings including primary care, emergency departments, social service agencies, home healthcare agencies, senior housing, and inpatient programmes.

The brief intervention protocol includes the following steps:

1 *Identification of future goals* for health, work, school, activities, hobbies, relationships, and financial stability. This step gives the service provider and the older adult information on what the older adult is interested in achieving and can help to target goals for the intervention.

2 *Summary of health habits*. Customized feedback on screening questions relating to drinking and/or drug use patterns and other health habits (may also include smoking, nutrition, tobacco use, seat belt use, safe sex, etc.). This health behaviours information can come from screening questionnaires or from the patient during this session.

3 *Discussion of standard drinks* (see Figure 26.1 for a picture representation of standard drink equivalents). All of these beverages containing alcohol are roughly equivalent in alcohol content (12 oz of beer or ale = 1.5 oz of distilled spirits = 4–5 oz of wine = 4 oz of sherry or liqueur).

4 *Discussion of the norms for alcohol/psychoactive medication use in the population*, and where the older adult's use fits into the population norms for his/her age group. This introduces drinking guidelines (e.g. in the US, women under 65: no more than one drink/day; men under 65: nor more than two drinks/day; women and men 65 and over: no more than one drink/day or seven drinks/week.It is important to avoid creating additional resistance. It is very important to 'roll with the individual's resistance' or reluctance to further examine his/her use in an empathetic manner.

5 *Consequences of at-risk and problem drinking and psychoactive medication use*. This discussion relates consequences to any potential or ongoing health problem that is currently important in the person's care (e.g. hypertension, pain management, anxiety, gastrointestinal problems, etc).This is particularly important because the service provider needs to understand both the positive and negative

roles of alcohol and medications in the context of the older patient's life, including coping with loss and loneliness. It provides a climate in which patients can obtain greater clarity of how alcohol and/or psychoactive medication are or could be negatively affecting their lives.

6 *Reasons to quit or cut down on use.* This is a very brief discussion of how changing their use could have important benefits for the individual. Note: Some older patients may experience problems in physical, psychological, or social functioning even though they are drinking below cut-off levels. This section of the workbook reviews the potential social, emotional, and physical benefits of changing their drinking.

7 *Negotiated agreement for alcohol and/or psychoactive medications.* Drinking limits or actions needed to address psychoactive medication use in the form of an agreement can be negotiated and signed by the older adult and the intervener. *The older adult takes the workbook, including the agreement, with them when they leave the office.*

8 *Coping with risky situations.* Social isolation, boredom, pain, and negative family interactions can present special problems for individuals trying to change their behaviour. It helps if the individual can identify situations and moods that can be risky and identify some individualized cognitive and behavioural coping alternatives. Note: This step may be done at the time of the initial intervention or can take place after the older adult has had a chance to try out cutting back or stopping, etc.

9 *Summary of the session.* The summary should include a review of the session, including a review of the drinking and/or psychoactive medication goals, a discussion of the drinking and medication diary cards (calendar) to be completed for the next four weeks (or longer, if needed and useful to the older adult), and the recommendation to refer back to the workbook materials given to patients during intervention sessions.

Brief interventions are one of a *spectrum* of approaches to address alcohol and psychoactive medication/drug use misuse and abuse. 'Real world' implementation strategies to address time and logistical barriers will be the key to their adaptation. The use of screening, brief interventions, brief therapies, and referral to substance abuse treatment, where appropriate, provides a state-of-the-art constellation of short, targeted approaches for use by provider and other healthcare staff that form an evidence-based practice for working with a vulnerable population to improve outcomes and manage costs.

IMPLICATIONS FOR PRACTICE

Identifying substance-related problems in older adults can take place in many healthcare-related settings, including primary care clinics, specialty care settings, home healthcare, elder housing, and senior centre programmes. The methods for working with older adults who are using alcohol and/or psychoactive medications/drugs depend on the level of risk each older adult is experiencing. Interventions, tailored to the level of use and the level of risk, include prevention messages, minimal advice, structured brief intervention protocols, formalized treatment for older persons with alcohol abuse/dependence. Through the use of standardized screening and intervention protocols, the use of technology to assist in the process (e.g. computer/tablet completion of screening instrument; computerized interventions, etc.), these techniques can be easily embedded into clinical practices. If these strategies are implemented successfully, it will help to ensure that current and future generations of older adults with substance misuse have the opportunity for improved physical and emotional quality in their lives.

SUMMARY

Strategies for working with older adults who are using alcohol and/or psychoactive medications/drugs at risk levels—minimal advice, structured brief intervention protocols, formalized treatment for older persons with alcohol abuse/dependence, and specialized relapse prevention programmes—provide useful tools to begin to address this growing issue. Both from a public health standpoint and from a clinical perspective, with the growing population of older adults, there is a critical need to implement effective screening and intervention strategies with older drinkers who are at risk for more serious health, social, and emotional problems.

There are a number of challenges to the healthcare system in addressing substance misuse in older adults. Working with older adults in rural and remote communities presents challenges in terms of training providers, provider turnover, and resources for substance abuse treatment, if needed. The use of technology can enhance the delivery of SBIRT services across areas (e.g. the use of standardized computer-based interventions and telemedicine to assist with screening and interventions). To meet the needs of a culturally diverse population: (1) screening and intervention materials have been and can be available in a number of languages; (2) screening and intervention materials can be adapted to various cultures and groups; and (3) translators and/or providers from the target culture can be trained to work with older adults facing problems related to substance use. In addition, a challenge to healthcare systems world-wide will be addressing the needs of members of the ageing population who are misusing alcohol and/or medications/drugs in the context of a managed care environment, where providers are expected to deliver quality medical care for a wide variety of health problems within greater time constraints.

The development of short, effective techniques to address substance use issues in the growing population of older adults is one of the current and future foci for the substance use field (Barry, Center for Substance Abuse Treatment 1999). Innovative screening, intervention, and treatment methods for alcohol and drug misuse among older adults, if successfully implemented, are steps in the process of assuring that current and future generations have the opportunity for improved physical and emotional quality in their lives.

KEY REFERENCES AND SOURCES FOR FURTHER READING

Babor, T. F., Higgins-Biddle, J. C., and Saunders J. B. (2001). *The Alcohol Use Disorders Identification Test: Guidelines for Use in Primary Care*. Geneva: World Health Organization.

Barry, K. L., Oslin, D., and Blow, F. C. (2001). *Alcohol Problems in Older Adults: Prevention and Management*. New York: Springer.

Blazer, D. G. and Wu, L. (2009). 'The Epidemiology of At-risk and Binge Drinking among Middle-aged and Elderly Community Adults: National Survey on Drug Use and Health'. *American Journal of Psychiatry* 166(10): 1162–1169. doi: 10.1176/appi.ajp.2009.09010016.

Blow, F. C., Center for Substance Abuse Treatment (1998). *Substance Abuse among Older Adults.* Treatment Improvement Protocol (TIP) Series 26. DHHS Publication No. (SMA) 98-3179. Rockville, MD: Substance Abuse and Mental Health Services Administration.

Blow, F. C., Bartels, S. J., Brockmann, L. M., and Van Citters, A. D. (2006). *Evidence-based Practices for Preventing Substance Abuse and Mental Health Problems in Older Adults.* Rockville, MD: Older American Substance Abuse and Mental Health Technical Assistance Center, SAMHSA.

Centers for Disease Control and Prevention (2007). *The State of Aging and Health in America, 2007.* http://www.cdc.gov/Aging/pdf/saha_2007.pdf. Whitehouse Station, NJ: Merck Company Foundation.

Fleming, M. F., Manwell, L. B., Barry, K. L., Adams, W., and Stauffacer, E. A. (1999). 'Brief Physician Advice for Alcohol Problems in Older Adults: A Randomized Community-based Trial'. *Journal of Family Practice* 48(5): 378–384.

National Institute on Alcohol Abuse and Alcoholism (2005). *Helping Patients who Drink Too Much. A Clinician's Guide, Updated 2005 Edition.* US Department of Health and Human Services, National Institute of Health. NIH Publication No. 07-3769.

National Institute for Health and Clinical Excellence (2010). Alcohol use disorders: Preventing harmful drinking. http://www.nice.org.uk/nicemedia/live/13001/48984/48984.pdf. Manchester: NICE.

REFERENCES

Adams, W. L., Barry, K. L., and Fleming, M. F. (1996). 'Screening for Problem Drinking in Older Primary Care Patients'. *Journal of the American Medical Association* 276(24): 1964–1967.

Adams, W. L., McIlvain, H. E., Lacy, N. L., Magsi, H., and Crabtree, B. F., et al. (2002). 'Primary Care for Elderly People: Why Do Doctors Find it so Hard?' *Gerontologist* 42(6): 835–842.

Administration on Aging (2010). *A Profile of Older Americans: 2010.* http://www.aoa.gov/aoaroot/aging_statistics/profile/2010/docs/2010profile.pdf. Washington, DC: Administration on Aging.

Agency for Healthcare Research and Quality (2010). 'Hospitalizations for Medication and Illicit Drug-related Conditions on the Rise among Americans Ages 45 and Older'. Press release. http://www.ahrq.gov/news/press/pr2010/hospmedpr.htm.

Babor, T. F., De La Fuente, J. R., Saunders, J., and Grant, M. (1989). *AUDIT: The Alcohol Use Disorders Identification Test. Guidelines for Use in Primary Health Care.* Geneva: World Health Organization.

Babor, T. F., Kranzler, H. R., and Lauerman, R. J. (1989). 'Early Detection of Harmful Alcohol Consumption: Comparison of Clinical, Laboratory, and Self-report Screening Procedures'. *Addictive Behaviors* 14(2): 139–157.

Babor, T. F. and Grant, M. (1992). *Project on Identification and Management of Alcohol-related Problems. Report on Phase II: A Randomized Clinical Trial of Brief Interventions in Primary Health Care.* Geneva: World Health Organization.

Babor, T. F., Higgins-Biddle, J. C., and Saunders, J. B. (2001). *The Alcohol Use Disorders Identification Test: Guidelines for Use in Primary Care*. Geneva: World Health Organization.

Barry, K. L. and Fleming, M. F. (1993). 'The Alcohol Use Disorders Identification Test (AUDIT) and the SMAST-13: Predictive Validity in a Rural Primary Care Sample'. *Alcohol and Alcoholism* 2(1): 33–42.

Barry, K. L. (1997). 'Alcohol and Drug Abuse'. In M. Mengel and W. Holleman (eds), *Fundamentals of Clinical Practice: A Textbook on the Patient, Doctor, and Society* (pp. 689–715). New York: Plenum.

Barry, K. L., Center for Substance Abuse Treatment (1999). *Brief Interventions and Brief Therapies for Substance Abuse*. Treatment Improvement Protocol (TIP) Series 34. DHHS Publication No. (SMA) 99-3353. Rockville, MD: Substance Abuse and Mental Health Services Administration.

Barry, K. L., Oslin, D., and Blow, F. C. (2001). *Alcohol Problems in Older Adults: Prevention and Management*. New York: Springer.

Barry, K. L. and Blow, F. C. (2009). 'Screening, Assessing and Intervening for Alcohol and Medication Misuse in Older Adults'. In P. Lichtenberg (ed.), *Handbook of Assessment in Clinical Gerontology* (2nd edn; 310–330). New York: Wiley.

Blazer, D. G. and Wu, L. (2009). 'The Epidemiology of At-risk and Binge Drinking among Middle-aged and Elderly Community Adults: National Survey on Drug Use and Health'. *American Journal of Psychiatry* 166(10): 1162–1169. doi:10.1176/appi.ajp.2009.09010016.

Blow, F. C., Center for Substance Abuse Treatment (1998). *Substance Abuse Among Older Adults*. Treatment Improvement Protocol (TIP) Series 26. DHHS Publication No. (SMA) 98–3179. Rockville, MD: Substance Abuse and Mental Health Services Administration.

Blow, F. C. and Barry K. L. (1999). 'Advances in Alcohol Screening and Brief Intervention with Older Adults'. In P. A. Lichtenberg (ed.), *Advances in Medical Psychotherapy* (Vol. 10; 107–124). Dubuque, IA: Kendall Hunt.

Blow, F. C., Walton, M. A., Chermack, S. T., Mudd, S. A., Brower, K. J., et al. (2000). 'Older Adult Treatment Outcome Following Elder-specific Inpatient Alcoholism Treatment'. *Journal of Substance Abuse Treatment* 19(1): 67–75.

Blow, F. C., Barry, K. L., Fuller, B., and Booth, B. M. (2002). 'Analysis of the National Health and Nutrition Examination Survey (NHANES): Longitudinal Analysis of Drinking over the Lifespan'. In S. P. Korper and C. L. Council (eds), *Substance Use by Older Adults: Estimates of Future Impact on the Treatment System* (pp. 125–141). Rockville, MD: Substance Abuse and Mental Health Services Administration, Office of Applied Studies. (DHHS Publication No. SMA 03-3763, Analytic Series A-21).

Blow, F. C., Oslin, D. W., and Barry, B. (2002). 'Misuse and Abuse of Alcohol, Illicit Drugs, and Psychoactive Medication among Older People'. *Generations* 26(1): 50–55.

Blow, F. C., Brockmann, L. M., and Barry, K. L. (2004). 'The Role of Alcohol in Late-life Suicide'. *Alcoholism: Clinical and Experimental Research* 28(5S): S48–S56.

Blow, F. C., Bartels, S. J., Brockmann, L. M., and Van Citters, A. D. (2006a). *Evidence-based Practices for Preventing Substance Abuse and Mental Health Problems in Older Adults*. Rockville, MD: Older American Substance Abuse and Mental Health Technical Assistance Center, SAMHSA.

Blow, F. C., Barry, K. L., Walton, M. A., Maio, R., Chermack, S. T., et al. (2006b). 'The Efficacy of Two Brief Intervention Strategies among Injured, At-risk Drinkers in the Emergency Department: Impact of Tailored Messaging and Brief Advice'. *Journal of Studies on Alcohol* 67(4): 568–578.

Blow, F. C., Gillespie, B. W., Barry. K. L, et al. (1998). 'Brief Screening for Alcohol Problems in an Elderly Population Using the Short Michigan Alcoholism Screening Test-Geriatric Version (SMAST-G)'. *Research Society on Alcoholism*, June 20–24.

Chermack, S. T., Blow, F. C., and Hill, E. M. (1996). 'The Relationship between Alcohol Symptoms and Consumption among Older Drinkers'. *Alcoholism: Clinical and Experimental Research* 20: 1153–1158.

Chick, J., Lloyd, G., and Crombie, E. (1985). 'Counseling Problem Drinkers in Medical Wards: A Controlled Study'. *British Medical Journal* 290: 965–967.

Compton, W. M. and Volkow, N. D. (2006). 'Commentary: Major Increases in Opioid Analgesic Abuse in the United States: Concerns and Strategies'. *Drug and Alcohol Dependence* 81(2): 103–107.

Culberson, J. and Ziska, M. (2008). 'Prescription Drug Misuse/Abuse in the Elderly'. *Geriatrics* 63(9): 22–31.

Dealberto, M. J., McAvay G. J., Seeman, T., and Berkman, L. (1997). 'Psychotropic Drug Use and Cognitive Decline among Older Men and Women'. *International Journal of Geriatric Psychiatry* 12(5): 567–574.

Fiellin, D. A., Reid, M. C., and O'Connor, P. G. (2000). 'Screening for Alcohol Problems in Primary Care: A Systematic Review'. *Archives of Internal Medicine* 160(13): 1977–1989.

Finlayson, R. E. and Davis, L. J. (1994). 'Prescription Drug Dependence in the Elderly Population: Demographic and Clinical Features of 100 Inpatients'. *Mayo Clinic Proceedings* 69(12): 1137–1145.

Fleming, M. F., Barry, K. L., and MacDonald, R. (1991). 'The Alcohol Use Disorders Identification Test'. *International Journal of the Addictions* 26(11): 1173–1185.

Fleming, M. F., Barry, K. L., Manwell, L. B., Johnson, K., and London, R. (1997). 'Brief Physician Advice for Problem Drinkers: A Randomized Controlled Trial in Community-based Primary Care Practices'. *Alcohol and Alcoholism* 277: 1039–1045.

Fleming, M. F., Manwell, L. B., Barry, K. L., Adams, W., and Stauffacer, E. A. (1999). 'Brief Physician Advice for Alcohol Problems in Older Adults: A Randomized Community-based Trial'. *Journal of Family Practice* 48(5): 378–384.

Hanlon, J. T., Horner, R. D., Schmader, K. E., Fillenbaum, G. G., Lewis, I. K., et al. (1998). 'Benzodiazepine Use and Cognitive Function among Community-dwelling Elderly'. *Clinical Pharmacology and Therapeutics* 64(6): 684–692.

Harris, K. B. and Miller, W. R. (1990). 'Behavioral Self-control Training for Problem Drinkers'. *Psychology of Addictive Behaviors* 4(2): 82–90.

Havard, A., Shakeshaft, A., and Sanson-Fisher, R. (2008). 'Systematic Review and Meta-analyses of Strategies Targeting Alcohol Problems in Emergency Departments: Interventions Reduce Alcohol-related Injuries'. *Addiction* 103(3): 368–376; discussion 377–378.

Health Development Agency and University of Wales College of Medicine (2002). *Manual for the Fast Alcohol Screening Test (FAST)*. http://www.nice.org.uk/niceMedia/documents/manual_fastalcohol.pdf. London: HDA.

Hogan, D., Maxwell, C., Fung, T. S., and Ebly, E. M. (2003). 'Prevalence and Potential Consequences of Benzodiazepine Use in Senior Citizens: Results from the Canadian Study of Health and Aging'. *Canadian Journal of Clinical Pharmacology* 10(2): 72–77.

Holmes, H. M., Hayley, D. C., Alexander, G. C., and Sachs, G. A. (2006). 'Reconsidering Medication Appropriateness for Patients Late in Life'. *Archives of Internal Medicine* 166: 605–609.

Huang, B., Dawson, D. A., Stinson, F. S., Hasin, D. S., Ruan, W. J., et al. (2006). 'Prevalence, Correlates, and Comorbidity of Nonmedical Prescription Drug Use and Drug Use Disorders in the United States: Results of the National Epidemiologic Survey on Alcohol and Related Conditions'. *Journal of Clinical Psychiatry* 67(7): 1062–1073.

Jinks, M. J. and Raschko, R. R. (1990). 'A Profile of Alcohol and Prescription Drug Abuse in a High-risk Community-based Elderly Population'. *Annals of Pharmacotherapy* 24(10): 971–975.

Korper, S. P. and Council, C. L. (eds) (2002). *Substance Use by Older Adults: Estimates of Future Impact on the Treatment System.* DHHS Publication No. SMA 03-3763, Analytic Series A-21). Rockville, MD: Substance Abuse and Mental Health Services Administration, Office of Applied Studies.

Leipzig, R. M., Cumming, R. G., and Tinetti, M. E. (1999). 'Drugs and Falls in Older People: A Systematic Review and Meta-analysis: I. Psychotropic Drugs'. *Journal of the American Geriatrics Society* 47(1): 30–39.

Lin, J. C., Karno, M. P., Barry, K. L., Blow, F. C., Davis, J. W., et al. (2010). 'Determinants of Early Reductions in Drinking in Older At-risk Drinkers Participating in the Intervention Arm of a Trial to Reduce At-risk Drinking in Primary Care'. *Journal of the American Geriatrics Society* 58: 227–233.

McLaughlin, D., Adams, J., Almeida, O., Brown, W., Byles, J., et al. (2011). 'Are the National Guidelines for Health Behaviour Appropriate for Older Australians? Evidence from the Men, Women and Ageing Project (Invited paper)'. *Australasian Journal on Ageing* 30(S2): 13–16.

Menninger, J. A. (2002). 'Assessment and Treatment of Alcoholism and Substance-related Disorders in the Elderly'. *Bulletin of the Menninger Clinic* 66(2): 166–183.

Moore, A. A., Morton, S. C., Beck, J. C., Hays, R. D., Oishi, S. M., et al. (1999). 'A New Paradigm for Alcohol Use in Older Persons'. *Medical Care* 37(2): 165–179.

Moore, A. A., Blow, F. C., Hoffing, M., Welgreen, S., Davis, J. W., et al. (2011). 'Primary Care-based Intervention to Reduce At-risk Drinking in Older Adults: A Randomized Controlled trial'. *Addiction* 106(1): 111–120.

National Institute on Alcohol Abuse and Alcoholism (NIAAA) (1995). *Diagnostic Criteria for Alcohol Abuse.* Alcohol Alert 30 (PH 359): 1–6.

National Institute on Alcohol Abuse and Alcoholism (2005). *Helping Patients who Drink too Much. A Clinician's Guide, Updated 2005 Edition.* Rockville, MD: US Department of Health and Human Services, National Institute of Health. NIH Publication No. 07-3769.

National Institute for Health and Clinical Excellence (2010). *Alcohol Use Disorders: Preventing Harmful Drinking.* http://www.nice.org.uk/nicemedia/live/13001/48984/48984.pdf. Manchester: NICE.

Office of Applied Studies (2004). Results from the 2003 National Survey on Drug Use and Health: National Findings. Rockville, MD: Substance Abuse and Mental Health Services Administration. DHHS Publication No. (SMA) 04-3964. NSDUH Series H–25.

Office of Applied Studies (2005). *The DASIS Report. Older Adults in Substance Abuse Treatment: Update.* Rockville, MD: Substance Abuse and Mental Health Services Administration. http://www.samhsa.gov/data/2k5/olderAdultsTX/olderAdultsTX.htm. Accessed 8 November 2013.

Oslin, D. W., Grantham, S., Coakley, E., Maxwell, J., Miles, K., et al. (2006). 'PRISM-E: Comparison of Integrated Care and Enhanced Specialty Referral in Managing At-risk Alcohol Use'. *Psychiatric Services* 57: 954–958.

Patterson, T. L. and Jeste, D. V. (1999). 'The Potential Impact of the Baby-boom Generation on Substance Abuse among Elderly Persons'. *Psychiatric Services* 50: 1184–1188.

Schmidt, A., Barry, K. L., and Fleming, M. F. (1995). 'Detection of Problem Drinkers: The Alcohol Use Disorders Identification Test (AUDIT)'. *Southern Medical Journal* 88(1): 52–59.

Schonfeld, L., King-Kallimanis, B., Duchene, D., Etheridge, R., Herrera. J., et al. (2010) 'Screening and Brief Intervention for Substance Misuse among Older Adults: The Florida BRITE Project'. *American Journal of Public Health* 100(1): 108–114. PMID: 19443821.

Scottish Health Action on Alcohol Problems (2007). *Alcohol: Price, Policy and Public Health. Report on the Findings of the Expert Workshop on Price Convened by SHAAP.* http://www. ias.org.uk/uploads/pdf/Price%20docs/Price%20Report%20-%20Full%20report.pdf. Edinburgh: SHAAP.

Simoni-Wastila, L. and Strickler, G. (2004). 'Risk Factors Associated with Problem Use of Prescription Drugs'. *American Journal of Public Health* 94 (2): 266–268.

Simoni-Wastila, L. I., Zuckerman, H., Singhal, P. K., Briesacher, B., and Hsu, V. D. (2005). 'National Estimates of Exposure to Prescription Drugs with Addiction Potential in Community-Dwelling Elders'. *Substance Abuse* 26(1): 33–42.

Simoni-Wastila, L. and Yang, H. K. (2006). 'Psychoactive Drug Abuse in Older Adults'. *American Journal of Geriatric Pharmacotherapy* 4: 380–394.

Solomon, K., Manepalli, J., Ireland, G. A., and Mahon, G. M. (1993). 'Alcoholism and Prescription Drug Abuse in the Elderly: St. Louis University Grand Rounds'. *Journal of the American Geriatrics Society* 41(1): 57–69.

Stein, C. and Moritz, I., on behalf of the World Health Organization (1999). *A Life Course Perspective of Maintaining Independence in Older Age.* whqlibdoc.who.int/hq/1999/WHO_HSC_AHE_99.2_life.pdf. Geneva: WHO.

Substance Abuse and Mental Health Services Administration (SAMHSA) (2007). Committee on Trauma Quick Guide. *Alcohol Screening and Brief Interventions (SBI) for Trauma Patients.* http://www.samhsa.gov/csatdisasterrecovery/featuredReports/01-alcohol%20SBI%20 for%20Trauma%20Patients.pdf

UNFPA (2012). *Ageing in the 21st Century: A Celebration and a Challenge.* http://unfpa.org/ageingreport/. New York and London: UNFPA and HelpAge International.

United Nations Department of Economic and Social Affairs/Population Division (2011). *World Mortality Report 2011.* http://www.un.org/en/development/desa/population/publications/pdf/mortality/worldMortalityReport2011.pdf.

United Nations Office on Drugs and Crime (2010). *World Drug Report.* Vienna: United Nations Office on Drugs and Crime.

United Nations Office on Drugs and Crime (2011). *The Nonmedical Use of Prescription Drugs: Policy Direction Issues.* https://www.unodc.org/docs/youthnet/Final_Prescription_Drugs_Paper.pdf. Vienna: United Nations Office on Drugs and Crime.

US Census Bureau (2008). *Projections of the Population by Age and Sex for the United States: 2010 to 2050* (NP2008-T12), Population Division. Release Date 14 August. Washington, DC: US Census Bureau.

Vestal, R. E., McGuire, E. A., Tobin, J. D., Andreas, R., Norris, A. H., et al. (1977). 'Aging and Ethanol Metabolism'. *Clinical Pharmacology & Therapeutics* 231: 343–354.

Wallace, P., Cutler, S., and Haines, A. (1988). 'Randomised Controlled Trial of General Practitioner Intervention in Patients with Excessive Alcohol Consumption'. *British Medical Journal* 297(6649): 663–668.

Whitlock, E. P., Polen, M. R., Green, C. A., Orleans, T., and Klein, J. (2004). 'Behavioral Counseling Interventions in Primary Care to Reduce Risky/Harmful Alcohol Use by Adults: A Summary of the Evidence for the U.S. Preventive Services Task Force'. *Annals of Internal Medicine* 140(7): 557–568.

CHAPTER 27

···

ELDER ABUSE

A Global Epidemic

···

NAGEEN MUSTAFA AND PAUL KINGSTON

INTRODUCTION

ELDER abuse is not a new phenomenon; it exists globally in both developing and developed countries. However, elder abuse can occur with little recognition or response and is often underreported (World Health Organization (WHO) 2011). Over the last two decades elder abuse has emerged as a serious social problem. Even in the second decade of the twenty-first century, reports suggest that elder abuse continues to be a 'taboo, mostly underestimated and ignored by societies across the world' (WHO 2011: 1). This compares unfavourably with child abuse and domestic violence—both issues that are fully recognized internationally, if not always effectively challenged.

In 2011 WHO reported that the global population of people aged 60 years and older will more than double, from 542 million in 1995 to about 1.2 billion in 2025. Therefore, it is likely that the issue of elder abuse will become a major political and welfare issue worldwide. Research to date has generally found that around 4–6% of older people have experienced some form of maltreatment in their own home (WHO 2011). However, the true incidence of elder abuse is still unknown, as prevalence rates exist only in selected developed countries across Europe.

Elder abuse has been found to lead to serious physical injuries and long-term psychological consequences (WHO 2011), and is suspected to be a major source of morbidity and mortality in older people (Chen and Koval 2002). For example, Lachs and colleagues (1998) assert that elder abuse is likely to lead to severe consequences for the individual involved, including mortality. Similarly, Mulroy and O'Neill (2011) report that elder abuse was directly accountable for 2500 deaths a year in countries on this continent. The risk of such negative outcomes as a result of elder abuse has been found to be more prevalent in the most vulnerable persons in the older adult population who are abused (Dong and Simon 2011). This includes those who have worsened functional status, progressive dependency, poorly rated self-health and increased social isolation, which in turn may lead to a multitude of medical issues (Wagenaar, Salois, and Komro 2009).

Elder abuse is associated with distress and an increased risk of mortality in older people (Dong 2005; Dong et al. 2009, 2010; Lachs et al. 1998) and psychological morbidity in care-givers (Compton et al., 1997). This should create a cause for concern in society and make it a priority in government policy. Moreover, Dong and Simon (2011) recently found that 'only a small fraction' of elder abuse may be reported. It is therefore not surprising that there have been calls for more extensive research on elder abuse due to the somewhat 'limited' current understanding of the consequences of elder abuse (Dong et al. 2010). Finally, determining the exact prevalence of elder abuse internationally can be very difficult because of the varying definitions of elder abuse utilized and varying sociocultural norms, particularly for the most common forms of elder abuse, namely psychological and financial abuse (Mulroy and O'Neill 2011).

DEFINITIONS OF ELDER ABUSE AND NEGLECT

In discussing elder abuse it is important first to establish the operational definitions of such acts and explore their meanings in relation to the context within which they are utilized.

In 1993 the UK group Action on Elder Abuse established the following definition of elder abuse: 'A single or repeated act or lack of appropriate action, occurring within any relationship where there is an expectation of trust, which causes harm or distress to an older person' (Action on Elder Abuse 2006). The main assertion of this definition is that there is an 'expectation of trust' established between an older person and another individual that is being violated (Action on Elder Abuse 2006). WHO (2011) adopted this definition in 2002, and it is promoted by the International Network for the Prevention of Elder Abuse.

More recently, elder abuse has been labelled as elder maltreatment (WHO 2011). WHO describes elder maltreatment as including various forms involving physical, mental, emotional, financial, and sexual abuse. In addition to this, elder maltreatment may also be manifested as neglect and/or loss of dignity (Dixon et al. 2009).

Elder abuse can occur in both private (the home) and institutional (nursing, residential homes and hospitals) settings (Biggs et al. 2009). Abusers may include family members, spouses, friends, care-givers or home care workers or professionals (WHO 2011). Elder abuse may involve intentional actions that cause harm or create a serious risk of harm (whether or not harm is intended) by a care-giver or other person who stands in a trust relationship to the older adult. It may involve failure by a care-giver to satisfy the elder's basic needs such as giving them food or first aid, or to protect the elder from harm such as a fall (National Research Council 2003). Finally, elder abuse could also include intimate partner violence, as well as the use of physical restraints and over-medication to control behaviour.

CHRONOLOGICAL AGE, AGEISM, AND ELDER ABUSE

Researchers have suggested that simply defining old age can be problematic. Dixon and colleagues (2010) propose that distinguishing the mistreatment of different groups of adults on the basis of their chronological age is 'arbitrary', and that the label 'elder mistreatment' makes the definition of old age problematic. Chappell and colleagues (2003) suggest that defining old age as beginning from the age of 65 years is the result of social construction. This age range has been implicated as 'old' because it coincides with the time individuals are expected to withdraw from the workforce as opposed to being based on any biological or physiological changes of the human body. Therefore, studies that discuss the experience of elder mistreatment should take into consideration that not all age-related factors impact upon or result in elder mistreatment. Furthermore, it has been suggested that factors related to elder mistreatment may be socially rather than biologically determined in the form of discriminatory attitudes (Dixon et al. 2010). However, age-related ill health has been consistently found in cases where there is evidence of elder mistreatment (Dixon et al. 2010).

In terms of societal status, age has been found to be an important factor in determining the context in which elder abuse occurs (Roscigno et al. 2007). For example, ageism has been found to help understand the societal levels within which elder abuse occurs (Bennett, Kingston, and Penhale 1997; Harbison, 1999). When society devalues older people it is argued that discrimination against the elderly may be justified because their devaluation in society is passed on through institutions such as hospitals (Roscigno et al. 2007; Schrank and Waring 1989). Moreover, if the devalutation is felt to be justified it may potentially manifest itself in professional practice (Angus and Reeves 2006).

In the context of human rights, it is suggested that the relationship between inequality and violence centres on lack of dignity and respect, and on low social status. Wilkinson (2004) has found that these three aspects are pivotal in relation to the occurrence of ageism and consequently abuse. Human rights legislation has been criticized, as it is believed that older people have benefited little from it. For example, it has been asserted that there is a fundamental flaw in such legislation because it marginalizes perceptions about ageism (Angus and Reeve 2006; Watson 2002). Socially constructed ageist attitudes may manifest themselves in socially acceptable practices such as a compulsory age of retirement in certain countries; an individual is thought to have to cease employment, potentially leading to younger candidates being a more favourable choice (Watson 2002). Watson (2002) has also found that older people are frequently subjected to infringements of their human rights, particularly with regard to aspects of dignity and respect. It has been suggested, therefore, that there should be an obligation on public institutions to defend and uphold the human rights of older people, particularly those who may be unable to articulate their rights themselves, such as those with dementia (Watson 2002).

PREVALENCE/INCIDENCE OF ELDER ABUSE

Internationally, elder abuse is being increasingly acknowledged as a social problem. Research and knowledge with regard to the extent of maltreatment has increased over the past twenty-five years with prevalence surveys having been carried out all over the world.

In 2005, the National Centre for Social Research and the Institute of Gerontology at King's College London were commissioned by the charity Comic Relief and the Department of Health to carry out the UK Study of Abuse and Neglect of Older People. This was reported to be the first dedicated study of its kind in the UK, and its aim was to provide representative prevalence estimates on elder abuse and neglect in the country. Results from this study showed that the estimated prevalence of elder abuse was 2.6%, which is equivalent to about one in forty of the older population (around 227,000 people in the UK aged 66 and over). Further, O'Keeffe and colleagues (2007) suggest that the statistical confidence limits indicate that the real figure will be somewhere between 159 200 and 322 600 based on assertions made by Lachs and Pillemer (2004). As a result, prevalence rates may be underestimated. Reasons for an underestimate in prevalence rates may be due to the conservative definitions used to measure mistreatment and the absence of people in the survey with severe dementia and those living in residential care. The absence of studies focusing on elder abuse among populations with dementia is a serious methodological challenge to the field.

This study also shows that there are a significant number of older people in the UK who have experienced or are continuing to experience abuse, which may have serious effects on their health and well-being. In support of this research, O'Keeffe and colleagues (2007) found that these UK rates of elder abuse were comparable to rates of abuse reported in other international research. Importantly, when rates of abuse in the form of social abuse (i.e. preventing a person from having contact with relatives, friends, service providers, and other people or restricting the person's activities) were added to family, friends and care workers as abusers, the prevalence rate increased from 2.6% to 4.0%. In summary, O'Keeffe and colleagues (2007) reported that neglect was the most predominant type of mistreatment, followed by financial abuse. This is in contrast to the commonly assumed notion of 'abuse' as physical violence.

In a study utilizing a systematic review of the literature surrounding the prevalence of elder abuse using standardized criteria of study quality, Cooper, Selwood, and Livingston (2008) found that elders, family, and professional care-givers were all willing to report abuse. In total, forty-nine studies met the inclusion criteria, and were therefore incorporated in the study. Results showed that the range of prevalence of abuse reported in general population studies was between 3.2% and 27.5%; the authors suggest that these findings may be representative of the variation in reported abuse rates across cultures as well as the differences in defining and measuring abuse. More specifically, nearly a quarter of older people dependent on carers reported significant psychological abuse, and a fifth reported neglect. In terms of the abuser, it was found that over a third of family carers reported perpetrating significant abuse.

As a result of these findings, it may be assumed that both the abused and abuser may be willing to report abuse and so should therefore be asked about it routinely, as the authors suggest this method may be more sensitive to detection of abuse than observer measures. However, this theory is said to be inapplicable to those who are nonverbal or too afraid to report abuse (Cooper et al. 2008). Nevertheless, Cooper and colleagues reported that one in four vulnerable adults is at risk of abuse, and that only a small proportion of these cases are ever detected. This may be due to the reporting and detection of only the most serious cases of abuse, which in turn reflects the isolated and secretive nature of the abusive act (Cooper et al. 2008). In addition, Cooper and colleagues (2008) recommend that greater efforts to address institutional abuse through improved detection strategies such as whistle-blowing schemes are urgently needed.

Daly, Merchant, and Jogerst (2011) found that 'prevalence studies are conducted in different settings, with different types and definitions of elder abuse and various instruments to measure the abuse. With such a variation, it is difficult to compare results, and comparisons should only be made across the same type of study' (361). Moreover, Cooper, Balamurali, Selwood, and Livingston (2007) found that the level and frequency of abusive acts considered to constitute an abuse case, and used in prevalence studies, vary, and so also impact upon rates reported. Overall, the prevalence rates that have been found across studies include: 2.6% in the UK (O'Keeffe et al. 2007); 3.2% in the US (Pillemer and Finkelhor 1989); 4% in Canada (Podnieks 1992); 5.4% in Finland (Kivela et al. 1992); 5.6% in Amsterdam (Comijs et al. 1998); 6.3% in Seoul (Oh et al. 2006); 8.8% in Britain (Ogg and Bennett 1992); and 14% in India (Chokkanathan and Lee 2005). In all these studies rates of abuse were calculated for people aged 65 years and over with the exception of Britain, where the age was 60, and the UK study, where the age was 66 years and over.

More recently, in a study measuring the twelve-month prevalence of elder abuse with 2021 participants in Ireland, Naughton and colleagues (2010) found that elder abuse and neglect rates were 2.2% over a twelve-month period. The types of mistreatment included financial abuse (1.3%), psychological abuse (1.2%), physical abuse (0.5%), neglect (0.3%), and sexual abuse (0.05%). In addition they found that women were more likely than men to report abuse and that those with a lower income, impaired physical health, mental health problems, and poor social support were associated with being at higher risk of mistreatment. In terms of perpetrators of abuse, adult children were found to be the most common abusers, and associated factors included unemployment and addiction.

Chompunud et al. (2010) reported that the prevalence of elder abuse in Thailand is greatly underreported. They found that approximately 14.6% of 240 participants had been victims of elder abuse. The selection criteria of participants included male and female Thais who were 60 years of age and older, lived within five randomly selected communities in one district of metropolitan Bangkok, were able to read and write Thai, and were not cognitively impaired. Factors associated with the prevalence of abuse included gender, adequacy of income, perceptions of health, personal health compared to the health of other elders, and family members' mental health, dependency, and relationship issues. Predictors of elder abuse included gender (female elders were approximately five times more likely to have been abused by family members than elderly males), family members' dependency on the older adult, and the reported nature (whether good or bad) of the relationship between the abuser and victim. Together, these factors predicted 28.6% of elder abuse.

Research conducted in Nigeria with 404 elderly women (aged 60 and over) found that the overall prevalence of any type of elder abuse was 30%. In this study physical abuse (14.6%) was the most frequently occurring type of abuse followed by financial abuse (13.1%) and emotional abuse (11.1%). Only 7 (1.2%) of the older participants reported neglect, while two (0.04%) respondents reported sexual abuse. In many instances, children were the most likely perpetrators of physical abuse (43.7%), emotional abuse (40.5%), and neglect (83.3%). Neighbours and co-tenants (47.6%), however, were the main perpetrators of financial abuse (Cadmus and Owoajea 2012).

What may be concluded from the overview of research surrounding the prevalence of elder abuse on an international level is that research on elder abuse is minimal and possibly under-representative of actual rates of abuse due to poor rates of detection and reporting. Moreover, estimates of the prevalence of elder abuse are thought to vary due to the survey methodology utilized to collect the information and the sample characteristics (Dong et al. 2010). Measures of abuse and a consensus on what constitutes an adequate measure of abuse are needed to improve the accuracy in the prevalence of abuse (Cooper et al. 2008). From the studies discussed in this section, prevalence rates vary by region which may also indicate differences on a sociocultural level.

Risk factors

Several risk factors for elder abuse have been identified (see Table 27.1). In addition to these findings, the care-giver stress framework suggests that to enable the older person to continue to reside in the community care-givers may have to compromise their own physical and mental health. Therefore, the care provided to older adults reduces in quality, potentially leading to abuse or neglect over time (Beach et al. 2005). Coyne and colleagues (1993) examined the relationship between dementia and abusive behaviour in 342 dementia patients and their care-givers (adult children, spouses, and other relatives). Results showed that thirty-three care-givers reported that they had abused the older adult in their care. Characteristics of these abusers included providing care for more years, caring for patients functioning at a lower level, displaying higher burden scores, and having higher depression scores than care-givers who reported no abuse towards the older adult in their care. However, Homer and Gilleard (1990) report a lack of association between abuse and the diagnosis of dementia or degree of mental impairment of the older adult.

Research that focuses on identifying the risk factors for elder abuse has often relied upon care-giver and/or family member interviews, with many studies examining abuse within the context of dementia care-giving (Beach et al. 2005). In terms of self-reported data, this may be unreliable, especially if the care recipient has cognitive deficits, and so reliance on only the carers' reports may reduce the reliability of the data. In support of the findings reported by Hildreth, Burke, and Golub (2011), studies have identified that problem behaviour, violence, or aggression towards the care-giver, and higher levels of physical and cognitive impairment of the elderly person, may act as risk factors for abuse (Compton, Flanagan, and Gregg 1997). In relation to characteristics of the abuser, depression, anxiety, low self-esteem, and substance abuse have been reported as risk factors for abuse, in addition to higher levels of care-giving involvement in the form of the length of time spent caring for the individual and the number of hours spent caring for the older adult on a continuous basis (Beach et al. 2005).

Lachs and Pillemer (2004) indicate that a shared living situation is a major risk factor for elder abuse and that people living alone are at lowest risk. The authors suggest that the reason for this is that a shared living situation allows increased opportunities for contact with a vulnerable person and also increases the conflict and tension between persons in a

Table 27.1 Risk factors associated with elder abuse

Risk factors related to the abuser	Risk factors related to the abused
Feeling overwhelmed	Memory problems
Feelings of resentment	Physical disabilities
Current or past substance abuse problem	Depression
History of abuse	Loneliness
Dependence on abused for needs	Lack of social support
	Alcohol/substance abuse
	Verbally/physically combative

shared living situation. However, those that live alone have been found to be more prone to financial abuse (Podnieks 1992). Social isolation has also been implicated in elder abuse, as the lack of other people allows the abuser to abuse without the intervention of others. In addition, Lachs and Pillemer (2004) found that people who commit elder abuse are likely to be heavily dependent on the person they are mistreating, including trying to obtain financial resources from the victim. Alternatively, those who have a physical disability may not be able to defend themselves or to escape an abusive situation and may therefore be more vulnerable to abuse (Lachs and Pillemer 2004).

It should be noted that abuse can take place with or without any of the reported risk factors being apparent. Nevertheless, the profiles of both the older person who may be at risk as well as the abuser may help to inform both the practitioner and researcher alike so that future incidences of abuse can be prevented.

Intervention studies

As a result of the potential consequences of elder abuse, it is vital that effective prevention and management strategies are developed. Unfortunately, there is little consensus around the most effective type of model of intervention in situations of elder abuse and neglect. As far back as 1999, Harbison pointed to six different models of intervention: the psychological model, the systems model, the hierarchical model, the quasi-legal model, the child welfare model, and the participatory model. As Harbison (1999) further states, it is unusual that one distinct model of intervention is used without recourse to elements of other models. To date, little attention has been focused on testing empirically the most effective 'model' of intervention.

Kalaga and Kingston (2007) offered an approach based on three intervention levels (primary, secondary, and tertiary). Protection and support for 'at risk' adults is available at three stages:

- *Primary intervention* aims to prevent abuse occurring in the first instance
- *Secondary intervention* aims to identify and respond directly to allegations of potential abuse
- *Tertiary intervention* aims to remedy any negative and harmful consequences of the abuse, and put in place measures to prevent future occurrences.

They then further analysed each level in response to types of abuse including discriminatory abuse, financial abuse, institutional abuse, sexual abuse, and physical abuse. Their final analysis repeats Harbison's (1999) claim that no one single intervention will likely prove to be totally effective.

However, Levine (2003) asserts that the reality of elder abuse is that interventions satisfactory to all parties rarely transpire. Moreover, individuals may prefer being at home—even in a potentially harmful situation—rather than being put into a strange environment. The Equality and Human Rights Commission reported that the reason for this is that:

> care in people's own homes allows older people to continue to live as they wish even once they
> can no longer carry out all their day-to-day tasks without support. As long as older people

have the good quality care they need to support them at home, they can keep their independence and control over their lives in familiar surroundings.

(Equality and Human Rights Commission 2011: 23)

Intervention studies suggest a variety of approaches for the detection, assessment, and management of elder abuse. Ploeg and colleagues (2009) conducted a systematic review of intervention studies of this type of abuse. Following the application of inclusion criterion, only eight studies were incorporated out of 1253. The inclusion criteria specified abuse of persons 60 and over; that the abuse involved related to physical, psychological, or financial abuse or neglect; and that the research described an intervention for abused persons or the abuser, professionals who care for the older person, or the community. The high exclusion rate indicates that a need remains for intervention studies in relation to elder abuse covering a wider area of investigation and intervention. Moreover, Ploeg and colleagues (2009) concluded that there was insufficient evidence to support any particular intervention related to elder abuse targeting clients, abusers, or healthcare professionals. Overall, they found that there may be negative consequences associated with some interventions for elder abuse.

McDonald (2011) has argued that in order to develop preventative programs and targeted interventions, there needs to be an established explanation for the abuse and neglect of older adults. It was asserted that the issue of elder abuse is evident; however, the barrier to prevention has been lack of knowledge in relation to this type of abuse. McDonald (2011) states that part of the reason is the lack of specific types of investigation that are urgently needed, including prevalence studies in the community and institutions, serious theory development, and random clinical trials to test interventions both socially and legally.

McDonald and Thomas (2012) assert that theory guides the scope and reach of a study, provides the basis for predicting causation, and influences how terms are conceptualized and operationalized. However, there is no overarching theoretical framework that has guided research in the field of elder abuse (McDonald 2011). Specifically, it is asserted that a life course perspective provides insight into existing theories and perspectives on elder mistreatment, in that it links the individual to their social structure. Furthermore, it is suggested that such a life course perspective provides a useful framework for understanding elder abuse and neglect (McDonald and Thomas 2012). In a study conducted by McDonald and Thomas (2012) it was found that childhood abuse was a deciding influence on abuse in later life. Therefore, they recommend that professionals should ask victims of elder abuse questions related to their previous experiences with abuse including the life stage during which any other abuse occurred, as well as the type of abuse.

In India the Eleventh Five-Year Plan (2007–2011) has brought attention to the marginalization of older adults and recommends a specific healthcare plan that may help to reduce the abuse of older people in that society (Shankardass 2013). It has been found that a lack of healthcare provision makes older people more vulnerable to neglect, mistreatment, and abuse in society, so care plans directed at older adults may help to prevent abuse (Shankardass 2013). Further, Shankardass (2013) has found that there is a need in India to recognize the burden on care-givers and develop support services for them in order to help minimize the prevalence of elder abuse. Specifically, respite care and day care centres are emerging as constructive factors that may be utilized in providing support to carers of older people, who in places such as India are usually family members. Moreover, it has been found that despite new government initiatives in India, building a system for the detection, treatment, and monitoring of abusive cases has still not been realized. Reasons for this may include there being a lack of specialized agencies and professionals from the social, legal, and health fields for dealing with elder abuse issues (Shankardass 2013).

What is clear is that the issue of elder abuse, and how to address the problem and create interventions by strengthening practice, are key concerns for countries not only in Asia but across the world. Brownell (2006) suggests that there is a need to address elder abuse from an interdisciplinary collaborative perspective that, although challenging, would be effective for successful intervention. In support of this idea, it was also found that intervention services should develop multidisciplinary expertise and resources for dealing with elder abuse following a study by Wang (2006) in Taiwan. The author carried out a study of psychological abuse and its characteristic correlates among older adult Taiwanese people and reported that psychological abuse in particular is common among older adult Taiwanese in community settings but that a multidisciplinary approach would help to tackle the problem.

In order to try to prevent abuse, Wang asserts that:

> caution against oversimplification of psychological abuse as a unitary problem should be activated. Nevertheless, attention should also be paid to the personal characteristics of the elderly, because the cognitive and physical function of the elderly was closely associated with level of abuse. The contextual factors related to psychological abuse of the elderly must be monitored to prevent abuse.
>
> (Wang 2006: 316)

Finally, in a study conducted in the US, Anetzberger and colleagues (2000) found that education and training for both older adults and carers can be effective in interventions in elder mistreatment. For example, educational curricula for cross-training, screening tools, and referral protocols were developed and tested for staff and volunteers in adult protective services and dementia care. A handbook for care-givers of persons with dementia was produced that enables care-givers to self-identify elder abuse risk and seek appropriate interventions to prevent abuse. The authors assert that the aim of their intervention for elder abuse and dementia was to increase case identification and promote prevention of abuse in persons with dementia who are suspected of being, or who are, at risk of elder abuse. They found that their intervention was effective in the prevention and treatment of elder abuse in situations involving persons with dementia. Further, results showed that their approach may be applied to other situations of abuse, such as elder abuse in other circumstances or domestic violence, which require intervention from diverse service systems. Joshi and Flaherty (2005) have also suggested that education for older adults and care-givers and other interventions targeted towards risk factors or types of abuse or neglect play an invaluable role in preventing elder abuse and mistreatment.

IMPLICATIONS FOR PRACTICE

Psychological interventions can be developed at a primary level, with psychologists assisting with the development of media campaigns, developing strategies in concert with public health agencies, and advancing education strategies for all health and welfare professionals. Previous studies have argued that inadequate attention is paid to family violence generally in the qualifying curricula of health and welfare students (Kingston, Penhale, and Bennett 1995).

At the secondary level, interventions that assist in managing situations where individuals are victims of abuse using psychological interventions are required. Designing psychological interventions to support and empower victims is essential, as are interventions with a family therapy focus. Psychological interventions to assist perpetrators are also an urgent requirement.

At the tertiary level, post-abuse support appears to be almost non-existent as an intervention in most countries. One suggestion would be to begin to consider interventions as a life course challenge, and to avoid focusing on particular generations (Kingston and Penhale 1995).

Summary

Elder abuse is an important issue within society that may occur in both informal and formal contexts. All those who have contact with older people have an obligation to protect them from perpetrators of abuse as well as abuse within systems of care.

Phelan (2008) suggests that 'a framework of universal rights [that] critically analyses systems for inherent ageist perspectives (attitudes, practices or actions) and reduces the possibility of providing stereotypical, unethical and inequitable care is needed…facilitating, maintaining and defending autonomy, integrity, dignity and respect' (7). However, whether or not this will ever emerge is as yet unknown.

Key References and Sources for Further Reading

Bennett, G., Kingston, P. and Penhale. B. (1997). *The Dimensions of Elder Abuse: Perspectives for Practitioners*. Basingstoke, UK: Macmillan.

Daly, J. M., Merchant, M. L., and Jogerst, G. J. (2011). 'Elder Abuse Research: A Systematic Review'. *Journal of Elder Abuse and Neglect* 23(4): 348–365.

Equality and Human Rights Commission (2011). *Close to Home. An Inquiry into Older People and Human Rights in Home Care*. http://www.equalityhumanrights.com/uploaded_files/homecareFI/home_care_report.pdf.

Harbison, J. (1999). 'Models for Intervention for "Elder Abuse and Neglect": A Canadian Perspective on Ageism, Participation and Empowerment'. *Journal of Elder Abuse and Neglect*. 10: 1–17.

Hildreth, C. J., Burke, A. E., and Golub, R. M. (2011). 'Elder Abuse'. *Journal of the American Medical Association* 306(5): 568.

Joseph Roundtree Foundation (2009). *A Better Life*. York: Joseph Rowntree Foundation.

World Health Organization (2011). *European Report on Preventing Elder Maltreatment*. Copenhagen: WHO.

References

Action on Elder Abuse (2006). *Action on Elder Abuse*. http://www.elderabuse.org.uk/.

Anetzberger, G., Palmisano, B. R., Eckert, S., and Schimer, M. R. (2000). 'A Model Intervention for Elder Abuse and Dementia'. *Gerontologist* 40(4): 492–497.

Angus, J. and Reeves, P. (2006). 'Ageism: A Threat to "Aging Well" in the 21st Century'. *Journal of Applied Gerontology* 25: 137–152.

Beach, S. R., Schulz, R., Williamson, G. M., Miller, L. S., and Weiner, M. E. (2005). 'Risk Factors for Potentially Harmful Informal Caregiver Behaviour'. *Journal of the American Geriatrics Society* 55: 255–261.

Bennett, G., Kingston, P., and Penhale. B. (1997). *The Dimensions of Elder Abuse: Perspectives for Practitioners*. Basingstoke: Macmillan.

Biggs, S., Doyle, M., Hall, J., and Sanchez, M. (2009). *Abuse and Neglect of Older People: Secondary Analysis of the UK Prevalence Survey*. London: NatCen.

Brownell, P. (2006). 'Introduction'. In M. J. Mellor and P. Brownell (eds), *Elder Abuse and Mistreatment: Policy, Practice and Research*. New York: Haworth Press

Cadmus, E. O., and Owoaje, E. T. (2012). 'Prevalence and Correlates of Elder Abuse among Older Women in Rural and Urban Communities in South Western Nigeria'. *Health Care Women International* 33(10): 973–984.

Chappell, N. L., Gee, E., MacDonald, L., and Stones, M. (2003). *Aging in Contemporary Canada*. Toronto, Canada: Prentice-Hall.

Chen, A. L. and Koval, K. J. (2002). 'Elder Abuse: The Role of the Orthopaedic Surgeon in Diagnosis and Management'. *Journal of Academy of Orthopaedic Surgeons* 10(1): 25–31.

Chokkanathan, S. and Lee, A. E. (2005). 'Elder Mistreatment in Urban India: A Community Based Study'. *Journal of Elder Abuse and Neglect* 17: 45–61.

Chompunud, M. L. S., Charoenyooth, C., Palmer, M. H., Pongthavornkamol, K., Vorapongsathorn, T., et al. (2010). 'Prevalence, Associated Factors and Predictors of Elder Abuse in Thailand'. *Pacific Rim International Journal of Nursing Research* 14(4): 283–296.

Comijs, H. C., Pot, A. M., Smit, H. H., and Jonker, C. (1998). 'Elder Abuse in the Community: Prevalence and Consequences'. *Journal of the American Geriatrics Society* 46: 885–888.

Compton, S. A., Flanagan, P., and Gregg, W. (1997). 'Elder Abuse in People with Dementia in Northern Ireland: Prevalence and Predictors in Cases Referred to a Psychiatry of Old Age Service'. *International Journal of Geriatric Psychiatry* 12: 632–635.

Cooper, C., Balamurali, T. B, Selwood, A., and Livingston, G. (2007). 'A Systematic Review of Intervention Studies about Anxiety in Caregivers of People with Dementia'. *International Journal of Geriatric Psychiatry* 22(3):181–188.

Cooper, C., Selwood, A., and Livingston, G. (2008). 'The Prevalence of Elder Abuse and Neglect: A Systematic Review'. *Age and Ageing* 37(2): 151–160.

Coyne, A. C., Reichmann, W. E., and Berbig L. J. (1993). 'The Relationship between Dementia and Elder Abuse'. *American Journal of Psychiatry* 150: 643–646.

Daly, J. M., Merchant, M. L., and Jogerst, G. J. (2011). 'Elder Abuse Research: A Systematic Review'. *Journal of Elder Abuse and Neglect* 23(4): 348–365.

Dixon, J., Biggs, S., Tinker, A., Stevens, M., and Lee, L. (2009). *Abuse, Neglect and Loss of Dignity in the Institutional Care of Older People*. London: King's College London. http://www.kcl.ac.uk/content/1/c6/06/75/83/Dixonetal2009Abuse.pdf.

Dixon, J., Manthorpe, J., Biggs, S., Mowlam, A., Tennant, R., et al. (2010). 'Defining Elder Mistreatment: Reflections on the United Kingdom Study of Abuse and Neglect of Older People'. *Ageing and Society* 30: 403–420.

Dong, X. (2005). 'Medical Implications of Elder Abuse and Neglect'. *Clinical Geriatric Medicine* 21: 293–313.

Dong, X., Simon, M. A., Mendes De Leon, C. F., Fulmer, T., Beck, T., et al. (2009). 'Elder Self-neglect and Abuse and Mortality Risk in a Community-dwelling Population'. *Journal of the American Medical Association* 302: 517–526.

Dong, X., Simon, M. A., Beck, T. T., Farran, C., McCann, J. J., et al. (2010). 'Elder Abuse and Mortality: The Role of Psychological and Social Wellbeing'. *Journal of Gerontology* 29(6): 720–739

Dong X. and Simon M. A. (2011). 'Enhancing National Policy and Programs to Address Elder Abuse'. *Journal of the American Medical Association* 305(23): 2460–2461.

Equality and Human Rights Commission (2011). *Close to Home: An Inquiry into Older People and Human Rights in Home Care.* http://www.equalityhumanrights.com/uploaded_files/homecareFI/home_care_report.pdf.

Harbison, J. (1999). 'Models for Intervention for "Elder Abuse and Neglect": A Canadian Perspective on Ageism, Participation and Empowerment'. *Journal of Elder Abuse and Neglect* 10: 1–17.

Hildreth, C. J., Burke, A. E., and Golub, R. M. (2011). 'Elder Abuse'. *Journal of the American Medical Association* 306(5): 568.

Homer, A. C. and Gilleard, C. (1990). 'Abuse of Elderly People by their Carers'. *British Medical Journal* 301: 1359–1362.

Joshi, S. and Flaherty, J. (2005). 'Elder Abuse and Neglect in Long-term Care'. *Clinics in Geriatric Medicine* 21(2): 333–354.

Kalaga, L. and Kingston, P. (2007). *A Review of Literature on Effective Interventions that Prevent and Respond to Harm Against Adults.* Edinburgh: Scottish Parliament.

Kingston, P. and Penhale, B. (1995). *Family Violence and the Caring Professions.* Basingstoke: Macmillan.

Kingston, P., Penhale, B., and Bennett, G. (1995). 'Is Elder Abuse on the Curriculum? The Relative Contribution of Child Abuse, Domestic Violence and Elder Abuse in Social Work, Nursing and Medicine Qualifying Curricula'. *Health and Social Care in the Community* 3(6): 353–362.

Kivela, S. L., Kongas-Saviaro, P., Kesti, E., Pahkala, K., and Ijas, M. L. (1992). 'Abuse in Old Age: Epidemiological Data from Finland'. *Journal of Elder Abuse and Neglect* 4(3): 1–18.

Lachs, M. S., Williams, C. S., O'Brien, S., Pillemer, K. A., and Charlson, M. E. (1998). 'The Mortality of Elder Mistreatment'. *Journal of the American Medical Association* 280: 428–432.

Lachs, M. S. and Pillemer, K. (2004). 'Elder Abuse'. *Lancet* 364(9441): 1263–1273.

Levine, J. M. (2003). 'Elder Neglect and Abuse'. *Geriatrics* 58(10): 37–42.

McDonald, L. (2011). 'Elder Abuse and Neglect in Canada: The Glass is Still Half Full'. *Canadian Journal on Ageing* 30(3): 437–465.

McDonald, L. and Thomas. C. (2012). 'Elder Abuse through a Life Course Lens'. *International Psychogeriatrics* 25(8): 1235–1243.

Mulroy, M. and O'Neill, D. (2011). 'Elder Abuse'. *British Medical Journal* 22: 343.

National Research Council, Panel to Review Risk and Prevalence of Elder Abuse and Neglect (2003). *Elder Mistreatment: Abuse, Neglect, and Exploitation in an Aging America.* Washington, DC: National Academies Press.

Naughton, C., Drennan, J., Treacy, P., Lafferty, A., Lyons, I., et al. (2010). *Abuse and Neglect of Older People in Ireland: Report of the National Study of Elder Abuse and Neglect.* Dublin: HSE and UCD.

Ogg, J. and Bennett, G. (1992). 'Elder Abuse in Britain'. *British Medical Journal* 305: 998–999.

Oh, J., Kim, H. S., Martins, D., and Kim, H. (2006). 'A Study of Elder Abuse in Korea'. *International Journal of Nursing Studies* 43: 203–214.

O'Keeffe, M., Hills, A., Doyle, M., McCreadie, C., Scholes, S., et al. (2007). *UK Study of the Abuse and Neglect of Older People*. London: NatCen.

Phelan, A. (2008). 'Elder Abuse, Ageism, Human Rights and Citizenship: Implications for Nursing Discourse'. *Nursing Inquiry* 15(4): 320–329.

Pillemer, K. and Finkelhor, D. (1989). 'Causes of Elder Abuse: Caregiver Stress versus Problem Relatives'. *American Journal of Orthopsychiatry* 59: 179–187.

Ploeg, J., Fear, J., Hutchison, B., MacMillan, H., and Bolan, G. (2009). 'A Systematic Review of Interventions for Elder Abuse'. *Journal of Elder Abuse and Neglect* 21(3): 187–210.

Podnieks, E. (1992). 'National Survey on Abuse of the Elderly in Canada'. *Journal of Elder Abuse and Neglect* 41(1/2): 5–58.

Roscigno, V. L., Mong, S., Byron, R., and Griff, T. (2007). 'Age Discrimination, Social Closure and Employment'. *Social Forces* 86: 313–334.

Shankardass, M. K. (2013). 'Addressing Elder Abuse: Review of Societal Responses in India and Selected Asian Countries'. *International Psychogeriatrics* 25(8): 1229–1234.

Schrank, H. T. and Waring, J. M. (1989). 'Older Workers: Ambivalence and Interventions'. *Annals of the American Academy of Political and Social Sciences* 503: 113–126.

Wagenaar, A. C., Salois, M. J., and Komro, K. A. (2009). 'Effects of Beverage Alcohol Price and Tax Levels on Drinking: A Meta-analysis of 1003 Estimates from 112 Studies'. *Addiction* 104: 179–190.

Wang, J. J. (2006). 'Psychological Abuse and its Characteristic Correlates among Elderly Taiwanese'. *Archives of Gerontology and Geriatrics* 42(3): 307–318.

Watson, J. (2002). *Something for Everyone: The Impact of the Human Rights Act and the Need for a Human Rights Commission*. London: British Institute of Human Rights.

Wilkinson, R. (2004). 'Linking Social Structure and Individual Vulnerability'. *Journal of Community Work and Development* 5: 31–47.

World Health Organization (2011). *European Report on Preventing Elder Maltreatment*. Copenhagen: World Health Organization.

CHAPTER 28

LIFE STYLE RISKS AND COGNITIVE HEALTH

YUNHWAN LEE

INTRODUCTION

WITH the ageing of the population worldwide, dementia is increasingly recognized as a major public health problem. In 2010, dementia prevalence was estimated to be 4.7%, with 35.6 million of the world's population being affected by the condition (Alzheimer's Disease International 2009). The number of people with dementia is projected to double every 20 years to reach 65.7 million in 2030 and 115.4 million by 2050 (Figure 28.1). The increase in dementia prevalence is observed across all regions, in both high- and low-income countries, driven mainly by population growth and demographic ageing.

Dementia is a progressively debilitating condition, contributing to a high disease burden on the person with dementia, their family, and their care-givers. Those with dementia live an average of 7.4 years with disability (Alzheimer's Disease International 2009). An extension of this analysis concluded that if dementia could be eliminated, 36% of the ageing population's dependence and disability could be avoided. Dementia imposes a huge economic burden on society, with the total cost of dementia worldwide being estimated at US$604 billion (Alzheimer's Disease International 2010).

Although pharmacological treatments have been developed to ameliorate its symptoms and delay its progression, there is currently no cure for dementia. In recent years, advances in diagnostic tools, including biomarkers and neuroimaging techniques, have paved the way for early detection and treatment of dementia. These therapeutic interventions may slow the disease's progress and help to lessen its severity, but preventive programmes that delay the onset would prove to be more effective in decreasing the overall prevalence of dementia (Sloane et al. 2002). Preventing dementia will bring huge public health benefits in the coming decades. It is estimated that preventive interventions that delay the onset of the disease by two years will result in 22.8 million fewer cases worldwide in 2050 (Brookmeyer et al. 2007).

With the increasing emphasis on prevention with regard to dementia specifically as well as in relation to cognitive health in later life more broadly, health behaviours and life-style risks have gained wide attention. These factors are potentially modifiable and amenable

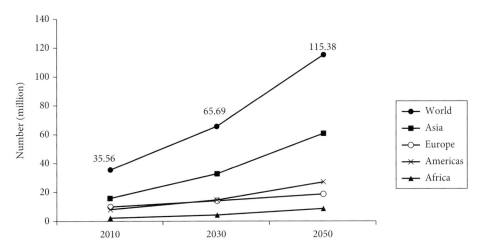

FIGURE 28.1 The projected increase in people with dementia worldwide.

Data from Alzheimer's Disease International *World Alzheimer Report 2009.*

to intervention. There has been accumulating evidence in recent years from prospective cohort studies that have examined the association of behavioural risk factors with cognitive decline and dementia in later years. More recently, based on these observational findings, randomized controlled trials have been conducted to identify life-style modifications effective in maintaining cognitive function in late-life.

This chapter presents current evidence on the relationship between life-style behavioural risk factors and cognitive health in older adults. An overview of major research findings will be provided in sections covering seven behavioural life-style factors: smoking, alcohol consumption, physical activity, body weight, nutrition and diet, social activity, and mental activity. Because of the heterogeneity of research on this topic, systematic reviews that have extracted and summarized mostly prospective cohort studies, complemented by more recent and ongoing clinical trials, will serve as the basis of this review.

LIFE-STYLE RISK FACTORS

Smoking

Although the association between smoking and dementia is not without controversy, recent evidence suggests that smoking increases the risk of dementia, particularly of the Alzheimer type. In the Rotterdam Study, 6868 people in the community aged 55 years and older were followed up for seven years (Reitz et al. 2007). Compared with non-smokers, current smokers showed a 40–50% elevated risk of developing dementia and Alzheimer's disease. Similar findings have been reported by Tyas et al. (2003) from the Honolulu-Asian Aging Study that followed middle-aged men over the course of twenty-five years.

These studies suggest that current smoking, compared with non-smoking, raises the risk of dementia. Past or former smoking has not been shown to increase dementia risk.

Moreover, smoking's adverse effects seem cumulative. Among smokers, levels of exposure to smoking contributed to higher dementia risk, showing a steady gradient between pack-years of smoking and increasing risk. There may, however, be a threshold at about twenty pack-years, above which the risk significantly rises.

There is less convincing evidence on smoking's effects on cognitive decline and vascular dementia. A recent meta-analysis reported higher, but non-significant, pooled odds for cognitive decline and vascular dementia in smokers than non-smokers (Peters et al. 2008b). More recently, however, a forty-year longitudinal study of a Swedish cohort found current smokers to have 1.6 times higher risk of vascular dementia (Rönnemaa et al. 2011). In the Whitehall II study from the UK, men who continued smoking for ten years in mid-life, compared with non-smokers, showed faster declines in global cognition, memory, and executive function in early old age (Sabia et al. 2012). Clinical trials would provide more supportive evidence, but due to ethical issues randomized controlled trials are not feasible. An alternative approach examining the impact of smoking cessation on cognition in older adults found those who quit smoking, compared with those who continued to smoke, to have slower rates of cognitive decline (Almeida et al. 2011).

Analysis stratified by apolipoprotein (APOE) ε4 allele, a well-known susceptibility gene for Alzheimer's disease, has revealed inconsistent findings with respect to smoking. Kivipelto et al. (2008) found the magnitude of the association between smoking and dementia to be elevated among APOE carriers. In contrast, Reitz et al. (2007) reported significant relationships only among non-carriers of the genotype. In this case, it has been hypothesized that the increased risk of dementia by APOE is so strong that smoking's influence was non-contributory. Smoking may also facilitate the release of acetylcholine and increase nicotinic receptor density, compensating for the APOE-induced impairment.

Many different mechanisms have been put forward to account for the increased risk of dementia from smoking. Smoking, mediated by oxidative stress, inflammation, and atherosclerosis, may increase the risk of neurodegeneration (Swan and Lessov-Schlaggar 2007). Cigarette smoking, both active and passive, contributes to oxidative stress, considered to play a major role in the onset and progression of Alzheimer's disease. Increased levels of inflammatory markers, such as C-reactive protein and interleukin-6, have been found in Alzheimer's disease. Smoking is also known to induce endothelial damage and increase vasodilatory dysfunction, hypertension, and blood coagulability, predisposing the individual to atherosclerosis. Moreover, preclinical brain changes, such as silent infarcts, white matter hyperintensities, and subcortical atrophy, observed among smokers may elevate the risk for cognitive decline. Cigarettes contain numerous neurotoxic compounds, such as lead and cadmium. However, nicotine, the main addictive chemical contained in cigarette smoke, also has cognitive enhancing effects (Herman and Sofuoglu 2010), which may, in part, explain the conflicting results between smoking and cognition.

Alcohol consumption

Numerous studies have reported the beneficial effect of moderate alcohol consumption on cognitive function and dementia. A recent systematic review (Peters et al. 2008a) has shown moderate alcohol consumption significantly to reduce overall risk of incident dementia by 38% and Alzheimer's disease by 32%, but did not find significant association with vascular dementia and cognitive decline. Some protective effects of moderate drinking against cognitive decline have been reported in nurse and community cohorts of older persons (Ganguli et al. 2005; Stampfer et al. 2005). In the Cardiovascular Risk Factors, Aging and Dementia (CAIDE) study, which examined Finnish men and women aged 65 to 79 years, those who drank less than once per month had a lower risk of mild cognitive impairment (Anttila et al. 2004). For vascular dementia, studies demonstrate contradictory results. While a study from China (Deng et al. 2006) demonstrated lower risk of vascular dementia among those who drank moderately, a Japanese study (Yoshitake et al. 1995) reported higher risk of vascular dementia among drinkers than non-drinkers.

The relationship between alcohol consumption and dementia and mild cognitive impairment risk appears to be U-shaped, with the greatest benefit accrued to those who drink moderately. Abstainers and heavy drinkers appear to be at higher risk. The optimal level of drinking, however, is less well established because of the heterogeneity in ways of measuring and defining moderate alcohol consumption. Benefits have been reported for one drink per day (McGuire, Ajani, and Ford 2007), from less than once a month to a frequency averaging daily to weekly (Ganguli et al. 2005), one to three servings of wine every day (Luchsinger et al. 2004), 1g to 14.9g per day (Stampfer et al. 2005), and one to twenty-eight drinks per week (Simons et al. 2006).

There is currently insufficient evidence to conclude whether certain types of alcohol confer more benefit. Several studies, however, lend support to the protective effects of wine. Consumption of wine, rather than beer and spirits, has been found significantly to reduce the risk of dementia (Luchsinger et al. 2004; Mehlig et al. 2008) and Alzheimer's disease (Lindsay et al. 2002). Interestingly, Deng et al. (2006) reported that whereas moderate consumption of wine lowered the risk of dementia, beer drinking increased its risk.

Although heavy drinking and chronic alcohol abuse are known to cause brain damage and neurodegeneration, moderate drinking may be protective against dementia through its beneficial haematological, cerebrovascular, and cardiovascular effects. Light to moderate alcohol consumption is associated with increased levels of HDL cholesterol and fibrinolytic factors, thus reducing risk of stroke and ischaemia (Peters et al. 2008a). Cardiovascular benefits derived from enhanced insulin sensitivity and reduced inflammatory response may engender some protection. Moreover, antioxidant properties in wine may help to reduce oxidative damage in the brain brought on by the disease. Recently, direct neuroprotective effects of alcohol have been observed in animal models and *in vivo* studies (Collins et al. 2009). Exposure to moderate alcohol levels has been found to protect against beta amyloid, a protein deposit found in the brains of patients with Alzheimer's disease. Moderate alcohol consumption may further trigger anti-inflammatory mechanisms in the brain that can lead to a preconditioned neuroprotective state.

Physical activity

There is a large body of evidence supporting the cognitive benefits of physical activity. A meta-analysis of fifteen prospective cohort studies examining physical activity's effect on cognitive decline among those without dementia has demonstrated a 38% reduction in risk for those who performed a high level of exercise, compared with a sedentary group (Sofi et al. 2011). A similarly reduced risk (35%) was observed among those participating in low- to moderate-level exercise. These findings were consistent across gender, sample size, duration of follow-up, and measures of cognitive performance. In a review of randomized controlled trials, eight out of eleven studies found aerobic exercise to enhance cognitive function, with a major effect on motor function and auditory attention, and moderate effects on processing speed and visual attention (Angevaren et al. 2008).

A growing amount of research suggests that mid-life exercise reduces the risk of late-life dementia and mild cognitive impairment (Ahlskog et al. 2011). The weight of the evidence favours some protective effects of physical activity on Alzheimer's disease and unspecified dementia (Lee et al. 2010). In a recent meta-analysis of five prospective cohort studies, there was a reduced pooled risk (OR = 0.62, 95% CI: 0.42–0.92) of vascular dementia among those who were physically active (Aarsland et al. 2010).

Despite the considerable amount of research demonstrating the positive influence of physical activity on cognitive health, there is much less agreement on how much exercise is actually effective. In the Nurses' Health Study, higher levels of activity measured by energy expenditure from participating in various types of physical activity, such as running, jogging, walking, hiking, bicycling, swimming, and gardening, were associated with better cognition (Weuve et al. 2004). Others have reported thresholds of four or more different activities (Podewils et al. 2005), three times or more per week of regular exercise (Larson et al. 2006), and more than 2.5 hours per week of moderate activity or more than one hour per week of vigorous activity (Singh-Manoux et al. 2005). Alternatively, even light-intensity activity, such as daily walking (Simons et al. 2006), walking at an easy pace of at least 1.5 hours per week (Weuve et al. 2004), and walking 2 miles per day (Abbott et al. 2004), was found to be associated with better cognitive performance and reduced risk of dementia. Mid-life work-related physical activity and commuting to work by walking or bicycling, however, did not show protective effects against dementia in later life (Rovio et al. 2007).

Recently, randomized controlled trials have demonstrated the beneficial effects of physical activity on cognitive health across diverse population groups. Six-month aerobic exercise programmes of moderate intensity (Lautenschlager et al. 2008) and high intensity (Baker et al. 2010) improved cognition in older adults with mild cognitive impairment. In the Lifestyle Interventions and Independence for Elders Pilot (LIFE-P) study that targeted older people with sedentary life style at risk of disability, improvements in physical function from moderate-intensity exercise were significantly correlated with cognitive improvements (Williamson et al. 2009). A recent clinical trial of Tai Chi on Chinese subjects at risk of dementia has shown some benefits on cognitive function (Lam et al. 2011). For dementia patients residing in residential care facilities, however, exercise programmes did not yield significant improvements in cognitive function (Littbrand, Stenvall, and Rosendahl 2011).

The protective effects of physical activity on the brain have been attributed to various mechanisms (Ahlskog et al. 2011). One plausible explanation is that exercise reduces cerebrovascular risks, such as diabetes mellitus and glucose intolerance, hypertension, hyperlipidaemia, and obesity, as well as mitigating small vessel disease. Exercise may also enhance brain vasculature by increasing the proliferation of brain endothelial cells and angiogenesis (Van Praag 2009). Animal studies show physical exercise promotes synaptogenesis and neurogenesis by upregulating the expression of brain-derived neutrophic factors. Moreover, structural and functional neuroimaging studies have reported a positive relationship between cardiorespiratory fitness and brain volume and white matter integrity among healthy older adults and those with mild Alzheimer's disease (Hayes et al. 2013). Cardiorespiratory fitness has been shown to be linked to enhanced cognitive performance. Executive functions tied to fronto-parietal regions and spatial memory tasks that are hippocampus-dependent were found to have a positive association with cardiorespiratory fitness.

Body weight

The relationship between body mass index (BMI) and dementia appears U-shaped, with increased dementia risk for those underweight and obese. A recent systematic review of prospective studies found that low BMI in mid-life, compared with normal BMI, was associated with a two times higher risk of developing Alzheimer's disease (Anstey et al. 2011). A subsequent meta-analysis revealed that being overweight was significantly associated with an elevated risk of Alzheimer's disease and vascular dementia, whereas obesity was significantly associated with only Alzheimer's disease. In a thirty-six-year follow-up study of 10 136 adults aged 40 to 45 years, compared with normal weight, those overweight had a two-fold increase in risk of Alzheimer's disease and vascular dementia, while obesity was associated with three times and five times higher risk of Alzheimer's disease and vascular dementia, respectively (Whitmer et al. 2007). In the Baltimore Longitudinal Study of Aging (BLSA), higher body composition was associated with more rapid decline in global function, executive function, and memory (Gunstad et al. 2010). There are reports, however, that higher BMI is protective of dementia (Atti et al. 2008; Luchsinger et al. 2007). Although obesity is reported to have a negative impact on the brain across the lifespan, its effect in late-life is still controversial, in part because BMI does not adequately reflect body composition in old age (Smith et al. 2011).

In this sense, a better measure to use may be weight change. Severe BMI loss of greater than 10% (Atti et al. 2008) and weight loss of more than 1kg per year (Luchsinger et al. 2007) were both associated with a higher risk of dementia. In a study of Catholic clergy members, an annual decline of one unit of BMI was associated with a 35% increase in Alzheimer's disease risk (Buchman et al. 2005). Other measures of adiposity, such as waist circumference and waist–hip ratio that assess central obesity, and skin-fold thickness have also been shown to predict dementia risk (Beydoun et al. 2008). This finding, however, is not without controversy. In a study of older Australian women, although weight gain or loss was associated with a poor visual memory performance, no significant association was found for other measures of adiposity (Lo et al. 2012b).

Obesity may have negative effects on the brain through pathways involving low-grade systemic inflammation, elevated triglycerides, and insulin resistance (Smith et al. 2011). Low BMI is likely due to weight loss, which precedes hyperinsulinaemia, a risk factor for dementia (Luchsinger et al. 2007). Weight loss may also be a preclinical marker of dementia caused by progressive structural changes in the brain (Buchman et al. 2005). For example, structural changes in the brain, such as atrophy of the medial temporal lobe and hippocampus, preceding overt Alzheimer's disease have been found to be associated with low body weight. Alternatively, weight loss may reflect change in eating habits and inadequate nutrition intake due to impaired memory, or an increase in anorectic adipokines and inflammatory cytokines associated with frailty brought on by dementia (Beydoun et al. 2008).

Diet and nutrition

In regard to research examining the relationship between life-style factors and cognitive function, nutrition has arguably received the most attention. Current evidence indicates that diets with higher intake of fruits, vegetables, fish, nuts, and legumes, but lower intake of meat and saturated fat are beneficial for cognitive function (Gu and Scarmeas 2011). For example, in the Three-City (3C) study, daily fruit and vegetable consumption was shown to lower the risk of dementia by 28%, and weekly fish intake was associated with a 35% reduced risk of Alzheimer's disease (Barberger-Gateau et al. 2007). In the CAIDE study, mid-life high polyunsaturated fat (PUFA) intake was associated with better semantic memory, whereas saturated fat (SFA) intake from dairy products was associated with poorer global cognitive function and prospective memory, and an increased risk of mild cognitive impairment, controlling for covariates and APOE (Eskelinen et al. 2008).

The influence of vitamins and other micronutrients on cognitive function, however, is still controversial. Deficiencies in vitamin B_6, B_{12}, and folic acid (B_9) are known to be associated with neuropsychological dysfunction and increased homocysteine concentrations that elevate the risk for Alzheimer's disease (Selhub, Troen, and Rosenberg 2010). Because poor nutritional status is quite prevalent in old age, older people are particularly vulnerable to cognitive impairment and dementia. Prospective epidemiological studies, however, have found conflicting results as to the relationship linking higher levels of B vitamins to lower risk of cognitive decline and dementia (Gillette Guyonnet et al. 2007). A recent comprehensive review of randomized controlled trials did not find strong evidence that supplementation of B vitamins alone or in combination improves cognitive function in those with or without cognitive impairment (Ford and Almeida 2012). Studies of antioxidant nutrients, such as vitamins C and E, carotenes, and flavonoids, have also provided mixed results (Lee et al. 2010). More recently, vitamin D has gained attention as having neuroprotective properties, with low levels found to be associated with a higher risk of cognitive decline (Dickens et al. 2011).

Apart from research examining individual food and nutrient intake on cognition, more attention has recently been paid to studying dietary patterns. This whole-diet or dietary pattern approach takes into account interactions among the different components of diet. It also reflects the way people actually eat. One of the most extensively studied dietary patterns is the Mediterranean diet (MeDi), comprising of high intakes of vegetables, fruits, nuts and legumes, cereals, fish, and olive oil as the primary source of monounsaturated fatty acids (MUFA), with low intakes of meat and dairy products, and moderate wine consumption. MeDi has been found to be associated with slower cognitive decline, reduced risk of conversion of mild cognitive impairment to dementia, and lower risk of Alzheimer's disease (Solfrizzi et al. 2011). Various mechanisms, such as lowering the risk of vascular risk factors, decreased insulin resistance, high antioxidant properties contained in the diet, and reduced inflammatory response, have been suggested to account for its modulating effect on cognitive function.

Social activity

Although studies on the association between social activity and cognitive function are still quite limited (Wang, Xu, and Pei 2012), there is growing evidence that older adults who have large and dense social networks are less likely to be at risk for cognitive decline and impairment. In the Health and Retirement Study (HRS) of people aged 50 years and older, higher levels of social integration, measured by marital status, volunteer activities, and contact with parents, children, and neighbours, were predictive of more gradual memory loss (Ertel, Glymour, and Berkman 2008). Using brain biopsy data, Bennett et al. (2006) showed that those having larger social network size maintained higher cognitive function at even severe levels of pathology, indicating that network size modified Alzheimer's disease pathology. The quality of the social relationships may also matter. Holtzman et al. (2004) reported that not only frequent contact in a larger social network, but higher levels of emotional support were associated with better cognitive function.

Engagement in various types of social activities has been found to lower the risk of dementia. In the Washington Heights-Inwood Columbia Aging Project (WHICAP), visiting friends or relatives and going to movies or restaurants were associated with a respective 40% and 38% reduced risk of incident dementia (Scarmeas et al. 2001). In the Paquid study, older French adults engaging in activities such as travelling, gardening, odd jobs, and knitting showed lower risk of dementia (Fabrigoule et al. 1995). Kåreholt et al. (2011) reported that mid-life participation in political activities, such as the delivery of a speech at a meeting and taking part in public demonstrations, were predictive of cognition more than two decades later. Interestingly, a decreased social engagement from mid-life to late-life was associated with an elevated risk of incident dementia (Saczynski et al. 2006).

Considering that brain plasticity, the ability of the brain to change with learning, to repair and compensate, is a lifelong process and is influenced by environmental stimulation, engagement in social activities might provide such a medium in forming more efficient neural networks (Scarmeas and Stern 2003). Social activity may play a critical role in increasing synaptic density, activity, and connectivity, and making efficient use of alternative networks. In addition, social engagement may enhance emotional well-being through decreased stress and cortisol levels, thus reducing vascular risks (Bielak 2010). Emotional support received from family, friends, and relatives may lessen adverse cardiovascular and neuroendocrine responses to stress and promote the adoption of healthy life styles, with both contributing to protect cognitive health (Holtzman et al. 2004).

Mental activity

Mental or cognitive activity has received considerable research attention in recent years. A number of prospective cohort studies have examined the relationship of mentally stimulating activity to incident dementia. For example, in the Bronx Aging Study, among the different cognitive activities frequent participation, defined as at least several times per week, in reading, playing board games, and playing musical instruments was associated with a reduced risk of dementia (Verghese et al. 2003). Among the CHAP participants, more frequent engagement in seven cognitive activities (viewing television; listening to radio; reading newspapers; reading magazines; reading books; playing games like cards, checkers, crosswords, or other puzzles; and going to a museum) were associated with a reduced cognitive decline (Wilson et al. 2003) and a lower risk of incident Alzheimer's disease (Wilson et al. 2002). Cognitive activity has been further suggested to compress cognitive morbidity, delaying the onset of dementia but hastening its progression once begun, thus shortening the total time spent with dementia (Wilson et al. 2010).

Randomized controlled trials have been utilized to examine the effects of brain exercise. Perhaps one of the largest studies to date has been the ACTIVE (Advanced Cognitive Training for Independent and Vital Elderly) study, in which 2832 older adults aged 65 to 94 years living independently in the community participated in ten-session group training over five to six weeks (Ball et al. 2002). Those who received cognitive training in memory, reasoning, and processing speed improved in targeted cognitive abilities (Ball et al. 2002), with less declines in daily functioning (Willis et al. 2006) and quality of life (Wolinsky et al. 2006). Besides targeting healthy older people, is cognitive activity beneficial for people who already have dementia? This question was addressed in a recent meta-analysis that examined the effectiveness of one form of mental exercise, cognitive stimulation (Woods et al. 2012). Cognitive stimulation involved older people with mild to moderate dementia participating in small-group activities, such as word games, puzzles, music, baking, and indoor gardening. Participation in cognitively engaging activities had positive effects on the patient's global cognitive function as well as on the quality of life.

As with physical and social activities, cognitive activities may be a part of life experiences that increases cognitive reserve, leading to the ability better to cope and compensate for acquired brain pathology (Yaakov 2009). Increased cerebral blood flows, synaptogenesis, and optimal neurochemical compositions may play a role (Bielak 2010). However, the 'use it or lose it' hypothesis that forms the theoretical basis of cognitive training, although intuitively appealing, still lacks convincing evidence (Salthouse 2006).

IMPLICATIONS FOR PRACTICE

There is an increasing recognition of the role of healthy life styles in improving cognitive health. Individual life styles of non-smoking, moderate alcohol consumption, physical activity, normal body weight, healthy diet, social activity, and mental activity appear to have a positive influence on cognitive function and may reduce the risk of dementia. Moreover, there are indications of synergistic effects among these behavioural factors and leisure activities. For example, in the Honolulu-Asia Aging Study, higher scores in the combinations of non-smoking, normal BMI, physical activity, and healthy diet were correlated with a lower risk of dementia (Gelber et al. 2012). There appears to be synergy between diet and exercise in enhancing neuroplasticity (van Praag 2009). In addition, an increased benefit of simultaneous engagement in physical activity, social activity, and cognitive activity in reducing dementia risk has been observed (Karp 2006). These results strongly suggest that multiple, rather than single, life-style modifications may have a greater impact on cognitive function in late-life.

It is well known that life-style factors tend to co-occur, with clustering of different combinations of life style behaviours such as non-smoking, no heavy alcohol consumption, and physical activity (Lee et al. 2012). In developing cognitive health promotion programmes for older adults, aiming for multiple behaviour changes would seem appropriate. However, it is still unknown whether multimodal interventions, such as simultaneous cognitive training and physical activity, are more effective than individual interventions (Kraft 2012). Targeting key life-style factors, such as smoking, that can trigger the adoption of other healthy behaviours may prove to be a more efficient strategy.

Increasing evidence suggests that maintaining an active life style in late-life is conducive to cognitive health. Engaging in diverse physical, mental, and social activities appears to offer the most promise in slowing cognitive decline (Lo et al. 2012a). However, it is unclear which of the individual components of life-style activities are most effective in generating cognitive benefits, because they are intrinsically linked to one another. For example, physical exercise and mentally stimulating activities often involve socialization, in that they occur in a group setting, such as in amateur dancing, and a socially interactive environment may turn out to be as important as the aerobic component of the physical activity (Kraft 2012). Delineating the effects of specific activities in individual and group settings may help to elucidate the role leisure activities play in preserving cognitive function in later life.

Although evidence continues to accumulate, the impact of healthy life styles on cognitive function and dementia are far from conclusive. A recent systematic review conducted by the US National Institutes of Health (Daviglus et al. 2011; Williams et al. 2010) has graded the quality of current evidence on the effects of life-style factors on cognitive decline and Alzheimer's disease to be 'low'. Reasons cited for this somewhat sceptical analysis were a small number of studies with limited evidence, heterogeneity, and imprecision in exposure and outcome measures, inconsistent results among studies, conflicting results across cognitive decline and Alzheimer's disease, modest effect sizes, and, perhaps more importantly, few randomized controlled trials. Clearly, there is a need for more research, particularly research that incorporates multiple life-style modifications in larger samples.

In order to help meet this challenge, large clinical trials of multicomponent life-style modifications are currently underway (Andrieu et al. 2011). The Finnish Geriatric Intervention study to prevent cognitive impairment and disability (FINGER) is a multi-domain intervention that includes dietary intervention, an exercise training programme, cognitive training, and monitoring and management of metabolic and vascular risk factors. In the Multi-domain Alzheimer Preventive Trial (MAPT) designed in France, investigators are examining the effects of treatment with omega-3 and/or multi-domain intervention (nutritional, physical, and cognitive training) on cognitive decline.

Meanwhile, a community experiment, with volunteerism and civic engagement at its core, provides a good example of how a broad social participation approach in a 'real-world' setting can be effective in promoting cognitive health. In the Experience Corps programme, older adults engaged in multi-modal cognitive activities as part of a volunteer service in elementary schools to assist teachers improve children's literacy and academic achievement (Fried et al. 2004). The participants showed not only improvements in physical activity and social support (Fried et al. 2004), but significant improvements in executive function and memory (Carlson et al. 2008), with intervention-specific increases in brain activities captured in the functional magnetic resonance imaging (Carlson et al. 2009).

At the national level, based on current knowledge and the evidence base, policies and strategies on dementia prevention are being developed. In the US, a comprehensive review of the evidence on risk factors of dementia led to the Healthy Brain Initiative, a public-private partnership to promote cognitive health, with the National Alzheimer's

Project Act being signed into law in 2011 (Centers for Disease Control and Prevention 2011). The UK's National Dementia Strategy includes raising public awareness about dementia prevention by means of promoting cerebrovascular health, focusing on public education messages on diet and life styles (UK Department of Health 2009). Alzheimer's Australia promotes life-style strategies to reduce the risk of dementia, setting the stage for the establishment of a National Dementia Preventative Health Strategy (Alzheimer's Australia 2010). In Korea, a public health recommendation for cognitive health, named PASCAL (an acronym for Physical activity, Anti-smoking, Social activity, Cognitive activity, Alcohol in moderation, and Lean body mass and healthy diet) has been put forward (Lee et al. 2009), and the Dementia Management Act, established in 2011, serves to advance preventive strategies at both national and regional levels.

SUMMARY

There is an increasing recognition of the role life styles may play in reducing the risk of cognitive decline and incident dementia in late-life. In recent years, substantial literatures documenting the benefits of healthy life styles on cognitive health have been accumulating. Prospective cohort studies have demonstrated a significant impact of non-smoking, moderate alcohol consumption, physical activity, normal body weight, healthy diet and nutrition, social activity, and mental activity on cognitive outcomes. There have been, however, relatively few efforts to conduct randomized controlled trials and investigate the combined effects of different life-style factors. More research is required to evaluate the effectiveness of life-style change on cognitive function, especially in larger and more diverse community populations.

Meanwhile, it may be prudent to initiate public health campaigns to promote healthy life styles, as the potential benefit of life-style change appears to outweigh any harm. Health education and counselling programmes need to be developed to raise awareness of the importance of engaging in healthy life styles for cognitive health. National policies should begin to address life-style modifications as a vital component of dementia prevention strategies.

ACKNOWLEDGEMENTS

The preparation of this manuscript was supported by a grant from the Korea Healthcare Technology R&D Project, Ministry of Health and Welfare, Republic of Korea (HI10C2020).

KEY REFERENCES AND SOURCES FOR FURTHER READING

Centers for Disease Control and Prevention. Healthy Brain Initiative. http://www.cdc.gov/aging/healthybrain/.

Lee, Y., Back, J. H., Kim, J., Kim, S. H., Na, D. L., et al. (2010). 'Systematic Review of Health Behavioral Risks and Cognitive Health in Older Adults'. *International Psychogeriatrics* 22(2): 174–187.

Lo, A. H. Y., Pachana, N. A., Byrne, G. J., and Sachdev, P. S. (2012). 'A Review of Tobacco, Alcohol, Adiposity, and Activity as Predictors of Cognitive Change'. *Clinical Gerontologist* 35(2): 148–194.

Williams, J. W., Plassman, B. L., Burke, J., Holsinger, T., and Benjamin, S. (2010). *Preventing Alzheimer's Disease and Cognitive Decline. Evidence Report/Technology Assessment No. 193.* Rockville, MD: Agency for Healthcare Research and Quality. http://www.ncbi.nlm.nih.gov/books/NBK47456/.

References

Aarsland, D., Sardahaee, F. S., Anderssen, S., Ballard, C., and the Alzheimer's Society Systematic Review Group (2010). 'Is Physical Activity a Potential Preventive Factor for Vascular Dementia? A Systematic Review'. *Aging & Mental Health* 14(4): 386–395.

Abbott, R. D., White, L. R., Ross, G. W., Masaki, K. H., Curb, J. D., et al. (2004). 'Walking and Dementia in Physically Capable Elderly Men'. *Journal of the American Medical Association* 292(12), 1447–1453.

Ahlskog, J. E., Geda, Y. E., Graff-Radford, N. R., and Petersen, R. C. (2011). 'Physical Exercise as a Preventive or Disease-modifying Treatment of Dementia and Brain Aging'. *Mayo Clinic Proceedings* 86 (9): 876–884.

Almeida, O. P., Garrido, G. J., Alfonso, H., Hulse, G., Lautenschlager, N. T., et al. (2011). '24-month Effect of Smoking Cessation on Cognitive Function and Brain Structure in Later Life'. *NeuroImage* 55 (4): 1480–1489.

Alzheimer's Australia (2010). *Towards a National Dementia Preventative Health Strategy.* Canberra: Alzheimer's Australia.

Alzheimer's Disease International (2009). *World Alzheimer Report 2009.* London: Alzheimer's Disease International.

Alzheimer's Disease International (2010). *World Alzheimer Report 2010: The Global Economic Impact of Dementia.* London: Alzheimer's Disease International.

Andrieu, S., Aboderin, I., Baeyens, J., Beard, J., Benetos, A., et al. (2011). 'IAGG Workshop: Health Promotion Program on Prevention of Late Onset Dementia'. *Journal of Nutrition, Health & Aging* 15 (7): 562–575.

Angevaren, M., Aufdemkampe, G., Verhaar, H. J., Aleman, A., and Vanhees, L. (2008). 'Physical Activity and Enhanced Fitness to Improve Cognitive Function in Older People without Known Cognitive Impairment'. *Cochrane Database of Systematic Reviews* 3, CD005381.

Anstey, K. J., Cherbuin, N., Budge, M., and Young, J. (2011). 'Body Mass Index in Midlife and Late-life as a Risk Factor for Dementia: A Meta-analysis of Prospective Studies'. *Obesity Reviews* 12 (5): e426–e37.

Anttila, T., Helkala, E. L., Viitanen, M., Kåreholt, I., Fratiglioni, L. et al. (2004). 'Alcohol Drinking in Middle Age and Subsequent Risk of Mild Cognitive Impairment and Dementia in Old Age: A Prospective Population Based Study'. *British Medical Journal* 329 (7465): 539.

Atti, A. R., Palmer, K., Volpato, S., Winblad, B., De Ronchi, D., et al. (2008). 'Late-life Body Mass Index and Dementia Incidence: Nine-year Follow-up Data from the Kungsholmen Project'. *Journal of the American Geriatrics Society* 56(1): 111–116.

Baker, L. D., Frank, L. L., Foster-Schubert, K., Green, P. S., Wilkinson, C. W., et al. (2010). 'Effects of Aerobic Exercise on Mild Cognitive Impairment: A Controlled Trial'. *Archives of Neurology* 67(1): 71–79.

Ball, K., Berch, D. B., Helmers, K. F., Jobe, J. B., Leveck, M. D., et al. (2002). 'Effects of Cognitive Training Interventions with Older Adults: A Randomized Controlled Trial'. *Journal of the American Medical Association* 288(18): 2271–2281.

Barberger-Gateau, P., Raffaitin, C., Letenneur, L., Berr, C., Tzourio, C., et al. (2007). 'Dietary Patterns and Risk of Dementia: The Three-City Cohort Study'. *Neurology* 69(20): 1921–1930.

Bennett, D. A., Schneider, J. A., Tang, Y., Arnold, S. E., and Wilson, R. S. (2006). 'The Effect of Social Networks on the Relation between Alzheimer's Disease Pathology and Level of Cognitive Function in Old People: A Longitudinal Cohort Study'. *Lancet Neurology* 5(5): 406–412.

Beydoun, M. A., Beydoun, H. A., and Wang, Y. (2008). 'Obesity and Central Obesity as Risk Factors for Incident Dementia and its Subtypes: A Systematic Review and Meta-analysis'. *Obesity Reviews* 9(3): 204–218.

Bielak, A. A. (2010). 'How Can We Not "Lose It" If We Still Don't Understand How To "Use It"? Unanswered Questions about the Influence of Activity Participation on Cognitive Performance in Older Age—A Mini-review'. *Gerontology* 56(5): 507–519.

Brookmeyer, R., Johnson, E., Ziegler-Graham, K., and Arrighi, H. M. (2007). 'Forecasting The Global Burden of Alzheimer's Disease'. *Alzheimer's & Dementia* 3(3): 186–191.

Buchman, A. S., Wilson, R. S., Bienias, J. L., Shah, R. C., Evans, D. A., et al. (2005). 'Change in Body Mass Index and Risk of Incident Alzheimer Disease'. *Neurology* 65(6): 892–897.

Carlson, M. C., Saczynski, J. S., Rebok, G. W., Seeman, T., Glass, T. A., et al. (2008). 'Exploring the Effects of an "Everyday" Activity Program on Executive Function and Memory in Older Adults: Experience Corps'. *Gerontologist* 48(6): 793–801.

Carlson, M. C., Erickson, K. I., Kramer, A. F., Voss, M. W., Bolean, N., et al. (2009). 'Evidence for Neurocognitive Plasticity in At-risk Older Adults: The Experience Corps Program'. *Journals of Gerontology, Series A: Biological Sciences and Medical Sciences* 64A(12): 1275–1282.

Centers for Disease Control and Prevention (2011). *The CDC Healthy Brain Initiative: Progress 2006–2011*. Atlanta, GA: Centers for Disease Control and Prevention .

Collins, M. A., Neafsey, E. J., Mukamal, K. J., Gray, M. O., Parks, D. L., et al. (2009). 'Alcohol in Moderation, Cardioprotection, and Neuroprotection: Epidemiological Considerations and Mechanistic Studies'. *Alcoholism* 33(2): 206–219.

Daviglus, M. L., Plassman, B. L., Pirzada, A., Bell, C. C., Bowen, P. E., et al. (2011). 'Risk Factors and Preventive Interventions for Alzheimer Disease: State of the Science'. *Archives of Neurology* 68(9): 1185–1190.

Deng, J., Zhou, D. H., Li, J., Wang, Y. J., Gao, C., et al. (2006). 'A 2-year Follow-up Study of Alcohol Consumption and Risk of Dementia'. *Clinical Neurology and Neurosurgery* 108(4): 378–383.

Dickens, A. P., Lang, I. A., Langa, K. M., Kos, K., and Llewellyn, D. J. (2011). 'Vitamin D, Cognitive Dysfunction and Dementia in Older Adults'. *CNS Drugs* 25 (8): 629–639.

Ertel, K. A., Glymour, M. M., and Berkman, L. F. (2008). 'Effects of Social Integration on Preserving Memory Function in a Nationally Representative US Elderly Population'. *American Journal of Public Health* 98(7): 1215–1220.

Eskelinen, M. H., Ngandu, T., Helkala, E. L., Tuomilehto, J., Nissinen, A., et al. (2008). 'Fat Intake at Midlife and Cognitive Impairment Later in Life: A Population-based CAIDE Study'. *International Journal of Geriatric Psychiatry* 23(7): 741–747.

Fabrigoule, C., Letenneur, L., Dartigues, J. F., Zarrouk, M., Commenges, D., and Barberger-Gateau, P. (1995). 'Social and Leisure Activities and Risk of Dementia: A Prospective Longitudinal Study'. *Journal of the American Geriatrics Society* 43(5): 485–490.

Ford, A. H. and Almeida, O. P. (2012). 'Effect of Homocysteine Lowering Treatment on Cognitive Function: A Systematic Review and Meta-analysis of Randomized Controlled Trials'. *Journal of Alzheimer's Disease* 29(1): 133–149.

Fried, L. P., Carlson, M. C., Freedman, M., Frick, K. D., Glass, T. A., et al. (2004). 'A Social Model for Health Promotion for an Aging Population: Initial Evidence on the Experience Corps Model'. *Journal of Urban Health* 81(1): 64–78.

Ganguli, M., Bilt, J. V., Saxton, J. A., Shen, C., and Dodge, H. H. (2005). 'Alcohol Consumption and Cognitive Function in Late Life: A Longitudinal Community Study'. *Neurology* 65(8): 1210–1217.

Gelber, R. P., Petrovitch, H., Masaki, K. H., Abbott, R. D., Ross, G. W., et al. (2012). 'Lifestyle and the Risk of Dementia in Japanese-American Men'. *Journal of the American Geriatrics Society* 60(1): 118–123.

Gillette Guyonnet, S., Abellan Van Kan, G., Andrieu, S., Barberger Gateau, P., Berr, C., et al. (2007). 'IANA Task Force on Nutrition and Cognitive Decline with Aging'. *Journal of Nutrition, Health & Aging* 11(2): 132–152.

Gu, Y. and Scarmeas, N. (2011). 'Dietary Patterns in Alzheimer's Disease and Cognitive Aging'. *Current Alzheimer Research* 8(5): 510–519.

Gunstad, J., Lhotsky, A., Wendell, C. R., Ferrucci, L., and Zonderman, A. B. (2010). 'Longitudinal Examination of Obesity and Cognitive Function: Results from the Baltimore Longitudinal Study of Aging'. *Neuroepidemiology* 34(4): 222–229.

Hayes, S. M., Hayes, J. P., Cadden, M., and Verfaellie, M. (2013). 'A Review of Cardiorespiratory Fitness-related Neuroplasticity in the Aging Brain'. *Frontiers in Aging Neuroscience* 5: 31.

Herman, A. I. and Sofuoglu, M. (2010). 'Cognitive Effects of Nicotine: Genetic Moderators'. *Addiction Biology* 15(3): 250–265.

Holtzman, R. E., Rebok, G. W., Saczynski, J. S., Kouzis, A. C., Wilcox Doyle, K., et al. (2004). 'Social Network Characteristics and Cognition in Middle-aged and Older Adults'. *Journals of Gerontology, Series B: Psychological Sciences and Social Sciences* 59(6): P278–P284.

Kåreholt, I., Lennartsson, C., Gatz, M., and Parker, M. G. (2011). 'Baseline Leisure Time Activity and Cognition More than Two Decades Later'. *International Journal of Geriatric Psychiatry* 26(1): 65–74.

Karp, A. (2006). 'Mental, Physical and Social Components in Leisure Activities Equally Contribute to Decrease Dementia Risk'. *Dementia and Geriatric Cognitive Disorders* 21(2): 65–73.

Kivipelto, M., Rovio, S., Ngandu, T., Kåreholt, I., Eskelinen, M., et al. (2008). 'Apolipoprotein E Epsilon4 Magnifies Lifestyle Risks for Dementia: A Population Based Study'. *Journal of Cellular and Molecular Medicine* 12(6B): 2762–2771.

Kraft, E. (2012). 'Cognitive Function, Physical Activity, and Aging: Possible Biological Links and Implications for Multimodal Interventions'. *Neuropsychology, Development, and Cognition, Section B: Aging, Neuropsychology, and Cognition* 19(1–2): 248–263.

Lam, L. C. W., Chau, R. C. M., Wong, B. M. L., Fung, A. W., Lui, V. W., et al. (2011). 'Interim Follow-up of a Randomized Controlled Trial Comparing Chinese Style Mind Body (Tai Chi) and Stretching Exercises on Cognitive Function in Subjects at Risk of Progressive Cognitive Decline'. *International Journal of Geriatric Psychiatry* 26(7): 733–740.

Larson, E. B., Wang, L., Bowen, J. D., McCormick, W. C., Teri, L., et al. (2006). 'Exercise is Associated with Reduced Risk for Incident Dementia among Persons 65 Years of Age and Older'. *Annals of Internal Medicine* 144(2): 73–81.

Lautenschlager, N. T., Cox, K. L., Flicker, L., Foster, J. K., van Bockxmeer, F. M., et al. (2008). 'Effect of Physical Activity on Cognitive Function in Older Adults at Risk for Alzheimer Disease: A Randomized Trial'. *Journal of the American Medical Association* 300(9): 1027–1037.

Lee, Y., Na, D. L., Cheong, H.-K., Hong, C. H., Back, J. H., et al. (2009). 'Lifestyle Recommendations for Dementia Prevention: PASCAL'. *Journal of the Korean Geriatrics Society* 13(2): 61–68.

Lee, Y., Back, J. H., Kim, J., Kim, S. H., Na, D. L., et al. (2010). 'Systematic Review of Health Behavioral Risks and Cognitive Health in Older Adults'. *International Psychogeriatrics* 22(2): 174–187.

Lee, Y., Back, J. H., Kim, J., Byeon, H., Kim, S., and Ryu, M. (2012). 'Clustering of Multiple Healthy Lifestyles among Older Korean Adults Living in the Community'. *Geriatrics & Gerontology International* 12(3): 515–523.

Lindsay, J., Laurin, D., Verreault, R., Hébert, R., Helliwell, B., et al. (2002). 'Risk Factors for Alzheimer's Disease: A Prospective Analysis from the Canadian Study of Health and Aging'. *American Journal of Epidemiology* 156(5): 445–453.

Littbrand, H., Stenvall, M., and Rosendahl, E. (2011). 'Applicability and Effects of Physical Exercise on Physical and Cognitive Functions and Activities of Daily Living among People with Dementia: A Systematic Review'. *American Journal of Physical Medicine & Rehabilitation* 90(6): 495–518.

Lo, A. H. Y., Pachana, N. A., Byrne, G. J., and Sachdev, P. S. (2012a). 'A Review of Tobacco, Alcohol, Adiposity, and Activity as Predictors of Cognitive Change'. *Clinical Gerontologist* 35(2): 148–194.

Lo, A. H. Y., Pachana, N. A., Byrne, G. J., Sachdev, P. S., and Woodman, R. J. (2012b). 'Relationship between Changes in Body Weight and Cognitive Function in Middle-aged and Older Women'. *International Journal of Geriatric Psychiatry* 27(8): 863–872.

Luchsinger, J. A., Tang, M. X., Siddiqui, M., Shea, S., and Mayeux, R. (2004). 'Alcohol Intake and Risk of Dementia'. *Journal of the American Geriatrics Society* 52(4): 540–546.

Luchsinger, J. A., Patel, B., Tang, M. X., Schupf, N., and Mayeux, R. (2007). 'Measures of Adiposity and Dementia Risk in Elderly Persons'. *Archives of Neurology* 64(3): 392–398.

McGuire, L. C., Ajani, U. A., and Ford, E. S. (2007). 'Cognitive Functioning in Late Life: The Impact of Moderate Alcohol Consumption'. *Annals of Epidemiology* 17(2): 93–99.

Mehlig, K., Skoog, I., Guo, X., Schütze, M., Gustafson, D., et al. (2008). 'Alcoholic Beverages and Incidence of Dementia: 34-year Follow-up of the Prospective Population Study of Women in Göteborg'. *American Journal of Epidemiology* 167(6): 684–691.

Peters, R., Peters, J., Warner, J., Beckett, N., and Bulpitt, C. (2008a). 'Alcohol, Dementia and Cognitive Decline in the Elderly: A Systematic Review'. *Age and Ageing* 37(5): 505–512.

Peters, R., Poulter, R., Warner, J., Beckett, N., Burch, L., and Bulpitt, C. (2008b). 'Smoking, Dementia and Cognitive Decline in the Elderly: a Systematic Review'. *BMC Geriatrics* 8(1): 36.

Podewils, L. J., Guallar, E., Kuller, L. H., Fried, L. H., Lopez, O. L., et al. (2005). 'Physical Activity, APOE Genotype, and Dementia Risk: Findings from the Cardiovascular Health Cognition Study'. *American Journal of Epidemiology* 161(7): 639–651.

Reitz, C., Den Heijer, T., Van Duijn, C., Hofman, A., and Breteler, M. M. B. (2007). 'Relation between Smoking and Risk of Dementia and Alzheimer Disease: The Rotterdam Study'. *Neurology* 69(10): 998–1005.

Rönnemaa, E., Zethelius, B., Lannfelt, L., and Kilander, L. (2011). 'Vascular Risk Factors and Dementia: 40-year Follow-up of a Population-based Cohort'. *Dementia and Geriatric Cognitive Disorders* 31(6): 460–466.

Rovio, S., Kareholt, I., Viitanen, M., Winblad, B., Tuomilehto, J., et al. (2007). 'Work-related Physical Activity and the Risk of Dementia and Alzheimer's Disease'. *International Journal of Geriatric Psychiatry* 22 (9): 874–882.

Sabia, S., Elbaz, A., Dugravot, A., Head, J., Shipley, M., et al. (2012). 'Impact of Smoking on Cognitive Decline in Early Old Age: The Whitehall II Cohort Study'. *Archives of General Psychiatry*. (epub).

Saczynski, J. S., Pfeifer, L. A., Masaki, K., Korf, D. S., Laurin, D., et al. (2006). 'The Effect of Social Engagement on Incident Dementia: The Honolulu-Asia Aging Study'. *American Journal of Epidemiology* 163(5): 433–440.

Salthouse, T. A. (2006). 'Mental Exercise and Mental Aging: Evaluating the Validity of the "Use It or Lose It" Hypothesis'. *Perspectives on Psychological Science* 1(1): 68–87.

Scarmeas, N. and Stern, Y. (2003). 'Cognitive Reserve and Lifestyle'. *Journal of Clinical and Experimental Neuropsychology* 25(5): 625–633.

Scarmeas, N., Levy, G., Tang, M. X., Manly, J., and Stern, Y. (2001). 'Influence of Leisure Activity on the Incidence of Alzheimer's Disease'. *Neurology* 57(12): 2236–2242.

Selhub, J., Troen, A., and Rosenberg, I. H. (2010). 'B Vitamins and the Aging Brain'. *Nutrition Reviews* 68: S112–S118.

Simons, L. A., Simons, J., McCallum, J., and Friedlander, Y. (2006). 'Lifestyle Factors and Risk of Dementia: Dubbo Study of the Elderly'. *Medical Journal of Australia* 184(2): 68–70.

Singh-Manoux, A., Hillsdon, M., Brunner, E., and Marmot, M. (2005). 'Effects of Physical Activity on Cognitive Functioning in Middle Age: Evidence from the Whitehall II Prospective Cohort Study'. *American Journal of Public Health* 95(12): 2252–2258.

Sloane, P. D., Zimmerman, S., Suchindran, C., Reed, P., Wang, L., et al. (2002). 'The Public Health Impact of Alzheimer's Disease 2000–2050: Potential Implication of Treatment Advances'. *Annual Review of Public Health* 23(1): 213–231.

Smith, E., Hay, P., Campbell, L., and Trollor, J. N. (2011). 'A Review of the Association between Obesity and Cognitive Function across the Lifespan: Implications for Novel Approaches to Prevention and Treatment'. *Obesity Reviews* 12(9): 740–755.

Sofi, F., Valecchi, D., Bacci, D., Abbate, R., Gensini, G. F., et al. (2011). 'Physical Activity and Risk of Cognitive Decline: A Meta-analysis of Prospective Studies'. *Journal of Internal Medicine* 269(1): 107–117.

Solfrizzi, V., Frisardi, V., Seripa, D., Logroscino, G., Imbimbo, B. P., et al. (2011). 'Mediterranean Diet in Predementia and Dementia Syndromes'. *Current Alzheimer Research* 8(5): 520–542.

Stampfer, M. J., Kang, J. H., Chen, J., Cherry, R., and Grodstein, F. (2005). 'Effects of Moderate Alcohol Consumption on Cognitive Function in Women'. *New England Journal of Medicine* 352(3): 245–253.

Swan, G. E. and Lessov-Schlaggar, C. N. (2007). 'The Effects of Tobacco Smoke and Nicotine on Cognition and the Brain'. *Neuropsychology Review* 17(3): 259–273.

Tyas, S. L., White, L. R., Petrovitch, H., Webster Ross, G., Foley, D. J., et al. (2003). 'Mid-life Smoking and Late-life Dementia: The Honolulu-Asia Aging Study'. *Neurobiology of Aging* 24(4): 589–596.

UK Department of Health (2009). *Living Well with Dementia: A National Dementia Strategy*. Leeds: UK Department of Health.

Van Praag, H. (2009). 'Exercise and the Brain: Something to Chew On'. *Trends in Neurosciences* 32(5): 283–290.

Verghese, J., Lipton, R. B., Katz, M. J., Hall, C. B., Derby, C. A., et al. (2003). 'Leisure Activities and the Risk of Dementia in the Elderly'. *New England Journal of Medicine* 348(25): 2508–2516.

Wang, H.-X., Xu, W., and Pei, J.-J. (2012). 'Leisure Activities, Cognition and Dementia'. *Biochimica et Biophysica Acta* 1822(3): 482–491.

Weuve, J., Kang, J. H., Manson, J. E., Breteler, M. M. B., Ware, J. H., et al. (2004). 'Physical Activity, Including Walking, and Cognitive Function in Older Women'. *Journal of the American Medical Association* 292(12): 1454–1461.

Whitmer, R. A., Gunderson, E. P., Quesenberry Jr, C. P., Zhou, J., and Yaffe, K. (2007). 'Body Mass Index in Midlife and Risk of Alzheimer Disease and Vascular Dementia'. *Current Alzheimer Research* 4(2): 103–109.

Williams, J. W., Plassman, B. L., Burke, J., Holsinger, T., and Benjamin, S. (2010). *Preventing Alzheimer's Disease and Cognitive Decline.* Evidence Report/Technology Assessment No. 193. Rockville, MD: Agency for Healthcare Research and Quality.

Williamson, J. D., Espeland, M., Kritchevsky, S. B., et al. (2009). 'Changes in Cognitive Function in a Randomized Trial of Physical Activity: Results of the Lifestyle Interventions and Independence for Elders Pilot Study'. *Journals of Gerontology, Series A: Biological Sciences and Medical Sciences* 64A(6): 688–694.

Willis, S. L., Tennstedt, S. L., Marsiske, M., Ball, K., Elias, J., et al. (2006). 'Long-term Effects of Cognitive Training on Everyday Functional Outcomes in Older Adults'. *Journal of the American Medical Association* 296(23): 2805–2814.

Wilson, R. S., Bennett, D. A., Bienias, J. L., Aggarwal, N. T., Mendes De Leon, C. F., et al. (2002). 'Cognitive Activity and Incident AD in a Population-based Sample of Older Persons'. *Neurology* 59(12): 1910–1914.

Wilson, R. S., Bennett, D. A., Bienias, J. L., Mendes de Leon, C. F., Morris, M. C., et al. (2003). 'Cognitive Activity and Cognitive Decline in a Biracial Community Population'. *Neurology* 61(6): 812–816.

Wilson, R. S., Barnes, L. L., Aggarwal, N. T., Boyle, P. A., Hebert, L. E., et al. (2010). 'Cognitive Activity and the Cognitive Morbidity of Alzheimer Disease'. *Neurology* 75 (11): 990–996.

Wolinsky, F. D., Unverzagt, F. W., Smith, D. M., Jones, R., Wright, E., et al. (2006). 'The Effects of the ACTIVE Cognitive Training Trial on Clinically Relevant Declines in Health-related Quality of Life'. *Journals of Gerontology, Series B: Psychological Sciences and Social Sciences* 61(5): S281–S287.

Woods, B., Aguirre, E., Spector, A. E., and Orrell, M. (2012). 'Cognitive Stimulation to Improve Cognitive Functioning in People with Dementia'. *Cochrane Database of Systematic Reviews* 2: CD005562.

Yaakov, S. (2009). 'Cognitive Reserve'. *Neuropsychologia* 47(10): 2015–2028.

Yoshitake, T., Kiyohara, Y., Kato, I., and Ohmura, T. (1995). 'Incidence and Risk Factors of Vascular Dementia and Alzheimer's Disease in a Defined Elderly Japanese Population: The Hisayama Study'. *Neurology* 45(6): 1161–1168.

PART IV

INTERVENTIONS

CHAPTER 29

COGNITIVE-BEHAVIOUR THERAPY WITH OLDER PEOPLE

KEN LAIDLAW AND
LARRY W. THOMPSON

THE DEMOGRAPHIC CONTEXT AND ACCESS TO PSYCHOLOGICAL THERAPY FOR OLDER PEOPLE

POPULATION ageing is unprecedented in the whole of human history (United Nations (UN) 2011). In July 2011, the world population peaked at 6.97 billion persons with close to 810 million aged 60 years and above. By 2050, the global population aged over 60 years will be two billion, representing 22% of the global population (UNFPA 2012). As the total population is projected to reach nine billion persons this means within the span of a single lifetime, over one-fifth of the world's population will be aged 60 years and above. This currently equates to two people celebrating their 60th birthday every second around the globe (UNFPA 2012).

Never before has the world witnessed the levels of longevity that people are achieving now, with virtually all nations experiencing growth in the relative numbers of older people within the population (Kinsella and Wan 2009). Although the relative numbers of older people is largest in developed societies, the developing world is witnessing the fastest progression of population ageing (UNFPA 2012). The demographic challenge is that while the developed world grew rich before it grew old, the developing world is growing old before it has had the chance to grow rich (Kinsella and Wan 2009). Meanwhile the US, still relatively young by the standards of Europe, is on the threshold of a boom in its older population, as the first of the baby boomers turned 65 in 2011 (Wan et al. 2005). By 2040, one in five people in North America will be aged 65 years (Kinsella and Wan 2009).

The oldest-old section of society is increasing the fastest. For example, in the UK in 1970, there were 1180 centenarians alive, whereas this figure increased almost twelve-fold to 12 640 in 2010 (ONS 2011). By mid 2040, according to UK population projections, the number of centenarians alive in the UK is estimated to reach 160 000 persons, a more than twelve-fold increase over 2010 figures (ONS 2011). These statistics are repeated in many other countries globally.

A consequence of demographic change is that many more psychotherapists will likely be expected to provide psychological therapy to and with older people seeking help. In all probability, the issues older people bring into therapy will change as longevity increases (Laidlaw and Pachana 2011; Laidlaw 2013a).

Contrary to many clinician's beliefs, rates of depression in older people are lower than one might expect when taking account of the challenges people can face as they age (Sadavoy, 2009). Blazer (2010) suggests lower rates if depression in later life can be attributed to three protective factors including enhanced emotion regulation competence, increased wisdom over a lifespan and resilience with older people coping better with stressful events as these are experienced as being 'on time'.

The need to consider the psychological needs of older people as distinct and specialist is recognized by the Department of Health (NHS England) commissioning a new older adult indicative curriculum for low- and high-intensity CBT therapists working in Increasing Access to Psychological Therapy (IAPT) services in England and also by the recent nascent development of specialist postgraduate training in CBT with older people in the UK (see Davies 2011 for an interesting perspective on increasing access to evidence-based psycho-logical therapy with older people).

The oldest-old are likely to be much higher consumers of healthcare and this may have important implications for healthcare models of provision. Similarly, CBT therapists coming into contact with the oldest-old have to take account of comorbidity, continuity of problems, chronicity of psychological and physical conditions (Sadavoy 2009). Therapists may be con-fronted with belief systems (cohort beliefs) that are out of step with their own when working with the oldest-old (Knight, 2004). Therefore the application of CBT and how we augment our treatment models to improve outcome is going to become a more crucially important issue. Consequently, psychotherapists coming into contact with older people in their practice may wish to appraise themselves of geropsychology competences (Karel, Gatz, and Smyer 2012; Knight et al. 2009). Engaging effectively with older people entails identifying and challeng-ing *erroneous* age-related negative cognitions (e.g. growing older is depressing) that may seem understandable and factual to people who are depressed, or otherwise realistic to therapists inexperienced in working with older people (Laidlaw and McAlpine 2008; Laidlaw 2013b).

Knight and colleagues (2009) helpfully summarize the competences and knowledge base that practitioners may require when working with older people. This paper is commonly known as the Pike's Peak model for training, as the group met to discuss these competencies in the valley below Pike's Peak in Colorado. Four broad areas of professional practice define the work of professionals specializing in work with older people: roots in lifespan develop-ment, knowledge of psychopathology in later life, understanding chronic medical comor-bidity and age-specific environmental contexts (Karel et al. 2012; Molinari 2011).

ACCESSING PSYCHOLOGICAL THERAPY FOR OLDER PEOPLE

Despite psychotherapy generally, and more specifically CBT, proving its worth as a treat-ment for late-life depression and anxiety, older people under-utilize mental health services

(Crabb and Hunsley 2006). Contrary to popular misconceptions, older people hold positive attitudes towards seeking help for mental health problems (MacKenzie et al. 2008).

When asked, older people rate psychotherapy for depression as acceptable and as effective as medication but with much fewer side-effects (more than half expect side-effects with medication but fewer than one in ten older people expect this for psychotherapies; Kuruvilla et al. 2006). If given a choice, older people prefer to receive psychotherapeutic treatments rather than psychotropic medication; nevertheless, older people are less likely to receive this option (Gum et al. 2006). Perhaps this may be explained by older people who seek out psychological help having to discuss treatment options with healthcare professionals lacking training in ageing and geriatrics (Burroughs et al. 2006: Murray et al. 2006). This may prove to be a substantial barrier in a number of ways. There may be a lack of awareness amongst primary care providers about levels of late-life depression and anxiety (Mitchell, Rao, and Vaze 2011), with less understanding of the existence of efficacious psychological treatments with older people, as well as reticence to investigate emotional distress in older people for fear of opening a 'pandora's box' of complex and challenging scenarios they fear being ill equipped to manage (Unutzer et al. 1999). Another explanation is that GPs are somewhat reticent to use terms like 'depression' with older people for fear of causing upset, partly because they assume older people are more concerned with somatic complaints than psychological symptoms. In an interesting and thoughtful evaluation, Murray et al. (2006) note that while GPs do not consider depression to be a normal consequence of ageing, most consider depression to be an understandable consequence of distressing experiences associated with later life.

Health professionals inexperienced in working with older people may also endorse more negative beliefs about ageing where depression is seen as 'justifiable' and 'understandable' (Burroughs et al. 2006). In a process described as the 'fallacy of good reasons' (Unutzer et al. 1999: 235), poor treatment outcomes are expected, as healthcare providers misattribute depression symptoms to be a consequence of ageing, with the effect that distress is normalized and diminished. It is possible that such a viewpoint will discount psychological therapies as a viable treatment option. Therapeutic nihilism endorsed by professionals may also find resonance in the beliefs of depressed older people themselves, as depressed older people attributing their depression to ageing were less likely to seek treatment for it (Sarkisian, Lee-Henderson, and Mangione 2003).

Given the foregoing, there is much need for geropsychologists using psychotherapy to engage with services and referrers to increase awareness of the availability of services and for older people to have better access to evidence-based treatment (Boddington 2011).

EFFICACY OF CBT WITH OLDER PEOPLE: A SHORT CONTEMPORARY ACCOUNT

Late-life Depression

The overall conclusion about CBT with older people is that there is good evidence for its efficacy as a treatment for depression and anxiety (Pinquart, Duberstein, and Lyness 2007), although the literature on psychotherapy outcome with the oldest-old remains insufficient (Cuijpers et al. 2009). Recent randomized controlled trials (RCTs) in the UK also attest to the efficacy of CBT for late-life depression in primary care settings (Laidlaw et al. 2008; Serfaty et al. 2009). Meta-analyses and systematic reviews suggest CBT is an effective treatment approach for reducing depression in later life (Shah and Scogin 2012; Wilson, Mottram, and Vassilas 2008), while others report a statistical advantage for CBT in comparison to other forms of psychosocial intervention (Pinquart et al. 2007). Overall, a consensus has emerged that CBT is a most efficacious treatment approach with older people (Laidlaw 2013b).

In the main, some general conclusions about the efficacy of CBT for late-life depression can be reached. They are outlined below (taken from Laidlaw 2013b):

- Evidence for the efficacy of CBT in late-life depression is stronger than for other forms of therapy, but there are insufficient studies of optimal quality to conclude definitively that CBT is superior to other forms of psychological therapy in older people.
- Individual CBT treatment appears to be superior to group CBT interventions.
- CBT appears comparable in efficacy to medication, in terms of both treatment outcome and dropout, but data are small as this comparison has rarely been directly tested under controlled conditions with older people with depression.
- There are limited data examining the effect of combination treatments (i.e. CBT plus medication vs medication or CBT alone) in late-life depression, and this is an area that needs further focus.
- CBT is as efficacious with older people as with working-age adults but the literature on psychotherapy outcome with the oldest-old remains insufficient since many of the earlier outcome studies tended to recruit very 'young-old' participants. The changing nature of demographics means this data may no longer be appropriate.
- Many of the earlier psychotherapy and CBT outcome studies tended to report data on completer samples rather than use intention to treat (ITT) designs, and hence results may be less conservative than would be optimal. Recent CBT outcome studies have reported efficacious outcomes when using ITT designs.

Late-life Anxiety

The evidence base for CBT for late-life anxiety suggests this treatment is efficacious but may not be as efficacious as with adults of working age, although this has not yet been established conclusively. Cognitive-behaviour therapy for generalized anxiety disorder (GAD) is twice as effective with adults of working age compared to older people, with attrition rates in GAD treatment trials twice as high in older people (Gorenstein and Papp 2007).

There have been a number of clinical trials in recent years, but these have tended to be conducted in the US and the evidence may need translation for it to be more directly applicable in NHS settings in the UK. There is a great deal of heterogeneity of CBT outcome studies looking at late-life anxiety, with some studies comparing CBT to an active control and others comparing CBT to a waiting list comparison. There is also a problem with the methodological quality of a number of the US-based anxiety outcome studies, as they have tended to recruit younger, relatively resource-rich participants. The applicability of the current data is therefore called into question.

In the main, criticisms of recent clinical trials focus on the following points:

- CBT appears less effective with older people in comparison to working-age adults (Gorenstein and Papp 2007).
- Treatment trials more commonly utilize group-based approaches than individualized treatment (Gorenstein and Papp 2007; Wetherell, Lenze, and Stanley 2005), despite indications that participants in group-based CBT for GAD are more likely to drop out of treatment (Hunot et al. 2007). This may dilute efficacy and appears inconsistent with working-age research studies.
- Many current RCTs are small, use younger, relatively healthy, and well-educated older adults, and appear to report completer data rather than intention-to-treat data (Hunot et al. 2007; Wetherell et al. 2005).
- Most trials have focused on GAD with much less concentration on simple phobias, obsessive compulsive disorder (OCD), post-traumatic stress disorder (PTSD), and Parkinson's disease (PD) (Wetherell et al. 2005; Wolitzky-Taylor et al. 2010).

DEPRESSION AND ANXIETY IN DEMENTIA

Many psychological therapists have shied away from working with older people with dementia as they assume that such clients will be unable to engage in the process of therapy. This is often a naive assumption, as many people diagnosed with dementia in the early stages will retain enough insight and enough capacity to engage in therapy and potentially benefit. The clinical literature on psychological treatment with people with dementia is rather sparse; however, a thoughtful review is provided by Bonder (1994), who recommends a sessional focus on post-diagnostic stress management, enhancing coping strategies, affirming the person's sense of identity, providing individualized support, affording expression of emotion, and restoring a sense of order by enhancing the person's intellectual abilities through retaining a sense of mastery. This approach is sympathetic and compatible with a CBT perspective.

An RCT comparing a brief psychodynamically oriented interpersonal psychotherapy (six sessions in total) to treatment as usual reported little benefit to participants (Burns et al. 2005). This finding is inconsistent with other psychotherapy studies, in which psychotherapy has been employed to good effect. An explanation for the lack of effect may be found in how brief this intervention was. It seems at odds with a clinical picture of, one would assume, a magnified level of complexity for depression and anxiety, to reduce treatment beyond that for a more 'standard' presentation of depression.

Evidence for the efficacy of CBT in anxiety and depression in dementia comes from a range of small intriguing clinical trials and case studies. In a small clinical trial by Koder (1998), CBT was shown to be promising with good outcome achieved in two individuals with moderate dementia and anxiety disorders. Scholey and Woods (2003) report a series of seven case studies of non-modified CBT for depression in dementia. The results were somewhat mixed, with two out of the seven participants evidencing clinically significant improvement in mood using standardized mood scales. Nonetheless, this provides a lot of optimism regarding the potential efficacy and utility of CBT for people with dementia.

More recently, a series of cases studies has shown that a modified and simplified CBT approach that recruited and trained family members to act as collateral therapists may hold promise for anxiety disorders in dementia. This treatment emphasizes active self-monitoring by the clients (i.e. keeping a notebook handy to remember homework tasks, enhanced use of checklists to remain oriented; Kraus et al. 2009). There is a stronger reliance on change through behaviour rather than cognitive means (e.g. less use of thought challenging) and specific strategies are employed to enhance recall (such as use of cues and other retrieval-based strategies). A small open trial of this intervention has produced positive results, although there remains a need for a more systematic evaluation (Paukert et al. 2010).

Other innovative approaches that are based on CBT include problem adaptation therapy (PATH: Kiosses et al. 2011), a twelve-session home-delivered intervention based on problem-solving therapy (a derivation of CBT) that again utilizes the primary care-giver as a collateral therapist. At the moment this intervention is in its early stages, with case studies reporting good outcome.

THE APPLICATION OF CBT WITH OLDER PEOPLE

Cognitive-behaviour therapy with older people is an active, directive, time-limited, and structured treatment approach whose primary aim is symptom reduction (Laidlaw et al. 2003). The most common form of CBT used in the UK is based upon the Beck et al. (1979) cognitive model of dysfunctional information processing in emotional disorders. CBT retains a strong scientific identity and lends itself especially well to evaluation and delivery by treatment protocols. Central to the application of CBT for people with depression or anxiety is the concept that an individual's appraisal of their experience, rather than the experience itself, is what determines its impact. This approach in CBT can be summed up by the writings of Greek philosophers such as Epictetus, who wrote, 'Men are disturbed not by things, but by the views which they take of them.'

CBT aims to be empowering of individuals and seeks to promote self-agency as it adopts a non-pathologizing stance to understanding how a client's problems may have developed. As such it can be a very attractive form of therapy for older people, who often endorse strong cohort beliefs about personal independence and problem-solving. To do CBT well requires great skill and ingenuity; one must be scientific and approachable and accessible. The goal is for clients to become their own therapists.

CBT is a uniquely structured format of psychological therapy. Each CBT session should share the same elements. These include agenda setting, review of previous homework tasks, focus on current problems/session targets involving both cognitive restructuring and behavioural experiments, and ending of session after agreement of new homework tasks. CBT can be differentiated from other forms of psychotherapy by its emphasis on the empirical investigation of the client's thoughts, appraisals, inferences, and assumptions (Laidlaw 2013a, 2013c).

CBT explicitly uses cognitive (thought monitoring and challenging) *and* behavioural (activity scheduling, graded exposure, etc.) techniques to help an individual confront their

---

Box 29.1 Philosophy value and practice in CBT

CBT can be differentiated from other forms of psychotherapy by the following elements:

- Sessions are structured according to an agenda.
- Collaborative empiricism is emphasized throughout treatment.
- Negative idiosyncratic interpretations are hypotheses requiring empirical testing.
- Homework tasks are essential to generalize learning outside of the session and to promote a sense of personal agency.
- The primary means of exploration is Socratic questioning, although...
- CBT is more a 'doing cure' than a 'talking cure' (enduring change comes from the client doing things differently).
- Interventions are linked to individualized case-conceptualizations.

---

primary presenting problems in a more systematic and effective way. The model of working in CBT with older people is that the therapist takes on the role of a 'coach', encouraging the client to try new ways to approach old problems, rather than an 'expert' who tells a client what to do. CBT is particularly appropriate as a treatment for the psychological problems and challenges experienced by older adults because it is skills enhancing, present-oriented, problem-focused, straightforward to use, and effective. Additionally, CBT is empowering of individuals as they learn new ways to cope with what may be old problems recurring over many years, and as such it can be effective in increasing positive affect as well as reducing negative affect (Laidlaw 2010).

THREE-PHASE MODEL OF TREATMENT IN CBT

Typically, CBT has at least three treatment phases: early, middle, and late (Laidlaw et al. 2003; Laidlaw 2010; Laidlaw 2013b; Laidlaw & Thompson, 2008). In the early phase of therapy, socialization of clients into the cognitive model and to the structure of sessions is very important. During this phase of therapy, gaining an understanding of the nature of the severity, frequency, and intensity of problems within the idiosyncratic point of view of the client is essential for developing a strong therapeutic alliance. How well understood clients feel by their therapist may be very important in the early stages of engagement with therapy.

While the famous quotation from Beck applies, i.e. that the therapeutic relationship is, 'Necessary but not sufficient' (Beck et al. 1979: 45), the nature of the relationship and the trust we engender in our therapy sessions is going to be important in determining how much our clients are willing to challenge themselves towards growth during treatment (Dryden 2012). It is also during the early phase of treatment that a lot of time is dedicated towards psychoeducation so that the client is able to approach their problems from a fresh perspective. At the end of the first phase of treatment, the therapist may be in a position to develop an initial conceptualization, or formulation, and present this interim understanding to the client. A formulation is a basic theory of the client's rules for living, understandings of the

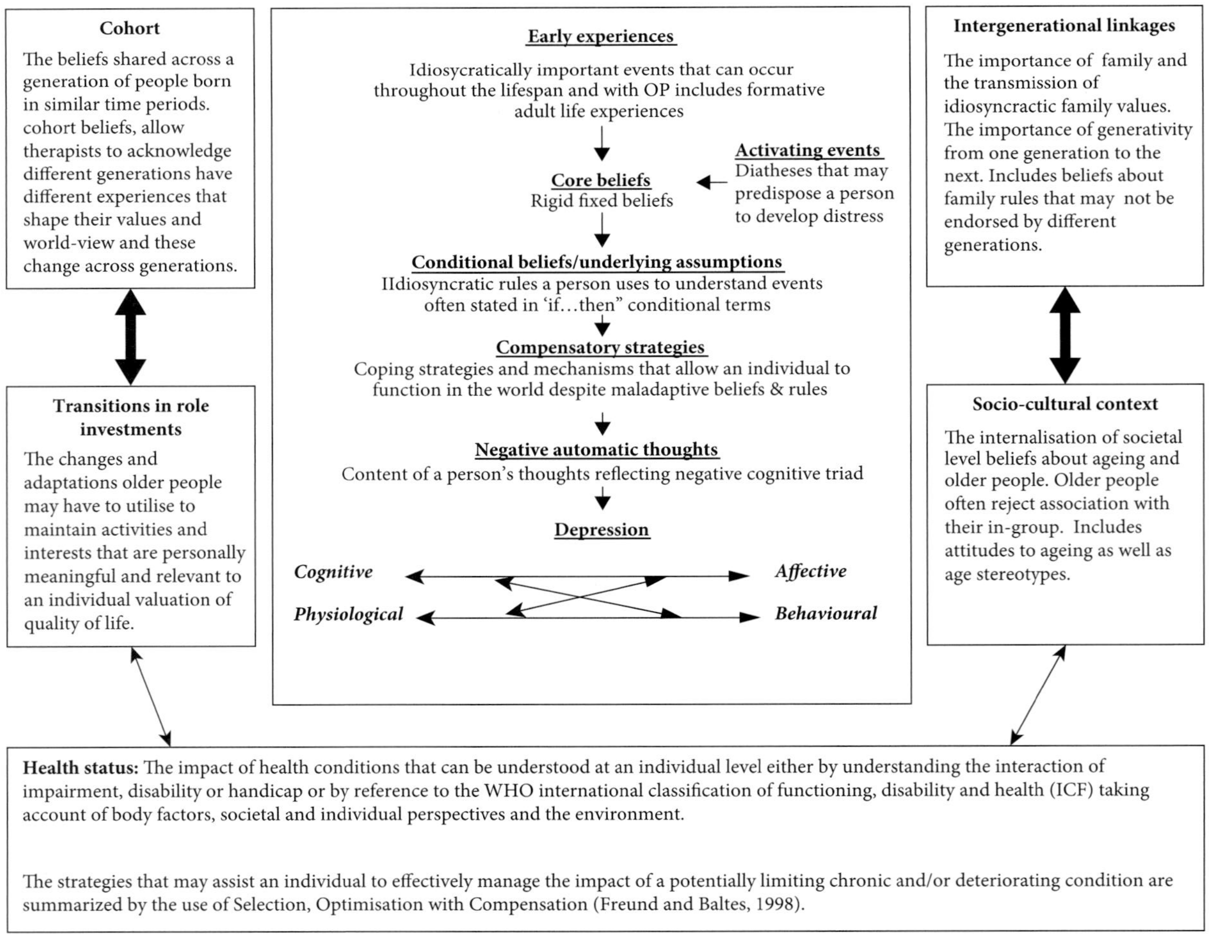

Intergenerational linkages

The importance of family and the transmission of idiosyncratic family values. The importance of generativity from one generation to the next. Includes beliefs about family rules that may not be endorsed by different generations.

Socio-cultural context

The internalisation of societal level beliefs about ageing and older people. Older people often reject association with their in-group. Includes attitudes to ageing as well as age stereotypes.

Early experiences

Idiosycratically important events that can occur throughout the lifespan and with OP includes formative adult life experiences

Activating events

Diatheses that may predispose a person to develop distress

Core beliefs

Rigid fixed beliefs

Conditional beliefs/underlying assumptions

Idiosyncratic rules a person uses to understand events often stated in "if...then" conditional terms

Compensatory strategies

Coping strategies and mechanisms that allow an individual to function in the world despite maladaptive beliefs & rules

Negative automatic thoughts

Content of a person's thoughts reflecting negative cognitive triad

Depression

Cognitive

Affective

Behavioural

Physiological

Cohort

The beliefs shared across a generation of people born in similar time periods. cohort beliefs, allow therapists to acknowledge different generations have different experiences that shape their values and world-view and these change across generations.

Transitions in role investments

The changes and adaptations older people may have to utilise to maintain activities and interests that are personally meaningful and relevant to an individual valuation of quality of life.

Health status: The impact of health conditions that can be understood at an individual level either by understanding the interaction of impairment, disability or handicap or by reference to the WHO international classification of functioning, disability and health (ICF) taking account of body factors, societal and individual perspectives and the environment.

The strategies that may assist an individual to effectively manage the impact of a potentially limiting chronic and/or deteriorating condition are summarized by the use of Selection, Optimisation with Compensation (Freund and Baltes, 1998).

FIGURE 29.1 Comprehensive Cognitive Formulation for CBT with older people (CCF).

world, appreciation of their own and other's motivations that assist in understanding how the current stressors in an individual's life are linked to depressive or anxious symptomatology. Understanding how an individual makes sense of their experience means understanding that individual in context. This may be in the context of their relationships with others or their relationship with themselves. With older people this can often mean that the CBT needs to be augmented by factors that influence people's experience of ageing (Laidlaw and McAlpine 2008; Laidlaw 2013c).

In the middle phase of therapy, the focus turns to the identification and restructuring of maladaptive cognitions termed negative automatic thoughts (NATs). In CBT, the specificity hypothesis suggests that the content of negative thoughts is different depending upon whether the client is depressed, anxious, or has psychosis. Thus therapists need to focus not only upon cognitive processing errors but also upon content errors when clients describe their current problems. In depression, content of thoughts are to do with perceived failings, and in anxiety, content of thoughts is to do with sense of threat and danger. Laidlaw (2010) has suggested that there may be age-related negative cognitions of which therapists should be aware when working with older people.

An example of age-related NAT comes from Mrs Rogers. She is a 74-year-old widow living on her own. She blames a lot of her problems on the fact that she is old now. She warns the therapist working with her that growing old is every bit as bad as she had feared and she is constantly reminded of how much her mother had told her that being old was unpleasant. Mrs Rogers considers her main problems to be caused by her age and wonders about whether it is worth living as it (life) is only likely to get worse as she gets older.

She explains 'ageing is a terrible experience' and warns the therapist that once age set in there was not a lot of joy in life. She states that she rarely smiles or laughs now and often feels on the verge of tears for no apparent reason. She also says, 'I forget a lot of things now. When I start talking I forget what I was going to say.'

Mrs Rogers goes on to say, 'I do a lot of sitting and not a lot of doing. I take a long time to get ready to go out now. When I do go out, I often can't be bothered and wish I were back home.' She also notes that she avoids people because 'If people talk to me, I cannot bear to answer them. I want to run away. I don't have the same interest [in people] as I had before. Sometimes I take the phone off the hook. I am more introverted now.' Finally she said, 'When I look in the mirror I just want to pack it in.'

Contained in this statement are a number of different age-related negative thoughts, such as that ageing is a terrible experience and that she forgets a lot of things now. These types of thought are conveyed by a powerful sense of conviction on the part of Mrs Rogers. It can seem disrespectful for therapists to attempt to dispute these statements as thoughts to be tested out for their veracity and utility. However, unless a therapist is able to understand that for the majority of older people this is neither factual nor true, they may become passive in helping Mrs Rogers to overcome her depression, and her hopelessness within it. In this example, using cognitive content strategies (e.g. what is the evidence for this thought?, what is an alternative way to think about this?. etc.) is unlikely to be successful. To Mrs Rogers her perception is that her current situation is not as bad as it gets, but unfortunately as good as it gets (and that's not good). This means that she will be very challenging for a therapist to work with and they may become as demoralized as their client. It is recommended that the therapist works with Mrs Rogers to reframe her cognitions. The data Mrs Rogers cites as evidence can actually be reframed as depression symptoms, and depression is a more changeable target than ageing.

In this phase of therapy, behavioural experiments are discussed within sessions and plans are made for understandings to be translated into practice exercises and completed as homework. As many older people will have successfully met and dealt with adversity throughout their lives, CBT provides a means of rediscovering old skills and competences that may have been forgotten by the client (Laidlaw 2013c).

As CBT is skills enhancing, clients are taught self-monitoring skills to identify thoughts that are associated with negative mood and maladaptive behavioural response (Laidlaw et al. 2003). Identifying and challenging negative automatic thoughts is termed cognitive restructuring and a common method of doing this is to use a dysfunctional thought record (DTR).

DTRs can be poorly complied with in therapy and sometimes they are used too soon. Asking your client to monitor, record, and challenge thoughts requires a very complex set of skills. As a minimum, it requires an individual to be reflective about their thoughts. Very often clients find the process of identifying thoughts in a specific testable way challenging. The requirement to record thoughts as verbatim as possible is also a challenging skill to develop. When asking clients to record their thought on diary forms, the difficulty is often far more than that of an individual finding it hard to write down their thoughts. Often thoughts are mixed up with affect and in the early stages clients can be quite confused in completing DTRs. As a rule, it is recommended that the therapist approaches the use of DTRs as a skill to be built up gradually in their client. This can usefully and more effectively be achieved when simpler formats of DTRs are used as interim steps. It is important to spend time within the session to help the client realize the skill of completing DTRs for them to achieve the full benefit of this intervention. Thoughts being recorded in a DTR ought to have the following characteristics:

- They should be specific and focused, often describing a discrete and identifiable situation that has provoked a strong emotional response.
- Emotions should be clearly identified with the event/situation and the associated thought.
- Thoughts ought to be written as close to verbatim as possible (in practice, the therapist may capture a negative thought by the patient in session and model the completion of a diary by writing their verbatim thought in the appropriate column in the DTR).
- Responses or challenges to the negative automatic thought should also be specific and focused and linked to the negative thought. They ought to reflect a more compassionate or helpful response.
- They ought to be a thought or response that the patient is happy to endorse. The response should result in a reduction in negative affect.

When helping people identify and challenge negative automatic thoughts, guided discovery can be useful. Guided discovery is a process of having a client mentally 'retrace their steps' when recalling an event that elicits strong emotion. All aspects of the distressing situation are recalled in order for the client to access thoughts or images they experienced prior to a change in their emotional state. The therapist can model the completion of a diary form by writing parts of the diary in the relevant sections (situation, thoughts, feelings, etc.) in front of the client and then discussing the usefulness of this technique. Guided discovery is often discussed in connection with a procedure known as *Socratic questioning*. Socratic questioning usually involves asking a patient a series of open-ended questions that facilitate meaning understanding and reveal maladaptive thought patterns.

In the final phase of therapy, two main tasks remain to be accomplished: (1) the agreement of an appropriate termination point for therapy and (2) the elaboration of a relapse prevention plan. Endings in CBT have often been minimized because of the de-emphasis of the importance of the therapist–client relationship (Ochoa and Muran 2008). However, for many people, sometimes including the therapist, deciding when to stop treatment is a big decision. It can be important to allow the client to have as much input into the ending as is possible once the final number of sessions has been agreed.

Michael was seen by his therapist for a long time, as he had experienced a number of loss experiences and age-related challenges that had changed the emphasis and goals for therapy. When discharge was agreed and set, Michael completed a relapse prevention diary, but also wrote a more personal 'end-of-term report' that outlined what he had gained in therapy and what he would miss. This is what he found helpful about therapy: 'always debating, and finding alternatives, never criticizing. Most of all the opportunity to talk and debate to an agenda that was always stimulating and intelligent.'

It can be useful when working with clients to discuss prior to the end of therapy what they have learned from therapy and how this may prepare them for dealing with any setbacks they may experience in the future. The therapist works with the client to anticipate how they might respond to certain stressors and to imagine possible strategies they may employ to help them manage. It may be helpful to role-play some of the identifiable challenges with the person prior to discharge. When role-playing, the therapist should take on the role of the client and the client can either act as the therapist or as a person being challenging to them in imagined stressful situations.

Many therapists are uncertain when therapy has reached a natural point for ending to be discussed. Jakobsons et al. (2007) have identified seven criteria that guide the decision as to whether therapists have reached the point at which the client can be discharged from therapy. However, a more parsimonious guide is provided by Ochoa and Muran (2008: 201): 'CBT ends when the goals of therapy identified at the beginning of treatment are met, and the patient has acquired the tools by which to function as his or her own therapist when future difficulties arise.'

It is not always possible to achieve a good ending, and sometimes endings with a client are agreed because they achieved insufficient progress despite the best efforts of both parties. In these circumstances, the therapist needs to ensure that ending in therapy is carried out as much as possible in tandem with the client's wishes. In such cases, the therapist ought to work with the client to agree possible options and make arrangements for follow-on treatment before therapy ends.

Age-appropriate Models of CBT with Older People

It is frequently asked whether therapists working with older people need to consider modifications to ensure CBT is maximally effective and applicable with older people. Modifications may be indicated and may be required in order to address normal age-related changes such as the presence of physical frailty or changes to cognitive processing and status (Grant and Casey 1995). Modifications to a treatment model are intended to enhance treatment outcome but seek to remain consistent with the values and core philosophy of the therapy modality (i.e. CBT), whereas adaptations are intended to alert clinicians to the possibility that the treatment model they have chosen may be inadequate for the circumstances or the population with which they intend to apply this model (Laidlaw 2013b). While there may be clinical necessity for the former in some instances, the evidence for the latter is still lacking.

In some regard, modifications could be said to be unnecessary as outcome studies of CBT for late-life depression have, by and large, applied standard models of CBT with relatively good outcome (Cuijpers et al. 2009). One cannot prescribe modifications to an already efficacious treatment approach solely on the basis of chronological age as this rarely provides the best basis for understanding or a particularly accurate description of an individual's difficulties or health status. Nevertheless, older people are part of a heterogeneous population that contains up to four different generations, and therefore the need for modifications may become more acute as mental health professionals work with much older clients than ever before.

Current models of CBT may need to take account of demographic changes so as to maximize therapeutic outcomes by augmenting CBT outcome with gerontological theory, as this provides for a conceptual approach to enhancing age-appropriate CBT treatment models. Possible 'candidate' theories from gerontology that may augment CBT with older people and are consistent with the values and orientation of CBT are theories focusing on optimal ageing (selection, optimization with compensation; Freund and Baltes 1998) that advocate an active problem-focused positive approach to meeting the challenges of ageing. Theories of negative age stereotypes that are long-held vulnerabilities that older people may have internalized from a younger age can act much like a stress-diathesis in the development of problems in later life (Laidlaw 2010, 2013b). Mrs Rogers' problems earlier on in this chapter can be understood as an internalization of negative age stereotypes (see Levy 2009; stereotype-embodiment theory). Finally, when working with older people who have a chronic history of depression, this can result in older people developing a negative narrative of themselves as weak or as failures.

Wisdom is a meta-theory in gerontology and it is a convenient 'vehicle for change' in CBT as it is a positively endorsed attribute of ageing consistent with the valuing, collaborative, and respectful philosophy of CBT (Knight and Laidlaw 2009). More theoretically, Baltes and colleagues (see Baltes and Smith 2008) characterize wisdom as representing the operation of expert knowledge about the conduct and planning of life. Importantly, wisdom is not simply intelligence but requires more complex interplay between intelligence, intuition, and pragmatic procedural strategies. This model of wisdom is a good fit with the Beck model of cognitive therapy.

In order for one to become wise, there is a need for a rich factual knowledge base as well as enriched procedural knowledge in order to know how to apply one's factual knowledge in ways that are helpful (Baltes and Smith 2008). This is akin to psychoeducation within CBT. In order for people to be wise about depression they need to understand it and understand how to apply their knowledge in helpful ways for their own benefit (Laidlaw 2013a, 2013c).

A useful technique for the therapist to employ when understanding an individual's personal narrative over the course of their lifetime without getting overwhelmed with negative recall is to ask clients to construct a 'timeline' within therapy (Laidlaw 2010. This allows important events to be highlighted. The timeline can be located on a vertical line that connects the client's birthdate at the start of the timeline with the current date at the end of the timeline, drawn as horizontal lines at either extreme end of the vertical timeline. The therapist should try to note down the client's strengths and resilience in difficult times throughout his/her life (Laidlaw 2013c). These should be brought to the attention of the client, so as to help empower them to deal with other current stressors. By employing this simple technique, the therapist gains an 'edited' and highly idiosyncratic summary of the high and low points of an individual's life.

The position advocated here is a simple and traditional idea within CBT: In order to enhance possibilities for treatment outcome in CBT, the person does not need to change to fit the model; the model needs to change to fit the person to ensure maximal effectiveness (Laidlaw 2013a, 2013c). CBT theorists have always focused on the development of theory-driven models to aid treatment. What is advocated here is that intervention strategies focused upon a problem-solving, explorative approach to understanding problems are retained, but the use of these strategies is contextualized in an age-appropriate conceptual frame of reference. In so doing, a wider canvas for considering interventions is drawn on in CBT with older people. Looking at the individual's level of beliefs and attributions about problems and possibility for change may be influenced by the individual's own beliefs about ageing. Thus, if a person believes themselves to have few remaining good years of life, their level of passivity and hopelessness will increase and a belief in the possibility of change may be reduced. For these reasons the augmentation of the cognitive theory of CBT with gerontology theories is likely to enhance treatment outcome. Interested readers can see a fuller elaboration of these concepts in Laidlaw (2013c).

An obvious place to start when considering an augmented approach to CBT that is age appropriate is to develop an age-appropriate formulation that takes account of the different experiences of older people and contextualizes a more nuanced approach to understanding the challenges of depression and anxiety in later life. Psychologists use the term *formulation* to describe the process of integrating knowledge of the person, their background, their culture, and their current circumstances (Persons 2008). Formulation can guide the selection of and focus of interventions in CBT (Kuyken, Padesky, and Dudley 2009). Formulation is a clinical theory pertaining to an individual linking the overt nature of symptoms presented with an acknowledgement that underlying, or covert, issues may explain long-standing vulnerability to the development of problems or the persistent and recurrent nature of presenting problems within the individual's own lifespan development.

Depression in later life may not necessarily be different symptomatologically in comparison to depression in adults of working age, but in order to work most effectively with older people it may be necessary to make use of a contextualization framework or specific formulation mode for CBT with older people (Laidlaw et al. 2004). There may be age-specific developmental factors to take into account when working with older people because loss (either through bereavement or loss of health) is a common experience in ageing that impacts upon the quality and quantity of social networks. In the experience of therapists working with older people, depression treatment can be complicated by the fact that the client may be the last surviving member of their age cohort (sociocultural context) and have an increased sense of their own mortality, simultaneously experiencing increased social isolation because they have diminished social capital older resources available to draw upon (Gray 2009). Thus, CBT with older people can be different with regard to the types of challenges that people may face as they age. This means that psychotherapists may need to understand a wider knowledge base around ageing, longevity, and cognitive and affective development.

The comprehensive conceptualization framework (CCF; Laidlaw et al. 2004) for CBT with older people helps therapists, particularly those inexperienced in working with older people, provide a way of framing contextualizing older adults' problems within the standard Beck model of CBT model (see Figure 29.1, Box 29.1). The main elements of the CCF are cohort beliefs, transition in role investments, inter-generational linkages, the sociocultural context, and health status. Each element serves to broaden the understanding that a therapist will draw on when working with elders. The CCF model is outlined in much more detail elsewhere (see Laidlaw et al. 2004).

The use of wisdom theories (Laidlaw 2013c) can help people become more accepting and compassionate towards themselves. Drawing on experience, and becoming 'wise' by reflecting upon and reframing narratives associated with past experiences may promote growth and potentiate the effectiveness of CBT. Wisdom retains a currency amongst many people as it constitutes a commonly understood 'folk theory' of ageing and emphasizes growth through adversity across the lifespan. It is commonly assumed that wisdom comes with age; however, wisdom is not an outcome of age per se. Personal wisdom may develop over a lifetime as individuals become adept at dealing with uncertainty and ambiguity, and responding as optimally as possible as circumstances dictate. Sternberg (2012) suggests that personal wisdom requires a desire on the part of the individual to change and to develop the skills inherent in personal wisdom—openness to experience and willingness to reflect and then to learn or profit from experience. It is personal wisdom, rather than more general wisdom, that is seen as a desirable outcome in psychotherapy with depressed or anxious older people.

Wisdom enhancement can be an important aim in CBT as it can be used to explicitly link people to their life experiences (good and bad), and thus contextualizes current episodes of depression within a lifespan perspective (Laidlaw 2013c). In adopting wisdom enhancement as a legitimate aim in the treatment of anxiety and depression in later life, the therapist encourages the client to use their past experiences to help them cope with current life challenges. Thus the here-and-now orientation of CBT is retained, as is a way of using the rich life experience of older people. As people construct personal narratives as a way of constructing meaning in relation to their life and experiences in depression, the autobiographical nature of recall becomes over-generalized and people see only failures. As people may have internalized negative self-stereotypes this may result in people erroneously considering their problems as unchangeable aspects of age (Laidlaw 2010, 2013c). If left unchallenged, personal narratives coloured by depressive affect engender a passive self-defeated perspective in an older person dealing with a current challenging episode in their life. By helping people reframe their personal narratives within CBT, resilience is acknowledged through having overcome past adversity. Thus CBT fosters positive affect while aiming to reduce negative affect.

Therefore a contemporary approach to psychotherapy with older people will be to develop an age-appropriate version of CBT that adheres to the evidence-based and theory-driven orientation of the therapy but does so in a way that results in a treatment model that equips therapists to be better placed to deal with the challenges the new cohort of older people may bring into therapy.

CONCLUSIONS

Many more therapists are likely to come into direct contact with older people as a result of the global demographic transition. When therapists work with this age group, it is important that they educate themselves about this new experience of ageing and about the new cohort of older people (Karel et al. 2012). This can be a very positive experience for therapist and client as emotional development trajectories suggest older people may be more emotionally ready to fully engage with the process of psychotherapy and more attuned to the benefits of emotional balance and flexibility.

With new cohorts of older people there may be reasons to consider whether there is a need to augment CBT by using models from the science of ageing (gerontology). If there are reasons to adapt CBT in order to augment its effectiveness with older people, this ought to be considered from a conceptual basis in order that practical and effective changes may improve the experience of therapy and its outcome. It is insufficient to suggest banal changes to therapy such as slowing sessions down, encouraging repetition of information, and ensuring that interviews are conducted in a quiet, well-ventilated, well-lit room (Laidlaw and McAlpine 2008).

There is a mature evidence base for the effectiveness of psychological treatments for older people. However, many gaps in knowledge remain and there is a need for future research into the effectiveness of psychological treatment for depression in older people in physical conditions with high levels of psychological distress, such as dementia. Many of these conditions are currently in the early stages of evaluation of efficacy in relation to psychological and physical treatments for depression. From a more personal perspective on developing evidence for psychological therapy with older people, it is exciting to see psychological researchers turning their attention to the emotional needs of people with dementia post-diagnostically. It is expected that CBT will have great potential in helping people with dementia reduce excess disability because of anxiety and depressive symptoms.

This is an interesting and stimulating time to work with older people, especially as the baby boomers are coming of age. It will be fascinating to see whether this new cohort of older people will push for more access to psychological therapies and whether they will usher in a new agenda. CBT continues to develop and mature in terms of its application with older people. This is an important endeavour because older people's needs have been ill served for too long. Perhaps this is in the process of becoming less possible, and if so there will be a greater need to train more therapists in the application of evidence-based approaches like CBT with older people. The IAPT agenda in England seems to suggest this may be a direction some policy makers may be willing to take.

KEY REFERENCES AND SOURCES FOR FURTHER READING

Useful websites and associated resources

A new curriculum for therapists working with older people is available for free at http://www.iapt.nhs.uk/workforce/iapt-older-peoples-training/.

The Department of Health (NHS England) in 2009 produced a very helpful positive practice guide to increasing access to psychological therapies with older people. It is available
online at http://www.iapt.nhs.uk/silo/files/older-people-positive-practice-guide.pdf.

The Faculty of Psychologists working with Older People in the UK, have also published a
number of helpful guides for clinicians working with older people. The Faculty now known
as FPOP (previously PSIGE) have published a comprehensive and very useful document
setting out good practice guidelines for UK clinical psychology training programmes for
training psychologists to work with older people in clinical practice. It is available online
at http://www.psige.org/public/files/PSIGE%20BPS%20Nov%202006%20Good%20
Practice%20Guidelines%20Training%20Providers.pdf.

Knight et al. (2009) and Molinari (2011) provide more in-depth analysis of the Pike's Peak
training model for clinical geropsychology competence. Additionally readers may also wish
to consult the website for the Council of Professional Geropsychology Training Programs
http://www.copgtp.org.

ADDITIONAL MAJOR SOURCES FOR FURTHER READING

Bengston, V., Silverstein, M., Putney, N. M., and Gans, D. (eds) (2008). *Handbook of Theories of
Aging* (2nd edn). New York: Springer.
Dryden, W. and Branch, R. (eds) (2011). *The CBT Handbook*. London: Sage.
NHS Education for Scotland (2011). *A Guide to Delivery of Evidence-based Psychological
Therapies in Scotland*. Edinburgh: NES.
Persons, J. B. (2008). *The Case Formulation Approach to Cognitive Behavior Therapy*.
New York: Guilford Press.
Scogin, F. and Shah, A. (eds) (2012). *Making Evidence-based Psychological Treatments Work
with Older Adults*. Washington DC: American Psychological Association.
United Nations, Department of Economic and Social Affairs, Population Division (2011). *World
Population Prospects: The 2010 Revision, Highlights and Advance Tables*. Working Paper No.
ESA/P/WP.220. New York: UN.

REFERENCES

Baltes, P. B. and Smith, J. (2008). 'The Fascination of Wisdom: Its Nature, Ontogeny, and
Function'. *Perspectives on Psychological Science* 3: 56–64.
Beck, A. T., Rush, A. J., Shaw, B. F., and Emery, G. (1979). *Cognitive Therapy of Depression*.
New York: Guilford Press.
Blazer, D. G. (2010). 'Protection from Depression'. *International Psychogeriatrics* 22: 171–173.
Boddington, S. (2011). 'Where Are All the Older People? Equality of Access to IAPT Services'.
PSIGE Newsletter 113: 11–14.
Bonder, B. R. (1994). 'Psychotherapy for Individuals with Alzheimer Disease'. *Alzheimer Disease
and Associated Disorders* 8(suppl. 3): 75–81.
Burns, A., Guthrie, E., Marino-Francis, F., Busby, C., Morris, J., et al. (2005). 'Brief Psychotherapy
in Alzheimer's Disease'. *British Journal of Psychiatry* 187: 143–147.
Burroughs, H., Lovell, K., Morley, M., Baldwin, R., Burns, A., et al. (2006). '"Justifiable
Depression": How Primary Care Professionals and Patients View Late Life Depression?
A Qualitative Study'. *Family Practice* 23: 369–377.

Crabb, R. and Hunsley, J. (2006). 'Utilization of Mental Health Care Services among Older Adults with Depression'. *Journal of Clinical Psychology* 62: 299–312.

Cuijpers, P., Van Straten, A., Smit, F., and Andersson, G. (2009). 'Is Psychotherapy for Depression Equally Effective in Younger and in Older Adults? A Meta-regression Analysis'. *International Psychogeriatrics* 21: 16–24.

Davies, S. (2011). 'IAPT and Older People: A Training Perspective'. *PSIGE Newsletter* 113: 22–24.

Dryden, W. (2012). 'The Therapeutic Relationship in CBT'. In W. Dryden and R. Branch (eds), *The CBT Handbook*. London: Sage.

Freund, A. M. and Baltes, P. B. (1998). 'Selection, Optimization, and Compensation as Strategies of Life Management: Correlations with Subjective Indicators of Successful Aging'. *Psychology and Aging* 13: 531–543.

Gorenstein, E. E. and Papp, L. A. (2007). 'Cognitive Behavior Therapy for Anxiety in the Elderly'. *Current Psychiatry Reports* 9: 20–25.

Grant, R. W. and Casey, D. A. (1995). 'Adapting Cognitive Behavioral Therapy for the Frail Elderly'. *International Psychogeriatrics* 7: 561–571.

Gray, A. (2009). 'The Social Capital of Older People'. *Aging and Society* 29: 5–31.

Gum, A., Arean, P., Hunkeler, E., Tang, L., Katon, W., et al. (2006). 'Depression Treatment Preferences in Older Primary Care Patients'. *Gerontologist* 46: 14–22.

Hunot, V., Churchill, R., Teixeira, V., and Silva de Lima, M. (2007). 'Psychological Therapies for Generalized Anxiety Disorder'. *Cochrane Database of Systematic Reviews* 1: CD001848. doi: 10.1002/14651858.CD001848.pub4.

Jakobsons, L. J., Brown, J. S., Gordon, K. H., and Joiner, T. E. (2007). 'When Are Clients Ready to Terminate?' *Cognitive & Behavioral Practice* 24(2): 218–230.

Karel, M. J., Gatz, M., and Smyer, M. A. (2012). 'Aging and Mental Health in the Decade Ahead: What Psychologists Need to Know'. *American Psychologist* 67: 184–198.

Kinsella, K. and Wan, H. (2009). *US Census Bureau, Series P95/09–1: An Aging World: 2008.* Washington DC: US Government Printing Office.

Kiosses, D., Teri, L., Velligan, D. I., and Alexopoulos, G. S. (2011). 'A Home-delivered Intervention for Depressed, Cognitively Impaired Disabled Elders'. *International Journal of Geriatric Psychiatry* 26: 256–262.

Knight, B. G. (2004). *Psychotherapy with Older Adults* (3rd edn). Thousand Oaks: Sage.

Knight, B., Karel, M. G., Hinrichsen, G. A., Qualls, S. H., and Duffy, M. (2009). 'Pikes Peak Model for Training in Professional Geropyschology'. *American Psychologist* 64: 205–214.

Knight, B. G. and Laidlaw, K. (2009). 'Translational Theory: A Wisdom-based Model for Psychological Interventions to Enhance Well-being in Later Life'. In V. Bengston, M. Silverstein, N. M. Putney, and D. Gans (eds), *Handbook of Theories of Aging* (2nd edn) (pp. 693–706). New York: Springer.

Koder, D. A. (1998). 'Treatment of Anxiety in the Cognitively Impaired Elderly: Can Cognitive-behavior Therapy Help?' *International Psychogeriatrics* 10: 173–182.

Kraus, C. A., Seignourel, P., Balasubramanyam, V., Snow, A. L., Wilson, N. L., et al. (2009). 'Cognitive-behavioral Treatment for Anxiety in Patients with Dementia: Two Case Studies'. *Journal of Psychiatric Practice* 14: 186–192.

Kuruvilla, T., Fenwick, C. D., Haque, M. S., and Vassilas, C. A. (2006). 'Elderly Depressed Patients: What Are their Views on Treatment Options?' *Aging & Mental Health* 10: 204–206.

Kuyken, W., Padesky, C. A., and Dudley, R. (2009). *Collaborative Case Conceptualization.* New York: Guilford Press.

Laidlaw, K., Thompson, L. W., Siskin-Dick, L., and Gallagher-Thompson, D. (2003). *Cognitive Behavioural Therapy with Older People*. Chichester: Wiley.

Laidlaw, K., Thompson, L., and Gallagher-Thompson, D. (2004). 'Comprehensive Conceptualisation of Cognitive Behaviour Therapy for Late Life Depression'. *Behavioural & Cognitive Psychotherapy* 32, 389–399.

Laidlaw, K., Davidson, K. M., Toner, H. L., Jackson, G., Clark, S., et al. (2008). 'A Randomised Controlled Trial of Cognitive Behaviour Therapy versus Treatment as Usual in the Treatment of Mild to Moderate Late Life Depression'. *International Journal of Geriatric Psychiatry* 23: 843–850.

Laidlaw, K. and McAlpine, S. (2008). 'Cognitive-behaviour Therapy: How Is It Different with Older People?' *Journal of Rational Emotive Cognitive Behaviour Therapy* 26(4): 250–262.

Laidlaw, K. and Thompson, L. W. (2008). 'Cognitive Behaviour Therapy with Older People'. In K. Laidlaw and B. G. Knight (eds), *Handbook of the Assessment and Treatment of Emotional Disorders in Later Life* (pp. 91–116). Oxford: Oxford University Press.

Laidlaw, K. (2010). 'Are Attitudes to Ageing and Wisdom Enhancement Legitimate Targets for CBT for Late Life Depression?' *Nordic Psychology* 62(2): 27–42.

Laidlaw, K. and Pachana, N. A. (2011). 'CE Corner: Aging with Grace'. *Monitor on Psychology* 42(10): 66–71.

Laidlaw, K. (2013a). 'A Deficit in Psychotherapeutic Care for Older People with Depression and Anxiety'. *Gerontology* 59: 549–556.

Laidlaw, K. (2013b). 'Depression in Older People: Cognitive Behaviour Therapy, Evidence & Practice'. In M. J. Power (ed.), *Mood Disorders: A Handbook of Science and Practice* (2nd edn) (pp. 463–484). Chichester: Wiley.

Laidlaw, K. (2013c). 'Self-Acceptance and Aging: Using Self-acceptance as a Mediator of Change in CBT with Depressed and Anxious Older People'. In M. E. Bernard (ed.), *The Strength of Self-acceptance* (pp. 263–280). Melbourne: Springer.

Levy, B. R. (2009). 'Stereotype Embodiment: A Psychosocial Approach to Aging'. *Current Directions in Psychological Science* 18: 332–336.

MacKenzie, C., Scott, T., Mather, A., and Sareen, J. (2008). 'Older Adults' Help-seeking Attitudes and Treatment Beliefs Concerning Mental Health Problems'. *American Journal of Geriatric Psychiatry* 16: 1010–1019.

Mitchell, A. J., Rao, S., and Vaze, A. (2011). 'Can General Practitioners Identify People with Distress and Mild Depression? A Meta Analysis of Clinical Accuracy'. *Journal of Affective Disorders* 130: 26–36.

Molinari, V. (ed.) (2011). *Speciality Competences in Geropsychology*. New York: Oxford University Press.

Murray, J., Banerjee, S., Byng, R., Tylee, A., Bhugra, D., et al. (2006). 'Primary Care Professionals' Perceptions of Depression in Older People: A Qualitative Study'. *Social Science & Medicine* 63: 1363–1373.

Ochoa, E. and Muran, J. C. (2008). 'A Relational Take on Termination in Cognitive-behavioral Therapy'. In W. T. O'Donohue and M. Cucciare (eds), *Terminating Psychotherapy: A Clinician's Guide* (pp. 183–204). New York: *Routledge*.

Office of National Statistics (2011). *Estimates of Centenarians in the UK, 2010. Population Aged 100 Years and Over, UK, 1965–2010*. Statistical Bulletin. London: ONS.

Paukert, A. L., Calleo, J., Kraus-Schuman, C., Snow, L., Wilson, N., et al. (2010). 'Peaceful Mind: An Open Trial of Cognitive-behavioral Therapy for Anxiety in Persons with Dementia'. *International Psychogeriatrics* 22: 1012–1021.

Pinquart, M. and Sörensen, S. (2001). 'How Effective Are Psychotherapeutic and Other Psychoscial Interventions with Older Adults? A Meta-analysis'. *Journal of Mental Health and Aging* 7: 207–243.

Pinquart, M., Duberstein, P., and Lyness, J. (2007). 'Effects of Psychotherapy and Other Behavioural Interventions on Clinically Depressed Older Adults: A Meta Analysis'. *Aging & Mental Health* 11: 645–657.

Sadavoy, J. (2009). 'An Integrated Model for Defining the Scope of Psychogeriatrics: The Five Cs'. *International Psychogeriatrics* 21: 805–812.

Sarkisian, C. A., Lee-Henderson, M. H., and Mangione, C. M. (2003). 'Do Depressed Older Adults Who Attribute Depression to "Old Age" Believe It Is Important to Seek Care?' *Journal of General Internal Medicine* 18: 1001–1005.

Scholey, K. A. and Woods, B. T. (2003). 'A Series of Brief Cognitive Therapy Interventions with People Experiencing both Dementia and Depression'. *Clinical Psychology and Psychotherapy* 10: 175–185.

Serfaty, M., Haworth, D., Blanchard, M., Buszewicz, M., Murad, S., et al. (2009). 'Clinical Effectiveness of Individual Cognitive Behavioural Therapy for Depressed Older People in Primary Care'. *Archives of General Psychiatry* 66: 1332–1340.

Shah, A. and Scogin, F. (2012). 'Evidence-Based Psychological Treatments for Depression in Older Adults'. In F. Scogin and A. Shah (eds), *Making Evidence-based Psychological Treatments Work with Older Adults* (pp. 87–130). Washington, DC: American Psychological Association.

Sternberg, R. J. (2012) 'The Science of Wisdom: Implications for Psychotherapy'. In C. K. Germer and R. D. Siegel (eds), *Wisdom and Compassion in Psychotherapy: Deepening Mindfulness in Clinical Practice.* New York: Guilford Press.

United Nations, Department of Economic and Social Affairs, Population Division (2011). *World Population Prospects: The 2010 Revision, Volume II: Demographic Profiles.* ST/ESA/SER.A/317. New York: UN.

United Nations Population Fund and HelpAge International; UNFPA (2012). *Ageing in the twenty-first century: A celebration and a challenge.* New York: UNFPA.

Unutzer, J., Katon, W., Sullivan, M., and Miranda, J. (1999). 'Treating Depressed Older Adults in Primary Care: Narrowing the Gap between Efficacy and Effectiveness'. *Milbank Quarterly* 77: 225–256.

Wan, H., Segupta, M., Velkoff, V. A., and Debarros, K. A. (2005). *65+ in the United States: 2005.* US Census Bureau, Current Population Reports, P23–209. Washington, DC: US Government Printing Office.

Wetherell, J. L., Lenze, E., and Stanley, M. A. (2005). 'Evidence-based Treatment of Geriatric Anxiety Disorders'. *Psychiatric Clinics of North America* 28: 871–896.

Wilson, K., Mottram, P., and Vassilas, C. (2008). 'Psychotherapeutic Treatments for Older Depressed People'. *Cochrane Database of Systematic Reviews* 1: CD004853. doi: 10.1002/14651858.CD0044853.pub2.

Wolitzky-Taylor, K. B., Castriotta, N., Lenze, E. J., Stanley, M. A., and Craske, M. G. (2010). 'Anxiety Disorders in Older Adults: A Comprehensive Review'. *Depression and Anxiety* 27: 190–211.

CHAPTER 30

INTERPERSONAL PSYCHOTHERAPY FOR THE TREATMENT OF LATE-LIFE DEPRESSION

GREGORY A. HINRICHSEN AND MARIE-GENEVIÈVE ISELIN

INTRODUCTION

INTERPERSONAL Psychotherapy (IPT) is an evidence-based psychotherapy originally developed in the US in the 1970s for the treatment of depression. IPT has been studied in numerous clinical research investigations of depression and other mental disorders. A recent review of IPT in the treatment of depression concluded: 'There is no doubt that IPT efficaciously treats depression, both as an independent treatment and in combination with pharmacotherapy. IPT deserves its place in treatment guidelines as one of the most empirically validated treatments for depression' (Cuijpers et al. 2011: 581). Along with cognitive-behavioural therapy, IPT is recommended in the US (American Psychiatric Association 2000), the UK (National Institute for Health and Clinical Excellence 2004), and New Zealand, Australia (Ellis 2004) in depression treatment guidelines as a psychotherapeutic treatment of choice because of established efficacy. Outside of the US, IPT has been used in clinical research studies on the treatment of depression (Markowitz and Weissman 2012) including with older adults (Van Schaik et al. 2006). The International Society for Interpersonal Psychotherapy draws its membership from throughout the world (http://interpersonalpsychotherapy.org/). The versatility of IPT is evident in its utility in the treatment of both mood and non-mood disorders, varied treatment formats (individual, group, conjoint), use across the age spectrum including adolescents, adults, and older adults, and adaptation to different cultures. Notably, IPT was used in the first randomized, clinical trials of psychotherapy in Africa in the treatment of depressed Ugandan adults (Bolton et al. 2003) and adolescents (Verdeli et al. 2008). A challenge of evidence-based psychotherapies, including IPT, is that only a minority of mental healthcare professionals has been formally trained in them and they are not commonly used in clinical practice (Weissman and Sanderson 2002). This is especially true for IPT in the treatment of late-life depression where, to our knowledge, only a handful of geropsychologists in the US have received training in IPT. However, as will be discussed later, the US Department of Veterans Affairs (VA) healthcare system is currently in the process of training VA clinicians in IPT; and some mental health professionals in the UK who work with older adults have likely been trained in IPT as part of National Health Service efforts to disseminate evidence-based psychotherapies. In this chapter, we review the structure, goals, and strategies of IPT, argue that IPT is especially well-suited to older adults, briefly discuss research that supports IPT in the treatment of late-life depression, and share our experience in providing IPT to older people, and in training students to do IPT with older people. We provide two IPT clinical cases to illustrate its use with older adults.

THE ORIGINS AND STRUCTURE OF IPT

IPT was developed by Gerald Klerman, Myrna Weissman, and their colleagues. IPT was one of the first efforts to manualize a psychotherapy so that it could be implemented in clinical research trials (Weissman 2006). IPT is predicated on the assumption that interpersonally relevant life events increase vulnerability to depression, and that depression itself can seed interpersonally relevant problems. For example, Weissman and Paykel did early work on the social role (e.g., parent, spouse, homemaker) impairments associated with serious depression in women (Weissman and Paykel 1974). Notably, after the depressive episode ended, women continued to have social role impairments, suggesting that depression may have damaged relationships. A body of research prior and subsequent to the development of IPT has documented the reciprocal relationship between interpersonal events and depression including the role of family relationships in increasing or decreasing the risk of relapse into another depressive episode (Dohrenwend and Dohrenwend 1974; Hooley, Orley, and Teasdale 1986). Considerable interest in IPT developed as a research intervention following its demonstrated efficacy in the US landmark multisite clinical treatment study, the National Institute of Mental Health (NIMH) Treatment of Depression Collaborative Research Study (Elkin et al. 1989).

In the treatment of depression, IPT is conducted in sixteen weekly, individual psychotherapy sessions. The clinical treatment manual for IPT is *Comprehensive Guide to Interpersonal Psychotherapy* (Weissman, Markowitz, and Klerman 2000).

The therapeutic ethos of IPT is:

- active collaboration
- client encouragement
- conveyance of hope
- provision of psychoeducation
- focus on the bidirectional link between interpersonally relevant events and mood
- facilitation of client problem-solving.

Key elements of the structure of IPT include:

- time-limited treatment typically conducted over sixteen weekly, individual sessions
- three phases of treatment: Initial Sessions, Intermediate Sessions, Termination

- one or two problem areas are the focus of Intermediate Sessions: Grief, Role Transitions, Interpersonal Role Disputes, Interpersonal Deficits
- therapeutic goals and strategies are outlined for each of the problem areas
- therapeutic techniques are used to implement goals and strategies
- sometimes initial IPT treatment is followed by less frequent, Maintenance IPT sessions.

There are three phases of IPT: Initial Sessions (weeks 1–3), Intermediate Sessions (4–13), and Termination (15–16). In the Initial Sessions the therapist reviews the client's depressive symptoms, provides education about depression and its treatment, does a broad review of past and current relationships (the 'Interpersonal Inventory'), and establishes an understanding of what interpersonally relevant events preceded the onset of depression. After a broad review of significant current and past relationships is conducted, the therapist provides an 'interpersonal formulation' to the client which conveys the therapist's understanding of the likely precipitants (or in some cases, consequences) of the depression, identifies one or two problem areas that will be the focus of treatment, and establishes goals of treatment. The therapist then reviews the structure and format of the therapy including its focus on current issues, time-limited format, and need for active engagement of the client in the therapy. Depending on client interest and need, the client may concurrently be taking an anti-depressant. With the client's assent, the therapy moves into the Intermediate Sessions.

Intermediate Sessions are conducted within one or two of the four IPT problem areas. The problem areas include Grief (complicated bereavement), Interpersonal Role Disputes (conflicts with a significant other), Role Transitions (major life change), and Interpersonal Deficits (individuals who want interpersonal connections but find it difficult to establish or sustain them). IPT outlines specific goals and strategies for each problem area. The therapist also utilizes IPT techniques, as needed, to implement goals and strategies.

Commonly used IPT techniques include:

- decision analysis
- communication analysis
- role-play
- interpersonal skills building
- between-session efforts to make changes related to the identified problem area ('work-at-home').

The status of the client's depressive symptoms is regularly monitored by the therapist, including use of a depression severity scale such as the Beck Depression Inventory or the Hamilton Depression Rating Scale for Depression (HRSD). The therapist focuses sessions on interpersonally relevant events from the preceding week and helps the client to identify the reciprocal relationship between recent events and current mood. The client is encouraged to make active efforts to address issues tied to the identified problem area(s). Throughout the Intermediate Sessions the therapist reminds the client of the number of remaining sessions.

During Termination, the therapist encourages the client to talk about feelings about the planned end of therapy. Some clients have feelings of loss or fear about the end of therapy. The therapist reviews with the client progress (or lack of progress) in achieving therapeutic goals, discusses changes in depressive symptoms during the course of treatment, emphasizes active efforts that the client has made to achieve goals, and helps to identify interpersonally relevant issues that the client will likely be confronting in the near future and ways to address them. The therapist discusses other treatment options for those clients who have not benefited (or minimally benefited) by IPT. Treatment options might include adding or changing an antidepressant, changing therapists, or changing to another treatment modality. Some clients—particularly those with recurrent depression—will benefit from 'maintenance IPT.' Maintenance IPT is less frequent IPT treatment that, in clinical treatment trials, has been found to reduce the likelihood of recurrence of another problem episode (Frank et al. 1991). Maintenance IPT is usually provided on a monthly basis, builds on skills acquired during the sixteen-week IPT treatment, and often focuses on the problem area(s) from the acute IPT treatment but may focus on other IPT problem areas that have emerged after the initial sixteen-week IPT treatment.

Two major treatment studies have established the efficacy of IPT in the treatment of acute depression in adults. These include the Boston-New Haven Collaborative Study of the Treatment of Acute Depression (DiMascio et al. 1979; Weissman et al. 1979) and the NIMH Treatment of Depression Collaborative Research Study (Elkin et al. 1989). Two maintenance studies have established the efficacy of IPT in reducing the likelihood of a recurrence of depression. These are the Boston-New Haven Collaborative Study (Klerman et al. 1974) and a continuation/maintenance treatment study conducted at the University of Pittsburgh (Frank et al. 1991; Kupfer et al. 1992). Other studies also provide support for the efficacy of IPT in the treatment of depression (see review by Cuijpers et al. 2011 that was noted earlier in this chapter).

IPT in the Treatment of Late-life Depression

Advantages of IPT in the treatment of late-life depression:

- Four IPT problem areas map on to those often seen among depressed older adults.
- Requires no substantive adaptation from original IPT framework.
- Collaborative, problem-focus of IPT is consistent with general recommendations in clinical work with older adults.
- Helps most clinicians build on previously used therapeutic skills.
- Can be flexibly applied yet helps clinicians to better develop treatment goals and identify therapeutic strategies.

As early as the 1980s, IPT researchers noted that this therapy seemed particularly well suited to older adults (Sholomskas et al. 1983). The four IPT problem areas encompass many of the issues for which older adults commonly seek psychotherapy in the treatment of depression. IPT is informed by broader principles of working clinically with older adults (e.g., active, collaborative, problem-focused; Knight 2004) but requires no substantive adaptation from the original framework. Our experience is that most clinicians find that IPT can be used flexibly, can draw upon previously developed psychotherapeutic skills, and helps build clarity in establishing treatment goals and choosing therapeutic interventions. Use of evidenced-based psychotherapies with older adults is consistent with larger efforts to implement psychotherapies whose efficacy is supported by clinical research studies (Molinari 2011). Studies of IPT with older adults have accumulated more slowly than with other age groups, but on the whole they have supported early suggestions that IPT would be efficacious in the treatment of late-life depression. What has lagged behind is dissemination of IPT into clinical practice with older people.

The first author's (Hinrichsen) initial interest in IPT was piqued by findings from his own research that select family issues were tied to longer-term clinical outcomes in older adults who had been hospitalized for major depression (Hinrichsen and Hernandez 1993). By extrapolation, it seemed that using a therapeutic modality that addressed interpersonal issues had the potential to improve clinical outcomes for depressed older adults. The experience of over twenty years of the provision of IPT to older adults by Hinrichsen and others supports early observations that IPT is an excellent therapeutic modality for older adults who have interpersonally relevant problems (Hinrichsen 1997; Miller and Silberman 1996). Informal clinical observations suggest that outcomes in clinical practice are similar to those found in IPT research (Hinrichsen and Clougherty 2006). In the delivery of IPT by the authors in an outpatient geriatric mental health clinic, the vast majority of IPT clients completed IPT and were generally enthusiastic about its structure and therapeutic ethos.

IPT requires little adaptation for older adults. However, as in the provision of any clinical services to older adults, the clinician needs to have familiarity with aging-related issues. The American Psychological Association's recently revised (in press) *Guidelines for Psychological Practice with Older Adults* delineates those attitudes, knowledge, and skills that are a foundation for good practice with this age group. Many excellent geropsychology organizations, articles, handbooks, clinical manuals, and textbooks exist to guide someone who is interested in providing clinical services to older people.

The most common IPT problem area seen in clinical practice and research studies with older adults is Role Transitions (Hinrichsen and Clougherty 2006; Reynolds et al. 1999). Late-life is a time of both role loss and role acquisition. Typical Role Transition issues seen with older adults in IPT include care for a spouse with health problems, onset of health problems (i.e., transitioning into the patient role because of onset or exacerbation of medical problems), residential move (e.g., to assisted living, long-term care, a new community), retirement, and care for a grandchild (e.g., acquisition of a parenting role). The other problem area often seen in IPT treatment with older adults is Role Disputes. Role disputes among older adults often include onset or exacerbation of conflict with a spouse/partner, adult child, sibling, or friend. Those issues often treated within the Grief problem area include contending with the loss of a spouse/partner, adult child, sibling, grandchild, or close friend. In our clinical practice and in research studies, Interpersonal Deficits is the least commonly treated problem area. We suspect this is because older adults often enter outpatient treatment or clinical studies at the urging of involved others. Those with Interpersonal Deficits, by definition, have fewer people in their lives than others to play such a facilitating role. Our colleagues who work in long-term care settings have noted to us that they provide services to a greater number of older adults who have a history of social isolation than are seen in outpatient practice.

A number of studies support the efficacy of IPT in the treatment of major depression and depressive symptoms. Older adults have been included in studies of 'mixed age' adults but fewer studies have specifically examined the utility of IPT in the treatment of only older persons (typically defined as 65 years of age or older). Two early pilot studies provided suggestive data that

IPT was useful in the treatment of late-life depression (Rothblum et al. 1982; Sloane, Staples, and Schneider 1985). Another study found that a brief form of IPT was useful in the treatment of depressive symptoms among older adults with medical problems compared to those who received 'usual care' (Mossey et al. 1996). A group of Dutch investigators reported that IPT was efficacious in treating moderately to severely depressed older adults with major depression in primary care but not for those with mild depression (Van Schaik et al. 2006). Researchers at the University of Pittsburgh have conducted two major 'continuation/maintenance' studies of IPT and anti-depressant medication in older adults with recurrent major depression. In their first study, IPT, medication, and the combination of the two significantly reduced the likelihood of another episode of major depression (Reynolds et al. 1999). In the second study, only anti-depressant medication reduced the likelihood of another episode (Reynolds et al. 2006). One possible explanation for the divergence of study outcomes is the fact that participants in the first study were on average ten years younger than participants in the second study. Later age is typically associated with more physical and cognitive frailty in older adults, which may have attenuated IPT treatment effects for participants in the second study.

Training Students and Clinicians in IPT for Depressed Older Adults

As noted earlier, dissemination of evidence-based treatments into general clinical practice has been a challenge. Militating against dissemination is that, despite the well-established efficacy of several psychotherapies, many graduate programmes in the mental health disciplines do not provide substantive training to their students in evidence-based treatments (Weissman and Sanderson 2002). As will be discussed later, efforts by the US Department of Veterans Affairs to train a large number of mental health clinicians in evidence-based psychotherapies including IPT are notable. Training VA staff will likely result in dissemination of evidence-based treatment skills to graduate students receiving training in the VA healthcare system. Both authors have had considerable experience in training psychology interns and postdoctoral fellows in IPT for the treatment of depression in older adults. Our experience is that although most psychology interns and fellows have at least some (and often considerable) familiarity with cognitive-behavioural therapy, few to none have had any education or training in IPT.

In an effort to build IPT skills in psychology interns and postdoctoral fellows, Hinrichsen established an older adult IPT training programme almost fifteen years ago at the Zucker Hillside Hospital, North Shore-Long Island Jewish Health System. Iselin subsequently assumed leadership of this training programme. Each year four to five psychology interns and fellows take part in this year-long training programme. Trainees are required to read *Comprehensive Guide to Interpersonal Psychotherapy* (Weissman et al. 2000) and encouraged to read *Interpersonal Psychotherapy for Depressed Older Adults* (Hinrichsen and Clougherty 2006). Trainees take part in the equivalent of a one day IPT workshop where they are introduced to the IPT structure, goals, strategies, and techniques, which includes review of videotaped sessions of older adults being treated with IPT. Each trainee is required to provide IPT to at least one depressed older adult during the course of the training year. All sessions are audiotaped and reviewed by the supervisor. Trainees also take part in a weekly group IPT supervision during which selected segments of trainees' audiotaped IPT sessions are played and discussed by participants. Concurrently, IPT trainees take part in a year-long seminar on clinical geropsychology.

Formal trainee evaluations of the training programme have been favourable and trainees informally report enthusiasm about the opportunity substantively to learn an evidence-based treatment. Despite the considerable investment of supervisory time in listening to all audiotaped sessions, this effort provides a substantive means to judge trainee IPT competence (vs. trainee self-report) and is a vehicle to give detailed feedback to trainees about their skills. We have found that most trainees develop solid skills in the delivery of IPT. Ideally, however, we believe that supervision of two to three cases is optimal for building proficiency in delivery of IPT.

The authors also have conducted from one- to three-day IPT professional workshops for post-licensure mental healthcare professionals in the US; and the senior author in other countries including Australia, New Zealand, the UK, Switzerland, and China. One-day workshops provide an opportunity for attendees to become broadly familiar with IPT and, in some cases, to begin to incorporate select aspects of IPT into their clinical work with depressed older adults. Three-day workshops are often the foundation upon which an ongoing training programme is built that includes subsequent experience of providing IPT treatment that is supervised. Notably, some healthcare systems have developed formal programmes to build evidence-based psychotherapy skills among mental health workers. In the last six years, the US Department of Veterans Affairs (VA), which has a nationwide system of healthcare services for military service veterans, has invested considerable resources in training VA clinicians in evidence-based treatments (EBT) including cognitive-behavioural therapy, cognitive-processing therapy, prolonged-exposure therapy, and acceptance and commitment therapy (Karlin et al. 2010). A three-day workshop is followed by six months of phone consultation to clinicians (including feedback on audiotaped sessions) who are providing the EBT to veterans. Formal evaluation of EBT competencies is conducted. In 2011, the VA launched a large IPT training programme. Both chapter authors are part of this effort. Multiple cohorts of VA clinicians are being trained over several years. This effort includes delivery of IPT to a substantial number of older veterans since older veterans constitute almost half of those who use services in the VA healthcare system

IPT Clinical Cases Examples

Note: Some of the IPT specific tasks, techniques, and strategies are emboldened in the case examples to illustrate their use.

Problem area: Grief

Initial Sessions

NH was an 86-year-old, Caucasian, Protestant retired widowed man who was self-referred for psychotherapy. NH had no prior psychiatric history. He came for treatment because he had felt depressed ever since his wife's death. He had been prescribed a low dose of an anti-depressant by his primary care physician four months prior to starting psychotherapy which helped reduce his symptoms. Nonetheless, the client obtained a score of 24 (moderate depression) on the Beck Depression Inventory-II. The therapist reviewed the *DSM-IV* criteria with the client and confirmed that he had a Major Depressive Disorder, single episode, and characterized depression as an illness (**psychoeducation about depression and its treatment**). The depressive episode appeared tied to his wife's death from Alzheimer's disease a year and a half earlier (**tying the onset of the depressive episode to an interpersonally relevant issue**). NH reported sixty years of 'blissful' marriage to his wife. His wife had been diagnosed with Alzheimer's disease eight years prior to her death during which time NH had been a devoted care-giver. NH's depression appeared to have been triggered by: (1) witnessing his wife's deterioration from being a beautiful, much admired, and socially adept person to a seriously impaired individual; (2) the contraction of NH's social life during the time that he cared for his wife; and (3) missing his wife's companionship. NH's most prominent symptoms were anhedonia, inappropriate guilt, fatigue, hopelessness, amotivation, sadness, and daily bouts of crying. Prior to taking an anti-depressant medication NH reported experiencing passive suicidal ideation. The therapist completed the **Interpersonal Inventory**, which documented a history of generally good relationships with friends and family except for his brother. NH had had a lifelong difficult relationship with his brother. NH had lost contact with his brother several years earlier and, in fact, did not know whether his brother was alive or dead. In the years prior to his wife's death, NH had also lost contact with many friends and family members due to their deaths, relocation, and limited opportunities to socialize because of caregiving responsibilities for his wife. His relationship with his wife had always been very intimate and loving, and continued to be so despite her increasingly severe functional and cognitive deficits. NH volunteered one day a week in a centre for people suffering from dementia, which he enjoyed. He also enjoyed a very close relationship with his granddaughter and two longtime friends, all of whom he saw often.

At the end of the Initial Sessions, the therapist provided a summary of her understanding of NH's difficulties and offered a plan for treatment. This summary (**Interpersonal Formulation**) included a restatement that NH was suffering from a major depressive illness and that his depression appeared to have been triggered by grief over his wife's passing. The therapist recommended that NH undergo a course of IPT, the goals of which would be a significant reduction in depressive symptoms, emotionally coming to terms with his wife's death, and reestablishing and/or possibly expanding meaningful relationships with others. Therefore, the problem area that would be addressed in IPT would be grief.

Intermediate Sessions

NH first worked on reviewing his relationship with his wife (**reconstruction of the relationship with the deceased**). The therapist encouraged him to bring in photos. NH brought pictures of his wife as a teenager when they first met, those of memorable family vacations, and photographs of her a few weeks before her death. These pictures served as catalysts for the client's **recounting of both positive and negative memories of their relationship**. The client also shared with the therapist the daily rituals tied to his mourning process including engaging in imaginary interactions with his wife, going through old letters from her, and reviewing condolence cards. These discussions helped facilitate NH's expression of profound feelings of loss.

As he thought more about the loss of his wife, he grew more interested in tracking down his brother. Via an internet search he learned his brother had died two years earlier. He was saddened but also angry at his brother's daughter for failing to notify him. The client weighed (**decision analysis**) whether or not to send an angry letter to his niece that he had written but not yet mailed. In session, he worked on redrafting the letter to better communicate his feelings to his niece so as to preserve an opportunity for a constructive dialogue with her.

Further facilitating the mourning process, the therapist encouraged him to discuss the events surrounding her death and his own complex feelings during that time (**describing the events prior to, during, and after the death**). At one point, NH discussed that he did not follow his wife's wishes regarding disposal of her remains. NH was guilt-ridden about not following her wishes. At session 8, the therapist reevaluated NH with the BDI-II on which he obtained a score of 12 (mild depression).

During sessions 9, 10, and 11, NH decided to send the redrafted letter to his niece. He reviewed her possible responses to this letter and how he would handle each of those responses. The client reported decreased feelings of guilt concerning disposal of his wife's remains. Although he said there were times when he sorely missed his wife, the frequency and intensity of these episodes lessened. In subsequent sessions, NH discussed his volunteer work at a dementia centre and his interest in deepening his relationships with co-workers and staff (**consider ways to increase involvement with others**). He thought about the possibility of another volunteer opportunity unrelated to dementia care. NH contemplated resuming more frequent contact with family members from whom he had isolated himself. The client also considered the possibility of discarding some of his wife's clothes, about which he expressed considerable emotion.

Toward the end of the Intermediate Sessions, NH received a response to the letter he sent to his niece. This led to the resumption of his relationship with her. Re-engagement with his niece also led to feelings of sadness over losing his brother, as well as regret over the difficulties with him. The client also decided to begin the process of disposing of his wife's clothes by starting with those that still had sales tags attached to them. The frequency of his imaginary conversations with his wife (as noted earlier) reduced over time.

At the end of Intermediate Sessions and in the early part of Termination, NH reported that now and then he found himself humming songs to himself for the first time in a very long time. He was enjoying his volunteer work and was more active and socially involved. Importantly, NH discussed ways of being loyal to his wife without feeling obligated to remain depressed and/or to think of her all the time. At that point in the treatment NH's memories of his wife started to focus more on happy, early times in his relationship with her.

Termination

In sessions 15 and 16 the therapist again administered the BDI-II to the client and he obtained a score of 4 (minimal depression). The therapist engaged NH in a review of the course of IPT including progress he had made in grieving his wife's loss, re-establishment of some relationships, increase in the scope and frequency of activities, and engagement in new relationships (**discussion of termination and feelings about it**). The therapist also reviewed with NH the significant improvement in depressive symptoms that had been evident during the course of treatment. The therapist emphasized that the client had achieved the primary goal of the psychotherapy, which was resolution of grief. The therapist discussed with NH the option that he take part in less frequent IPT sessions ('Maintenance IPT'; **discussion of continuation/maintenance treatment**) but he did not feel he wanted to do that.

Seven months later, however, NH contacted the therapist because of an increase in depression symptoms. Although his symptoms were neither as numerous nor severe as they had been when he had begun the course of IPT treatment the previous year, NH suffered a recurrence of depression. NH was engaged in a new course of IPT treatment (ten sessions), which further focused on grief and also on role transitions. At the end of this second IPT treatment he evidenced a full remission of symptoms. This second course of IPT was followed by monthly Maintenance IPT.

Problem area: Interpersonal Role Disputes

Initial Sessions

BT was a 79-year-old Catholic, Hispanic, divorced woman who sought treatment for symptoms of depressed mood, guilt, difficulty sleeping and concentrating, constant sadness and hopelessness, anxiety, and passive suicidal ideation. She was initially referred to a partial psychiatric hospitalization programme, at the end of which she evidenced a significant reduction of symptoms. She was referred to an outpatient clinic for medication management and subsequently referred for a course of IPT. At the start of IPT her Hamilton Depression Scale score was 12 ('mild depression') but she continued to meet criteria for Major Depressive Disorder, recurrent.

The **Interpersonal Inventory** revealed that BT had long been divorced from her husband, had raised a son almost entirely by herself, and had supported herself by often working more than one job at a time before retiring at the age of 65. Over the years she had had fewer and fewer social connections. BT had one friend with whom she was still in touch, but she found her friendship to be more dissatisfying than satisfying. The client's mother suffered from Alzheimer's disease and had been living in a nursing home for the past twelve months. Prior to moving her mother to a nursing home, BT had lived with her mother and had been her primary care-giver. Care-giving responsibilities further contributed to the contraction of her social world. One important cause of the client's depression appeared to be lack of daily structure since her mother moved to the nursing home and she no longer provided daily, hands-on care to her mother (**tying the onset of the depressive episode to an interpersonally relevant issue**). In IPT parlance, her role as care-giver had transitioned from the role of a day-to-day care-giver to that of a care-giver with general oversight of care that was provided to her mother by others in an institutional setting.

Six months before starting treatment, BT had moved to her divorced son's multifamily house, in which she now had her own apartment. Her son had a teenage daughter with whom she had a fair relationship. What appeared to be most closely tied to her depression was a conflictual relationship with her son. BT said she had decided to renovate the house she owned and no longer lived in, and that the renovation led to frequent arguments with her son. After arguments with her son she often had suicidal thoughts. As a result she tried to avoid arguments with him but felt that not speaking up also made her depressed. Further, sometimes she felt neglected by her son and by her granddaughter.

In the third session the therapist offered her understanding of BT's current difficulties (**Interpersonal Formulation**). She explained to BT that she was suffering from depression that started after her mother moved to the nursing home, her own move to a new residence, and increasing arguments with her son over renovation of her former home. The primary IPT problem area was thus determined to be interpersonal role disputes with her son. The secondary IPT problem area was role transition from living with her mother as primary care-giver to someone who provided secondary care (i.e. oversight of her mother's care in the nursing home) and with considerable unstructured time.

Intermediate Sessions

The therapist first helped BT clarify the **current stage of the dispute** with her son. Relationship problems seemed to alternate between conflictual episodes during which they sometimes tried to resolve difficulties, and periods in which there was very little communication or time spent together. In one of the earlier Intermediate Sessions, BT said she slept all day due to mistakenly taking twice her usual dose of a psychotropic medication. She denied that this medication mistake was in any way a suicide attempt. BT was disappointed that no one in the house had checked on her that day. She did not bring up this issue with her son for fear of an argument. The therapist engaged BT in a discussion of the pros and cons of discussing this matter with her son (**decision analysis**). The client agreed to consider having a conversation with him about the recent episode of oversleeping. BT and the therapist **role-played** a conversation between herself and her son during which she asked him to check on her more often. During the next session, BT reported that she had talked to her son, and that he had agreed to more frequent 'check-ins'. The client expressed relief that this discussion had not led to any tension.

Around session 6, BT reported a decreased frequency of conflicts with her son. The therapist wanted to clarify if this was because of BT's enhanced ability to manage conflict or avoidance of issues of concern. She felt she had improved her skills in conflict resolution, but reported that there was also an important problem with her son that she had been very reluctant to bring up with him. BT explained that she relied on her son to organize and supervise the renovation work on her former home. Because of his important role in the project BT had put her son's name on all of her bank accounts so that housing renovations could be easily paid. BT had asked her son only to use her business bank account to pay for the renovation expenses. However, she learned that her son was taking out large sums of money from another bank account that seemed unrelated to the renovations. BT expressed great frustration, disappointment, and sadness that her son was doing this.

BT said she was hesitant to bring up this matter with her son because of fear about the repercussions on their long-term relationship. She feared that if she raised the issue of funds being withdrawn from her account she would 'lose him'. Nonetheless BT wanted to consider ways in which she might bring up this issue with her son (**decision analysis**), since she was aware that her frustration and sadness were contributing to her depression. The therapist engaged her in several **role-plays** during which she practised (**interpersonal skills building**) confronting her son in a calm but assertive way and setting boundaries regarding her son's use of her money.

By session 8, BT obtained a Hamilton score of 7, which indicated that she was suffering from minimal depressive symptoms. Most interestingly, although BT had first announced to the therapist that she was not ready to talk to her son about the financial issue, she subsequently reported with pride that she had gone ahead and had that conversation with her son, and that it did not escalate into an argument (**review of work-at-home**). After this seminal event, BT reported being more assertive with her son while also choosing which battles she wanted to fight.

Towards the end of the Intermediate Sessions, BT and the therapist conducted a **communication analysis** about a conversation she had recently had with her son regarding their respective plans for their future lives. Her son said that in the future he thought about relocating to the southern part of the US. She tried to make her son feel guilty about this rather than directly sharing her own feelings of disappointment and fear should her son actually move. The therapist asked whether she handled differences with other people in the same way (**exploration of parallels in other relationships**). BT acknowledged that she sometimes tried to make others feel guilty rather than directly communicate her own views or preferences. She provided recent examples of communication with her granddaughter and a friend. BT considered pros and cons of changing her communication style to being more assertive with others (**decision analysis**).

Concurrent with her work on role disputes, BT was also making strides in resolving her difficulties transitioning from being her mother's primary care-giver to living alone and having more time for herself. **Exploring the positive and negative aspects of her old role** as a primary care-giver, BT reported loving the feeling that she provided such good care to her mother and that someone needed her so much. By relinquishing that role she experienced guilt that she had 'abandoned' her mother to a nursing home. The therapist encouraged BT to think about the difficulties associated with care of her mother (**review of positive and negative aspects of old role**). She acknowledged the stresses of providing ongoing assistance to her at home. She recalled that as her mother's dementia became more severe, her mother had bouts of sometimes uncontrollable anger and night-time wandering. Now that her mother was in the nursing home she no longer had to contend with these stresses. Yet she struggled with ambivalence about reaching out to friends or forming new connections. However, by the end of the Intermediate Phase, BT agreed to resume singing lessons and join a Bible-reading group at her church (**exploration of opportunities in the new role**).

Termination

During Termination, the therapist reviewed with BT the course of her treatment (**discussion of termination**). This included BT's conclusion that she needed to be more assertive with her son and others. The therapist praised BT for being more direct in making requests to her son and others, and showing evidence of improved communication skills. The therapist also underlined how BT had worked on identifying possibilities of enlarging her social relationships, and on considering resuming activities she had once enjoyed. The therapist pointed out how the changes BT had made resulted in significant improvements in the Major Depression that was, in fact, in remission. Reflecting this, BT's HRSD score was 7 ('normal') at session 16. BT and her therapist also reviewed possible future triggers for depression, strategies to use in response to these triggers, and symptoms that would indicate that BT would need additional mental healthcare. During the discussion about the planned end of therapy BT expressed interest in taking part in group therapy, which she subsequently began.

Implications for Practice

Efforts by the US Department of Veterans Affairs will likely have a lasting impact on the development of IPT expertise among VA clinicians and likely among graduate students receiving training within the VA. More work is needed to disseminate IPT into graduate school curricula, post-licensure continuing education venues, and into everyday clinical practice. Geropsychologists can contribute to this effort by building expertise in one or more evidence-based psychotherapies including IPT, teaching them to graduate students, clinical trainees, and colleagues, and advocating for their inclusion in professional organizations' treatment guidelines and training requirements related to older adults. Those interested in learning more about IPT are encouraged to read resources listed below. IPT training workshops are intermittently offered in the US and abroad, and in-person or telephone-based supervised training is available from those who have substantive IPT expertise (i.e. review of audiotaped IPT sessions, treatment consultation, formal assessment of IPT competencies). IPT training opportunities are listed on the website of the International Society for Interpersonal Psychotherapy (http://interpersonalpsychotherapy.org/), the Council of the Professional Geropsychology Training Programs (http://www.copgtp.org/), or can be identified by contacting the senior author (geropsychgah@aol.com). Clinicians working for the US Department of Veterans Affairs can check with their facility evidence-based training coordinator about IPT training options.

Summary

IPT is especially well suited to older adults. Its problem-focused, collaborative, time-limited format is appealing to many older adults and its interpersonal problem areas reflect many of the issues commonly addressed in outpatient treatment of late-life depression. A large compendium of research supports the utility of IPT in the treatment of depression and other mental disorders. A smaller body of research provides evidence for its efficacy with older people. Professional clinical treatment guidelines commonly recommend IPT as psychotherapeutic modality in the treatment of depression. Most psychology students appear to obtain solid grounding in the provision of IPT during a one-year training course.

Key References and Sources for Further Reading

Hinrichsen, G. A. (2008). 'Interpersonal Psychotherapy as a Treatment for Depression in Late Life'. *Professional Psychology: Research and Practice* 39: 306–312.

Hinrichsen, G. A. and Clougherty, K. F. (2006). *Interpersonal Psychotherapy for Depressed Older Adults*. Washington, DC: American Psychological Association.

Markowitz, J. C. and Weissman, M. M. (2012). 'Interpersonal Psychotherapy: Past, Present, and Future'. *Clinical Psychology and Psychotherapy* 19: 99–105.

Scogin, F. and Shah, A. (eds) (2012). *Making Evidence-based Psychological Treatments Work with Older Adults*. Washington, DC: American Psychological Association.

Weissman, M. M., Markowitz, J. C., and Klerman, G. L. (2000). *Comprehensive Guide to Interpersonal Psychotherapy*. New York: Basic Books.

REFERENCES

American Psychiatric Association (2000). 'Practice Guideline for the Treatment of Patients with Major Depressive Disorder' (2nd edn). *American Journal of Psychiatry* 157 (April suppl.).

American Psychological Association (in press). Guidelines for psychological practice with older adults. *American Psychologist*.

Bolton, P., Bass, J., Neugebauer, R., Verdeli, H., Clougherty, K. F., et al. (2003). 'A Clinical Trial of Group Interpersonal Psychotherapy for Depression in Rural Uganda'. *Journal of the American Medical Association* 289: 3117–3124.

Cuijpers, P., Geraedts, A. S., van Oppen, P., Andersson, G., Markowitz, J. C., et al. (2011). 'Interpersonal Psychotherapy for Depression: A Meta-analysis'. *American Journal of Psychiatry* 168: 581–592.

DiMascio, A., Weissman, M. M., Prusoff, B. A., Neu, C., Zwilling, M., et al. (1979). 'Differential Symptom Reduction by Drugs and Psychotherapy in Acute Depression'. *Archives of General Psychiatry* 36: 1450–1456.

Dohrenwend, B. S. and Dohrenwend, B. P. (eds) (1974). *Stressful Life Events: Their Nature and Effects*. New York: Wiley.

Elkin, I., Shea, M. T., Watkins, J. T., Imber, S. D., Sotsky, S. M., et al. (1989). 'National Institute of Mental Health Treatment of Depression Collaborative Research Program: General Effectiveness of Treatments'. *Archives of General Psychiatry* 46: 971–982.

Ellis, P. (2004). 'Royal Australian and New Zealand College of Psychiatrists Clinical Practice Guidelines Team for Depression: Australian and New Zealand Clinical Practice Guidelines for the Treatment of Depression'. *Australian and New Zealand Journal of Psychiatry* 38: 389–407.

Frank, E., Kupfer, D. J., Wagner, E. F., McEachran, A. B., and Cornes, C. (1991). 'Efficacy of Interpersonal Psychotherapy as a Maintenance Treatment of Recurrent Depression: Contributing Factors'. *Archives of General Psychiatry* 48: 1053–1059.

Hinrichsen, G. A. and Hernandez, N. A. (1993). 'Factors Associated with Recovery from and Relapse into Major Depressive Disorder in the Elderly'. *American Journal of Psychiatry* 150: 1820–1825.

Hinrichsen, G. A. (1997). 'Interpersonal Psychotherapy for Depressed Older Adults'. *Journal of Geriatric Psychiatry* 30: 239–257.

Hinrichsen, G. A. and Clougherty, K. F. (2006). *Interpersonal Psychotherapy for Depressed Older Adults*. Washington, DC: American Psychological Association.

Hooley, J. M., Orley, J., and Teasdale, D. J. (1986). 'Levels of Expressed Emotion and Relapse in Depressed Patients'. *British Journal of Psychiatry* 148: 642–647.

Karlin, B. E., Ruzek, J. I., Chard, K. M., Eftekhari, A., Monson, C. M., et al. (2010). 'Dissemination of Evidence-based Psychological Treatments for Posttraumatic Stress Disorder in the Veterans Health Administration'. *Journal of Traumatic Stress* 23: 663–673.

Klerman, G., Dimascio, A., Weissman, M., Prusoff, B., and Paykel, E. (1974). 'Treatment of Depression by Drugs and Psychotherapy'. *American Journal of Psychiatry* 131: 186–191.

Knight, B. G. (2004). *Psychotherapy with Older Adults* (3rd edn). Thousand Oaks, CA: Sage Publications.

Kupfer, D. J., Frank, E., Perel, J. M., Cornes, C., and Mallinger, V. J. (1992). 'Five-year Outcome for Maintenance Therapies in Recurrent Depression'. *Archives of General Psychiatry* 49: 769–773.

Markowitz, J. C. and Weissman, M. M. (2012). 'Interpersonal Psychotherapy: Past, Present, and Future'. *Clinical Psychology and Psychotherapy* 19: 99–105.

Miller, M. D. and Silberman, R. L. (1996). 'Using Interpersonal Psychotherapy with Depressed Elders'. In S. H. Zarit and B. G. Knight (eds), *A Guide to Psychotherapy and Aging* (pp. 83–99). Washington, DC: American Psychological Association.

Molinari, V. (ed.) (2011). *Specialty Competencies in Geropsychology*. New York: Oxford University Press.

Mossey, J. M., Knott, K. A., Higgins, M., and Talerico, K. (1996). 'Effectiveness of a Psychosocial Intervention, Interpersonal Counseling, for Subdysthymic Depression in Medically Ill Elderly'. *Journal of Gerontology: Medical Sciences* 51A: M172–M178.

National Institute for Clinical Excellence (2004; amended 2007). *Depression: Management of Depression in Primary and Secondary Care* (National Clinical Practice Guideline 23). London: NICE.

Reynolds, C. F., III, Frank E., Perel, J. M., Imber, S. D., Cornes, C., et al. (1999). 'Nortriptyline and Interpersonal Psychotherapy as Maintenance Therapies for Recurrent Major Depression: A Randomized Controlled Trial in Patients Older than 59 Years'. *Journal of the American Medical Association* 281: 39–45.

Reynolds, C. F., III, Dew, M. A., Pollack, B. G., Mulsant, B. H., Frank, E., et al. (2006). 'Maintenance Treatment of Major Depression in Old Age'. *New England Journal of Medicine* 354: 1130–1138.

Rothblum, E. D., Sholomskas, A. J., Berry, C., and Prusoff, B. A. (1982). 'Issues in Clinical Trials with the Depressed Elderly'. *Journal of the American Geriatrics Society* 30: 694–699.

Sholomskas, A. J., Chevron, E. S., Prusoff, B. A., and Berry, C. (1983). 'Short-term Interpersonal Therapy (IPT) with the Depressed Elderly: Case Reports and Discussion'. *American Journal of Psychotherapy* 37: 552–566.

Sloane, R. B., Staples, F. R., and Schneider, L. S. (1985). 'Interpersonal Psychotherapy versus Nortriptyline for Depression in the Elderly'. In G. Burrows, T. R. Norman, and L. Dennerstein (eds), *Clinical and Pharmacological Studies in Psychiatric Disorders* (pp. 344–346). London: John Libbey.

Van Schaik, A., van Marwijk, H., Ader, H., van Dyck, R., de Hann, M., et al. (2006). 'Interpersonal Psychotherapy for Elderly Patients in Primary Care'. *American Journal of Geriatric Psychiatry* 14: 777–786.

Verdeli, H., Clougherty K., Onyango, G., Lewandowski, E., Speelman, L., et al. (2008). 'Group Interpersonal Psychotherapy for Depressed Youth in IDP camps in Northern Uganda: Adaptation and Training'. *Child and Adolescent Psychiatry Clinics of North America* 17(8): 605–624.

Weissman, M. M. and Paykel, E. (1974). *The Depressed Woman*. Chicago: University of Chicago Press.

Weissman M. M., Prusoff, B. A., DiMascio, A., Neu, C., Goklaney, M., et al. (1979). 'The Efficacy of Drugs and Psychotherapy in the Treatment of Acute Depressive Episodes'. *American Journal of Psychiatry* 134: 555–558.

Weissman, M. M., Markowitz, J. C., and Klerman, G. L. (2000). *Comprehensive Guide to Interpersonal Psychotherapy*. New York: Basic Books.

Weissman, M. M. and Sanderson, W. C. (2002). 'Problems and Promises in Modern Psychotherapy: The Need for Increased Training in Evidence Based Treatments'. In B. Hamburg (ed.), *Modern Psychiatry: Challenges in Educating Health Professionals to Meet New Needs*. New York: Josiah Macy Foundation.

Weissman, M. M. (2006). 'A Brief History of Interpersonal Psychotherapy'. *Psychiatric Annals* 36: 553–557.

....

CHAPTER 31

ACT AND CBT IN OLDER AGE

Towards a Wise Synthesis

....

DAVID GILLANDERS AND KEN LAIDLAW

INTRODUCTION

DESPITE prevalent negative age stereotypes (Cuddy, Norton, and Fiske 2005), ageing is *not* an inevitably negative experience (Carstensen et al. 2011). In a longitudinal survey, older people report better emotional stability and are more competent at emotional regulation in comparison to adults of working age (Carstensen et al. 2011). The current cohort of older people experiences a more positive quality of life than previous ageing cohorts (Rohr and Lang 2009), with ageing well entailing an individual becoming active in shaping and responding to their environment. This may be especially important in the complex and dynamic social context of ageing (Rohr and Lang 2009). Ageing can be a time of continued growth, mastery, and feelings of accomplishment, connection with others, and of leaving a legacy for future generations (Scheibe and Carstensen 2010). Research evidence suggests that ageing can result in an enriched positive emotional trajectory of development. Emotion-regulation skill translates into older people being more resilient than younger adults (Gooding et al. 2012). As older people become aware of their finite lifespan, they are motivated to foster better emotional relationships and enhanced affect regulation in the moment (Scheibe and Carstensen 2010). This is a point not lost on others in the field, with Knight (2004) observing:

> The more traditional, largely pessimistic, view has been that adult development and increased experience make people rigid and set in their ways. Yet some clinicians working with the elderly have felt that the effect is quite the reverse: that growth and experience teaches adults to be more flexible, less dogmatic, and more aware that there are different ways of looking at life.
>
> (Knight 2004: 46)

If this view is accepted as reflective of the 'normal' experience of ageing, then older people may make better candidates for psychological therapy (Laidlaw 2013a).

The 'ageing paradox' exists to challenge a model of ageing solely in terms of loss and deficit, although it is also acknowledged that age can bring with it many challenges at an individual level. The ageing paradox is that whilst resources may diminish and threats may increase with age, empirical studies show well-being and life satisfaction (for the majority) are surprisingly high and remain so until the last stages of life (Westerhof, Dittmann-Kohli, and Bode 2003). The ageing paradox is understood to involve successful adaptation, redefinition of values and goals, engaging in new behaviours and seeking out new resources, and a lowering or changing of aspirations (Dittmann-Kohli 2005).

Subjective well-being also remains relatively stable and invariant to age, but less stable when physical health is compromised (Kunzmann et al. 2000). However even in these circumstances, reductions in positive affect are balanced by negative affect remaining stable (Kunzmann et al. 2000). Therefore, well-being in later life appears to be subjective and dependent upon one's frame of reference. George (2010) suggests older people make more 'downward social comparisons' in that they compare themselves with others they perceive to be less fortunate than themselves, and hence well-being remains relatively stable even during times of loss, transition, and change. Ageing, however, is more of a process than a state and as such is complex and multifactorial with Diehl and Werner-Wahl (2010) proposing that awareness of age-related change (AARC) may capture the personal multidimensional experience of ageing. An individual's idiosyncratic awareness of aging results in a perception that life has changed, and attributions about the nature of that change are due to some consequence of ageing, or of the passing of time. Changes attributed to age are therefore perceived as either positive or negative. This integrative model acknowledges that awareness of age-related change may serve an important motivational factor in terms of an individual lifespan developmental trajectory. Perception of increased vulnerability may serve to trigger the use of self-regulation strategies and as such may moderate effects of loss deficits associated with ageing. The AARC model therefore places a central role for psychological processing of the experience of ageing, with cognitive, affective, and behavioural responses predicated upon the apprehension and appraisal of the individual.

Growing older can nevertheless be associated with acute and chronic physical illnesses, comorbid conditions such as depression and anxiety, or subclinical depression/chronic dysthymia. Medical conditions increase rates of depression in later life, with a greater burden of illness resulting in an increased risk of depression, but most older people who develop physical problems do not develop depression. In a systematic review of community-based studies assessing prevalence of late-life depression, Beekman et al., (1999) calculated an average prevalence rate of 13.5% for clinically relevant depression symptoms. More recently, McDougall et al. (2007) reporting findings from a large epidemiological study looking at the prevalence of depression in people aged 65 years and older from across England and Wales, estimated prevalence of depression among older people to be 8.7%, with a prevalence rate for severe depression of 2.7%. McDougall et al. (2007) report no association between age and prevalence of depression. Factors more associated with depression were being female, medical comorbidity and disability, and social deprivation. These factors are more universally present than related to age challenges. Anxiety disorders are more common than depressive conditions, with Generalized Anxiety Disorder (GAD) and specific phobias being the most common sources of emotional distress in later life, and anxiety symptoms being more common still (Worlitzky-Taylor et al. 2010).

Blazer (2010) notes that depression rates in later life are lower than most professionals expect and that this may be because of three protective factors in later life. First is that older people have an appreciation of having lived longer than they have left to live and therefore tend to prioritize goals that are more meaningful in the present. As such, they tend selectively to optimize the positive aspects of the present. Indeed, research indicates nondepressed older people have a positivity bias for recall of memories (Carstensen and Mickels 2005), so Blazer (2010) may have a point here. The second factor is wisdom, with research suggesting age itself is irrelevant to the development of wisdom; rather, dealing with ambiguity and adversity develops greater wisdom, and as older people have an abundance of life experience they have more opportunities to develop competence in this domain. With longitudinal studies evidencing richer emotional development in later life (Carstensen et al. 2011), Blazer again seems to have an interesting explanation for the low rate of distress in later life. The third protective factor is that people adapt and accept events in later life partly because of the first two factors, but also because events such as the loss of a spouse are not unanticipated; these are events that are 'on time' and as such older people accept them as part of life. This is an interesting idea and it seems intuitively right and consistent with clinical practice as many older patients talk of having thought in advance of what they would do if their spouse were to die before them. It is an education for younger therapists to see older men and women learning to live alone, often for the first time in their adult lives, especially after marriages lasting close to fifty years and sometimes more.

The needs of older people with mental health problems such as depression and anxiety remain under-recognized and inadequately met, with access to psychological therapy frequently being insufficiently supported and available (Laidlaw 2013a). Despite anxiety symptoms and disorders being risk factors for disability and death (Bryant, Jackson, and Ames 2008) anxiety remains under-treated, tending to go 'under the radar' of mental health professionals and older people themselves, perhaps because of the presumed 'common currency' of the universal experience of anxiety and stress symptoms (Laidlaw 2013a). Older people may experience social isolation, withdrawing from others due to their own and other's stigmatization and stereotyping of older people. Furthermore, older people may fear further illness or deterioration of existing conditions. They may experience a range of cognitive difficulties with attention, concentration, judgment, inhibition of behaviour, and memory problems. Old age can be a time of multiple losses in terms of physical and mental functioning, valued roles, and bereavements.

Individuals with long histories of poor health or mental well-being are likely to carry these lifelong struggles into their third and fourth age and will likely be at greater risk of developing further later-life-related problems due to impoverished social support, poorly developed coping responses, and multiple comorbidities. People with chronic histories of depression are likely to get an especially poor deal from mental health services and are at risk of becoming 'revolving door' patients, referred in and out of services (McCullough 2012). Older people, in particular female spouses, may have significant burdens of caring for others with physical health needs, dementias, and mental health problems (Pinquart and Sörensen 2011). In summary, later life, in common with other stages of adulthood, can bring with it significant struggles, burdens, and threats to well-being. Psychological therapies exist that have been shown to be useful to older people in managing these challenges. Cognitive-behavioural therapy (CBT) is one such intervention that has a strong evidence base in addressing the needs and issues frequently faced by older people (Laidlaw et al. 2003; Pinquart, Duberstein, and Lyness 2007).

Characteristics of CBT for Older People

Several of the structural features of CBT make it especially well suited to address the psychological issues frequently seen in later life. CBT is highly structured, involving planning, agenda setting, and both in-session and between-session goals. There is an emphasis on therapist and client developing a shared understanding of the client's problems and the meaning of these in the client's phenomenological world. CBT therapists seek to achieve this via a highly collaborative relationship, where both parties view themselves as working together as a team to help the client. The combination of collaborative relationship and shared understanding of the client's problems, and in particular the here and now factors that maintain them, are particularly helpful in 'remoralizing' the client. Problems that were previously experienced as hopeless, isolating, and inevitable can become understandable, shared, and solvable.

CBT is explicit in sharing a formulation or case conceptualization with the client, at a level of detail that is accessible and meaningful to them. The joint development of a collaborative case conceptualization is part of the process of relationship building, socializing the client into the cognitive model, and developing shared understanding. The case formulation also helps the therapist to guide and plan treatment, from strategies to specific tasks and interventions. The formulation helps the therapist to anticipate the client's likely responses to interventions and can help to reduce roadblocks and resistance. Laidlaw et al. (Laidlaw, Thompson, and Gallagher-Thompson 2004) developed a comprehensive case conceptualization framework (CCF) that can accommodate the broader age context when working with older people.

In terms of specific interventions, CBT for older people draws heavily on cognitive *and* behavioural aspects of treatment. Behaviour activation/activity scheduling is useful when an older person has stopped doing things that would previously have been a source of positive reinforcement. Often this strategy is supplemented with asking the client to rate activities for the degree to which they bring a sense of pleasure or achievement. Such ratings can be helpful in refuting a depressed client's typically pervasive pessimism regarding the point of setting goals. In addition, older people who have stopped doing certain activities may find their resumption associated with fear, or loss of confidence, particularly fear of falling or injury. Behavioural tools such as collaboratively constructed graded exposure hierarchies can be useful ways of approaching such behaviour change.

While these tools derive primarily from the behavioural approach, within CBT their use is also designed to potentiate cognitive change. Just as the rating of a planned activity for pleasure or mastery can bring a powerful behavioural refutation of pessimistic appraisals, so can progressing through a gradually increasing fear hierarchy lead to changes in appraisal of the self as capable and the world as less threatening. Such exposure sessions can be delivered either with or without emotion-regulation strategies, such as breathing relaxation. Diverse relaxation strategies, such as Applied Relaxation (Öst 1987) or guided imagery (Arena and Blanchard 1996) can also be used to help clients who experience persistent over-arousal to reduce the physiological sensations and emotions associated with this.

Finally, the shared construction of meaning and narrative, and the development of explicit strategies for managing and responding to negative thinking, facilitates the problem changing from unknowable and inevitable to understandable and potentially changeable.

Examples include using automatic thought records to 'catch' thoughts and to modify these to be more realistic, less catastrophic, and less pessimistic. Over time, therapist and client will detect recurring themes in such work and will explore and modify the underlying beliefs that 'support' or drive problematic responding, such as 'Being old means that I am redundant and no use to my family.' Such techniques are effective in helping older people to regain control over their behaviour, emotions, and their thinking and by doing so, break the maladaptive patterns that maintain problems.

CBT is applicable when circumstances facing individuals have no easy solution such as when physical health problems are likely to be long-standing and may even be degenerative. As CBT with older people is still developing an evidence base when dealing with situations of a more chronic and complex presentation in longer-term conditions, this can be very challenging for therapists. A particularly acute challenge for novice CBT practitioners is where individual appraisals are seemingly relatively realistic, or where cure or remission of a problem is unlikely. A fundamental misapprehension of the applicability and utility of CBT with older people is that CBT will be less effective when negative thoughts are associated with 'realistic' challenges. Of central importance in using CBT in these conditions is the concept that it is the individual's appraisal of their experience rather than the experience itself that is important in understanding how well they cope with an event. As famously put by the Stoic Epictetus, 'People are not disturbed by things, but by the view they take of them.' A more modern CBT maxim may be, 'It's not what happens to you, but how you react to it that matters.' Thus cognitive restructuring and behavioural modification retain important utility when older people are confronted with age-related challenges. Evidence consistent with this point is clinical trials showing good outcomes for CBT when applied to people with depression and anxiety in Parkinson's disease (Dobkin et al. 2011), the utility of an augmented approach to CBT for post-stroke depression (Broomfield et al. 2011), and the potential applicability of CBT to people with dementia (Wilkins, Kiosses, and Raudin 2010).

However, when a person has experience of using cognitive strategies and these have not worked, or when the client's pursuit of emotional, physiological, or cognitive control results in them avoiding important parts of their life, a possible psychological therapy alternative to more traditional forms of CBT is acceptance and commitment therapy (ACT, said as one word, not three letters). A particularly useful strategy in helping people to manage age-specific challenges is a focus on 'experiential avoidance', and this is at the heart of ACT (Hayes, Strosahl, and Wilson 2012). ACT may therefore become part of a range of efficacious therapeutic alternatives available to older people. This is an important aim as it will seldom be the case that any single format of psychological therapy will work in all circumstances and with all populations. Hence we welcome the entry of ACT as a new opportunity to increase access to psychological therapy for older people.

ACT is part of the cognitive and behavioural therapies. It is distinct from cognitive therapy in placing less emphasis on cognitive change or cognitive mediation of psychological disorders. ACT is part of behaviour analysis and draws its historical roots from the radical behaviourism of B. F. Skinner (e.g. Skinner 1974). In radical behaviourism, all psychological events including thoughts, urges, sensations, and feelings are viewed as forms of behaviour. The goal of such a stance is to construct an applied behaviour analysis of such 'private events' and their influence on overt behaviours, within specified contexts, with the same kind of rigour and precision that behaviour analysis has traditionally brought to overt behaviour.

The empirical literature for ACT shows promise (e.g. Hayes et al. 2006; Hayes et al. 2010; Powers et al. 2009; Ruiz 2010). There are now over seventy trials of ACT, of which many are randomized controlled trials, across a very wide range of clinical and subclinical problems. ACT interventions have been used successfully to treat psychiatric disorders such as major depression, generalized anxiety, psychosis, eating disorders, and substance misuse problems. In the physical health arena, ACT interventions have been used successfully with people with diabetes, epilepsy, obesity, and for smoking cessation. When compared to waiting list controls and to treatment as usual, ACT interventions typically show large effect sizes. In comparison to well-established psychological interventions such as cognitive therapy, the picture is more controversial. While a number of meta-analyses have found that ACT interventions show a modest effect size *in favour* of ACT, these trials have been criticized as being of methodologically poorer quality on a range of factors that *could* lead to inflated effect sizes (e.g. Öst 2008).

There have been robust responses to such critiques (e.g. Gaudiano 2009), suggesting that the Öst analysis is unfair as it fails to take account of the level of funding received by the ACT trials and the stage of development of the ACT work in comparison to cognitive therapy. The state of the empirical evidence is further reviewed by Powers et al. (2009), who, while also finding a large effect comparing ACT to waiting lists or to treatment as usual, find no difference between ACT and established treatments in terms of outcome. The picture is made more complicated, however, by Levin and Hayes (2009), who argue that Powers et al.'s meta-analysis was incorrect, having labelled some measures as primary outcomes when in fact they were secondary, and vice versa. In addition, they suggest that Powers et al.'s grouping of treatments in the treatment as usual group puts active well-established treatments in that group, inflating the effect size for that comparison. When Levin and Hayes (2009) correct these 'errors', they find that the effect size for ACT in comparison to active treatments favours ACT. Finally, at least one early ACT study (Bach and Hayes 2002) was included in a critical review of reporting practices (Cook et al. 2002), suggesting that the reporting of trials could be improved and that the results of such trials should be treated with caution.

It is of note that in the US, the Department of Health and Human Services Substance Abuse and Mental Health Services Administration (www.samhsa.gov) has recently entered ACT into its National Registry of Evidence Based Programmes and Practices (SAMHSA 2010). In addition, in the field of major depression, ACT has been designated by the American Psychological Association as a 'probably efficacious treatment' (APA 2011). The APA also describe ACT for Chronic Pain as having 'Strong Research Support' (APA, 2011). Further, more recent randomized controlled trials, directly comparing ACT and CBT, have shown that these treatments appear equally effective and credible, certainly in the anxiety and depressive disorders (Arch et al. 2012; Forman et al. 2007; 2012).

A balanced perspective suggests that the ACT literature shows promise as an intervention, but that the work is continuing to mature and that future clinical studies of ACT could benefit from the methodological recommendations set out by earlier critical reviews. What is particularly notable is the wide range of mental and physical health problems to which the same functional technology has been applied. In addition, much ACT work has focused on disorders that are notably hard to treat due to chronicity. Whether ACT is superior to other well-established treatments is perhaps less important than finding that ACT appears *at least* as effective as other active psychological treatments, giving therapists an alternate choice of intervention, particularly under circumstances when cognitively oriented or control-based interventions have been tried and found to be insufficient.

An ACT Approach to the Problems of Older People

An ACT approach is at its heart a *functional contextual* behavioural approach. While in CBT we might emphasize the meaning structures and understandings that older people make as they age and encounter life's challenges, in ACT the focus is upon what the older person *does* in a specific context. ACT further specifies six overlapping behavioural processes that help a therapist to conceptualize the functions of a person's behaviour. These six processes can be represented in a hexagonal diagram sometimes called the 'ACT Hexaflex' (Figure 31.1). The ACT Hexaflex model describes six overlapping and interdependent processes that lead to either psychological inflexibility or psychological flexibility. In Figure 31.1, the hexagon on the left represents the inflexibility processes, whilst the one on the right represents the other side of the same coin: the six psychological flexibility processes.

Briefly, the six inflexibility processes are: experiential avoidance (efforts to avoid private events such as feelings, memories, and thoughts); cognitive fusion (taking thoughts literally, being excessively entangled in thinking, behaviour being dominated by cognition); lack of contact with the present moment (worrying about the future or brooding on the past); attachment to a narrowly defined conceptualized self (being dominated by a narrow vision of who we are and what is possible); lack of contact or clarity of values (not being in touch with what is important to us, being guided instead by 'oughts, shoulds'. etc.); and lack of committed action (inactivity, impulsivity, or acting to avoid difficult experiences). When combinations of these six processes are in operation, behaviour is relatively more rigid, inflexible, and oriented towards threat and avoidance.

The six processes of psychological flexibility are: willingness (choosing to take in whatever life is offering, both in the world outside and in the world of private events); defusion (stepping back from the dominance of cognitive events over behaviour, seeing thoughts as thoughts); present-moment awareness (being in touch with now, as each moment unfolds); a repertoire of flexible perspective-taking skills known as 'self as context' (e.g. seeing the self as the context in which psychological events happen, or as an observer of psychological content, rather than identifying with that content); values (knowing and connecting with what matters most to us); and committed action (taking steps and making commitments to behaviours that lead us in the direction of our values). When combinations of these six processes are active, a person has greater capacity to be present to what is happening now and, given what the situation affords, to choose to persist or change behaviour in the service of their own overarching life goals or values.

Using this model we can begin to develop functional analyses of the kinds of problems faced by some people as they age. Increasing physical health problems, for example, may lead to activity limitations, which in turn makes it hard for a person to maintain committed actions to things that they value, such as providing childcare for their grandchildren. In this context, the degree to which a person is 'fused' or 'entangled' with thoughts that equate

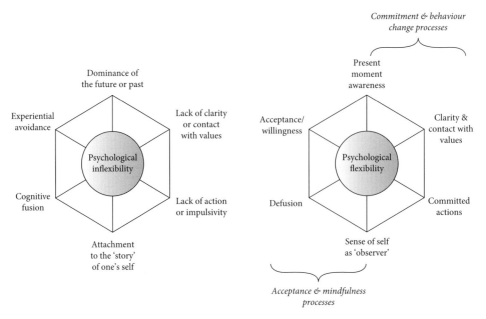

FIGURE 31.1 The acceptance and commitment therapy model—processes of inflexibility and psychological flexibility.

this caring role to their worth as a person will predict the degree of psychological flexibility they have to persist or change behaviour in the service of their values. In CBT we might explore the meaning of being a carer and use strategies to institute more balanced thinking, for instance seeing a caring role as only one element of self-worth. In an ACT model, by contrast, we would focus less effort on changing the meaning of such self-statements, preferring instead to use strategies that encourage seeing thoughts and beliefs as mental events only and instituting valued behaviour even in the presence of negative thinking.

The ACT therapist may use mindfulness techniques as part of such 'stepping back' from thinking and establishing direct control over behaviour, while letting go of the need to control thoughts, feelings, and physiological sensations. Further 'defusion' exercises include visualizing what a difficult thought or feeling would 'look like' if it could be seen in the room (Hayes et al. 2012). In using these kinds of intervention, therapists negotiate moment by moment what the client is willing to experience and what they are not, thereby creating a therapeutic context in which acceptance/willingness is fostered. Levy (2003, 2009) suggests that awareness of ageing may not always be a positively welcome experience, as negative stereotypes of ageing may make people fearful of growing older. Ageist societal attitudes internalized from a very young age and reinforced throughout adulthood can become negative age stereotypes reinforced by an attentional bias towards negative information about ageing (Levy 2003). ACT may be useful when working with an older person's future fears. In this context thoughts and feelings are examined not for their truth value but for the degree to which they are useful guides to behaviour. By examining the functional consequences of doing as thoughts suggest, their power to control behavioural responding is reduced.

One element that ACT emphasizes in this shared examination is an analysis of the 'work-ability' of currently employed strategies for dealing with whatever problem a person is seeking help for. In this early phase of ACT work, the client is typically struck by the discovery that much of their behaviour is in the service of reducing, controlling, or avoiding the problem (be that difficult thoughts, feelings, or physiological sensations). It is also usually evident that many of these avoidance-based strategies are maintained *precisely because* they provide short-term relief or reduction of discomfort, but that in the long term they do not help the client to live a full, vital, purposeful, meaningful life.

The older person who has experienced a fall, for example, becomes entangled with anxious thoughts and feelings regarding leaving the house, likely more so when the weather is icy. Their deciding not to go out temporarily reduces their anxiety about going out and gives a brief respite from the 'what if I fall?' thinking. In ACT, we might help the person to make deep experiential contact with the things they would leave the house for. Using eyes-closed exercises, a therapist might help the person to contact images and memories of a valued social contact, or a family event. Using imagery and metaphor the therapist works with the client to develop willingness to experience anxiety and anxious thoughts, in the service of taking specific steps in the direction of these valued life goals.

The explicit focus on values in ACT is a part of the model that is currently poorly developed in relation to issues of ageing considered by other psychological therapies. Consistent with evidence from socio-emotional selectivity theory (SST; Carstensen, Isaacowitz, and Charles 1999; Scheibe and Carstensen 2010), a person's values change as they age. Values of work and productivity may become de-emphasized, while those of community and connection may remain high. Additionally, some values (such as family) may remain important, though the specific steps and goals that make up this valued direction are likely to change in older age. The value of being a parent at the age of 75 is likely to involve different specific behaviours than the same value at the age of 30. This is, of course, not specific to old age: a person who has valued being a parent will have changed the specific ways in which they live this value many times over many years. The behaviours involved in parenting a six-month-old baby are different from those needed when a child is 3 or 10 or 17. Importantly, these ideas are theorized and more research is needed examining how values and their associated committed actions change and develop in response to ageing and age-related challenges. One study that does provide a preliminary investigation of these issues is described by Ferssizidis et al. (2010). In this study, a group of older adults and college students were compared on their responses to measures of values, well-being, and life satisfaction. After writing their own ideographic values of how they would most like to be in relationships (friendships, family, and romantic relationships), participants rated their agreement with statements related to their own self-reported behavioural commitment to living in accordance with that value: e.g. 'I am committed to living this value and acting consistently towards this value'. Commitment to values was associated with greater well-being and life satisfaction for both age groups. Interestingly, there was no difference between the younger and older adults in their commitment to values. In addition, life satisfaction was higher in the older adult group.

An element of the ACT model that may be particularly useful to therapists working with older people is the 'attachment to the self story'. This might be useful on several levels. First, given the cultural context in which most therapists in the Western world have grown up, we are highly likely to have been exposed to age-related stereotypes. The attachment to the self-story may be a particular form of age-related stereotype that may become a trap for therapists. While it is true that clients in psychological therapy may well be 'wed' to the story of themselves (e.g. 'I cannot form good relationships because of my childhood'), there is no evidence that older people are any more or less vulnerable to this process than younger adults. The belief that 'older people's psychology is more rigid and less amenable to change' may be exactly the kind of attachment to a story that could work against therapists and health professionals. Laidlaw (2010, 2013b) has pointed out that a potential therapeutic gap exists when CBT therapists do not make use of the individual's life-story information. In short, we need to figure out how to use the life experience of older people yet retain the here and now orientation of cognitive-behavioural therapies so the person can use this new information to help themselves address their current problems in a more personally empowered way. Laidlaw (2010, 2013b) suggests the use of timelines, and the use of life experience to help people reframe their self-story as one of resilience and survival enhancing compassionate self-acceptance in a move consistent with ACT philosophy and values.

Of course, the other level at which this element of the ACT model may be useful to therapists working with older people is that older people (just as younger people) *may well be* fused with such stories about themselves! Indeed, evidence suggests that older people's own negative attitudes to ageing are associated with poorer outcomes in relation to mental health and quality of life (Kalfoss, Low, and Molzahn 2010; Laidlaw et al. 2007). The ACT model is explicit that the six psychological processes that apply to those we term 'clients' also apply to the therapist. Our own discomfort may lead us to avoid important issues or moves with a client, our own 'stories' about ageing may hook us in to behaving in ways that are not in the service of the client's valued living. Such an explicit recognition is reflected in the high degree of experiential learning and participation encountered in good-quality ACT training and is designed to help therapists to hold their own age (and other group) stereotypes simply as mental events, acquired due to a particular history of cultural reinforcement. Such 'ideas' need not govern behaviour—providing one experiences these ideas *as ideas* flexibly, in a detached and open manner, and one commits to actions that are not consistent with 'the story'.

Given this explicit focus on awareness of the psychological processes involved in treatment from both the patient and the therapist's side of the interaction, it is reasonable to suggest that an ACT-based approach may also be a useful perspective to bring to clinical multidisciplinary teams, multi-agency working, and working with the systems in which older people live. These systems include healthcare systems, housing systems, and family systems. Such systems can unwittingly add to the burdens faced by older people in how the system responds to the behaviour and distress experienced by the older person. Systemic responses are highly influenced by the individual and collective appraisals that are made of the older person, their distress, and their behaviour. An ACT-based perspective may help a team or other system to hold such appraisals flexibly and to reduce their impact upon both clinical behaviour and practitioner well-being (Gauntlett-Gilbert 2011; Kangas and Shapiro 2011).

For instance, as multidisciplinary teams discuss a particularly challenging presentation of a client's distress, it can be evident that 'the story' the team forms around this patient and their problems can then influence subsequent clinician behaviour. Words such as 'frail' or 'fragile' may make a team less likely to be active in setting activity goals. Stories that involve long histories of psychological difficulty also tend to make clinicians pessimistic about change and less likely to offer change-oriented therapies. Two important elements in ACT may be useful in such situations: first, it is likely that previous attempts at therapy may have been focused on symptom reduction. ACT's focus on valued living in the presence of symptoms, thoughts, feelings, and so on is likely to be experienced as radically different by the patient and the team. Second, the explicit defusion of team members from their 'stories' about the patient may allow them to see the effect of 'the story' upon their clinical behaviour and therefore have greater choice over how they respond.

SIMILARITIES AND DIFFERENCES BETWEEN ACT AND COGNITIVE THERAPY

There are substantial areas of overlap between ACT and cognitive therapy (CT), though also some notable differences. At the level of principle; both tend to be highly structured, involve a high degree of collaboration and participation from both client and therapist, involve goals often expressed in terms of here and now behaviours and aim to establish more reliable control over the things a person does—their behaviour. Furthermore, they share a focus on cognition and emotion as important factors that influence behaviour. Both ACT and CT allow for the person's learning history to have shaped their behaviour, their beliefs, and their moment-to-moment patterns of thinking and feeling. Both approaches focus more explicitly on disrupting maladaptive patterns of responding to historical events and their psychological sequelae *in the here and now*, rather than uncovering hidden or unconscious meanings that have their roots in experiences *there and then*. Both approaches allow therapists to focus on historical material in the service of current change strategies.

CBT is perhaps more explicit in using such historical work as a means to 'heal' (e.g. Janoff-Bulman 1992), reducing the power or emotion of traumatic memories and trauma-related beliefs. Cognitive therapists are also more likely to use direct cognitive-modification strategies as a means to emotion or behaviour change. ACT therapists, in contrast work with a less explicit focus on changing such private cognitive and emotional events, but seek to help an individual respond to them with greater choice and flexibility. Both approaches use 'exposure-based' methods of treatment, though the function and purpose of exposure is thought of differently in these two approaches. In CBT (and in classical behaviour therapy), exposure is conceptualized as bringing someone into contact with a feared stimulus and preventing avoidance behaviour, such that extinction of fear occurs. In addition, emotional processing is thought to occur during prolonged exposure (Rachman 1980). From a cognitive therapy perspective, exposure also leads to changes in beliefs, such that the feared stimulus is reappraised as less threatening. In essence, exposure is engaged in to reduce fear and to change fear-related appraisals. In ACT, by contrast, exposure is seen as encouraging more flexible behaviour in the presence of a fear-eliciting stimulus. Whether or not fear diminishes or a person's appraisal of the stimulus changes is not considered to be especially relevant in an ACT conceptualization. Modelling, shaping, instigating, and reinforcing more flexible forms of behaviour in the presence of the feared stimulus are the goal. Interestingly, a recent empirical review by Craske et al. (2008) suggests that fear reduction during exposure does not predict therapy outcome.

Where ACT and CBT most diverge is in their concepts and their underpinning philosophical assumptions. CBT remains an approach that is specific to disorder. Indeed, significant scientific and clinical progress has been made when cognitive models of disorder allow more precise targeting of treatment, such as in the development of specific cognitive models of panic disorder (Clark 1986), obsessive compulsive disorder (Salkovskis 1985), and social phobia (Clark and Wells 1995). The specificity hypothesis suggests that specific cognitive distortions are implicated in specific conditions, and hence the more specific the model, the more targeted the treatment can be at the postulated mechanism of the disorder. By targeting the 'mechanism', the disorder will be treated, other symptoms of the disorder will reduce and the individual will function in more adaptive and healthy ways.

ACT, by contrast, has taken a trans-diagnostic approach to behavioural flexibility. The same functional technology has been shown to be useful across a wide range of problems by focusing on the function of acts in context, rather than the form of psychological events. Second, the goal in ACT is not to 'treat disorder' in an eliminative manner, but to focus on promoting valued goal-directed behaviour in the presence of the symptoms, thoughts, and feelings that are typical of the 'disorder'.

A further distinction is at the level of philosophical assumption. CBT takes an approach to the philosophy of science that could be described as 'elemental realism' (Hayes 2009). An elemental realist view of science could be described as typical of most science-based approaches in the natural sciences. In this view, the behaviour of the scientist is to 'uncover' the workings of the phenomenon that is being studied. They analyse the phenomenon into its parts, observe how the parts influence each other, and determine reliable, replicable patterns and predictions based upon these analyses. The success of their endeavour is reflected in the degree of match between theorized mechanisms and empirical observation, and the truth value of the scientist's analysis is in how 'accurately' they are able to describe the workings of the phenomenon they are investigating. The applied scientist then uses this understanding of mechanism to intervene in the postulated causal mechanism, thereby bringing about change.

ACT has chosen a different path in the development of its treatment. Based on the philosophical position of pragmatism (James 1907), ACT has adopted a functional contextual approach to science (Hayes, Hayes, and Reece 1988). The scientist working from a functional contextual position seeks to understand the function of a whole act in a given context. It is the functions of that act within that context that govern the act, rather than the act being caused by or governed by specific aspects such as thoughts, urges, or drives. From this point of view, the scientist seeks to understand what features of the context (including things such as thoughts, feelings, history of responding in that context) are antecedent to and consequent upon a given behaviour (both overt behaviours and private events), and how these consequences are instrumental in shaping future responses to those antecedents in that context and other contexts. For the functional contextual based scientist, their analysis of a phenomenon does not 'uncover' a truth about the universe. Functional contextualism is 'aontological'. It makes no assumptions that there is a universe 'out there' to be uncovered. Instead, the functional contextual scientist specifies in advance the goals of their investigation, and the analysis is said to be 'true' to the degree to which it provides progress towards that scientific goal. This is known as the truth criterion of successful working or 'workability'. The goal of contextual behavioural science (of which ACT is a part) has been stated as, 'The prediction and influence of psychological events, with precision, scope and depth' (Vilardaga, Hayes, and Levin 2009).

Such a way of talking about thoughts, feelings, and urges as 'private behaviours' is odd, given the 'common sense' way in which these things are dealt with in CBT. The value of the functional contextual approach is, however, that it keeps a clearer separation of what is a dependant variable and what is an independent variable, to use the terminology of science. This distinction is important, because the scientist needs to be able reliably to manipulate the independent variable and observe the effects on the dependent variables. From the functional contextual perspective, the only reliably manipulable independent variable is context: the antecedents and consequences surrounding an act, be that act overt or private, and the functional relationships these antecedents and consequences have upon the act.

ADAPTING ACT TO THE SPECIFIC ISSUES OF AGEING

The central message of ACT (that attempts to control may be part of the problem, rather than the solution) is relatively counter-cultural. Many people struggle with the basic stance in ACT, due to our long histories of reinforcement by the 'verbal community' of controlling our expression of emotion, regulating our behaviour, and behaving in a consistent and rational manner. It is because of this difficulty that ACT gives emphasis to facing the struggle and closely examining the workability of control-based strategies. Older people are likely to be *no different* from younger people in this regard. It is possible, however, that a longer history of investing in control-based strategies *may* make this shift in stance towards acceptance more difficult for some older people. Consistent with lifespan developmental thinking, older people experiencing many challenges and adversity over their lifespan develop an increased adaptive capacity to optimize function despite declining capacity (Heckhausen, Wrosch, and Schulz 2010). In this regard, the ACT philosophy of giving up control may resonate with an older person's experience, with the paradoxical outcome that giving up former means of engaging control may result in enhanced well-being and reduce discrepancy between a sense of achievement and false fixed beliefs about control.

Other ways in which ACT can be tailored to older people include ensuring that the metaphors and imagery techniques used in ACT are culturally accessible to this cohort. For instance, in one exercise (designed to increase experiential contact with values), clients are guided to visualize their own funeral and what they *would most wish* to be said about them and their lives in their eulogy (Hayes et al. 1999: 215). Petkus and Wetherell (2013) describe a case study in which this exercise is used successfully with a 69-year-old man. However, for some older people, this kind of imagery may already be well rehearsed in a relatively unhelpful way and it would then be easy for this exercise to have a variety of unintended consequences. Instead, therapists could focus on a shorter time scale: for example, imagining that through the therapeutic work some small but important changes begin to take place in how the client is living with their problems, imagining that it is their birthday in one year's time and that someone they care about is giving a speech about this previous year and how the person had been acting during that time.

Just as in some chronic health work, there may be activities that are no longer accessible to a client for reasons of physical ability or reduced independence. Therapists will need to explore with the client what values were being served by previously valued activities and try to incorporate small steps in these directions, or creatively work out alternative ways to pursue those values.

Importantly, when considering how ACT should be tailored to older people, therapists should beware of falling into stereotypes about what older people can and cannot do, and what they will or will not relate to. In tailoring metaphors for adolescents, for instance, we might do a piece of values work around the metaphor of 'if you got to choose the playlist that was your life, what "tracks" would you choose to have on it?' Or an adaptation of the classic 'Soldiers in the Parade' exercise (Hayes et al. 1999: 158) can be to visualize thoughts as 'Twitter feeds' scrolling up the screen. While it might be the case that older people might find the playlist or Twitter feed metaphor harder to relate to, this should not be assumed! The key issue is that the function of a metaphor (contacting values, seeing thoughts as thoughts, etc.) is the important part, but that the content of the metaphor needs to be accessible to the specific client, in order that the intended function can operate. Age and cohort effects *may* be a factor that influences this accessibility, though there is likely to be as much intra-cohort variability as there is inter-cohort. Petkus and Wetherell (2013) give further ideas about adapting ACT to older people.

EVIDENCE THAT ACT IS EFFECTIVE FOR OLDER PEOPLE

As described above, the ACT literature is maturing, with one small pilot study of ACT vs CBT for generalized anxiety disorder in older adults reporting potentially positive results (Wetherell et al. 2011). Furthermore, McCracken and Jones (2012) show that intensive ACT for chronic pain has similar efficacy for people over the age of 60 as it does for younger people. Karlin et al. (2013) show that ACT treatment for depression in former combat veterans is effective, and that older veterans respond just as well as younger ones. Interestingly, older veterans were also less likely to drop out of therapy. In addition, there are some case studies describing the use of ACT for chronic pain in older people (e.g. Lunde and Nordus 2009). Butler and Ciarrochi (2007) report a study of psychological acceptance and its relationship with quality of life in older people. As the ACT model predicts, psychological acceptance is associated with greater quality of life, particularly for those individuals whose productivity (hours spent in work, study, childcare, leisure time) was lower. Although cross-sectional, this study supports the concept that increasing psychological acceptance (particularly in those whose activity has been impaired due to age-related factors) should be a useful therapeutic target.

These early-stage investigations suggest that ACT is acceptable to older people, and the effects seen in these studies suggest ACT for older people is worthy of further investigation. This is in contrast to a relatively strong evidence base for cognitive-behavioural therapy (e.g. Laidlaw et al. 2008). Several of the existing controlled trials for ACT have, however, included people over the age of 65 (e.g. Bohlmeijer et al. 2011; Butryn et al. 2011; Gifford et al. 2004; Johnston et al. 2010; Twohig et al. 2010; Wetherell et al. 2011). These papers have not specified differential treatment response, acceptability, or attrition in relation to age. This is an encouraging sign, though specific applications of ACT for older people are needed to be fully confident of its usefulness with this cohort.

On a related note, a number of studies have investigated mindfulness or mindfulness-based cognitive therapy interventions with people over the age of 65 for a variety of conditions (e.g. dementia care-giving, Mackenzie and Poulin 2006; recurring depression, Smith, Graham, and Senthinathan 2007; chronic pain, Morone, Greco, and Weiner 2008, Wang and Feinstein 2011; emotional distress, Splevins, Smith, and Sampson 2009; and a particular type of cognitive deficit known as over-selectivity, McHugh, Simpson, and Reed 2010). These studies show that older people can develop mindfulness skills as well as younger people and can benefit from this intervention. This is another encouraging sign for the further investigation of ACT for older people.

A Strategy for the Development of ACT for Older People

Clearly the ACT model has the potential to be a credible and useful alternative method for intervening in the psychological issues often encountered in older age. There is some preliminary evidence supporting its utility; in addition, ACT could benefit from clinical development work targeted specifically at these issues. Practitioners in this area should be encouraged to use standardized outcome measures, as well as the growing number of useful process measures available, to track changes on ACT-relevant processes in response to interventions. Such a case-study approach can develop into single-case experimental designs, which not only help establish efficacy in cost-effective ways, but can also provide insight into mechanisms of treatment. Larger group-based designs are also needed. These often develop in a step-like manner with uncontrolled trials followed by randomized controlled trials.

Alongside such clinical development work, a programme of basic research is needed, investigating specific aspects of ageing and ACT concepts. For instance, how does 'valuing' change in later life? Are there age-related limits to cognitive defusion (or indeed, does age enhance defusion)? What adaptations are required to ACT in the presence of cognitive impairment? How does ageing affect the 'story' of oneself and one's attachment to or liberation from self-limiting stories? There is a role to play for qualitative, experimental, and cross-sectional work using a variety of methods, as well as the clinical development work suggested. Finally, issues relating to the stress of caring for older relatives, particularly in the context of dementia, deserve careful attention from an ACT perspective (see chapter in this Handbook).

Summary

Whilst ageing is not inevitably a time of difficulty, the kinds of issue that can be problematic for people as they age (e.g. loss, cognitive problems, health issues, role transitions) can usefully be considered from the perspective of ACT and CBT. Whilst there is a degree of overlap between these approaches at the level of technique, and even some shared concepts, they diverge more completely when we consider the conceptual and philosophical assumptions of each approach. There is growing evidence of the applicability and efficacy of acceptance-based approaches for older people's issues and a host of unanswered research questions in this area.

Given the global demographic transition, with an increase in the relative numbers of older people within societies and a welcome increase in longevity (United Nations Population Fund and HelpAge International 2012), people facing challenges associated with ageing, or those wishing to improve their well-being may come forward for psychological therapy. Behavioural scientists can be very useful to society by exploring this relatively less well-charted territory with increasing older populations, both clinically and scientifically. Our goal must be to continue to develop a range of alternative workable, practical solutions for problems and issues that will likely visit many of us and those we care about.

Key References and Sources for Further Reading

Bernard, M. E. (ed.) (2013). *The Strength of Self-acceptance, Theory, Practice and Research*. New York: Springer.

Hayes, S. C., Luoma, J. B., Bond, F. W., Masuda, A., and Lillis, J. (2006). 'Acceptance and Commitment Therapy: Model, Processes and Outcomes'. *Behaviour Research and Therapy* 44(1): 1–25. doi:10.1016/j.brat.2005.06.006.

Hayes, S. C., Strosahl, K. D., and Wilson, K. G. (2012). *Acceptance and Commitment Therapy: The Process and Practice of Mindful Change* (2nd edn). New York: Guilford Press.

Scogin, F. and Shah, A. (eds) (2012). *Making Evidence-based Psychological Treatments Work with Older Adults*. Washington DC: American Psychological Association.

Vengston, V. L., Gans, D., Putney, N. M., and Silverstein, M. (2009). *Handbook of the Theories of Aging* (2nd edn). New York: Springer.

References

American Psychological Association (2011). *Acceptance and Commitment Therapy for Chronic Pain*. http://www.div12.org/PsychologicalTreatments/treatments/chronicpain_act.html (accessed 2 August 2011).

American Psychological Association (2011). *Acceptance and Commitment Therapy for Depression*. http://www.psychology.sunysb.edu/eklonsky-division12/treatments/depression_acceptance.html (accessed 2 August 2011).

Arch, J. J., Eifert, G. H., Davies, C., Vilardaga, J. C. P., Rose, R. D., et al. (2012). 'Randomized Clinical Trial of Cognitive Behavioral Therapy (CBT) versus Acceptance and Commitment Therapy (ACT) for Mixed Anxiety Disorders'. *Journal of Consulting and Clinical Psychology* 80: 750–765. doi: 10.1037/a0028310.

Arena, J. G. and Blanchard, E. B. (1996). 'Biofeedback and Relaxation Therapy for Chronic Pain Disorders'. In R. J. Gatchel and D. C. Turk (eds), *Chronic Pain: Psychological Perspectives on Treatment*. New York: Guilford Press.

Bach, P. and Hayes, S. C. (2002). 'The Use of Acceptance and Commitment Therapy to Prevent the Rehospitalization of Psychotic Patients: A Randomized Controlled Trial'. *Journal of Consulting and Clinical Psychology* 70(5) 1129–1139. doi:10.1037//0022–006X.70.5.1129.

Beekman, A. T., Copeland, J. R. and Prince, M. J. (1999). 'Review of Community Prevalence of Depression in Later Life'. *British Journal of Psychiatry* 174: 307–311.

Blazer, D. G. (2010). 'Protection from Late Life Depression'. *International Psychogeriatrics* 22: 171–173.

Bohlmeijer, E. T., Fledderus, M., Rokx, T. A., and Pieterse, M. E. (2011). 'Efficacy of an Early Intervention Based on Acceptance and Commitment Therapy for Adults with Depressive Symptomatology: Evaluation in a Randomized Controlled Trial'. *Behaviour Research and Therapy* 49(1) 62–67. doi:10.1016/j.brat.2010.10.003.

Broomfield, N. M., Laidlaw, K., Hickabottom, E., Murray, M., Pendrey, R., Whittick, J., and Gillespie, D. C. (2011). 'Post-stroke Depression: The Case for Augmented, Individually Tailored Cognitive Behavioural Therapy'. *Clinical Psychology and Psychotherapy* 18: 202–217.

Bryant, C., Jackson, H., and Ames, D. (2008). 'The Prevalence of Anxiety in Older Adults: Methodological Issues and a Review of the Literature'. *Journal of Affective Disorders* 109: 233–250.

Butler, J. and Ciarrochi, J. (2007). 'Psychological Acceptance and Quality of Life in the Elderly'. *Quality of Life Research* 16: 607–615. doi:10.1007/s11136–006-9149–1.

Butryn, M. L., Forman, E., Hoffman, K., Shaw, J., and Juarascio, A. (2011). 'A Pilot Study of Acceptance and Commitment Therapy for Promotion of Physical Activity'. *Journal of Physical Activity and Health* 8(4): 516–22. http://www.ncbi.nlm.nih.gov/pubmed/21597124.

Carstensen, L., Isaacowitz, D., and Charles, S. T. (1999). 'Taking Time Seriously: A Theory of Socioemotional Selectivity'. *American Psychologist* 54: 165–181.

Carstensen, L. and Mickels, J. A. (2005). 'At the Intersection of Emotion and Cognition: Aging and the Positivity Effect'. *Current Directions in Psychological Science* 14: 117–121.

Carstensen, L. L., Turan, B., Scheibe, S., Ram, N., Erser-Hershfeld, H., et al. (2011). 'Emotional Experience Improves with Age: Evidence Based on over 10 Years of Experience Sampling'. *Psychology and Aging* 26: 21–33.

Clark, D. M. (1986). 'A Cognitive Approach to Panic Disorder'. *Behaviour Research and Therapy* 24: 461–470.

Clark, D. M. and Wells, A. (1995). 'A Cognitive Model of Social Phobia'. In R. Heimberg, M. Leibowitz, D. A. Hope, and F. R. Schneier (eds), *Social Phobia: Diagnosis, Assessment and Treatment*. New York: Guilford Press.

Cook, J. M., Hoffmann, K., Coyne, J. C., and Palmer, S. C. (2002). 'Reporting of Randomized Clinical Trials in the Journal of Consulting and Clinical Psychology 1992 and 2002: Before Consort and Beyond'. *Scientific Review of Mental Health Practice* 5(1): 69–80.

Craske, M. G., Kircanski, K., Zelikowsky, M., Mystkowski, J., Chowdhury, N., et al. (2008). 'Optimizing Inhibitory Learning during Exposure Therapy'. *Behaviour Research and Therapy* 46(1): 5–27. doi:10.1016/j.brat.2007.10.003.

Cuddy, A. J. C, Norton, M. I., and Fiske, S. T. (2005). 'This Old Stereotype: The Pervasiveness and Persistence of the Elderly Stereotype'. *Journal of Social Issues* 61: 265–283.

Diehl, M. K. and Werner-Wahl, H. (2010). 'Awareness of Age-related Change: Examination of a (Mostly) Unexplored Concept'. *Journal of Gerontology, Series B: Psychological Sciences* 65B: 340–350.

Dittmann-Kohli, F. (2005). 'Self and Identity'. In M. L. Johnson (ed.), *The Cambridge Handbook of Age and Ageing* (pp. 275–291). Cambridge: Cambridge University Press.

Dobkin, R. D., Menza, M. Allen, L. A., Gara, M. A., Mark, M. H., et al. (2011). 'Cognitive-behavioral Therapy for Depression in Parkinson's Disease: A Randomized, Controlled Trial'. *American Journal of Psychiatry* 168: 1066–1074.

Ferssizidis, P., Adams, L. M., Kashdan, T. B., Plummer, C., Mishra, A., et al. (2010). 'Motivation for and Commitment to Social Values: The Roles of Age and Gender'. *Motivation and Emotion* 34(4): 354–362. doi:10.1007/s11031-010-9187-4.

Forman, E. M., Herbert, J. D., Moitra, E., Yeomans, P. D., and Geller, P. A. (2007). 'A Randomized Controlled Effectiveness Trial of Acceptance and Commitment Therapy and Cognitive Therapy for Anxiety and Depression'. *Behavior Modification* 31: 772–799. http://dx.doi.org/10.1177/0145445507302202.

Forman, E. M., Shaw, J. A., Goetter, E. M., Herbert, J. D., Park, J. A., et al. (2012). 'Long-term Follow-up of a Randomized Controlled Trial Comparing Acceptance and Commitment Therapy and Standard Cognitive Behavior Therapy for Anxiety and Depression'. *Behavior Therapy* 43: 801–811.

Gaudiano, B. A. (2009). 'Öst's (2008) Methodological Comparison of Clinical Trials of Acceptance and Commitment Therapy versus Cognitive Behavior Therapy: Matching Apples with Oranges?' *Behaviour Research and Therapy* 47(12): 1066–1070. doi:10.1016/j.brat.2009.07.020

Gauntlett-Gilbert, J. (2011). 'Team Working and the Social Contexts of Health Care'. In L. McCracken (ed.), *Mindfulness and Acceptance in Behavioral Medicine: Current Theory and Practice*. Oakland, CA: New Harbinger.

George, L. K. (2010). 'Still Happy after All These Years: Research Frontiers on Subjective Well-being in Later Life'. *Journal of Gerontology, Series B: Psychological Sciences* 65B: 331–339.

Gifford, E., Kohlenberg, B., Hayes, S. C., Antonuccio, D., Piasecki, M., et al. (2004). 'Acceptance-based Treatment for Smoking Cessation'. *Behavior Therapy* 35(4): 689–705. doi:10.1016/S0005-7894(04)80015-7.

Gooding, P. A., Hurst, A, Johnson, J., and Tarrier, N. (2012). 'Psychological Resilience in Young and Older Adults'. *International Journal of Geriatric Psychiatry* 27: 262–270. doi: 10/1002/gps.2712.

Hayes, S. C., Hayes, L. J., and Reece, H. W. (1988). 'Finding the Philosophical Core: A Review of Stephen C. Pepper's World Hypotheses'. *Journal of the Experimental Analysis of Behavior* 50: 97–111.

Hayes, S. C., Strosahl, K. D., and Wilson, K. G. (1999). *Acceptance and Commitment Therapy: An Experiential Approach to Behavior Change*. New York: Guilford Press.

Hayes, S. C. (2009). 'The Importance of RFT to the Development of Contextual Behavioral Science'. Presidential address, Association for Contextual Behavioral Science World Conference, Enschede, Netherlands.

Hayes, S. C., Villatte, M., Levin, M., and Hildebrandt, M. (2010). 'Open, Aware, and Active: Contextual Approaches as an Emerging Trend in the Behavioral and Cognitive Therapies'. *Annual Review of Clinical Psychology* 7: 141–168. doi:10.1146/annurev-clinpsy-032210-104449.

Hayes, S. C., Strosahl, K. D., and Wilson, K. G. (2012). *Acceptance and Commitment Therapy: The Process and Practice of Mindful Change* (2nd edn). New York: Guilford Press.

Hayes, S. C., Luoma, J. B., Bond, F. W., Masuda, A., and Lillis, J. (2006). 'Acceptance and Commitment Therapy: Model, Processes and Outcomes'. *Behaviour Research and Therapy* 44(1): 1–25. doi:10.1016/j.brat.2005.06.006.

Heckhausen, J., Wrosch, C., and Schulz, R. (2010). 'A Motivational Theory of Life-span Development'. *Psychological Review* 117: 32–60. doi: 10.1037/a0017668.

James, W. (1907). *Pragmatism*. New York: Dover Publications.

Janoff-Bulman, R. (1992). *Shattered Assumptions: Towards a New Psychology of Trauma*. New York: Free Press.

Johnston, M., Foster, M., Shennan, J., Starkey, N. J., and Johnson, A. (2010). 'The Effectiveness of an Acceptance and Commitment Therapy Self-help Intervention for Chronic Pain'. *Clinical Journal of Pain* 26(5): 393–402. doi:10.1097/AJP.0b013e3181cf59ce.

Kalfoss, M. H., Low, G., and Molzahn, A. E. (2010). 'Reliability and Validity of the Attitudes to Ageing Questionnaire for Canadian and Norwegian Older Adults'. *Scandinavian Journal of Caring Sciences* 24(5):75–85. doi:10.1111/j.1471-6712.2010.00786.x.

Kangas, N. L. and Shapiro, S. L. (2011). 'Mindfulness-based Training for Health Care Professionals'. In L. McCracken (ed.), *Mindfulness and Acceptance in Behavioral Medicine: Current Theory and Practice*. Oakland, CA: New Harbinger.

Karlin, B. E., Walser, R. D., Yesavage, J., Zhang, A., Trockel, M., et al. (2013). 'Effectiveness of Acceptance and Commitment Therapy for Depression: Comparison among Older and Younger Veterans'. *Aging & Mental Health* 17: 555–563. doi:10.1080/13607863.2013.789002.

Knight, B. G. (2004). *Psychotherapy with Older Adults* (3rd edn). Thousand Oaks, CA: Sage.

Kunzmann, U., Little, T. D., and Smith, J. (2000). 'Is Age-related Stability of Subjective Well-being a Paradox? Cross-sectional and Longitudinal Evidence from the Berlin Ageing Study'. *Psychology and Aging* 15: 511–526.

Laidlaw, K., Thompson, L. W., Gallagher-Thompson, D., and Dick-Siskin, L. (2003). *Cognitive Behaviour Therapy with Older People*. Chichester: Wiley-Blackwell.

Laidlaw, K., Thompson, L., and Gallagher-Thompson, D. (2004). 'Comprehensive Conceptualisation of Cognitive Behaviour Therapy for Late Life Depression'. *Behavioural and Cognitive Psychotherapy* 32: 1–8.

Laidlaw, K., Power, M. J., Schmidt, S., and WHOQOL-OLD Group (2007). 'The Attitudes to Ageing Questionnaire (AAQ): Development and Psychometric Properties'. *International Journal of Geriatric Psychiatry* 22: 367–379. doi:10.1002/gps.

Laidlaw, K., Davidson, K., Toner, H., Jackson, G., Clark, S., et al. (2008). 'A Randomised Controlled Trial of Cognitive Behaviour Therapy vs Treatment as Usual in the Treatment of Mild to Moderate Late Life Depression'. *International Journal of Geriatric Psychiatry* 23: 843–850. doi:10.1002/gps.

Laidlaw, K. (2010). 'Enhancing Cognitive Behaviour Therapy with Older People Using Gerontological Theories as Vehicles for Change'. In N. A. Pachana, K. Laidlaw, and B. G. Knight (eds), *Casebook of Clinical Geropsychology: International Perspectives on Practice*. Oxford: Oxford University Press.

Laidlaw, K. (2013a). 'ViewPoint: A Deficit in Psychotherapeutic Care for Older People with Depression and Anxiety'. *Gerontology* 59(6): 549–556. doi:10.1159/000351439.

Laidlaw, K. (2013b). 'Self-Acceptance and Aging: Using Self-acceptance as a Mediator of Change in CBT with Depressed and Anxious Older People'. In M. E. Bernard (ed.), *The Strength of Self-acceptance*. Melbourne: Springer.

Levin, M. and Hayes, S. C. (2009). 'Is Acceptance and Commitment Therapy Superior to Established Treatment Comparisons?' *Psychotherapy and Psychosomatics* 78(6): 380–380. doi:10.1159/000235978.

Levy, B. R. (2003). 'Mind Matters: Cognitive and Physical Effects of Aging Self-Stereotypes'. *Journal of Gerontology: Psychological Science* 58: 203–211.

Levy, B. R. (2009). 'Stereotype Embodiment: A Psychosocial Approach to Aging'. *Current Directions in Psychological Science* 18: 332–336.

Lunde L.-H. and Nordhus I. H. (2009). 'Combining Acceptance and Commitment Therapy and Cognitive Behavioral Therapy for the Treatment of Chronic Pain in Older Adults'. *Clinical Case Studies* 8: 296–308. doi:10.1177/1534650109337527.

McCracken, L. M. and Jones, R. (2012). 'Treatment for Chronic Pain for Adults in the Seventh and Eighth Decades of Life: A Preliminary Study of Acceptance and Commitment Therapy (ACT)'. *Pain Medicine* 13: 861–867.

McDougall, F. A., Kvaal, K. Matthews, F. E., Paykel, E., Jones, P. B., et al. (2007). 'Prevalence of Depression in Older People in England and Wales: The MRC CFAS Study'. *Psychological Medicine* 37: 1787–1795.

McCullough, J. P. (2012). 'The Way Early-onset Chronically Depressed Patients are Treated Today Makes Me Sad'. *Open Journal of Psychiatry* 2: 9–11.

McHugh, L., Simpson, A., and Reed, P. (2010). 'Mindfulness as a Potential Intervention for Stimulus Over-selectivity in Older Adults'. *Research in Developmental Disabilities* 31: 178–184. doi:10.1016/j.ridd.2009.08.009.

Mackenzie, C. S. and Poulin, P. A. (2006). 'Living with the Dying: Using the Wisdom of Mindfulness to Support Caregivers of Older Adults with Dementia'. *International Journal of Health Promotion and Education* 44(1): 43–47.

Márquez-González, M., Romero-Moreno, R., and Losada, A. (2010). 'Caregiving Issues in a Therapeutic Context: New Insights from the Acceptance and Commitment Therapy Approach'. In K. Laidlaw and N. Pachana (eds), *Casebook of Clinical Geropsychology: International Perspectives on Practice* (pp. 33–51). New York: Oxford University Press.

Morone, N. E., Greco, C. M., and Weiner D. K. (2008). 'Mindfulness Meditation for the Treatment of Chronic Low Back Pain in Older Adults: A Randomized Controlled Pilot Study'. *Pain* 134: 310–319. doi:10.1016/j.pain.2007.04.038.

Petkus, A. J. and Wetherell, J. L. (2013). 'Acceptance and Commitment Therapy with Older Adults: Rationale and Considerations'. *Cognitive and Behavioral Practice* 20: 47–56.

Pinquart, M., Duberstein, P., and Lyness, J. (2007). 'Effects of Psychotherapy and Other Behavioural Interventions on Clinically Depressed Older Adults: A Meta-analysis'. *Aging & Mental Health* 11: 645–657.

Powers, M. B., Zum Vorde Sive Vording, M. B., and Emmelkamp, P. M. G. (2009). 'Acceptance and Commitment Therapy: A Meta-analytic Review'. *Psychotherapy and Psychosomatics* 78(2): 73–80. doi:10.1159/000190790.

Öst, L.-G. (1987). 'Applied Relaxation: Description of a Coping Technique and Review of Controlled Studies'. *Behaviour Research and Therapy* 25(5): 397–409. http://www.ncbi.nlm.nih.gov/pubmed/3318800.

Öst, L.-G. (2008). 'Efficacy of the Third Wave of Behavioral Therapies: A Systematic Review and Meta-analysis'. *Behaviour Research and Therapy* 46(3): 296–321. doi:10.1016/j.brat.2007.12.005.

Pinquart, M. and Sörensen, S. (2011). 'Spouses, Adult Children, and Children-in-law as Caregivers of Older Adults: A Meta-analytic Comparison'. *Psychology and Aging* 26: 1–14.

Rachman, S. (1980). 'Emotional Processing'. *Behaviour Research and Therapy* 18(1): 51–60. http://www.ncbi.nlm.nih.gov/pubmed/7369988.

Rohr, M. K. and Lang, F. R. (2009). 'Aging Well Together: A Mini Review'. *Gerontology* 55: 333–343. doi:10.1159/000212161.

Ruiz, F. J. (2010). 'A Review of Acceptance and Commitment Therapy (ACT) Empirical Evidence: Correlational, Experimental Psychopathology, Component and Outcome Studies'. *International Journal of Psychology and Psychological Therapy* 10(1): 125–162.

Salkovskis, P. M. (1985). 'Obsessional-compulsive Problems: A Cognitive-behavioural Analysis'. *Behaviour Research and Therapy* 23(5): 571–583.

Scheibe, S. and Carstensen, L. L. (2010). 'Emotional Aging: Recent Findings and Future Trends'. *Journal of Gerontology, Series B: Psychological Sciences* 65B: 135–144.

Skinner, B. F. (1974). *About Behaviourism*. New York: Random House.

Smith, A., Graham, L., and Senthinathan, S. (2007). 'Mindfulness-based Cognitive Therapy for Recurring Depression in Older People: A Qualitative Study'. *Aging & Mental Health* 11: 346–357. doi:10.1080/13607860601086256.

Splevins, K., Smith, A., and Simpson, J. (2009). 'Do Improvements in Emotional Distress Correlate with Becoming More Mindful? A Study of Older Adults'. *Aging & Mental Health* 13: 328–335. doi:10.1080/13607860802459807.

Substance Abuse and Mental Health Services Administration National Registry of Evidence Based Programs and Practices (2010). 'Acceptance and Commitment Therapy'. http://174.140.153.167/ViewIntervention.aspx?id=191.

Twohig, M. P., Hayes, S. C., Plumb, J. C., Pruitt, L. D., Collins, A. B., et al. (2010). 'A Randomized Clinical Trial of Acceptance and Commitment Therapy versus Progressive Relaxation Training for Obsessive-compulsive Disorder'. *Journal of Consulting and Clinical Psychology* 78(5): 705–716. doi:10.1037/a0020508.

United Nations Population Fund and HelpAge International (2012). *Ageing in the Twenty-first Century: A Celebration and a Challenge*. New York: UNFPA.

Vilardaga, R., Hayes, S. C., and Levin, M. E. (2009). 'Creating a Strategy for Progress: A Contextual Behavioral Science Approach'. *Behavior Analyst* 1(1): 105–133.

Wang, D. and Feinstein, A. (2011). 'Managing Pain in Older Adults: The Benefits of Yoga Postures, Meditation and Mindfulness'. *Topics in Geriatric Rehabilitation* 27: 104–109. doi:10.1097/TGR.0b013e31821bfffa.

Westerhof, G., Dittman-Kohli, F., and Bode, C. (2003). 'The Aging Paradox: Toward Personal Meaning in Gerontological Theory'. In S. Biggs, A. Lowenstein, and J. Hendricks (eds), *The Need for Theory: Critical Approaches to Social Gerontology* (pp. 127–144). Amityville, NY: Baywood.

Wetherell J. L., Liu L., Patterson T. L., Afari N., Ayers C. R., et al. (2011). 'Acceptance and Commitment Therapy for Generalized Anxiety Disorder in Older Adults: A Preliminary Report'. *Behavior Therapy* 42: 127–134. doi:10.1016/j.beth.2010.07.002.

Wilkins, V. Kiosses, D., and Ravdin, L. (2010). 'Late-life Depression with Comorbid Cognitive Impairment and Disability: Nonpharmacological Interventions'. *Clinical Interventions in Aging* 5: 323–331.

Worlitzky-Taylor, K. B., Castriotta, N., Lenze, E. J., Stanley, M. A., and Craske, M. G. (2010). 'Anxiety Disorders in Older Adults: A Comprehensive Review'. *Depression and Anxiety* 27: 190–211.

CHAPTER 32

ACCEPTANCE AND COMMITMENT THERAPY WITH DEMENTIA CARE-GIVERS

MARÍA MÁRQUEZ-GONZÁLEZ, ANDRÉS LOSADA BALTAR, AND ROSA ROMERO-MORENO

INTRODUCTION

FAMILY care-giving for older dependents is a common phenomenon in western countries, and it seems that in the near future there will be a significant increase in the number of people caring for a dependent family member. Caring for a dependent person, especially if they have dementia, is associated with substantial negative consequences for carers' psychological and physical health (Knight and Losada 2011). In order to understand why care-giving is associated with negative health consequences, researchers have turned to empirically supported theoretical models such as the Stress and Coping model (e.g. Knight and Sayegh 2010). According to this model, the demands and problematic situations that care-givers have to face (e.g. devoting many hours a day to care-giving, over many years, and having to deal with problematic behaviours from the family member), considered as stressors, do not affect all care-givers in the same way, since there are many variables—such as social support or coping strategies—that can influence whether care-givers deal with their task more or less adaptively.

Much of the research on care-givers aims to identify variables contributing to their distress, with a view to providing information that would allow the design of interventions to reduce such distress. The majority of initiatives with the greatest efficacy in the reduction of distress have been those of a multicomponent, behavioural, and psychotherapeutic nature, most notably cognitive-behavioural therapies (CBT; e.g. Gallagher-Thompson and Coon 2007; Pinquart and Sörensen 2006). Although the specific content and strategies of each initiative depend on its objectives, in general, such interventions are aimed at providing training in coping strategies for reducing the frequency or intensity of the problems faced by care-givers, training them in more flexible or realistic ways of thinking about care-giving (e.g. through cognitive restructuring), and increasing the number of pleasurable activities they undertake (e.g. Coon et al. 2003; Losada, Márquez-González, and Romero-Moreno 2011).

Despite the fact that, as pointed out, these types of intervention have proven effective in reducing care-giver distress, their effect size has in most cases been no more than moderate (Pinquart and Sörensen 2006). There are many explanations for the fact that interventions have not been as effective as might be expected. In this regard, the literature refers to the importance of considering care-givers' profiles in order to adapt interventions to the specific needs of each care-giver (Zarit and Femia 2008), as well as the need to pay more attention to the assessment of the implementation of the interventions (Márquez-González et al. 2007). On the other hand, as Zarit and Femia (2008: 7) stress, 'treating people for a problem they do not have may actually worsen their situation'. In this sense, it may not be advisable to apply psychological interventions indiscriminately to all those caring for people with dementia, as though the act of care-giving in and of itself were pathological. Thus, at present it is recommended to target those care-givers displaying high levels of distress (e.g. significant depressive symptomatology; Zarit and Femia, 2008).

The main objective of CBT interventions, then, is to achieve a change in the care-giver in some dimension (behaviours, emotions, or thoughts). However, as we discussed in a previous work (Márquez-González et al. 2010), in situations of caring for persons with dementia there are many circumstances and elements that cannot be changed, with respect to both events and situations external to the care-giver (e.g. the family member's memory and attention problems) as well as the care-giver's internal experiences (e.g. emotions—sadness—or thoughts—e.g. 'I feel overwhelmed, and I need this to end...'). In these situations, many people make considerable efforts to try to escape from, avoid, or control such experiences through cognitive, emotional, or behavioural mechanisms. Such mechanisms, though providing initial relief, may instead become factors that maintain or increase the individual's distress and, moreover, hinder the performance of important activities related to their values and life goals. This tendency has been called *experiential avoidance*, and has been linked to psychological distress in both the general psychological literature (for a review, see Hayes et al. 1996) and research specifically on care-givers (Márquez-González et al. 2010; Spira et al. 2007).

CBT, aimed largely at changing care-givers' thoughts and emotions, may not always be the most advisable approach to address internal experiences that are difficult to modify, or to modify the person's tendency to control such emotions and experiences. Alternatively, we may expect beneficial effects from interventions that encourage care-givers to accept such experiences and, having done so, to focus more on pursuing lines of action coherent with values or motives central to their well-being, the pursuit of which were blocked by the care-giving situation. An increase in consistency with one's own values is expected to increase care-givers' well-being and satisfaction or care-givers' reactions and avoidant coping strategies and, in the medium to long term, contribute to reducing the intensity and perceived 'aversiveness' of certain internal experiences.

These are some of the reasons for inquiring into the utility of the so-called 'third-generation' psychological therapies, and specifically acceptance and commitment therapy (ACT; Hayes, Strosahl, and Wilson 1999), for assisting people in the difficult task of caring for a family member with dementia.

APPLYING ACCEPTANCE AND COMMITMENT THERAPY PRINCIPLES TO UNDERSTAND AND ALLEVIATE DEMENTIA CARE-GIVERS' DISTRESS: BENEFITS AND CHALLENGES

The main objective of acceptance and commitment therapy is to help people with emotional difficulties to develop *psychological flexibility*, which is defined as the ability to act in chosen directions, in line with one's personal values, regardless of the uncomfortable internal experiences (thoughts, emotions, or sensations) one is having at that moment, and in contact with the present moment (Hayes et al. 2012). Hence, values, goals, and objectives constitute the essential framework of ACT intervention, and this makes the ACT approach highly compatible with the most relevant theoretical models about human development across the lifespan, such as the Selective Optimization with Compensation Model of successful ageing (SOC; Baltes and Baltes 1990) or the Motivational Theory of Life-Span Development (Heckhausen, Wrosch, and Schulz 2010). These models consider the person as an active and goal-oriented agent in lifespan development, who strives for adaptation to losses and changes throughout the lifespan, displaying motivational processes in the form of goal selection, goal pursuit, and goal disengagement. These characteristics make such approaches, together with ACT, very helpful frameworks from which to develop psychological interventions aimed at helping people adapt to changes, losses, and life transitions, which are the defining features of most care-giving situations.

According to the ACT perspective, psychological inflexibility is at the root of human psychopathology, and manifests itself in the following six processes (hexaflex model; Hayes, Strosahl, and Wilson 2012): (1) experiential avoidance; (2) low clarity of personal values or loss of contact with them; (3) lack of consistency with personal values (inaction); (4) loss of contact with the present moment; (5) conceptualized self; and (6) cognitive fusion or the excessive or improper regulation of behaviour by verbal processes.

ACT techniques mainly include metaphors and experiential exercises to foster acceptance of internal experiences, deliteralization, or cognitive defusion with the verbal content of thought, clarification of, and commitment with personal values through the performance of actions oriented to them, and mindfulness techniques.

So far, very little research has been conducted on the effectiveness of ACT for helping dementia care-givers. Since Spira et al. (2007) found experiential avoidance in care-givers to be associated with depression even when controlling care-givers' negative affect and care recipients' behaviour problems, no systematic research or randomized clinical trials (RCTs) have been conducted or published on the efficacy of ACT for addressing care-givers' distress. Only three pilot studies with very small samples have so far examined the efficacy of ACT (Márquez-Gonzalez, Romero-Moreno, and Losada 2012) and mindfulness-based interventions (Epstein-Lubow et al. 2011; McBee 2003) in alleviating Alzheimer's disease care-giver burden, providing at least preliminary support for the utility of this approach, especially its component of mindfulness, in improving care-givers' psychological well-being. Preliminary data from an RCT (N = 44) conducted by our research group to analyse the differential efficacy of ACT and CBT vs a minimal support control group to lessen care-givers' distress show that both types of psychological intervention are highly effective to reduce both depression and anxiety, with large effect sizes (ACT Cohen's d = 1.35; CBT Cohen's d: 1.35) (Losada et al. 2012). Specifically in the ACT condition, a 78.6% of care-givers (vs a 58.8% in the CBT one) showed CES-D scores lower than 16 at post-intervention. No significant changes in the outcome variables were found in the control group.

As can be deduced, it is too soon to assume that ACT is an effective and useful treatment to help dementia care-givers. However, the ACT perspective presents very interesting insights that make it particularly promising and worthy of empirical study in order to analyse its potential as a useful and effective therapeutic approach to help dementia care-givers. Indeed, the ACT component of fostering values of clarification and commitment is a central element of the existential psychological paradigm to dementia care-giving known as finding meaning through care-giving (Farran et al. 1991), which is clearly related to the concepts of post-traumatic growth (Tedeschi, Park, and Calhoun, 1998), and is empirically supported by qualitative (Motenko, 1989) and quantitative (Farran et al. 1997; Noonan and Tennstedt, 1997) data revealing the importance of the variable *finding meaning* in order to explain care-givers' depression.

Having accepted the need of further research in order to consider ACT as an empirically validated therapy for dementia care-givers, in the rest of the chapter we analyse, in the context of care-giver distress, the psychological processes highlighted in the ACT hexaflex model of psychopathology (Hayes et al. 2011), describing examples of them in cases of care-givers we have assisted in our clinical work, and outlining ACT-based therapeutic strategies that we have found useful on a clinical basis for modifying them.

Experiential Avoidance

As already outlined above, experiential avoidance is the tendency to display diverse cognitive-emotional and behavioural strategies for avoiding exposure to or escaping from disturbing private experiences (thoughts, including memories, as well as emotions or bodily sensations) (Hayes et al. 1996). This tendency is now widely accepted to be involved in the maintenance of anxiety and mood disorders (Barlow, Allen, and Choate 2004), since, while such avoidance may apparently be 'helpful' for the person in the immediate term by decreasing distress, it may eventually become maladaptive. Specifically, such avoidance may be undesirable: (1) when it leads to a paradoxical increase in distress ('boomerang effect') and the avoided material comes back reinforced and stronger, because it is not amenable to being controlled in a direct way; and/or (2) when it interferes with commitment to valued life directions and the performance of important activities which are crucial for the person's adaptation. The question in this regard would be: which internal experiences might a care-giver try to avoid? In the following section we provide examples of experiential avoidance in dementia care-givers.

Avoidance of positive emotions and the associated guilt

Box 32.1 describes the case of Jane.

Which experiences might Jane be avoiding or trying to control? Jane is likely trying to avoid feeling good, having fun, or just having some relief. Many care-givers assume that

---

Box 32.1 Jane's case

The centre of Jane's life is her mother, who was diagnosed with Alzheimer's disease six years ago and lives with her because she currently needs help in many activities of daily living (ADLs). All of Jane's activities are related to her caring, and her role as a housewife and mother of three children. Jane never pursues any leisure activities, which could bring her positive emotions or relief from her busy life as a care-giver, mother and daughter. She rejects help from friends and brothers: 'It's my duty. Now it's time for her well-being, not mine. I don't feel like having fun myself, given my situation... I'm sure I wouldn't be able to enjoy myself.'

---

care-giving implies necessarily putting aside positive emotions (fun, rest, respite, joy, etc.) for themselves, and feel guilty if they perform activities aimed at activating these positive emotional experiences ('I should not be enjoying myself' is an example of *dirty discomfort*; Hayes et al. 1999). Hence, experiential avoidance in care-givers may focus on positive experiences as a way to prevent feeling guilt. This style of experiential avoidance is likely to be related to *verbal rules*,[1] such as 'dementia care-givers are not supposed to have fun, to enjoy themselves or to look after their own well-being', which might lead care-givers to feel guilt (secondary emotion) if they engage in leisure and gratifying activities. These types of verbal rules related to the care-giver role may be linked to a strong attachment to a conceptualized self (the care-giving role), and are likely to lead care-givers to develop maladaptive behaviours, such as rejecting help from others and/or refusing to engage in pleasant activities which would help increase their well-being. This style of experiential avoidance brings about a situation whereby care-givers reject or show little or no interest at all in participating in psychological interventions aimed at helping them to feel better. In this line, we have found care-givers who deny having negative emotions or thoughts, and who only ask for help in order to learn how to manage direct care-giving situations (e.g. how to provide care). When the therapist tries to explore their private experiences (emotions/feelings/thoughts), they may become uncomfortable (e.g. 'I do not need this type of help you're giving me; I only need you to tell me what to do with my relative, not with me'), and at times may discontinue therapy.

Hence, the avoidance style illustrated by the case of Jane (Box 32.1) is closely related to rigid verbal rules which control the person's behaviour, and to attachment to a conceptualized self. Care-givers displaying this type of experiential avoidance may benefit in significant ways from therapeutic work on cognitive defusion (deliteralization), the promotion of self-as-context, and clarification and commitment to non-care-related values (see below, 'Loss of contact with present moment, cognitive fusion, and conceptualized self in care-givers').

It is important to make a subtle and complex distinction between care-givers who fail to engage in gratifying activities or ask for help due to a dysfunctional experiential avoidance style, and those who fail to attend to or address their own needs and interests, but without this being dysfunctional for them, as they have never really attended to or considered those needs as important, or because they consider their 'sacrifice' as a core set of actions in accordance with how much they love their loved ones. This latter profile of care-givers, in the Spanish cultural context, is likely to be common among older women with a low level of education who, throughout their lives, have played roles related to care-giving (housewife, spouse, mother), and who consider the caring role an essential part of their identity (self-as-content), a source of meaning and purpose in their lives. This profile is not infrequent in societies that still retain strong traditional gender roles (based on the notion of *machismo* in the case of Spain).

Avoidance of events (situations, thoughts, feelings) related to dementia

Box 32.2 describes the case of John.

What is John potentially avoiding or trying to control? John is likely to be avoiding the acceptance of: (1) facts: his wife has a chronic illness that severely affects her behaviour, cognition (memory and reasoning), and personality. She has changed, and she will never behave in the same way as she did in the past; (2) thoughts: related to his wife's change and the irreversibility of her illness; and (3) emotions: rage and grief related to his wife's changes, anger about some of her behaviours, sadness and fear about having to live his life without his wife 'as he once knew her'. For care-givers, it is very difficult to accept that an illness can make their loved ones almost 'disappear' or at least become an almost completely different person from the one they once knew.

Hence, the case of John illustrates another type of care-giving avoiding style: the resistance to accept illness itself and the changes it involves—namely the loved one no longer being 'the same' as they once knew her. This type of experiential avoidance implies a resistance to assume objective and hard-to-accept facts related to dementia, and, consequently, to face the sadness, fear, and other painful emotions that the acceptance of this diagnosis and its associated changes in the ill person involves. This style is usually associated with a mixture of angry outbursts in care-givers—who get mad at their relatives for behaving as they do, followed by guilt at having these 'losses of control'—and compassion and sadness with regard to their loved ones. Dementia is characterized by a pronounced instability in patients' behaviour, mood, and mental status (cognitive functioning), which implies a great degree of uncertainty and may easily lead care-givers to feel anxiety and emotional ambivalence towards their relatives. Dementia patients' behaviour is also highly changeable. Although problem behaviours (such as agitation, aggression, hallucination, or paranoia) are quite common, there can be many moments when they seem to have no cognitive impairment at all—moments of lucidity in which they 'connect' with care-givers (e.g. they can communicate with and understand them) or they behave as they did in the past, as if they were not ill at all. Thus, for example, they may remember specific things or events from the past and make rich and detailed descriptions of them, or their care-givers may notice that they realize

---

Box 32.2 John's case

John usually gets very irritated with his wife Mary, who constantly asks the same questions and forgets important things about her life and their family. 'How can she forget our daughter's name? She was always so clever, so bright...I can't believe she's the same person...If only she paid more attention!' Sometimes he gets really mad at her: 'I sometimes lose my temper and shout at her, or say bad words...and later I feel so mean and wretched...I should be able to control myself and have more patience.'

or become aware of what is happening to them. This instability of care recipients' behaviour leads many care-givers to ask themselves, for example, 'How is it possible that sometimes he clearly remember some things, and other times he doesn't even recognize close relatives? I don't understand this illness.' The moments of lucidity in dementia patients are also related to an attribution that many care-givers frequently make with regard to some of their relatives' problem behaviours. 'He does it on purpose! He is cruel and wants to drive me mad!' It is not difficult to understand how this kind of misinterpretation of care recipients' behaviour usually leads to heightened levels of distress, anxiety, and anger in care-givers.

When difficulties associated with this pattern of experiential avoidance are present, the main objectives of psychological intervention will be to help care-givers: (1) integrate their loved ones' different 'sides' or modes of functioning; (2) accept the instability as part of the illness; and (3) allow themselves to experience the emotional ambivalence which may arise as a natural consequence of the circumstances in which they are living. Useful therapeutic strategies in this regard are the following: (1) the application of the *self-as-context* component of ACT to their perception of their relatives, in order to be able to see the person who is beyond all those different behaviours and modes of functioning, the person 'in-there' (Castleman, Gallagher-Thompson, and Naythons 1999), their loved one; (2) providing care-givers with information about dementia symptoms and the progression of the disease, which includes an appropriate explanation of the cognitive, emotional, and behavioural instability that is a part of the illness; and (3) helping care-givers to make the *transition to a new relationship* with their loved ones.

Avoidance of 'failure' as a care-giver: the challenge of working with care-givers' guilt for not being 'perfect' care-givers

Many care-givers' goals revolve around how to be 'the best' care-givers for their relatives, with some of them implicitly taking on the mission of becoming *perfect* care-givers (as if such a thing existed), and, consequently, suffering the associated negative costs of this perfectionist attitude on their lives. These care-givers may have dysfunctional *verbal rules* with regard to what 'being a good care-giver' means (e.g. 'a good care-giver should never get mad or lose control with the person they are caring for'), and usually report high levels of guilt when they make a mistake or have negative thoughts about their relative (e.g. 'I feel bad when I get angry with my relative') (Losada et al. 2010). This was the case of Antonia (see Box 32.3).

Dementia care-givers' therapists should pay special attention to helping care-givers accept their mistakes or 'failures' and to working on their associated feelings of guilt, which are

---

Box 32.3 Antonia's case

Antonia is a 48-year-old woman who is caring for her mother, diagnosed with Alzheimer's disease. Antonia felt very anxious and expressed feelings of guilt due to, in her own words, 'that terrible mistake that I made one day with my mother…since that day, she seems to be deteriorating at a fast pace'. Specifically, her mother broke her hip due to a fall 'It was my fault', says Antonia, 'because I closed my car door so abruptly that it hit my mother, who fell down…and broke her hip.' Since that day, Antonia says she cannot look her mother in the eye, due to her feelings of guilt.

quite common. In this regard, we have found the therapeutic guidelines included in Hayes et al. (1999, 2011) to be very useful. These guidelines are aimed at helping clients distinguish between *paralysing* blame/guilt and *proactive* responsibility. Also useful is the exercise 'responsibility versus response-ability' (Hayes, Strosahl, and Wilson 1999: 103). For his part, Somov (2010), in his mindfulness approach to addressing *perfectionism*, suggests some helpful and practical strategies for helping clients manage guilt arising after a mistake, for developing skills to become more self-forgiving, and to learn from whatever happened without *self-loathing*, as a path towards self-acceptance. For example, it may be useful to teach care-givers to distinguish between guilt and regret, using the 'Shrug off undue responsibility' exercise (Somov 2010: 84): 'I did the best I could in this situation. If my best wasn't good enough for a successful outcome, then that's just how it is. It's a matter of regret, not guilt.'

Another useful strategy suggested by Somov (2010: 54) is teaching care-givers to use *motive-focused judgment*, which involves judging their behaviours on the basis of the motives behind the behaviour, rather than on its consequences. In the case of Antonia, this exercise was very helpful, as she was able to realize that the day the incident took place she had not slept well, and felt extremely tired and angry at her mother, as she was bothering her while she was driving. After the exercise, she realized that she had been judging her behaviour on the basis of the consequences ('Because of me she broke her hip and her illness has got worse') and not the motive (she was burnt out, had hardly slept, and unluckily, without her intending it, the incident with the car made her mother fall and break her hip). Finally, the 'reverse-empathy method' (Somov 2010: 89) is also helpful for addressing feelings of guilt. This exercise consists of the following steps: (1) first, the care-giver is asked to think of a mistake that he/she thinks he/she has made; (2) then, the care-giver is invited to ask him/herself: 'Would I forgive someone else for this mistake?'; (3) if the care-giver's answer is 'yes', the next question is: 'then, why wouldn't I forgive myself for this mistake?'

General avoidance of aversive internal events through lack of acknowledgement of emotions/thoughts or emotion/thought suppression

Gloria's situation, described in Box 32.4, is another case of a care-giver showing high levels of experiential avoidance.

Box 32.4 Gloria's case

Gloria is doing her best as the care-giver of her mother, diagnosed with dementia. She says that the first thing she does when she wakes up in the morning is to 'put on my smiling face' in order to dissipate negativity and bring positivity to her life. She is proud that she never 'complains or expresses any negative emotion'. With a huge smile on her face, she says 'I don't even stop to notice or analyse how I feel. That would not help me at all. It makes no sense to look at one's feelings. I prefer to focus on reality, on what I have to do as a care-giver, which, by the way, is a lot!'

A subtle form of experiential avoidance may involve the tendency to ignore or put aside one's own emotional experiences through diverse mechanisms: (1) not even noticing or paying attention to them; (2) voluntarily trying to suppress them, acting as if one were not having those experiences; or (3) not expressing them. This subtle style of experiential avoidance may thus involve a lack of acknowledgement of the experience of uncomfortable or painful emotions (pain, grief, rage, anger, etc.), or the avoidance of attending to one's internal experiences or talking to other people about one's feelings. This tendency may be related to lack of emotional clarity or alexithymia (Taylor, Bagby, and Parker 1997). While trying to focus on the positive, rather than the negative side of life may be a very helpful emotion-regulation strategy (e.g. positive reinterpretation), and focusing excessive attention on one's emotions has been related to rumination and emotional discomfort (anxiety and depression) (Salovey et al. 2002), the acceptance of painful emotions (noticing them, facing them, accepting them, or expressing them) does appear to be a necessary step for regulating them and behaving adaptively. For example, noticing that one is tired or exhausted is necessary so that one seeks the appropriate rest and recovers energy in order to keep on functioning properly as a care-giver. Therapeutic work with care-givers showing this type of experiential avoidance could be aimed at fostering their emotional self-awareness and, very relatedly, their self-compassion, which involves accepting themselves as human beings who naturally experience uncomfortable and difficult emotions and thoughts. Although this is not specifically related to care-givers, there is an important body of research supporting the benefits of potentiating these two aspects for emotional health and well-being (Boisseau et al. 2010; Neff, Kirkpatrick, and Rude, 2007).

Loss of Contact with the Present Moment, Cognitive Fusion, and Conceptualized Self in Care-givers

A loss of contact with the present moment is frequently observed in care-givers, many of whom are predominantly oriented to either a conceptualized past (e.g. 'Everything was better before the illness') or the future ('e.g. 'Oh my God, when I think of all that's to come with this illness... I don't think I'll be able to cope'). Processes of rumination and worry are closely related, respectively, to these tendencies to focus more on the past or on the future. Also closely bound up with these tendencies are cognitive fusion with negative thoughts and conceptualized self, commonly found in care-givers' experience of care. We shall look at this in more detail in the following sections.

When rumination and worry prevent care-givers from maintaining contact with the present moment

Many care-givers tend to remember their past in ways that highlight the *blessings* of their life before the dementia, as compared to the trials and suffering of their present lives. It is common for them to be constantly making comparisons between their relative's current and past behaviour/psychological state. Many of them also tend to have regrets with regard to past actions or some aspects of their former life (e.g. 'I should have been kinder to her when she was healthy', 'I should have enjoyed myself more in the past, because it is no longer possible'). These constant comparisons between the 'wonderful' past and the 'terrible' present (relational frame of comparison) may well hamper their sensitivity to and appropriate experience of current potentially gratifying or pleasurable contingencies, and it may also result in the generation and maintenance of painful emotions, such as sadness, rage, or frustration. When care-givers continually focus on these negative emotions, on their causes and consequences, through ruminative thinking (e.g. 'Why do I feel so lonely and depressed?', 'I should have managed to overcome these feelings'), their emotional distress is likely to be maintained or strengthened, as rumination means that people dwell on distressing stimuli, and a depressive state biases thinking processes in a negative way. Rumination has been considered as related to experiential avoidance of emotionally threatening material, and thus as interference in the normal processing of emotional experiences (Giorgio et al. 2010; Lyubomirsky et al. 2006).

Care-givers may also be continually focusing on the future, either distant or immediate. Many care-givers tend to anticipate the 'fatal' outcomes to be expected in Alzheimer's disease patients as the dementia progresses, and their potential lack of ability to cope with them (e.g. 'I'm afraid that I will not be able to help my relative if something serious happens'). These care-givers may express fears and worries about what the dementia will bring with it: 'How will things change in the future?', 'Will I be able to cope with these changes?', and so on. It is also very common for care-givers, given their busy agenda and the many different demands and tasks they have to deal with in their everyday life, to concentrate on the immediate future, constantly thinking what to do next (e.g. 'I have to do this, and then that...'), and thus spending a large part of their day running on 'automatic pilot'. As was the case with the relational frame of comparison between the past and present, this 'automatic pilot' (top-down-processing) mode may hinder care-givers from living in the 'here and now', and interfere with the appropriate experience of positive contingencies of their behaviour occurring in the present. Furthermore, in the same way as rumination, worry has been considered a subtle form of avoidance, as it serves the function of blunting the fear of uncertainty and preparing the care-giver for any bad things that might happen: the constant vigilance it implies is somehow expected by ruminators to be an effective way of preventing anything bad from happening (McKay, Fanning, and Zurita 2011).

When rumination style or excessive worry are significantly present in care-givers, it may be helpful to train them in the acceptance of uncertainty through exposure techniques and mindfulness exercises, which allow them to experience the present moment and come off their 'automatic pilot' (Somov 2010), while activating their personal values and committed actions based on those values (for mindfulness interventions, see Epstein-Lubow et al. 2011; McBee, 2003).

Cognitive fusion and conceptualized self in care-givers

The loss of contact with the here-and-now experience and the associated limitations in sensitivity to present contingencies are closely related to rigid adherence to verbal rules, which

---

Box 32.5 Pedro's case

Pedro is very worried: since his wife became ill, he cannot do anything because his wife 'doesn't let him'. He frequently has thoughts such as 'Now that my wife is ill, I can't enjoy activities. It's very difficult for me. I'm depressed. My depression doesn't allow me to do anything. I'm not emotion-ally relaxed, as I know my life has changed, and with this situation it is impossible. When I try to do things, I start thinking I shouldn't.' He sees his thoughts as literally true, and seems to be permanently fused with them. Furthermore, he tends to make great efforts to defend the certainty of his convictions. As he is caught up in the content of his cognitive activity, he is unable to move toward his valued life goals.

---

control a significant proportion of human behaviour (Skinner 1966). Many dysfunctional thoughts frequently found in care-givers (Losada et al. 2010) take the form of verbal rules which, when activated, are likely to interfere with the processing of stimuli and information inconsistent with the rule. For example, in the case of a care-giver adhering to the verbal rule 'I should help my mother in all activities of daily living, as she is no longer able to do any-thing by herself', it may happen that the person with dementia shows some signs of ability to perform some tasks on their own, but it is unlikely that the care-giver will notice these signs. The rigid compliance with verbal rules is closely linked to a human tendency that arises as a consequence of language becoming the dominant source of regulation of human behaviour, namely 'cognitive fusion'. It can be defined as the tendency to believe in the literal content of thoughts and feelings, and react to thoughts as if they were literal reality (Gillanders et al. in press; Hayes, Follette, and Linhan 2004). To be cognitively fused implies that one's attention and behaviour are dominated by the content of thoughts and that they are less influenced by direct contact with environmental contingencies. Cognitive fusion in care-givers may man-ifest itself in strong emotional reactions and/or dysfunctional behaviours that are activated by specific thoughts. These thoughts can thus act as conditioned stimuli for intense aver-sive emotions and, together with the emotional reactions, may function as discriminative stimuli for behaviours aimed at escaping or avoiding those thoughts/emotions (experiential avoidance).

Bearing the above in mind, it might be expected that many care-givers could benefit sig-nificantly from learning and applying cognitive defusion exercises in their everyday lives, as well as from fostering their *self-as-context*. A case which illustrates this is that of Pedro, a 78-year-old man who cares for his wife, diagnosed with Alzheimer's disease two years ago (see Box 32.5).

In cases similar to this one, we consider that therapists should focus on mindfulness and cognitive defusion or *deliteralization* techniques. Specifically, in the case of Pedro, it was very useful to work with the 'Passengers on the bus' cognitive defusion exercise (Hayes et al. 1999: 157), as he learned to distinguish between those passengers (thoughts) that helped him to get closer to his personal values, and those which hindered or blocked his progress towards them, and which he learned to *ignore*. In addition, the *bodyscan* (Kabat-Zinn 1990) and *breathing mindfully* (McKay et al., 2011) mindfulness techniques helped him to begin orienting his behaviour towards valued life goals.

Personal Values: Low Clarity and/or Low Consistency and one's Connection with Them

Care-giving is closely related to core values for most care-givers, such as love towards their relative, filial piety, reciprocity, or spirituality. In fact, many care-givers obtain significant meaning and purpose from caring for their loved ones. However, time constraints and the constant demands of the care-giving situation, together with the associated 'automatic pilot' mode that can predominate in many care-givers' daily functioning, may have certain consequences. Such consequences might include: (1) care-givers may lose contact with core values (love, gratitude, or sacrifice) that are at the root of their chosen manner of caring for their loved ones, in such a way that they are not consciously aware of them, which can lead to the feeling of being 'lost in the jungle' of caring (Márquez-González et al. 2010); and (2) the priority of care-giving tasks makes it difficult for care-givers to devote time to and activities based on commitment to other important values in their lives, unrelated to care-giving.

In many cases, care-givers may report that dementia has blocked their access to and enjoyment of the most important aspects of their relationship with their loved ones, and assume that this highly valued area of their lives has come to an end. Even when it is a matter of fact that many objectives and goals related to the value of love towards that person are no longer attainable, this valued direction is still there and is, in fact, what gives care-givers the strength to keep on caring for their loved ones. Important therapeutic work can be done in this regard to help care-givers flexibly adjust their objectives and goals (committed actions) related to this value to the present circumstances, restructuring their relationship with their loved one, exploring new possibilities of enjoying their relationship with them, in ways that help them to perceive coherence and consistency in this important area of their life.

It is also likely that care-givers have failed to clarify some of their non-care-related values, perhaps because they have never considered the possibility that areas such as work, personal growth or leisure might be important in their lives. Others may even deny that they have any values at all, as they might have a learning history full of failure experiences, which has led to feelings of helplessness. Therapeutic work on discovering values would seem to be especially relevant in these cases. Some questions that may guide a therapeutic dialogue with this objective are shown in Box 32.6: Helping care-givers to clarify their values and gain awareness

---

Box 32.6 Helping care-givers to clarify their values and gain awareness

The following questions are useful to explore and activate care-givers' values:

In an ideal world in which you could choose the conditions and circumstances of your life, what would you choose?

Is there anything in your life that you would not change at all? Why? This is an important aspect of your life, isn't it?

In what sense would it be helpful for you to feel better? Why do you want to feel better? What doors would open for you? What would your life be like?

Did you have any dreams or 'wish list' when you were a child…an adolescent…a young boy/girl?

Is there any person you admire? Any person you would like to look like?

of them, and training them in the identification, planning, and performance of behaviours that can help them move in their valued directions (committed actions) may be powerful therapeutic strategies for improving their quality of life and well-being.

Some Potential Limitations of ACT Interventions for Care-givers

By definition, ACT-based interventions may be useful for those care-givers with high levels of experiential avoidance. However, the different experiential avoidance levels and styles displayed by care-givers lead to peculiarities that must be addressed in interventions. For example, the presence of very high levels of experiential avoidance in some care-givers may make it extremely difficult to explore and access their private events, so that it will be necessary to devote more time to the initial phase of establishing the therapeutic relationship, and to expect a slower pace for the therapy. Even so, the rigour and experimental control required in applying the scientific method to testing the efficacy of psychological interventions (e.g. protocolized and manualized treatments, with a specific structure, the same number of treatment modules, same length for the different exercises) may make it difficult to appropriately address the specific needs and peculiarities of different care-givers. We also believe that the very nature of ACT is somehow at odds with treatment manualization. In this sense, a substantial limitation in developing an ACT-based intervention which involves promoting all the different components of the hexaflex model (Hayes et al. 2011) (acceptance of negative internal events, mindfulness, cognitive defusion, self-as-context, and clarification of and commitment to valued life directions) is that it does not easily allow therapists to take into account and respect the different rhythms and specific needs of care-givers, which is essential for adequately meeting their diverse needs (Gallagher-Thompson et al. 2012). However, the manualization of treatments appears to be a condition for the demonstration of their efficacy. A challenge for researchers and clinicians is to strike a balance between the use of experimental control and serving the specific needs of carers.

Summary

This aim of this chapter was to provide an overview of what ACT can bring to the current landscape of potential psychological interventions with depressed care-givers of persons with dementia. Starting out from an analysis of the limitations of CBT interventions with care-givers, the ACT model of psychopathology (hexaflex) was used to analyse some of the core processes involved in the maintenance of their psychological distress. Diverse types of experiential avoidance, as well as manifestations of cognitive fusion, conceptualized self, loss of contact with the present moment, and low clarity of or commitment to personal values—all of which are commonly found in care-givers—were illustrated with clinical examples. We also suggested some specific applications of ACT therapeutic strategies to address these pathological processes and help care-givers develop acceptance, mindfulness, clarity of and commitment to their values, cognitive defusion and a perspective of self-as-context. Finally, some limitations of ACT as an approach to relieve care-giver distress were acknowledged, mainly with regard to suitability of such programmes for manualization. Although it is still early to draw definitive conclusions, we can postulate that difficulties in accepting diverse care-related events (both external and private) seem to play a major role in the maintenance of distress in many care-givers, and should thus be taken into account in both assessment and intervention. ACT-based interventions may constitute a promising route to help 'experiential avoidant' care-givers stay committed to their care-giving role in a way that allows them to remain involved in their life projects, able to consciously pursue and enjoy valued life directions.

ACKNOWLEDGEMENTS

This work was supported by a grant from the Spanish Ministry of Science and Innovation (PSI2009-08132).

NOTE

1. Verbal rules are considered to be verbal stimuli that influence behaviour by describing the potential outcomes of engaging in a particular behaviour. This construct is similar to that of 'belief' in the cognitive framework. In our previous work from a CBT paradigm, we called this type of private stimulus with the capacity to influence behaviour 'dysfunctional thoughts'.

KEY REFERENCES AND SOURCES FOR FURTHER READING

Hayes, S. C., Strosahl, K. D., and Wilson, K. G. (1999). *Acceptance and Commitment Therapy: An Experiential Approach to Behavior Change*. New York: Guilford Press.

Hayes, S. C. and Smith, S. (2005). *Get Out of Your Mind and into Your Life: The New Acceptance and Commitment Therapy*. Oakland, CA: New Harbinger.

Márquez-González, M., Romero-Moreno, R., and Losada, A. (2010). 'Caregiving Issues in a Therapeutic Context: New Insights from the Acceptance and Commitment Therapy Approach'. In N. Pachana, K. Laidlaw, and B. Knight (eds), *Casebook of Clinical Geropsychology: International Perspectives on Practice* (pp. 33–53). New York: Oxford University Press.

REFERENCES

Baltes, P. B. and Baltes, M. M. (1990). 'Psychological Perspectives on Successful Aging: the Model of Selective Optimization with Compensation'. In P. B. Baltes and M. M. Baltes (eds), *Successful Aging: Perspectives from the Behavioral Sciences* (pp. 1–34). New York: Cambridge University Press.

Barlow, D. H., Allen, L. B., and Choate, M. L. (2004). 'Toward a Unified Treatment for Emotional Disorders'. *Behavior Therapy* 35: 205–230.

Boisseau, C. L., Farchione, T. J., Fairholme, C. P., Ellard, K. K., and Barlow, D. H. (2010). 'The Development of the Unified Protocol for the Transdiagnostic Treatment of Emotional Disorders: A Case Study'. *Cognitive and Behavioral Practice* 17: 102-113.

Castleman, M., Gallagher-Thompson, D., and Naythons, M. (1999). *There's Still a Person in There*. New York: Putnam.

Coon, D. W., Thompson, L., Steffen, A., Sorocco, K., and Gallagher-Thompson, D. (2003). 'Anger and Depression Management: Psychoeducational Skill Training Interventions for Women Caregivers of a Relative with Dementia'. *Gerontologist* 43: 678–689.

Epstein-Lubow, G., McBee, L., Darling, E., Armey, A., and Miller, I. W. (2011). 'A Pilot Investigation of MindfulnessBased Stress Reduction for Caregivers of Frail Elderly'. *Mindfulness* 2: 95–102.

Farran, C. J., Keane-Hagerty, E., Salloway, S., Kupferer, S., and Wilken, C. S. (1991). 'Finding Meaning: An Alternative Paradigm for Alzheimer's Disease Family Caregivers'. *Gerontologist* 31: 483–489.

Farran, C. J., Miller, B. H., Kaufman, J. E., and Davis, L. (1997). 'Race, Finding Meaning and Caregiver Distress'. *Journal of Aging and Health* 9: 316–313.

Gallagher-Thompson, D., and Coon, D. W. (2007). 'Evidence-based Psychological Treatments for Distress in Family Caregivers of Older Adults'. *Psychology and Aging* 22: 37–51.

Gallagher-Thompson, D., Tzuang, Y. M., Au, A., Brodaty, H., Charlesworth, G., et al. (2012). 'International Perspectives on Non-Pharmacological Best Practices for Dementia Family Caregivers: A Review'. *Clinical Gerontologist* 35: 316–355.

Gillanders, D. T., Boderston, H., Bond, F. W., Dempster, M., Flaxman, P. E., et al. (in press). 'The Development and Initial Validation of the Cognitive Fusion Questionnaire'. *Behavior Therapy*.

Giorgio, J. M., Sanflippo, J., Kleiman, E., Reilly, D., Bender, R. E., et al. (2010). 'An Experiential Avoidance Conceptualization of Depressive Rumination: Three Tests of the Model'. *Behaviour Research and Therapy* 48: 1021–1031.

Hayes, S. C., Wilson, K. W., Gifford, E. V., Follette, V. M., and Strosahl, K. (1996). 'Experiential Avoidance and Behavioral Disorders: A Functional Dimensional Approach to Diagnosis and Treatment'. *Journal of Consulting and Clinical Psychology* 64: 1152–1168.

Hayes, S. C., Strosahl, K. D., and Wilson, K. G. (1999). *Acceptance and Commitment Therapy: An Experiential Approach to Behavior Change*. New York: Guilford Press.

Hayes, S. C., Follette, V. M., and Linehan, M. M. (2004). *Mindfulness and Acceptance: Expanding the Cognitive-behavioral Tradition*. New York: Guilford Press.

Hayes, S. C., Strosahl, K., and Wilson, K. G. (2012). *Acceptance and Commitment Therapy: the Process and Practice of Mindful Change* (2nd edn). New York: Guilford Press.

Heckhausen, J., Wrosch, C., and Schulz, R. (2010). 'A Motivational Theory of Lifespan Development'. *Psychological Review* 117: 32–60.

Kabat-Zinn, J. (1990). *Full Catastrophe Living: Using the Wisdom of Your Body and Mind to Face Stress, Pain, and Illness*. New York: Dell.

Knight, B. and Sayegh, P. (2010). 'Cultural Values and Caregiving: The Updated Sociocultural Stress and Coping Model'. *Journal of Gerontology: Psychological Sciences* 65: 5–13.

Knight, B. and Losada, A. (2011). 'Family Caregiving for Cognitively or Physically Frail Older Adults: Theory, Research, and Practice'. In K. W. Schaie and S. L. Willis (eds), *Handbook of the Psychology of Aging* (7th ed) (pp. 353–365). New York: Academic Press.

Losada, A., Márquez-González, M. and Peñacoba, C., and Romero-Moreno, R. (2010). 'Development and Validation of the Caregiver Guilt Questionnaire'. *International Psychogeriatrics* 22: 650–660.

Losada, A., Márquez-González, M., and Romero-Moreno, R. (2011). 'Mechanisms of Action of a Psychological Intervention for Dementia Caregivers: Effects of Behavioral Activation and Modification of Dysfunctional Thoughts'. *International Journal of Geriatric Psychiatry* 26: 1119–1127.

Losada, A., Márquez-González, M., Romero-Moreno, R., López, J., Fernández-Fernández, V., et al. (2012). 'Acceptance and Commitment Therapy vs. Cognitive Behavioural Therapy for Dementia Family Caregivers: Outcomes of a Randomized Individual Treatment Study'. *Gerontologist* 52 (S1): 300.

Lyubomirsky, S., Kasri, F., Chang, O., and Chung, I. (2006). 'Ruminative Response Styles and Delay of Seeking Diagnosis for Breast Cancer Symptoms'. *Journal of Social and Clinical Psychology* 25: 276–304.

McBee, L. (2003). 'Mindfulness Practice with the Frail Elderly and Their Caregivers: Changing the Practitioner-Patient Relationship'. *Topics in Geriatric Rehabilitation* 19: 257–264.

McKay, M., Fanning, P., and Zurita, P. (2011). *Mind and Emotions: A Universal Treatment for Emotional Disorders.* Oakland, CA: New Harbinger.

Márquez-González, M., Losada, A., Izal, M., Pérez-Rojo, G., and Montorio, I. (2007). 'Modification of Dysfunctional Thoughts about Caregiving in Dementia Family Caregivers: Description and Outcomes of an Intervention Programme'. *Aging & Mental Health* 11: 616–625.

Márquez-González, M., Romero-Moreno, R., and Losada, A. (2010). 'Caregiving Issues in a Therapeutic Context: New Insights from the Acceptance and Commitment Therapy Approach'. In N. Pachana, K. Laidlaw, and Bob Knight (eds), *Casebook of Clinical Geropsychology: International Perspectives on Practice* (pp. 33–53). New York: Oxford University Press.

Motenko, A. K. (1989). 'The Frustrations, Gratifications, and Well-Being of Dementia Caregivers'. *The Gerontologist* 29: 166–172.

Neff, K., Kirkpatrick, K., and Rude, S. (2007). 'Self-compassion and Adaptive Psychological Functioning'. *Journal of Research in Personality* 41: 139–154.

Noonan, A. E. and Tennstedt, S. L. (1997). 'Meaning in Caregiving and its Contributions to Caregiver Well-being'. *Gerontologist* 37: 785–794.

Pinquart, M. and Sörensen, S. (2006). 'Gender Differences in Caregiver Stressors, Social Resources, and Health: An Updated Meta-analysis'. *Journal of Gerontology: Psychological Sciences* 61: 33–45.

Salovey, P., Stroud, L. R., Woolery, A., and Epel, E. S. (2002). 'Perceived Emotional Intelligence, Stress Reactivity, and Symptom Reports: Further Explorations Using the Trait Meta-mood Scale'. *Psychology and Health* 17: 611–627.

Skinner, B. F. (1966). 'An Operant Analysis of Problem Solving'. In B. Kleinmuntz (ed.), *Problem Solving: Research, Method and Theory* (pp. 133–171). New York: Wiley.

Somov, P. (2010). *Present Perfect: A Mindfulness Approach to Letting Go of Perfectionism and the Need for Control.* Oakland, CA: New Harbinger.

Spira, A. P., Beaudreau, S. A., Jimenez, D., Kierod, K., Cusing, M. M., et al. (2007). 'Experiential Avoidance, Acceptance, and Depression in Dementia Family Caregivers'. *Clinical Gerontologist* 30: 55–64.

Taylor, G. J., Bagby, R. M., and Parker, J. D. A. (1997). *Disorders of Affect Regulation: Alexithymia in Medical and Psychiatric Illness.* Cambridge: Cambridge University Press.

Tedeschi, R. G., Park, C. L., and Calhoun, L. G. (1998). *Posttraumatic Growth: Positive Changes in the Aftermath of Crisis*. Mahwah, NJ: Lawrence Erlbaum.

Zarit, S. H. and Femia, E. E. (2008). 'A Future for Family Care and Dementia Intervention Research? Challenges and Strategies'. *Aging & Mental Health* 12: 5–13.

···

CHAPTER 33

REMINISCENCE THERAPY
A Review

···

SUNIL S. BHAR[1]

INTRODUCTION

REMINISCENCE was considered indicative of dementia and cognitive decline in older adults. However, since Butler's (1963, 1974) proposal that reviewing one's life reflects an adaptive means for integrating and resolving experiences in preparation for death, reminiscence has come to be considered by many clinicians and researchers as a normal experience of healthy ageing, rather than as a sign of senility or poor mental health. Therapeutic uses of reminiscence have now been subjected to more than thirty randomized controlled trials (Pinquart and Forstmeier 2012). Reminiscence therapy—that is, interventions that principally use reminiscence—is considered an evidence-based intervention for depression in older adults (Scogin et al. 2005), and promising for other problems such as low cognitive functioning (Cotelli, Manenti, and Zanetti 2012; Woods et al. 2009). Such therapy is now frequently employed across community, hospital, and residential care settings for improving the well-being of older adults (Hendrix and Haight 2002).

Despite the widespread use of reminiscence therapy, terms such as 'reminiscence', 'storytelling', 'life review', and 'life review therapy' remain poorly defined; the same term is used to refer to a wide array of activities, while different terms are used to refer to similar concepts and procedures (Burnside and Haight 1992; Haight 1988; Thornton and Brotchie 1987). The literature on the efficacy of reminiscence therapy refers to various treatment protocols, populations, and outcomes, with few attempts by researchers to synthesize such heterogeneity. Given the growing number of studies investigating reminiscence as a therapy, it is timely to present an overview of activities and interventions that are called reminiscence therapy.

This chapter begins by reviewing the definition of reminiscence and its therapeutic applications. Second, it reviews the evidence of the efficacy of reminiscence therapy protocols. Third, it identifies the purported mechanisms of treatment. Finally, the chapter identifies gaps in the empirical literature that remain to be investigated. The intended purposes of this chapter are (1) to assist clinicians to use reminiscence-based strategies in an empirically informed manner—that is, to be able to identify which protocol may be warranted for a particular population—and (2) to direct future investigative efforts towards gaps in the empirical literature on reminiscence therapy.

What is Reminiscence?

Consider what you did yesterday or this morning. Are you reminiscing? Definitions of reminiscence have tended to emphasize the involvement of memories about more remote autobiographical experiences (Butler 1963). Perrotta and Meacham (1981) described reminiscence as the 'recall of events that happened in . . . early adulthood and childhood' (24). Indeed, when older adults are asked to reminisce, they tend to recall experiences that occurred mostly between the ages of 10 and 30 (Demiray, Gülgöz, and Bluck 2009)—a phenomenon, labelled the 'reminiscence bump' (708). Such memories are rated as significantly more novel, distinctive, important for identity formation, and more likely to reflect life transitions than memories from other life phases (Demiray et al. 2009).

What *types* of memories do individuals recall during reminiscence? Studies that have examined spontaneous reminiscence have found that adults often reminisce about what they have enjoyed in the past. Some gender differences have been noted: women have been found to reminisce about situations involving friends, children, and husbands, rather than about objects, places, or events (Bryant, Smart, and King 2005; Field 1981); men have been found to reminisce about events involving their careers and hobbies (Field 1981).

Reminiscence and Therapy

Reminiscence has been considered therapeutic in one of three contexts—when it occurs spontaneously, when it is used as a component as an established psychosocial treatment, and when it is used as therapy in its own right. Each position is outlined below.

Spontaneous reminiscence

A developing literature has cast reminiscence as a natural activity that is spontaneous, unstructured, and triggered by a range of prompts such as pictures, music, mementos, cultural icons, and other people (Webster and Haight 2002). For example, Cosley et al. (2009) asked individuals aged between 25 and 60 about a recent experience of reminiscence. These individuals described reminiscence as involuntarily triggered by external prompts such as photos, other people, or sounds. Such spontaneous reminiscence has been purported as therapeutic. Researchers have found that older and younger adults who spend more time reminiscing about positive memories report greater positive affect than those who spend less time reminiscing (Bryant et al. 2005).

However, some researchers have also suggested that not all types of reminiscence are beneficial. Wong and Watt (1991) proposed a taxonomy of functions associated with reminiscence. They suggested that reminiscence involving pleasurable experiences may provide a feeling of escapism to the individual, thus allowing relief from current preoccupations. Similarly, memories involving past problem-solving successes may strengthen personal appraisals of mastery, thus improving mood and hope. In contrast, ruminations about past mistakes or regrets may have a detrimental effect on mood.

Reminiscence as a component of therapy

Arguably, most therapeutic approaches include a reference to the individuals' past, even if this is not the focus of the therapy (Knight, Nordhus, and Satre 2003). Thus, reminiscence has been considered to constitute a component of therapies such as cognitive-behavioural therapy, psychodynamic approaches, and narrative therapy.

   For example, in psychodynamic therapies, the client is encouraged to reminisce about early childhood experiences in order to develop insight about the interplay between current difficulties and past experiences (Mills and Coleman 2002). In narrative therapy, autobiographical accounts of problems are placed in the context of stronger and more embellished recollections of personal experiences of mastery (Bohlmeijer, Westerhof, and Emmerik-de Jong 2008). In cognitive-behavioural therapy (CBT), the client is asked to locate their current difficulties in the context of their personal history or life story, in order to identify formative factors to dysfunctional beliefs and to modify such beliefs (Watt and Cappeliez 2000). Examples of such protocols are found in Bhar and Brown's description of CBT for suicide prevention (Bhar and Brown 2012; Brown et al. 2008) and Edwards' (1990) case studies of the use of guided imagery in restructuring early memories. Although reminiscence is utilized in such treatments, studies are needed to disentangle the specific benefits of reminiscence compared to the other components of the treatments.

Reminiscence as therapy

Reminiscence therapies have also proliferated as models of therapy distinct from other schools of therapy. The focus of such therapies has been to deliberately encourage the client to reminisce. Reminiscence therapies have been primarily designed for older adults on the assumption that such adults find reminiscence enjoyable, would benefit from sharing retrospective accounts of their past, and would be motivated to reflect on past experiences as a way of clarifying their personal identity and meaning in life. Webster, Bohlmeijer, and Westerhof (2010) have proposed that such therapies can be delineated into three broad types: Simple reminiscence, life review, and life review therapy.

Simple reminiscence

Simple reminiscence involves autobiographical storytelling that activates the social function of reminiscence—that is, it aims to 'enhance social contacts and short-term well-being' (Webster et al. 2010: 550). Positive memories may be prompted by tangible objects such as photographs, past household items, music, or archived sound recordings (Burnside 1995). In groups, participants usually share personal memories relating to particular topics, developmental stages, music, or memorabilia. For example, participants in a group may be asked to reflect on memories related to the war, holidays, school days, marriages, births of children, a particular song, or photographs. Participants are not asked to provide an integrated narrative of their life experiences or to revise beliefs about the self or the past. Rather, the aim of this intervention is to assist individuals to engage socially with other group members and to enjoy recalling past experiences.

For example, in one study (Ito et al. 2007), participants were encouraged to share childhood memories related to toys, schooldays, and textbooks, as well as memories related to seasonal events such as flowers, harvesting rice, and new-year greetings. In another, participants were asked to bring memorabilia that related to a different life stage each week, to facilitate discussion (Klausner et al. 1998). Similarly, Cook's protocol (Cook 1991; Cook 1984) involved the recollection of positive and pleasant experiences including holidays, school days, marriages, births of children, and happy events. Evocative materials, such as recordings of old songs, old pictures, and other memorabilia, were used to stimulate memories. In Burnside (1995), the most discussed themes were 'favourite holiday', 'first pet', and 'first job'. Some protocols for simple reminiscence have been designed for one-on-one discussions (Haslam et al. 2010; Lai, Chi, and Kayser-Jones 2004), or self-reflection (Bryant et al. 2005), but many are group based, and thus leverage shared experiences to improve social relationships among group members (Tadaka and Kanagawa 2004; Wang 2007; Youssef 1990).

Life review

Life review is 'much more structured', 'focuses on the integration of both positive and negative life events', and is 'evaluative' (Webster et al. 2010: 550). Individuals participating in life review are asked to recollect meaningful events and experiences from various stages of their life (childhood, adolescence, adulthood) in chronological order. The goals of such activity are to allow the individual to examine the significance of past experiences—both those that are felt to be positive and those that are felt to be negative—and to consolidate and integrate these experiences into a coherent narrative (Haight 1991; Haight and Burnside 1993; Haight and Dias 1992; Webster et al. 2010). This intervention purportedly allows individuals to gain insight into how they have developed throughout their lives to become the person they are now, to recognize and express what they have learnt from their positive and negative experiences, and to recall the coping repertoire and values that have guided them in their lives (Westerhof, Bohlmeijer, and Webster 2010).

Life review has been implemented as individual interviews (Haight 1989), and as group activities (Arean et al. 1993), usually lasting between six and twelve sessions. Memories of the past are typically primed by specific questions relating to specific life stages. One example of such a protocol is found in Haight (1989), where participants are guided to discuss experiences of childhood, adolescence, and adulthood, and to examine successes, disappointments, and feelings while growing up. Another example is found in a study by Bohlmeijer et al (2008), where participants are encouraged to discuss a different theme in weekly sessions, such as youth, work, difficult times, social relations, turning points, metaphors and meaning, and future. In the life review protocol of Pot et al. (2010), each session was centred on a topic related to the course of life, making explicit the link between the past and present. Participants were invited to discuss specific topics each week, such as houses they had lived in, friendships, and turning points. In Arean et al., weekly topics were used to guide each participant through a life history review and to stimulate discussion of the major positive and negative events in their lives.

Life review therapy

Life review therapy guides an individual to recall specific positive memories, rather than to review both positive and negative memories. The goal of life review *therapy* is to assist individuals replace negative beliefs about self and the past with more helpful beliefs for the purpose of improving mood, efficacy and hopefulness (Webster et al. 2010). An example of this model is found in Watt and Cappeliez (2000). In this study, reminiscence was combined with cognitive therapy to help individuals reappraise past self-defining events and to identify past coping successes. Six group sessions were conducted with two to four participants per group. Participants were prompted to recall past problem-solving successes, goal-directed activities, the attainment of goals, and experiences of helping others solve problems. Another example is found in the intervention protocol employed by Korte et al. (2012). The protocol involved eight structured group sessions with four to six participants. The sessions aimed to assist participants draw attention to specific positive memories and to integrate difficult life events into a therapeutic framework that emphasized the individual's identity and agency. Specific questions were asked to elicit 'agentic stories' (3):

> How were you able to cope with this situation? Were there any pleasant moments in this difficult time? Now, at a much later date, can you say that you have also learned from that period ... What does this say about the person you are ... What can you do in the near future to live by this value or meaning?

An illustration of life review therapy is presented in Bhar and Brown (2012) through the case of 'Jim', a 77-year-old retired widower who felt isolated, hopeless, and suicidal following the death of his spouse ten years previously. Life review therapy was employed in two ways: First, Jim was asked to construct a collection of items that reminded him of his accomplishments or acceptance. He compiled letters from friends and family, invitation cards to social gatherings, and a positive assessment report of his physical health from his primary care physician. He also included an essay that he had written some years ago for a class, in which he had received an A+ grade. This collection of memorabilia helped him remember that he was loved and valued. Second, Jim was encouraged to reflect on the activities that provided him with self-value. He was asked, 'What did you do in the past that made you feel worthwhile and useful?' He talked about his job as a teacher and reflected on the sense of purpose this job provided him. This conversation led him to decide to join a volunteer organization for teaching English to migrants. Jim was able to use such reminiscence to induce self-worth and efficacy, and to recall experiences that contributed to such feelings, which in turn assisted him in taking actions to reinstate purposeful activities such as teaching.

Efficacy of Reminiscence Therapies

Meta-analyses and systematic reviews of the reminiscence therapy literature have found mixed results regarding the efficacy of reminiscence therapy (Table 33.1). Some reviewers

Table 33.1 Systematic reviews and meta-analyses of the efficacy of reminiscence therapy for older adults

Study	Review	Eligibility criteria	n studies	Finding regarding the efficacy of RT
Bohlmeijer, Smit, and Cuijpers (2003)	MA	Controlled pre-post-test studies examining the effects of RT on depressive symptoms. Sufficient data had to be reported for the calculation of standardized effect sizes.	20	An overall effect size of 0.84 was found indicating a statistically and clinically significant effect of RT on depressive symptomology
Bohlmeijer et al. (2007)	MA	Studies that examined the effects of RT on well-being or life satisfaction	15	An overall effect of 0.54 was found indicating a moderate influence of RT on life satisfaction and emotional well-being in older adults
Buchanar et al. (2002)	SYS	Research studies involving participants aged 65+ focusing on reminiscing or life review and published in English	11	Mixed findings
Chin (2007)	MA	Controlled pre-post-test trials investigating the effect of RT on life satisfaction, happiness, self-esteem, and depression. Included studies had to have at least 5 participants at post-test.	15	RT showed significant benefits on happiness and depression, but not for life satisfaction, and self-esteem
Forsman, Nordmyr, and Wahlbeck (2011)	MA	Prospective controlled studies on older adults diagnosed with depressive disorder without comorbid psychiatric disorders	30	RT had no significant effect on depressive symptoms
Hill and Brettle (2005)	SYS	Studies on the effectiveness, appropriateness, or feasibility of counselling with older populations	47	Mixed findings
Hsieh and Wang (2003)	SYS	RCTs of the effects of RT on depression with adults aged 55+ living in residential care or retirement settings	9	Six of nine (67%) studies showed that RT resulted in a statistical significantly decrease in depression compared with a placebo or usual care conditions
Lin, Dai and Hwang (2003)	SYS	Qualitative, correlational, and experimental studies involving reminiscence with participants aged 65+ or with those living in residential aged care, and using outcome measures of depression, quality of life, self-esteem and SWB	13	Mixed findings

Study	Type	Eligibility criteria	N	Results
Pinquart and Forstmeier (2012)	MA	Controlled trials of RT contrasted against non-treatment control conditions, examining one of more of the following outcomes: Depression, other psychological symptoms, positive psychological well-being, ego-integrity, purpose in life, mastery, cognitive performance, social integration, and preparation for death. Studies needed to have provided sufficient information for computing effect sizes and be published or presented before November 2011	128	Compared with control conditions, at post-test, RT was associated with improved results for all outcomes. Largest improvements were found for ego-integrity, depression, purpose in life, death preparation, mastery, mental health, positive well-being, social integration, and cognitive performance. Intervention effects on depressive symptoms and positive well-being varied by the form of reminiscence. Stronger effects were found in life-review therapy than life review and simple reminiscence
Pinquart and Sörensen (2001)	MA	Controlled trials of RT on depression or SWB, where the control condition was an untreated control group and statistics could be converted to effect sizes; Participants' age 55+	122	RT did not significantly improve clinician-rated depression, and was less effective than cognitive therapy in improving SWB
Scogin and McElreath (1994)	MA	Controlled studies on depression	17	Cognitive therapy and RT were more effective than control conditions for reducing depression
Scogin et al. (2005)	SYS	RCTs of psychological treatments for depressed older adults	20	RT met criteria as evidence-based treatment for depression in older adults
Subramanian and Woods (2012)	SYS	RCTs of individual-based RT for people with dementia	5	Effects were stronger for life review, than for simple reminiscence.
Woods et al. (2009)	MA	Randomized and quasi-randomized trials of RT for dementia, which included at least 6 sessions led by professional staff. Comparisons were made to no-treatment or attention control conditions	5	RT was associated with significant benefits for cognition, mood, and behavioural function. However, studies were found to be of low quality

Note: RT = reminiscence therapy; SWB = subjective well-being; RCTs = randomized controlled trials; SYS = systematic reviews, that is, reviews that provide eligibility criteria and search strategy for the sample of studies included in the review; MA = meta-analysis.

have concluded that reminiscence therapy is not associated with improvement in mental health outcomes (Forsman, Nordmyr, and Wahlbeck 2011; Hsieh and Wang 2003; Pinquart and Sörensen 2001).

Conversely, other reviewers have found positive effects for reminiscence therapy (e.g. Pinquart and Forstmeier 2012), but have also suggested that the effects of therapy vary depending on the type of therapy and problem domain. For example, in their review of reminiscence therapies for individuals with dementia, Subramanian and Woods (2012) found that life review, rather than simple reminiscence, was beneficial for improving mood and cognitive functioning. Other reviews of the literature suggest that while all three types of reminiscence therapy are beneficial for improving mood and well-being for older adults without dementia, the benefits of reminiscence increase as the therapy becomes more structured—that is, from simple reminiscence to life review and to life review therapy (Bohlmeijer et al. 2007; Bohlmeijer, Smit, and Cuijpers 2003; Pinquart, Duberstein, and Lyness 2007).

Based on criteria for empirically supported psychological therapies (Chambless and Hollon 1998), Scogin and colleagues concluded that life review and life review therapy were evidence-based treatments (EBT) for depression in older adults (Scogin et al. 2005). Insufficient evidence exists about the status of such approaches or simple reminiscence as EBT for other problem domains in older adults, such as late-life anxiety (Ayers et al. 2007), memory problems, and dementia-related disruptive behaviours (Logsdon, McCurry, and Teri 2007; Woods et al. 2009).

MECHANISMS OF TREATMENT

The mechanisms of reminiscence therapy that account for outcomes remain unclear. With very few exceptions (Korte, Westerhof, and Bohlmeijer 2012), studies that have alluded to mechanisms of outcome have relied on anecdotal and correlational data, rather than on an analysis of the sequence of changes that occur in reminiscence therapy. Thus, assertions regarding purported mechanisms are, at best, hypotheses, rather than conclusive research-based findings.

Social engagement

Butler (1980) hypothesized that through reminiscing, 'People get much out of the opportunity to express their thought and feeling to someone willing to listen' (37). Similarly, Hsu and Wang (2009) suggest that the positive effects of reminiscence are due to social connectedness—'By sharing past memories and experiences during reminiscence sessions, elders obtain support and empathy from other residents' (297). In a cleverly designed study, Haslam et al. (2010) compared the effects of group-based reminiscence, individually administered reminiscence, and a group-based social activity (playing skittles). Each session was conducted weekly for thirty minutes over six weeks. They found both group-based interventions produced significantly greater positive outcomes (cognitive performance and well-being) than individual reminiscence. They suggest that group membership and associated social interaction, rather than reminiscence per se, produce benefits.

Reducing negative mood states

Individuals may feel better because of the elicitation of positive memories (Butler 1963). Such memories may be a source of pleasure and enjoyment, due to the immersive reverie associated with such retrospection. Indeed, such reminiscence has been linked with pleasure and positive mood (Alea, Vick, and Hyatt 2010; Elford et al. 2005).

Positive beliefs of self

Some researchers have suggested that reminiscence therapy may improve depression in individuals because it promotes greater recall of autobiographical memories (Gonçalves, Albuquerque, and Paul 2009; Serrano et al. 2004). Through the systematic questions, creation of life-story books, prompts (e.g. photographs) and social interaction, individuals may be assisted to recall more specific and detailed accounts of the past. Indeed, an improved ability to retrieve specific autobiographical memories in individuals with and without dementia undergoing life review has been found to be associated with improvements in depression (Gonçalves et al. 2009; Morgan and Woods 2012; Serrano et al. 2004). Two reasons have been forwarded for why increased autobiographical specificity improves mood.

First, reminiscence may assist the individual to remember strategies employed for past problem-solving successes, and thus, to improve their perception of self-mastery for solving problems (Bohlmeijer et al. 2008; Cappeliez and O'Rourke 2006; Cappeliez and Robitaille 2010; Watt and Cappeliez 2000). An early empirical study examining the role of reminiscence in healthy ageing found that improved mental and physical health in older adults was associated with more extensive retrospection about past problem-solving strategies (Watt and Wong 1991). Thus, the recollection of past coping activities may serve to facilitate confidence and strategies for solving current problems, which in turn promotes positive mental health outcomes.

Second, through increased autobiographical specificity, the individual may remember evidence against defeatist beliefs. Through the evaluation of a wide range of experiences, individuals may thus 'disconfirm global, negative evaluations of the self that are associated with depression and begin to develop a realistic, adaptive view of the self that incorporates both positive and negative attributes' (Watt and Cappeliez 2000: 167). In a recent analysis of mediators of the effects of life review on late-life depression and anxiety, Korte, Westerhof, and Bohlmeijer (2012b) found that improvement in positive thoughts about self was a key mechanism in explaining the effectiveness of life review.

Ego integrity

According to Erikson (1963), the developmental task of the final stage of life is to obtain ego-integrity—that is to accept one's life as 'something that had to be and that, by necessity, permitted...no substitutions' (232). The task involves an integration of past experiences in a way that enables one to have a view of one's life as purposeful and meaningful. A review of life events is purported to allow individuals to clarify one's values, uniqueness, and identity. The life review process is thus put forward as a method for achieving such ego integrity, which in turn is believed to prevent despair and to allow the older adult to accept the ending of life with self-esteem. A number of studies have supported the relationship between reminiscing and ego integrity (Afonso et al. 2011; Westerhof et al. 2010).

Summary of the literature of mechanisms in reminiscence therapy

In summary, various mechanisms have been purported to explain positive outcomes of reminiscence therapy. None of these are necessarily mutually exclusive, and in fact are likely to be closely interrelated. For example, it is possible that through social engagement, individuals feel less depressed, and are able to recall more pleasant and specific memories about the past. Furthermore, through such retrieval, individuals may develop a more coherent and acceptable representation of self and the past. The sequence by which such mechanisms unfold in treatment is yet to be empirically examined.

FURTHER RESEARCH

Much is yet to be investigated about reminiscence therapy. Three gaps in the empirical literature on the therapy remain particularly open for empirical investigation.

First, there is much scope for improving the methodological rigour of this literature base. Many randomized controlled trials (RCTs) of reminiscence therapy are underpowered, do not use manualized treatment protocols, fail to assess for treatment integrity, and do not include follow-up assessments. Thus, despite the proliferation of RCTs in this field, many cannot verify if therapy was delivered as intended, was sufficiently different from comparison treatments, or resulted in durable improved outcomes (see Pinquart and Forstmeier 2012).

Second, little is known about the moderators of treatment effects. Some researchers have suggested that a minimum of six sessions is needed to obtain therapeutic effects (Haight and Dias 1992), while others have found positive results after two sessions (Ando et al. 2010). Researchers have suggested that clarity and specificity of memories moderate outcomes (Sutin and Robins 2007), but this suggestion is yet to be fully empirically examined.

Third, as older adults become more technology and computer literate, technology-mediated reminiscence has become more readily available. The use of the telephone and social media such as Facebook and internet-based video sharing websites such as YouTube have enabled peer-to-peer reminiscence initiatives, particularly for individuals who are geographically dispersed (Davis, Guyker, and Persky 2012; Rourke et al. 2011). A number of online applications and commercial software products have emerged over the last decade to prompt reflection and reminiscence (Crete-Nishihata et al. 2012). Some have encouraged the audio recording of personal histories (www.storycorps.com), while others (www.mylifesoftware.com; Alm et al. 2007) have used personal or public digital media to stimulate reminiscence about past events, to trigger positive emotions, and to prompt conversations between family members (Etchemendy et al. 2011). Mobile smartphones have also increasingly allowed for logging, sharing, and reflecting on daily experiences (Isaacs et al. 2013). Despite the proliferation of such offerings, evidence for their feasibility and efficacy with older adults remains to be subjected to rigorous empirical examination.

CLINICAL IMPLICATIONS

Reminiscence therapy can be implemented by clinicians from various theoretical and professional orientations. It relies heavily on common skill sets such as basic counselling and interviewing methods, and does not require specialist knowledge in specific techniques such as socratic questioning, process comments, or behavioural activation. Furthermore, the rationale for such therapy may be readily accepted by both clinician and clients—that is, both may be likely to accept the premise that talking about past events can be a useful means of inducing a positive mood, triggering efficacious self-representations, and developing strategies for solving current problems.

While the therapy is used to improve various problem domains (e.g. depression, life-satisfaction, social engagement, dementia-related problems), clearly more research is warranted on the evidence base of the therapy for problems other than depression. Furthermore, while simple reminiscence is easier to implement given its unstructured format and applicability across contexts, its utility for assisting with mental health problems such as depression has not been well established. Hence, clinicians may need to become familiar with more structured and evidence-based reminiscence protocols such as those found in Haight (1989) and Watt and Cappeliez (2000).

Finally, a common concern for clinicians employing reminiscence therapy is the fear of triggering unwanted memories and feelings in clients. This possibility must be acknowledged, and therefore provisions should be made to minimize or address the emergence of such negative experiences. Such provisions include asking the client for permission to talk about the past, being sensitive to the client's desire to avoid talking about negative past experiences, showing curiosity about the meaning that has been reached about past challenges and adversity, and deliberately focusing on experiences of triumph and success (Gibson 2011). Such efforts will provide a therapeutic context for the client to reminisce about the past.

SUMMARY

Reminiscence therapy has been subjected to much research and is now considered an evidence-based treatment for late-life depression. Although ambiguity about the definition of such therapy persists, recent models have emerged to clarify the strategies and goals relevant to the different forms of reminiscence therapy. Empirical research on the efficacy of each form for different problem domains is beginning to emerge in the literature, although more research is clearly needed. Research is also indicated to elucidate treatment mechanisms and to explore the efficacy of reminiscence when mediated by technology. However, over the last forty years, a growing literature base has amassed to support reminiscence therapy as a promising and relevant intervention for older adults.

Notes

1. Correspondence concerning this article should be addressed to Sunil S. Bhar, Faculty of Health, Arts and Design, Swinburne University of Technology, H99, PO Box 218 Hawthorn, VIC 3122, Australia. Telephone +613 9214 8371; Fax +613 9214 8912, Email: sbhar@swin.edu.au.

Key References and Sources for Further Reading

Readings

Gibson, F. (2011). *Reminiscence and Life Story Work: A Practice Guide*. London: Jessica Kingsley.
Haight, B. K and Webster, J. D. (eds). (2002). *Critical Advances in Reminiscence Work: From Theory to Application*. New York: Springer.
Webster, J., Bohlmeijer, E. T., and Westerhof, G. J. (2010). 'Mapping the Future of Reminiscence: A Conceptual Guide for Research and Practice'. *Research on Aging* 32(4): 527–564.

Professional and non-profit organizations that promote reminiscence

International Institute for Reminiscence and Life review. http://69.195.124.63/~reminis8/.
Association of Personal Historians. http://www.personalhistorians.org/.
StoryCorps. http://storycorps.org/.

References

Afonso, R. M., Bueno, B., Loureiro, M. J., and Pereira, H. (2011). 'Reminiscence, Psychological Well-being, and Ego Integrity in Portuguese Elderly People'. *Educational Gerontology* 37(12): 1063–1080.
Alea, N., Vick, S., and Hyatt, A. (2010). 'The Content of Older Adults' Autobiographical Memories Predicts the Beneficial Outcomes of Reminiscence Group Participation'. *Journal of Adult Development* 17(3): 135–145.
Alm, N., Dye, R., Gowans, G., Campbell, J., Astell, A., and Ellis, M. (2007). 'A Communication Support System for Older People with Dementia'. *Computer* (May): 60–66.

Ando, M., Morita, T., Akechi, T., and Okamoto, T. (2010). 'Efficacy of Short-term Life-review Interviews on the Spiritual Well-Being of Terminally Ill Cancer Patients'. *Journal of Pain and Symptom Management* 39(6): 993–1002.

Arean, P. A., Perri, M. G., Nezu, A. M., Schein, R. L., Christopher, F., and Joseph, T. X. (1993). 'Comparative Effectiveness of Social Problem-solving Therapy and Reminiscence Therapy as Treatments for Depression in Older Adults'. *Journal of Consulting and Clinical Psychology* 61(6): 1003–1010.

Ayers, C. R., Sorrell, J. T., Thorp, S. R., and Wetherell, J. L. (2007). 'Evidence-based psychological treatments for late-life anxiety'. *Psychology and Aging* 22(1): 8–17.

Bhar, S. S. and Brown, G. (2012). 'Treatment of Depression and Suicide in Older Adults'. *Cognitive and Behavioral Practice* 19: 116–125.

Bohlmeijer, E., Smit, F., and Cuijpers, P. (2003). 'Effects of Reminiscence and Life Review on Late-life Depression: A Meta-analysis'. *International Journal of Geriatric Psychiatry* 18(12): 1088–1094.

Bohlmeijer, E., Roemer, M., Cuijpers, P., and Smit, F. (2007). 'The Effects of Reminiscence on Psychological Well-being in Older Adults: A Meta-analysis'. *Aging & Mental Health* 11(3): 291–300.

Bohlmeijer, E. T., Westerhof, G. J., and Emmerik-de Jong, M. (2008). 'The Effects of Integrative Reminiscence on Meaning in Life: Results of a Quasi-experimental Study'. *Aging & Mental Health* 12(5): 639–646.

Brown, G. K., Brown, L. M., Bhar, S. S., and Beck, A. T. (2008). 'Cognitive Therapy for Suicidal Older Adults'. In A. Steffen, L. W. Thompson, and D. Gallagher-Thompson (eds), *Handbook of Behavioral and Cognitive Therapies with Older Adults* (pp. 135–150). New York: Springer.

Bryant, F. B., Smart, C. M., and King, S. P. (2005). 'Using the Past to Enhance the Present: Boosting Happiness through Positive Reminiscence'. *Journal of Happiness Studies* 6(3): 227–260.

Buchanan, D., Moorhouse, A., Cabico, L., Krock, M., Campbell, H., and Spevakow, D. (2002). 'A Critical Review and Synthesis of Literature on Reminiscing with Older Adults'. *Canadian Journal of Nursing Research* 34(3): 123–139.

Burnside, I. (1995). 'Themes and props: Adjuncts for Reminiscence Therapy Groups'. In B. K. Haight and J. D. Webster (eds), *The Art and Science of Reminiscing: Theory, Research, Methods, and Applications* (pp. 153–163). Philadelphia, PA: Taylor and Francis.

Burnside, I. and Haight, B. K. (1992). 'Reminiscence and Life Review: Analysing each Concept'. *Journal of Advanced Nursing* 17(7): 855–862.

Butler, R. N. (1963). 'The Life Review: An Interpretation of Reminscence in the Aged'. *Psychiatry* 26: 65–76.

Butler, R. N. (1974). 'Successful Aging and the Role of the Life Review'. *Journal of the American Geriatrics Society* 22(12): 529–535.

Butler, R. N. (1980). 'The Life Review: An Unrecognized Bonanza'. *International Journal of Aging and Human Development* 12(1): 35–38.

Cappeliez, P. and O'Rourke, N. (2006). 'Empirical Validation of a Model of Reminiscence and Health in Later Life'. *Journals of Gerontology: Series B: Psychological Sciences and Social Sciences* 61B(4): P237–P244.

Cappeliez, P. and Robitaille, A. (2010). 'Coping Mediates the Relationships between Reminiscence and Psychological Well-being among Older Adults'. *Aging & Mental Health* 14(7): 807–818.

Chambless, D. L. and Hollon, S. D. (1998). 'Defining Empirically Supported Therapies'. *Journal of Consulting and Clinical Psychology* 66(1): 7–18.

Chin, A. M. (2007). 'Clinical Effects of Reminiscence Therapy in Older Adults: A Meta-analysis of Controlled Trials'. *Hong Kong Journal of Occupational Therapy* 17(1): 10–22.

Cook, E. A. (1991). 'The Effects of Reminiscence on Psychological Measures of Ego Integrity in Elderly Nursing Home Residents'. *Archives of Psychiatric Nursing* 5(5): 292–298.

Cook, J. B. (1984). 'Reminiscing: How it Can Help Confused Nursing Home Residents'. *Social Casework* 65(2): 90–93.

Cosley, D., Akey, K., Alson, B., Baxter, J., Broomfield, M., et al. (2009). 'Using Technologies to Support Reminscence'. Paper presented at the BCS HCI, Cambridge, UK.

Cotelli, M., Manenti, R., and Zanetti, O. (2012). 'Reminiscence Therapy in Dementia: A Review'. *Maturitas* 72(3): 203–205.

Crete-Nishihata, M., Baecker, R. M., Massimi, M., Ptak, D., Campigotto, R., et al. (2012). 'Reconstructing the Past: Personal Memory Technologies Are Not Just Personal and Not Just for Memory'. *Human–Computer Interaction* 27(1–2): 92–123.

Davis, M., Guyker, W., and Persky, I. (2012). 'Uniting Veterans across Distance through a Telephone-based Reminiscence Group Therapy Intervention'. *Psychological Services* 9(2): 206–208.

Demiray, B., Gülgöz, S., and Bluck, S. (2009). 'Examining the Life Story Account of the Reminiscence Bump: Why We Remember More from Young Adulthood'. *Memory* 17(7): 708–723.

Edwards, D. J. (1990). 'Cognitive Therapy and the Restructuring of Early Memories through Guided Imagery'. *Journal of Cognitive Psychotherapy* 4(1): 33–50.

Elford, H., Wilson, F., McKee, K. J., Chung, M. C., Bolton, G., et al. (2005). 'Psychosocial Benefits of Solitary Reminiscence Writing: An Exploratory Study'. *Aging & Mental Health* 9(4): 305–314.

Erikson, E. (1963). *Childhood and Society*. New York: Norton.

Etchemendy, E., Baños, R. M., Botella, C., Castilla, D., Alcañiz, M., et al. (2011). 'An e-health Platform for the Elderly Population: The Butler System'. *Computers and Education* 56(1): 275–279.

Field, D. (1981). *That's What We Enjoyed in the Old Days: Retrospective Reports*. Paper presented at the Joint Annual Meeting of the Scientific Gerontological Society (34th) and the Scientific & Educational Canadian Association on Gerontology (10th), (Toronto, Ontario, Canada, November 8–12, 1981).

Forsman, A. K., Nordmyr, J., and Wahlbeck, K. (2011). 'Psychosocial Interventions for the Promotion of Mental Health and the Prevention of Depression among Older Adults'. *Health Promotion International* 26(suppl. 1): i85–i107.

Gibson, F. (2011). *Reminiscence and Life Story Work: A Practice Guide*. London: Jessica Kingsley.

Gonçalves, D. C., Albuquerque, P. B., and Paul, C. (2009). 'Life Review with Older Women: An Intervention to Reduce Depression and Improve Autobiographical Memory'. *Aging—Clinical and Experimental Research* 21(4–5): 369–371.

Haight, B. K. (1988). 'The Therapeutic Role of a Structured Life Review Process in Homebound Elderly Subjects'. *Journals of Gerontology* 43(2): P40–P44.

Haight, B. K. (1989). 'Life Review: A Method For Pastoral Counselling: Part 1'. *Journal of Religion and Aging* 5(3): 17–29.

Haight, B. K. (1991). 'Reminiscing: The State of the Art as a Basis for Practice'. *International Journal of Aging and Human Development* 33(1): 1–32.

Haight, B. K. and Burnside, I. (1993). 'Reminiscence and Life Review: Explaining the Differences'. *Archives of Psychiatric Nursing* 7(2): 91–98.

Haight, B. K. and Dias, J. K. (1992). 'Examining Key Variables in Selected Reminiscing Modalities'. *International Psychogeriatrics* 4(Suppl. 2): 279–290.

Haslam, C., Haslam, S. A., Jetten, J., Bevins, A., Ravenscroft, S., et al. (2010). 'The Social Treatment: The Benefits of Group Interventions in Residential Care Settings'. *Psychology and Aging* 25(1): 157–167.

Hendrix, S. and Haight, B. K. (2002). *A Continued Review of Reminiscence*. New York: Springer.

Hill, A. and Brettle, A. (2005). 'The Effectiveness of Counselling with Older People: Results of a Systematic Review'. *Counselling and Psychotherapy Research* 5(4): 265–272.

Hsieh, H. and Wang, J. (2003). 'Effect of Reminiscence Therapy on Depression in Older Adults: A Systematic Review'. *International Journal of Nursing Studies* 40(4): 335.

Hsu, Y. and Wang, J. (2009). 'Physical, Affective, and Behavioral Effects of Group Reminiscence on Depressed Institutionalized Elders in Taiwan'. *Nursing Research* 58(4): 294–299.

Isaacs, E., Konrad, A., Walendowski, A., Lennig, T., Hollis, V., et al. (2013). *Echoes from the Past: How Technology Mediated Reflection Improves Well-being*. Paper presented at the CHI, Paris, France.

Ito, T., Meguro, K., Akanuma, K., Ishii, H., and Mori, E. (2007). 'A Randomized Controlled Trial of the Group Reminiscence Approach in Patients with Vascular Dementia'. *Dementia and Geriatric Cognitive Disorders* 24(1): 48–54.

Klausner, E. J., Clarkin, J. F., Spielman, L., Pupo, C., and Abrams, R. (1998). 'Late-life Depression and Functional Disability: The Role of Goal-focused Group Psychotherapy'. *International Journal of Geriatric Psychiatry* 13(10): 707–716.

Knight, B. G., Nordhus, I. H., and Satre, D. D. (2003). 'Psychotherapy with Older Adults'. In G. Stricker, T. A. Widiger, and I. B. Weiner (eds), *Handbook of Psychology: Clinical Psychology* (*Vol. 8*, pp. 453–468). Hoboken, NJ: Wiley.

Korte, J., Bohlmeijer, E. T., Cappeliez, P., Smit, F., and Westerhof, G. J. (2012a). 'Life Review Therapy for Older Adults with Moderate Depressive Symptomatology: A Pragmatic Randomized Controlled Trial'. *Psychological Medicine* 42(06): 1163–1173.

Korte, J., Westerhof, G. J., and Bohlmeijer, E. T. (2012b). 'Mediating Processes in an Effective Life-review Intervention'. *Psychology and Aging* 27(4): 1172–1181.

Lai, C. K. Y., Chi, I., and Kayser-Jones, J. (2004). 'A Randomized Controlled Trial of a Specific Reminiscence Approach to Promote the Well-being of Nursing Home Residents with Dementia'. *International Psychogeriatrics* 16(1): 33–49.

Lin, Y. C., Dai, Y. T., and Hwang, S. L. (2003). 'The Effect of Reminiscence on the Elderly Population: A Systematic Review'. *Public Health Nursing* 20(4): 297–306.

Logsdon, R. G., McCurry, S. M., and Teri, L. (2007). 'Evidence-based Psychological Treatments for Disruptive Behaviors in Individuals with Dementia'. *Psychology and Aging* 22(1): 28–36.

Mills, M. A. and Coleman, P. G. (2002). 'Using Reminiscence and Life Review Interventions with Older People: A Psychodynamic Approach'. *Journal of Geriatric Psychiatry* 35(1): 63–76.

Morgan, S. and Woods, R., T. (2012). 'Life Review with People with Dementia in Care Homes: A Preliminary Randomized Controlled Trial'. *Non-pharmacological Therapies in Dementia* 1(1): 43–59.

Perrotta, P. and Meacham, J. A. (1981). 'Can a Reminiscing Intervention Alter Depression and Self-esteem?' *International Journal of Aging and Human Development* 14(1): 23–30.

Pinquart, M. and Sörensen, S. (2001). 'How Effective are Psychotherapeutic and Other Psychosocial Interventions with Older Adults? A Meta-analysis'. *Journal of Mental Health and Aging* 7(2): 207–243.

Pinquart, M., Duberstein, P. R., and Lyness, J. M. (2007). 'Effects of Psychotherapy and Other Behavioral Interventions on Clinically Depressed Older Adults: A Meta-analysis'. *Aging & Mental Health* 11(6): 645–657.

Pinquart, M. and Forstmeier, S. (2012). 'Effects of Reminiscence Interventions on Psychosocial Outcomes: A Meta-analysis'. *Aging & Mental Health* 16(5): 541–558.

Pot, A. M., Bohlmeijer, E. T., Onrust, S., Melenhorst, A.-S., Veerbeek, M., et al. (2010). 'The Impact of Life Review on Depression in Older Adults: A Randomized Controlled Trial'. *International Psychogeriatrics* 22(4): 572–581.

Rourke, J., Tobin, F., O'Callaghan, S., Sowman, R., and Collins, D. (2011). '"YouTube": A Useful Tool for Reminiscence Therapy in Dementia'. *Age and Ageing Advance Access* 40: 1–3.

Scogin, F. and McElreath, L. (1994). 'Efficacy of Psychosocial Treatments for Geriatric Depression: A Quantitative Review'. *Journal of Consulting and Clinical Psychology* 62(1): 69–74.

Scogin, F., Welsh, D., Hanson, A., Stump, J., and Coates, A. (2005). 'Evidence-based Psychotherapies for Depression in Older Adults'. *Clinical Psychology: Science and Practice* 12(3): 222–237.

Serrano, J. P., Latorre, J. M., Gatz, M., and Montanes, J. (2004). 'Life Review Therapy Using Autobiographical Retrieval Practice for Older Adults with Depressive Symptomatology'. *Psychology and Aging* 19(2): 272–277.

Subramaniam, P. and Woods, B. (2012). 'The Impact of Individual Reminiscence Therapy for People with Dementia: Systematic Review'. *Expert Review of Neurotherapeutics* 12(5): 545–555.

Sutin, A. R. and Robins, R. W. (2007). 'Phenomenology of Autobiographical Memories: The Memory Experiences Questionnaire'. *Memory* 15(4): 390–411.

Tadaka, E. and Kanagawa, K. (2004). 'Randomized Controlled Trial of a Group Care Program for Community-dwelling Elderly People with Dementia'. *Japan Journal of Nursing Science* 1(1): 19–25.

Thornton, S. and Brotchie, J. (1987). 'Reminiscence: A Critical Review of the Empirical Literature'. *British Journal of Clinical Psychology* 26(2): 93–111.

Wang, J. J. (2007). 'Group Reminiscence Therapy for Cognitive and Affective Function of Demented Elderly in Taiwan'. *International Journal of Geriatric Psychiatry* 22(12): 1235–1240.

Watt, L. M. and Wong, P. T. (1991). 'A Taxonomy of Reminiscence and Therapeutic Implications'. *Journal of Gerontological Social Work* 16(1/2): 37–56.

Watt, L. M. and Cappeliez, P. (2000). 'Integrative and Instrumental Reminiscence Therapies for Depression in Older Adults: Intervention Strategies and Treatment Effectiveness'. *Aging & Mental Health* 4(2): 166–177.

Webster, J., Bohlmeijer, E. T., and Westerhof, G. J. (2010). 'Mapping the Future of Reminiscence: A Conceptual Guide for Research and Practice'. *Research on Aging* 32(4): 527–564.

Webster, J. D. and Haight, B. K. (2002). *Critical Advances in Reminiscence Work: From Theory to Application*. New York: Springer.

Westerhof, G. J., Bohlmeijer, E., and Webster, J. D. (2010). 'Reminiscence and Mental Health: A Review of Recent Progress in Theory, Research and Interventions'. *Ageing & Society* 30(4): 697–721.

Westerhof, G. J., Bohlmeijer, E. T., van Beljouw, I. M. J., and Pot, A. M. (2010). 'Improvement in Personal Meaning Mediates the Effects of a Life Review Intervention on Depressive Symptoms in a Randomized Controlled Trial'. *Gerontologist* 50(4): 541–549.

Wong, P. T. and Watt, L. M. (1991). 'What Types of Reminiscence are Associated with Successful Aging?' *Psychology and Aging* 6(2): 272–279.

Woods, B., Spector, A. E., Jones, C. A., Orrell, M., and Davis, S. P. (2009). 'Reminiscence Therapy for Dementia'. *Cochrane Database of Systematic Reviews* 2. Hoboken, NJ: Wiley.

Youssef, F. A. (1990). 'The Impact of Group Reminiscence Counseling on a Depressed Elderly Population'. *Nurse Practitioner* 15(4): 3237.

CHAPTER 34

COGNITIVE ANALYTIC THERAPY AND LATER LIFE

MICHELLE HAMILL AND ALISTAIR GASKELL

INTRODUCTION

> The self remains permeable throughout life, generating and responding to other selves.
>
> Ryle (2001: 4)

COGNITIVE-ANALYTIC therapy (CAT) was developed by Dr Anthony Ryle in an attempt to deliver effective, time-limited psychotherapy to clients being seen in the UK National Health Service. CAT is now also practised internationally in countries including Australia, Finland, Ireland, Spain, Greece, France, Italy, New Zealand, Poland, India, and Hong Kong. CAT is proposed as a safe and accessible intervention for a wide variety of psychological and mental health problems in many different clinical settings. As a relatively new model, CAT continues to require research to evaluate its comparative validity and effectiveness although it conforms fully to what is known of the characteristics of effective therapies (Kerr 2005). CAT has a strong commitment to research and several controlled trials are under way in various areas, which will augment its existing evidence base (Chanen et al. 2008; Fosbury et al. 1997; Hepple and Sutton 2004; Margison 2000; Marriott and Kellett 2010). For a full review and critique of the development of the theoretical model and its growing evidence and research base see the references and links at the end of chapter.

> Personality and relationships are not adequately described in terms of objects, conflicts or assumptions. They are sustained through an ongoing conversation within ourselves and with others—a conversation with roots in the past and pointing to the future.
>
> (Ryle 2000)

CAT is an integrative and relational model of human development and psychotherapy, bringing together understandings from cognitive and psychoanalytic approaches, activity theory, and dialogism. It focuses on the concerns that a person brings to therapy, and the deeper patterns of relating and cultural formation that underlie these, making it suitable for clients interested in exploring their relational patterns within the context of their lives and experiences. CAT can be applied to a wide range of psychological problems, from depression and anxiety with antecedents in earlier life experiences to more complex personality disorders. However, CAT is not primarily concerned with traditional psychiatric symptoms, syndromes or diagnoses. Rather, it aims to help clients find their own language for what appears to go wrong and set manageable goals to bring about change (Ryle and Kerr 2002). CAT has also been used where there is no definitive recommendation for a specific therapy in treatment guidelines or where a recommended approach has not proved suitable.

Influenced by developmental studies (Rutter et al. 1997; Stern 1985; Trevarthen 1993; Winnicott 1971), CAT's central theory is based on a clearly defined and social concept of the self, which is developed through a process of reciprocal interaction between an individual's inherited characteristics, evolutionary predispositions, and care-givers, in a given society and culture (Ryle and Kerr 2002). CAT is active and collaborative, usually consisting of sixteen or twenty-four sessions. It aims to enable people to gain an understanding of how their difficulties may be made worse by habitual coping strategies, which despite their contribution to distress were once effective (albeit maladaptive) solutions to painful earlier life experiences. Specific questionnaires and self-monitoring methods are used to explore mood shifts and commonly experienced difficulties. Drawing on these, the early sessions focus on developing a shared understanding ('reformulation') of the client's problems in terms of long-established learned patterns of relationships (called 'reciprocal roles'), which evolve from internalizing perceived outer experiences between care-givers and infants (Leiman 1994). It is the internalized relationships rather than the individuals involved that act as templates for future social interaction (Hepple 2002). These roles describe intra- and interpersonal relational patterns in which the self and other take up complementary roles within a defining relationship (Denman 2001): 'a dance into which others are continually invited as a known and predictable way of being in the world' (Hepple 2006: 21). These roles can be functional or dysfunctional, for example 'nurturing to nurtured' or 'abusing to abused'.

These patterns of relating are also inevitably enacted within the therapeutic relationship and it is the open and honest discussion of these in therapy that guides both client and therapist alike. This is considered especially important in the case of complex trauma, where therapists may be at risk of being either overwhelmed or numbed when confronted with intensity of emotions (Robbins and Sutton 2004). In CAT, the therapeutic relationship becomes the medium that enables clients to become aware of their own processes, and use their strength to let go of unhelpful patterns of relating, thinking, and responding to bring about change and reduce distress.

Written descriptions, called a 'reformulation letter', typically read by the therapist in session 4 or 5 (see case examples that follow for excerpts from these letters), and diagrams, in the form of 'sequential diagrammatic reformulation'—the 'SDR' (Figures 34.1–6)—are developed in collaboration between the client and the therapist. These tools are used within, outside, and after therapy ends to enhance self-reflection, thus helping to recognize, challenge, and revise old patterns (usually termed 'procedures') that do not work well and contribute to distress. Alternative possibilities ('exits') and strategies are discussed, practised, and monitored for effectiveness, using standardized or self-report measures. Endings are openly acknowledged and attended to as CAT recognizes that finishing therapy can be distressing, especially if endings have been difficult for clients in the past, or if future endings loom large in the client's mind. The final sessions are used to think back over the course of therapy and plan ahead for after its completion. The therapist writes a 'goodbye letter' and invites clients to do the same, typically read out in the final session reflecting on the experience of therapy, what has been learned, what has been gained, and any disappointments. A follow-up appointment is usually offered two to three months later, where further evaluation of change can be made.

Although there are no formal trials of CAT with older adults, in their edited book *Cognitive Analytic Therapy and Later Life*, Jason Hepple and Laura Sutton (2004), in conjunction with other CAT therapists, outline how CAT is well suited to working therapeutically in later life. They describe how CAT offers a coherent way of linking past and present, emphasizing the interpersonal and finding shared meaning and understanding across generational and cultural boundaries to manage distress. The early sessions of CAT have been found to be effective at engaging older adults who may feel that no one has the time to listen and understand their life story (Hepple 2002). The collaborative and relational nature of CAT, which uses the therapeutic relationship to bring about change and improve well-being, makes it especially suitable to working with this client group when considering theories of emotional regulation in later life. Specifically, as people age, their values change towards emotional balance and the achievement of intimacy with a few valued others (Carstensen and Mikels 2005; Scheibe and Carstensen 2010). Furthermore, with its explicit focus on endings, CAT can sensitively address issues of intimacy and loss related to completion of therapy. The case examples that follow aim to illustrate what CAT can offer in terms of the treatment of difficulties in later life, primarily related to complex and earlier or more distant traumatic life events.

NEGLECT AND TRAUMA IN EARLY LIFE, AND THE EMERGENCE OF DISTRESS IN LATER LIFE

The empirical connection between adverse experience in early life and psychological distress in later life has increasingly been drawn (Kasen et al. 2010; Kraaij and de Wildea 2001). However, the mechanisms by which this connection occurs are not well understood. CAT theory, with its emphasis on the internalization of important relational experiences, provides a powerful means to theorize this connection in a way that gives clients an understanding of their distress, which has the potential to reduce feelings of self-blame and can open the opportunity for changes in both self-to-self and self-to-other relationships.

Sutton and Gaskell (2009) have looked at the situation of children growing up in the absence of adequate emotional care, leading to emotional neglect. For the people presenting to their practices that grew up in the 1940s and 1950s in Britain, there were many reasons that such absences of emotional care occurred, including premature deaths of parents, evacuations, social dislocation, and parental trauma. The absence of emotional care on an individual level may have been mirrored by the lack of social priority for emotional development at a time of national trauma and struggle. Both influences can contribute to the establishment of a reciprocal role of non-attending, neglecting to neglected and needy.

Attachment theory (Bowlby 1969/1982) suggests two main responses to this situation. One might be for a child to amplify expressions of need, in an attempt to secure the attention of an unreliably attending other (such as a depressed mother) while simultaneously neglecting the child's own ability to cater for their own emotional needs. Another is to develop a self-to-self reciprocal role that is controlling, and denying emotional need in an attempt to elicit the protection and approval of care-givers (which in some cultures may be reinforced by a cultural value accorded to non-expression of emotion). In such a situation, a child may develop patterns of caring for others (sometimes in a 'compulsive' way), while at the same time neglecting their own emotional needs.

Sutton and Gaskell argue that self-controlling/self-neglecting reciprocal roles are often manageable in working-age adult life, as non-attention to emotional needs may be adaptive when the priorities are earning a living or the practical tasks of home-making and child-rearing. These reciprocal roles may become more problematic when one or more 'crises' of later life, such as retirement from work, the loss of a significant other they have cared for, or the loss of health enabling a person to look after others, forces a person's emotional needs to come to the fore once again. In such a situation, the person may be in a type of procedure known in CAT as a 'dilemma'. For example:

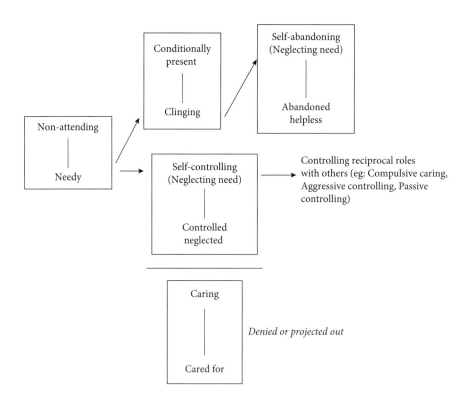

FIGURE 34.1 Responses to absence of adequate emotional care.

EITHER
  I deny my emotional needs and suffer in silence and confusion
  OR
  I experience terrifying feelings of neediness, shame and guilt, which seem to have no solution.

Understanding this kind of procedure can be useful when an older person is referred for therapy (particularly when the impetus for the referral comes from someone other than the person themselves), as this type of dilemma can be acted out in relationship to the therapist. The potential client may be initially reluctant to acknowledge emotional distress and they may oscillate between a wish to communicate and share grief and a wish to deny and withdraw from potential help. The therapist needs to be alert to such processes and not prematurely close off the option of psychological therapy because of an initial reluctance to talk about the experience of distress.

For the clients referred to in Figure 34.2, a sensitive and thorough reformulation letter can help a client to conceptualize their distress as an 'understandable' response to adversity, which is no longer working, and work to develop and build on alternative reciprocal roles. One key idea is often the development of self-compassion. Paul Gilbert (2009) has elaborated a very useful framework for the conceptualization and promotion of compassion and his ideas are commonly used within a CAT model, although CAT might additionally place emphasis on a reformulation letter as a compassionate intervention, and stress the importance of the experience of a compassionate therapeutic relationship in the development of self-compassion.

A CAT conceptualization of the processes surrounding neglect can also illustrate the way in which societal/cultural discourses can influence an interaction. The danger of a therapist unwittingly recreating an experience of neglect of emotional need is reinforced both by cultural discourses about need which a client may have internalized (e.g. 'it's wrong to make a fuss') and contemporary discourse about ageing (e.g. 'you can't teach an old dog new tricks').

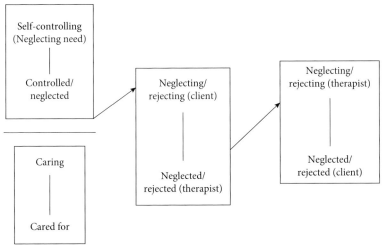

FIGURE 34.2 The process by which a self-controlling reciprocal role can lead to rejection of therapy.

CASE EXAMPLE: 'ALICE'

Alice was an 80-year-old woman who presented with recurrent depression, which had worsened two to three years prior to referral following the death of her husband. At assessment she described long-standing low self-esteem and a history of difficult relationships with other people, in which she often felt rejected or used and responded to this by withdrawal. She was initially very ambivalent about whether talking could possibly help.

She described, rather unemotionally, a troubled childhood living in a seaside town in the south of England. She was an only child who had had a good relationship with her 'adored' mother but not with her father, whom she described as teasing and tormenting her, repeatedly calling her names. She was evacuated to protect her from wartime bombing at the age of 9 and did not return until she was 13, when she found out that her mother had died. Following this there were several further traumas such as an attempt at sexual abuse from her father, his subsequent death, and her going to live with an aunt who did not want her and made her sleep under the stairs. Despite this difficult start in life, Alice was in many ways successful in her adult life—working for many years in a department store, rising through the ranks to a management position, and maintaining a long relationship with her husband, albeit one in which she felt extremely 'let down' in several important ways.

In the fifth therapy session, Alice's therapist retold her story in a reformulation letter, which attempted to draw connections between early and later experiences. An extract is presented below.

> From a young age, you experienced multiple separations from loved ones and a deprecating father and aunt. It is not surprising that you have been left feeling 'worthless' 'unloved ' and 'insecure' and that other people cannot be trusted and will let you down, abandon you or reject you...I wonder whether any indications that other people will not care for you perfectly as you remember your mum doing, triggers a fear that they will treat you terribly like your father did. It's understandable then that you are highly sensitive to potential indications of rejection or criticism in others.

The letter went on to describe the procedure by which she had tried to cope with the years of lack of care either by cutting herself off and trying to control her feeling of need, or by trying to attach to an idealized other and inevitably feeling let down.

The process of therapy was of trying to help her to understand and tolerate her distress and to cut off from other people less when she did feel distressed. She made considerable progress over sixteen sessions of CAT, which was reflected both in self-rating scales and in the description of her change, which was written as part of the exchange of letters between client and therapist at the end of therapy.

> All that had occurred in my life, all the separations and changes left me feeling that I was not worth much...I was held in a kind of 'captivity', the thoughts about myself being controlled by the unpleasant incidents that I had endured through many years...
>
> I feel very different now. I am able to recognize that I must have had some talent to be able to work for the same company for 45 years, with so many promotions during that time...
>
> When I read your letter again [the reformulation letter] just recently, my reaction was of great sympathy for this poor woman who had experienced a sad and difficult life, I felt real sympathy for her. Her name was Alice, like mine, but as I read through the letter it was as if

I was reading about someone else and not me. The compassion I felt for her was real…I've become my friend and not my accuser like some kind of enemy. Hope that makes sense.

It seems that Alice had been able to modify her self-to-self reciprocal roles from what Hepple (2006) describes as the position of a judge to that of a witness to the traumas and losses of her life.

COMPLEX PRESENTATIONS

Across the lifespan, CAT has been seen as a particularly helpful method of conceptualizing the long-term effects of past trauma persisting into later life and intervening in more complex cases, such as with people who might either be diagnosed with a personality disorder or might not reach the threshold for diagnosis, but have similar long-term interpersonal difficulties (Chanen et al. 2008; Ryle et al. 1997). The strength of CAT in working with such presentations lies in building links between current distress and past experiences and in formulating the abrupt changes in mood states in response to intra- or interpersonal processes that particularly characterize borderline presentations. Ryle et al. (1997) describe the 'multiple self-states' model of borderline personality disorder in which therapist and client work together to create a 'Self States Sequential Diagram' which maps out each self-state and the conditions that lead to shifts between states. In addition to helping the client understand the apparently random fluctuation of their moods, this can also help the therapist to understand the way in which negative reciprocal roles occur in the therapeutic relationship and avoid unhelpful enactments of procedures in response to them, such as the potential for collusion in reciprocal roles such as ideal client to ideally caring therapist.

Working with older people two particular types of presentation have been noted in the CAT literature; these are described in more detail below.

Borderline presentations

Hepple (2004b) has described an 'unmasking' theory of the emergence of borderline states in later life. Losses such as bereavement, retirement, sensory health problems, and reduced coping abilities combine to challenge usual coping mechanisms and produce the possibility of adoption of more 'borderline' defences, where these are part of an individual's underlying character. He argues that such defences can present themselves in different ways in older people compared to younger adults, which can cause their meaning to be misinterpreted, particularly as the diagnostic criteria for personality disorders have been formulated with younger people in mind.

So an older person may be more inclined to act out a search for ideal care through adhesive attachments or demanding behaviour towards a care-giver, or may enact an abusing-to-abused reciprocal role through less obvious forms of self-harm than a younger adult, such as abuse of prescription medication or self-neglect. In extreme cases the retreat from distress into a cut-off state may include a retreat into confusion or 'pseudodementia'. One of the strengths of CAT is the ability to represent these processes in diagrammatic form, which provides a basis for a client's self-reflection but can also be used to promote understanding in the system around a client who is experienced as 'difficult'.

Narcissistic presentations

Ennis (2004) and Loates (2004) have described the way in which narcissistic organizations of personality, which often have a dissociation between desired admiring-to-admired and contemptuous-to-contemptible reciprocal roles, are challenged by adverse health and the losses of later life which make it harder to maintain the desired roles. Hepple (2004c) describes how individuals may not be able to maintain the admiring-to-admired roles based on intellect, looks, or talent and may suffer a 'narcissistic collapse' and a sense of emptiness, despair, and unfocused rage. Working with people who have this kind of personality organization can be uncomfortable for therapists and other services. Therapy has the aim of helping the client to develop a more varied repertoire of roles, in particular the development or reinforcement of a 'good-enough' self-state in which reciprocal roles such as tolerance of or compassion towards emotional need are encouraged.

CASE EXAMPLE: 'WILLIAM'

William was a divorced man, originally from northern England, who lived alone and was referred by his GP shortly after his 65th birthday. He had experienced persistent low-level depression for many years and had begun to think about the possibility of ending his life. He would sometimes set dates in his mind when he might end his life, but always found a reason to delay for a while longer. He had a horror of growing old and spoke about how disgusting he thought old people and his own ageing body were. He was initially very unsure about undertaking therapy. He came for an assessment and was offered CAT but cancelled his sessions following a sudden apparent recovery. But the improvement did not last and he agreed to come for sessions.

When he wrote his goodbye letter at the end of therapy he described his earlier state:

> When they [the sessions] began I was in a bit of a mess! I was extremely self-critical; suffering from lack of self-esteem; fearful of getting old; not in control of my emotions especially anger; overly proud and perfectionist; riddled with guilt and shame, some of it over events I hardly remembered; fearful of and always expecting rejection, wary of other people; unable to cope with situations which I felt I could not resolve; fiercely independent, yet at the same time lacking confidence in my own ability sometimes (panicking!) and of course suicidal (in thoughts anyway!).

From his therapist's point of view, his presentation seemed complex too and much time was spent in mapping out his different states of mind and the transitions between them. Particularly noticeable was the role of shame/humiliation—when he faced a problem that he was not immediately able to solve he experienced shame and panic and either responded aggressively or gave up completely. This seemed to be connected to his early-life experiences. His mother was critical of William and worried that he would embarrass her with the neighbours. His father was a 'strong silent type', whom he looked up to but who was also largely emotionally absent. With both of his parents there was a powerful avoidance of emotion and he internalized a need to control his emotions. He was a bright boy who won a place at grammar school but was severely bullied and felt unable to ask either parents or teachers for help. In telling his story his experience of shame was very strong.

A Sequential Diagrammatic Reformulation (Figure 34.3) was produced collaboratively, which mapped out the split between very painful reciprocal roles and an 'in-control' detached and safe place that was associated with an admiring-to-admired reciprocal role. He called the detached, safe state 'Homo Reasonablis', in which he temporarily felt safe and 'super tolerant, logical and humble'.

The therapy was about him finding a middle ground in which he was 'allowed' to have emotions, make mistakes, and make more emotional contact. A breakthrough came when he was able to talk about his feeling that he was not a proper 'man' and that he found extreme difficulty in even using the word 'man'. In view of the more complex presentation the therapy lasted twenty-four sessions and progress was uneven, especially initially. Trust in the therapeutic relationship seemed fragile, and periods of connection alternated with withdrawal and at times criticism of the therapeutic process, although this aspect was perhaps less marked than in other people with a similar personality organization.

He described the change in him in another extract from his 'goodbye' letter.

> I feel that most of the issues, defects, call them what you will that I list in my opening paragraph have been resolved, or very nearly anyway, I feel more relaxed about things, more able to cope, more comfortable with people. The feelings of guilt and shame have receded and I don't

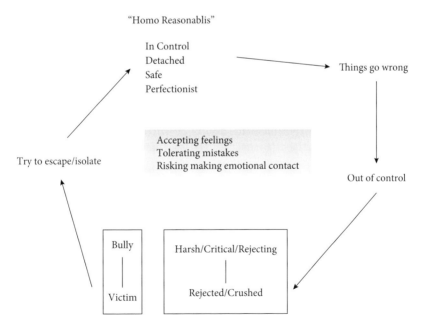

FIGURE 34.3 William's SDR.

worry so much about getting things perfect. I don't get as futilely angry as I used to or try to escape from situations that I would have previously found humiliating—I just go with the flow and laugh them off. I even believe I can now accept getting older (though I wouldn't say I was looking forward to it!).

After discharge he did re-present to the service about nine months later, following a problem in his relationship with his daughter, but was able to find a strategy to address this problem with just a single extra session.

CAT with Long-term Disabling Conditions

The challenges of working with long-term disabling conditions of later life, including dementia, have led CAT into new areas. The relational context surrounding people with such conditions is crucial to high-quality care. CAT concepts can help to create an understanding to manage problematic patterns, at both an individual and a systemic level, in order to enhance the quality of life of people with such conditions and those around them.

Individual work following dementia and stroke

The *World Alzheimer Report* (Alzheimer Disease International 2009) estimated that in 2010 35.6 million people worldwide would be living with dementia. People who have been given the diagnosis of dementia can face major issues of loss, especially as the illness progresses, from communication difficulties to memory loss, confusion, and loss of control over their lives and relationships. Often this can result in anxiety and depression. Adjusting to the certainty of future deterioration is made all the more difficult due to the failing capacity to use words to express feelings and make sense of the world (Cheston 1998). CAT has been used to benefit individuals in the early stages of dementia to address and contain feelings of loss within the context of a person's life while also improving familial relationships associated with this transition (Sutton 1997). Similarly, there are issues of loss and adjustment, in addition to cognitive difficulties, as a consequence of stroke (Yeates et al. 2008). Writing about unresolved mourning, Ryle and Kerr (2002) reflect that coping requires the acceptance of the loss followed by assimilation of its meaning. The time limit of CAT, its intensity, and the direct focus on loss at termination, which is recorded in the 'goodbye letter' make it a suitable intervention for clients with such problems.

Case Example: 'Jim'

Jim was a 68-year-old male living in a nursing home following two strokes. Jim experienced suicidal ideation in response to his overwhelming sense of loss and resultant dependency on others due to his inability to carry out the activities of daily living. Neuropsychological assessment revealed memory and organizational difficulties, further compromising his ability to make sense of his situation. Jim reported that 'my mind is in a terrible state' and described feeling 'in pieces', shifting quickly between a range of emotional states including fear, confusion, persecution, and idealization. He felt that the staff overestimated his abilities, and living with people twenty years his senior with dementia frustrated him. Staff recounted how Jim often became angry, lashing out at them and other residents. They felt at a loss as to how to help him. Jim's confusing and emotional state shifts were described and mapped out in twenty-four sessions of CAT. A prominent coping mechanism of his was to deal with trauma and pain by wanting to forget things. Jim frequently read over his reformulation letter, which enhanced his reflective capacity and functioned as a containment tool (Bion 1962). His Sequential Diagrammatic Reformulation (Figure 34.4) functioned as an insight tool that helped him to recognize his various emotional states by acting as a visual means of integration, which he could hold onto when switching between these. Jim's experience of loss and the meaning of this in light of the changes he had experienced were explored.

NeuroPage®, an assistive technology that uses text message technology via a pager to send reminders of things to do, was subsequently introduced. Although mistrustful of this, Jim agreed to try it, within the safety of the therapeutic relationship. The reminders initially focused on activities of daily living, such as having a shave, and then moved on to facilitate recognition of self-states by using his thoughts associated with unified states as further prompts (e.g. 'I've got the strength, faith and belief to get through this'). These latter prompts were aimed to function as triggering a temporary internal meta-commentary, integrating the fragmented self-states and unhelpful coping strategies. With Jim's permission some sessions took place with care staff where Jim and his therapist talked through his diagram to help them to understand his difficulties in adjusting, in light of his past

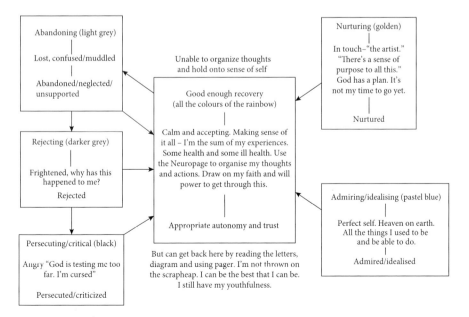

FIGURE 34.4 Jim's SDR.

need for independence. This helped staff to manage their confusion at his switches in presentation.

As therapy progressed Jim regained a sense of independence and unity again. He was carrying out activities of daily living without prompting and eventually without the pager. Staff perceptions changed over time: both Jim and the staff noted the improvement in relations in the home, and he began to tell them when he was feeling angry or upset rather than bottling these feelings up or taking them out on the others. Eight months after finishing therapy, Jim successfully moved into sheltered accommodation, continuing to feel more settled in his mood overall. Central to the work was the use of the therapeutic relationship to co-construct new facets of psychological functioning using cultural tools, which in this case included technology.

CARERS OF PEOPLE WITH DEMENTIA

Given the focus on relationships, both in terms of how a person self-manages and interacts with others within the social context, CAT can provide a useful and sensitive framework when working with carers of people with dementia (Hamill and Mahony 2011). Clinical and research evidence indicates that the maintenance of a person with dementia in the community has more to do with the well-being and attitudes of family carers than factors such as the severity of the disease (Mittelman et al. 2006), highlighting the importance of attending to the relational world of the person with dementia and the environment of care-giving in service provision. Care-givers often report feeling very alone and left to cope with a wide range of feelings towards the person they are caring for, including compassion, disgust, and resentment, which can arouse significant guilt and anxiety (Davenhill 2007) and grief associated with their changing role within the relationship.

By integrating cognitive and analytic models of understanding CAT lends itself to focusing on both the conscious and unconscious conflicts associated with the caring role. CAT can help to make sense of how the caring role can trigger unhelpful coping patterns in the carer that can be linked to early experiences as well as the wider social and cultural environment, while keeping the person with dementia in mind. Drawing on Kitwood's (1997) ideas of 'task-oriented' and 'relationship-oriented' cultures of care, CAT lends itself to working psychotherapeutically with carers who are trying to balance the provision of practical day-to-day care with the emotional and unconscious struggles that can arise as a result of changes in their relationships and role when caring (Wood 2007).

A number of commonly elicited carer roles triggered by caring for someone with dementia across age and cultural backgrounds have been reported (Hamill and Mahony 2011). These include managing (or not) the caring role to the neglect of their own needs, feeling controlled by the progressive and deteriorating nature of the illness, being told by others what is best, or being ignored and overlooked, including by services, while striving to provide perfect care. CAT has been found to help provide a therapeutic space to make sense of these patterns in the context of carers' lives, to find some new possibilities, and adapt to the caring role, and, through its sensitivity to endings, to acknowledge and facilitate the associated grieving process in dementia. The therapist aims to recognize and not collude with the re-enactment of limiting or harmful relational patterns within and between the carer, the person with dementia, and the wider society.

Case Example: 'Susan'

Susan, who was in her late 70s, was referred for therapy due to her depressed mood. She related this to the burden of care of her husband, who had advanced dementia, as well as her own poor health. Her husband was often suspicious, restless, and agitated. She had decided to care for him at home rather than place him in residential care, against the recommendation of social services. Consequently, she had been labelled as 'difficult' by services who attributed her depression solely to the practical burden of caring for her husband, something that could be 'sorted out' by placing him in long-term care. Some of her children agreed that their father should move into residential care while others agreed with Susan's wishes for him to remain at home. Various splitting arose within and between Susan's family and the professionals involved in their care in response to their increasing vulnerability and dependency. She felt unheard and stuck in the middle. She agreed to sixteen sessions of CAT.

Susan explained that she had 'never been one to look after herself' and expected little from men as husbands or fathers. She had multiple physical health problems but seemed indifferent to attending to these and was poorly compliant with her medication. Exploration of her life revealed that, having grown up in a large family, Susan had learnt to rely on herself and keep her feelings to herself. She described hating having to rely on others for fear that they would take over. She appeared to have taken after her mother, putting others' needs ahead of her own, deriving her self-esteem from caring, to the neglect of her own needs and wishes. She recounted feeling as if 'in prison', trapped by her own failing health and that of her husband, as well as her family and other professionals, with everyone telling her what to do and taking over.

An excerpt from her reformulation letter:

> It seems that your dilemma is that either you are independent, in control but ultimately neglected (always put others' needs ahead of your own) or dependent, controlled and helpless (others making decisions for you but it may not be what you want); either way your needs go unmet. It is as though you are the young child again struggling to be heard, invisible and lacking control... My hope for you in this therapy is to create a space for you, about you, where you feel heard and work towards you finding a balance between others doing for you and looking after your own needs as well as exploring the feelings of loss, which surround you at present.

It was the manifestations of these patterns within the therapeutic relationship that formed the focus of the work: recognizing the therapist's identification of feeling helpless, frustrated, and experiencing lack of control in the face of a progressive illness and the organizational system's response to this profound need—in addition to Susan's projections of sadness due to her need to 'soldier on' and keep her feelings initially buried inside for fear of losing control. Susan began to recognize these patterns in her daily life by using her diagram (Figure 34.5), and alternative strategies were developed that she began to internalize and implement. She began to attend to her own needs, learning to receive support from others as well as

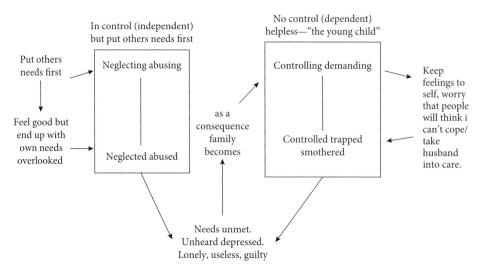

FIGURE 34.5 Susan's SDR.

speaking up more for herself. She expressed surprise at how she was beginning to feel less overlooked and more in control, contrary to her fears of being taken over, in addition to attending to her feelings of loss.

Susan reported how therapy helped her to become aware of how she was neglecting her own needs, and feeling smothered and controlled by her family and professionals telling her what was best for both of them. Through the telling of her life story, a shared understanding of these long-held patterns was reached, thus enhancing her reflective capacity. She began finding new possibilities for her to attend to her own needs, 'find her voice' in relation to others and facilitate her grieving process in relation to her husband as well as her own life. Her goodbye letter to her therapist read: 'When I first came to you I couldn't see how talking to someone would make me feel better…but you have helped me to see things differently and to care about myself more.' Susan's mood, appetite, and sleeping improved and although she was still experiencing psychological distress, this was at an understandable level given her situation. These gains were maintained at her three-month follow-up.

CAT IN CONSULTATION

As highlighted in Jim's therapy, CAT can be used in consultation with staff to help make sense of complex presentations, especially where emotional state shifts occur that may be confusing and challenging for staff, resulting in splitting and demoralization. Behavioural difficulties are often solely attributed to the client but can be understood as a systemic phenomenon in which wider systemic and organizational issues can contribute to the perpetuation of disability and distress. The feelings and emotional reactions generated by the system—for example the staff in a nursing home or the community mental health team and carers—can be used to make sense of how individuals are involved in perpetuating

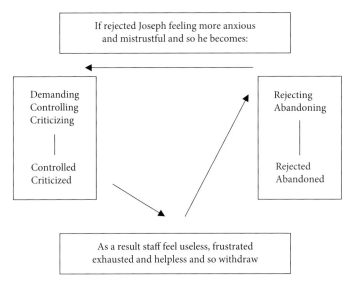

FIGURE 34.6 The team's SDR.

unhelpful dynamics, and to come up with more helpful alternatives to reduce the level of distress and damage caused by destructive behaviour. CAT can help to make sense of staff, client, and system dynamics resulting in containment of powerful feelings and enable staff to respond therapeutically and empathically rather than simply reacting to such clients (Ryle and Kerr 2002). Co-developing an SDR can be containing and educative for staff and permits ownership of negative emotions and responses (e.g. anger) that may not feel permissible professionally by locating these in a non-judgmental system of causality. The case of Joseph is illustrative.

Joseph, in his 80s, had been living in a care home for many years. He had a diagnosis of paranoid schizophrenia and OCD. The care staff experienced Joseph as demanding and critical and they felt worn out, frustrated, and helpless. Some consultation sessions took place with the staff as a result of which the issue of control (or lack of control), resulting from Joseph's perceived sense of personal threat and the anxiety that this provoked, appeared to underlie many of the problems they were having in relation to caring for him. Staff feelings and responses to Joseph were mapped out together (Figure 34.6), with the result that they were able to see how their responses could exacerbate his sense of having no control and increase his anxiety and subsequent demands. Staff worked to develop new strategies including focusing on Joseph's emotions and explaining to him the rationale behind why they were taking a break or getting on with other tasks. This helped staff to feel less helpless and frustrated and maintain a sense of empathy, while helping Joseph to feel less anxious.

SUMMARY

We have given an overview of some applications of CAT to address psychological distress in later life, including the long-term effects of early trauma and organic conditions, as well as its use in consultation in residential care settings. CAT is a developing model and open to revision and integration of ideas through its commitment to further research and practice, which is required to further develop evidence of its effectiveness across the lifespan. For CAT, maintaining a dialogical perspective of the self and therapy is an ongoing work in progress of shared discussion and reflection across and among different schools of thought and cultures. In embracing the breadth of socially and culturally mediated development, CAT offers hope for the development of new meanings, and enables the possibility of a reparative internal dialogue to facilitate more adaptive ways of being in the world, regardless of age (Hepple 2006).

ACKNOWLEDGEMENTS

The authors would like to thank Dr Laura Sutton for her comments on an earlier draft of this chapter, Marian Quinn who was the therapist for one of the case examples, and the clients who generously gave us permission to write about their therapy.

KEY REFERENCES AND SOURCES FOR FURTHER READING

Readings

Hepple, J., Pearce, J., and Wilkinson, P. (eds) (2002). *Psychological Therapies with Older People: Developing Treatments for Effective Practice*. Hove: Brunner Routledge.

Hepple, J. and Sutton, L. (eds) (2004). *Cognitive Analytic Therapy and Later Life*. Hove: Brunner Routledge.

McCormick, E. (2012). *Change for the Better: Self Help through Practical Psychotherapy* (4th edn). London: Sage.

Pollock, P. (2001). *Cognitive Analytic Therapy for Adult Survivors of Childhood Abuse: Approaches to Treatment and Case Management*. Chichester: Wiley-Blackwell.

Ryle, A. and Kerr, I. (2002). *Introducing Cognitive Analytic Therapy: Principles and Practice*. Chichester: Wiley.

Ryle, A., Leighton, T., and Pollock, P. (1997). *Cognitive Analytic Therapy of Borderline Personality Disorder: The Model and the Method*. Chichester: Wiley-Blackwell.

Websites and resources

Association of Cognitive Analytic Therapy (ACAT). http://www.acat.me.uk/page/home.

International Association of Cognitive Analytic Therapy (ICATA). http://www.international cat.org.

Research projects and evidence in CAT. http://www.acat.me.uk/page/key+references.

Books, chapters and journal articles. http://www.acat.me.uk/page/full+bibliography.

Research in progress. http://www.acat.me.uk/page/research+in+the+pipeline.

REFERENCES

Alzheimer's Disease International. (2009). *World Alzheimer Report 2009*. London: Alzheimer's Disease International.

Bion, W. R. (1962). 'Learning from Experience'. *International Journal of Psychoanalysis* 43: 306–310.

Bowlby, J. (1969/1982). *Attachment and Loss, Vol. 1: Attachment*. New York: Basic Books.

Carstensen, L. L. and Mikels, J. A. (2005). 'At the Intersection of Emotion and Cognition: Aging and the Positivity Effect'. *Current Directions in Psychological Science* 14: 117–121.

Chanen, A., Jackson, H. J., McCutcheon, L., Jovev, M., Dudgeon, D., et al. (2008). 'Early Intervention for Adolescents with Borderline Personality Disorder Using Cognitive Analytic Therapy: Randomized Controlled Trial'. *British Journal of Psychiatry* 193: 477–84.

Cheston, R. (1998). 'Psychotherapeutic Work with People with Dementia: A Review of the Literature'. *British Journal of Medical Psychology* 71: 211–231.

Davenhill, R. (ed.) (2007). *Looking into Later Life: A Psychoanalytic Approach to Depression and Dementia in Old Age*. London: Karnac.

Denman, C. (2001). 'Cognitive Analytic Therapy'. *Advances in Psychiatric Treatment* 7: 243–252.

Ennis, S. (2004). 'King Lear: The Mirror Cracked'. In J. Hepple and L. Sutton (eds), *Cognitive Analytic Therapy and Later Life*. Hove: Brunner Routledge.

Fosbury, J. A., Bosley, C. M., Ryle, A., Sönksen, P. H., and Judd, S. L. A. (1997). 'A Trial of Cognitive Analytic Therapy in Poorly Controlled Type I Patients'. *Diabetes Care* 20: 959–964.

Gilbert, P. (2009). *The Compassionate Mind*. London: Constable.

Hamill, M. and Mahony, K. (2011). 'The Long Goodbye: Cognitive Analytic Therapy with Carers of People with Dementia'. *British Journal of Psychotherapy* 27: 292–304.

Hepple, J. (2002). 'Cognitive Analytic Therapy'. In J. Hepple, J. Pearce, and P. Wilkinson (eds), *Psychological Therapies with Older People: Developing Treatments for Effective Practice* (pp. 128–160). Hove: Brunner Routledge.

Hepple, J. (2004a). 'Psychotherapies with Older People: An Overview'. *Advances in Psychiatric Treatment* 10: 371–377.

Hepple, J. (2004b). 'Borderline Traits and Dissociated States in Later Life'. In J. Hepple and L. Sutton (eds), *Cognitive Analytic Therapy and Later Life* (pp. 177–200). Hove: Brunner Routledge.

Hepple, J. (2004c). 'Introduction to the Developmental Conditions of Later Life from a CAT Perspective'. In J. Hepple and L. Sutton (eds), *Cognitive Analytic Therapy and Later Life* (pp. 101–108). Hove: Brunner Routledge.

Hepple, J. and Sutton, L. (eds) (2004). *Cognitive Analytic Therapy and Later Life*. Hove: Brunner Routledge.

Hepple, J. (2006). 'The Witness and the Judge, Cognitive Analytic Therapy in Later Life: the case of Maureen'. *British Journal of Psychotherapy Integration* 2(2): 21–27.

Kasen, S., Henian, C., Sneed, J. R., and Cohen, P. (2010). 'Earlier Stress Exposure and Subsequent Major Depression in Aging Women'. *International Journal of Geriatric Psychiatry* 25(1): 91–99.

Kerr, I. J. (2005). 'Cognitive Analytic Therapy'. *Psychiatry* 4(5): 28–32.

Kitwood, T. (1997). *Dementia Reconsidered: The Person Comes First*. Buckingham: Open University Press.

Kraaij, V. and de Wildea, E. J. (2001). 'Negative Life Events and Depressive Symptoms in the Elderly: A Life Span Perspective'. *Aging & Mental Health* 5(1): 84–91.

Leiman, M. (1994). 'The Development of Cognitive Analytic Therapy'. *International Journal of Short Term Psychotherapy* 9(2–3): 67–82.

Loates, M. (2004). 'The Case of Michael'. In J. Hepple and L. Sutton (eds), *Cognitive Analytic Therapy and Later Life*. Hove: Brunner Routledge.

Margison, F. (2000). 'Cognitive Analytic Therapy: A Case Study in Treatment Development (editorial)'. *British Journal of Medical Psychology* 73: 145–149.

Marriott, M. and Kellett, S. (2010). 'Evaluating a Cognitive Analytic Therapy Service; Practice-based Outcomes and Comparisons with Person-centred and Cognitive-behavioural Therapies'. *Psychology and Psychotherapy: Theory, Research and Practice* 82: 1, 57–72.

Mittelman, M., Haley, W. E, Clay, O. J., and Roth, D. L. (2006). 'Improving Caregiver Well-being Delays Nursing Home Placement of Patients with Alzheimer Disease'. *Neurology* 67: 1592–1599.

Potter, S. and Sutton, L. (2006). 'Making the Dialogic Clearer in the Practice of Cognitive Analytic Therapy'. Keynote speech, 2nd International Conference for Cognitive Analytic Therapy. Maynooth, Ireland. http://www.acat.me.uk/page/full+bibliography.

Robbins, I. and Sutton, L. (2004). 'A Coming Together of CBT and CAT'. In J. Hepple and L. Sutton (eds), *Cognitive Analytic Therapy and Later Life*. Hove: Brunner Routledge.

Rutter, M., Dunn, J., Plomin, R., Simonoff, E., Pickles, A., et al. (1997). 'Integrating Nature and Nurture: Implications of Person–Environment Correlations and Interactions for Developmental Psychopathology'. *Development and Psychopathology* 9: 335–364.

Ryle, A. (2000). *What Theory is CAT Based on? Origins of CAT*. Text from ACAT website quoted in Hepple, J. (2002). 'Cognitive Analytic Therapy'. p. 130. In J. Hepple, J. Pearce, and P. Wilkinson (eds), *Psychological Therapies with Older People: Developing Treatments for Effective Practice* (pp. 128–160). Hove: Brunner Routledge.

Ryle, A. (2001). 'CAT's Dialogic Perspective on the Self'. *Reformulation*. http://www.acat.me.uk/reformulation.php?issue_id=33&article_id=385.

Ryle, A. and Kerr, I. B. (2002). *Introducing Cognitive Analytic Therapy: Principles and Practice*. Chichester: Wiley.

Ryle, A., Leighton, T. and Pollock, P. (1997). *Cognitive Analytic Therapy and Borderline Personality Disorder: The Model and the Method*. Chichester: Wiley.

Scheibe, S. and Carstensen, L. L. (2010). 'Emotional Aging: Recent Findings and Future Trends'. *Journal of Gerontology: Series B: Psychological Sciences* 65(2): 135–144.

Stern, D. N. (1985). *The Interpersonal World of the Infant: A View from Psychoanalysis and Developmental Psychology*. New York: Basic Books.

Sutton, L. and Cheston, R. (1997). 'Rewriting the Story of Dementia: A Narrative Approach to Psychotherapy with People with Dementia'. In M. Marshall (ed.), *State of the Art in Dementia Care*. London: Centre for Policy on Ageing.

Sutton, L. (1997). "Out of the Silence." When People Can't Talk About It'. In L. Hunt, M. Marshall and C. Rowlings (eds), *Past Trauma in Later Life: European Perspectives on Therapeutic Work with Older People*. London: Jessica Kingsley.

Sutton, L. (2004). 'Cultures of Care in Severe Depression and Dementia'. In J. Hepple and L. Sutton (eds), *Cognitive Analytic Therapy and Later Life* (pp. 201–220). Hove: Brunner Routledge.

Sutton, L. S. and Leiman, M. (2004). 'The Development of the Dialogic Self in CAT. A Fresh Perspective on Ageing'. In J. Hepple and L. Sutton (eds), *Cognitive Analytic Therapy and Later Life*. Hove: Brunner Routledge.

Sutton, L. and Gaskell, A. (2009). 'Meeting with Older People as CAT Practitioners: Attending to Neglect'. *Reformulation* (Summer): 6–13.

Trevarthen, C. (1993). 'Playing into Reality: Conversations with Infant Communicator'. *Journal of the Squiggle Foundation, Winnicott Studies* 7: 67–84.

Winnicott, D. W. (1971). *Playing and Reality*. London. Tavistock.

Wood, H. (2007). 'Caring for a Relative with Dementia—Who Is the Sufferer?' In R. Davenhill (ed.), *Looking into Later Life: A Psychoanalytic Approach to Depression and Dementia in Old Age* (pp. 269–282). London: Karnac.

Yeates, G., Hamill, M., Sutton, L., Psaila, K., Gracey, F., et al. (2008). 'Dysexecutive Problems and Interpersonal Relating Following Frontal Brain Injury: Reformulation and Compensation in Cognitive Analytic Therapy'. *Neuro-psychoanalysis: An Interdisciplinary Journal of Psychoanalysis and the Neurosciences* 10(1): 43–58.

CHAPTER 35

FAMILY THERAPY WITH AGEING FAMILIES

SARA HONN QUALLS

INTRODUCTION

FAMILY therapy interventions are relatively rare in clinical geropsychology despite the strong involvement of families in the social lives and care support of older adults. Care systems frequently interact with families but geropsychologists are rarely prepared theoretically or clinically to intervene with family systems and so lack a powerful tool that could be useful. Families are the primary social context (Fingerman, Miller, and Seidel 2009) as well as the primary care-giving resource for older adults (Stephens and Franks 2009). As such, older adults usually transition through normal developmental processes in later life within the context of a social convoy or network that travels through life with them, dominated by family (Kahn and Antonucci 1980). As with adults of any age, therapeutic interventions for clinical difficulties need to fit into the life context, suggesting that family is relevant to the assessment of clinical conditions in older adults. Interventions may engage family in various instrumental or emotional support roles for the individual's therapeutic work. In some circumstances, family structures and processes become the focus of possible interventions, among which family therapy is an option.

Family therapies are most commonly considered when some aspect of family structure or patterns of functioning interfere with, or need to adapt to, changes in the well-being of the older family member who is the focus of concern. The older person may become the *identified patient* (IP) if functional well-being declines due to changes in biological, psychological, or social functioning. Changes in any one domain tend to have reverberating effects on other domains, as outlined in the biopsychosocial model (Engel 1980; Frankel, Quill, and McDaniel 2003). By virtue of its important role in social well-being, family functioning is a relevant factor to consider in any investigation of clinical care for older adults due to shifts in biological or psychological functioning. Just as biological and psychological domains of function can be the focus of intervention, so the social domain offers opportunities to impact all aspects of well-being, including the use of family interventions. Family interventions, specifically interventions that alter family structures or functioning, are one social intervention that can have powerful effects on individual well-being.

> Carter Weems, a retired attorney, requested an appointment for himself and his wife, Millie, to help them address the tension between them. In the first session, he shared that he was struggling to support his wife through her frustrations with daily tasks that were now more difficult due to dementia, and she seemed irritated by that. She was obviously annoyed at his use of the word 'dementia'. She did not believe there was anything wrong with her, and was angry that he would say that. He gently but firmly reminded her of the series of evaluations that led her physician to give that diagnosis. She remained miffed, and thought it was silly they were in my office. Mr Weems was obviously worried about her and distressed at her denial. I reassured them that couples dealing with dementia often viewed the problem differently, and that they could learn to work out the problems in their communication even if they didn't share the same view of the cause.

This chapter offers a rationale for the value of family-level interventions with ageing families, reviews theories of family therapy, summarizes applications with ageing adults, and suggests implications for practice in clinical geropsychology.

THE ROLES OF FAMILIES IN GEROPSYCHOLOGY

As a highly salient social context for older adults, families may become relevant to practice for geropsychologists in assessment and intervention. Although some family roles are primarily supportive of individual-level interventions, other interventions target the family system itself, its basic role structure, or patterns of functioning, as the focus of the intervention. The distinction between individual-level intervention with family members, and family-level intervention (whether with one or multiple family members participating) is a critical distinguishing factor in what can be defined as family therapy.

The role of family in clinical geropsychology assessment and intervention may be simply a contextual factor that enriches the clinician's understanding of the person and/or disorder. Knowledge of the family context may help the clinician tailor an intervention to the specific life context in a way that enhances success. For example, interventions for depression often involve increasing the frequency of engagement in pleasant events such as social interactions. Some family members might provide consistent mood-enhancing interactions whereas others would generate more distress than positive mood. Knowledge of the role and meaning of family relationships is often relevant, and at times key, to effective treatment planning.

For some older adults, family dynamics are an aetiological factor for mental disorder. Family circumstances and stresses can precipitate significant anxiety, grief, and low mood, which contribute to a downward spiral of psychological functioning (Hammen et al. 2012). For example, when an adult child experiences a highly conflicted divorce, a grandchild commits suicide, or a late-life marital conflict is not resolved, distress is an expected response. In some cases, the strategies used to manage the distress contribute to the development of a clinical disorder. Extended periods of social disruption or distress can wear the person down physically or psychologically and thus increase the risk for clinical syndromes, as occurs in long-term care-giving for a spouse with dementia (Kiecolt-Glaser et al. 1991).

Table 35.1 Choosing family-level interventions

Individual-level problem	Examples of problems that may warrant family involvement	Family-level strategies
Dementia diagnosis was made by primary care provider without thorough evaluation, and neither family nor patient believes it	Family members refuse to help patient based on their belief the patient is being lazy, regardless of the diagnosis.	Patient invites family to session with psychologist who builds consensus among family about care plan after – detailed review of test results with relevant family members – values clarification exercise regarding health choices and the balance between autonomy and safety.
Challenges with activities of daily living	Older adult with legal decision-making capacity continues to drive after medical documentation validates inappropriateness due to mild cognitive impairment.	Family members build consensus about decision and announce it to patient together, using carefully planned strategy for roles each will play in persuasive conversation.
	Housekeeper repeatedly finds pills on the floor that patient claims to have ingested; patient agrees to talk with family about help but refuses assistance from paid carers.	Concerned family members engage in problem-solving discussion to share medication oversight that would be too heavy a burden for any single person to manage.
Care-giver provides less service than is needed	Care-giver has too many work and family responsibilities to provide the level of care needed by the older person.	Family meeting is held to review all of the care needs and position primary care-giver to be manager of multiple family members providing service.
	Care-giver wants to micro-manage care services and pushes away persons who could help.	Family genogram shows many members in position to help so roles are restructured to position primary care-giver in charge of emotional support and another family member in charge of instrumental support
Care-giver provides more service than is needed	Family member provides so much assistance that older adult becomes passive and sedentary.	Assessment of capabilities provides basis for planning the activities for which older adult should maintain responsibility. Care-giver is assigned alternative tasks so she will not interfere with independent actions.
	Daughter brings food every night and stays to help her mother with her father's care. Mother is exhausted by daughter's constant nagging and complaining during the daily visits.	Mother is coached to communicate with daughter differently, detailing the desired supportive services that are truly helpful. Mother asks her other daughter to communicate more regularly with the daughter needing more emotional support.
Care-giver is distressed and at risk	Frail wife cares for husband with Parkinson's Disease in their home. She rarely sees other people and feels trapped by the burdens of 24/7 care. She is growing depressed.	Wife invites larger family network to session for purpose of creating a distributed care plan over which she will retain control. A strong support programme for the primary care-giver is implemented with regular family meetings to handle disruptions in the plan.

Although it is not always valuable, in some cases engagement of the family in the intervention is helpful. Table 35.1 offers a framework for the contexts in which clinical services might engage family members and may target family interactions as the focus of the work.

Family dynamics may also be the venue in which older adults display their psychological disorder. Elder abuse is an extreme example of a family dynamic that may be rooted in the psychological disorders of the perpetrator (Pillemer 1985; Schiamberg 2000). Even in less dramatic situations, a depressed or anxious older adult who is the primary care-giver for another person may place the care recipient at risk if the disorder undermines the quality of care or imposes psychological distress on the care recipient. Yet another example occurs in families in which a personality disorder in a frail older adult care-giver leads him or her to make inappropriate demands on adult children when the care-giver's sense of control is threatened. In each of these cases, family therapy adds to the intervention alternatives that can help the family manage difficult interpersonal interactions that result from problems in one or more individual family members.

Difficult family dynamics may also interrupt implementation of healthcare services (Rolland 1994). Family conflicts, as well as over-involved or under-involved families can all interfere with implementation of a treatment or care plan for any aspect of healthcare, including psychological services. Examples include interruptions in care the family promises to provide (e.g. monitoring of medication or nutritional intake, transportation to social outings) and encouragement of non-compliance with treatment recommendations (e.g. delivering doughnuts daily to a person with diabetes). Frail older adults who rely on family for proxy decision-making authority about health or legal matters are particularly vulnerable to difficult family dynamics. Elder abuse can occur in the context of family relationships in which multiple family members know or suspect the abuse but long-term dynamics deter them from intervening.

In sum, family is the highly salient social and care-giving context for most older adults. As such, families can be viewed as on a continuum from very minimal to intensive involvement. They may be merely relevant bystanders to psychological work with older adults, or may be key participants in interventions that target the interpersonal dynamics themselves.

The daily activities in which frustration and conflict arose were explored in the first session with the Weems couple. I attended closely to the timing, frequency, triggers, and contexts of conflict. I also noticed that Millie faded out quite often, obviously losing track of the conversation. Carter tried to pull her back in, usually without success. At one point, Millie put her face in her hands and described her sense of hopelessness that 'this will ever be better'. I asked Carter to attend the next session alone, and Millie was visibly relieved that she would not have to come. I also asked for, and received, permission from both of them to gather her medical records. He was her health durable power of attorney so could sign legally; I also asked for her assent which she gave.

In the second session, with Carter alone, I gathered more history. Millie showed subtle changes in cognition about five years previously. Carter had not been concerned initially because he thought it was another bout of depression. Millie had battled recurrent Major Depressive Disorder her whole life, with multiple hospitalizations in her history. Between episodes, Carter described her as a devoted housewife and mother who produced beautiful quilts, caring mothering, and excellent meals. This long history had impacted the family significantly. Carter's personality preferred predictability and order, so he responded to her absence by structuring the family tightly. He noted that their sons had missed out on a lot from their mother, and resented him for taking over her roles so 'poorly'. Carter described their older son as a financially successful but cold person who had interacted with his parents rarely since he left home. This son called on holidays but travelled the 1000 miles from his home only every few years to visit in person. The younger son lived in a remote wilderness region, working as a forest ranger, without partner or children. On his annual visits, he was warmer with his parents, especially his mother. Both sons were obviously a disappointment to Carter, and relatively estranged. Yet he insisted he wanted them kept apprised of Millie's status. He could not quite figure out how to do that, however, because the older son got so agitated and angry at Carter when dementia was mentioned because he did not believe his mother had any problems other than having to live with Carter's controlling personality.

Effectiveness of Family Therapy with Ageing Families

Family care-givers are at significantly elevated risk for physical and mental health problems, especially during extended periods of care-giving (Haley et al. 2010; Pinquart and Sörensen 2005; Schulz and Martire 2004). Family members provide the vast majority of care for older adults, engaging in an average of 20.4 hours per week of emotional and instrumental support tasks (National Alliance for Caregiving 2009). Care-giving interventions have proliferated within various geriatric health disciplines and among gerontologists (e.g. nursing, occupational therapy, psychology, social work, adult developmentalists), ranging from awareness-building and education to intensive interventions (Coon, Gallagher-Thompson, and Thompson 2003; Coon et al. 2012; Pinquart and Sörensen 2006).

Among the varied approaches to reducing distress and burden in family care-givers is a wide variation in the focus on family relationships (Zarit 2009). Some models explicitly address family relationship patterns, primarily for the purpose of increasing perceived support for the primary care-giver (Eisdorfer et al. 2003; Mittelman et al. 1993). Most appreciate the distinctions between spousal care-givers and adult children, for example, even if the intervention is not explicitly focused on the relationship structure itself. Research on cultural variations in care-giving burdens make clear the importance of family structures, roles, and acculturation processes in shaping the nature and impact of care-giving on the care-giver (Knight and Sayengh 2010). As the context for care, families are the conduit through which broader cultural factors (e.g. norms, definitions of family) influence care-giving structures and experiences, norms and obligations, along with specific strategies and patterns of care.

Several care-giving interventions now focus explicitly on family roles, particularly emotional support for the primary care-giver. The current preferred paradigm seems to be a flexible approach that values the diverse points in the care-giving journey of help-seeking clients, the care-givers' varied needs, and the varied contexts of care including diverse family structures.

The evidence base for use of family therapy with later life families is still developing; training programmes rarely prepare students to work or conduct intervention research at the level of the family and this, among other reasons, has slowed the development of the literature in this area. With a focus on the interaction among family members, family therapy interventions seek to interrupt familiar communication patterns so new patterns can emerge. The idiosyncratic nature of those patterns within each family have also been a sub-stantial barrier to efforts to study the effects of family therapy in randomized clinical trials (RCTs). Later-life families pose particular challenges because the membership of the family varies substantially across families. In contrast to child-rearing families in which the basic family roles (e.g. parent and child) can be presumed to be needed in all families, the lines of authority among generations of adults are not as simply aligned along parent/child lines. Even the membership in the family is highly variable, with sisters caring for each other, nieces stepping in to support an aunt who lacks children of her own, and siblings collabo-rating with one parent in care of the other parent. Simple reliance upon blood lineages or even cohabitation are not likely to be appropriate, and the growing variations in family and family-alternative structures are likely to increase in future decades. In essence, later-life families provide substantial ambiguity regarding who is in the family, what structures and roles would benefit the family's functioning, and the desired outcomes.

Another challenge to conducting RCTs with family therapy is the wide variation in the focus of the intervention. As will be seen in the outcome studies detailed below, tremendous flexibility is needed in implementation of family interventions due to the wide variation in who participates, the focus of the problem, and existing role structures within the family. For example, decision-making authority may be a key issue in one family, whereas another family may struggle to engage enough care support to meet the needs of a medically fragile older member. Modularized approaches to intervention are sometimes used to handle this variation (Zarit 2009), requiring a different methodology from a traditional RCT. In this approach, assessments are used to identify the intervention goals, and goal-specific modules are selected from a broader set of module options. Intervention outcomes may include eval-uation of the impact of particular modules, as well as assessment of measures of individual well-being. Despite the focus on family functioning in family therapy, outcome measures almost exclusively assess individual well-being rather than evaluating the family-level struc-ture or functioning.

In addition to clinical case studies, two intervention studies included a family-level inter-vention within a multicomponent clinical trial. In the New York University intervention with care-givers of persons with dementia, four family counselling sessions were combined with two individual sessions for the primary care-giver, weekly support-group participation by the primary care-giver, and ongoing ad hoc counselling on an as-needed basis (Mittelman et al. 2004). When compared with usual care (referral to support groups and education), the multicomponent intervention showed greater impact on depressive symptoms that was sustained over a three-year period (Mittelman et al. 2004) along with delays in institutional placement of the person with dementia (Mittelman et al. 1996, 2004). A second outcome study was conducted at the Miami site of the original REACH (Resources for Enhancing Alzheimer's Caregiver Health) study. The family intervention used at this site was a com-bination of family therapy following Szapoznik's family intervention model designed spe-cifically for Cuban-American families along with use of a conference-calling telephone that was installed in the home of the primary care-giver to encourage social support from other family members (Eisdorfer et al. 2003). The Family-based Structure Multi-system In-home Intervention model focused on restructuring relationships within the family and those between family and other institutions that cause distress for the care-giver. Specifically, problematic and supportive interactions were identified, the relationships between care-giving functions and those interactions were analysed, and therapists intervened to 'enhance supportive and reduce maladaptive interactions' (Belle et al. 2006: 525). The technology intervention provided a mechanism to support enhanced multiperson interactions by allowing conferencing among multiple individuals. When compared with controls, the family intervention combined with the teleconferencing technology yielded reductions of 5–6 points on the Center for Epidemiological Studies Depression scale (Radloff 1977) over a six-month period, which were among the strongest effects across the six sites (Schulz et al. 2003). The intervention benefits were greatest for Cuban-American husbands and daughters and White non-Hispanic daughters (Belle et al. 2006).

Interventions with family care-givers are encouraged to be multicomponent in order to address the wide range of concerns that arise in the context of caring for a person with significant physical or mental health problems. An example of a clinical trial (with family care-givers of people with dementia) of a multicomponent model is REACH II (Resources for Enhancing Adult Caregiver Health), a multisite study that integrated findings from the original REACH project into a multicomponent protocol. REACH II combined the most potent ingredients from the six original REACH sites into a flexibly structured multicomponent intervention. The interventionists sequenced the components specifically for each family, to address the needs of each specific family. REACH II tested the multicomponent intervention with over 600 family care-givers from three major ethnic groups (Latino-Hispanic, Black-African-American, Non-Hispanic White-Caucasian). Offered in English or Spanish, the intervention consisted of twelve individual sessions with the primary care-giver (nine delivered in-home, three via telephone), along with five structured telephone sessions. Intervention strategies included provision of information, skills training, problem solving, stress management, role-playing, and telephone support (Belle et al. 2006). Among the many intervention strategies implemented in those contacts were efforts to increase the rate of social support from families to the primary care-giver. When compared with controls, care-givers receiving the total intervention package showed significant benefits to their overall quality of life and depression, although the size of the effects varied considerably across ethnic groups (Belle et al. 2006). Only the overall effects of the intervention could be evaluated; a component analysis was not part of the design so the impact of the family component cannot be presumed from the findings.

At this time, the state of family interventions in geropsychology is that models of family development are being articulated, existing models of family therapy are being adapted as theoretical foundations for interventions, and case studies illustrate the key ingredients in those models. Within the care-giving intervention literature, family-level interventions are being integrated into multicomponent models as one portion of intervention packages but no analysis of the impact of that particular ingredient can be ferreted out for its specific effects on the family or the older adult who is the IP.

FAMILY THERAPY: THEORY AND CLINICAL APPROACHES

Family therapy is a modality that focuses on family structure or functioning as the focal point for intervention, with the goal of improving the context for meeting individual family members' developmental needs. As described briefly above, family is often a relevant back-drop for clinical work with older adults, but this level of engagement of family is not considered family therapy. Family therapy interventions are used when shifts in the family structure and function are needed to improve the well-being of the older adult and/or other family members.

Family systems

Family therapy with later-life families draws upon approaches originally developed for child-rearing families, such as structural (Minuchin 1974) and strategic (Haley and Richeport-Haley 2007) models, as well as broader frameworks such as family systems (Seaburn, Landau-Stanton, and Horwitz 1995) and family development (Walsh 2003; Rodgers and White 1993). Each framework or theory offers an explanatory model of human behaviour, and the distinction among them is far beyond the state of the field in geropsychology, which is still working to integrate basic systems frameworks into clinical work, research, and training. For the purposes of this chapter, the overarching framework is emphasized, which in general can be viewed as the commonalities that constitute the systemic paradigm.

Family therapy views behaviour in terms of its communication function within relationships (Watzlawick, Beavin, and Jackson 1967). Behaviour is viewed as occurring in a stream of circular, recursive sequences rather than as a point in a linear antecedent-behaviour-consequent sequence, as illustrated in Figure 35.1. A particular problematic behaviour is conceptualized as but a point in a non-linear series of highly redundant interaction sequences that can be labelled by observers as rules of automatic or procedural action sequences. The behaviours associated with mental disorders are identified as having a particular function within an interpersonal context, and thus the relationship is a potential point for intervention. Traditional family therapy models address problems with family structures, such as poor boundaries around the parental role structures in child-rearing families (Minuchin 1974) or ineffective communication patterns (Watzlawick, Beavin, and Jackson 1967) that disrupt the basic functions of the family. Guilt, forgiveness, and a life history of mutual hurts also often come to the fore in later life (Hargrave and Anderson 1992). The common theme in family therapy is the focus on shaping family interactions as a mechanism to improve the functioning or well-being of one or more family members. For example, adult children who compete for power or control over a parent's finances or health decisions can disrupt the quality of care from providers who feel trapped between warring camps within the family. A family intervention to clarify roles, communication processes, and authority with external providers helps ensure that providers can meet the need of the older adult while reducing stress on care-giving family members that is caused by interpersonal conflict.

Family development

Family development theory explains shifts in family structures and dynamics as products of the entry and exit of family members across the lifespan (Gerson 1995) and gains and losses

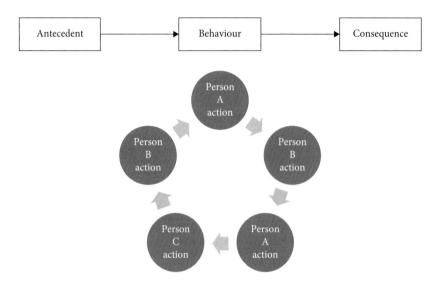

FIGURE 35.1 Circular versus linear causality.

in the developmental capabilities and needs of individual family members (McGoldrick, Carter, and Garcia-Preto 2010). Individual development propels families into a new stage of family life that typically involves subtle or significant changes in family structure and function. For example, the emerging walking capabilities of a toddler require new parenting (and often sibling) roles, as does the emerging social independence experienced during adolescence in most cultures. Parents often notice differences in their beliefs about how to support both safety and autonomy during these phases, with the potential of risks to the previously strong alliance between parents. Although development occurs at the individual level, periods of great transition in the capabilities of individuals (e.g. adolescence) require significant shifts in family roles as well.

The timing and dimensions of developmental transitions are ambiguous at best. In early toddlerhood, for example, families must figure out how to respond to cues about the needs of the child almost on a daily basis, without explicit cultural norms for handling the often confusing and inconsistent patterns of behaviour. On successive days, a toddler may insist on doing a task on her own or on needing complete assistance to accomplish the same task. To complicate matters further, the behavioural cues are often highly emotionally evocative (e.g. verbal outbursts, non-compliance with family rules), and can easily surpass the capacity of any adult to maintain emotional self-control and wise decision-making. Developmental transitions with high rates of ambiguity (e.g. adolescence, parent is missing in action during war) offer significant stress that can produce disruptions in individual and family well-being (Boss and Greenberg 1984). Parents who cannot 'get on the same page' with respect to parenting strategies are likely to suffer losses within the quality or integrity of their marriage or partnership.

In later life, developmental shifts also provoke changes in family structures as members enter and exit literally or figuratively through retirement, divorce, death, or illness (McGoldrick, Carter, and Garcia-Preto 2010). Individual transitions often reverberate through the close social network, which is made up primarily of family members (Kahn and Antonucci 1980). Adult children may engage in new roles with a parent after the death of his or her spouse. Functional declines that accompany later stages of chronic disease affect the daily lives of persons who are yoked socially to someone suffering with the disease. Retirement increases discretionary time in daily life patterns that may also reverberate through the close social network, generating changes in the structure or function of family. Although most individuals and families navigate normative developmental transitions effectively, some have low tolerance for change or poor adaptation skills that position individuals to be at risk for distress or disorder. For example, siblings that refuse to communicate with each other, or whose only communication strategy is escalation of verbal accusations, are poorly positioned to collaborate on care of, or decisions about, older family members. Ineffective structures prior to the transition may add to the risk of low psychological functioning or poor family functioning (Shields, King, and Wynne 1995).

Families often view the challenges associated with developmental transitions as problems within the individual (e.g. the person), whereas family systems frameworks view the entire system as in transition because role changes are needed in multiple persons to accommodate the gains or losses in any one member. The individual-focused explanation easily leads to pathologizing of the individual (e.g. as lazy, depressed, oppositional, narcissistic). Systems frameworks examine the function of the behaviour in a particular context, and how the interaction sequences among members of the system maintain the difficult behaviour.

Consider the case of Mary, whose declining cognitive functioning due to dementia impairs her ability to recall why her husband insists that she bathe on a particular day. It always seems to Mary that she just took a bath, and certainly, she feels that another person should not tell her when to take a bath. John, Mary's husband, gets so frustrated with her that he yells at her every morning before bath time in hopes that she will not fight with him about whether it is time for a bath. Their only son dreads visiting the couple in their home, yet faithfully visits several evenings a week during which he consistently expresses displeasure if his mother's hair and hygiene are not kept up to the level she always used to maintain. John also dreads his visits, knowing their son will be disappointed and upset to see Mary dishevelled. As a result, almost every morning John ends up upset at Mary about 'not caring' about her appearance.

This case illustrates how a behaviour (reduced frequency of bathing) can be caused by a disease (dementia) that reduces memory and awareness of self-presentation, but the distress and problematic social interactions are within the family system. Education of each family member is needed, but for some families, education will be insufficient to prompt them to make fundamental role changes. In this family example, John's role now includes prompting and cueing of basic self-care, but he needs to create a role structure that does not set him up to yell or speak derisively towards Mary. John and their son need to clarify their expectations of John's role and of the son's role vis-à-vis each parent. A systems analysis examines the thoughts, feelings, and action sequences that maintain the recursive, redundant behaviour sequence.

Medical family therapy

Medical family therapy helps families adapt to the extraordinary challenges of illness or disability that disrupt previous patterns of functioning (McDaniel, Hepworth, and Doherty

1992; McDaniel et al. 2005; Rolland 1994). Family systems form relationships with the illness or disability as well as with health providers and health systems (McDaniel et al. 1992). Illnesses and disabilities are almost like new members of the system with demands and challenges posed by the illness itself. Thus, members of the family form a relationship with the entity that shapes the family system and is sometimes shaped by it.

Clinical geropsychologists are familiar with the cases in which the family system has shaped the illness or disability through interaction patterns that communicate important messages about functional ability or disability, role limitations or expectations, and rules for giving and receiving nurturance, for example.

> You have cancer; we can't go on vacation!
> Women with Down's Syndrome cannot live safely on their own.
> I can't get mad at my husband because he does so much for me.
> Here, let me do that for you.

The meanings of illnesses or disabilities for family members as well as for the family system itself are explored in medical family therapy (McDaniel, Hepworth, and Doherty 1997; Rolland 1994). Meanings may be embedded in historical experience such as can occur when an older adult's intensive reaction to personal care in a hospital evokes PTSD responses rooted in early childhood sexual abuse. They may also be shaped by (mis)understanding of the meaning and course of illnesses, which are rarely well understood. The proximal environment may also shape meaning, such as often occurs in long-term care settings where limitations in control over small decisions such as the timing of a bath or the choice to open window coverings to the light may be regulated by others who lack knowledge of personal preferences or the time to learn them.

Although the experience of illness and disability is shared within the family (McDaniel et al. 1997), the intersections of the illness with particular family roles during specific periods of individual and family development yield very individualized experiences among family members. The impact of an ageing parent's cancer on a particular son or daughter is likely to be quite distinct, as is the impact of dementia on a spouse as opposed to a child of the patient. Role differences as well as variations in meaning of the illness lead towards varied vantage points that are expressed in interactions and individualized well-being. Illness provokes shifts in interaction dynamics among members that can warrant family therapy to address disruptions of well-being (McDaniel et al. 1997; Rolland 1994).

Families often find themselves working with larger systems that can also disrupt or exaggerate long-term family dynamics as they respond to the meaning of illness or disability within the realities of the care environment (Qualls 2000; Rolland 1994). In acute care settings, families are challenged to form a relationship that exceeds the time-frame of a day because rarely will the family encounter the same nurse or aide on a daily basis. Long-term care staff may have more predictable schedules, but families are rarely privy to the plan. In the course of a year, the direct care staff who provide the intimate care hour by hour are highly likely to have been replaced at least once in an industry with turnover rates that exceed 100% per year. Furthermore, facilities rarely make explicit their preferred roles for families. Beyond the basics of attendance at care conferences, families are given little instruction about what they can, should, or are expected to do with residents or staff. In the absence of information about their roles, family members engage with each other and with the facility in patterns that are familiar to that family. Examples include low rates of positive communication and high rates of negative statements, passive aggressive strategies, placating behaviour, critical communication with direct care staff, and splitting staff to obtain desirable responses.

Staff are rarely trained to engage in explicit communication with families, and so rely on what they experienced within their own families of origin for guidance about how to handle interpersonal challenges. Assisted-living or nursing home managers and staff view themselves as professionals who should be trusted by families. 'Why won't she leave me alone to do my job with her mother instead of telling me every little detail that I have heard 1000 times?' Managers sometimes avoid telling messy details they believe might upset families. Care staff are justifiably baffled by the inherent conflict in the message that direct care staff should treat residents as if they were their own grandparents but wear gloves whenever they touch their bodies (Smyer, Cohn, and Brannon 1988).

Some families struggle to partner with staff. Manuel was such a man. He visited his mother frequently, much to the chagrin of the assisted-living facility staff. He seemed to take delight in finding something amiss, and wasted no time in pointing it out loudly and forcefully to the nearest staff member. The administrator and nurse met with him on two occasions to discuss his concerns and encouraged him to talk with them rather than staff, offering the rationale that the specific staff person on duty may not be the only one who needed proper direction to address his concerns. Nothing worked. He continued to accost staff with loud, angry directives on almost every visit. Staff began to withdraw from his mother as well as from him, in fear that they would be targeted next. The administrator grew concerned about protecting both the resident's quality of care and the staff's well-being.

I listened to staff and administrative concerns, and documented his pattern of visits and frequency of berating behaviour. When I met with Manuel to discuss his obvious displeasure with the facility, I was surprised to find that he was complimentary about it. He was more interested in talking about his agony in deciding to place her there, and his frustration that he could not provide personal care at home. He also commented disdainfully about his siblings 'abandoning' their mother because they 'couldn't stand to see her like this'. This familiar description of guilt about placement was framed as a family role challenge: Manuel wanted desperately to be a good son, and felt like a failure every time he entered the facility. I talked with Manuel about what he wanted for his mother, and how he viewed his responsibility as her son. Manuel openly wept in sadness and frustration about the impossibility of being a good son of a mother in a facility. Good sons provided hands-on care, but he simply could not do that and maintain his job. After much conversation about his values, I worked out a role definition for 'good son of a mother in a facility' that included roles as advocate, emotional support for his mother, keeper of her personal pre-placement history, and reporter to siblings. Manuel acknowledged the legitimacy and importance of these roles, and worked with me to lay out specific strategies for implementing them. He noticed that he could apply skills from other parts of his life to these roles. That month I taught an in-service for staff on partnering with family that addressed these issues, but without specifically referencing Manuel. Staff used Manuel as an example of an 'impossible family', which offered me an opportunity to build empathy by exploring the family's experience of placement. I did a role-play with staff (staff had fun being the 'impossible family member') to demonstrate skills in partnering with families. The administrator and Manuel agreed to meet every few months to check on Manuel's partnership with staff. This case illustrates the importance of helping families clarify and implement roles appropriate to the family contexts of later life, including partnership with paid care-givers.

In short, rarely do healthcare systems have a systematic programme to build true partnerships between family members and professionals, staff, or the care system as a whole. The absence of an explicit model or process to engage families and care systems positions families to replicate their internal dynamics with external providers. Add in the complexities of system reorganization to include the pragmatics and meanings of illness and disabilities, and families seem quite likely to experience distress and/or dysfunction as they navigate acute or long-term illnesses. Medical family therapy appears to have a healthy future, with a high likelihood of encountering ageing families, given the epidemiology of illness and disability. Awareness of later-life tasks and dilemmas in family development will be inherently useful.

My conceptualization of the Weems family introduced early in the chapter was shaped by my understanding of their system, their developmental history and current stage, and the challenges that dementia imposes on families. I viewed them as struggling with communication patterns in the marital subsystem and the parent–child subsystem that were long term. The launching of their sons had not been a smooth process and, subsequently, the sons used geographic distance and low frequency of contact to manage the poor interpersonal emotion regulation between father and each son. The developmental task at hand was to adapt to Millie's dementia with added structure to foster maximum independence in her, while shifting the marriage from a balance based on equal voice in decisions to an unequal balance appropriate to the added responsibilities Carter held for overseeing Millie's health and safety needs. Although willing to accept that role, Carter abdicated it when decisions were needed, demanding that Millie participate beyond her capacity. Similarly, Carter insisted that the boys shared decision-making authority with him yet could not provide them with sufficient information, and they could not sustain engagement with him to make joint decision-making a viable option. The long-term absence of nurturance and emotional safety during conflict left all family members anxious when communication was needed.

I used the Caregiver Family Therapy (CFT) model (Qualls and Williams 2013) with the Weems family. As seen in Figure 35.2, the CFT model walks the therapist through a series of steps to consider the range of needs of the family. The initial step is to investigate issues related to how the problem is named. Dementias often provoke conflict within families related to naming the problem. Early signs are confusing, so families often interpret them within the context of their personal history, attributing early symptoms to problems with personality, roles, other illnesses, depression, or intention behaviour (often called manipulation). The process of obtaining a diagnosis may require multiple visits with multiple providers, sometimes over years, as the early symptoms blossom into more blatant cognitive difficulties. Family members have varied schemas about members' behaviour and variations in it; those early signs are later recognized as part of the emerging dementia.

> The Weems family needed to get clear information about the aetiology of Millie's behaviour, attempt to come to consensus on how to understand those problems, and accept differences in viewpoints without being paralysed in making decisions. A neuropsychological evaluation provided a clear new diagnosis: vascular dementia. Millie had struggled with Major Depressive Disorder throughout adulthood, so her current depression symptoms were produced by some combination of this lifelong condition and the depression that can accompany vascular dementia. Carter reported that his older son flatly rejected the diagnosis, insisting

on a second opinion. His younger son was hesitant and sad to hear the news, and scheduled a flight to visit his mother. I asked Carter if he thought a telephone conference call in which we reviewed the neuropsychological report together might be helpful. He was excited to arrange this, and his sons agreed, although with some reluctance on the part of the older son who clearly questioned the expertise of this clinic. Carter shared his copy of the report with both sons by fax prior to the call. A ninety-minute phone call provided time to (1) review expectations and goals for the call; (2) review Millie's cognitive strengths and weaknesses as well as the diagnostic findings and recommendations; and (3) discuss how they wanted to work together to support Millie during the journey ahead. The level of detail in the report seemed to help the older son accept that the diagnosis was appropriate and he backed off from the demand for a second opinion, although his level of suspicion about the clinic's credibility remained high. The older son also was consistently and vocally hostile to Carter, in a style that suggested a very long history of conflict between them. By the conclusion of the call, Carter was satisfied that both sons were well informed, and that his older son would not be a meaningful source of support to him. Carter was touched by his younger son's obvious distress over his mother's condition, and was grateful he planned to visit within a few weeks. The phone call seemed to solidify Carter's understanding and acceptance of the findings of the report, while clarifying the impossibility of achieving consensus in the understanding or framing of the problem with his two sons. The problem now had a clear name, a clear identity, and the sons' openness to working together (or not) was clearer.

CFT's second step is to address practical problems faced by families. Many care-giving families must learn many new skills, and/or adapt their day-to-day life style significantly. For example, families may need to learn how to implement complex medical regimens at home, schedule and transport the patient to multiple appointments, develop strategies for distraction from unsafe behaviour, or alter diet significantly to address medical conditions. Families are sometimes stuck in a problem for which they can see no solutions simply because they lack knowledge or understanding of care strategies or available services. CFT may involve some degree of case management to link care-givers with resources that can calm down major family drama. Some families need to learn problem-solving strategies, although among later-life families I always want to understand how they got to later life without knowing simple problem-solving approaches. My work is quite different with families who have never understood them vs those who have strong skills they just have not yet applied to this novel situation.

> Practical problems in structuring daily life with Millie needed to be addressed to ensure an appropriate balance in supporting both her independence and her safety. Because Carter was an excellent problem solver, my major therapeutic input with him was to help identify the full range of problems in daily life. He struggled, for example, to decide if Millie's refusal to bathe more than twice a week was a problem, or if her desire to sit for hours watching television was a problem. I educated him about the effects of her dementia on daily functioning, and we proceeded to distinguish between the problems that required solution to maintain her safety, and those that represented his expectations that needed to be realigned to match her capabilities.

Implementation of problem-solving strategies in new health situations often requires changes in roles among family members (Step 3). A care recipient must learn to receive assistance, retaining as much control over his or her own life style, body, and daily routines as possible. Other members need to learn how to initiate care respectfully, listen for preferences, or cajole a resistant or confused care recipient into partnering in care. Previous

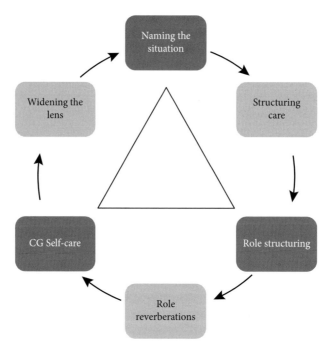

FIGURE 35.2 Care-giver family therapy process components.

interpersonal balances of power and nurturance are disrupted and new patterns must be formed around new roles, hopefully with all parties participating in the choice of how those will be structured. Resistance to care among care recipients presents care-givers with emotionally challenging moments in which coercive strategies must be avoided, care preferences must be respected, and yet sometimes the care simply has to be provided even if the recipient does not like the process. In dementia care, bathing is a notorious battleground for care-givers who dread forcing a highly resistant loved one to maintain at least basic hygiene standards. Roles also must be negotiated among care-givers, with the goal of having a clearly identifiable primary care-giver who is supported by other family members (Lieberman and Fisher 1999). Grief over the loss of former roles between care-giver and care recipient are also important. Spouses or partners, adult children, and friends have very different losses to process, and each distinct relationship has idiosyncratic losses that become evident over time. Role changes thus involve letting go, learning new skills and rhythms, and significant processing of the meaning of changes that may appear subtle to others but are loaded with relational meaning (Jacobs 2006; Qualls 2003).

> Carter needed to figure out how to proceed with truly necessary daily life structures despite Millie's consistent protest on almost all daily tasks (e.g. she resisted dressing, bathing, moving from one room to another, eating meals). Given his long history of working with Millie's low motivational state during episodes of severe depression, Carter was familiar with having to prod, persuade, cajole, and insist on some basic self-care or hygiene. He hated that role, and was loath to think that he was now in this position for life. After clarifying the difference between the current situation, in which Millie could not remember to do self-care behaviour, and past experiences, where the depression made them seem impossible or irrelevant, Carter

was able to specify ways in which his role could be structured to his satisfaction. He worked through the list of 'must do' daily activities to discriminate between those he considered truly critical vs those he preferred. With a shorter list of tasks he would need to structure with and for Millie, we reviewed strategies for communicating with her in ways that sustained respect for her preferences while pushing through the tasks in a timely way to ensure her basic safety and well-being. He was also happy to add some paid staff time to engage Millie in some tasks, and he was gratified to note that she actually resisted a paid provider far less than she resisted him. The fundamental relationship implications of these role changes also required some significant adjustment for Carter. I helped him process the meaning of being a spouse of a long-time, intimate, familiar partner who is now a shadow of her former self. He had to work through the loneliness, guilt for having a life in which she could no longer participate, and the almost complete absence of initiation of affection or warmth from her.

Once care-giving roles are structured in ways that meet the needs of the care recipient, CFT therapists need to guide the care-giver through a review of the impact of these roles on the rest of the care-giver's roles (Step 4). Does implementation of the roles as structured interfere with other aspects of the person's volunteer or job roles, friendships or other family relationships, and basic self-care?

As he reviewed the impact of care-giving on his other roles, Carter also needed to consider how he would fulfil his many volunteer responsibilities in the community, given that Millie needed nearly constant oversight. Carter had transitioned in retirement into several significant volunteer leadership roles. He served on multiple nonprofit organization boards and was active in his Rotary Club. He recognized that his friendships as well as his sense of personal accomplishment were all structured within those leadership roles. He chose to reduce the number of roles, but retain his favourite board memberships, regular church attendance, and his weekly Rotary breakfast meeting. Those commitments required him again to engage in problem solving to work out a plan whereby he could attend meetings with some assurance that Millie had oversight. He investigated respite care alternatives, including two day programmes and two in-home respite care providers. Millie disliked all of those options, claiming she was fine to stay alone, and almost had him convinced until she left the stove on one day after heating water for tea while he was home with her. He chose in-home respite care for Millie so she could retain her preferred sleeping-in pattern, a strategy that had the added advantages that he would not have to push her to get around early and that a home care aide would actually assist her with hygiene and dressing three mornings each week.

When care needs are settled, and the care-giver's roles are balanced, CFT therapists attend to self-care (Step 5). The therapists in our programme consistently find that care-givers resist focusing on self-care until the care recipient's needs are met. So despite the high priority we place on care-giver self-care, we wait to address this therapeutically until the care-giver roles are settled and the care-giver can implement the needed care strategies successfully.

Self-care requires the care-giver to prioritize some time and attention to what maintains his or her quality of life and well-being. Some care-givers have never really managed self-care well while others just need to figure out how to implement familiar self-care activities in this new context of care-giving. For the latter, problem-solving skills are brought to bear again to create space, time, and opportunity for engaging in successful self-care even in the midst of the demands of family care. Men and women who have never cared for themselves well may find the work they do in CFT to be life-transforming. Crises really do provide us with opportunities to review our lives and think about our most fundamental choices. Some care-givers seek assistance only at the point when they are overwhelmed with distress, perhaps with a strong sense of burden, depression, or of being trapped and over-whelmed. The critical tasks for Steps 1–3 of CFT get the objective burdens of care under con-trol. Step 4 helps the care-giver integrate the care-giving role into the rest of life. Now, in Step 5, care-givers are educated about the literature on morbidity and mortality risks brought on by care-giving. Self-care is also presented as critical to the care-giver's capacity to main-tain responsibility for the care recipient. We developed a series of strategies for enhancing a sense of urgency for engaging in self-care (see Qualls and Williams 2013 for fuller dis-cussion) that emphasize the risks to the care recipient of any lapse in the well-being of the care-giver. Hence, self-care by the care-giver serves the double duty of maintaining his or her well-being while protecting the loved one from the complete loss of care structures that would occur if the care-giver became unable to oversee them due to illness or accident.

Self-care involves all dimensions of wellness: physical health promotion, management of medical conditions, psychological, social, and spiritual. Care-givers often let therapists know which dimensions of their self-care have been sacrificed to meet the needs of the care recipient. However, CFT therapists are also encouraged to review systematically less obvi-ous domains such as nutrition, exercise, intellectual engagement, social relationships, as well as participation in cultural and arts, volunteer, or employment roles, and community or civic engagement. The strategies used in cognitive-behavioural therapy for depression are often helpful to implement here—tracking mood, identifying pleasant events, planning and tracking activity, and linking mood and activity tracking data to see which forms of behav-ioural activation have which kind of effect.

> As he accepted greater responsibility as Millie's care-giver, Carter needed to plan more explic-itly to care for himself (Step 5). He needed to develop a wider social support network to meet his psychosocial needs because Millie's companionship no longer offered him even simple social benefits like conversation. He also needed to figure out how to get exercise, which he knew was key to both his physical and mental health. Carter's decision to stay involved in community volunteer roles, his church, and service club offered him meaningful and familiar patterns of social participation that also addressed his sense of personal meaning and spir-ituality. The decision to hire in-home respite care now paid off handsomely as he established a daily routine of early morning exercise at home while she slept, after which he could go out to breakfast meetings with organizations or even just arrange breakfast with a friend. Carter appreciated the tracking data I encouraged him to collect because it was consistent with his long-term commitment to data-driven decisions. He readily recognized the importance to his overall well-being of the various self-care activities that sustained his mood and resilience so he could provide the quality of care he wanted to give Millie. He even noticed that his good moods were somewhat contagious, such that she was often in a better mood if he had been out and about engaging in activities that nurtured him.

CFT recognizes that family systems rarely consist of only the care-giver and care recipient, so the final step in the CFT cycle used to guide an episode of services is to 'widen the lens' (Step 6). Stepping back from the daily life structures of primary care-giver and care recipi-ent, the CFT therapist guides the client(s) to review how the now-working structures impact other members of the family. A care-giver may be able to sustain a particular care-giving approach and may even be able to care for herself, but if she has withdrawn from her chil-dren or other key persons in her world to make these new care-giving structures work, unin-tended consequences may ensue. A teenage child who has less oversight or more burdens may not be getting his or her needs met. A valued relationship with a friend or sister, or a marriage, may starve from lack of nurturance as the demands of care-giving increase. Before completing an episode of work with a care-giver or family, I pause to look at the wider family system for the reverberating effects of care-giving.

> Carter's relationships with his sons and their families was impacted by his lack of freedom to travel. His older son's family was unwilling to travel to see Carter and Millie, citing competing demands of work and sports activities. Although he noted that less frequent contact with his older son was not going to impact their strained relationship, he really missed seeing his grandson and had a genuine fear that he would not know his grandson if he did not see him regularly until after Millie died. No other reverberations of his care-giving role were obvious, other than those already addressed in his self-care plan. With encouragement, Carter upgraded his computer and learned how to do video calls via Skype, and set a regular time to talk with his grandson. Later, he chose to use a brief residential respite stay for Millie so he could travel to one of his grandson's special sporting events. Many months later, Carter reported that he had a growing appreciation of the investment in this relationship with his grandson, and that the weekend respite experience was teaching him that Millie would be OK without him so he could entertain the possibility of leaving for four- to five-day brief vacations to the family cabin that had always been so meaningful to him.

A final task in an episode of CFT is to anticipate the types of change that may face the care-giver down the road. Some trajectories of care are hard to map, but even a very general sense of how an illness, disability, or condition are going to unfold are very helpful to the care-giver. At a minimum, care-givers can be guided to consider the types of problem that emerge in the near future, and to anticipate solutions to those. As with any psychotherapy, helping a client name out loud the signs that their coping strategies are not working well can help with early identification of psychological symptoms that might benefit from intervention.

> Carter consistently asked for a script for what lay ahead for Millie. Unable to provide the level of detail he sought, I still offered broad brushstrokes for the future trajectory of most dementias. I noted common signs of functional decline from her current state, and I foreshadowed the need for quite different care structures in the future. Although he could not imagine it now, Carter acknowledged that placement in a facility likely lay ahead in their future. We also anticipated future versions of Carter's pattern of over-extending himself before he recognized the need for additional help. We noticed the symptoms that arose in him that could inform him that he was at or past his limits: fatigue, resentment, depressed mood, social withdrawal, irritability at Millie. I framed these as useful signals that the current care structure was no longer meeting their needs, and invited him to view that as informative rather than as failure. I also invited him to call for a booster session at any time, and to recognize that in the future we were likely to do another episode or two of CFT, working our way around the cycle of steps as he adapted to a new phase of the journey.

IMPLICATIONS FOR PRACTICE

Clinicians working with older adults experiencing illness and disability need to recognize the key role families have in supporting well-being both emotionally and instrumentally. Particularly salient for frail older adults, clinical care follows a trajectory of chronic care interspersed with intermittent interruptions in functional health. Families are the constant source of care that follows a frail older adult through hospitalizations, home health rehabilitative care, and back into primary care oversight of stable long-term care services. Once the family's central role in managing care over time is acknowledged, clinicians will naturally begin to seek ways to engage families in the ongoing trajectory of care, with a particular focus on navigating the transitions in care that represent such a risk period for exacerbation of ongoing frailties.

Although clinicians and counsellors can be encouraged to always 'think family', the option of when and how to include family members always rests with the patient or his/her legal decision-maker. Adults of any age, including older adults, have full responsibility and choice about whether to include family members, and in what ways. Clinicians who ask whether and how patients want family involved will find rich opportunities to engage the primary social network of older adults in powerful and creative ways. The theoretical frameworks described above offer rich alternative ways to explore the intersection of ageing, individual development, family development, and clinical care. Adaptations of the models for primary care (McDaniel et al. 2005) and long-term care (Qualls 2000) offer frameworks for the distinct issues that arise when engaging families in particular healthcare settings.

In the past decade, we have worked to create an integrative model to help clinicians organize their work with care-giving families of frail older adults. CFT (Qualls 2008; Qualls and Williams 2013) organizes common factors across other interventions to engage families in common practices that aid the well-being of family members. These are organized in a circular image (Figure 35.2) to illustrate how the same questions and work can be done with care-giving families in any stage or form of care-giving. For example, almost all models of family intervention start with clarifying understanding of the older adult's health and functional status and sharing educational materials to enhance family understanding, so the top of the figure begins with the task of 'Naming the Problem'. Practical problem solving is another common component, along with care-giver self-care. Family therapy models typically examine the family structure with a focus on structuring roles to support the many functions of care-giving, including communication, decision-making, emotional support, and instrumental service sharing. The family therapy paradigm is reflected in the emphasis on the broad examination of family roles to ensure that strategies for providing care to the older adult do not interfere with support for individual development in all family members, including those distal to the care-giving itself. The goal of CFT is to assist the family in structuring care so the needs of the older adult(s) are met while protecting the individual well-being of all family members.

Summary

Family therapy is powerful because families are critical and highly valued members of the social context of older adults with a long history of reciprocally meaningful emotional and instrumental exchanges. Families are important factors in the aetiology and treatment of mental disorders as well as key members of the team of providers of healthcare more generally, so they can be useful to engage in intervention or may become the focus of intervention. Family therapy strategies are designed to address changes in family systems that occur during transitions caused by family developmental processes or non-normative events such as illnesses. Specific models for intervening with late-life families have emerged in the medical family therapy and family care-giving intervention literature, although few clinical trials have been conducted to test efficacy of interventions focused on family structures and processes. The CFT model is detailed here to demonstrate how multiple approaches can be used in a systematic approach to family-level care-giver intervention.

KEY REFERENCES AND SOURCES FOR FURTHER READING

Aneshensel, C. S., Pearlin, L. I., Mullan, J. T., Zarit, S. H., and Whitlatch, C. J. (1995). *Profiles in Caregiving: The Unexpected Career*. San Diego, CA: Academic Press.

Hargrave, T. D. and Anderson, W. T. (1992). *Finishing Well: Aging and Reparation in the Intergenerational Family*. New York: Brunner/Mazel.

Qualls, S. H. and Williams, A. A. (2013). *Caregiver Family Therapy*. Washington, DC: American Psychological Association.

Qualls, S. H., and Zarit, S. H. (eds) (2008). *Aging Families and Caregiving: A Clinician's Guide to Research, Practice, and Technology*. Hoboken, NJ: Wiley.

Rolland, J. S. (1994). *Families, Illness, & Disability: An Integrative Treatment Model*. New York: Basic Books.

WEB SITES

National Alliance for Caregiving. http://www.caregiving.org/.

APA Caregiver Briefcase. http://www.apa.org/pi/about/publications/caregivers/.

Collaborative Family Healthcare Association. http://www.cfha.net/.

American Association of Marriage and Family Therapy. www.aamft.org.

REFERENCES

Belle, S. H., Burgio, L., Burns, R., Coon, D., Czaja, S. J., et al. (2006). 'Enhancing the Quality of Life of Dementia Caregivers from Different Ethnic or Racial Groups'. *Annals of Internal Medicine* 145: 727–738.

Boss, P. and Greenberg, J. S. (1984). 'Family Boundary Ambiguity: A New Variable in Family Stress Theory'. *Family Process* 23: 535–546.

Coon, D. W., Gallagher-Thompson, D., and Thompson, L. (eds) (2003). *Innovative Interventions to Reduce Dementia Caregiver Distress: A Clinical Guide*. New York: Springer.

Coon, D. W., Keaveny, M., Valverde, I. R., Dadvar, S., and Gallagher-Thompson, D. (2012). 'Evidence-based Psychological Treatments for Distress in Family Caregivers of Older Adults'. In F. Scogin and A. Shah (eds), *Making Evidence-based Psychological Treatments Work with Older Adults* (pp. 225–284). Washington DC: American Psychological Association.

Eisdorfer, C. Szaja, S. J., Loewenstein, D. A., Robert, M. P., Argüelles, S., et al. (2003). 'The Effect of a Family Therapy and Technology-based Intervention on Caregiver Depression'. *Gerontologist* 43: 521–531.

Engel, G. L. (1980). 'The Clinical Application of the Biopsychosocial Model'. *American Journal of Psychiatry* 137: 535–544.

Fingerman, K., Miller, L., and Seidel, A. (2009). 'Functions Families Serve in Old Age'. In S. H. Qualls and S. H. Zarit (eds), *Aging Families and Caregiving* (pp. 19–43). Hoboken, NJ: Wiley.

Frankel, R. M., Quill, T. E., and McDaniel, S. H. (2003). *The Biopsychosocial Approach: Past, Present, and Future*. Rochester, NY: University of Rochester Press.

Gerson, R. (1995). 'The Family Life Cycle: Phases, Stages, and Crises'. In R. H. Mikesell, D. D. Lusterman, and S. H. McDaniel (eds), *Integrating Family Therapy: Handbook of Family Psychology and Systems Theory* (pp. 91–111). Washington, DC: American Psychological Association.

Haley, J. and Richeport-Haley, M. (2007). *Directive Family Therapy*. New York: Taylor and Francis.

Haley, W. E., Roth, D. L., Howard, G., and Stafford, M. M. (2010). 'Caregiving Strain Estimated Risk for Stroke and Coronary Heart Disease among Spouse Caregivers: Differential Effects by Race and Sex'. *Stroke 41*: 331–336.

Hammen, C. C., Hazel, N. A., Brennan, P. A., and Najman, J. J. (2012). 'Intergenerational Transmission and Continuity of Stress and Depression: Depressed Women and their Offspring in 20 Years of Follow-up'. *Psychological Medicine* 42(5): 931–942. doi:10.1017/S0033291711001978.

Hargrave, T. D. and Anderson, W. T. (1992). *Finishing Well: Aging and Reparation in the Intergenerational Family*. New York: Brunner/Mazel.

Jacobs, B. J. (2006). *The Emotional Survival Guide for Caregivers: Looking After Yourself and Your Family while Helping an Aging Parent*. New York: Guilford Press.

Kahn, R. L. and Antonucci, T. C. (1980). 'Convoys over the life course: Attachment, roles, and social support'. In P. B. Baltes, and O. G. Brim (eds), *Life-span Development and Behavior* (Vol. 3, pp. 253–286). New York: Academic Press.

Kiecolt-Glaser, J. K., Dura, J. R., Speicher, C. E., Trask, O. J., and Glaser, R. (1991). 'Spousal Caregivers of Dementia Victims: Longitudinal Changes in Immunity and Health'. *Psychosomatic Medicine* 53: 345–362.

Knight, B. G. and Sayengh, P. (2010). 'Cultural Values and Caregiving: The Updated Sociocultural Stress and Coping Model'. *Journals of Gerontology: Series B: Psychological Sciences* 65B: 5–13.

Lieberman, M. A. and Fisher, L. (1999). 'The Effects of Family Conflict Resolution and Decision Making on the Provision of Help for an Elder with Alzheimer's Disease'. *Gerontologist* 39: 159–166.

McDaniel, S. H., Hepworth, J., and Doherty, W. J. (1992). *Medical Family Therapy: A Biopsychosocial Approach to Families with Health Problems*. New York: Basic Books.

McDaniel, S. H., Hepworth, J., and Doherty, W. J. (1997). *The Shared Experience of Illness*. New York: Basic Books.

McDaniel, S. H., Campbell, T. L., Hepworth, J., and Lorenz, A. (2005). *Family-oriented Primary Care* (2nd edn). New York: Springer.

McGoldrick, M., Carter, B., and Garcia-Preto, N. (2010). *The Expanded Family Life Cycle: Individual, Family, and Social Perspectives* (4th edn). New York: Pearson.

Minuchin, S. (1974). *Families and Family Therapy*. Cambridge, MA: Harvard University Press.

Mittelman, M. S., Ferris, S. H., Shulman, E., Steinberg, G., and Levin, B. (1996). 'A Family Intervention to Delay Nursing Home Placement of Patients with Alzheimer Disease'. *Journal of the American Medical Association* 276: 1725–1731.

Mittelman, M. S., Ferris, S. H., Steinberg, G., Shulman, E., Mackell, J. A., Ambinder, A., and Cohen, J. (1993). 'An Intervention that Delays Institutionalization of Alzheimer's Disease Patients: Treatment of Spouse-Caregivers'. *The Gerontologist* 33: 730–740.

Mittelman, M. S., Roth, D. L., Coon, D. W., and Haley, W. E. (2004). 'Sustained Benefit of Supportive Intervention for Depressive Symptoms in Caregivers of Patients with Alzheimer's Disease'. *American Journal of Psychiatry* 161: 850–856.

National Alliance for Caregiving (2009). *Caregiving in the US*. National Alliance for Caregiving and American Association of Retired Persons. http://www.caregiving.org/data/Caregiving_in_the_US_2009_full_report.pdf.

Nezu, D., Palmatier, A., and Nezu, A. (2004). 'Problem-solving Therapy for Caregivers'. In E. C. Chang, T. J. D'Zurilla, and L. J. Sanna (eds), *Social Problem Solving: Theory, Research, and Training.* (pp. 223–238). Washington, DC: American Psychological Association.

Pillemer, K. (1985). 'The Dangers of Dependency: New Findings on Domestic Violence against the Elderly'. *Social Problems* 33(2): 146–158.

Pinquart, M. and Sörensen, S. (2005). 'Caregiving Distress and Psychological Health of Caregivers'. In K. V. Oxington (ed.), *Psychology of Stress* (pp. 165–206). Hauppauge: Nova Biomedical Books.

Pinquart, M. and Sörensen, S. (2006). 'Helping Caregivers of Persons with Dementia: Which Interventions Work and How Large are their Effects?' *International Psychogeriatrics* 18: 577–595.

Qualls, S. H. (2000). 'Working with Families in Nursing Homes'. In V. Molinari (ed.), *Professional Psychology in Long Term Care* (pp. 91–112). New York: Hatherleigh.

Qualls, S. H. (2003). 'Aging and Cognitive Impairment'. In D. K. Snyder and M. A. Whisman (eds), *Treating Difficult Couples: Managing Emotional, Behavioral, and Health Problems in Couples Therapy* (pp. 370–391). New York: Guilford Press.

Qualls, S. H. (2008). 'Caregiver Family Therapy'. In B. Knight and K. Laidlaw (eds), *Handbook of Emotional Disorders in Older Adults* (pp. 183–209). Oxford: Oxford University Press.

Qualls, S. H. and Williams, A. A. (2013). *Caregiver Family Therapy*. Washington, DC: American Psychological Association.

Radloff, L. S. (1977). 'The CES-D scale: A Self-report Depression Scale for Research in the General Population'. *Applied Psychological Measures* 1: 385–401.

Rodgers, R. H. and White, J. W. (1993). 'Family Development Theory'. In P. G. Boss, W. J. Doherty, R. LaRossa, W. R. Schumm, and S. K. Steinmetz (eds), *Sourcebook of Family Theories and Methods* (pp. 225–254). New York: Plenum.

Rolland, J. S. (1994). *Families, Illness, and Disability: An Integrative Treatment Model.* New York: Basic Books.

Schiamberg, L. D. (2000). 'Elder Abuse by Adult Children: An Applied Ecological Framework for Understanding Contextual Risk Factors and the Intergenerational Character of Quality of Life'. *International Journal of Aging and Human Development* 50: 329–359.

Schulz, R., Burgio, L., Burns, R., Eisdorfer, C., Gallagher-Thompson, D., and Gitlin, L. N. (2003). 'Resources for Enhancing Alzheimer's Caregiver Health (REACH): Overview, Site-specific Outcomes, and Future Directions'. *Gerontologist* 43: 514–520.

Schulz, R. and Martire, L. M. (2004). 'Family Caregiving of Persons with Dementia: Prevalence, Health Effects, and Support Strategies'. *American Journal of Geriatric Psychiatry* 12: 240–249.

Seaburn, D., Landau-Stanton, J., and Horwitz, S. (1995). 'Core Techniques in Family Therapy'. In R. H. Mikesell, D. D. Lusterman, and S. H. McDaniel (eds), *Integrating Family Therapy: Handbook of Family Psychology and Systems Theory* (pp. 5–26). Washington, DC: American Psychological Association.

Shields, C. G., King, D. A., and Wynne, L. C. (1995). 'Interventions with Later Life Families'. In R. H. Mikesell, D. D. Lusterman, and S. H. McDaniel (eds), *Integrating Family Therapy: Handbook of Family Psychology and Systems Theory* (pp. 141–158). Washington, DC: American Psychological Association.

Smyer, M. A., Cohn, M. D., and Brannon, D. (1988). '*Mental Health Consultation in Nursing Homes*'. New York: NYU Press.

Stephens, M. A. P. and Franks, M. (2009). 'All in the Family: Providing Care to Chronically Ill and Disabled Older Adults'. In S. H. Qualls and S. H. Zarit (eds), *Aging Families and Caregiving* (pp. 61–84). Hoboken, NJ: Wiley.

Walsh, F. (2003). *Normal Family Processes: Growing Diversity and Complexity* (3rd edn). New York: Guilford Press.

Watzlawick, P., Beavin, J. H., and Jackson, D. D. (1967). *Pragmatics of Human Communication*. New York: Norton.

Zarit, S. H. (2009). 'Empirically Supported Treatment for Family Caregivers'. In S. H. Qualls and S. H. Zarit (eds), *Aging Families and Caregiving* (pp. 131–154). Hoboken, NJ: Wiley.

CHAPTER 36

INTERPROFESSIONAL GERIATRIC HEALTHCARE

Competencies and Resources for Teamwork

ANN M. STEFFEN, ANTONETTE M. ZEISS, AND
MICHELE J. KAREL

INTRODUCTION

Mʀ Brent Simpson is a second-year trainee in a Doctor of Clinical Psychology (DClinPsychol) programme in the UK. Upon completion, he will be eligible for registration as a practitioner psychologist with the Health & Care Professions Council (HCPC) which is the accrediting body for clinical psychologists in the UK. As Brent considers the options for his third-year elective clinical placement, he is torn between a centre providing outpatient cognitive-behavioural psychotherapy for a variety of mental health problems, and a health clinic treating middle-aged and older adults with chronic health conditions. In addition to providing supervised clinical experiences with cognitive-behavioural interventions for pain management and depression, this placement would involve working with an interprofessional team. As he weighs these options, Brent wonders 'How would this specific interprofessional team be similar to, or different from, the other clinical placements I've had that involve interprofessional consultation? Would this be a good placement for me at this point in my career?'

Dr Maria Sanchez received her cedula (licence from the Direccion General de Profesiones) for independent practice in Mexico. She has just accepted a prestigious position as the psychologist in the Geriatric Evaluation and Management unit (GEM) of a hospital run by the public health service (IMSS; Instituto Mexicano de Seguro Social). Dr Sanchez assessed and treated chronic pain conditions while completing the social service for her licenciatura; later, she gained additional experiences in geriatric mental health. She does not, however, consider herself to be an expert in interdisciplinary healthcare team development. She wonders 'How can I advance my knowledge and skills to help this GEM team function well? Where should I begin?'

Questions similar to those raised by Mr Simpson and Dr Sanchez are increasingly common due to the growing number of psychologists working with older adults in healthcare settings (see also Armento and Stanley this volume; Konnert and Petrovic-Poljak this volume). Some mental health providers know early in their professional development that they want to specialize in clinical work with older adults, and select their training experiences accordingly. Far more, however, encounter opportunities and challenges in geriatric care that stretch their existing knowledge and skills. Interdisciplinary collaboration, which includes working with interprofessional healthcare teams, involves an essential set of competencies for healthcare professionals whose clinical practice includes older adults.

In this chapter, we aim to provide a broad overview of interprofessional teams as the sine qua non of geriatric healthcare and professional collaboration. We begin by defining key terms and briefly summarize the empirical support for interprofessional geriatric healthcare. A conceptual model of interprofessional healthcare team performance is described which frames such teams within their larger organizations and national healthcare systems. We then return to the issue of interprofessional team competencies and suggest resources for training and development. Although this chapter is written from the disciplinary perspective of psychology and the specialty of clinical geropsychology, we believe that much of this discussion is relevant (and, hopefully, helpful) for our colleagues in the many healthcare professions needed by the older adults whom we jointly serve.

Definitional Issues in Healthcare Teams

Any discussion of team approaches within healthcare raises definitional concerns. In what ways are 'interprofessional collaboration', 'interprofessional care', 'interdisciplinary teams', and 'multidisciplinary teams' referring to similar or different practices? Does 'interprofessional' or 'interdisciplinary' refer to a specific set of professions/disciplines? Because interprofessional teams may not always be labelled as such, providers and trainees do not necessarily differentiate between interprofessional and other multidisciplinary care strategies within specific healthcare settings. The published literature on healthcare teams also includes confusing terminology. Although there are no final answers to these questions, consensus among those in the field provides some progress toward shared terminology.

Within any healthcare unit that provides care by different professional disciplines, the exact range of disciplines involved depends upon the nature of the patients served and organizational factors. In some healthcare systems and for some health concerns this might be regulated (e.g. in the US, the Medicare system requires physical rehabilitation teams to have a minimum of physician, registered nurse, and physical therapist). In many healthcare settings, the most common core disciplines are nursing, medicine, and social work, with additions from varying others depending upon the needs of a specific patient population (e.g. audiologists, chaplains, dentists, dieticians, occupational therapists, optometrists, pharmacists, physical therapists, podiatrists, psychologists, recreation/music therapists, speech pathologists). In the majority of interprofessional healthcare teams, members from various disciplines are employed by the same organization to work within a specific unit/department that serves a common population. Interprofessional healthcare teams may function within one treatment setting with team members and patients geographically co-located (e.g. long-term care) or teams can serve patients as they move across a continuum of care settings (including home-based care). Advances in communication technologies have facilitated the development of virtual teams that are especially valuable in serving the needs of rural populations (Emery et al. 2012; Sekerak et al. 2009).

Language about coordinated healthcare services provided by teams of more than one discipline/profession is often confused and misleading. We have found published articles on healthcare teams in which the terms interprofessional, interdisciplinary, and multidisciplinary are used interchangeably. On occasion, these terms are incorrectly used when professionals from two disciplines simply consult with each other on a specific case. In too many instances, the meanings are not clarified or terms are used incorrectly, leading to the continued 'terminological quagmire' surrounding healthcare teams (Leathard 2003). The following section of this chapter will explore the differences among these various kinds of healthcare teams in terms of the way they function, and the attitudes, knowledge, and skills required of team members.

Within the international literature on 'interprofessional care', the *majority* of published works refer to the same approach and processes as the 'interdisciplinary' term more commonly used within the US (although in the US there is also a growing trend for adoption of 'interprofessional' language). So in many cases 'interprofessional' and 'interdisciplinary' are appropriately used interchangeably. In other reports and articles, 'interprofessional' and 'interdisciplinary' are also used to include collaborative relationships between professionals who are functioning outside a formally specified healthcare team. We believe that the use of 'interprofessional team' to connote a high level of coordinated interprofessional collaboration remains the best option. For the remainder of this chapter, we will refer to interprofessional teams and mean that to subsume work in teams that previously might have been appropriately described as either interprofessional or interdisciplinary.

The interprofessional framework delineated by Reeves, Zwarenstein, and Goldman (2011) describes such healthcare teams as a specific type of interprofessional practice intervention in which team members from different professional disciplines work together interdependently to collaborate in planning and providing care. Interprofessional teams develop a unified plan for patient assessment and treatment, and all team members are considered to be colleagues who have a range of both unique and overlapping skills that contribute to patient care and team functioning (Zeiss and Steffen 1998). Therefore, members of interprofessional teams are required to have extensive knowledge about the professional training and competencies of the disciplines represented on the team. Team members share responsibility for the effective functioning of the team, and share leadership functions. In multidisciplinary teams, on the other hand, patient care is provided by professionals from various disciplines who each develop an independent assessment and treatment plan, and then share this plan and patient outcomes with other members of the healthcare team.

INTERPROFESSIONAL VS MULTIDISCIPLINARY HEALTHCARE TEAMS

The contrasting functionality of interprofessional vs multidisciplinary healthcare teams reflects differences in the attitudes, knowledge, and skills required of their team members.

Members of multidisciplinary teams take responsibility for and focus on patient outcomes, with little to no attention given to the effectiveness of team functioning.

Table 36.1 Essential differences between interprofessional and multidisciplinary healthcare teams

	Multidisciplinary	Interprofessional
Attitudes	Assessment and treatment plans formed by other disciplines are peripherally relevant for one's own discipline-specific care plan. Team discussions optimally focus on specific cases. Some disciplines are inherently more appropriate for team leadership role due to knowledge and organizational prestige.	A biopsychosocial model provides best understanding of the patient, clinical problems, health factors, and overall team goals. Quality care of complex/chronic cases requires coordination among various disciplines with overlapping and unique contributions. Team discussions should address group process and functioning in addition to issues of patient care. Team development must be supported—hiring staff with needed clinical skills is essential but placing them in a common setting will not enable effective collaboration. The organization and team must support time and resources to develop effective team functioning over time. All team members have the capacity to develop and exercise team leadership functions which are best shared across team members.
Knowledge	Able to describe the core patient care functions performed by the other disciplines. Thorough understanding of roles and responsibilities for one's own discipline within a specific team. Recognition of designated team leader and that individual's responsibilities for managing the team.	Able to describe the training, professional milestones, and competencies of other disciplines. Able to articulate areas of role overlap vs unique contributions among the disciplines and how team collaboration and interdependence can make optimal use of all contributions. Knowledge of team process and development issues.
Behaviours	Each discipline generates own assessment and treatment plan, evaluates progress, and refines independently.	Team collaborates on joint plan for patient assessment and treatment. Members acknowledge areas of role overlap with aim to prevent duplication, and enhance coverage of key areas. Members can handle disagreement as a valuable resource for understanding a breadth of information that no single team member could obtain; team can use such complementary and conflicting information to craft a coherent, holistic understanding of the patient/family and how to best address overall problems.

Multidisciplinary teams are also typically hierarchically organized, with the individual from the highest status discipline most commonly identified as the team leader. An examination of these differences may help Mr Simpson and Dr Sanchez determine if the 'interprofessional' teams they join are multidisciplinary or truly functioning at a higher level of collaboration that can be characterized as interprofessional.

As shown in Table 36.1, when compared to multidisciplinary teams, interprofessional teams call for more flexible attitudes towards discipline-specific roles and responsibilities. Beliefs about the value of attending to team process and functioning, as well as shared leadership, are important in such team settings. In addition to the professional knowledge base for work on multidisciplinary teams, interprofessional teamwork requires a deeper understanding of the training and skill sets of other team members—as well as knowledge about team developmental processes. These differences in attitudes and knowledge then provide the foundation for effective interprofessional skills in joint assessment and treatment planning, creation of team role maps, group processing, and advanced communication skills to navigate areas of conflict.

There are good reasons why interprofessional teams are considered the international gold standard of healthcare for medically frail older adults. Interprofessional teams are important for treating complex patients with chronic health conditions; for this reason, they play a prominent role in best practices for geriatric care. Not all health conditions require the time and effort required of interprofessional teams, so psychologists are most likely to become involved in such teams within organizations serving medically complex and/or chronic patient populations. Although geriatric primary care within some healthcare systems has integrated psychological services or is moving towards such integration (Armento and Stanley, this volume; Speer and Schneider 2003), countries vary in whether a formalized interprofessional team approach is used in primary care. For patients assessed and treated by an interprofessional team, there may be occasions on which a straightforward concern develops that can be fully addressed by a single discipline. Thus, part of the challenge within an interprofessional team is determining the match between identified patient problems and the degree of collaboration called for at any given time (Drinka and Clark 2000).

Empirical Support for Interprofessional Healthcare Teams

Why are interprofessional teams considered the gold standard for the treatment of older adults with complex or chronic medical conditions? An exhaustive review of the empirical support for interprofessional teams is beyond the scope of this chapter and complicated by a number of methodological issues. For example, most intervention studies involve more than the addition of an interprofessional team approach (e.g. team care plus more frequent appointments, team care plus home health visits). Because so few randomized controlled trials involve treatment conditions varying solely in team functioning, it is difficult to attribute differences in patient outcomes directly to the team approach. Few published studies have a sufficient sample size of teams to generalize beyond a small number of specific groups. Research conducted in different countries is also impacted by the differing national models for healthcare delivery and financing; such organizational and contextual differences frame the nature of the team functioning. It should also be noted that professionals from behavioural/mental health disciplines, including psychologists, psychiatrists, psychiatric nurse practitioners, and mental health social workers, have not always been part of the geriatric healthcare teams that have been studied to date. We are mindful of these caveats as we provide readers with key reviews and a sense of the overall empirical support for interprofessional healthcare teams serving older adults.

Across inpatient and outpatient team settings, outcomes for interprofessional teams cited in the literature have included better continuity and quality of care, and improved health outcomes without increasing costs (Callahan, Boutstani, and Unverzagt 2006; Counsell, Callahan, and Clark 2007; Famadas, Frick, and Haydar 2008; Mion, Odegard, and Resnick 2006; Rubenstein 2004). Research that did not show improved mortality or medical outcomes has demonstrated improved daily functioning and decreased hospital readmissions (Caplan, Williams, and Daly 2004). Additional important patient outcomes of interprofessional teams include improved patient safety (Baker et al. 2005), along with better medication adherence and fewer adverse drug reactions (Farris, Cote, and Feeny 2004; Schmader, Hanlon, and Pieper 2004). Geriatric Evaluation and Mangement (GEM) units, which are a special type of inpatient interprofessional team focused on medically frail older adults, have received perhaps the most attention in the literature. Research on GEM units conducted in the US, UK, Canada, and Australia is also important because the same team structure and assessment/treatment approach has been applied across multiple healthcare systems and in different countries. The GEM interprofessional team approach has been demonstrated to improve patient functioning and decrease mortality (Mion et al. 2006; Rubenstein 2004) and benefit family carers (Silliman, McGarvey, and Raymong 1990).

THE INTERNATIONAL MODEL OF HEALTHCARE TEAM PERFORMANCE

As psychologists, we value clinical practices that are empirically tested and grounded in theory. Theory helps us consolidate research findings, improve healthcare practices, and identify relationships among variables that need further examination. Because so many factors influence team processes and outcomes, it is important to have a solid conceptual framework for understanding interprofessional healthcare teams. In this chapter addressing an international audience, we present and expand upon the Model of Team Performance (Heinemann and Zeiss 2002) which was utilized within the Interprofessional Team Training and Development (ITT&D) Program of the US Department of Veterans Affairs.

This conceptual framework combines organizational theory with the Developmental Model of Small-group Processes (Tuckman 1965; Tuckman and Jensen 1977). In the Model of Team Performance (Heinemann and Zeiss 2002), teams develop over time and function at different levels due to factors both within and external to the team. Teams are part of a complex organization, so the structure and context of the larger organization can benefit or hinder team functioning. Within the team, four domains of team performance—structure, context, process, and productivity—form the overarching components of team performance (Heinemann and Zeiss 2002). These dimensions are not independent—each one is a necessary but insufficient building block for the next. Thus, teams must be organized with good structure in order to develop a positive, constructive context that will generate effectively interdependent team work processes that will lead to productive work outcomes. The following sections provide more information about this original conception of team dimensions and how they are interconnected. Measurement tools that have been developed to assess various facets within these dimensions are also described by Heinemann and Zeiss (2002).

Two types of *structure* are important with regard to team performance: the structure of the organization in which the team is working and the structure of the team itself: what do the organization (e.g. the hospital, nursing home, or other healthcare facility) and the team or work group 'look like' in terms of how are they linked and how they relate to one another—i.e. what is the role of the team within the organization? Optimally, the team will be understood, appreciated, and utilized throughout various levels of the organization. Similarly, the structure within the team influences its performance and optimally the team will have (1) a mission that is clear to all members; (2) well-defined member roles and responsibilities; and (3) a well-developed culture with norms, values, rules, and procedures for operating. Team structure includes attention to leadership roles and responsibilities, and established procedures for designating/sharing these functions. Structure is related to team development (Farrell, Heinemann, and Schmitt 1986; Wheelan 1993); over time and with good management, members come to have a shared understanding of the team's mission, goals, and objectives—a positive team climate develops, with interdependent team processes, such that members participate more equally in the team's tasks. The team's structure becomes a 'coalition of colleagues' (Farrell et al. 1986).

Context refers to how it 'feels' to work in a particular organization and team: the atmosphere or environmental affect in which employees function. Context is strongly influenced by leadership style and the quality of interpersonal relationships. Leadership within well-functioning interprofessional teams is not held by a single individual; rather, leadership is shared and various team members may take leadership for various roles, such as guiding decision-making, drawing out more quiet team members, handling disagreements effectively, and leading in organizational tasks that must be completed. Some of these roles are more formal (e.g. generating reports to the larger organization of which the team is a part, as the identified 'clinical coordinator' of the team), and others are more informal (e.g. helping with process at key moments in team discussions). These leadership issues are well explored in Drinka and Clark (2000). Optimally, organizational management (1) creates a climate of collaboration and respect that engender empowerment, enthusiasm, and job pride and satisfaction; and (2) is flexible, offers opportunities for career and personal development, and is not rigid with regard to time and cost constraints or established performance guidelines. Similarly, context within the team refers to perceptions and feelings regarding the team's socio-emotional atmosphere. Team context is also influenced by the stage of a team's development, and by styles of relating among team members and the interpersonal skills of team leaders (Dimock 1987; Farrell et al. 1986). During optimal team development, as team members participate in the team's tasks more equally, the atmosphere in the team becomes one of high trust. Trust allows members to communicate openly with one another without fear of negative responses, and team members build upon each other's strengths, complete tasks efficiently, and develop pride and satisfaction with their own and the team's work. Team leadership crucially affects the tone or climate of the team, and optimally, leadership will be shared among various team members who take on leadership responsibilities in relation to both their official roles and their personal strengths and interests. Leaders who are warm and caring as well as task-oriented, and who readily share leadership with other team members, create a comfortable team climate in which members share and participate effectively (Drinka and Clark, 2000).

Process refers to increasingly integrative activities used by teams to accomplish tasks and achieve goals, along two dimensions: (1) increased interdependence of team member (the key to interprofessional teamwork), and (2) growth and development of team members. Interdependent process develops over time, from a possible worst-case scenario analogous to young children in parallel play who share space but do 'their own thing' and are unable to share activities, leading to conflict. As any team matures, team process improves: members learn from one another; they better understand each other's perspectives; and they understand unique professional roles as well as areas of overlap. When team members depend upon one another to accomplish tasks and goals, productivity increases. The ability to grow and mature applies to both team members and the team itself. As trust, cohesion, and a sense of unity develop, team members, individually and jointly, can be more flexible, try new ways of doing things, and take risks. They share their perceptions of one another and the team, and utilize this information to improve individual and team performance. Team members take advantage of education, training, and consultation to become better clinicians and healthcare providers, more highly skilled employees, and better team members.

Productivity includes (1) strategies used to be productive and (2) accomplishments of sustained workload, quality outcomes, and impact on the organization. Teams must create strategies to document results and collect, store, manage, analyse, and present information documenting productivity and accomplishments. Mature teams accept responsibility for monitoring and evaluating their own performance and they use incentives, celebrations, and rewards within the team to energize and motivate team members. Achieving such task-oriented goals can result in expansion of the team's mission, so potential accomplishments of the team become more numerous. For example, some well-functioning teams providing excellent care to their patient population may add to their mission the education of medical and health profession trainees, an additional area that must be monitored and accomplished successfully. When a team becomes mature and well performing, as demonstrated by the outcomes shown in Figure 36.1, it will be better integrated with other parts of the healthcare organization; such relationships with customers and other teams in the organization are important accomplishments. Conducting effective team meetings is a key step, demonstrating time management, good communication, and use of new technologies. The ultimate measure of productivity is positive patient health outcomes, along multiple dimensions, especially when considering geriatric patients. Such outcomes include (1) healthier lifestyles, disease prevention, and involvement in planned care; (2) cure, maintenance, or a slowed decline in health status (including decreased hospitalization episodes/days, and prevention of more intensive and expensive care); (3) maintaining quality of life, ensuring death with dignity, and supporting the family throughout the duration of a patient's involvement with the team. Documentation of such positive outcomes should lead to support and resources from management and can be used as the basis for rewards to teams and their members.

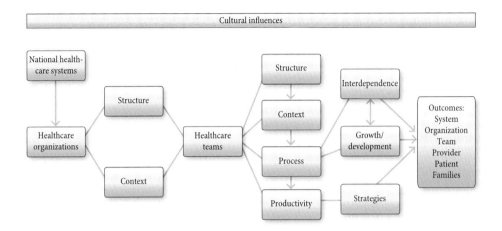

FIGURE 36.1 International Model of Healthcare Team Performance.

Reproduced from 'A model of team performance', In GD Heinemann & AM Zeiss (eds.) Team performance in health care: Assessment and development, © 2002, Springer Science and Business Media. With kind permission from Springer Science and Business Media.

As we considered the international audience of this volume, we found the need to revise and expand this model in Figure 36.1 by adding Cultural Factors and Healthcare Delivery Systems which both influence specific healthcare organizations. We have also clarified the implied relationships among the dimensions to reflect the causal relationships between organizational and team domains and a host of possible outcomes. Within this International Model of Healthcare Team Performance, outcomes are framed as multifaceted. Team-level domains of structure, context, process, and productivity impact patients (e.g. health conditions, functioning) and their families (e.g. satisfaction with quality of care, perceived stress), but also the providers on the team (e.g. work satisfaction, staff turnover), the team itself (e.g. quality care indices), and the larger healthcare organization (e.g. horizontal models of healthcare management and quality improvement practices). When enough teams across enough healthcare organizations show important benefits, these cumulatively have the power to impact entire national healthcare systems.

The strength of this model is in its attention to the nature of specific collaborative practices within interprofessional teams; the model reflects a deep well of different dimensions, facets, and elements of team practice and specific assessment tools to measure them. This model attends to team processes and structural/contextual aspects of both the team and the larger healthcare organization in which it is embedded. This formal acknowledgement of environmental factors that influence team process is relatively rare in the literature on interprofessional collaboration. Readers will, however, note the absence of patient-level variables in this model; this is for a practical reason rather than a theoretical one. It would certainly be possible to build consideration of patient-level factors into the model, but the reality is that patients are only peripherally involved in the treatment planning process within most interprofessional teams. Many patients may currently remain unaware of the team. An important future goal for interprofessional care will be to move towards 'visible team care' (D'amour et al. 2005) that reflects growing attention to the values and practices of patient-centred care.

NATIONAL POSITION STATEMENTS ON INTERPROFESSIONAL CARE AND EDUCATION

National statements on the importance of interprofessional education (IPE) for health-care professionals abound, with systematic reviews available from the Australian Capital Territory (ACT) Department of Health (Braithwaite and Travaglia 2005), Health Canada (2012), the Cochrane Collaboration in the UK (Reeves et al. 2001), and the US Agency for Healthcare Research and Quality (Baker et al. 2005). In addition, in the US, the Institute of Medicine (2010) report, *Redesigning Continuing Education in the Health Professions*, emphasized the importance of interprofessional education in one of its major recommendations: 'Continuing education efforts should bring health professionals from various disciplines together in carefully tailored learning environments. As team-based healthcare delivery becomes increasingly important, such interprofessional efforts will enable participants to learn both individually and as collaborative members of a team, with a common goal of improving patient outcomes.' (2).

For healthcare educators who would like to explore models and practical strategies for interprofessional team education and training, readers are encouraged to see the edited work by Royeen, Jensen, and Harvan (2009) that emerged from a working conference on rural health interprofessional education. Educators will also find it helpful to explore the work by Siegler et al. (1998), which describes the John A. Hartford Foundation Geriatric Interdisciplinary Team Training Program (GITT) in the US. Clark (2011, 2013) reviews institutional, systemic, and funding challenges for implementing and sustaining interprofessional education, and proposes a trans-theoretical model of institutional change that may help educational leaders to facilitate and maintain change supportive of IPE.

POLICY IMPLICATIONS

Interprofessional teams are not generally supported in countries and in healthcare systems when the financing of medical care is linked to a specific unit of direct clinical service delivered by a specific healthcare provider. In the US, fragmented fee-for-service funding of outpatient and most inpatient services has historically limited the spread of interprofessional teams because only direct patient care is reimbursed and time spent for team discussion and coordination of care is not reimbursed. Different funding models within the US's Department of Veterans Affairs healthcare system, coordinated by the Veterans Health Administration—VHA (Karlin and Zeiss 2010; Zeiss and Karlin 2008), and in the two Medicare programs for frail (PACE) or terminally ill (hospice) beneficiaries have supported and encouraged the development of interprofessional teams. Thus, professionals from these programmes have served as national leaders for interprofessional team training in geriatrics within the USA.

In all healthcare, including care offered in VHA, it is essential that policy decisions lead to adequate workload credit for team interaction time for clinical planning and team development, not just for direct clinical care. Healthcare procedure codes used to track clinical activities and to guide billing in the US (current procedural terminology—CPT—codes) exist but have minimal or no weighted value in terms of relative value units (RVUs), which are typically used for monitoring workload and ensuring productivity of team members. Thus, team members can note activities related to coordination of care, but this data is not captured in the workload summaries that are reviewed by many supervisors. It is essential that this be corrected in order to support staff in devoting adequate time to develop expertise as a team and to use that expertise to guide patient care, with workload encompassing a range of activities including patient care coordination and team planning.

In addition, there are policy implications for the training of healthcare professionals. Currently in the US, each healthcare profession sets their own training requirements, accredits training programmes, and focuses on discipline-specific skills in such training. Consequently, there are no national healthcare policy requirements ensuring that healthcare professionals will also be trained in interprofessional skills and articulating the reasons why these are essential for optimal care. Many disciplines have endorsed such a policy shift, but to date we are not aware of any concrete actions that would result in changed clinical curriculum requirements.

IMPLICATIONS FOR PRACTICE: COMPETENCIES IN TEAMWORK FOR PSYCHOLOGISTS

Let's return to Brent and Maria and how their upcoming opportunities call for specialized knowledge and skills. What can Brent hope to learn through a clinical placement that requires his participation on an interprofessional team? What competencies might Maria look to develop to increase her confidence and effectiveness in participating in and guiding her GEM team? Within professional psychology, which historically has not emphasized interprofessional care as part of its training curriculum, there is increasing attention to the role that psychologists can play in healthcare settings around the world. Across national guidelines for general and specialized practice of psychologists, the need for competencies to work within interprofessional teams is increasingly apparent. The Partnership for Health in Aging in the USA, a coalition of twenty-two organizations representing healthcare professions caring for older adults, developed a position statement emphasizing that interprofessional teamwork must be a core component of training for all health professionals working with older adults. The position statement was supported by professional associations representing dentists, geriatric care managers, nurses, occupational therapists, pharmacists, physicians, physical therapists, psychiatrists, psychologists, social workers, and others (Partnership for Health in Aging Workgroup on Interdisciplinary Team Training 2011). Table 36.2 shows the nine teamwork-specific interprofessional competencies endorsed in this position statement.

In the US, the Pikes Peak Model for Training in Professional Geropsychology details competencies for teamwork that are important for psychological practice with older adults (Knight et al. 2009). A foundational competency for professional geropsychology functioning is to '[a]ddress complex biopsychosocial issues among many older adults by collaborating with other disciplines in multi-and inter-disciplinary teams' (Knight et al. 2009).

Behavioural indicators of this competency include the need to understand the theory and science of geriatric team building and value the role that other providers play in the assessment and treatment of older clients (Karel et al. 2010a; see http://gerocentral.org/competencies/). Likewise, a core consultation competency for professional geropsychology practice is to 'participate in interprofessional teams that serve older adults' (Knight et al. 2009). Behavioural anchors for this competency are the ability to (1) work with professionals in other disciplines to incorporate geropsychological information into team treatment planning and implementation; (2) communicate psychological conceptualizations clearly and respectfully to other providers; (3) appreciate and integrate feedback from interprofessional team members into case conceptualizations; (4) work to build consensus on treatment plans and goals of care, to invite various perspectives, and to negotiate conflict constructively; and (5) demonstrate ability to work with diverse team structures (e.g. hierarchical, lateral, virtual) and team members (e.g. including the ethics board, chaplains, and families in palliative care teams) (Karel et al. 2010b).

Developing a Psychologist's Role on Interprofessional Teams

The focus of activities of a psychologist on an interprofessional team varies by the clinical population being served, the team's level of functioning, and the extent to which the team is familiar with and values the perspectives of a psychologist. Maria will need to evaluate these aspects of her GEM team in order to guide her approach. For example, how cohesive is the team? To what extent does the team incorporate mental health issues into treatment planning? What services is she most likely to provide to patients, families, and/or the team to

---

Table 36.2 Professional competencies for interdisciplinary healthcare teamwork

Ideally, all members of an interdisciplinary healthcare team will have sufficient didactic and clinical training to enable them to:

1 Understand their respective roles and responsibilities on the team.
2 Establish common goals for the team.
3 Agree on rules for conducting team meetings.
4 Communicate well with other members of the team.
5 Identify and resolve conflict.
6 Share decision-making and execute defined tasks when consensus is reached.
7 Provide support for one another, including the development of leadership roles.
8 Be flexible in response to changing circumstances.
9 Participate in periodic team performance reviews to ensure that the team is functioning well and that its goals are being met.

Data from: PHA/AGS Position Statement on Interdisciplinary Team Training (2011). See http://www.americangeriatrics.org/files/documents/pha/PHA_IDTStatement.pdf.

enhance overall interprofessional care? Likewise, Brent may find himself warmly welcomed into a team that values his perspectives as a psychology trainee or, potentially, into a team that is not quite sure what he does.

In already functioning teams, psychologists educate other team members about the roles and responsibilities of psychology and how these approaches are optimally integrated within the team's practice. Other contexts require psychologists to provide more education about their disciplinary training and licensure to practise independently, help team members identify cases that will most benefit from psychological services, or make steps to move the team towards a more truly interprofessional approach (Zeiss and Gallagher-Thompson 2003). For example, psychologists can help the team become more aware of behavioural/mental health issues while advancing a biopsychosocial conceptualization of patients. This approach ensures that mental health issues are addressed in a unified manner by the entire team, as appropriate (i.e. the psychologist's job is not to independently 'fix' complex problems without support of the entire team).

Psychologists have skills by virtue of our professional training that are extremely useful for modelling and facilitating interprofessional team process and functioning. These skills include active listening and verbal/nonverbal communication skills, the ability to tolerate and respond constructively to a range of emotional expression (by patients, families, and colleagues), and problem-solving skills, as well as systematic conceptualization—of people and systems. Psychologists can model and encourage respectful communication, facilitate negotiation of conflict, as well as encourage expression and recognition of the wide range of strengths on the team.

Interprofessional Team Training for Psychologists

What types of training experiences can help professionals, and psychologists in particular, to develop competence for interprofessional practice? For Brent, what type of training and supervision might he hope for to become an effective participant in interprofessional care? For Maria, who no longer has the freedom to devote all of her time to training and professional development, what resources are available to her to learn more? We recommend the framework provided by D'Amour and Oandasan (2005), which emphasizes the interdependencies between health professional education and interprofessional collaborative practice. Reeves and colleagues (2011) also highlight the intersections in the literature between interprofessional education (IPE) and interprofessional collaboration (IPC).

The World Health Organization *Framework for Action on Interprofessional Education and Collaborative Practice* (2010) summarizes the link between IPE and outcomes of effective interprofessional collaborative practice. Per the WHO report, 'Interprofessional education occurs when two or more professions learn about, from and with each other to enable effective collaboration and improve health outcomes. Professional is an all-encompassing term that includes individuals with the knowledge and/or skills to contribute to the physical, mental and social well-being of a community' (13). To develop skills for interprofessional practice, it is critical to have these opportunities to learn with and from people from different professional backgrounds. Historically, psychology training has focused on intraprofessional training, that is, training focused on education by and with psychologists. One of the core features of training in geropsychology, per the Pikes Peak model in the US (Knight et al., 2009), is interprofessional team training: 'Interprofessional team training is an essential part of professional geropsychology training. Trainees must learn about the knowledge base, scope of practice, and distinct professional work styles of other disciplines' (Knight et al. 2009, 210). Trainees need to learn about different professional training models and socialization practices that affect professional values and assumptions (Qualls and Czirr 1988). The specific methods for interprofessional team training will certainly vary by national training models for clinical psychology, and by national healthcare models. For example, psychologists newly exposed to team practice in the US may encounter a medical model where psychological services are considered either a non-essential luxury or an adjunctive treatment to be offered in isolation from the rest of medical care. Trainees often struggle to clarify their own role on the team—to themselves and then to the team (Karel and Moye 2005). Ideally, trainees will have the opportunity to see other psychologists (ideally their own supervisors) 'in action' in team settings, as role models and to have their own contributions to team discussion/practice observed.

In addition to actual participation on an interprofessional team, other individual and group learning exercises can be very helpful. Discussion of cases in seminars or group supervision settings, including trainees from different disciplines, can be very effective. Case discussion may be based on actual cases in the clinical setting or cases developed for instructional purposes. For example, learners may discuss cases published in books (e.g. Mezey et al. 2002) or via online geriatric training websites (e.g. see http://shp.missouri. edu/vhct/studies.htm). Further, encouraging learners to reflect about their experiences and observations in team contexts, through journal writing or other assignments requiring self-assessment or interpretation of one's observations, can be very helpful (Clark 2009). It is important for developing professionals to have a sense of their own styles of communication, conflict resolution, and leadership, as well to appreciate the variety of such styles in others, and the impact of individual styles and their interaction on team performance.

Using our case examples, Brent would be well advised to prioritize opportunities for a placement in which he could work directly with physicians, nurses, pharmacists, social workers, and/or other health professionals, and learn from them about their perspectives towards patient care while sharing his own. Maria, in her own continuing professional development, will want to seek written and experiential continuing education related to interprofessional team practice. A number of institutions and associations are offering online education and resources regarding team practice (see Table 36.3). It will also be important for Maria to seek a mentor (or mentors) with interprofessional team/leadership experience—who may or may not be a psychologist—to discuss her own programme, how to think about needs assessment and team development, and strategies for prioritizing her professional activities. When such mentors are not available within a specific healthcare setting, consultations with other members of a professional organization may be helpful (Zimmerman, Fiske, and Scogin 2011). For example, in the US, both the American Psychological Association's Society of Clinical Geropsychology and the organization Psychologists in Long Term Care (http://www.pltcweb.org/index.php) have mentoring/consultation programmes.

Table 36.3 Resources for interprofessional team training and development

Books

Drinka, T. and Clark, P. (2000). *Healthcare Teamwork: Interdisciplinary Practice and Teaching.* Westport, CT: Auburn House.

Heinemann, G. and Zeiss, A. M. (eds) (2002). *Team Performance in Health Care: Assessment and Development.* New York: Kluwer Academic/Plenum Press.

Speciality journals

Journal of Interdisciplinary Healthcare Education

Journal of Interprofessional Care. http://informahealthcare.com/jic.

Journal of Research in Interprofessional Practice and Education. http://www.jripe.org.

Reports

American Psychological Association (2008). *Blueprint for Change: Achieving Integrated Health Care for an Aging Population.* Washington, DC: APA Press. http://www.apa.org/pi/aging/blueprint.html.

Institute of Medicine (2012). *The Mental Health and Substance Use Workforce for Older Adults: In Whose Hands?* Washington, DC: National Academies Press.

Interprofessional Education Collaborative Expert Panel (2011). *Core Competencies for Interprofessional Collaborative Practice: Report of an Expert Panel.* Washington, DC: Interprofessional Education Collaborative.

Partnership for Health in Aging Workgroup on Interdisciplinary Team Training (2011). *Position Statement on Interdisciplinary Team Training in Geriatrics: An Essential Component of Quality Healthcare for Older Adults.* New York: American Geriatrics Society. http://www. americangeriatrics.org/pha.

World Health Organization (2010). *Statement on Interprofessional Education and Collaborative Practice.* Geneva: WHO. http://www.who.int/hrh/resources/framework_action/en/index.html.

Professional associations and organizations

American Interprofessional Health Collaborative (AIHC). http://www.aihc-us.org/.

American Psychological Association (APA). http://www.apa.org/ed/graduate/competency.aspx.

Australasian Interprofessional Practice and Education Network (AIPPEN). http://www.aippen.net/.

Centre for the Advancement of Interprofessional Education—United Kingdom (CAIPE). http://www. caipe.org.uk/.

Canadian Interprofessional Health Collaborative (CIHC). http://www.cihc.ca/.

European Association for Psychotherapy (EAP). http://www.psychotherapy-competency.eu/ Competencies/Core/core_competencies_domain7.php.

European Interprofessional Practice and Education Network in Health and Social Care (EIPEN). http://www.eipen.eu/.

Nordic Interprofessional Network (NIPNET). http://nipnet.org/.

Training resources

http://americangeriatrics.org/about_us/partnership_for_health_in_aging/ interdisciplinary_team_training_statement/

http://www.ipe.umn.edu

http://www.nynj.va.gov/grecccurriculum.asp

http://www.macyfoundation.org/

http://collaborate.uw.edu/educators-toolkit/educators-toolkit.html

Another important point to mention is that psychologists can have very important roles in interprofessional education. Psychologists can teach in nursing, medical, and other professional programmes, and offer interprofessional continuing education regarding team functioning and the integration of mental and behavioural healthcare into geriatric care teams.

Future Directions for Research on Interprofessional Teams

The future of interprofessional team healthcare for older people is heavily dependent upon the demonstrated cost effectiveness of this approach. Changes in healthcare are dependent upon institutional resources for specific practices; resources means financing, and policy mandates. Thus, we strongly encourage cost-effectiveness research on interprofessional teams across a range of settings, but especially for serving the needs of older adults.

Although different regions of the world vary in the use of specific technologies for team communication, the use of technology continues to grow. As a result, there is a need for research in how technological advances in communication impact team functioning. We are particularly struck by the challenges of cross-cultural research in this area, and hope that this chapter might be the impetus for readers to frame questions that could be addressed (Berry, Pandey, and Poortinga 1996). One of the merits of the edited book by Royeen and colleagues (2009) is the strong emphasis on cultural competencies needed by healthcare professionals, and how these specifically strengthen the function of interprofessional teams working to address health disparities in underserved communities. The literature on GEM units, which has strong international contributions in the literature, is another excellent entry into cross-cultural research on interprofessional healthcare teams, given the similar approach to identifying frail elders and similar components for GEM services. More research is also needed on dissemination of interprofessional team structures and processes, with need for use of theory to guide evaluation of dissemination practices (Davies, Walker, and Grimshaw 2010).

Summary

As national healthcare systems shift towards models of care that integrate mental and physical health, clinical psychologists find themselves working in an expanded range of healthcare settings and with an increasing number of older adults. Interprofessional teams constitute *the* best practice for treating older patients with chronic health conditions—such teams lead to improved health outcomes and quality care without increasing costs. Interprofessional teams engage in a high level of collaborative care; team members from different professional disciplines work interdependently to develop a unified plan for patient assessment and treatment. Interprofessional team members acquire knowledge about team developmental processes and share responsibility for both the effective functioning of the team and leadership functions. Within this chapter, the International Model of Healthcare Team Performance describes four within-team domains (i.e. structure, context, process, and productivity) that are framed by healthcare systems (organizational, national) and broader cultural influences. Interprofessional teamwork calls for a wide range of professional competencies, with a number of international resources available for the necessary training and continuing education of psychologists. Organizational as well as national systems and policies that facilitate team-based care will hopefully continue to develop, so that we may effectively work together to meet the physical and mental healthcare needs of our ageing population.

KEY REFERENCES AND SOURCES FOR FURTHER READING

Please refer to Table 36.3 for resources for interested readers.

REFERENCES

Baker, D., Gustafson, S., Beaubien, J., Salas, E., and Barach, P. (2005). *Medical Teamwork and Patient Safety: The Evidence-based Relation.* AHRQ Publication No. 05-0053. Rockville, MD: Agency for Healthcare Research and Quality.

Berry, J. W., Pandey, J., and Poortinga, Y. H. (eds) (1996). *Handbook of Cross-cultural Psychology: Volume 1: Theory and Method* (2nd edn). Needham Heights, MA: Allyn and Bacon.

Braithwaite, J. and Travaglia, J. F. (2005). *Inter-professional Learning and Clinical Education: An Overview of the Literature.* Canberra: Braithwaite and Associates, ACT Health Department,.

Canadian Psychological Association (2011). *Accreditation Standards and Procedures for Doctoral Programmes and Internships in Professional Psychology* (5th edn). Ottawa, ON: Canadian Psychological Association.

Callahan, C. M., Boustani, M. A., and Unverzagt, F. W. (2005). 'Effectiveness of Collaborative Care for Older Adults with Alzheimer's Disease in Primary Care'. *Journal of the American Medical Association* 295: 2148–2157.

Caplan, G. A., Williams, A. J., and Daly, B. (2004). 'A Randomized Controlled Trial of Comprehensive Geriatric Assessment and Multidisciplinary Intervention after Discharge of Elderly from the Emergency Department—the DEED II Study'. *Journal of the American Geriatrics Society* 52: 1417–1423.

Clark, P. G. (2009). 'Reflection on Reflection in Interprofessional Education: Implications for Theory and Practice'. *Journal of Interprofessional Care* 23: 213–223.

Clark, P. G. (2011). 'The Devil is in the Details: The Seven Deadly Sins of Organizing and Continuing Interprofessional Education in the US'. *Journal of Interprofessional Care* 25: 321–327.

Clark, P. G. (2013). 'Toward a Transtheoretical Model of Interprofessional Education: Stages, Processes, and Forces Supporting Institutional Change'. *Journal of Interprofessional Care* 27: 43–49.

Counsell, S. R., Callahan, C. M., and Clark, D. O. (2007). 'Geriatric Care Management for Low Income Seniors: A Randomized Controlled Trial'. *Journal of the American Medical Association* 298: 2623–2633.

D'Amour, D., Ferrada-Videla, M., San Martin Rodriguez, L., and Beaulieu, M. D. (2005). 'The Conceptual Basis for Interprofessional Collaboration: Core Concepts and Theoretical Frameworks'. *Journal of Interprofessional Care* 19(suppl. 1): 116–131.

D'Amour, D. and Oandasan, I. (2005). 'Interprofessionality as the Field of Interprofessional Practice and Interprofessional Education: An Emerging Concept'. *Journal of Interprofessional Care* 19(suppl. 1): 8–20.

Davies, P., Walker, A. E., and Grimshaw, J. M. (2010). 'A Systematic Review of the Use of Theory in the Design of Guideline Dissemination and Implementation Strategies and Interpretation of the Results of Rigorous Evaluations'. *Implementation Science* 5: 14.

Dimock, H. G. (1987). *Groups: Leadership and Group Development*. San Diego, CA: University Associates.

Drinka, T. and Clark, P. (2000). *Healthcare Teamwork: Interdisciplinary Practice and Teaching*. Westport, CT: Auburn House.

Emery, E. E., Lapidos, S., Eisenstein, A. R., Ivan, I. I., and Golden, R. L. (2012). 'The BRIGHTEN Program: Implementation and Evaluation of a Program to Bridge Resources of an Interdisciplinary Geriatric Health Team via Electronic Networking'. *Gerontologist* 52: 857–865.

Famadas, J. C., Frick, K. D., and Haydar, Z. R. (2008). 'The Effects of Interdisciplinary Outpatient Geriatrics On the Use, Costs, and Quality of Health Services in the Fee-for-service Environment'. *Aging Clinical and Experimental Research* 20: 556–561.

Farrell, M. P., Heinemann, G. D., and Schmitt, M. H. (1986). 'Informal Roles, Rituals and Styles of Humor in Interdisciplinary Health Care Teams: Their Relationship to Stages of Group Development'. *International Journal of Small Group Research* 2: 143–162.

Farris, K. B., Cote, I., and Feeny, D. (2004). 'Enhancing Primary Care for Complex Patients: Demonstration Project Using Multidisciplinary Teams'. *Canadian Family Physician* 50: 1009–1003.

Health Canada (2012). *Interprofessional Education for Collaborative Patient-centered Care: Final Report*. http://www.hc-sc.gc.ca/hcs-sss/pubs/hhrhs/2006-iecps-fipccp-workatel/index-eng.php. Accessed 8 December 2012.

Heinemann, G. D. and Zeiss, A. M. (2002). 'A Model of Team Performance'. In G. D. Heinemann and A. M. Zeiss (eds), *Team Performance in Health Care: Assessment and Development*. New York: Springer.

Institute of Medicine (2010). *Redesigning Continuing Education in the Health Professions*. Washington, DC: National Academies Press.

Interprofessional Education Collaborative Expert Panel (2011). *Core Competencies for Interprofessional Collaborative Practice: Report of an Expert Panel*. Washington, DC: Interprofessional Education Collaborative.

Karel, M. J. and Moye, J. (2005). 'Geropsychology Training in a VA Nursing Home Setting'. *Gerontology and Geriatrics Education* 25: 83–105.

Karel, M. J., Emery, E. E., Molinari, V., and CoPGTP Task Force on the Assessment of Geropsychology Competencies (2010a). 'Development of a Tool to Evaluate Geropsychology Knowledge and Skill Competencies'. *International Psychogeriatrics* 22: 886–896.

Karel, M. J., Knight, B. G., Duffy, M., Hinrichsen, G., and Zeiss, A. M. (2010b). 'Attitude, Knowledge, and Skill Competencies for Practice in Professional Geropsychology: Implications for Training and Building a Geropsychology Workforce'. *Training and Education in Professional Psychology* 4: 75–84.

Karlin, B. E. and Zeiss, A. M. (2010). 'Transforming Mental Healthcare for Older Veterans in the Veterans Health Administration'. *Generations* 34(2): 74–83.

Knight, B. G., Karel, M. J., Hinrichsen, G. A., Qualls, S. H., and Duffy, M. (2009). 'Pikes Peak Model for Training in Professional Geropsychology'. *American Psychologist* 64: 205–214.

Leathard, A. (2003). *Interprofessional Collaboration: From Policy to Practice in Health and Social Care*. Hove: Brunner Routledge.

Mezey, M. D., Cassel, C. K., Bottrell, M. M., Hyer, K., Howe, J. L., et al. (eds) (2002). *Ethical Patient Care: A Casebook for Geriatric Health Care Teams*. Baltimore, MD: Johns Hopkins University Press.

Mion, L., Odegard, P. S., and Resnick, B. (2005). 'Interdisciplinary Care for Older Adults with Complex Needs: American Geriatrics Society Position Statement'. *Journal of the American Geriatrics Society* 54: 849–852.

Partnership for Health in Aging Workgroup on Interdisciplinary Team Training (2011). *Position Statement on Interdisciplinary Team Training in Geriatrics: An Essential Component of Quality Healthcare for Older Adults*. New York: American Geriatrics Society. http://www.american geriatrics.org/pha.

Qualls, S. H. and Czirr, R. (1988). 'Geriatric Health Teams: Classifying Models of Professional and Team Functioning'. *Gerontologist* 28: 372–376.

Reeves, S., Zwarenstein, M., and Goldman, J. (2001). 'Interprofessional Education: Effects on Professional Practice and Health Care Outcomes'. *Cochrane Database of Systematic Reviews* 1: CD002213.

Reeves, S., Goldman, J., Gilbert, J., Tepper, J., Silver, I., et al. (2011) 'A Scoping Review to Improve Conceptual Clarity of Interprofessional Interventions'. *Journal of Interprofessional Care* 25: 167–174.

Royeen, C. B., Jensen, G. M., and Harvan, R. A. (2009). *Leadership in Interprofessional Health Education and Practice*. Sudbury, MA: Jones and Bartlett.

Rubenstein, L. Z. (2004). 'Joseph T. Freeman Award Lecture: Comprehensive Geriatric Assessment: From Miracle to Reality'. *Journal of the Gerontological Association for Science in Medicine* 59: 473–477.

Schmader, K. E., Hanlon, J. T., and Pieper, C. F. (2004). 'Effects of Geriatric Evaluation and Management on Adverse Drug Reactions and Suboptimal Prescribing in the Frail Elderly'. *American Journal of Medicine* 116: 394–401.

Sekerak, D., Wakeford, L., Cochran, K., and Alexander, J. (2009). 'Interprofessional Training in Telehealth Technologies for Service Delivery and Development of Rural Communities of Practice'. In C. B. Royeen, G. M. Jensen, and R. A. Harvan (eds), *Leadership in Interprofessional Health Education and Practice*. Sudbury, MA: Jones and Bartlett.

Siegler, E., Hyer, K., Fulmer, T., and Mezey, M. (1998). *Geriatric Interdisciplinary Team Training*. New York: Springer.

Silliman, R. A., McGarvey, S. T., and Raymong, P. M. (1990). 'The Senior Care Study. Does Inpatient Interdisciplinary Geriatric Assessment Help Family Caregivers of Acutely Ill Older Patients?' *Journal of the American Geriatrics Society* 38: 1163.

Speer, D. C. and Schneider, M. G. (2003). 'Mental Health Needs of Older Adults and Primary Care: Opportunity for Interdisciplinary Geriatric Team Practice'. *Clinical Psychology: Science and Practice* 10(1): 85–101.

Tuckman, B. W. (1965). 'Developmental Sequences in Small Groups'. *Psychological Bulletin* 63: 384–399.

Tuckman, B. W. and Jensen, M. A. (1977). 'Stages of Small Group Development Revisited'. *Group and Organizational Studies* 2: 419–427.

Wheelan, S. A. (1993). *The Group Development Questionnaire: A Manual for Professionals*. Philadelphia, PA: GDQ Associates.

World Health Organization (2010). *Framework for Action on Interprofessional Education and Collaborative Practice*. Geneva: World Health Organization.

Zeiss, A. M. and Steffen, A. M. (1998). 'Interdisciplinary Health Care Teams in Geriatrics: An International Model'. In A. S. Bellack and M. Hersen (eds), *Comprehensive Clinical Psychology 7: Clinical Geropsychology* (pp. 551–570). Oxford: Pergamon Press.

Zeiss, A. M. and Gallagher-Thompson, D. (2003). 'Providing Interdisciplinary Geriatric Team Care: What Does It Really Take?' *Clinical Psychology: Science and Practice* 10: 115–119.

Zeiss, A. M. and Karlin, B. E. (2008). 'Integrating Mental Health and Primary Care Services in the Department of Veterans Affairs Health Care System'. *Journal of Clinical Psychology in Medical Settings* 15(1): 73–78.

Zimmerman, J. A., Fiske, A., and Scogin, F. (2011) 'Mentoring in Clinical Geropsychology: Across the Stages of Professional Development'. *Educational Gerontology* 37: 355–369.

CHAPTER 37

THE USE OF CBT FOR BEHAVIOURS THAT CHALLENGE IN DEMENTIA

IAN A. JAMES

INTRODUCTION

THERE is considerable interest in the potential of psychosocial interventions for the treatment of behaviours that challenge (BC) (Bird and Moniz-Cook 2008; Gitlin, Kales, and Lyketsos 2012). In the US and Europe there is consensus that non-pharmacological interventions should be the first-line treatments in most situations rather than medication (Banerjee 2009; Doody et al. 2001; Salzman et al. 2008). Systematic reviews of treatments tend to favour multicomponent interventions, rather than standalone therapies, such as aromatherapy, music, or reminiscence. The multicomponent interventions are often guided via idiographic formulations, incorporating features of functional analysis (Moniz-Cook et al. 2012), carer training (Marriot et al. 2000) and sometimes exercise (Teri et al., this volume). The current chapter will not review the latter treatments in detail because comprehensive reviews are readily accessible (Hulme et al. 2010; Olazarán et al. 2010). Rather this chapter examines the use of cognitive-behaviour therapy (CBT) and the application of some of its principles in the treatment of BC in dementia. Further, the content focuses on those people with moderate to severe cognitive impairment—those who would struggle to use standardized CBT approaches.

BCs are defined as actions that detract from the well-being of individuals due to the physical or psychological distress they cause within the settings they are performed. The individuals affected may be either the instigators of the acts or those in the immediate surroundings (James 2011). Common BCs include: screaming, hitting, excessive inactivity, or pacing (see Table 37.1). The BCs often have multiple causes (e.g. physical, mental, environmental, neurological), which are moderated by people's emotions and beliefs. BCs are common, and generally managed well by carers, and many resolve with time. However, some problems can become chronic or risky, and on these occasions specialist assistance is required in the form of biopsychosocial approaches (i.e. medical and non-pharmacological). Good practice suggests such approaches require a thorough assessment of the situation, and then effective targeting of the causal factors underlying the behaviours (Brechin et al. 2013). If there are no obvious physical causes (infection, pain, etc.), non-pharmacological strategies are recommended prior to the use of psychotropics (i.e. sedatives and tranquillizers). In the past, psychotropics, particularly antipsychotics, have been prescribed too readily. This has resulted in many serious side-effects and premature deaths, with limited benefits in 80% of the recipients of antipsychotics (Banerjee 2009). The features and issues raised above will be unpacked in this chapter, and the following aspects emphasized:

- Behaviours perceived to be 'challenging' will differ between settings, with some onlookers being more tolerant than others. For this reason, the term 'BC' can be viewed as a 'social construct'.
- They often reflect some form of need that is either driven by a belief (e.g. the person thinks she needs to collect her children from school), or is related to distress (e.g. signalling or coping with discomfort/boredom)
- BCs have multiple causes, and the neurological impairment associated with dementia is just one of the numerous factors
- Owing to the complexities involved in treating chronic BC, formulations are critical in delivering effective treatments. CBT conceptualizations have been helpful in understanding the needs of people with dementia.
- Standard CBT treatment methods are effective in the treatment of carers.

A list of behaviours termed as challenging is presented in Table 37.1. It is worth noting that there are many difficulties associated with defining BC in terms of behaviour. This is in part because it encourages clinicians to think of people's difficulties in terms of their outward signs (i.e. the actions) rather than their underlying cause(s). For example, by labelling a BC as 'aggression', one might be distracted from identifying its true cause which could be either pain or paranoia. The actions listed in Table 37.1 are divided into aggressive and non-aggressive forms; their ordering does not reflect frequency of occurrence. Frequency counts repeatedly suggest that apathy-related behaviours are the most common forms of BC (33–56% of problematic behaviours observed—see Aalten et al. 2008; Selbaeck et al. 2007). However, the apathy-related BCs often go under-reported and untreated owing to the lack of disruption and passivity associated with apathy. The latter is particularly true for twenty-four-hour communal settings.

When reading Table 37.1, it becomes apparent that BCs are not solely a feature of dementia. Indeed, the behaviours described in the table are frequently displayed on the high streets of many towns by younger people, particularly on alcohol-fuelled weekends. In truth, the behaviours are often exhibited by all of us when we are emotional, distressed, and/or confused. Thus when devising treatments for BCs, it is important to acknowledge that one is dealing with a basic range of activities for people with and without dementia.

Figure 37.1 is a diagram that serves to remind us about the links between behaviours and their causes. The triangle represents an iceberg and below the surface are all the things about the person that we cannot see. This is a biopsychosocial conceptualization and illustrates the complexities occurring within an individual, with the behavioural aspect being only one feature of the person's overall experience at a given moment. As a clinician, it is important not to see the behaviour as a meaningful diagnostic label (e.g. aggression, wandering, vocalizing, etc.), treatable via medication alone. That said, within the person's presentation there may well be real diagnostic conditions requiring treatment: depression, anxiety,

Table 37.1 List of behaviours that challenge (BC)

Aggressive forms of BC	Non-aggressive forms of BC
Hitting	Apathy and depression
Kicking	Repetitive noise
Grabbing	Repetitive questions
Pushing	Making strange noises
Nipping	Constant requests for help
Scratching	Eating/drinking excessively
Biting	Over-activity
Spitting	Pacing
Choking	General agitation
Hair pulling	Following others/trailing
Tripping someone	Inappropriate exposure of parts of body
Throwing objects	Masturbating in public areas
Stick prodding	Urinating in inappropriate places
Stabbing	Smearing
Swearing	Handling things inappropriately
Screaming	Dismantling objects
Shouting	Hoarding things
Physical sexual assault	Hiding items
Verbal sexual advances	Falling intentionally
Acts of self harm	Eating inappropriate substances
	Non-compliance
	Misidentifying

psychosis, bipolar disorder. The latter are common comorbid conditions found in people with dementia.

As can be seen from the diagram, the link between the behaviours and their causes is often via some form of belief. Such beliefs are often emotionally charged by fear, anger, pride, or despair. Beliefs are also related to 'needs', whereby a person who is time-shifted may believe she is unmarried, not recognizing the man next to her as her husband, and thus perceiving she needs to protect herself from the old man (i.e. husband) trying to hold her hand.

Action scripts also play an important role in activating belief systems. These scripts (aka schemas, James 2011) are outdated proceduralized activities and patterns of behaving: for example, an ex-miner attempting to leave the house very early in order to start a shift at work, or a retired plumber repeatedly dismantling the central heating system. It is suggested that it is the role of a competent therapist to obtain an understanding of such cognitions, via a formulation, in order to direct appropriate treatment. Hence, with such an emphasis on thoughts and cognitions, it is an obvious step to employ CBT conceptual models and tools in the treatment of people who challenge, whether or not they have dementia.

An overview of the sorts of dimensions for which treatment is offered by therapists is presented in Figure 37.2 and Table 37.2.

Traditional psychotherapy methods (CBT, interpersonal therapy, behavioural therapy) may be used to treat BC arising from 3–4 presentations. However, the focus of this chapter is the presentations displayed by patients described in Cells 5–8. Within these latter domains psychotherapy can serve two functions: (1) to maintain well-being in those with good

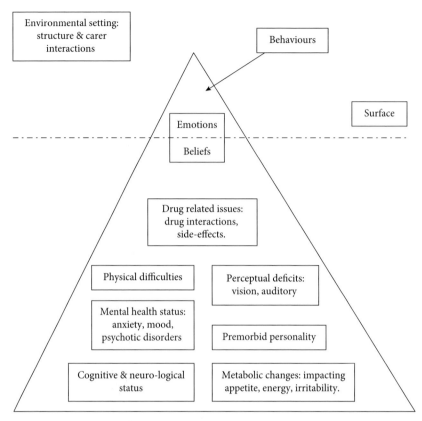

FIGURE 37.1 Iceberg analogy Reproduced from James, I. (2011). *Understanding Behaviour in Dementia that Challenges: A Guide to Assessment and Treatment.* London and Philadelphia: Jessica Kingsley Publishers.

Reproduced from James, I. (2011). Understanding Behaviour in Dementia that Challenges: A Guide to Assessment and Treatment. Jessica Kingsley Publishers, London and Philadelphia. Reprinted with permission of Jessica Kingsley Publishers.

Table 37.2 Grid outlining the eight cells of the three–axes model

	No to little cognitive impairment		Moderate to severe cognitive impairment	
Good physical health	1 Good mental health	3 Poor mental health	5 Good mental health	7 Poor mental health
Poor physical health	2 Good mental health	4 Poor mental health	6 Good mental health	8 Poor mental health

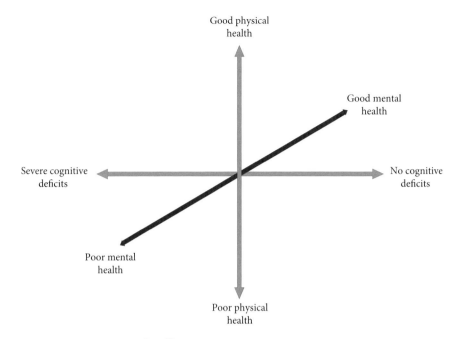

FIGURE 37.2 Dimensions of wellbeing: a 3-D perspective.

mental health (i.e. to prevent people moving from Cells 5 and 6 to 7 and 8, respectively); (2) to promote well-being in those with poor mental health (i.e. to facilitate the move from 7 and 8 to 5 and 6, respectively). In previous articles these two aims have been discussed in terms of preventative and intervention approaches (Fossey et al. 2006; James and Fossey 2008)—see Table 37.3.

The preventative approaches have been presented as separate standalone therapies. However, in many respects it is useful to see them as techniques that can be applied alone or in combination. In truth, many of the preventative approaches are frequently recommended as targeted strategies (e.g. life review, music, aromatherapy, etc.) via a formulation. The difference in their employment in the latter case concerns the 'rationale' underpinning their use. For example, when using music therapy via a formulation-led intervention it is tailored to the individual and his/her context in terms of the type of music selected, when and where it is played, the monitoring of effectiveness, etc.

As with all therapeutic work, a vital ingredient of delivering these therapies and techniques is the use of good communication skills. A systematic review of communication strategies for people with dementia was conducted by Vasse et al. (2010) for residents in care settings. To Vasse et al.'s surprise, while they demonstrated that staff-communication skills could be improved, this was not found to be related to incidence of BC. Those working with people with dementia will be familiar with the controversial topic of the use of therapeutic lies as methods of communication. The current author has done a lot of work in this area, and has shown that paid carers use lies frequently (James et al. 2006). It has been noted that the benefits and problems concerning their use are well recognized by professionals and older people with and without dementia (Day et al. 2011). In many cases people recognize

Table 37.3 Non-pharmacological approaches in dementia and their evidence base

Therapies	Systematic reviews and empirical status in dementia	KEY ARTICLES
I—Preventative approaches: These are generally designed to promote a positive therapeutic milieu and positive well-being. It is suggested that improving people's general levels of contentment serves to improve mood, and reduces anxiety and the incidences of problematic behaviours.		
Reality orientation: uses rehearsal and physical prompts to improve cognitive functioning related to personal orientation.	A Cochrane review by Spector et al. (2000) identified six RCTs. The reviewers concluded there was evidence of improvements in terms of cognitive and behavioural features. RO is now assessed under cognitive stimulation therapy.	Scanland and Emershaw (1993); Woods et al. (2012)
Reminiscence therapy: involves discussion of past experiences individually or in a group format. Photographs, familiar objects, or sensory items used to prompt recall and discussion.	A Cochrane review by Woods et al. (2005b, updated 2009) identified five RCTs, four containing extractable data. The reviewers reported significant results in terms of cognitions, mood, care-giver strain, and functional abilities. However, the quality of the studies was perceived to be poor.	Bohlmeijer et al. (2003); Brooker and Duce (2000); Lin, Dai, and Hwang (2003)
Validation therapy: based on the general principle of acceptance of the reality of the person and validation of his/her experience.	A Cochrane Review by Neal and Barton Wright (2003, updated 2009) identified three studies, two showing positive effects. However, the reviewers concluded there was insufficient evidence to view the approach as effective.	Feil and de Klerk-Rubin (2002); Schrijnemaekers (2002)
Psychomotor therapy: exercises (e.g. walking and ball games) are used to target depression and behavioural difficulties.	A Cochrane Review by Montgomery and Denis (2002) examining the impact of exercise on sleep problems identified one trial that demonstrated significant effects on a range of sleep variables. Forbes et al. (2008) found limited evidence that physical exercise slowed down cognitive decline.	Eggermont and Scherder 2006; Teri et al. (this volume)
Multi-sensory stimulation: stimuli such as light, sound, and tactile sensations, often in specially designed rooms, used to increase the opportunity for communication and improved quality of experience.	A Cochrane Review by Chung and Lai (2002, updated 2009) identified two RCTs. Despite some favourable results, the studies were so different that they could not be pooled. As such, the reviewers concluded there was insufficient evidence to view the approach as effective.	Baker et al. (2001) Van Weert et al. (2006)
Cognitive stimulation therapy: derived from Reality Orientation, focuses on information processing rather than rehearsal of factual knowledge. Used with all presentation, Cells 1–8, although developed for Cells 5–8. In people with dementia it tends to improve skills only in those areas that training has been given, otherwise limited generalization.	Awaiting findings of a new review by Woods et al. (2012). The two previous reviews (Clare et al. 2003; Woods et al. 2005a) concluded that despite positive evidence there was insufficient evidence to view the approach as effective.	Spector et al. (2003, 2006)

Aromatherapy: use of essential oils to provide sensory experiences and interactions with staff. The oils can be administered via massage techniques or in patients' baths.

A Cochrane Review by Holt et al. (2003) identified two RCTs, but only Ballard et al. (2002) trial reviewed. This trial, despite flaws, was viewed favourably in terms of reducing agitation and neuropsychiatric symptoms. Quynh-anh and Paton's (2008) work showed equivocal results.

Ballard et al. (2002); Holmes et al. (2002)

Music therapy: includes playing and/or listening to music as a way of generally enhancing well-being. Can be used in movement therapies.

A Cochrane Review by Vink et al. (2004) identified five studies. However, the quality of the studies was poor. As such, the reviewers concluded there was insufficient evidence to view the approach as effective.

Gotell, Brown, Ekman (2002); Sherrat, Thornton, and Hatton (2004)

Environmental manipulation: use of environmental cues, signage, and appropriate building layout in order to facilitate communication, exercise, and pleasure and to reduce disorientation.

A Cochrane review by Forbes et al. (2009) on the use of bright light therapy in terms of mood, sleep, and behaviour reviewed three trials. However, the quality of the studies was poor. As such, the reviewers concluded there was insufficient evidence to view the approach as effective. A Cochrane Review by Price et al. (2001, updated 2009) on the use of environmental and social barriers to prevent wandering failed to identify suitable trials.

Day et al. (2000); Zuidema et al. (2010)

II—Intervention strategies (formulation-led approaches): These are reactive strategies, responding to difficulties that have already been diagnosed (depression, anxiety) or observed (agitation, shouting, wandering) and the procedures are specifically targeted to intervene with the problem or its causes. These approaches routinely involve the development of a formulation to help understand the triggering and maintaining features of the problem.

Behavioural management techniques/functional analysis (FA): based on learning theory and utilizing the antecedents and consequences of behaviour to devise and execute interventions. The approach has a long therapeutic tradition and can be applied to all people, no matter the level of cognitive impairment.

A systematic review by Spira and Edelstein (2006) reported twenty-three studies. These tended to be of poor to moderate quality, and many were single-case design. Moniz-Cook et al.'s recent Cochrane Review(2012) has identified eighteen studies with weak but favourable evidence.

Moniz-Cook et al. (2012)

Psychotherapies: adaptions for 1:1 therapy with people with dementia are recent developments, and limited to people with mild dementia. However, use of the underlying principles of CBT, IPT, and psychodynamic approaches is widespread, particularly in programmes aimed at promoting improved carer interactions.

Teri et al. (1997) demonstrated the positive impact of CBT on mood and problem solving abilities in people with dementia. Teri and Gallagher-Thompson's (1991) RCT revealed significant reduction in depression for both people with dementia and their carers. Scholey and Woods (2003) undertook CBT with seven people with dementia and depression, and identified key themes in such work.

Miller and Reynolds (2007); Teri, Logsdon, and Uomoto (1991) that lies can be helpful when they 'fit with the person's current reality' and serve to reduce distress (e.g. telling an increasingly distressed ex-miner that he does not need to leave for the pit, because today is a holiday).

Before focusing specifically on CBT perspectives, it is worth noting that there have been a number of important reviews on non-pharmacological strategies conducted over the last ten years (including Cohen-Mansfield 2001; Hulme et al. 2010; James 2011; Livingston et al. 2005; Olazarán et al. 2010). The largest current review has just been completed by Ballard and his team via the WHELD project (Improving Well-being and Health for People with Dementia); this major National Institute Health Research UK programme will present its findings over the next twelve months (Whitaker et al. 2013). This group is also completing the final stages of a pilot study which is examining Person Centred Care training either alone or in combination with Antipsychotic Review, Exercise, and Social Interaction. The main aim of the study is to determine whether the combination of Person Centred Care and Antipsychotic Review results in the reduction of antipsychotic prescribing and improvement of participant outcomes compared to Person Centred Care training alone. The secondary objective is to establish the specific impact of each therapy (Antipsychotic Review, Social Intervention, and Pleasant Activities, Exercise) in addition to Person Centred Care training.

USE OF CBT WITH PEOPLE WITH DEMENTIA WHO CHALLENGE

Safran and Segal's (1990) suitability criteria make it clear that CBT is not appropriate for everyone. In the present author's experience, the following list describes the specific skills generally required of a client in order to work well with a CBT model. The person needs to be able to:

- recognize and accept the need for change
- identify, differentiate, and monitor specific thoughts, emotions, and behaviours
- recognize the links between thoughts, emotions, behaviours, and sensations
- weigh up evidence and identify pros and cons
- recognize and re-evaluate biased thoughts and the associated emotions
- concentrate
- problem solve
- be the agent of change
- engage in a collaborative therapeutic relationship
- appreciate the perspective of others (i.e. adopt a theory of mind perspective)
- work with a simple conceptual model
- work within a structured one-to-one session, which will include agreeing and executing out-of-session tasks.

In those situations where the client does not have some of the abilities outlined above, an adapted form of CBT must be used (Kipling, Bailey, and Charlesworth 1999; Paukert et al.

2010). For example, Charlesworth and Reichelt (2004) discussed the value of employing two-stage and three-stage formulations in order to simplify the conceptual features of the therapy. Scholey and Woods (2003) identified several principles for using CBT with people with dementia, including the need to:

- investigate clients' beliefs about the causes of their cognitive impairment, because such reasoning often leads to distress and anger
- examine feelings of loss of control and hopelessness, and feelings of insecurity
- check out whether the impact of earlier traumas have resurfaced owing to a dislocation between memory and the use of previously effective coping strategies
- take account of comorbid problems, particularly physical difficulties
- take account of the systemic nature of the clients' presentations (Teri and Gallagher-Thompson 1991).
- exercise flexibility, patience, and tolerance with the client, providing the additional structures that will be required (Teri et al. 1997). Coon, Thompson, and Gallagher-Thompson (2007) give some good advice about how to structure homework tasks appropriately.

However, when working with someone with dementia a point will be reached whereby the adaptations will be so great that the approach may no longer be badged as a true form of CBT with respect to the client. In such circumstances, distinctions need to be made and therefore an acknowledgement that the treatments are actually carer-mediated in nature rather than direct client work. Typical carer-mediated interventions may aim at improving the carers' coping and include: (1) in-the-moment CBT; (2) cognitive triads; (3) CBT formulation-led frameworks; (4) CBT for carers; (5) mindfulness techniques.

In-the-moment CBT

As the term suggests, the interventions in this form of CBT deal with problems arising 'in the moment' and there is no intention that the impact of the approaches will generalize across time or situation because of clients' memory and cognitive difficulties. The methodology exploits the CBT cycles' guidance in helping us to understand other people's experiences. Indeed, one of the helpful things about CBT is that the simple 'hot-cross bun' cycle is a useful and elegant way of representing someone's experience of distress. Although clearly an artificial construct, it breaks down experiences into simple accessible units (thoughts, feelings, behaviours, physiology). These units can be targeted for both assessment and treatment purposes (James 2010). In traditional CBT, these are the units that the client is socialized to and works with throughout therapy. However, in the case of the person with dementia, the cycle can become the carers' template to help them understand what might be going on for the person. From a 'normalizing' perspective, it highlights that there is continuity in how distress is experienced whether or not there is cognitive impairment present. As such, the construct helps to guide therapists' responses to BC by stressing the need to try to understand the perpetrator's thinking and feeling states that may have triggered their actions. For example, consider Mary, who was referred for pulling the hair of her carer. Based on initial discussions with her carer, the scenario illustrated in Figure 37.3 appeared

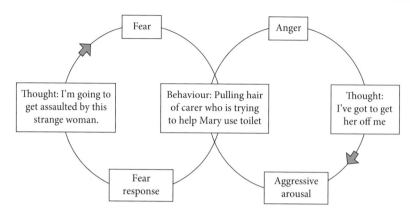

FIGURE 37.3 Mary's interlocking CBT cycles of fear and aggression.

to have occurred. In discussion, it became apparent that the two-cycle model best fitted the event, with the anxiety-led cycle preceding the aggression. In such cases, it is the prevention of the anxiety that is the easiest and most effective to achieve—for example by improving the carer's interaction and communication style.

Over recent years we have simplified the four-item cycle to a triadic model based on Beck's (1976) notion of cognitive specificity. Consequently, the triads have been used with carers to help them understand how their emotional reactions interact with those of the person with dementia—see below.

Cognitive triads

From Charles Darwin's (1872) work it is evident that humans are good at distinguishing between emotions, and are able to empathize with the states of other people displaying such feelings. Darwin noted that across all cultures of the world, people are able to recognize six basic emotional expressions: anger, depression, anxiety, disgust, surprise, happiness (Ekman 1973). Beck moved this area further forward from a psychotherapy perspective with his models of content specificity (Beck 1976). He suggested that people's appearance is linked to certain types of thought, which were best illustrated via a cognitive triad (Table 37.4). For the present purpose, the themes associated with three key emotions are discussed—depression, anxiety, and anger.

For example, a typical triad for depression would be: 'I'm worthless', 'The world is punishing', 'The future is bleak', whereas the corresponding triad for anxiety would be 'I'm vulnerable', 'The world is threatening/chaotic', 'The future is unpredictable'. The cognitive triad format can also be used to elucidate the typical thoughts associated with the emotion of anger: for example 'It shouldn't happen to me', 'The world is hostile', 'The future is dangerous' (James 2001a, 2010).

These triads are particularly useful in the area of BC, especially in situations where one's clients may have poor communication skills. In such circumstances, one is often unable to ask them how they are feeling or what they are thinking. However, by simply looking at their expressions, one can gain some insight into the themes of their distress. Further, the triad is

Table 37.4 Cognitive themes and their relationships to emotional appearance

Appearance	Cognitive themes
Depressed	The person has self-perception of being worthless or inadequate, perceiving the world as hostile or uncaring, and viewing the future as being hopeless.
Anxious	The person has self-perception of being vulnerable, perceiving her environment to be chaotic, and the future as unpredictable.
Angry	The person perceives that someone is acting unjustly towards him and his rights, and is being hostile; there is a need to act immediately to protect his self-esteem from future harm.

helpful as a treatment template—thus if a therapist sees someone looking anxious, he should simply ask himself: (1) What is making Mrs Smith feel vulnerable—is there anything I can do to change this?; (2) Is there anything I can do to make things more predictable—by the use of cues, signage, routines?; (3) What can I do to reduce the chaos within the environment—improve the structure?

These triads are also useful when examining the dynamics occurring during BC episodes, providing an opportunity for carers to explore their own reactions to difficult situations. A typical carer example is given below (Figure 37.4). It highlights the way in which triadic models can be used to help carers learn to empathize with the experience of the person with dementia through monitoring the care recipient's mood and behaviour.

CBT formulation frameworks

There are a number of conceptual models directing the treatment of BC (Cohen-Mansfield 2000; Kitwood 1997; Volicer and Hurley 2003—see James 2011 for a review). The best developed of these is the Cohen-Mansfield 'unmet needs' perspective, which has a satisfactory evidence base (Cohen-Mansfield, Libin, and Marx 2007). The Newcastle model (James 1999, 2011) is also well respected and has received some empirical support (Fossey and James 2007). The production of these frameworks serves at least two functions, one summative and the other formative. The *summative function* is the establishment of an idiosyncractic formulation of the person and his/her presentation. To obtain this, a therapist typically works with carers to collect personal and contextual information, including data about physical and mental health status, medication, social environment. A detailed analysis of the behaviours is also undertaken using ABC charts. The *formative function* occurs in those carers who participate in the data collection. Their monitoring and careful observation facilitates their own pattern recognition and hypothesis development with respect to the BC, and can result in the development of a more positive attitude towards the person with dementia. Thus the process of collecting data to inform the conceptual model frequently enhances carer attitude, leading to a process termed 're-personalization' (Kitwood 1997). It is important to recognize that much skill is required to facilitate carer participation in the above work. The relevant competences have been previously compared to the skills outlined in the Cognitive Therapy Scale (CTS, Young and Beck 1988) and the CTS-revised

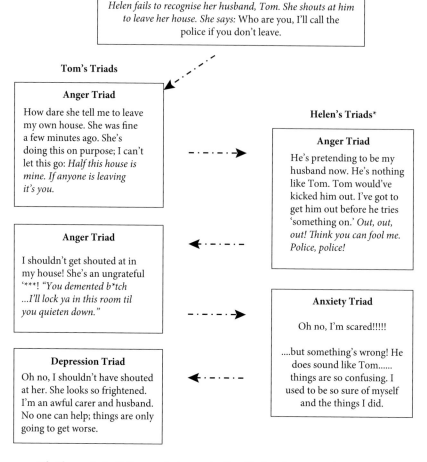

Triggering Behaviour
Helen fails to recognise her husband, Tom. She shouts at him to leave her house. She says: Who are you, I'll call the police if you don't leave.

Tom's Triads

Anger Triad

How dare she tell me to leave my own house. She was fine a few minutes ago. She's doing this on purpose; I can't let this go: *Half this house is mine. If anyone is leaving it's you.*

Helen's Triads*

Anger Triad

He's pretending to be my husband now. He's nothing like Tom. Tom would've kicked him out. I've got to get him out before he tries 'something on.' *Out, out, out! Think you can fool me. Police, police!*

Anger Triad

I shouldn't get shouted at in my house! She's an ungrateful '***'! *"You demented b*tch ...I'll lock ya in this room til you quieten down."*

Anxiety Triad

Oh no, I'm scared!!!!!

....but something's wrong! He does sound like Tom...... things are so confusing. I used to be so sure of myself and the things I did.

Depression Triad

Oh no, I shouldn't have shouted at her. She looks so frightened. I'm an awful carer and husband. No one can help; things are only going to get worse.

Nb. The quotes in italics are what was actually said, the other material are examples of internal dialogue

*Owing to Helen's cognitive difficulties, she was unable to provide details of her thoughts about the incidents. Hence, in a clinical setting, her triads would be derived collaboratively between the therapist and the carer. In this example, the therapist would use specific questions to help Tom gain better insight and to to generate his wife's triads (e.g., If you were in your wife's position, how might you respond to what was said and how you said it?).

FIGURE 37.4 Mapping the triads for Mr and Mrs Smith.

(Blackburn et al. 2001), with a future intention of developing a competence scale for assessing BC therapists (James 2011).

The BC conceptual model that is most firmly situated within a CBT framework is the Roseberry Park (RP) framework (Dexter-Smith 2007, 2010). This is a straightforward diathesis stress model, collecting information about early history and life experiences, as well as details of the 'here and now' via a hot-cross bun cycle. The model makes explicit that

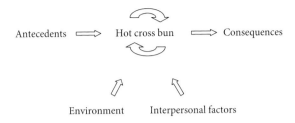

FIGURE 37.5 Representation of Roseberry Park model.

environmental features and interpersonal processes influence clients' behaviour. The RP is well explained in terms of structural and process features in a series of articles (Craven-Staines, Dexter-Smith, and Li 2010; Dexter-Smith 2010; Dexter-Smith, Hopper, and Sharpe 2010), noting that often in dementia one starts from the hot-cross bun cycle and works one's way backwards to the more distal features (core beliefs, early history, etc.). Another interesting tool with respect to the RP is the development of ABC assessment charts which incorporate the hot-cross bun cycle (Figure 37.5).

The interventions for BC are often practical and not CBT in nature, but the conceptual models provide the rationale for selecting and directing them. And once one has a rationale, the interventions can be appropriately tweaked, or if found not to be effective, replaced by a sensible alternative which is also in keeping with the rationale. Some of the techniques that may be employed have been discussed previously in the table of therapies (Table 37.3).

CBT for family and paid carers

According to the World Alzheimer Report (2010) the vast majority of people with dementia are cared for by their families; this is also the case in most 'high income countries'. In the UK one-third of people live in care, while two-thirds are cared for at home. Hence, supporting family carers is an essential part of any treatment regimen in BC. By keeping carers fit and mentally healthy, they are enabled to deal better with the tasks of supporting and caring for the person through any challenging period. Moniz-Cook et al.'s (2012) recent Cochrane Review on the use of behaviour therapy (functional analysis, FA) of BC has shown that 66% of the fifteen quality studies have been conducted within 'own-home' settings. The overall findings of this systematic review demonstrated that the use of FA behavioural methodologies significantly reduced care-giver burden.

Carer interventions take various forms. The psychotherapeutic approaches may use either a formal one-to-one therapy or a group format, while education and training approaches can be used to enhance skills and improve knowledge and attitudes (see McCabe, Davison, and George 2007; Mittelman et al. 2004, 2007). It is relevant to note that each of the approaches has a different goal. The formal therapeutic approaches tend to be used to tackle psychiatric disorders, such as depression and anxiety. The teaching methods enhance coping abilities, and help the carers to develop practical caring skills. One of the few approaches to have an empirically validated manual for the treatment of BC is Teri's STAR programme (Staff Training in Assisted Residences, Teri et al. 2005a, 2005b). STAR teaches staff to understand and modify their interactions with residents by identifying ABCs. The programme also involves teaching on dementia, communication skills, and use of activities. Teri has conducted two RCTs using STAR; one for families and one in an assisted-living setting (Teri et al. 2005a, 2005b). Both of these studies are included in Moniz-Cook's Cochrane Review. This Cochrane Review shows that of the five quality studies conducted into residential care settings, none employed CBT, despite all aiming to change staff attitudes (Chenoweth et al. 2009; Fossey et al. 2006; Proctor et al. 1999; Teri et al. 2005b; Visser et al. 2008).

In recent years there have been a number of systematic reviews regarding care-giver training and support programmes (Cooper et al. 2006; Pinquart and Sörensen 2006; Sörensen, Pinquart, and Duberstein 2002). Despite Cooper's review examining only anxiety in care-givers of people with dementia, her categorization of the types of intervention is a helpful summary of the approaches used. Here are the types of projects she identified, together with the number of trials she found under each heading: *five* CBT trials (Akkerman and Ostwald 2004; Gendron, Poitras, and Dastoor 1996; Gendron et al. 1986; Hebert et al. 2003; Wilkins et al. 1999); *four* coping strategy/professional support; *four* alternative placements; *three* behavioural interventions; *three* respite; *two* relaxation/yoga; *two* exercise; *one* group counselling; *one* information technology support. Her conclusion from the review was somewhat disappointing, with only Akkerman and Ostwald's CBT study showing significant effects in terms of anxiety. This was a nine-week CBT intervention which reduced anxiety in family carers of people with dementia. Their approach also included training in relaxation when appropriate.

In relation to carer depression, Marriott et al.'s (2000) CBT study of fourteen families demonstrated significant effects on measures of affect for the carers, and improvements in 'activities of daily living' for the clients. Over the fourteen weeks of this RCT there were three sessions of care-giver education, six sessions of stress management, and five sessions of coping skills training. Moderate effects have also been observed by Buchanan (2004) in terms of family carers' self-reported anger and depression. A well-described study was also undertaken by Secker and Brown (2005), who conducted a successful RCT using a twelve-to-fourteen-week programme of CBT designed to alleviate strain and burden in carers of patients with Parkinson's disease (patients presenting in Cell 8 of Table 37.2). The content of the programme is summarized in Table 37.5. The positive effects were evident over a three-month follow-up period compared to controls. The modules of this programme are currently being employed in our own work, but with carers of people displaying BC.

This study was modelled on the work of Marriot et al. (2000), and emphasized the importance of carers stepping back and taking stock of their situations, creating time and space for themselves, seeking support from other sources, tackling unhelpful cognitions and rationalizing guilt and other problematic emotions.

Exciting work is currently being done using acceptance and commitment therapy (ACT) for carers of people displaying BC (Marquez-Gonzalez, Romero-Moreno, and Losada 2010). The Spanish group of researchers are employing this third-wave form of CBT to help carers recognize their emotions, accept change and discomfort, and commit to valued goals and 'life directions'. This team are currently engaged in a research trial using ACT and will publish their findings over the next two years.

While it is evident that carers need support, it is demonstrable that not all forms of help are effective. Aakhus et al.'s (2009) small RCT showed that a single session educational programme for care-givers of psychogeriatric inpatients resulted in increased distress. They accounted for this finding by suggesting that the knowledge given may have served to increase anxiety. Such an effect was previously observed by Graham, Ballard, and Sham

Table 37.5 Modules used in the trial of CBT for carers of people with Parkinson's disease

Education and introduction to cognitive-behavioural therapy
Questions about Parkinson's disease were discussed and relevant information was given. There was also a discussion about the therapy itself, and a review of the carer's goals and expectations.

Accessing community resources and supports:
In this module, the carer's support network was reviewed and information provided where necessary. The carer worked on how to access and communicate effectively with available services.

Pleasant activity scheduling:
This module consisted primarily of (a) encouraging the carer to make designated times for recreation without the person they cared for, doing things they themselves enjoyed and (b) designating time to engage in enjoyable things with the person they cared for that did not involve normal care duties.

Relaxation training:
This module focused on practical strategies for the relief of anxiety and tension.

Sleep improvement:
This module covered sleep-preparation behaviour and also ways to manage the sleep problems of the individual with Parkinson's disease.

Identifying and challenging negative thoughts and feelings:
This module targeted those carers with recurrent negative thinking patterns. This was most suitable for carers presenting with depression, anxiety, and persistent worry. Skills taught in this module included identifying and rating negative feelings, automatic thought recording, and rationalizing guilt.

Challenging maladaptive rules and core beliefs:
This was a more complex level of CBT, which included teaching awareness of (a) rules and conditional assumptions around caring, and (b) the restructuring of core schematic beliefs (e.g. 'I am a bad carer', and 'There is no future').

Review, planning for the future, and ending of treatment:
This final module reviewed all of the previous modules and prepared the carer for ending therapy.

(1997), who found that a higher degree of knowledge about dementia was associated with greater anxiety.

Mindfulness-based approaches with carers

Mindfulness meditation approaches were synthesized with CBT approximately ten years ago (Segal, Williams, and Teasdale 2002), and have proved to be particularly effective for CBT-treatment-resistant depression. Mindfulness-based cognitive therapy (MBCT) is now a well established member of the CBT family of treatments. Unlike traditional CBT, clients are taught to develop a different relationship with their thoughts. Indeed, instead of trying to re-evaluate negative thoughts, people are trained to accept them without engaging with them. The lack of attention paid to the cognitions prevents the spiralling of negative and biased thinking, which often characterizes depression. Singh (and colleagues 2008), in the field of learning disability, has demonstrated that these approaches can also be adapted for carers. In numerous studies he has demonstrated that mindfulness can assist care staff to deal better with challenging behaviours. He has shown that training staff in mindfulness can lead to increases in their own well-being and improve the quality of life of clients with profound multiple disabilities.

Trials have also been conducted with older people and their carers, and the latter has been described well by McBee (2008) in her book on mindfulness-based elder care (MBEC). Useful work has also been carried out by Epstein-Lubow et al. (2011) for care-givers with dementia. Typically the carers are taught how not to ruminate on events, thereby preventing them getting stuck in cycles of negativity. Being less negative, the carers tend not to engage in emotional thinking and thus their problem-solving abilities are preserved and used to develop solutions quicker.

Conclusion

Many traditional models in dementia have been guilty of failing to address cognitions adequately. This has been a major oversight because thoughts and beliefs are fundamental to our experiences, regardless of one's level of cognitive impairment. As such this chapter has demonstrated that CBT approaches are helpful in understanding both ill-being and well-being in people with dementia, and especially in the treatment of BC. Notwithstanding such oversights, methodologies in the BC specialty have much to contribute to standard CBT. Indeed, having treated working-aged adults for many years, I am struck by how 'dementia work' reaffirms the value of using all elements of the client's presentation in understanding his/her experience. For example, due to dementia clients' communication problems and disordered thinking, a close analysis of patterns of behaviour and outward displays of emotion becomes key to populating their formulations. It is suggested that such valuable behavioural analysis (functional analysis) is less common in CBT when working with many other presentations, apart from those with learning disabilities. In addition to this micro level of assessment, BC work requires one to examine the important roles of social systems and the impact of key advocates. It could be argued that mainstream CBT fails to address these micro and macro levels adequately, with a tendency of modern CBT to focus excessively on cognitions from the distant past (i.e. core beliefs), using the diathesis-stress perspective with its attendant problems (James 2001b).

Implications for Practice

Over the last ten years many countries have become aware of the tsunami of dementia-related conditions that will affect us all in the future; many states have written national dementia strategies in preparation for the health and social impacts. In relation to BC, our understanding has increased, in part due to improved standards of research. For example, good quality randomized controlled trials are becoming more common (Fossey et al. 2006; Moniz-Cook et al. 2012). Thus far, it appears that effective treatments are multicomponent in nature, with little evidence of a single therapeutic intervention being effective across all settings and presentations. As such, in terms of people with dementia, CBT has proved useful in conceptualizing distress and theorizing about beliefs associated with emotions. More research is required in this area, building on exciting work being conducted by Spector et al. (2012) and Mohlam (Mohlam and Gorman 2005) using CBT with people experiencing executive difficulties. CBT already has a good evidence base in relation to the treatment of carers, both using traditional formats and third-wave ACT perspectives (Marquez-Gonzalez, Romero-Moreno, and Losada 2010). Finally, on a more global level, it is important that CBT plays an important role in reducing people's negative attitudes concerning dementia. Such negativity reduces both quality of life as well as access to appropriate physical and mental health services. Improving attitudes and reducing stigma was the focus of the World Alzheimer Report in 2012. This publication stated that:

> Symptoms of dementia are perceived differently in different parts of the world. This includes considering dementia as a normal part of ageing, mental illness, something metaphysical linked to supernatural or spiritual beliefs or as an irreversible disease of the brain. It is very important that there is better public awareness and understanding to reduce the stigma associated with dementia.

Key References

Brechin, D., Murphy. G., James I., and Codner, J. (2013). *Alternatives to Antipsychotic Medication: Psychological Approaches in Managing Psychological and Behavioural Distress in People with Dementia,* 207, pp. 1–38. London: British Psychological Society Publications. www.bps.org.uk.

Gitlin, L., Kales, H., and Lyketsos, C. (2012). 'Nonpharmacologic Management of Behavioural Symptoms in Dementia'. *Journal of the American Medical Association* 308(19): 2020–2029.

James, I. A. (2010). *Cognitive Behaviour Therapy for People With and Without Dementia.* London: Jessica Kingsley.

Moniz-Cook, E., Roberts-Stride, K., James, I., Maluf, R., De Vugt, M., et al. (2012). 'Functional Analysis-based Interventions in Challenging Behavior in Dementia'. *Cochrane Database* 1: CD006929. doi: 0.1002/14651858.CD006929.

Vernooij-Dassen, M., Vasse, E., Zuidema, S., Cohen-Mansfield, J., and Moyle, W. (2010). 'Psychosocial Interventions for Dementia Patients in Long-term Care'. *International Psychogeriatrics* 22(7): 1121–1128.

References

Aakhus, E., Engedal, K., Aspelund, T., and Selbaek, G. (2009). 'Single Session Educational Programme for Caregivers of Psychogeriatric In-patients—Results from a Randomized Controlled Pilot Study'. *International Journal of Geriatric Psychiatry* 24: 269–274.

Aalten P., Verhey, F. R. J., Boziki, M., Brugnolo, A., Bullock, R., et al. (2008). 'Consistency of Neuropsychiatric Syndromes across Dementias: Results from the European Alzheimer Disease Consortium'. *Dementia Geriatric Cognitive Disorders* 25: 1–8.

Akkerman, R., and Ostwald, S. K. (2004). 'Reducing Anxiety in Alzheimer's Disease Family Caregivers: Effectiveness of a Nine-week Cognitive Behavioural Intervention'. *American Journal of Alzheimer's Disease and Other Disorders* 19(2): 117–123.

American Academy of Neurology (2001). 'Detection, Diagnosis and Management of Dementia'. http://tools.aan.com/professionals/practice/pdfs/dementia_guideline.pdf.

Baker, R., Bell, S., Baker, E., Gibson, S., Holloway, J., et al. (2001). 'A Randomised Controlled Trial of the Effects of Multi-sensory Stimulation for People with Dementia'. *British Journal of Clinical Psychology* 40: 81–96.

Ballard, C. G., O'Brien, J. T., Reichelt, K., and Perry, E. K. (2002). 'Aromatherapy as a Safe and Effective Treatment for the Management of Agitation in Severe Dementia: The Results of a Double-blind, Placebo-controlled Trial with Melissa'. *Journal of Clinical Psychiatry* 63(7): 553–558.

Banerjee, S. (2009). *The Use of Antipsychotic Medication for People with Dementia: Time for Action*. London: Department of Health.

Beck, A. T. (1976). *Cognitive Therapy and the Emotional Disorders*. New York: International University Press.

Bird, M. and Moniz-Cook, E. (2008). 'Challenging Behaviour in Dementia: A Psychosocial Approach to Intervention'. In B. Woods and L. Clare (eds), *Handbook of the Clinical Psychology of Ageing* (2nd edn). London: Wiley.

Blackburn, I. M., James, I. A., Milne, D. L., Baker, C., Standart, S., et al. (2001). 'The Revised Cognitive Therapy Scale (CTS-R): Psychometric Properties'. *Behavioural and Cognitive Psychotherapy* 29(4): 431–447.

Bohlmeijer, E., Smit, F., and Cuipers, P. (2003). 'Effects of Reminiscence and Life Review on Late-life Depression: A Meta-analysis'. *International Journal of Geriatric Psychiatry* 18: 1088–1094.

Brechin, D., Murphy. G., James I., and Codner, J. (2013). *Alternatives to Antipsychotic Medication: Psychological Approaches in Managing Psychological and Behavioural Distress in People with Dementia,* 207, pp. 1–38. London: British Psychological Society Publications. www.bps.org.uk.

Brooker, D. and Duce, L. (2000). 'Wellbeing and Activity in Dementia: A Comparison of Group Reminiscence Therapy, Structured Goal-directed Group Activity and Unstructured Time'. *Aging & Mental Health* 4(4): 354–358.

Buchanan, J. (2004). 'Generalization of the Effects of a Cognitive-behavioral Intervention for Family Caregivers of Individuals with Dementia'. *Dissertation Abstracts International: Section B: The Sciences and Engineering* 65, US.

Charlesworth, G. and Reichelt, F. K. (2004). 'Keeping Conceptualisations Simple: Examples with Family Carers of People with Dementia'. *Behaviour and Cognitive Psychotherapy* 32: 401–409.

Chenoweth, L., King, M. T., Jeon, Y. H., Brodaty, H., Stein-Parbury, J., et al. (2009). 'Caring for Aged Dementia Care Resident Study (CADRES) of Person-centred Care, Dementia-care Mapping, and Usual Care in Dementia: A Cluster-Randomised Trial'. *Lancet Neurology* 8(4): 317–325.

Chung, J. and Lai, C. (2002). 'Snoezelen for Dementia'. *Cochrane Database of Systematic Reviews* Reviews 4.

Clare, L., Woods, B., Moniz-Cooke, E., Orrell, M., and Spector, A. (2003). 'Cognitive Rehabilitation and Cognitive Training Interventions Targeting Memory Functioning in Early Stage Dementia and Vascular Dementia'. *Cochrane Database of Systematic Reviews* 4.

Cohen-Mansfield, J. (2000). 'Nonpharmacological Management of Behavioural Problems in Persons with Dementia: The TREA Model'. *Alzheimer Care Quarterly* 1: 22–34.

Cohen-Mansfield, J. (2001). 'Nonpharmacological Interventions for Inappropriate Behaviors in Dementia: A Review, Summary and Critique'. *American Journal of Geriatric Psychiatry* 9: 381–391.

Cohen-Mansfield, J., Libin, A., and Marx M. (2007). 'Nonpharmacological Treatment of Agitation: A Controlled Trial of Systematic Individualized Intervention'. *Journal of Gerontology: Medical Sciences* 62A(8): 906–918.

Coon, D., Thompson, L., and Gallagher-Thompson, D. (2007). 'Adapting Homework for an Older Adult Client with Cognitive Impairment'. *Cognitive and Behavioral Practice* 14(3): 252–260.

Cooper, C., Katona, C., Orrell, M., and Livingston, G. (2006). 'Coping Strategies and Anxiety in Caregivers of People with Alzheimer's Disease: The LASER-AD Study'. *Journal of Affective Disorders* 90(1): 15–20.

Cooper, C., Balamurali, T. B., Selwood, A., and Livingston, G. (2007). 'A Systematic Review of Intervention Studies about Anxiety in Caregivers of People with Dementia'. *International Journal of Geriatric Psychiatry* 22(3): 181–188.

Craven Staines, S., Dexter-Smith, S., and Li, C. (2010). 'Integrating Psychological Formulations into Older People's Services—Three Years On (Part 3): Staff Perception of Formulation Meetings'. *PSIGE Newsletter, British Psychological Society* 112: 16–22.

Darwin, C. (1872). *The Expression of the Emotions in Man and Animals*. London: Murray.

Day, A., James, I., Meyer, T., and Lee, D. (2011). 'Do People with Dementia Find Lies and Deception in Dementia Care Acceptable'. *Ageing & Mental Health* 15(7): 822–829.

Day, K., Carreon, D., and Stump, C. (2000). 'Therapeutic Design of Environments for People with Dementia: A Review of the Empirical Research'. *Gerontologist* 40: 397–416.

Dexter-Smith, S. (2007). 'Integrating Psychological Formulations into Inpatient Services'. *PSIGE Newsletter, British Psychological Society* 97: 38–42.

Dexter-Smith, S. (2010). 'Integrating Psychological Formulations into Older People's Services—Three Years On (Part 1)'. *PSIGE Newsletter, British Psychological Society* 112: 8–11.

Dexter-Smith, S., Hopper, S., and Sharpe, P. (2010). 'Integrating Psychological Formulations into Older People's Services: Evaluation of the Formulation Training Programme'. *PSIGE Newsletter, British Psychological Society* 12–15.

Doody, R. S., Stevens, J. C., Beck, C., Dubinsky, R. M., Kaye, J. A., Gwyther, L., Mohs, R. C., Thal, L. J., Whitehouse, P. J., DeKosky, S. T., and Cummings,, J. L. (2001). 'Practice Parameter: Management of Dementia (an Evidence-based Review). Report of the Quality Standards Subcommittee of the American Academy of Neurology'. *Neurology* 8; 56(9): 1154–66.

Eggermont, L. and Scherder, E. (2006). 'Physical Activity and Behaviour in Dementia: A Review of the Literature and Implications for Psychosocial Interventions in Primary Care'. *Dementia* 5(3): 411–428.

Ekman, P. (1973). 'Cross Cultural Studies of Facial Expression'. In P. Ekman (ed.), *Darwin and Facial Expressions: A Century of Research in Review*. New York: Academic Press.

Epstein-Lubow, G., McBee, L., Darling, E., Armey, M., and Miller, I. (2011). 'A Pilot Investigation of Mindfulness-based Stress Reduction for Caregivers of Frail Elderly'. *Mindfulness* 2: 95–102.

Feil, N. and de Klerk-Rubin, V. (2002). *The Validation Breakthrough: Simple Techniques for Communicating with People with Alzheimer-Type-Dementia*. Baltimore, MD: Health Professions Press.

Forbes, D., Forbes, S., Morgan, M., Markle-Reid, M., Wood, J., et al. (2008) 'Physical Activity Programs for Persons with Dementia'. *Cochrane Database of Systematic Reviews*, 3.

Forbes, D., Culum, I., and Lischka, A. (2009) 'Light Therapy for Managing Cognitive, Sleep, Functional, Behavioural or Psychiatric Disturbances in Dementia'. *Cochrane Database of Systematic Reviews*, 4.

Fossey, J., Ballard, C., Juszczak, E., James, I., et al. (2006). 'Effect of Enhanced Psychosocial Care on Antipsychotic Use in Nursing Home Residents with Severe Dementia: Cluster Randomised Trial'. *British Medical Journal* 332: 756–758.

Fossey, J. and James, I. A. (2007). *Evidence-based Approaches for Improving Dementia Care in Care Homes*. London: Alzheimer's Society.

Gendron, C., Poitras, L., and Dastoor, D. P. (1996). 'Cognitive-behavioural Group Intervention for Spouse Caregivers: Findings and Clinical Considerations'. *Clinical Gerontology* 17(1): 3–19.

Gendron, C., Poitras, L., Engels, M., Dastoor, D. Sirota, S., et al. (1986). 'Skills Training with Supporters of the Demented'. *Journal of the American Geriatrics Society* 30(12): 875–880.

Gitlin, L., Kales, H., and Lyketsos, C. (2012). 'Nonpharmacologic Management of Behavioural Symptoms in Dementia'. *Journal of the American Medical Association* 308(19): 2020–2029.

Gotell. E., Brown, S., and Ekman, S. (2002). 'Caregiver Singing and Background Music in Dementia Care'. *Western Journal Nursing Research* 24(2): 195–216.

Graham, C., Ballard, C., and Sham, P. (1997). 'Carers' Knowledge of Dementia, their Coping Strategies and Morbidity'. *International Journal of Geriatric Psychiatry* 12: 931–936.

Hébert, R., Lévesque, L., Vézina, J., Lavoie, J., Ducharme, F., et al. (2003). 'Efficacy of a Psychoeducative Group Program for Caregivers of Demented Persons Living at Home: A Randomized Controlled Trial'. *Journals of Gerontology, Series B: Psychological Sciences and Social Sciences* 58(1): S58–S67.

Holmes, C., Hopkins, V. Hensford, C., MacLaughlin, V., Wilkinson, D., et al. (2002). 'Lavender Oil as a Treatment for Agitated Behaviour in Severe Dementia: A Placebo Controlled Study'. *International Journal of Geriatric Psychiatry* 17(4): 305–308.

Holt, F., Birks, T., Thorgrimsen, L., Spector, E., Wiles, A., et al. (2003) 'Aromatherapy for Dementia'. *Cochrane Database of Systematic Reviews*, 3 (updated 2009).

Hulme, C., Wright, J., Crocker, T., Oluboyeded, Y, and House, A. (2010). 'Non-pharmacological Approaches for Dementia that Informal Carers Might Try to Access: A Systematic Review'. *International Journal of Geriatric Psychiatry* 25: 756–763.

James, I. A. (1999). 'Using a Cognitive Rationale to Conceptualise Anxiety in People with Dementia'. *Behavioural and Cognitive Psychotherapy* 27(4): 345–351.

James, I. A. (2001a). 'The Anger Triad and Its Use with People with Severe Dementia'. *PSIGE Newsletter, British Psychological Society* 76: 45–47.

James, I. A. (2001b). 'Schema Therapy: The Next Generation, but Should it Carry a Health Warning?' *Behavioural and Cognitive Psychotherapy* 29(4): 401–407.

James, I. A., Wood-Mitchell, A., Waterworth, A. M., Mackenzie, L., and Cunningham, J. (2006). 'Lying to People with Dementia: Developing Ethical Guidelines for Care Settings'. *International Journal of Geriatric Psychiatry* 21: 800–801.

James, I. A. and Fossey, J. (2008). 'Non-pharmacological Intervention in Care Homes'. In R. Jacoby, C. Oppenheimer, T. Dening, and A. Thomas (eds), *Oxford Textbook of Old Age Psychiatry* (pp. 285–298). Oxford: Oxford University Press.

James, I. A. (2010). *Cognitive Behavioural Therapy with Older People: Interventions for Those with and without Dementia*. London: Jessica Kingsley.

James, I. A. (2011). *Understanding Behaviour in Dementia that Challenges*. London: Jessica Kingsley.

Kipling, T., Bailey, M., and Charlesworth, G. (1999). 'The Feasibility of a Cognitive Behavioural Therapy Group for Men with Mild/Moderate Cognitive Impairment'. *Behavioural and Cognitive Psychotherapy* 27: 189–193.

Kitwood, T. (1997). *Dementia Reconsidered*. Buckingham: Open University Press.

Lin, Y., Dai, Y., and Hwang, S. (2003). 'The Effect of Reminiscence on the Elderly Population: A Systematic Review'. *Public Health Nursing* 20(4): 297–306.

Livingston, G., Johnston, K., Katona, C., Paton, J., and Lyketsos, C. (2005). 'Systematic Review of Psychological Approaches to the Management of Neuropsychiatric Symptoms of Dementia'. *American Journal of Psychiatry* 162(11): 1996–2021.

McBee, L.(2008). *Mindfulness-based Elder Care*. New York: Springer Publishing.

McCabe, M. P., Davison, T. E., and George, K. (2007). 'Effectiveness of Staff Training Programs for Behavioral Problems among Older People with Dementia'. *Aging & Mental Health* 11(5): 505–519.

Marquez-Gonzalez, M., Romero-Moreno, R., and Losada, A. (2010). 'Caregiving Issues in a Therapeutic Context: New Insights from Acceptance and Commitment Therapy Approach'. In N. Pachana, K. Laidlaw, and B. Knight (eds), *Casebook of Clinical Geropsychology* (pp. 33–53). Oxford: Oxford University Press.

Marriott, A., Donaldson, C., Tarrier, N., and Burns, A. (2000). 'Effectiveness of Cognitive-behavioural Family Intervention in Reducing the Burden of Care in Carers of Patients with Alzheimer's Disease'. *British Journal of Psychiatry* 176: 557–562.

Miller, M. and Reynolds, C. (2007). 'Expanding the Usefulness of Interpersonal Psychotherapy (IPT) for Depressed Elders with Comorbid Cognitive Impairment'. *International Journal of Geriatric Psychiatry* 11: 97–102.

Mittelman, M. S., Roth, D., Haley, W., and Zarit, S. (2004). 'Effects of Caregiver Intervention on Negative Caregiver Appraisals of Behaviour Problems in Patients with Alzheimer's Disease: Results of a Randomised Trial'. *Journal of Gerontology* 59B(1): 27–34.

Mittelman, M. S., Roth, D., Clay, O., and Haley, W. (2007). 'Preserving the Health of Alzheimer's Caregivers: Impact of a Spouse Caregiver Intervention'. *American Journal of Geriatric Psychiatry* 15: 780–789.

Mohlam, J. and Gorman, J. (2005). 'The Role of Executive Functioning in CBT: A Pilot Study with Anxious Older Adults'. *Behavior Research and Therapy* 43(4): 447–465.

Moniz-Cook, E., Roberts-Stride, K., James, I., Maluf, R., De Vugt, M., et al. (2012). 'Functional Analysis-based Interventions in Challenging Behavior in Dementia'. *Cochrane Database* 1: CD006929. doi:0.1002/14651858.CD006929.

Montgomery, P. and Dennis, J. (2002). 'Physical Exercise for Sleep Problems in Adults Aged 60+'. *Cochrane Database of Systematic Reviews* 4: CD003404.

Neal, M., and Barton Wright, P. (2003). 'Validation Therapy for Dementia'. *Cochrane Database of Systematic Reviews* 3: CD001394. doi:10.1002/14651858 (updated 2009).

Olazarán, J., Reisberg, B., Clare, L., Cruz, I., Peña-Casanova, J., et al. (2010). 'Nonpharmacological Therapies in Alzheimer's Disease: A Systematic Review of Efficacy'. *Dementia and Geriatric Cognitive Disorders* 30: 161–178. doi: 10.1159/000316119.

Orgeta, V., Spector, A., and Orrell, M. (2011). 'Psychological Treatments for Depression and Anxiety in Dementia and Mild Cognitive Impairment (Protocol)'. *Cochrane Database of Systematic Reviews* 5: CD009125.

Paukert, A., Calleo, J., Kraus-Schuman, C., Snow, L, Wilson, N., et al. (2010). 'Peaceful Mind: An Open Trial of Cognitive-behavioural Therapy for Anxiety in Persons with Dementia'. *International Psychogeriatrics* 22(6): 1012–1021.

Price, J., Hermans, D., and Grimley Evans, J. (2001). 'Subjective Barriers to Prevent Wandering of Cognitive Impaired People'. *Cochrane Database of Systematic Reviews* 4: CD001932 (updated 2009).

Proctor, R., Burns, A., Powell, H., Tarrier, N., Faragher, B., et al. (1999). 'Behavioural Management in Nursing And Residential Homes: A Randomized Controlled Trial'. *Lancet* 354: 26–29.

Quynh-anh, N. and Paton, C. (2008). 'The Use of Aromatherapy to Treat Behaviour Problems in Dementia'. *International Journal of Geriatric Psychiatry* 27(4): 337–346.

Safran, J. D. and Segal, Z. V. (1990). *Interpersonal Processes in Cognitive Therapy*. New York: Basic Books.

Salzman, C., Jeste, D. V., Meyer, R. E., Cohen-Mansfield, J., Cummings, J., et al. (2008). 'Elderly Patients with Dementia-related Symptoms of Severe Agitation and Aggression: Consensus Statement on Treatment Options, Clinical Trials Methodology, and Policy'. *Journal of Clinical Psychiatry* 69(6): 889–898.

Scanland, S. and Emershaw, L. (1993). 'Reality Orientation and Validation Therapy'. *Journal of Gerontological Nursing* 19: 7–11.

Schrijnemaekers, V., Vanrossum, E., Candel, M., Fredricks, C., Derix, M., et al. (2002). 'Effects of Emotion Oriented Care on Elderly People with Cognitive Impairment and Behavioural Problems'. *International Journal of Geriatric Psychiatry* 17: 926–937.

Scholey, K. A., and Woods, B. T. (2003). 'A Series of Brief Cognitive Therapy Interventions with People Experiencing both Dementia and Depression: A Description of Techniques and Common Themes'. *Clinical Psychology and Psychotherapy* 10(3): 175–185.

Secker, D. and Brown, R. G. (2005). 'Cognitive Behavioural Therapy (CBT) for Carers of Patients with Parkinson's Disease: A Preliminary Randomised Control Trial'. *Journal of Neurological Neurosurgery and Psychiatry* 76: 491–497.

Segal, Z., Williams, M., and Teasdale, J. (2002). *Mindfulness-based Cognitive Therapy for Depression: A New Approach to Preventing Relapse*. New York: Guilford Press.

Sherrat, K., Thornton, A., and Hatton, C. (2004). 'Music Interventions for People with Dementia: A Review of the Literature'. *Journal of Mental Health and Aging* 8(1): 3–12.

Singh, N., Lancioni, G. E., Wahler, R. G., Winton, A. S., and Singh, J. (2008). 'Mindfulness Approaches in Cognitive Behavior Therapy'. *Behavioural and Cognitive Psychotherapy* 36(6): 659–666.

Sörensen, S., Pinquart, M., and Duberstein, P. (2002). 'How Effective are Interventions with Caregivers? An Updated Meta-analysis'. *Gerontologist* 42(3): 356–372.

Spector, A., Orrell, M., Davies, S., and Woods, R. T. (2000) 'Reality Orientation for Dementia'. *Cochrane Database System Reviews* 4: CD001119.

Spector, A., Thorgrimsen, L., Woods, B., Royan, L., Davies, S., et al. (2003). 'Efficacy of an Evidence-based Cognitive Stimulation Programme for People with Dementia: Randomised Controlled Trial'. *British Journal of Psychiatry* 183: 248–254.

Spector, A., Thorgrimsen, L., Woods, B., and Orrell, M. (2006). *Making a Difference: An Evidence-based Group Programme to Offer Cognitive Stimulation Therapy (CST) to People with Dementia*. London: Hawker Publications.

Spector, A., Orrell, M., Lattimer, M., Hoe, J., King, M., et al. (2012). 'Cognitive Behavioural Therapy (CBT) for Anxiety in People with Dementia: Study Protocol for a Randomised Controlled Trial'. *Trials* 13: 197. doi:10.1186/1745–6215–13–197.

Spira, A. and Edelstein, B. (2006). 'Behavioral Interventions for Agitation in Older Adults with Dementia: An Evaluative Review'. *International Psychogeriatrics* 18(2): 195–225.

Teri, L. and Gallagher-Thompson, D. (1991). 'Cognitive-behavioural Interventions for Treatment of Depression in Alzheimer's Patients'. *Gerontologist* 31(3): 413–416.

Teri, L., Logsdon, R., and Uomoto, J. (1991). *Treatment of Depression in Patients with Alzheimer's Disease. Therapist Manual*. Seattle: University of Washington School of Medicine.

Teri, L., Logsdon, R. G., Uomoto, J., and McCurry, S. M. (1997). 'Behavioural Treatment of Depression in Dementia Patients: A Controlled Clinical Trial'. *Journal of Gerontology: Psychological Sciences* 52B(4): 159–166.

Teri, L., McCurry, S., Logsdon, R. Gibbons, L. (2005a). 'Training Community Consultants to Help Family Members Improve Dementia Care: A Randomised Controlled Trial'. *Gerontologist* 45: 802–811.

Teri, L., Huda, P., Gibbons, L., Young, H., and Van Leynseele, J. (2005b). 'STAR: A Dementia—Specific Training Program for Staff in Assisted Living Residences'. *Gerontologist* 45(5): 686–693.

Van Weert, J., Janssen, B., Van Dulmen, A., Spreeuwenberg, P., Ribbe, M., et al. (2006). 'Nursing Assistants' Behaviour during Morning Care: Effects of the Implementation of Snoezelen, Integrated in 24 hr Dementia Care'. *Journal of Advanced Nursing* 53: 656–668.

Vasse, E., Vernooij-Dassen, M., Spijker, A., Rikket, M. O., and Koopmans, R. (2010). 'A Systematic Review of Communication Strategies for People with Dementia in Residential and Nursing Homes'. *International Psychogeriatrics* 22(2): 189–200.

Vernooij-Dassen, M., Vasse, E., Zuidema, S., Cohen-Mansfield, J., and Moyle, W. (2010). 'Psychosocial Interventions for Dementia Patients in Long-term Care'. *International Psychogeriatrics* 22(7): 1121–1128.

Vink, A., Birks, J., Bruinsma, M. and Scholten, R. (2004). 'Music Therapy for People with Dementia'. *Cochrane Database of Systematic Reviews* 3: CD003477 (updated 2009).

Visser, S., McCabe, M., Hudgson, C., Buchanan, G., Davison, T, et al. (2008). 'Managing Behavioural Symptoms of Dementia: Effectiveness of Staff Education and Peer Support'. *Aging & Mental Health* 1: 47–55.

Volicer, L. and Hurley, A. (2003). 'Management of Behavioural Symptoms in Progressive Degenerative Dementias'. *Journal of Gerontology* 58A(9): 837–845.

Whitaker, R., Ballard, C., Stafford, J., Orrell, M., Moniz-Cook, E., et al. (2013). 'Feasibility Study of an Optimised Person-centred Intervention To Improve Mental Health and Reduce Antipsychotics amongst People with Dementia in Care Homes: Study Protocol for a Randomised Controlled Trial'. *Trials* 14: 13.

Wilkins, S., Castle, S., Heck, E., Tanzy, K., and Fahey, J. (1999). 'Immune Function, Mood, and Perceived Burden among Caregivers Participating in a Psychoeducational Intervention'. *Psychiatric Services* 50(6): 747–749.

Woods, B., Spector, A., Prendergast, L., and Orrell, M. (2005a). 'Cognitive Stimulation to Improve Cognitive Functioning in People with Dementia'. *Cochrane Database of Systematic Reviews* 4: CD005562.

Woods, B., Spector, A., Jones, C., Orrell, M., and Davies. S. (2005b). 'Reminiscence Therapy for Dementia'. *Cochrane Database of Systematic Reviews* 2: CD001120.

Woods, B., Aquirre, E., Spector, A., and Orrell, M. (2012). 'Cognitive Stimulation to Improve Cognitive Functioning in People with Dementia'. *Cochrane Database of Systematic Reviews* 2: CD005562pub2. doi.10.1002.14651858.

World Alzheimer Report (2010). *The Global Economic Impact of Dementia*. London: Alzheimer's Disease International.

World Alzheimer Report (2012). *Overcoming the Stigma of Dementia*. London: Alzheimer's Disease International.

Young, J. and Beck, A. T. (1988). '*Cognitive Therapy Scale*'. Unpublished manuscript, University of Pennsylvania, Philadelphia, PA.

Zuidema, S., de Jonghe, J., Verhey, F., and Koopmans, R. (2010). 'Environmental Correlates of Neuropsychiatric Symptoms in Nursing Home Patients with Dementia'. *International Journal of Geriatric Psychiatry* 25(1): 14–22.

CHAPTER 38

LESBIAN, GAY, BISEXUAL, AND TRANSGENDER AGEING

Considerations for Interventions

LINDA A. TRAVIS AND DOUGLAS C. KIMMEL

INTRODUCTION

DURING the lifespan of older adults the characterization of homosexual, bisexual, and transgender individuals has changed dramatically. When they were children and young adults, homosexuality was regarded as a mental illness and was a severe stigma that could result in loss of employment, social ruin, imprisonment, and sometimes death. In many countries it was a crime, an illness, and a sin. Gradually over the last half of the twentieth century homosexuality was decriminalized, the stigma of mental illness was removed by psychiatric organizations, and same-sex marriage became legal in some places and often more accepted by society even when not legal. This historical period has also seen increasing awareness of bisexual and transgender individuals. The movement towards pride and increased legal rights, social acceptance, and recognition of diverse sexual minorities ushered in the current use of the terms lesbian, gay, bisexual, and transgender (LGBT).

This chapter is written for psychologists and all other healthcare professionals working with older adults, as it can be assumed that ageing LGBT individuals are clients in all geriatric healthcare settings. There are widespread assumptions about the universality and normality of heterosexual relationships, and professionals are not immune to these assumptions. The assumptions permeate, indirectly or directly, all facets of communication and service delivery to older adults and thereby compromise the effectiveness of interventions with LGBT older adults. Many practitioners feel ill prepared or uninformed about considerations in working with LGBT older adults. Others may hold biased attitudes towards the LGBT population, whereas other professionals are eager to make system-wide changes in their settings so that LGBT older adults can be better served. The chapter addresses each of these groups and begins with an overview of key information about LGBT older adult culture as well as the diversity within this community. Following the overview, recommendations are offered for how psychologists can prepare themselves to work with LGBT older adults and for how healthcare settings can become more welcoming to LGBT older adults. Finally, several types of integrated healthcare settings are briefly discussed with attention to considerations for interventions with LGBT older adults.

Basic Information about LGBT Older Adult Culture

To understand the social-cultural and psychosocial dimensions in the lives of older LGBT adults, psychologists must not ignore the long-standing and pervasive impact of the historical mistreatment of LGBT individuals. Simply put, older LGBT individuals grew up in a hostile environment and received explicit declarations of their immoral, pathological, or criminal status (Kimmel, Rose, and David 2006). To ensure safety and survival, older adults often elected to remain invisible to others. Many older LGBT individuals did not disclose their sexual identity except to friends 'in the know' until they retired and often not to their extended family, preferring to be known as the unmarried aunt or uncle. In contrast, many older LGBT individuals involved in the gay rights movement beginning in the 1960s may have been open and demanding of gay-affirmative services throughout their adult lives. Therefore, there are both cohort and period effects involved in the extent to which older LGBT individuals are open (Grossman, Frank, and McCutcheon 2012).

> Practitioners are advised to recognize likely differences in disclosure and openness across age groups of LGBT older adults.

Due to varying degrees of estrangement from families of origin either from conflict in relationships or from concealment of one's identity, members of the LGBT community often created *families of choice* to experience a sense of belonging, acceptance, and support (LGBT Movement Advancement Project (MAP) and Services and Advocacy for Gay, Lesbian, Bisexual, and Transgender Elders (SAGE) 2010). Family of choice members may include friends, partners, former partners, co-workers, neighbours, and family of origin members. Although friendships are important to all older adults, there are differences in the function and meaning of friends for LGBT older adults as compared with heterosexual older adults. In a MetLife study (2010) comparing the two groups, LGBT older adults were more likely to live with friends, receive emotional support from friends, talk over end-of-life preferences with friends, and rely on friends as care-givers. As family of choice members are likely to be of the same generation as LGBT older adults, there may be less intergenerational exchange in care and support than is the case for heterosexual older adults. This lack of intergenerational exchange presents potential care-giving challenges (MAP and SAGE 2010). Contemporary cohorts of LGBT older adults, or at least those participating in research studies, are less likely to have children to rely upon for care-giving while heterosexual older adults are more likely to rely on children for care-giving (MAP and SAGE 2010). Family of choice members and partners are not granted the same legal rights or authority to make urgent or end-of-life medical decisions in the same way as a heterosexual spouse or biological family members, however. This lack of 'automatic' legal protection for families of choice presents a considerable vulnerability for LGBT older adults with regard to medical decisions. Some LGBT older adults take extraordinary measures to secure adequate legal protection and documentation while others simply cannot afford such legal services or may be unaware of the vulnerability facing family of choice members, especially in emergency situations. The individual, interpersonal, organizational, community, and policy barriers for LGBT care-givers warrant significant attention (Coon 2003).

> Practitioners are advised to ask questions about important people in the lives of LGBT older adults and recognize the central role of families of choice in social support and care-giving situations. Additionally, practitioners may need to refer LGBT older adults to colleagues in the legal profession for review and/or development of relevant legal documents pertaining to the role of family of choice members.

Significant gaps in legal rights and protections are only one area of unfair treatment encountered by LGBT older adults. The lack of legal recognition for LGBT couple relationships spirals into exclusion from some government ageing-related programmes, including programmes operating as primary or secondary sources of income for older adults. The resulting financial strain further burdens couples. In many healthcare situations, older LGBT individuals can secure rights via documentation (such as preferences for end-of-life care). The reader is reminded: for LGBT older adults, every country will vary as to legal rights and limitations, the applicability of government ageing-related programmes, and even the structure of entire healthcare systems. These three factors must be considered for effective interventions in healthcare settings. For example, consider the situation of a bi-national LGBT couple. Psychologists seeking greater understanding of the international considerations for LGBT individuals may explore resources through the International Network of LGBT Issues in Psychology (http://www.apa.org/pi/lgbt/resources/international-network.aspx). Members of this International Network include South Africa, Australia, Hong Kong, Brazil, and the Netherlands. Of note, position statements are available from psychological associations (e.g. Hong Kong Psychological Society 2012) regarding psychologists' work with sexual minority individuals.

At the time of writing this chapter, countries such as New Zealand and Uruguay (CNN 2013) have enacted legislation recognizing same-sex marriages. However, citizens may not experience the impact of such change for a considerable period of time, even years. LGBT older adults may not feel safe in accessing services, benefits, or even relevant legal support. Unfortunately, legislation may be enacted in such a way that the changes are not universally recognized or enforced within a particular country. For example, the 2013 US Supreme Court decision declaring the Defense of Marriage Act (DOMA) as unconstitutional (see the Lambda Legal website) raises complex questions about federal vs state rights for LGBT couples. Real change regarding federal programmes, such as social security benefits, may vary across states for several years.

> Practitioners are advised to become knowledgeable about the legal parameters, both protections and exclusions, for LGBT couples' eligibility in government-sponsored retirement, health, and ageing programmes. Practitioners must distinguish between areas where legal rights can be secured vs areas where no actions can be taken for equitable treatment. Furthermore, practitioners should consult with local, state, and federal professionals

regarding how LGBT legal rights are enacted, secured, and enforced in specific communities. Recognizing that legal rights vary within a country and across countries are critical steps in recognizing the national and international contexts for older LGBT individuals and couples. Finally, legal recognition of same-sex marriage and the rights and benefits that accompany that status is a prominent issue in many nations. Practitioners are encouraged to consult with local legal professionals to learn of legal resources for clients.

In addition to legal and financial inequities, LGBT older adults experience significant barriers when interfacing with healthcare systems. LGBT older adults have often experienced bias and discrimination by healthcare providers (Lambda Legal 2010). Fears of additional mistreatment by providers result in delays in seeking help, a lack of full disclosure regarding health-related concerns, or discussion of one's relationships (Institute of Medicine (IOM) 2011). Additionally, too many providers may lack the training and awareness to gain their patient's trust and to deliver adequate care to the ageing community (MAP and SAGE 2010). As a result, there are health and behavioural health disparities for LGBT older adults (Fredriksen-Goldsen et al. 2011).

> Practitioners are advised to become aware of the negative history and fear that often accompany the ageing LGBT person upon entering any part of the healthcare system.

The above factors place LGBT older adults at risk for a host of interpersonal, social, legal, financial, and health problems. Nevertheless, any discussion of *risk factors* among LGBT older adults must be balanced with equal attention to *resilience factors* among LGBT older adults. It is important to note that older persons are all survivors who lived long enough to grow old. The more disadvantaged the group has been during their young adult years, the greater the risk that they will not grow old. Therefore, today's older LGBT individuals are doubly survivors and this very fact attests to the resilience often noted among sexual minorities of all ages.

There are two resilience factors of note. *Families of choice* are an important area of resilience for LGBT older adults, and such networks offer particularly strong social support and care-giving resources for LGBT older adults. Second, scholarship on *crisis competence* (Kimmel 1978) suggests that a lifetime of dealing with one minority identity (LGBT) may ultimately be helpful in navigating another minority identity (such as ageing). Interestingly, nearly 75% of ageing LGBT respondents in the MetLife study (2010) identified benefits from their LGBT status towards preparation for ageing. The two major themes of these benefits were the development of personal/interpersonal strengths and the ability to overcome adversity (MetLife 2010). Thus, LGBT older adults bring resilience to the challenges of ageing.

> Practitioners are advised to recognize resilience and protective factors over the life course and future trajectory of LGBT older adults.

In summary, it is vital that psychologists understand key differences in the lives of LGBT older adults as compared with the lives of heterosexual older adults. Additionally, comprehending LGBT culture is also critical as providers can gain credibility with LGBT older adults when they are informed and aware of LGBT history and inequalities (Travis 2011). The recommendations offered here are concrete ways to improve the quality and effectiveness of interventions with LGBT older adults.

DIVERSITY WITHIN THE LGBT OLDER
ADULT COMMUNITY

The previous section focused on distinctions between LGBT and heterosexual older adults. In that discussion, the LGBT community was discussed as a group unto itself—one that suffers from a variety of legal and financial inequalities. These inequalities present unique challenges in LGBT ageing and contrast with the legal rights or financial benefits afforded heterosexual couples and individuals.

These are important distinctions that must not be forgotten in working with LGBT older adults in geriatric healthcare settings. Nonetheless, it is impossible to define the experiences, meanings, and life course of LGBT older adults through the *single* spotlight of lesbian, gay, bisexual, or transgender identity. Knowing that someone is lesbian, gay, bisexual, or transgender reveals relatively little about the person. The effect of that label is similar to knowing only that someone is over age 65, or Catholic, or from Asia.

At this time, it is estimated that there are about 1.5 million LGBT older adults in the US, and this number is expected to grow to between two and six million by the year 2030 (Fredriksen-Goldsen and Muraco 2010). It is important to better understand this minority population in the coming years in order to provide quality healthcare. In this section, diversity *within* the LGBT community is discussed, from the perspective of *multiple minority identities*, from a *life course* perspective, and finally from the perspective of *diversity among the subgroups* of older lesbians, gay men, bisexual individuals, and transgender individuals.

Multiple minority identities

The first area of diversity within the LGBT community involves recognition of multiple identities, or statuses, for LGBT older adults. Examples of additional minority statuses might include age, race, ethnicity, and socio-economic status. Multiple minority statuses may result in worse physical and mental health for LGBT individuals (Kim and Fredriksen-Goldsen 2012). However, experience in navigating one stigmatized identity may actually assist in navigating another minority identity (American Psychological Association (APA) 2011; MetLife 2010; Kimmel 1978). Researchers are only beginning to investigate the impact of multiple and intersecting identities for LGBT older adults. Thus, our discussion below will briefly examine the possible impact of specific additional identities in relation to the LGBT identity for older persons.

Age and cohort

By definition, all LGBT older adults navigate at least two identities: being LGBT and being older. There is risk of marginalization in each identity, as the older adult community may not accept ageing LGBT individuals and the LGBT community itself may not be welcoming of an older LGBT individual. Furthermore, younger LGBT generations may not grasp the impact of living in a time when homosexuality was regarded as a despicable perversion and social disgrace. Younger people today are more familiar with sexual and gender identities that shift over time, so they may also be puzzled by the categories used by their elders, such as 'butch' or 'fem'; 'gay' instead of 'lesbian'; and 'in the life' instead of 'gay.' They may be surprised to find that someone told no one until late in life, or that a husband returned to his wife after a same-sex relationship of significant duration. Likewise, they may fail to understand why some older LGBT individuals are reluctant to be open about their sexual identity or object to the term 'queer'. Such differences need to be understood as unique generational experiences and suggest that intergenerational programmes within the LGBT community might benefit each of the cohorts. Research is needed to better understand possible benefits of intergenerational programmes within the LGBT community.

Socio-economic status

Socio-economic status is closely related to many other factors, such as education, income, insurance, healthcare, housing, and neighbourhoods. Although the socioe-conomic status of LGBT communities varies widely, recent research illuminates concerns about the socio-economic well-being of LGBT older adults. Fredriksen-Goldsen et al. (2011) found household incomes at or below 200% of the Federal Poverty level for 31% of LGBT older adults in the study. These individuals were at higher risk for poorer health, were less likely to engage in health-promoting activities (e.g. PSA test, Pap smear), were more likely to smoke, and had higher levels of victimization related to their LGBT identity (Fredriksen-Goldsen et al. 2011). These results contradict the myth about LGBT people being more educated and having higher incomes than heterosexuals; Badgett (2001) has noted that this assumption is untrue and reflects the sampling bias of the limited studies of volunteer and snowball samples.

Race and ethnicity

Racism, in its many forms, impacts people of colour throughout the lifespan. Discrimination and unfair treatment in education, employment, housing, financial, and health arenas continue to exist. For example, racially and ethnically diverse older adults suffer a disproportionately higher rate of poverty as compared with white older persons (APA 2009a). The LGBT community is not immune to racism and the image of white LGBT activists or media personalities is retained as the modal face for the LGBT community. However, there is a growing recognition of ethnic and racial diversity in the sexual and gender minority community. For example, a Gallup survey of 120,000 US adults indicates that: 'African-Americans and other racial and ethnic minorities are more likely than white Americans to identify as LGBT. The results show that 4.6% of African-Americans identify as LGBT along with 4.0% of Hispanics and 4.3% of Asians. Among white Americans, the figure was 3.2%' (Gates and Newport 2012). It may be assumed that these reports are lower than actual incidence, however, due to a reluctance to disclose.

Racially and ethnically diverse LGBT individuals are likely to experience marginalization from individuals sharing their race and/or ethnic identification as well as from the LGBT community. Conflicting values between each minority identity may result in the LGBT person of colour not experiencing a sense of belonging to either group (APA 2011).

In addition to race and ethnicity status, the *acculturation status* of an LGBT older adult must be considered throughout interventions to ensure relevancy to one's worldview and beliefs about healthcare. In-person and written communication must consider language and word preferences in light of acculturation identities. In our rapidly shrinking world, practitioners must be cognizant of migration, immigration, and acculturation realities for older LGBT individuals and couples.

International status

An international perspective on LGBT issues and ageing broadens the view from the Western countries where dramatic changes have taken place in the last sixty years. There can be significant differences in LGBT issues across regions and between adjacent countries. For example, Canada offers national same-sex marriage and appropriate medical care for transgender individuals, while this remains the exceptional case in the US today. Likewise, the ability for same-sex couples to obtain immigration rights similar to heterosexual couples is available in Canada and some European countries, but is a severe problem in the US.

The pattern of rights and marriage for same-sex couples differs widely within the EU, other European countries, and South America. With the exception of South Africa, same-sex relationships are unrecognized and unprotected in Africa; in some countries, they are severely stigmatized and Uganda has proposed draconian laws resulting in death penalties (Kron 2012).

Although Japan and China have removed homosexuality from their list of medical diseases, the Confucian expectation of heterosexual marriage and childbearing is widely accepted as the norm and homosexuality is regarded as an individual aberration worthy of no special protection or consideration. While individuals may live a relatively openly adult gay life, they are generally outside the mainstream employment and social settings and, if needing care in old age, typically expect to need to hide their sexual orientation.

Middle Eastern countries, especially those that are predominantly Muslim, often have strongly negatively attitudes and laws about homosexuality, as well as restrictive attitudes and laws about women, which provide for challenging conditions for LGBT individuals. Israel is the exceptional case, with similar attitudes to those of the US (Smith 2011).

Since many older LGBT individuals travel or move to other countries, or have immigrated from other countries, the experiences from their earlier years may leave lasting expectations. Similarly, variations in healthcare across different countries may affect expatriates as well as prompt older LGBT individuals to immigrate or leave their home country. An excellent resource offering current information on international LGBT news is located through the Williams Institute (see link in the Key References section).

The focus of this chapter is on older LGBT individuals. However, it should be noted that in some nations, the laws, advocacy groups, or organizations may recognize LGB individuals but *not* transgender individuals. Alternatively, some countries (e.g. Australia) may demonstrate greater inclusiveness regarding intersex people and refer to 'LGBTI' in laws and programmes. Thus, it is essential to recognize the international differences in the subgroups defined as sexual and/or gender minorities.

Military status

Military status or identity is often carried far past the last dates of active duty. A particular national military system may or may not recognize LGBT couples, thereby compromising financial benefits that are afforded to heterosexual couples. Additionally, discovery of a person's LGBT identity may have resulted in discharge from the military, loss of benefits, and long-term stigma. Electing to serve and protect one's country while being rejected by that country places LGBT older adult veterans in an untenable position. Although recent changes in some countries, such as the US, are removing LGBT discrimination in the military, injustices from the past still exist for older veterans as well as for younger LGBT veterans who may be marginalized by veterans' groups.

Spirituality and religion

Gerontologists often note that religion and spirituality become more important in later life (APA 2009a), but it is also assumed that the negative attitudes of many religious institutions have alienated older LGBT individuals. It is likely that both statements are correct, but the result has often been that those religions that welcome sexual and gender minorities have attracted LGBT adults from those religions that are less welcoming or openly hostile. Moreover, churches that focus on gay-affirmative beliefs have developed in some communities. As spirituality is another important aspect of diversity in the LGBT community, providers are encouraged to explore both harmful and satisfying experiences of older LGBT adults regarding spirituality and religion.

Life course perspective

LGBT older adults, like all older adults, engage in many meaningful relationships over the life course. Specific types of relationship (e.g. such as those with parents and siblings, partners/spouses, children/stepchildren/grandchildren, friends and family of choice members) often take on more or less importance at various points of the life cycle. For older LGBT individuals, it is useful to examine the interactions among these types of relationship in accordance with the life stage in which one's LGBT identity became public.

It is critical to understand that an *LGBT identity* may not be openly carried throughout all of one's life. An equally likely pathway is that a shift in acceptance of an erotic preference or a gender identity may become more apparent at mid-life or even later in life. Some older LGBT individuals related to and married persons of the other sex because of a lack of awareness of an affirmative LGBT community, or because their erotic feelings were ambivalent or unacceptable. This was especially true during the last century and must be recognized as a substantial force for many LGBT older persons in the timing and openness of an LGBT identity.

Self-acceptance of an LGBT identity early in one's life may bring about stigma and disapproval from family and community, but it also allows the possibility of clarity, an accepting family of choice, and a new community. A shift in sexual or gender identity at mid-life or late-life may instigate a tidal wave of crises and restructuring of established relationships and rejection by a formerly welcoming community. Spouses, partners, children, family members, and friends may be confused and feel betrayed. An entire life may have to be dismantled and reassembled. Yet there is courage and freedom in making decisions congruent with one's gender identity and/or sexual orientation. Living out mid-life and late-life years with self-acceptance in a social community can bring peace.

Relationships in turmoil at one life stage might become harmonious and cherished at other life stages. Some older LGBT individuals enjoy contact and even close relationships with former spouses from a heterosexual marriage or with in-laws and extended family members from that network. Other older LGBT persons have little interest in or access to their spouses and children. Some lost custody and were not allowed any contact with their children. At times, there may be a reconciliation of the relationship with a child once the child reaches adulthood and is able independently to relate to the LGBT parent. The arrival of grandchildren into families also prompts changes, often in the direction of connections across generations.

LGBT older adult couples span the same wide spectrum of longevity as do heterosexual older couples. Some have been a couple for decades, others elected to have a few long-term relationships over the decades, and others have had brief relationships. Some older LGBT individuals do not wish to be partnered and prefer being single, but have an extensive friendship network. For all, connecting with families of choice and the LGBT community is key in accessing needed support and validation from the outside world.

One unique characteristic in LGBT couple relationships involves potentially different degrees of openness about LGBT identity. The couple will need to discuss how to manage successfully such differences across interactions with families, friends, neighbours, and co-workers. As noted throughout the chapter, many older LGBT individuals express understandable fears about coming out. However, there are intrapersonal and interpersonal gains in electing greater openness with others. Clearly, the choice of coming out is best made by the couple, and practitioners are advised to understand that choices regarding openness may vary over time.

> Practitioners are advised to understand that claiming an LGBT identity is not a 'neutral' life event, especially for LGBT older adults. The LGBT identity places one at risk for possible family rejection as well as for probable discrimination, stigma, and victimization from society at large. Older LGBT persons often encountered substantial pressures to 'change back' to being heterosexual, and some sought help from professionals for this reason. In fact, sexual orientation change efforts (SOCE) are ineffective and may cause harm, including depression, anxiety, and suicidality (APA 2011). Psychologists are strongly encouraged to adhere to current assessment and treatment recommendations should clients seek changes in sexual orientation (APA 2011; APA 2009b; British Psychological Society 2012).

DIVERSITY WITHIN THE SUBGROUPS OF L-G-B-T

Thus far we have examined critical differences within the lives of LGBT older adults from the perspective of multiple minority identities as well as from the perspective of claiming an LGBT identity at various life stages. There is also diversity among the particular subgroups of L-G-B-T older adults, although research is at a very early stage in exploring such differences. For example, in terms of healthcare, the *historical context* is somewhat different for each subgroup. Many lesbian older adults identified with the social equality movements of the 1960s and 1970s. The pursuit of equal rights for women and people of colour helped launch a Women's Health Movement. Some older gay men are survivors of decimated friendship networks due to the HIV/AIDS epidemic in the 1980s and 1990s, and have had to reconstruct lives after severe bereavement and extraordinary grief experiences.

We have all witnessed this fatal illness become transformed into a chronic illness, and people who did not expect to grow old are now doing so. Sero-positive individuals will express their concerns about HIV/AIDS with providers, but the comorbidity of age-related chronic illnesses is likely to raise concerns about the successful management of multiple conditions. In addition, the long-term effects of anti-retroviral therapy are unknown. The 'culture' of HIV/AIDS healthcare is likely to be more gay-friendly than much of the 'culture' of geriatric care, and *families of choice* and care-givers will need to help sero-positive gay and bisexual men be proactive within geriatric care settings.

Older bisexual individuals are more likely than gay men or lesbians to have been legally married and be assumed to be heterosexual; but in the last century they were often thought to be confused about their sexuality and still today may experience marginalization from both the LGBT and heterosexual communities. Bisexual older adults are less likely to disclose their sexual minority identity to healthcare professionals than are LGBT older adults (Fredriksen-Goldsen et al. 2011). In addition, bisexual older adults are more guarded in their overall disclosure rates to others (e.g. co-workers, neighbours) compared to LGBT older adults (MetLife 2010). Their social support networks often include more heterosexual individuals (Grossman, D'Augelli, and Herschberger 2000). Compared to older lesbians, *older bisexual women* are less likely to have a primary healthcare provider and report greater fear in seeking healthcare within the LGBT community at nearly three times the rate of older lesbian women (Fredriksen-Goldsen et al. 2011). *Older bisexual men* are more likely than gay men to have children and are significantly more likely to attend spiritual or religious activities (Fredriksen-Goldsen et al. 2011). However, their children are unlikely to live in the household and older bisexual men are more likely to live alone (Fredriksen-Goldsen et al. 2011). The optimal group of care-givers and *families of choice* for older bisexual women and men is likely to be a mixture of heterosexual and LGBT individuals. The nature of their support network would be an important area to explore with the older bisexual individual.

Transgender individuals must disclose their identity to providers in order to secure hormonal supports and pursue additional physical modifications (Coleman et al. 2011). However, older transsexual individuals often fear the need for emergency healthcare, hospitalization, and nursing home situations since they feel vulnerable about staff or healthcare providers seeing their bodies. Transgender older adults are also very diverse. For example, they vary as to their degree of physical transition, and the extent to which their bodies may remain incongruent with their public gender identity. Some do not reveal their gender identity to family or friends. Care-givers may need to be proactive in working with healthcare providers and staff to manage these concerns, especially during a health crisis or in a long-term care setting (Cook-Daniels 2006). Compared to other sexual-minority groups, transgender older persons are more likely to attend religious and spiritual activities (Fredriksen-Goldsen et al. 2011).

Lesbians and gay men tend to be equally involved in care-giving within the LGBT community. However, Cohen and Murray (2006) found that gay men are more likely to provide care for individuals with HIV/AIDS, whereas lesbians are more likely to provide care to individuals with physical problems. *Gay men* provide significantly more care to others than do heterosexual men and often report the care-giving to be a meaningful activity (De Vries and Herdt 2012).

Of course, some of the care-giving is with partners, parents, or other members of their *family of origin*. Care-giving for older gay men may also involve an acknowledgement of a continuing interest in sexual relationships and connections with gay male friends (Wierzalis et al. 2006).

Given concerns about finances, poor health insurance coverage, and mistrust of providers, lesbians are less likely to seek healthcare. Like heterosexual women, older lesbians may continue to perform the traditional women's role of care-taking for the ageing members of their own *family of origin* (Cohen and Murray 2006). *Older lesbians* have been shown to have large social networks (Grossman et al. 2000) and often enjoy social involvement with both *family of choice* members and with children and grandchildren from previous heterosexual relationships. It bears mentioning here, that because women live longer than men, it is predicted that lesbians will constitute a much larger proportion of the older LGBT community (MAP and SAGE 2010).

In summary, families of choice, care-givers, and social relationships are important supports for all LGBT older adults. However, there is diversity in the composition of these support structures. Likewise, each subgroup of the LGBT community demonstrates its own forms of resilience. For example, researchers have documented the importance of religious and spiritual involvement for bisexual men and transgender individuals. Gay men and transgender individuals demonstrate a great deal of self-efficacy in navigating complex healthcare systems. For gay men, helping others is meaningful and there may be an existential outlook about life, having survived the death of so many peers. Lesbians typically enjoy social connection within the LGBT community and are involved in social relationships with a variety of people across the lifespan. Older bisexual women also have large and complex social networks across communities. The degree of importance of the LGBT community appears most variable for older bisexual women and men. Care-giving and interventions must be guided by all of these differences.

> Practitioners are advised to consider the variations within the LGBT community or risk failing or offending the LGBT older adult. Understanding diversity as expressed through multiple minority identities, all through the life course, and through each of the four subgroups of L-G-B-T are essential aspects of effective work with LGBT older adults. The research presented here is in the very early stages of examining diversity within the LGBT community and it is possible that future studies will refute these findings or perhaps more closely hone in on differences. Nonetheless, unique areas of challenge and unique areas of resilience seem to exist for each group.

Effective work with LGBT older adults requires more than obtaining knowledge. We shift in the next section to offer recommendations for working with LGBT older adults in healthcare settings.

PREPARING PSYCHOLOGISTS TO ADDRESS LGBT AGEING WITHIN HEALTHCARE SETTINGS

The importance of developing psychologists' multicultural competence with minority groups across the lifespan is a critical topic across psychology and specifically within geropsychology (e.g. APA 2009a). The expectation for multicultural competence is also underscored within psychologists' ethical principles and code of conduct (e.g. APA 2002; Australian Psychological Society 2012; Psychological Association of the Philippines 2010). Sue, Arredondo, and McDavis (1992) proposed a model of multicultural competency consisting of three domains: *awareness, knowledge, and skills.* At the center of the model is the recognition that multicultural competency does not involve a singular focus on knowledge, awareness, or skills but instead that it is the interplay among these domains that facilitates multicultural competency (Sue et al. 1992; Sue and Sue 2008).

Awareness

Readers are invited to reflect on the scenarios below. Please consider reactions to each scenario to become more aware of personal assumptions, attitudes, as well as possible biases related to LGBT ageing. It may also be useful to reflect on the scenarios from the perspective of LGBT older adults.

1A Reflect on your thoughts and feelings upon hearing comments from friends, colleagues, or clients/patients, such as:
> 'These LGBT people think they are special—there is a reason they don't have rights.'
> 'It's just not normal and it's that simple.'
> 'It is fine with me as there are no differences between us—we are all humans.'
> 'I don't mind but I don't think they should talk about it.'

1B Further reflect on situations when friends, colleagues, or clients/patients have expressed the above sentiments nonverbally. Then consider the times where verbal expressions did not match nonverbal expressions on an LGBT topic.

2A Examine your comfort level when envisioning an LGBT couple holding hands or kissing in your presence.

2B Now imagine the couple holding hands or kissing at a community social event as well as in a geriatric healthcare setting (an outpatient clinic, a hospital, or a long-term care setting). Examine your comfort level in these situations.

In considering reactions to these four scenarios, perhaps you have become aware of the need to review assumptions or attitudes regarding older LGBT persons.

Knowledge

Local, state, or national psychological organizations, LGBT ageing services, and online resources provide opportunities for psychologists to broaden peer and professional networks for ongoing learning about LGBT ageing. Some readers may experience distress, shock, frustration, or disappointment upon reading the statements or envisioning nonverbal expressions that might be received by LGBT older adults. Unlike in relation to some other minority groups, many people find it quite acceptable to convey overt or covert homophobic or heterosexist assumptions in conversations. These unfiltered and 'raw' expressions have been experienced by many LGBT older adults. Finally, the scenario about an LGBT couple holding hands or kissing may evoke a more 'real-life' awareness of LGBT older adults and the potential challenges in social settings with peers or in healthcare settings with providers. Some have termed this the 'yuck factor'.

Skills

To further extend awareness of attitudes and beliefs about LGBT ageing, think about possible reactions of healthcare colleagues and team members to each of those scenarios. What might LGBT older adults experience during and after their interactions with healthcare colleagues? What are some suggested improvements for interactions between LGBT older adults and healthcare providers to expand multicultural competency with LGBT older adults?

Healthcare providers and psychologists are increasingly working together on integrated healthcare teams that serve older adults. Integrated healthcare is characterized by interdisciplinary team members collaborating to address the biological, psychological, and social needs of older adults (APA 2008). The *biopsychosocial* framework challenges both health providers and behavioural health providers to broaden their perspectives on illness and encourages collaboration among professionals of different disciplines (Seaburn et al. 2003). For example, psychologists and behavioural health providers might begin learning more about the biological or biomedical aspects of care for LGBT older adults. Healthcare providers might seek guidance from psychologists to understand LGBT older adults' personal, relationship, and social support networks. Psychologists should be prepared for such collaboration with health providers. In fact, it has been specifically recommended that psychologists in integrated care become knowledgeable about 'gender and sexual orientation diversity among older adults' (e.g. APA 2008: 20) and that 'healthcare teams and psychologists need to increase their multicultural competency for those with a gay, lesbian, or transgender orientation' (e.g. APA 2008: 33). Healthcare teams and healthcare systems, as well as LGBT older adults, would benefit greatly from psychologists' contributions as direct service providers and as consultants on LGBT ageing.

How might psychologists move forward as members of integrated healthcare teams to improve care for LGBT older adults? To prepare psychologists to address these issues, two sets of recommendations are offered (Box 38.1).

Lifelong learning

Recognizing that there is a significant lack of knowledge about LGBT ageing at this time, psychologists are advised to adopt a stance of lifelong learning. Consultation with colleagues is a critical component of lifelong learning and this learning may take the form of knowledge, awareness, and skills. Note that the area of LGBT ageing requires learning on the part of the psychologist with expertise in ageing as well as on the part of the psychologist with expertise in LGBT psychology. For those specialists in clinical gerospsychology, a starting point includes reflection on previous LGBT older adult clients. What could have been

---

Box 38.1 Recommendations to address LGBT ageing within healthcare settings

---

1 Psychologists engage in lifelong learning about:
  (a) LGBT culture
      i Historical context
      ii Families of choice
      iii Care-giving challenges
      iv Legal rights and protections, or lack thereof
      v Exclusion from government ageing-related programmes and subsequent financial burden
      vi Stigma and fears of discrimination from healthcare providers
      vii Resilience factors

  (b) Key intersections of LGBT identity with:
      i Multiple minority identities (e.g. race, ethnicity, and socio-economic status)
      ii Life course process and life cycle stages
      iii Diversity within each subgroup of L-G-B-T

2 Psychologists work with healthcare providers and healthcare systems to create a welcoming environment for LGBT older adults as demonstrated by:
  (a) LGBT friendly websites and brochures, both in words and in images
  (b) Non-discrimination policies posted and enforced
  (c) Paperwork and forms contain LGBT sensitive language
  (d) Consultation on LGBT ageing topics for integrated care providers and staff

---

different in those cases? Were there heterosexist assumptions being made when listening to clients' life stories? What actions or interventions, either directly with the client or indirectly with colleagues, might the psychologist initiate to increase awareness and support of an ageing LGBT client? Does the healthcare team or healthcare setting know how to welcome LGBT clients? Just as the psychologist with expertise in geropsychology is encouraged to access LGBT psychology resources and to examine heterosexist assumptions, the psychologist with expertise in LGBT psychology is encouraged to access geropsychology resources and examine ageist assumptions. The LGBT community is often viewed as holding its own strong biases of ageism (Kimmel et al. 2006). Reflecting back on prior cases is a useful starting point to consider if or how the topic of ageing was addressed with LGBT clients. Did the psychologist, client, or both avoid the topic of ageing? What could have been different in those cases?

Specific recommendations for psychologists' learning were offered earlier in the chapter for the following aspects of LGBT culture: historical context, families of choice, care-giving challenges, legal rights (or lack thereof), exclusion from government-sponsored ageing programmes, financial burden, fears of discrimination from healthcare providers, and resilience factors.

It is vital that providers understand key differences in the lives of LGBT older adults as compared to the lives of heterosexual older adults. Additionally, psychologists must grasp diversity *within* the LGBT community—from the perspective of multiple minority identities, from a life course perspective, and finally from the perspectives of the subgroups of older lesbians, gay men, bisexual individuals, and transgender individuals. We are at the very early stages of investigation into LGBT ageing. However, it is clear that limited scholarship and research should not translate into limited or delayed action on the part of psychologists. An opposite strategy is called for. Healthcare settings need to be more welcoming and comfortable for LGBT older adults and there are specific actions to take on this front.

Creating a welcoming environment

Psychologists can assess the degree to which the overall environment of the healthcare office, or system, is welcoming to LGBT older adults. Initial areas to examine are websites, brochures, the waiting room, paperwork, and forms. Are images of older adults exclusively those of heterosexual couples? LGBT older adults may feel less welcome. If the language used on websites and brochures contains words like 'spouse' or 'husband' and 'wife' then LGBT older adults may feel excluded. Instead, words such as 'partner' and 'significant other' are recommended. On forms, questions asking about 'relationship status' instead of 'marital status' are advised, along with inclusion of questions inquiring if current sexual partners are female, male, or both and if past sexual partners are female, male, or both. Asking transgender individuals for their pronoun preferences (e.g. to be called 'he' or 'she') and offering options of female, male, and transgender across all paperwork is essential. Staff and healthcare practitioners must become comfortable using the language as well as modifying forms. As a reminder about multiple identities, it is equally important to include images of LGBT individuals of different races and to incorporate culture-specific language and meanings about healthcare for various ethnic minority groups.

A clear display of non-discrimination policies is essential. Displaying LGBT stickers or symbols is a way to welcome LGBT older adults. Inclusion of LGBT magazines, newsletters, and community flyers is yet another form of communicating awareness to LGBT older adults. There are an increasing number of resources available to assist healthcare practitioners in developing forms with questions about sexual orientation and gender diversity across the lifespan (Gay and Lesbian Medical Association 2006) and specific to LGBT older adults (National Resource Center on LGBT Aging 2013). Discussion of these resources among team members is another useful starting point when considering changes in paperwork and forms. Of particular concern, providers must be clear about the limits of confidentiality on any and all paperwork and electronic records.

Since healthcare providers often lack training in LGBT healthcare (IOM 2011), psychologists can offer training that addresses the interpersonal and social context of healthcare for LGBT older adults. Training formats might include case-based consultation, brief didactic seminars, team meetings, or impromptu discussions on specific topics (e.g. the significance of families of choice). In summary, building trust and improving communication among team members and LGBT older adult patients is a central step in providing a welcoming environment.

CONSIDERATIONS FOR INTERVENTIONS IN SPECIFIC INTEGRATED HEALTHCARE SETTINGS

This section will address a wide range of healthcare settings where older LGBT individuals have special concerns or issues that may be expected to differ from those older people who are, or are assumed to be, heterosexual. Essentially no research has been done on many of these settings, so our discussion will be brief and do little more than point out some important considerations and call for additional research. It is evident that health and behavioural health data collection on LGBT older adults is extremely difficult. Efforts to improve data collection on LGBT health are beginning and should provide a clearer picture of the scope of health and behavioural health disparities in ageing LGBT people as well as guide the development of best practices for clinical decisions.

Primary care settings are characterized by ongoing provider–client relationships, and this feature is fairly distinct from the acute or time-limited provider–client relationships often found in specialty care, hospital care, or emergency care settings. Psychologists in primary care teams are likely to help providers work towards patient-centred care (McDaniel and Fogarty 2009). Yet it is well known that older LGBT individuals are less likely to have a satisfactory relationship with a primary care provider (IOM 2011). Thus, psychologists can be instrumental in helping colleagues recognize and understand the psychological and social functioning of LGBT elders. Additionally, primary care practitioners can inquire about important people in the life of the LGBT older adult and assist the older adult in gradually disclosing such relationships, as these are standard topics within the primary care setting. Furthermore, information about partners and family of choice members in the life of an LGBT older adult sets the stage for discussions about healthcare directives, power of attorney, and other legal documents advised to be in place for older adults. In addition, primary care providers should assume that LGBT older adults are sexually active and initiate discussions about sexual health and risks, including HIV tests, as part of standard care.

Specialty care settings (such as surgery) often require referrals from primary care providers. As referrals may include information about an LGBT identity of a client, both primary care and specialty care providers must be in clear communication with one another and with the LGBT client. Is the client aware of the contents of the medical record? What wishes and control does the client have for communication of personal information? Even in those cases where providers automatically share information via electronic medical records, the psychologist might assist the LGBT client in thinking through options when meeting with the specialist provider.

In acute care settings, such as *emergency rooms*, there may be no time for thought as to how to proceed with disclosure to a healthcare team. For transgender clients, this type of situation may be particularly terrifying to contemplate. The psychologist working in acute care settings may need to work with interdisciplinary team members about their reactions in reconciling differences in gender identity and physical anatomy of a transgender client. Ethical codes and institutional policy are vital to guide interactions in such settings, and healthcare institutions should prepare all levels of staff and providers for LGBT clients. Acute care settings should train providers to be competent and comfortable with LGBT clients.

Hospitals can be unfriendly places for families of choice to visit LGBT loved ones. Although policies regarding hospital visitation are changing in many healthcare systems, too often there is a time gap between policy change and practice change. Seeing an LGBT couple holding hands in a hospital may elicit varying responses from staff and other visitors. Perceiving this rejecting or disapproving response has a negative impact on LGBT older adults and their loved ones. For LGBT older adults, family of origin members (e.g. siblings, nieces, and nephews) may appear and attempt to assume a role of authority in medical decision-making causing staff to become confused. Therefore, family of choice members are advised to bring legal documents to the hospital in order to expedite any urgent medical decisions so as to clarify roles and relationships with the hospital staff.

As a transition from an acute care setting or as part of ongoing care for chronic health, LGBT older adults might receive *home care*. Like so many older adults, LGBT older adults wish to stay in their homes and communities for as long as possible. There is a large variation in the type and length of home care services yet it is clear that this is one of the fastest-growing segments of the healthcare industry (Niles 2011). Particular vulnerabilities for LGBT older adults receiving home care include the personal and social nature of home care in contrast to the more formal atmosphere of office care. Psychologists on interdisciplinary home healthcare teams might help LGBT older adults decide about the nature and scope of conversation with home care workers.

Partners, family of choice members, and care-givers may also experience unique concerns when considering loved ones' admittance to *long-term care facilities*, including assisted living and skilled nursing facilities. Their concerns are primarily focused on the safety and care of the LGBT older adult client, especially if the LGBT older adult suffers from physical and/or cognitive impairment and cannot fully advocate for him/herself or may be cared for by staff not competent to care for LGBT older adults (MAP and SAGE 2010). Unlike in the case of heterosexual couples, many long-term care facilities do not allow LGBT couples to cohabit and this can be devastating for the LGBT couple. On a hopeful note, Project Visibility is a training programme designed to develop competencies in caring for LGBT older adults (see resource section for website).

Hospice care may occur in the older adult's home or in a healthcare setting. Many urgent and planned medical decisions might be required by a partner or family of choice member and these individuals are not typically recognized as having the 'natural' authority to make those decisions. Hence, documents such as power of attorney and advance care directives are extremely important to have in order. Psychologists can work with integrated care team members to ensure that the LGBT older adult's wishes are respected at all stages of care. Partners, family of choice members, and care-givers might also need support from psychologists, both in relation to the dying process and in relation to any legal issues or healthcare system barriers encountered within the hospice. Hospice professionals may also need support and training for dealing with their emotional reactions to grieving LGBT *families of choice* and their expressions of love and loss.

Summary

In their lifetimes, LGBT older adults have witnessed substantial changes in larger social-cultural attitudes, with a gradual shift towards acceptance of sexual minorities. This increased acceptance, however, did not alter the reality of health, legal, and financial disparities for older LGBT individuals. In spite of these disparities, older LGBT individuals demonstrate resilience through the channels of *crisis competence* and *families of choice* as friends and care-givers. There is widespread diversity within the LGBT community that can be understood from the perspective of multiple minority identities, from a life course perspective, and from the perspective of diversity among the subgroups of older lesbians, gay men, bisexual, and transgender older persons.

Psychologists on integrated teams in a range of geriatric settings are in a unique position to help healthcare providers and healthcare settings move towards more effective care for LGBT older adults. Specifically, more effective care must include attention to the relationships and social networks of older LGBT individuals. Psychologists can assist healthcare providers understand the social and emotional aspects of caring for older LGBT persons. Interventions that consider the diversity and resilience in the lives of LGBT elders are then more likely to be most relevant. Psychologists also bring expertise in communication and relationship building to integrated teams, along with awareness of the importance of creating a welcoming environment for the LGBT older adult community. In summary, we remain optimistic about LGBT older adults receiving better care in healthcare systems, and in psychologists' pivotal role in creating such change.

KEY REFERENCES AND SOURCES FOR FURTHER READING

Key resources

Diverse Elders Coalition. http://www.diverseelders.org/.

Kimmel, D., Rose, T., and David, S. (eds) (2006). *Lesbian, Gay, Bisexual, and Transgender Aging: Research and Clinical Perspectives.* New York: Columbia University Press.

National Resource Center on LGBT Aging. http://www.lgbtagingcenter.org/.

Services and Advocacy for GLBT Elders (SAGE). http://www.sageusa.org/.

Witten, T. M. and Eyler, A. E. (eds) (2012). *Gay, Lesbian, Bisexual, and Transgender Aging.* Baltimore, MD: Johns Hopkins University Press.

Internet resources

Diverse Elders Coalition. http://www.diverseelders.org/.

International Network on Lesbian, Gay, & Bisexual Concerns & Transgender Issues in Psychology. http://www.apa.org/pi/lgbt/resources/international-network.aspx.

Intersex Society of North America. www.isna.org.

Lambda Legal. http://www.lambdalegal.org/search/node/aging.

LGBT Aging Project. http://www.lgbtagingproject.org/.

National Center for Lesbian Rights. http://www.nclrights.org/.

National Center for Transgender Equality. http://transequality.org/.

National Gay and Lesbian Task Force. http://www.ngltf.org/our_work/public_policy/lgbt_aging_initiative.

National Resource Center on LGBT Aging. http://www.lgbtagingcenter.org/.

National Senior Citizens Law Center. http://www.nsclc.org/.

OpenHouse. http://openhouse-sf.org/.

Opening Doors London. http://www.openingdoorslondon.org.uk/.

Project Visibility. http://www.bouldercounty.org/family/seniors/pages/projvis.aspx.

Services and Advocacy for GLBT Elders (SAGE). http://www.sageusa.org/.

Williams Institute. http://williamsinstitute.law.ucla.edu/category/research/international/.

World Professional Organization for Transgender Health (WPATH). www.wpath.org.

References

American Psychological Association (2002). 'Ethical Principles of Psychologists and Code of Conduct'. *American Psychologist* 57: 1060–1073.

American Psychological Association (2011). *Guidelines for Psychological Practice with Lesbian, Gay, and Bisexual Clients*. Washington DC: American Psychological Association. http://www.apa.org/pi/lgbt/resources/guidelines.aspx.

American Psychological Association, Committee on Aging (2009a). *Multicultural Competency in Gerospsychology*. Washington DC: American Psychological Association.

American Psychological Association, Presidential Task Force on Integrated Health Care for an Aging Population (2008). *Blueprint for Change: Achieving Integrated Health Care for an Aging Population*. Washington DC: American Psychological Association. http://www.apa.org/pi/aging/resources/guides/exec-summary.aspx.

American Psychological Association, Task Force on Appropriate Therapeutic Responses to Sexual Orientation (2009b). *Report of the Task Force on Appropriate Therapeutic Responses to Sexual Orientation*. Washington, DC: American Psychological Association. http://www.apa.org/pi/lgbt/resources/sexual-orientation.aspx.

Australian Psychological Society (2012). *APS Code of Ethics*. https://www.psychology.org.au/about/ethics/#s1.

Badgett, M. V. L. (2001). *Money, Myths, and Change: The Economic Lives of Lesbians and Gay Men*. Chicago: University of Chicago Press.

British Psychological Society (2012). *Position Statement: Therapies Attempting to Change Sexual Orientation*. http://www.bps.org.uk/.

CNN (2013). 'New Zealand's Parliament Votes to Legalize Same-sex Marriage', 17 April. http://www.cnn.com/2013/04/17/world/new-zealand-same-sex-marriage/.

Cohen, H. L. and Murray, Y. (2006). 'Older Lesbian and Gay Caregivers: Caring for Families of Choice and Caring for Families of Origin'. *Journal of Human Behavior in the Social Environment* 14(1/2): 275–298. doi:10.1300/J137v14n01_14.

Coleman, E., Bocktin, W., Botzer, M., Cohen-Kettenis, P., DeCuypere, G., et al. (2011). 'Standards of Care for the Health of Transsexual, Transgender, and Gender-nonconforming People, Version 7'. *International Journal of Transgenderism*, 13: 165–232. doi: 10.1080/15532739.2011.700873.

Cook-Daniels, L. (2006). 'Trans Aging'. In D. Kimmel, T. Rose, and S. David (eds), *Lesbian, Gay, Bisexual, and Transgender Aging: Research and Clinical Perspectives* (pp. 20–36). New York: Columbia University Press.

Coon, D. W. (2003). *Lesbian, Gay, Bisexual, and Transgender Issues and Family Caregiving*. San Francisco: Family Caregiver Alliance, National Center on Caregiving.

De Vries, B. and Herdt, G. (2012). 'Aging in the Gay Community'. In T. M. Witten and A. E. Eyler (eds), *Gay, Lesbian, Bisexual, and Transgender Aging* (pp. 84–129). Baltimore, MD: Johns Hopkins University Press.

Fredriksen-Goldsen, K. I. and Muraco, A. (2010). 'Aging and Sexual Orientation: A 25-year Review of the Literature'. *Research on Aging* 32: 372–413. doi:10.1177/0164027509360355.

Fredriksen-Goldsen, K. I., Kim, H. J., Emlet, C. A., Muraco, A., Erosheva, E. A., et al. (2011). *The Aging and Health Report: Disparities and Resilience among Lesbian, Gay, Bisexual, and Transgender Older Adults*. Seattle, WA: Institute for Multigenerational Health. http://carin gandaging.org/.

Gates, G. G. and Newport, R. (2012). *Gallup Special Report: The U.S. Adult LGBT Population*. http://williamsinstitute.law.ucla.edu/research/census-lgbt-demographics-studies/ gallup-specialreport-18oct-2012/.

Gay and Lesbian Medical Association (2006). *Guidelines for the Care of Lesbian, Gay, Bisexual, and Transgender Patients*. San Francisco: Gay and Lesbian Medical Association. http://glma. org/_data/n_0001/resources/live/GLMA%20guidelines%202006%20FINAL.pdf.

Grossman, A. H., D'Augelli, A. R., and Hershberger, S. L. (2000). 'Social Support Networks of Lesbian, Gay, and Bisexual Adults 60 Years of Age and Older'. *Journal of Gerontology, Series B: Psychological Sciences* 55B(3): P171–P179.

Grossman, A. H., Frank, J. A., and McCutcheon, M. J. (2012). 'Sexual Orientation and Aging in Western Society'. In C. J. Patterson and A. R. D'Augelli (eds), *Handbook of Psychology and Sexual Orientation* (pp. 132–148). New York: Oxford University Press.

Hong Kong Psychological Society, Division of Clinical Psychology (2012). *Position Paper for Psychologists Working with Lesbians, Gays, and Bisexual Individuals*. http://www.hkps.org. hk/padmin/upload/wpage1_26download2_Position%20Paper%20on%20LGB.pdf.

Institute of Medicine (2011). *The Health of Lesbian, Gay, Bisexual, and Transgender People: Building a Foundation for Better Understanding*. Washington, DC: National Academy of Sciences. http://www.iom.edu/lgbthealth.

Kim, H-J. and Fredriksen-Goldsen, K. I. (2012). 'Hispanic Lesbians and Bisexual Women at Heightened Risk for Health Disparities'. *American Journal of Public Health* 102(1): E9–E15.

Kimmel, D. (1978). 'Adult Development and Aging: A Gay Perspective'. *Journal of Social Issues* 34(3): 113–130.

Kimmel, D., Rose, T., and David, S. (eds) (2006). *Lesbian, Gay, Bisexual, and Transgender Aging: Research and Clinical Perspectives*. New York: Columbia University Press.

Kron. J. (2012). 'Resentment toward the West Bolsters Uganda's New Anti-gay Bill'. *New York Times*, 28 February.

Lambda Legal (2010). *When Health Care isn't Caring: Lambda Legal's Survey of Discrimination against LGBT People and People with HIV*. New York: Lambda Legal. http://www.lambdale gal.org/health-care-report.

LGBT Movement Advancement Project and Services and Advocacy for Gay, Lesbian, Bisexual and Transgender Elders (2010). *Improving the Lives of LGBT Older Adults*. http://www. sageusa.org/resources/publications.cfm?ID=21.

McDaniel, S. H. and Fogarty, C. T. (2009). 'What Primary Care Psychology Has to Offer the Patient-centered Medical Home'. *Professional Psychology: Research and Practice* 40(5): 483–492.

Met-Life (2010). *Still Out, Sill Aging: The MetLife Study of Lesbian, Gay, Bisexual, and Transgender Baby Boomers*. Westport, CT: MetLife Mature Market Institute. http://sageusa. org/resources/publications.cfm?ID=23.

National Resource Center on LGBT Aging (2013). *Inclusive Questions for Older Adults: A Practical Guide to Collecting Data on Sexual Orientation and Gender Identity*. New York: Services and Advocacy for GLBT Elders. http://www.sageusa.org/resources/publications.cfm?ID=161.

Niles, N. J. (2011). *Basics of the U.S. Health Care System*. Sudbury, MA: Jones and Barlett Publishers.

Psychological Association of the Philippines (2010). *Code of Ethics for Philippine Psychologists*. http://www.pap.org.ph/includes/view/default/uploads/code_of_ethics_pdf.pdf.

Seaburn, D. B., Lorenz, A. D., Gunn, W. B., Jr Gawinski, B. A., and Mauksch, L. B. (2003). *Models of Collaboration: A Guide for Mental Health Professionals Working with Health Care Practitioners*. New York: Basic Books.

Smith, T. W. (2013). 'Cross-national Differences in Attitudes toward Homosexuality'. http://williamsinstitute.law.ucla.edu/wp-content/uploads/Smith-CrossNational-NORC-May-2011.pdf.

Sue, D. W., Arredondo, P., and McDavis, R. J. (1992). 'Multicultural Counseling Competencies and Standards: A Call to the Profession'. *Journal of Counseling and Development* 70: 477–486.

Sue, D. W. and Sue, D. (2008). *Counseling the Culturally Diverse: Theory and Practice*, (5th edn). Hoboken, NJ: Wiley.

Travis, L. (2011). *Elder Care: A Resource for Interprofessional Providers: What You Should Know about LGBT Older Adults*. Tucson, AZ: Donald W. Reynolds Foundation, Arizona Geriatric Education Center, and the Arizona Center on Aging. http://www.reynolds.med.arizona.edu/EduProducts/providerSheets/LGBT.pdf.

Wierzalis, E. A., Barret, B., Pope, M., and Rankins, M. (2006). 'Gay Men and Aging: Sex and Intimacy'. In D. Kimmel, T. Rose, and S. David (eds), *Lesbian, Gay, Bisexual, and Transgender Aging: Research and Clinical Perspectives* (pp. 91–109). New York: Columbia University Press.

....

CHAPTER 39

CARING FOR CARE-GIVERS OF A PERSON WITH DEMENTIA

....

MARIAN TZUANG AND DOLORES GALLAGHER-THOMPSON

INTRODUCTION

As the number of older persons increases worldwide, dementia is becoming an increasingly challenging global public health concern. A recent Alzheimer's Disease International (2009) report estimated that about thirty-six million people worldwide are currently living with dementia, with numbers doubling every twenty years to sixty-six million by 2030, and 115 million by 2050. In this chapter, we use the term 'dementia' to refer to Alzheimer's disease (AD) and related disorders (e.g. frontal temporal dementia, vascular dementia), unless otherwise specified. Please note that most research has been conducted with patients with known AD, which is the most prevalent type of dementia.

The loss of independence and functioning typically associated with chronic illnesses or disabilities cause care-giving and care receiving to occur at any point in the course of life. All over the world, the costs and burdens of providing care for dementia patients rest primarily on the shoulders of one critical resource—the family members of the patient (World Health Organization and Alzheimer's Disease International 2012). For example, over 15 million Americans provided on average 21.9 hours of unpaid care per week to persons debilitated by dementia in the US (Alzheimer's Association 2012). Globally, it is estimated that there were 35.6 million people living with dementia in 2010; nearly two-thirds live in low and middle income countries where the sharpest increases in numbers are expected to occur (Alzheimer's Disease International 2011). However, fewer than a dozen countries worldwide currently have national plans or programmes in place to address dementia. Such programmes focus on improving early diagnosis, raising public awareness about the disease and reducing barriers to care, and providing better services and support to care-givers, according to WHO (World Health Organization and Alzheimer's Disease International 2012). In this same report, it was noted that even in high income countries having more comprehensive health and social care systems, the role of families and their need for support is often overlooked; whereas in lower-to-middle income countries, the reliability and universality of the family care system is often overestimated.

The rising number of adults with dementia creates a growing demand for care-givers (CGs) around the world. In this chapter the term 'care-giver' is used to describe family members who provide informal unpaid care to an older relative with Alzheimer's disease or another form of dementia. There is also an increase in diversity of that segment of the population in some countries, for example, in the US. As a result, there is considerable interest worldwide in helping CGs from divergent sociocultural contexts to decrease the stress and negative impacts associated with care-giving. The primary reasons to develop and disseminate cost-effective interventions for CGs are both to ease psychological (and other forms of) distress that are common in this situation, and to enable them to remain in the care-giving role longer (thus avoiding or delaying costly institutional placement) and in a more productive manner (avoiding lost time at work and/or reduced productivity) (Gallagher-Thompson et al. 2012).

We will begin first with a snapshot of who the CGs are and what they do. An overview of the consequences of care-giving is discussed next, followed by our conceptual model of the various outcomes (both positive and negative) that are associated with dementia care-giving, and our observations as to what key variables impact those outcomes. We will then present recommendations for assessment tools that can be used both in clinical and in research settings. Next, we will identify various evidence-based interventions designed to reduce dementia CG distress. Also discussed are some 'promising' interventions that are currently in the pipeline. We will then address some barriers and challenges for implementing interventions. And lastly, a summary of the key points addressed in this chapter will be provided, along with implications for practice and for future research in the field.

WHO ARE THE CARE-GIVERS?

Family CGs can be defined in several ways: by their relationship to the care-recipient (spouse, adult children, daughters- and sons-in-law, etc.), by whether or not they are the primary or secondary care-giver; type of living arrangements (co-resident with the care recipient or living separately); and extent of care input (regular, occasional or routine). CGs can be involved in providing 'hands-on' care or—also a very significant role—in organizing care delivered by others, even from a distance. Primary CGs are 'persons who spend most of the time with the person with dementia', and secondary CGs are those family and friends who 'play a supplementary role to the care of a relative' (Gaugler et al. 2003).

In the US, when compared with CGs of individuals with other conditions, dementia care-givers were more likely to be older (average of 52 years of age), female (70.3%), married (72.8%), and white (80%). Moreover, they tend to be the primary breadwinners of their household (55%); nearly half are employed full or part time; half of these CGs live under the same roof with the care recipient; 30% had children under 18; and almost half take care of their parents, with about 20% taking care of a spouse (Alzheimer's Association 2012).

In studies outside the US women are again found to outnumber men as primary CGs, but most CGs were spouses (rather than adult children) in the European studies (Schneider et al. 1999). Similar results were reported for the multi-centre study by the 10/66 Dementia

Research Group (10/66 Dementia Research Group 2004) that included dementia CGs in Latin America and some Asian countries as well. With the inevitable demographic shift as the population ages, countries will see an impact on the size of family network as well as its availability and willingness to provide care for frail older relatives (Kaneda 2011).

WHAT DO CARE-GIVERS DO?

Family CGs are confronted with multiple tasks that evolve throughout the stages of dementia.

Typically, the list of tasks increases as the disease progresses, starting with support for instrumental activities of daily living (grocery shopping, preparing meals, providing transportation, managing finances) and expanding to include personal care (bathing, feeding, toileting), and eventually almost constant supervision to avoid unsafe activities such as wandering. The extent of need and the types of care needed, and their progression over time, depend on many factors such as the clinical profile (types and severity of cognitive impairments and behavioural and psychological symptoms, which may vary by subtype of dementia), the presence of comorbid physical and psychological problems, the custom and habits of the person with dementia (PWD), his/her personality and prior coping skills, and, most importantly, their relationship history with the CG (World Health Organization and Alzheimer's Disease International 2012). In the later stages, CGs usually need the assistance of professional carers if the PWD continues living in the community, or is moved to an assisted-living facility or nursing home. Yet many CGs still continue to assist with both instrumental activities of daily living (e.g. making arrangements for medical care, managing legal affairs, and providing emotional support) and personal care tasks (bathing or dressing their loved one) even after he/she is placed in a nursing home or other extended care facility (Garity 2006; Port et al. 2005; Schulz et al. 2004).

CONSEQUENCES OF DEMENTIA CARE-GIVING

Caring for a person with dementia poses special challenges. Studies have shown that dementia CGs often provide more hours of care, have a greater number of care-giving tasks, and longer duration of care-giving compared to CGs of persons with other chronic illness such as cancer or heart disease (Ory et al. 1999; Steadman, Tremon, and Davis 2007; Tremont, Davis, and Bishop 2006). Although care-giving can be (and often is) rewarding in some ways to the primary CG, there is a well-documented set of negative effects that are typically found in long-term care-giving across a variety of ethnic, cultural, and racial groups that have been studied. These negative impacts include: depressive symptoms and other negative emotions (e.g. anxiety, frustration, and guilt); poor self-rated health; poor actual health (e.g. compromised immune function and dysregulated cortisol function); social isolation; and possibly heightened rates of mortality (Akkerman and Ostwald 2004; Andren and Elmstahl 2005; Beach et al. 2005; Brodaty and Hadzi-Pavlovic 1990; Coon et al. 2004; Pinquart and Sörensen 2003; Prince et al. 2011; Shaw et al. 1997; Sörensen et al. 2006). In addition to these effects on the primary CG, the challenges of caring for a demented person on a day-to-day basis can also have profound negative impacts on family dynamics and role functioning (Qualls 1997; Qualls and Vair 2013). Thus, CGs are often regarded as society's 'hidden patients' whose need for adequate support and intervention is very real, yet is often overlooked in the process of evaluating and treating the PWD. Clearly, the emphasis needs to shift to include *both* CG and PWD in assessment and intervention programmes.

Psychological well-being

Prevalence of depressive symptoms is high in virtually all groups studied, averaging 30–50%, depending on methodology and measures used (Ballard et al. 1996; Cuijpers 2005; Gallagher et al. 1989; Pinquart and Sörensen 2003; Schulz and Beach 1999; Schulz et al. 1995; Spector and Tampi 2005). Women CGs have higher levels of depressive and anxiety symptoms and lower life satisfaction compared to men (Miller and Cafasso 1992; Yee and Schulz 2000). The risk of developing an affective disorder is higher for CGs after many years of care-giving and even after care-giving ends, following the death of the care recipient (Robinson-Whelen et al. 2001; Schulz and Beach 1999; Schulz et al. 2006). A similar trend is present in studies done outside of the US. The 10/66 Dementia Research Group found that the levels of psychological morbidity among 706 CGs of people with dementia were at least as high as those seen in studies conducted in high-income countries (Prince 2004).

Studies have also found reduced quality of life (Markowitz et al. 2003; Pinquart and Sörensen 2003). On the other hand, several studies have also found that care-giving can be a very positive experience for the primary CG, despite the stress that is associated with it (Aranda and Knight 1997; Cohen, Colantonio, and Vernich 2002; Coon, Ory, and Schulz 2004; Dilworth-Anderson et al. 2004; Roff et al. 2004).

Physical health

Negative physical health impacts include: compromised immune function (e.g. greater susceptibility to colds and infections and longer time to heal) (Kiecolt-Glaser et al. 1991; Vitaliano et al. 2003), high blood pressure and related heart problems) (King, Oka, and Young 1994; Shaw et al. 1997), and dysregulated cortisol (e.g. in contrast to the normal diurnal rhythm seen in non-highly stressed persons, this physiological marker of stress remains high over a period of time—this situation is implicated in many health problems) (see Holland et al. 2010; 2011 for studies specifically on CG stress and cortisol). In addition, reduced engagement in preventive health behaviours (Schulz et al. 1997; Vitaliano et al. 2003) and poorer health maintenance practices (Rabinowitz et al. 2007) have also been found. Thus, evidence is accumulating that the chronic stress associated with dementia care-giving may increase susceptibility to a host of illnesses; although clearly more research is needed to demonstrate any causal links. Furthermore, women and ethnic minority CGs report poorer health than men and Caucasian CGs (Pinquart and Sörensen 2005). Unique to dementia CGs, patient problem behaviours are consistently linked to both psychiatric and physical morbidity of the care-giver, and patient cognitive impairment is consistently related to physical morbidity of the care-giver (Majerovitz 1995; Moritz et al. 1992; Schulz et al. 1995).

Finally, we would like to call the reader's attention to an issue that is currently receiving a great deal of research attention—that is, availability of other family members to support the primary CG. Although the general assumption is that CGs who have large inter-generational families (typically found in more traditional societies and among ethnic minority groups) will cope better with dementia and are relatively immune from care-giver distress, this does not seem to actually be the case. Pilot studies across twenty-five sites of the 10/66 Dementia Research Group in Africa, Latin America, China, and India revealed levels of care-giver strain comparable to those seen in European and Northern American studies (Prince 2004). Similar US studies and reviews have also made this point (Dilworth-Anderson and Gibson 2002; Dilworth-Anderson et al. 2002; Neary and Mahoney 2005; Scharlach et al. 2006; Torti et al. 2004), suggesting that many times the primary CG is not able to rely on informal support from within the family. The changing role of family members regarding their engagement in care for a relative with dementia needs to be taken into account in the design and implementation of CG intervention programmes.

THEORETICAL MODELS OF CARE-GIVER DISTRESS

Care-giving is a complex and ever-changing process. There are certainly positive aspects of care-giving that have been well-documented, but for the most part, disparities in the CGs' social and financial resources, psychological coping capabilities, and wide variance in the care recipients' degree of impairment and the frequency and intensity of their problem behaviours make it very difficult to infer causal relationships. Often the 'stress' in care-giving comes from multiple sources, so CGs must adopt different strategies to deal with these multiple problems. Over the past two decades, several models have been proposed to guide our understanding of CGs and their psychosocial needs. The one that has been predominantly used is by Pearlin et al. (Pearlin et al. 1990). This was an elaboration of Folkman's original 'stress process' model (Folkman 1984). Pearlin's model focuses on the ways in which CGs use personal and social resources (both internal and external) to respond to care-giving demands. Perceived stress is defined as the extent to which demands exceed resources, *and* the requisite coping skills to cope with these demands are no longer adequate. Furthermore, Pearlin et al. and later, Schulz and Martire (Schulz and Martire 2004) extended this theoretical work by distinguishing between *primary* and *secondary* stressors: the former refers to the multiple demands that CGs experience—such as employment demands; family needs (e.g. most CGs are married and are raising young or teenaged children), and level of care required by the PWD (a function of their diagnosis and the extent of their cognitive and behavioural problems). The latter refers to stressors that are often less obvious to clinicians (e.g. relationship strain such as competing time demands between child care and caring for the frail parent; lack of support from other family members; and disputes over financial matters related to care). When CGs perceive these demands as potential threats, and see themselves as without sufficient coping capacities or strategies to meet these demands, they experience stress. According to these models, the greater the stress (defined in these terms), the more likely the CG is to be at risk for physical and psychiatric illnesses. At the same time, this model shows how multifaceted coping resources and external supports might alleviate the impact of these stressors and potentially reduce negative outcomes down the road.

Conceptual models that include 'cultural context' and diversity as key components

Over the years, as more care-giving research was done in ethnic minority populations in the US (as well as other parts of the world), the importance of recognizing and appreciating both diversity and the 'cultural context of care-giving' have become more widely recognized (Dilworth-Anderson et al. 2002). We define 'diversity' here to include differences in beliefs about dementia, care-giving, family role expectations, and help-seeking beliefs and actions that are based on race, ethnicity, culture, and/or sexual orientation. Within the last decade 'cultural diversity' has been added as an important dimension to the 'stress process' model. Simply put, this means recognizing and appreciating the fact that each ethnic/racial/cultural/sexually diverse group presents a different set of strengths and vulnerabilities that can guide CG assessment and treatment (Aranda and Knight 1997; Connell and Gibson 1997; Dilworth-Anderson et al. 2002; Hilgeman et al. 2009; Knight et al. 2000; Pinquart and Sörensen 2005; Zeiss et al. 2010).

Specifically, Aranda and Knight (1997) proposed a sociocultural stress and coping model that acknowledges that cultural differences can affect the appraisal of care-giving, what is considered 'stressful', and what coping skills might be used to handle that stress. Other models have also been introduced that examine the role of culturally situated factors as mediators of CG outcomes (Hilgeman et al. 2009; Montoro-Rodriguez and Gallagher-Thompson 2009). It is important that while some cultural beliefs and practices, such as religiosity and/or spirituality, can buffer and protect CGs from negative mental and physical health outcomes associated with care-giving, other cultural beliefs—such as filial obligation (referred to as 'filial piety' in most Asian cultures and 'familism' in Hispanic/Latino cultures, which is the belief that the needs of the collective, in this case the family, comes first and take precedence over the needs of the CG)—may work in the opposite way and actually prevent CGs from 'reaching out' to get the help they need. How these cultural beliefs may serve as facilitators *or* barriers to care will be explored further, below. To date, few models have attempted to integrate both 'stress process' concepts and cultural diversity issues into one comprehensive model. In Figure 39.1 we present such a model.

ASSESSMENT APPROACHES WITH DEMENTIA FAMILY CARE-GIVERS

In order to use this model to guide research and practice it is necessary to be able to assess or evaluate its various components in reliable ways. This section (referring to Figure 39.1) is a review of measures that we believe tap into these constructs.

Background variables and cultural context

To assess cultural context, we recommend (besides the obvious indices of age, relationship to care recipient, length of time as a care-giver, etc.) inquiring about his/her immigration

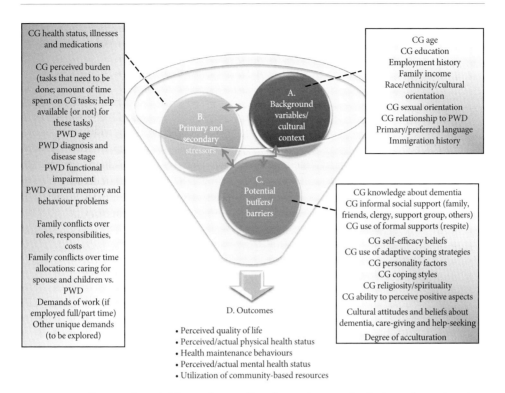

CG health status, illnesses and medications

CG perceived burden (tasks that need to be done; amount of time spent on CG tasks; help available {or not} for these tasks)
PWD age
PWD diagnosis and disease stage
PWD functional impairment
PWD current memory and behaviour problems

Family conflicts over roles, responsibilities, costs
Family conflicts over time allocations: caring for spouse and children vs. PWD
Demands of work (if employed full/part time)
Other unique demands (to be explored)

A. Background variables/ cultural context

B. Primary and secondary stressors

C. Potential buffers/ barriers

D. Outcomes
• Perceived quality of life
• Perceived/actual physical health status
• Health maintenance behaviours
• Perceived/actual mental health status
• Utilization of community-based resources

CG age
CG education
Employment history
Family income
Race/ethnicity/cultural orientation
CG sexual orientation
CG relationship to PWD
Primary/preferred language
Immigration history

CG knowledge about dementia
CG informal social support (family, friends, clergy, support group, others)
CG use of formal supports (respite)
CG self-efficacy beliefs
CG use of adaptive coping strategies
CG personality factors
CG coping styles
CG religiosity/spirituality
CG ability to perceive positive aspects

Cultural attitudes and beliefs about dementia, care-giving and help-seeking
Degree of acculturation

FIGURE 39.1 Proposed model for understanding dementia care-giver's strengths and strains.

history (where the person was born and educated, number of years in host country), preferred language for thinking, speaking, reading, and writing; and preferences for friends, foods, cultural celebrations, etc. that are important to the individual. Based on responses, one might want to ask additional questions related to the extent to which the person describes him/herself as aware of the common belief systems operating in western medicine. A useful tool for this is the LEARN model, a cross-cultural communication tool to help practitioners overcome communication and cultural barriers to successful patient education. There are five steps: (1) L: Listen with sympathy and understanding to the patient's perception of the problem; (2) E: Explain your perceptions of the problem; (3) A: Acknowledge and discuss the differences and similarities; (4) R: Recommend treatment; (5) N: Negotiate agreement (Berlin and Fowkes 1983).

Primary and secondary stressors

1 It is crucial to assess for basic safety needs of both care-giver and care recipient: Safety issues for both CG and the PWD may include (but are not limited to): (1) care recipient's continued driving, which can potentially pose danger to him/herself and others in the car; (2) home environmental safety (presence of throw rugs, steep steps instead of ramps for those using a wheelchair or walker, and easy access to household cleaning products which the PWD may not recognize as such); and finally,

(3) abuse and neglect—although these remain problems largely hidden and under-reported (Cooney, Howard, and Lawlor 2006; Cooper et al. 2009; Wiglesworth et al. 2010; Yan and Kwok 2010). When abuse is detected, clinicians should be aware of any legal requirements in their own region and country to make referrals to local authorities to further investigate and resolve the situation.

2 The Revised Memory and Behavior Problems Checklist (RMBPC) is a twenty-four-item, self-report measure specifically designed to assess the frequency of behavioural problems in dementia patients, as well as how the CG reacted to each of the problems. CGs indicate how much they were 'stressed' or 'bothered' by each problem in the past week (Teri et al. 1992). Clinically, it helps guide the clinician to identify the nature of the behavioural problems exhibited by the PWD, while learning which of these behavioural problems bring the most distress to the CG. This allows the clinician to give specific recommendations for behaviour management and/or to refer the CG to appropriate community resources. The authors also suggest that it can be used to monitor changes in the PWD over time and as a treatment evaluation tool for CGs who presumably would report less distress following participation in a successful intervention programme.

Potential buffers and barriers

1 Care-giver's knowledge of dementia: It is helpful when care-givers accurately understand what dementia is (and is not), what the likely progression of a disease like Alzheimer's will be, and what treatment options are available. A commonly used measure is the Knowledge of Alzheimer's Disease (KAD) (Gray et al. 2009; Roberts and Connell 2000). KAD has four subscales with a total of fourteen-item true/false questions that assess respondents' knowledge, attitudes, and beliefs regarding Alzheimer's disease. In our experience, CGs with low education (below eighth grade) and with low 'health literacy' defined by the Institute of Medicine report (Nielsen-Bohlman et al. 2004) as 'the degree to which individuals have the capacity to obtain, process, and understand basic health information and services needed to make appropriate health decision') have less accurate knowledge of what dementia is all about, what treatments are available, and how to cope with common problems (Gray et al. 2009).

In addition, many websites (governmental and professional) have educational materials available for download with information (some translated into other languages). Three such sites in the US are, first, the national website of the Alzheimer's Association (www.alz.org), with several 'language portals' (e.g. Spanish, Chinese), which provides carefully translated print information and other resources such as DVDs and video clips. In addition, the Family Caregiver Alliance website (www.caregiver.org) and the Alzheimer's Disease Education and Referral Center (ADEAR, sponsored by the National Institute on Aging in the US) (www.nia.nih.gov/alzheimers/) are excellent sources with up-to-date accurate information for both professionals and family members. Information about Alzheimer's Associations in other countries can be found on the Alzheimer's Disease International website (www.alz.co.uk/). We recommend ordering some of these materials and having them available to hand to CGs, as well as developing a local resource list, so that gaps in CGs' knowledge can be addressed.

2 Social support:

- Lubben's Social Support Network Scale (LSNS): This is a widely used scale for measuring the social aspect of quality of life in older adults. It measures three dimensions of social networks and support: family, friends, and mutual support; and in each of the dimensions, items inquire about the size and closeness of the network, as well as frequency of contact (Lubben and Gironda 1996). Tracking an individual's social support level over time can be achieved by administering this measure at initial assessment, and at various intervals during the encounters.

- Abbreviated Duke Social Support Index (DSSI): The DSSI is an eleven-item measure to assess perceived social support (Koenig et al. 1993). The scale consists of two subscales: social satisfaction and social interaction and has been validated with older adults over age 60 (n = 1394). It asks questions such as: How many persons in this area within one hour's travel do you feel you can depend on or feel very close to?; Does it seem that your family and friends understand you most of the time, some of the time, or hardly ever?; When you are talking with your family and friends, do you feel you are being listened to most of the time, some of the time, or hardly ever?

3 Positive Aspects of Caregiving scale was developed fairly recently and has been demonstrated to be a valid and reliable instrument (Tarlow et al. 2004). This nine-item questionnaire assesses the extent to which the CG is satisfied with their role and derives pleasure from it. This is an important construct to include in a comprehensive assessment since many CGs experience both positive and negative feelings that change over time.

4 Self-Efficacy Measure (Steffen et al. 2002): This measure has three subscales: self-efficacy for obtaining respite; for controlling upsetting thoughts; and for responding to disruptive behaviour. CGs rate the extent to which they feel confident that they can do the specific behaviours mentioned which were selected and honed from earlier pilot work. Although an interviewer-administered, rather than a self-report measure (and therefore more time consuming to give), this has proved to be a valuable moderator variable in explaining why some CGs benefit from interventions and some do not (Rabinowitz et al. 2006). It is also useful for identifying CGs who are most vulnerable for depression (Rabinowitz et al. 2009).

5 Sense of Mastery: A commonly used tool to measure one's global sense of personal control is the seven-item scale developed by Pearlin and Schooler (Pearlin and Schooler 1978). When applied to CGs, it asks how strongly they agree or disagree on statements such as 'I have little control over the things that happen to me,' 'I often feel helpless in dealing with the problems of life,' and 'I can do just about anything I really set my mind to do.' A higher score indicates higher levels of mastery.

Culturally related constructs are discussed next. These include:

6 Acculturation: Degree of acculturation plays an important role in various health issues among ethnic minority individuals. In the context of care-giving, it has been associated with illness perception and help-seeking—both its likelihood and the type of help sought. Acculturation measures intend to capture the psychological, behavioural, and

attitudinal changes that occur when an individual comes in continuous contact with another culture different from their original culture (Cabassa 2003).

- Measuring acculturation in Latino Americans: Two rating scales have been developed for Hispanic/Latinos in the United States: Bidimensional Acculturation Scale for Hispanics (BAS) (Marín and Gamba 1996) and Acculturation Rating Scale for Mexican Americans-Revised (ARSMA-II) (Cuellar, Arnold, and Maldonado 1995). Both measures have flaws that have been raised (Cabassa 2003), namely their non-continuous design, and BAS moreover for all its items being language-based. ARSMA-II is considered to be a stronger measure that includes different cultural domains inherent in the acculturation process (such as changes in attitudes and values) rather than relying solely on language-based items. ARSMA-II has been validated in older adult and care-giver populations (Haan et al. 2003, Jimenez et al. 2010). A modification of ARSMA-II was made for geriatric population, the Geriatric Acculturation Ratings Scale for Mexican Americans (G-ARSMA) (Gonzalez, Haan, and Hinton 2001).
- Measuring acculturation in Asian populations: The twenty-one-item Suinn-Lew Self Identity Acculturation Scale (SL-ASIA) assesses the degree of acculturation of Asian Americans. It has been used successfully with people in various age groups (Suinn, Ahuna, and Khoo 1992).
- It is recommended that clinicians and researchers become familiar with this construct so that they can measure it and include that information when selecting the most appropriate intervention programme for a particular individual CG.

7 Familism: This is one of the core cultural values in Hispanic/Latino groups. Although there are several existing scales that measure this construct, we recommend the Attitudinal Familism Scale which consists of eighteen items assessing familial support, familial interconnectedness, familial honour, and subjugation of self to family (Lugo Steidel and Contreras 2003). Assessing the CGs' strength of belief in familism may help clinicians identify whether or not it serves as a protective factor (buffering the CG against stress) or whether it seems to contribute to the degree of stress experienced (Gallagher-Thompson et al. 2006; Kim, Knight, and Longmire 2007; Knight et al. 2002).

8 Filial Piety: Filial piety, or 'xiao' in Mandarin Chinese, is a Confucian concept which encompasses a broad range of attitudes, behaviours, obligations, and expectations, for each individual in the family. Several studies have examined the effects of filial piety on the appraisal of care-giving burden by family care-givers, mostly done with Chinese American or Canadian care-givers, and care-givers in some Asian countries (Chou, Lamontage, and Hepworth 1999; Lai 2010; Zhan and Montgomery 2003). A number of measures examining filial concepts across cultures are available and are introduced in Jones, Lee, and Zhang (2011). We have not found universal agreement in terms of the best scale to recommend at this time.

9 Spiritual/Religious Beliefs: Religion and/or spirituality can be important coping resources for care-givers. For many, expressing their religious beliefs and participating in religious practices (going to church, reading the Bible) provide comfort and solace during times of stress. For others who do not identify with a particular religion but who are spiritually oriented, beliefs and practices that stem from their spiritual orientation towards life can also be a source of strength and serve

to buffer against possible negative outcomes from care-giving. For a review of the research on this topic please see Hebert et al. (2006). Here we introduce two measures: Duke University Religion Index and the Santa Clara Strength of Religious Faith Questionnaire. The Duke University Religion Index is a five-item scale that asks questions about an individual's religious beliefs and religious involvements (Koenig, Parkerson, and Meador 1997). It has been used in large cross-sectional and longitudinal observational studies, and included in epidemiological surveys to examine relationships between religion and health outcomes (Koenig and Büssing 2010). It is now available in ten languages.

Santa Clara Strength of Religious Faith Questionnaire: The SCSRF questionnaire is a ten-item measure that asks about the strength and importance of religious faith regardless of denomination. This instrument is quick and easy to administer and score, and has the ability to assess the core behaviours and beliefs associated with many organized religions (Plante and Boccaccini 1997).

Outcomes

A variety of measures exist to assess the impact of care-giving; here we recommend several that are widely used in both clinical and research settings.

1 WHOQOL-BREF: This scale is based on the WHOQOL-100, a rigorously tested scale on quality of life that was developed simultaneously in fifteen field centres around the world and that takes into account inputs from patients and health professionals in a variety of cultures. It is an abbreviated version, with just twenty-six items that measure the following broad domains: physical health, psychological health, social relationships, and environment (World Health Organization 2012). This shortened version allows for easier utilization in research studies, clinical trials, and clinical practices. This instrument is now available in seven languages other than English, and can be downloaded from www.who.int/substance_abuse/research_tools/whoqolbref/en/.

2 To assess depressive symptoms, one reliable measure is the Center for Epidemiologic Studies Depression Scale (CES-D). This is a twenty-item self-report that asks about the frequency of occurrence of common depression symptoms in the past week (Radloff 1977). CES-D is not copyrighted and is available by doing a Google search. It is also easily scored by hand. Individuals having a score of 16 and above are likely to be clinically depressed, as established in numerous studies in the US and other countries. For more information, visit cesd-r.com/.

The Geriatric Depression Scale (GDS) is another reliable measure to screen for depression that has also been widely used around the world. It was designed to incorporate more psychological aspects of depression and purposively reduced somatic items (Sheikh and Yesavage 1986). The simple 'yes/no' response format makes it easier for CGs with limited education or low health literacy to understand. All language versions as well as several short forms of the GDS are downloadable from the website: www.stanford.edu/~yesavage/GDS.html. The latest development is that it now has free iPhone and Android apps that allow subscribers to do the fifteen-item GDS (the short form) on the phone and have it automatically scored for them. However, it has not been widely used with care-givers, probably since so many care-givers are younger or middle-aged.

3 In addition to assessing mental distress, we recommend assessment of several key indices of physical health. The most common one used is overall perceived physical health status, which generally ranges from 'excellent' to 'poor' on a 4- or 5-point Likert-type scale. For more in-depth assessment, we suggest inquiries about current health symptoms, actual diagnosed health problems, current medications, health maintenance behaviours, and extent of functional limitations (if any). No one single scale exists at present that taps into all of these dimensions. The extent and depth of these inquiries will depend to some extent on the amount of time available, and the purpose for collecting the information. If only one self-report can be used (and no actual measures of physical health, such as blood pressure, lipids, heart rate, immune system function or HPA axis function can be collected, for whatever reason), then we recommend the SF-36 or its briefer version, the SF-12, both of which have been extensively researched. The SF-36 Health Survey is a comprehensive tool that assesses both physical and mental components of health including physical functioning, role limitations due to physical health problems, social functioning, emotional well-being, pain, energy and/or fatigue, and general health perceptions (Ware 1998). Results can be used in screening and monitoring individuals over time. More information can be found at the website: www.sf-36.org/tools/SF36.shtml. This measure is copyrighted. Requests for permission to use can be sent to sfinfo@qualitymetric.com.

Multi-dimensional measures: These were developed to be quick, effective ways to get a general sense of how distressed the CG is, overall. They give only a 'broad brush' overview, and no fine-grained detail, as would the measures previously discussed. That said, they can be very useful in busy clinical practices where there is not sufficient time to do an in-depth assessment. These two can be recommended for their brevity, as well as their good psychometric properties.

The 16-item Risk Appraisal Measure (RAM) is a brief screen that helps identify risk areas and guide interventions. Originally developed as part of the multi-site randomized clinical intervention project called 'Resources for Enhancing Alzheimer's Caregiver Health' (REACH II), and specifically for ethnically diverse dementia care-givers, this particular measure evaluates a range of care-giving stressors (depression, burden, self-care and health behaviours, social support, safety, and patient problem behaviours) while remaining short enough to be administered during a typical patient doctor's visit or in the waiting room. This measure can be used in research, clinical and community settings to guide, prioritize, and target efforts to reduce care-giver distress (Czaja et al. 2009). RAM is also available in Spanish; copies can be obtained from the study authors.

The Caregiver Self-Assessment Questionnaire developed by the American Medical Association is a brief questionnaire that was developed and tested for distribution in physician's offices. CGs are encouraged to complete the form when they accompany the PWD to the doctor's visit. Scores serve as an index of care-giver distress which the physician can then use to make appropriate referrals or discuss other services. It should be noted that this measure was not specifically developed for dementia CGs, and its use and effectiveness in settings outside the physician's offices has not yet been demonstrated. This screening tool can be downloaded from www.ama-assn.org/ama/pub/physician-resources/public-health/promoting-healthy-lifestyles/geriatric-health/care-giver-health/care-giver-self-assessment.page and is also available in Spanish.

In summary, depending upon different practice settings (i.e. mental health outpatient clinic or a support group vs an academic research study or a community-based translational study), the clinician or investigator will want to focus more or less on specific domains of interest, and will be limited by available time and resources. Interested readers may find more information on various care-giver assessment measures from the Family Caregiver Alliance website (www.caregiver.org), in particular, the 'Caregivers Count Too!' toolkit for practitioners. The toolkit is nicely organized to include general literature on care-giver assessment, reviews of care-giver assessment measures, as well as international literature on this topic. Alternatively, readers can refer to several recently published review articles on measures for research in dementia care-giving (Brodaty 2007; Moniz-Cook et al. 2008; Van Durme et al. 2011) which contain some measures in addition to the ones discussed here.

EVIDENCE-BASED INTERVENTIONS FOR DEMENTIA CARE-GIVERS

Over the years there have been a number of reviews published on evidence-based interventions for dementia family CGs. In a recent one by Coon et al. (2012), the authors provided a detailed review of studies grounded in psychological theories or models of behaviour change. They classified them into three overarching categories, namely psychoeducational skill building, psychotherapy-counselling, and multicomponent interventions. These categories are consistent with the established care-giving intervention literature (e.g. Bourgeois, Schulz, and Burgio 1996; Coon et al. 2003a; Gatz et al. 1998; Schulz, Martire, and Klinger 2005; Sörensen et al. 2002). While their review was based primarily on studies conducted in the US, a subsequent paper expanded the review to include interventions carried out in other parts of the world (Gallagher-Thompson et al. 2012). Details on each of these interventions are presented below.

Table 39.1 summarizes information from the review by Coon et al. (2012). It includes research on culturally or ethnically diverse samples within the US and some studies carried out in other countries. Some studies in this table appear more than once because multiple interventions were reported. Of special note is that while other approaches (e.g. support groups, case management, and respite care) also showed promising results, these types of intervention have not yet met the stringent criteria used to establish an intervention as 'evidence-based'. In other words, they are not empirically tested as standalone treatments for care-giver distress.

Psychoeducational skill-building interventions

An example is the Coping with Caregiving programme (CWC). Table 39.2 presents an overview of the design of a CWC programme. The original CWC format, which typically

Table 39.1 Examples of evidence-based interventions for dementia family care-givers

Interventions	Brief description	Key citations
Psychoeducational Skill-Building CG Intervention Studies	Aim is to increase CGs' knowledge of the disease and teach them to build coping skills such as dealing with their own complex feelings, reduce their care-giver-related stress, and learning to manage the common emotional and/or behavioural problems associated with dementia.	
1 Behavioural management skill training	Focuses on teaching behaviour management skills to CGs so they can respond more effectively to care recipient behaviour problems and other care-giving challenges.	Beauchamp et al. (2005); Bourgeois et al. (2002); Davis et al. (2004); Farran et al. (2004); Gonyea, O'Connor, and Boyle (2006); Graff et al. (2006); Perren, Schmid, and Wettstein (2006); Teri et al. (1997; 2005).
2 Depression management skill training	Teaches care-givers a set of cognitive and behavioural skills (e.g. challenging negative thinking patterns; increasing engagement in everyday positive activities) shown in prior research to improve depressed mood and well-being.	Au et al. (2010a); Burgio et al. (2009); Coon et al. (2003b); Gallagher-Thompson et al. (2000; 2003; 2007b; 2008); Hepburn et al. (2007); Losada et al. (2011); Márquez-González et al. (2007); Martin-Carrasco et al. (2009).
3 Progressively lowered stress threshold model	A model that focuses on modifying environmental demands to alleviate the stress experienced by persons with dementia.	Buckwalter et al. (1999); Gitlin et al. (2003a); Gitlin et al. (2005; 2008); Huang et al. (2003); Kuo et al. (2012); Teri et al. (1997).
4 Anger management skill training	Emphasizes the multiple sources of CG frustration and uses a variety of behavioural and cognitive skills to reduce anger and hostility.	Coon et al. (2003b); Steffen (2000).
5 Health maintenance training	Focuses on specific skill training for health maintenance, i.e. managing sleep disruption, frustration, or managing stress through exercise.	Castro et al. (2002); King et al. (2002); McCurry et al. (2005); Teri et al. (2003).
6 Mixed	Place greater emphasis on education and support in comparison to the skill-building components than other interventions in this category	Chien and Lee (2008); Fung and Chien (2002); Hepburn et al. (2001); Ostwald et al. (1999); Smith and Toseland (2006); Toseland, Rossiter, and Labrecque (1989).
Psychotherapy-Counselling CG Intervention Studies	Individual, or group, or family counselling provided by trained mental health providers. In contrast to psychoeducational skill-building interventions, these place more emphasis on the development and use of the therapeutic relationship in the treatment process. Both CBT and psychodynamic therapies have been used effectively with family CGs. Newer approaches, such as Acceptance and Commitment Therapy, are just now starting to be used with CGs to decrease CG depression and manage stress.	Akkerman and Ostwald (2004); Charlesworth and Reichel (2004); Gallagher-Thompson and Steffen (1994); López and Crespo (2008); Márquez-González et al. (2010); Marriott et al. (2000).
Multicomponent CG Intervention Studies	Interventions that incorporate two or more conceptually different approaches into one intervention package.	Belle et al. (2006); Brodaty and Gresham (1989); Brodaty, Gresham, and Luscombe (1997); Eisdorfer et al. (2003); Gallagher-Thompson et al. (2003; 2008); Gitlin et al. (2003b); Hilgeman et al. (2009); Holland, Currier, and Gallagher-Thompson (2009); Mittelman et al. (1993; 1996; 2004; 2006; 2007; 2008); Schulz et al. (2003).

involves face-to-face contact in a small group for a period between eight and twelve weeks, was culturally adapted and used successfully in Hong Kong (Au et al. 2010a) and Spain (Losada et al. 2004). It is currently being adapted to the needs of Australian CGs of PWD, and recently a significant revision was completed so that basic CWC skills could be taught to grandparents providing primary care to grandchildren. This work is 'in progress' and at present there are no published reports on its effectiveness; however, verbal communications with that project's team leader indicate that the flexibility of the CWC approach has been well received by this new population.

Modifications have been made to the CWC, using different formats for presentation of the basic concepts and skills, and these may be of interest here. For example, in order to address stress and depression in Chinese American CGs (who, we learned from several focus groups with professionals serving this community, were reluctant to attend the group version of CWC), a DVD and an accompanying workbook (in Mandarin Chinese with a choice of English or Chinese subtitles) were developed. Then we conducted a randomized controlled trial to test the efficacy of this novel approach. We found that CGs who received the DVD and workbook were less stressed compared to those received only a purely educational DVD (also in Mandarin Chinese) that did not have a skill-training focus (Gallagher-Thompson et al. 2007b; Gallagher-Thompson et al. 2010).

Another adaptation of CWC is the *fotonovela* (FN) called 'Together We Can! Facing Memory Loss as a Family', which is a pamphlet akin to a colourful small book that uses a dramatic story line to impart health information. Although often used by the Centers for Disease Control to relay information on such chronic illnesses as diabetes and heart disease to the Latino community, only one other FN in Spanish exists on the topic of dementia. It focuses on recognition of the disease, but not on care-giver stress management. The new FN depicts some of the same skills taught in the CWC programme. Its development is detailed in Turner et al. (under review). This twenty-page FN 'tells the story' of how a Latino family learned coping skills to manage their own care-giving stress more effectively, as well as the everyday memory and behaviour problems of their loved one. An accompanying community teaching guide (aimed at clinicians or support group leaders) was also developed to explain how to use the FN to stimulate discussion. Both are available for download from the authors upon request or from http://www.alz.org/espanol/downloads/novella_span ish_081213.pdf. After materials were developed, a randomized trial was conducted in which Latino CGs who received the FN were compared to others who only received existing educational pamphlets (in Spanish or English, as preferred). Initial findings suggest that the FN improved Latino CGs' quality of life, and decreased depressive symptoms and stress. However, of note is that the FN alone was not the only factor that resulted in these positive changes. More of the CGs receiving the FN attended discussion groups (led by programme staff) to learn more about the materials provided, compared to those in the comparison condition. This may also have contributed to their positive responses (manuscript currently in preparation).

A more recent modification of the CWC is the iCare study, which to the authors' knowledge is the first internet-based programme for dementia care-givers that was derived from an evidence-based intervention (Kajiyama et al. 2013). It built in several action-oriented components and video segments that illustrate skills from the CWC. It was compared to a website with educational information culled from several national sources but without the interactive skill-building components. Results showed a decrease in the level of reported

Table 39.2 Coping with care-giving: general structure of intervention phases, class goals, and home practice that can be adapted, modified and 'tailored' as needed to fit specific needs

Classes	Goals of the class/group meeting	Home practice
Initial phase		
Class 1	Introduction, and overview of dementia, learn about the sources of frustration and anger, practice relaxation, start pleasant activities.	Daily relaxation diary.
Class 2–3	Learn the relationship between pleasant events and mood, identify pleasant events and activities, and understand and overcome personal barriers to increasing or infusing pleasant events in one's life.	Relaxation diary; pleasant events tracking form.
Second phase		
Classes 4–6	Learn cognitive skills to identify unhelpful thoughts about care-giving, change unhelpful thoughts into more helpful or adaptive ways of thinking. In class 6, start behaviour management; ABC approach.	Daily mood rating; daily thought record.
Third phase		
Classes 6–8	Learn to see how there often are antecedents to problem behaviours that can be identified and modified, as well as becoming aware of the consequences—mainly, how the CG reacts to the problem behaviour. While we may not be able to change the antecedent, we can often change how the CG responds. Using relaxation techniques and challenging unhelpful thoughts are important tools to reinforce in this process.	Daily mood rating; pleasant events tracking form/ adding: behaviour log to complete daily.
Classes 9–10	Understand types of communication (passive, assertive or effective, and aggressive) and role-play how to be more effective in asking for help with care-giving: particularly from family members and from healthcare providers.	Practice effective communication/add Communication Diary.
Class 11	Complete communication skills. Start reviewing skills learned in previous class/group meetings. Start to develop Action Plans for the future.	Relaxation diary; daily thought record; pleasant events tracking form; behaviour log and communication diary are all reviewed and CGs are encouraged to think about which ones are likely to be used in the future.
Class 12	Review skills covered in previous class/group meetings. Care-givers are encouraged to think about difficult situations that they can foresee in the next 3–6 months and are asked how they will apply the specific skills learned to those situations. When possible, these Action Plans are written in their workbooks, for future reference. At this class, a celebration or graduation ceremony is held and a certificate of completion is given out.	
Fourth phase (if necessary)		
Booster sessions as needed	Maintain and continue to fine tune skills and transfer these skills to daily care-giving situations. Typically these are held two, four, and six months later.	Transfer and practise skills in everyday life.

stress specifically related to care-giving, as well as a decrease in general perceived stress and depressive symptoms, along with improved quality of life. These positive changes were found for CGs enrolled in the iCare web-based programme compared to those who received the comparison condition.

The most recent modification of CWC that is currently under way is Project Mirela. Its aim is to create a *webnovela* that teaches the core CWC skills in a dramatic 'soap opera' fashion. This online drama will consist of eighteen episodes of fifteen to twenty minutes each that teach cognitive and behavioural skills to the whole family through dramatic enactments of how the grandmother's memory declines over time, and how the family can work together to manage their own stress and improve Mirela's quality of life. As of winter 2013, eighteen episodes were filmed and work is completed on the pilot (feasibility) study. This method of presentation has received considerable support from Latino professionals and CGs who have worked with the research team to develop and translate the materials, so it is anticipated that this type of outreach to a larger audience (though the use of the World Wide Web) will enable more Latino CGs to be helped to cope with care-giving stress.

Smaller pilot studies have been done in Farsi (with Iranian American CGs) (Azar et al. 2007) and with a group of primarily monolingual Japanese-speaking Japanese American care-givers (Gallagher-Thompson, Eto-Iwase, and Haneishi 2007a). Although these pilot studies were not randomized clinical trials, they did obtain similar positive results in terms of reducing CG stress, burden, and depression. To us this suggests that the CWC approach is both flexible and relevant to CGs from very diverse ethnic and linguistic backgrounds— assuming appropriate modifications are made in the content, and that trained bilingual and bicultural leaders are available to implement the programme.

Taken together, these results from the various CWC adaptations and changes in format suggest that at least for some culturally diverse groups (who may prefer alternatives to face-to-face individual or small group programmes) positive outcomes can still be achieved. Variations of the CWC, as well as key publications for each, are summarized in Table 39.3.

Psychotherapy-counselling care-giver interventions

The studies in this category implement individual, group, or family counselling provided by trained providers. In contrast to the psychoeducational skill-building interventions, these studies place more emphasis on development and use of the therapeutic relationship in the treatment process. All but one of them used cognitive-behavioural therapy (CBT) or was based strongly on CBT. The other study used a brief psychodynamic therapy (Gallagher-Thompson and Steffen 1994). On average, the clinicians who conducted these interventions are more professionally trained (doctoral-level psychologists, master's-level clinicians, or supervised interns or graduate-level trainees) than those in the other two categories (Coon et al. 2012). The relatively small number of studies in this category should be noted. Newer approaches, such as Acceptance and Commitment Therapy (which has been successfully used to treat depression) are just beginning to be studied in family CGs (see the chapter on ACT with Dementia Care-givers in this Handbook). Clearly, more research is needed to help clarify which CGs really require this level of intervention, since it is more costly and time-consuming to provide. However, for those CGs with a history of mental health problems and/or significant current distress (e.g. diagnosed depression, substance

Table 39.3 Variations of the Coping with Caregiving programme

Programme title	Primary language/ cultural group	Objectives and target population	Key publication
Coping with Caregiving (CWC) (original version)	English	Aims to teach a core set of coping skills to manage stress and mood, using a small group/workshop format, over 8–12 weeks.	Gallagher-Thompson et al. (2003; 2008).
iCare Project	English	CWC content and delivery mode were modified to create an internet-based programme consisting of several action-oriented components, including videotaped segments illustrating specific skills for stress management taken from the CWC protocol.	Kajiyama et al. (2013).
REACH I*	English and Spanish/ Caucasian, Black and Hispanic Americans	Six centres collaborated to develop a set of common core measures that were used in the intervention research programmes carried out (uniquely) at each site. At the Palo Alto site, the focus was on evaluation of the CWC programme, compared to an enhanced support group and a telephone counselling condition. CWC was superior to the two comparison conditions.	Gallagher-Thompson et al. (2003; 2008); Gitlin et al. (2003b); Holland et al. (2009); Schulz et al. (2003).
REACH II*	English and Spanish/ Caucasian, Black and Hispanic Americans	Parts of the active intervention protocol used at all REACH II study sites were derived from CWC. The length of treatment was extended to include nine home visits, six phone calls, and five telephone support groups. This active intervention was compared to a minimal contact control condition. Two unique features of REACH II were: CGs were included only if they reported care-related distress, and the treatments were more flexible and tailored to the needs of individual care-givers through the use of the Risk Appraisal process.	Belle et al. (2006).
Cognitive-behavioural training for dementia family care-givers	Spanish/CGs in Spain	CWC was modified and adapted for use for Spanish-speaking dementia family care-givers in Spain. The training emphasized modification of dysfunctional thoughts about care-giving.	Losada et al. (2011); Losada et al., (2004).
The Fotonovela Project	English and Spanish/ Hispanic/Latino Americans	This is a recent adaptation of CWC for Latino, Spanish-speaking care-givers. A fotonovela was developed that depicted most of the core CWC skills in an illustrated booklet showing successful ways to handle common stressful care-giving situations.	Manuscript in preparation.

Programme	Population	Description	Reference
Webnovela: Project Mirela	Spanish/Hispanic/Latino Americans	A new intervention called Webnovela, a short online Telenovela in Spanish, is specifically designed for Hispanic care-givers to teach them how to cope with dementia care-giving, reduce burden of care, decrease stress, and alleviate depression. It is based on CWC. A DVD will also be created for non-internet users.	Study currently in progress.
In-home programme for Chinese Dementia Caregivers	Mandarin Chinese/Chinese Americans	CWC was modified into an in-home behavioural management programme that taught psychological skills to deal with care-giving stress.	Gallagher-Thompson et al. (2007b).
The Chinese Caregiver DVD Project	Mandarin Chinese/Chinese Americans	With input from an Advisory Board consisting of Chinese-American bilingual/bicultural healthcare providers, a DVD (filmed in Mandarin Chinese with English subtitles) and an accompanying workbook were created to illustrate the core skills of CWC.	Gallagher-Thompson et al. (2007b; 2010).
Coping with Caregiving Group Programme	Cantonese/Chinese in Hong Kong	CWC was modified and adapted for use for Chinese family care-givers of PWD in Hong Kong. They participated in thirteen weekly training sessions, at which specific cognitive-behavioural strategies were taught to handle care-giving stress.	Au et al. (2010a).
Pilot programmes			
CWC for Iranian Americans	Farsi/Iranian Americans	CWC was simplified to have less text, more illustrations, and fewer home practice assignments. Portions of this manual have been pilot-tested with Farsi-speaking care-givers in the San Francisco Bay Area.	Azar et al. (2007).
CWC for Japanese Americans	Japanese/Japanese Americans	The original CWC was modified, implemented, and fully translated into Japanese for a primarily Japanese-speaking care-giver group recruited at and hosted by the San Jose, CA non-profit organization, Yu-Ai Kai Japanese American Community Senior Service Center.	Gallagher-Thompson et al. (2007a).

* REACH stands for Resources for Enhancing Alzheimer's Caregiver Health.

abuse problem, or chronic mental health problems they take medications for), individual therapy of one form or another, and/or pharmacotherapy, may well be the treatment(s) of choice.

Multicomponent intervention programmes

Multicomponent interventions incorporate two or more conceptually different approaches into one intervention package with the goal being to enhance effectiveness. The REACH II multisite study is one significant example: it used a combination of home visits, telephone follow-up calls, and telephone-based support groups, provided over a four-month period, to a sample of over six hundred CGs (African American, Hispanic/Latino American, and Caucasian). REACH II is the largest randomized trial for dementia CGs conducted in the US. The study found that on a number of 'quality of life' indices, CGs who received the active intervention improved to a significantly greater extent than those in the minimal contact control condition. Another well-known approach is that developed by Mittelman et al. which included comprehensive assessment and counselling for both CGs and other family members. Counselling was conducted by trained social workers and it aimed to reduce conflict and improve communication among family members. Additional counselling and support were provided by telephone on an as-needed basis for up to one year (Mittelman et al. 1996; 1993). Results indicated improved psychological well-being on several outcome measures along with delay in institutional placement for those in the active intervention compared to those in the control condition. Finally, a very different kind of multicomponent programme was developed by Gitlin and colleagues. It uses occupational therapists to do a comprehensive assessment of CG needs and the strengths and capabilities of the care recipient. Based on those assessments, a variety of interventions are implemented. In general, they focus on enabling CGs and their families to better manage care-giving tasks such as communication with the care recipient, home modifications, establishing daily routines, and engaging the PWD in meaningful activities (Gitlin et al. 2008). It is one of the few current multicomponent programmes to target both the CG and the PWD.

Reviews of multicomponent programmes generally support their efficacy (Acton and Kang 2001; Bourgeois et al. 1996; Pinquart and Sörensen 2006; Schulz 2000; Sörensen et al. 2002; Zarit and Femia 2008). However, one should note that due to the relatively small number of rigorous trials conducted to evaluate the effectiveness of multicomponent interventions, this is an area that needs further study and replication by other investigators.

Effects of these interventions

A number of reviews and meta-analyses were published in the past decade that focused on the mental and physical health—as well as social (and at times financial)—benefits of care-giver interventions (Brodaty, Green, and Koschera 2003; Gallagher-Thompson et al. 2012; Lee and Cameron 2006; Olazaran et al. 2010; Pinquart and Sörensen 2006; Smits et al. 2007; Spijker et al. 2008). Interventions reviewed included the three main categories of psychological/psychosocial (or non-pharmacological) programmes described earlier, as well as some on case management, support groups, and respite. Although some authors have raised concerns that overall effect sizes are moderate and variable, psychosocial interventions are generally considered to be positive for reducing care-giver stress, increasing CG knowledge and coping skills, strengthening social supports, and improving general well-being (Coon et al. 2012; Gallagher-Thompson et al. 2012; Knight, Lutzky, and Macofsky-Urban 1993; Pinquart and Sörensen 2006; Smits et al. 2007; Sörensen et al. 2002). Interested readers can learn more about factors that may contribute to the mixed effect sizes and variability of outcomes from such authors as Brodaty et al. (2003) and Spijker et al. (2008), who point out that many important variables that could have a major impact on CG intervention outcomes are not systematically studied. These include: heterogeneity in age, gender, relationship, living arrangements, type and severity of dementia, and degree of behavioural and psychological problems evidenced by the PWD. In addition, there may be differences in intervention effectiveness depending on the 'stage' of dementia that the PWD has reached. This has rarely been studied as a possible moderator of outcomes in the existing research reviewed here.

Also noteworthy is that a few studies have shown delayed institutional placement as a beneficial effect of care-giver interventions. However, in order to evaluate the impact of specific interventions on delay or avoidance of nursing home placement, longitudinal studies are required. These are the exception rather than the rule in care-giving research to date.

OTHER PROMISING INTERVENTIONS FOR DEMENTIA CARE-GIVERS

Although no strong evidence base exists at the moment, we wish to point to some interventions targeting dementia CGs that are being developed and studied as communications and other innovative forms of technology continue to advance. Given the rapid projected increase of the older population and the increasing demands on family CGs, it is reasonable to consider technology-based interventions as having the potential to reach a larger number of CGs (especially those living in rural or other areas where formal resources are limited) in a very cost-effective manner. A recent review described several interventions that used technology (Gallagher-Thompson et al. 2012), including:

1 Telephone/videophone consultation and/or treatment: This is the most frequently used and studied application of technology to clinical situations. It is usually carried out by clinicians for counselling and supportive services, with the goal of reducing stress and promoting optimal coping (Magnusson et al. 2004). Studies of this kind of intervention with CGs were conducted in the US (Archbold, Stewart, and Miller 1995; Finkel et al. 2007; Mahoney, Tarlow, and Jones 2003; Weiner, Rossetti, and Harrah 2011), Hong Kong (Au et al. 2010b), and Canada (Marziali and Garcia 2011).

2 Telehealth: In some parts of the world, both clinicians and their patients and CGs are offered access to electronic health records (Hassol et al. 2004; Weingart et al. 2006; Zhao et al. 2010). A novel programme in Malaysia used a text messaging reminder system (Leong et al. 2006). The most extensive one probably is the 3millionlives programme recently launched in the UK (www.3millionlives.co.uk). These

implementations could be helpful for a dementia family CG to arrange medical care for the care recipient, and improve the quality of life for both.

3 Applications using smartphones: Many apps have been developed for patients and CGs to monitor various aspects of care (i.e. medical adherence, monitoring of biometrics), though little has been done to date specifically for the dementia CG (Sarasohn-Kahn 2010). The emerging interdisciplinary field of *gerontechnology* is addressing some common health problems among older adults such as falling, wandering, depression, visual impairment, and memory failure through collaborative efforts between gerontologists and engineers (Fozard et al. 2000). Gallagher-Thompson et al. (2012) argue that use of smartphone apps for care-giving has the potential to become an attractive treatment delivery platform for dementia CGs as well.

4 Assistive technologies: Many assistive devices have been developed to improve the safety and autonomy of PWD (usually in the home environment) and bring 'peace of mind' to their CGs (Magnusson, Hanson, and Borg 2004; Magnusson, Hanson, and Nolan 2005; Topo 2009). To name a few of these technologies, there are alarm sensors that prevent dementia patients from wandering away; other sensors turn off the gas or stove automatically; etc. Whether these technologies are effective in improving CGs' quality of life, or reducing their depressive symptoms remains to be seen, since little controlled research exists at present.

5 DVD products: Several studies have used DVDs or videotapes as the format to deliver psychoeducational training to dementia family care-givers. One example is a DVD that was developed for Chinese American care-givers that taught a variety of cognitive and behavioural skills for coping with the stress of care-giving, and was presented in Mandarin Chinese (Gallagher-Thompson et al. 2010). It was evaluated in a randomized trial; results were described earlier. This approach was tailored to distribution in some regions of China, and is now currently undergoing modifications in Australia/New Zealand. Many other DVD products exist to educate dementia family CGs, and can be sought from the websites of credible sources, i.e. the Alzheimer's Association. However, few DVDs have been evaluated in randomized trials or other forms of controlled research studies.

6 Web-based service delivery programmes: As more and more people become 'computer savvy' and with the rapidly increasing availability of the internet, a number of web-based intervention programmes have appeared for dementia CGs (Bass et al. 1998; Beauchamp et al. 2005; Hepburn et al. 2003; Hepburn et al. 2007; Lewis, Hobday, and Hepburn 2010). There is also the previously mentioned iCare programme (Kajiyama et al. 2013), which was derived from an evidence-based programme and then tested in a randomized trial. Note that most of these studies were conducted in North America; other regions of the world with significant internet presence have not yet been involved in this type of research. Note also that the growth of social media and various virtual communities can be fertile ground for CGs who are motivated to seek their own sources of information. Again, these kinds of programme have not been rigorously tested or subjected to much empirical research.

Although many of the above-mentioned programmes reported favourable results, caution should be exercised before interpreting findings, as the effects were found to vary considerably among CGs with different characteristics (Powell, Chiu, and Eysenbach 2008; Topo

2009). More research and programme evaluation are needed to assess the effectiveness of technology-based programmes, and their potential to reach out to care-givers who may otherwise be 'untapped.'

UTILIZATION OF CARE-GIVER INTERVENTIONS ACROSS THE GLOBE

As identified earlier in the chapter, most CG intervention research was conducted in North America and Europe: the high-income countries, according to the World Health Organization (2012). Very few empirical studies have yet been carried out in other areas of the world, like the Asia Pacific region, some poorer regions in Europe, and the continents of India and Africa. Our search of the English-language published literature on care-giving did locate several intervention studies conducted in some of these underserved regions, including: Goa, India (Dias et al. 2008), Russia (Gavrilova et al. 2009), Taiwan (Huang et al. 2003; Kuo et al. 2012), Spain (Etxeberria et al. 2011; López, Crespo, and Zarit 2007; Losada, Márquez-González and Romero-Moreno 2011; Losada et al. 2004; Márquez-González et al. 2007), and Peru and Russia—as described in publications from the 10/66 Dementia Research Group (Gavrilova et al. 2009; Prince et al. 2009). For an overview of current best practices to support dementia CGs in different parts of the world, please see Gallagher-Thompson et al. (2012).

BARRIERS TO ACCESSING CARE-GIVER INTERVENTIONS

Unfortunately, even when evidence-based programmes exist, there is unequal access to them around the world (Alzheimer's Disease International 2011; Prince et al. 2011; WHO and Alzheimer's Disease International 2012). Barriers to access are not only found in low to middle-income countries, but also in higher-income countries (EUROFAMCARE 2006). In addition to systems barriers (lack of governmental policy planning and funding, lack of infrastructure and adequate human resources, and lack of funds for services, research, and training), other barriers pertain to individual, societal, and cultural level attitudes. They are discussed briefly below.

- Lack of knowledge among patients, CGs, and providers: There is a global shortage (both currently and in the predicted future) of physicians and other healthcare providers that have the skill set to screen, diagnose, and provide appropriate treatment or interventions for dementia patients and their CGs (Chen, Foo, and Ury 2002; MICINN 2011; Nielsen-Bohlman et al. 2004; Shaji et al. 2010; Tsolaki et al. 2010; Zarcadoolas, Pleasant, and Greer 2005). Take the IMPACT study, for example: survey results from five countries in Europe found that early signs and symptoms of dementia are difficult to detect in primary care settings as physicians lack necessary knowledge and also have negative attitudes towards dementia (Wortmann et al. 2010).

- Low health literacy and/or poor language proficiency: Poor literacy and poor health literacy (including dementia literacy), also present as barriers to accessing dementia care and services (Kwon and Kim 2011; Low and Anstey 2009; Nielsen-Bohlman et al. 2004; Zarcadoolas et al. 2005). Proficiency in health literacy includes a range of skills that are developed over a lifetime, so that individuals are able to understand medical information and follow healthcare plans. When patients and especially their CGs have low health literacy, it affects their attitudes and behaviours. In the US, low health literacy is more common in older adults and among ethnic minority older adults with poor English proficiency (Family Caregiver Alliance 2007; Paasche-Orlow et al. 2005). Similar findings have been reported in Taiwan and Spain (Lee et al. 2010; MICINN 2011). It is very likely that these problems are currently present but underreported in many parts of the world.
- Cultural beliefs and dementia: Different cultural beliefs are found to have significant influences on how dementia is perceived and on attitudes towards the medical establishment (Lai and Chung 2011; Nielsen-Bohlman et al. 2004; Nikmat, Hawthorne, and Ahmad Al-Mashoor 2011; Parry and Weiyuan 2011). Cultural beliefs also affect attitudes regarding seeking or receiving support from both within and outside the family. For example, if dementia is viewed as part of normal ageing instead of as a type of illness, and if healthcare providers are viewed with mistrust or suspicion, then there likely will also be beliefs that 'little or nothing can or should be done' (Gallagher-Thompson et al. 2012).
- More specifically to care-giving, cultural beliefs affect how care-giving itself is viewed, appraised, and dealt with (Yeo and Gallagher-Thompson 2006). For example, families in many areas of the world (particularly in Asian cultures, i.e. Chinese, Korean, Malaysian, and Asian Indian, and in some southern European countries), take on the primary care-giving responsibility for their family member with dementia without much resistance—if they value interdependence more than their own independence and if they were raised to put family needs ahead of their own. In cultures where strong *familism* or *filial piety* are present, families are also reluctant to ask for help outside the home (Alzheimer's Disease International 1999; Au et al. 2013; Etters, Goodall, and Harrison 2008; Hwang and Han 2010; Kwon and Kim 2011; Losada et al. 2010; Low et al. 2009). This can result in the delay of diagnosis and treatment for the PWD and less social and emotional support for CGs.

In summary, when these individual, systemic, and cultural barriers come into play, there is likely to be a lack of understanding about the importance of dementia diagnosis and treatment, as well as recognizing the importance of providing supportive care to the CG (Alzheimer's Australia 2008; Bond et al. 2005; Low and Anstey 2009).

IMPLICATIONS FOR PRACTICE

There are three key characteristics that can improve the effectiveness of intervention delivery in clinical practice. These are: (1) the intervention selected should be evidence-based and it should require active participation from the CG (such as role playing and developing 'action plans' to reinforce learning); (2) the intervention needs to be tailored to the specific needs of that particular CG—this is done by synthesizing information from a comprehensive initial assessment, and incorporating monitoring of change over time to see if the intervention is having the desired effects; (3) the programme needs to be delivered by trained providers who are 'faithful' to the original evidence-based approach; and (4) it needs to be of adequate duration to produce meaningful change. In many cases, bilingual/bicultural providers are needed in order to facilitate CGs having access to the services. Culturally appropriate outreach is needed to engage CGs in the programmes. Finally, programmes need to change with the progression of the care recipient's dementia decline (Woods 2010; World Health Organization and Alzheimer's Disease International 2012). Clearly, one size does *not* fit all when it comes to interventions for distressed CGs.

SUMMARY

In summary, we hope that this chapter provides the reader with a comprehensive conceptual framework for understanding not only care-giver distress but also positive aspects of care-giving, and how certain cultural and psychosocial factors can serve either as buffers against stress, or can greatly augment the stress that dementia CGs experience. We recommend specific tools for use in assessment (which we think should occur before any intervention is initiated) and we provide an understanding of the educational components that are now incorporated into many treatment protocols (such as teaching CGs behavioural approaches to manage the patient's difficult behaviours and cognitive/behavioural strategies that the CGs can apply to improve their own physical and psychological health). We encourage research that builds upon our conceptual model (which gives serious consideration to one's cultural context and associated constructs) and believe that future research that attempts to specify both moderators and mediators of treatment response will be invaluable to the field.

Clearly, this is a growing field, and we are seeing a growing number of empirical studies showing the effectiveness of various interventions for dementia CGs. However, much remains to be addressed in future research. For example, we need to be asking some new questions: Why do some CGs respond less favourably to certain interventions? What are the long-term impacts of these interventions, for example, on nursing-home placement and cost-effectiveness? And on the practice level, at what point in the care-giving process should an intervention be introduced for maximum effectiveness? How do practitioners incorporate evidence-based interventions into the overall care plan, whether the client is the patient with dementia or the care-giver? How can we disseminate more effectively and widely these proven interventions? Can technology play a greater (but also as effective) a role in increasing the accessibility of training to practitioners in rural or otherwise resource-limited areas, or even for CGs directly to receive interventions? Are there ways to scale up any of these interventions in our existing healthcare systems? Identifying and addressing potential resources as well as barriers to finding answers to these questions will need collaborative efforts from practitioners, researchers, and patients and their care-givers. This is the considerable challenge we face in the next decade!

ACKNOWLEDGEMENT

This work was supported by a grant to the Stanford Geriatric Education Center, from the Health Resources and Services Administration, US Department of Health and Human Services (UB4HP19049).

KEY REFERENCES AND SOURCES FOR FURTHER READING

Coon, D. W., Keaveny, M., Valverde, I., Dadvar, S., and Gallagher-Thompson, D. (2012). 'Providing Evidence-based Psychological Treatments for Distress in Family Caregivers of Older Adults'. In F. Scogin and A. Shah (eds), *Making Evidence-based Psychological Treatments Work with Older Adults* (pp. 225–284). Washington, DC: American Psychological Association.

Gallagher-Thompson, D., Tzuang, M., Au, A., Brodaty, H., Charlesworth, G., et al. (2012). 'International Perspectives on Nonpharmacological Best Practices for Dementia Family Caregivers: A Review'. *Clinical Gerontologist* 35: 316–355.

World Health Organization and Alzheimer's Disease International (2012). *Dementia: A Public Health Priority*. http://www.who.int/mental_health/publications/dementia_report_2012/en/index.html.

WEBSITES AND OTHER RESOURCES

Alzheimer's Association (United States). http://www.alz.org/.

Alzheimer's Disease Education and Referral Center (ADEAR). http://www.nia.nih.gov/alzheimers.

Alzheimer's Disease International. http://www.alz.co.uk/.

Eldercare Locator, US Administration on Aging. http://www.eldercare.gov/Eldercare.NET/Public/Index.aspx.

Family Caregiver Alliance. http://www.caregiver.org/.

iCare Family (Online Information and Stress Management Training for Family Caregivers). http://www.icarefamily.com/.

Older Adult and Family Center, Stanford University School of Medicine. http://oafc.stanford.edu/.

Rosalynn Carter Institute for Caregiving. http://www.rosalynncarter.org/.

Stanford Geriatric Education Center. http://sgec.stanford.edu.

REFERENCES

10/66 Dementia Research Group (2004). 'Behavioral and Psychological Symptoms of Dementia in Developing Countries'. *International Psychogeriatrics/IPA* 16: 441–459.

Acton, G. and Kang, J. (2001). 'Interventions to Reduce the Burden of Caregiving for an Adult with Dementia: A Meta-analysis'. *Research in Nursing and Health* 24: 349–360.

Akkerman, R. and Ostwald, S. (2004). 'Reducing Anxiety in Alzheimer's Disease Family Caregivers: Effectiveness of a Nine-week Cognitive Behavioral Intervention'. *American Journal of Alzheimer's Disease & Other Dementias* 19: 117–123.

Alzheimer's Association (2012). 'Alzheimer's Facts and Figures'. *Alzheimer's & Dementia* 9(2). http://www.alz.org/downloads/facts_figures_2012.pdf.

Alzheimer's Australia (2008). *Perceptions of Dementia in Ethnic Communities*. http://www.fight-dementia.org.au/common/files/NAT/20101201-Nat-CALD-Perceptions-of-dementia-in-ethnic-communities-Oct08.pdf.

Alzheimer's Disease International (1999). *Caring for People with Dementia around the World: Factsheet 5*. London: Alzheimer's Disease International. http://www.alz.co.uk/adi/pdf/5caring.pdf.

Alzheimer's Disease International (2009). *World Alzheimer Report 2009*. London: Alzheimer's Disease International. http://www.alz.co.uk/research/files/WorldAlzheimerReport.pdf.

Alzheimer's Disease International (2011). *World Alzheimer Report 2011: The Benefits of Early Diagnosis and Intervention*. London: Alzheimer's Disease International. http://www.alz.co.uk/research/WorldAlzheimerReport2011.pdf.

Andren, S. and Elmstahl, S. (2005). 'Family Caregivers' Subjective Experience of Satisfaction in Dementia Care: Aspects of Burden, Subjective Health and Sense of Coherence'. *Scandinavian Journal of Caring Science* 19: 157–168.

Aranda, M. and Knight, B. (1997). 'The Influence of Ethnicity and Culture on the Caregivers of Stress and Coping Process: A Sociocultural Review and Analysis'. *Gerontologist* 37: 342–354.

Archbold, P., Stewart, B., and Miller, L. (1995). 'The PREP System of Nursing Interventions: A Pilot Test with Families Caring for Older Members'. *Research in Nursing & Health* 18: 1–16.

Au, A., Li, S., Lee, K., Leung, P., Cheung, G., Pan, P.-C., et al. (2010a). 'The Coping with Caregiving Group Program for Chinese Caregivers of Patients with Alzheimer's Disease in Hong Kong'. *Patient Education and Counseling* 78: 256–260.

Au, A., Wong, M. K., Leung, L. M., Thompson, L., and Gallagher-Thompson, D. (2010b). 'Telephone Assisted Pleasant Event Scheduling (TAPES) for Enhancing the Well-being of Dementia Care-givers'. Health and Health Services Research Committee of the Hong Kong Special Administrative Region Government.

Au, A., Shardlow, S. M., Teng, Y., Tsien, T. and Chan, C. (2013). 'Coping Strategies and Social Support-seeking Behavior among Chinese Caring for Older People with Dementia'. *Aging and Society* 33(8): 1422–1441.

Azar, A., Dadvar, F., Wilson-Arias, E., Jimenez, D., Dupart, T., et al. (2007). 'Coping with Caregiving: An Intervention Manual for Caregivers where English is Not their First Language' (Unpublished).

Ballard, C., Eastwood, C., Gahir, M., and Wilcock, G. (1996). 'A Follow Up Study of Depression in the Carers of Dementia Sufferers'. *British Medical Journal* 312: 947.

Bass, D., McClendon, M., Brennan, P., and McCarthy, C. (1998). 'The Buffering Effect of a Computer Support Network on Caregiver Strain'. *Journal of Aging and Health* 10: 20–43.

Beach, S. R., Schulz, R., Williamson, G. M., Miller, L. S., Weiner, M. F., et al. (2005). 'Risk Factors for Potentially Harmful Informal Caregiver Behavior'. *Journal of the American Geriatrics Society* 53: 255–261.

Beauchamp, N., Irvine, A., Seeley, J., and Johnson, B. (2005). 'Worksite-based Internet Multimedia Program for Family Caregivers of Persons with Dementia'. *Gerontologist* 45: 793–801.

Belle, S., Burgio, L., Burns, R., Coon, D., Czaja, S., et al. (2006). 'Enhancing the Quality of Life of Dementia Caregivers from Different Ethnic or Racial Groups: A Randomized, Controlled Trial'. *Annals of Internal Medicine* 145: 727–738.

Berlin, E. and Fowkes, W. (1983). 'A Teaching Framework for Cross-cultural Health Care'. *Western Journal of Medicine* 139: 934–938.

Bond, C., Stave, A., Sganga, O., Vincenzino, B., O'Connell, B., et al. (2005). 'Inequalitites in Dementia Care across Europe: Key Findings of the Facing Dementia Survey'. *Journal of Clinical Practice* 59: 8–14.

Bourgeois, M., Schulz, R., and Burgio, L. (1996). 'Interventions for Caregivers of Patients with Alzheimer's Disease: A Review and Analysis of Content, Process, and Outcomes'. *International Journal of Aging and Human Development* 43: 35–92.

Bourgeois, M., Schulz, R., Burgio, L., and Beach, S. (2002). 'Skills Training for Spouses of Patients with Alzheimer's Disease: Outcomes of an Intervention Study'. *Journal of Clinical Geropsychology* 8: 53–73.

Brodaty, H. and Gresham, M. (1989). 'Effect of a Training Programme to Reduce Stress in Carers of Patients with Dementia'. *British Medical Journal* 299: 1375–1379.

Brodaty, H. and Hadzi-Pavlovic, D. (1990). 'Psychosocial Effects on Carers of Living with Persons with Dementia'. *Australian and New Zealand Journal of Psychiatry* 24: 351–361.

Brodaty, H., Gresham, M., and Luscombe, G. (1997). 'The Prince Henry Hospital Dementia Caregivers' Training Program'. *International Journal of Geriatric Psychiatry* 12: 183–192.

Brodaty, H., Green, A., and Koschera, A. (2003). 'Meta-analysis of Psychosocial Interventions for Caregivers of People with Dementia'. *Journal of the American Geriatrics Society* 51: 657–664.

Brodaty, H. (2007). 'Meaning and Measurement or Caregiver Outcomes'. *International Psychogeriatrics* 19: 363–381.

Buckwalter, K., Gerdner, L., Kohout, F., Richards Hall, G., Kelly, A., et al. (1999). 'A Nursing Intervention to Decrease Depression in Family Caregivers of Persons with Dementia'. *Archives of Psychiatric Nursing* 13: 80–88.

Burgio, L., Collins, I., Schmid, B., Wharton, T., McCallum, D., et al. (2009). 'Translating the REACH Caregiver Intervention for Use by Area Agency on Aging Personnel: The REACH OUT Program'. *Gerontologist* 49: 103–116.

Cabassa, L. J. (2003). 'Measuring Acculturation: Where We Are and Where We Need To Go'. *Hispanic Journal of Behavioral Sciences* 25: 127–146.

Castro, C., Wilcox, S., O'Sullivan, P., Baumann, B., and King, A. (2002). 'An Exercise Program for Women Who Are Caring for Relatives with Dementia'. *Psychosomatic Medicine* 64: 458–468.

Charlesworth, G. and Reichel, K. (2004). 'Keeping Conceptualizations Simple: Examples with Family Carers of People with Dementia'. *Behavioural and Cognitive Psychotherapy* 32: 401–409.

Chen, H., Foo, S., and Ury, W. (2002). 'Recognizing Dementia'. *Western Journal of Medicine* 176: 267–270.

Chien, W. and Lee, Y. (2008). 'A Disease Management Program for Families of Persons in Hong Kong with Dementia'. *Psychiatric Services* 59: 433–436.

Chou, K., Lamontagne, L., and Hepworth, J. (1999). 'Burden Experienced by Caregivers of Relatives with Dementia in Taiwan'. *Nursing Research* 48: 206–214.

Cohen, C., Colantonio, A., and Vernich, L. (2002). 'Positive Aspects of Caregiving: Rounding Out the Caregiver Experience'. *International Journal of Geriatric Psychiatry* 17: 184–188.

Connell, C. and Gibson, G. (1997). 'Racial, Ethnic, Cultural Differences in Dementia Caregiving: Review and Analysis'. *Gerontologist* 37: 355–364.

Coon, D., Ory, M., and Schulz, R. (eds) (2003a). *Family Caregivers: Enduring and Emergent Themes*. New York: Springer.

Coon, D., Thompson, L., Steffen, A., Sorocco, K., and Gallagher-Thompson, D. (2003b). 'Anger and Depression Management: Psychoeducational Skill Training Interventions for Women Caregivers of a Relative with Dementia'. *Gerontologist* 43: 678–689.

Coon, D. W., Rubert, M., Solano, N., Mausbach, B., Kraemer, H., et al. (2004). 'Well-being, Appraisal, and Coping in Latina and Caucasian Female Dementia Caregivers: Findings from the REACH Study'. *Aging & Mental Health* 8: 330–345.

Coon, D. W., Keaveny, M., Valverde, I., Dadvar, S., and Gallagher-Thompson, D. (eds) (2012). *Providing Evidence-based Psychological Treatments for Distress in Family Caregivers of Older Adults*. Washington, DC: American Psychological Association.

Cooney, C., Howard, R., and Lawlor, B. (2006). 'Abuse of Vulnerable People with Dementia by their Carers: Can We Identify those Most at Risk?' *International Journal of Geriatric Psychiatry* 21: 564–571.

Cooper, C., Selwood, A., Blanchard, M., Walker, Z., Blizard, G., et al. (2009). 'Abuse of People with Dementia by Family Carers: Representative Cross Sectional Survey'. *British Medical Journal* 339: 1–5.

Cuellar, I., Arnold, B., and Maldonado, R. (1995). 'Acculturation Rating Scale for Mexican Americans-II: A Revision of the Original ARSMA Scale'. *Hispanic Journal of Behavioral Sciences* 17: 275–304.

Cuijpers, P. (2005). 'Depressive Disorders in Caregivers of Dementia Patients: A Systematic Review'. *Aging & Mental Health* 9: 325–330.

Czaja, S., Gitlin, L., Zhang, S., Schulz, R., and Gallagher-Thompson, D. (2009). 'Development of the Risk Appraisal Measure (RAM): A Brief Screen to Identify Risk Areas and Guide Interventions for Dementia Caregivers'. *Journal of the American Geriatrics Society* 57: 1064–1072.

Davis, L., Burgio, L., Buckwalter, K., and Weaver, M. (2004). 'A Comparison of In-home and Telephone-based Skill Training Interventions with Caregivers of Persons with Dementia'. *Journal of Mental Health and Aging* 10: 31–44.

Dias, A., Dewey, M., D'Souza, J., Dhume, R., Motghare, D., et al. (2008). 'The Effectiveness of a Home Care Program for Supporting Caregivers of Persons with Dementia in Developing Countries: A Randomised Controlled Trial from Goa, India'. *PLoS One* 3(6): e2333. doi:10.1371/journal.pone.0002333.

Dilworth-Anderson, P. and Gibson, B. (2002). 'The Cultural Influence of Values, Norms, Meanings, and Perceptions in Understanding Dementia in Ethnic Minorities'. *Alzheimer Disease and Associated Disorders* 16: S56–S63.

Dilworth-Anderson, P., Williams, I., and Gibson, B. (2002). 'Issues of Race, Ethnicity, and Culture in Caregiving Research: A 20-year review (1980–2000)'. *Gerontologist* 42: 237–272.

Dilworth-Anderson, P., Goodwin, P., and Williams, S. (2004). 'Can Culture Help Explain the Physical Health Effects of Caregiving over Time among African American Caregivers?' *Journals of Gerontology, Series B: Social Sciences* 59: S135–S145.

Eisdorfer, C., Czaja, S., Loewenstein, D., Rubert, M., Arguelles, S., et al. (2003). 'The Effect of a Family Therapy and Technology-based Intervention on Caregiver Depression'. *Gerontologist* 43: 521–531.

Etters, L., Goodall, D., and Harrison, B. (2008). 'Caregiver Burden among Dementia Patient Caregivers: A Review of the Literature'. *Journal of the American Academy of Nurse Practitioners* 20: 423–428.

Etxeberria, I., García, A., Iglesias, A., Urdaneta, E., Lorea, I., et al. (2011). 'Effects of Training in Emotional Regulation Strategies on the Well-being of Carers of Alzheimer Patients'. *Revista Española de Geriatría y Gerontología* 46: 206–212.

EUROFAMCARE (2006). *Services for Supporting Family Carers of Elderly People in Europe: Characteristics, Coverage and Usage: Summary of Main Findings from EUROFAMCARE.* Hamburg: EUROFAMCARE. http://www.uke.de/extern/eurofamcare/ documents/deliverables/summary_of_findings.pdf.

Family Caregiver Alliance (2007). *Family Caregiving: State of the Art, Future Trends.* Report from a National Conference. San Francisco: Family Caregiver Alliance.

Farran, C., Gilley, D., McCann, J., Bienias, J., Lindeman, D., et al. (2004). 'Psychosocial Interventions to Reduce Depressive Symptoms of Dementia Caregivers: A Randomized Clinical Trial Comparing two Approaches'. *Journal of Mental Health and Aging* 10: 337–350.

Finkel, S., Czaja, S., Shulz, R., Martinovich, Z., Harris, C., et al. (2007). 'E-Care: a Telecommunications Technology Intervention for Family Caregivers of Dementia Patients'. *American Journal of Geriatric Psychiatry* 15: 443–448.

Folkman, S. (1984). 'Personal Control and Stress and Coping Processes: A Theoretical Analysis'. *Journal of Personality and Social Psychology* 46: 839–852.

Fozard, J., Rietsema, J., Bouma, H., and Graafmans, J. (2000). 'Gerontechnology: Creating Enabling Environments for the Challenges and Opportunities of Aging'. *Educational Gerontology* 26: 331–344.

Fung, W. and Chien, W. (2002). 'The Effectiveness of a Mutual Support Group for Family Caregivers of a Relative with Dementia'. *Archives of Psychiatric Nursing* 26: 134–144.

Gallagher, D., Rose, J., Rivera, P., Lovett, S., and Thompson, L. W. (1989). 'Prevalence of Depression in Family Caregivers'. *Gerontologist* 29: 449–456.

Gallagher-Thompson, D. and Steffen, A. (1994). 'Comparative Effects of Cognitive/Behavioral and Brief Psychodynamic Psychotherapies for Depressed Family Caregivers'. *Journal of Consulting and Clinical Psychology* 62: 543–549.

Gallagher-Thompson, D., Lovett, S., Rose, J., McKibbon, C., Coon, D., et al. (2000). 'Impact of Psychoeducational Interventions on Distressed Family Caregivers'. *Journal of Clinical Geropsychology* 6: 91–110.

Gallagher-Thompson, D., Coon, D., Solano, N., Ambler, C., Rabinowitz, Y., et al. (2003). 'Change in Indices of Distress among Latino and Anglo Female Caregivers of Elderly Relatives with Dementia: Site-specific Results from the REACH National Collaborative Study'. *Gerontologist* 43: 580–591.

Gallagher-Thompson, D., Shurgot, G., Rider, K., Gray, H., McKibbin, C., et al. (2006). 'Ethnicity, Stress, and Cortisol Function in Hispanic and Non-Hispanic White Women: A Preliminary Study of Family Dementia Caregivers and Noncaregivers'. *American Journal of Geriatric Psychiatry* 14: 334–342.

Gallagher-Thompson, D., Eto-Iwase, T., and Haneishi, Y. (2007a). *A Useful Guide in Dementia Caregiving: Building Skills and Reducing Stress.* San Jose, CA: Yu-AiKai and Older Adult and Family Center.

Gallagher-Thompson, D., Gray, H., Tang, P., Pu, C.-Y., Tse, C., et al. (2007b). 'Impact of In-home Intervention versus Telephone Support in Reducing Depression and Stress of Chinese Caregivers: Results of a Pilot Study'. *American Journal of Geriatric Psychiatry* 15: 425–434.

Gallagher-Thompson, D., Gray, H., Dupart, T., Jimenez, D., and Thompson, L. (2008). 'Effectiveness of Cognitive/Behavioral Small Group Intervention for Reduction of Depression and Stress in Non Hispanic White and Hispanic/Latino Women Dementia

Family Caregivers: Outcomes and Mediators of Change'. *Journal of Rational-Emotive and Cognitive-Behavior Therapy* 26: 286–303.

Gallagher-Thompson, D., Wang, P.-C., Liu, W., Cheung, V., Peng, R., et al. (2010). 'Effectiveness of a Psychoeducational Skill Training DVD Program to Reduce Stress in Chinese American Dementia Caregivers'. *Aging & Mental Health* 14: 263–273.

Gallagher-Thompson, D., Tzuang, M., Au, A., Brodaty, H., Charlesworth, G., et al. (2012). 'International Perspectives on Nonpharmacological Best Practices for Dementia Family Caregivers: A Review'. *Clinical Gerontologist* 35: 316–355.

Gallagher-Thompson, D., Tzuang, M., Hinton, L., Alvarez, P., Nevarez, J.R., et al. (2013). 'Effectiveness of a Fotonovela for Reducing Depression and Stress in Latino Dementia Family Caregivers'. *Alzheimer's & Dementia* 4: 325.

Garity, J. (2006). 'Caring for a Family Member with Alzheimer's Disease: Coping with Caregiver Burden Post-nursing Home Placement'. *Journal of Gerontological Nursing* 32: 39–48.

Gatz, M., Fiske, A., Fox, L., Kaskie, B., Kasl-Godley, J., et al. (1998). 'Empirically Validated Psychological Treatments for Older Adults'. *Journal of Mental Health and Aging* 4: 9–46.

Gaugler, J., Kane, R., Kane, R., Clay, T., and Newcomer, R. (2003). 'Caregiving and Institutionalization of Cognitively Impaired Older People: Utilizing Dynamic Predictors of Change'. *Gerontologist* 43: 219–229.

Gavrilova, S., Ferri, C., Mikhaylova, N., Sokolova, O., Banerjee, S., et al. (2009). 'Helping Carers to Care—the 10/66 Dementia Research Group's Randomized Control Trial of a Caregiver Intervention in Russia'. *International Journal of Geriatric Psychiatry* 24: 347–354.

Gitlin, L., Belle, S., Burgio, L., Czaja, S., Mahoney, D., et al. (2003a). 'Effect of Multicomponent Interventions on Caregiver Burden and Depression: The REACH Multisite Initiative at 6-month Follow-up'. *Psychology and Aging* 18: 361–374.

Gitlin, L., Winter, L., Corcoran, M., Dennis, M., Schinfeld, S., et al. (2003b). 'Effects of the Home Environmental Skill-building Program on the Caregiver–Care Recipient Dyad: 6-month Outcomes from the Philadelphia REACH Initiative'. *Gerontologist* 43: 532–546.

Gitlin, L., Hauck, W., Dennis, M., and Winter, L. (2005). 'Maintenance of Effects of the Home Environmental Skill-building Program for Family Caregivers and Individuals with Alzheimer's Disease and Related Disorders'. *Journals of Gerontology Series A: Biological Sciences and Medical Sciences* 60: 368–374.

Gitlin, L., Winter, L., Burke, J., Chernett, N., Dennis, M., et al. (2008). 'Tailored Activities to Manage Neuropsychiatric Behaviors in Persons with Dementia and Reduce Caregiver Burden: A Randomized Pilot Study'. *American Journal of Geriatric Psychiatry* 16: 229–239.

Gonyea, J., O'Connor, M., and Boyle, P. (2006). 'Project CARE: A Randomized Controlled Trial of a Behavioral Intervention Group for Alzheimer's Disease Caregivers'. *Gerontologist* 46: 827–832.

Gonzalez, H., Haan, M., and Hinton, L. (2001). 'Acculturation and the Prevalence of Depression in Older Mexican Americans: Baseline Results of the Sacramento Area Latino Study on Aging'. *Journal of the American Geriatrics Society* 49: 948–953.

Graff, M. J. L., Adang, E. M. M., Vernooij-Dassen, M. J. M., Dekker, J., Jöbsson, L., et al. (2006). 'Community Based Occupational Therapy for Patients with Dementia and their Care Givers: Randomised Controlled Trial'. *British Medical Journal* 333: 1196.

Gray, H., Jimenez, D., Cucciare, M., Tong, H.-Q., and Gallagher-Thompson, D. (2009). 'Ethnic Differences in Beliefs Regarding Alzheimer Disease among Dementia Family Caregivers'. *American Journal of Geriatric Psychiatry* 17: 925–933.

Haan, M., Mungas, D., Gonzalez, H., Ortiz, T., Acharya, A., et al. (2003). 'Prevalence of Dementia in Older Latinos: The Influence of Type 2 Diabetes Mellitus, Stroke, and Genetic Factors'. *Journal of the American Geriatrics Society* 51: 169–177.

Hassol, A., Walker, J., Kidder, D., Rokita, K., Young, D., et al. (2004). 'Patient Experiences and Attitudes about Access to a Patient Electronic Health Care Record and Linked Web Messaging'. *Journal of the American Medical Informatics Association* 11: 505–513.

Hebert, R., Weinstein, E., Martire, L., and Schulz, R. (2006). 'Religion, Spirituality and the Well-being of Informal Caregivers: A Review, Critique, and Research Prospectus'. *Aging & Mental Health* 10: 497–520.

Hepburn, K., Tornatore, J., Center, B., and Ostwald, S. (2001). 'Dementia Family Caregiver Training: Affecting Beliefs about Caregiving and Caregiver Outcomes'. *Journal of the American Geriatrics Society* 49: 450–457.

Hepburn, K., Lewis, M., Sherman, C., and Tornatore, J. (2003). 'The Savvy Caregiver Program: Developing and Testing a Transportable Dementia Family Caregiver Training Program'. *Gerontologist* 43: 908–915.

Hepburn, K., Lewis, M., Tornatore, J., Sherman, C., and Bremer, K. (2007). 'The Savvy Caregiver Program: The Demonstrated Effectiveness of a Transportable Dementia Caregiver Psychoeducation Program'. *Journal of Gerontological Nursing* 33: 30–36.

Hilgeman, M. M., Durkin, D., Sun, F., Decoster, J., Allen, R. S., et al. (2009). 'Testing a Theoretical Model of the Stress Process in Alzheimer's Caregivers with Race as a Moderator'. *Gerontologist* 49: 248–261.

Holland, J., Currier, J., and Gallagher-Thompson, D. (2009). 'Outcomes from the Resources for Enhancing Alzheimer's Caregiver Health (REACH) Program for Bereaved Caregivers'. *Psychology and Aging* 24: 190–202.

Holland, J., Thompson, L. W., Tzuang, M., and Gallagher-Thompson, D. (2010). 'Psychosocial Factors among Chinese American Women Dementia Caregivers and their Association with Salivary Cortisol: Results of an Exploratory Study'. *Ageing International* 35: 109–127.

Holland, J. M., Thompson, L. W., Cucciare, M. A., Tsuda, A., Okamura, H., et al. (2011). 'Cortisol Outcomes among Caucasian and Latina/Hispanic Women Caring for a Family Member with Dementia: A Preliminary Examination of Psychosocial Predictors and Effects of a Psychoeducational Intervention'. *Stress and Health* 27(4): 334–346.

Huang, H. L., Shyu, Y. I., Chen, M. C., Chen, S. T., and Lin, L. C. (2003). 'A Pilot Study on a Home-based Caregiver Training Program for Improving Caregiver Self-efficacy and Decreasing the Behavioral Problems of Elders with Dementia in Taiwan'. *International Journal of Geriatric Psychiatry* 18: 337–345.

Hwang, K. K. and Han, K. H. (2010). 'Face and Morality in Confucian Society'. In M. H. Bond (ed.), *The Oxford Handbook of Chinese Psychology* (pp. 265–295). Hong Kong: Oxford University Press.

Jimenez, D., Gray, H., Cucciare, M., Kumbhani, S., and Gallagher-Thompson, D. (2010). 'Using the Revised Acculturation Rating Scale for Mexican Americans (ARSMA-II) with Older Adults'. *Hispanic Health Care International* 8: 14–22.

Jones, P., Lee, J., and Zhang, X. (2011). 'Clarifying and Measuring Filial Concepts across Five Cultural Groups'. *Research in Nursing and Health* 34: 310–326.

Kajiyama, B., Thompson, L., Eto-Iwase, T., Yamashita, M., Di Mario, J., et al. (2013). 'Exploring the Effectiveness of an Internet-based Program for Reducing Caregivers' Distress Using the iCare Stress Management e-Training Program'. *Aging & Mental Health* 17(5): 544–554.

Kaneda, T. (2011). *Health Care Challenges for Developing Countries with Aging Populations.* Washington, DC: Population Reference Bureau. http://www.prb.org/Articles/2006/ HealthCareChallengesforDevelopingCountrieswithAgingPopulations.aspx.

Kiecolt-Glaser, J., Dura, J., Speicher, C., Trask, O., and Glaser, R. (1991). 'Spousal Caregivers of Dementia Victims: Longitudinal Changes in Immunity and Health'. *Psychosomatic Medicine* 53: 345–362.

Kim, J.-H., Knight, B., and Longmire, C. (2007). 'The Role of Familism in Stress and Coping Processes among African American and White Dementia Caregivers: Effects on Mental and Physical Health'. *Health Psychology* 26: 564–576.

King, A., Oka, R., and Young, D. (1994). 'Ambulatory Blood Pressure and Heart Rate Responses to the Stress of Work and Caregiving in Older Women'. *Journal of Gerontology* 49: M239–M245.

King, A., Baumann, K., O'Sullivan, P., Wilcox, S., and Castro, C. (2002). 'Effects of Moderate-intensity Exercise on Physiological, Behavioral, and Emotional Responses to Family Caregiving: A Randomized Controlled Trial'. *Journals of Gerontology Series A: Biological Sciences and Medical Sciences* 57: M26–M36.

Knight, B., Lutzky, S., and Macofsky-Urban, F. (1993). 'A Meta-analytic Review of Interventions for Caregiver Distress: Recommendations for Future Research'. *Gerontologist* 33: 240–248.

Knight, B., Silverstein, M., McCullum, T., and Fox, L. (2000). 'A Sociocultural Stress and Coping Model for Mental Health Outcomes among African American Caregivers in Southern California'. *Journal of Gerontology: Psychological Sciences* 55: 142–150.

Knight, B., Robinson, G., Longmire, C., Chun, M., Nakao, K., et al. (2002). 'Cross Cultural Issues in Caregiving for Persons with Dementia: Do Familism Values Reduce Burden and Distress?' *Ageing International* 27: 70–94.

Koenig, H. G., Westlund, R. E., George, L. K., Hughes, D. C., Blazer, D. G., et al. (1993). 'Abbreviating the Duke Social Support Index for Use in Chronically Ill Elderly Individuals'. *Psychosomatics* 34: 61–69.

Koenig, H., Parkerson, G., Jr, and Meador, K. (1997). 'Religion Index for Psychiatric Research: A 5-item Measure for Use in Health Outcome Studies'. *American Journal of Geriatric Psychiatry* 154: 885–886.

Koenig, H. and Büssing, A. (2010). 'The Duke University Religion Index (DUREL): A Five-item Measure for Use in Epidemiological Studies'. *Religions* 1: 78–85.

Kuo, L.-M., Huang, H.-L., Huang, H.-L., Liang, J., Chiu, Y.-C., et al. (2012). 'A Home-based Training Program Improves Taiwanese Family Caregivers' Quality of Life and Decreases their Risk for Depression: A Randomized Controlled Trial'. *International Journal of Geriatric Psychiatry* 28: 504–513.

Kwon, Y. and Kim, E. (2011). 'Korean Americans in Dementia Caregiving Research: Inclusive Strategies to Barriers in Recruitment'. *Clinical Gerontologist* 34: 335–352.

Lai, C. and Chung, J. (2011). 'Caregivers' Informational Needs on Dementia and Dementia Care'. *Asian Journal of Gerontology & Geriatrics* 2: 78–87.

Lai, D. (2010). 'Filial Piety, Caregiving Appraisal, and Caregiving Burden'. *Research on Aging* 32: 200–233.

Lee, H. and Cameron, M. (2006). 'Respite Care for People with Dementia and their Carers'. *Cochrane Database of Systematic Reviews* 2(1): 1–16. http://ot.creighton.edu/community/EBLP/Question5/Question%205%20Lee%20and%20Cameron%20Respite%20Care.pdf.

Lee, S. Y., Tsai, T. I., Tsai, Y. W., and Kuo, K. N. (2010). 'Health Literacy, Health Status, and Healthcare Utilization of Taiwanese Adults: Results from a National Survey'. *BMC Public Health* 10: 614.

Leong, K., Chen, W., Leong, K., Mastura, I., Mimi, O., et al. (2006). 'The Use of Text Messaging to Improve Attendance in Primary Care: A Randomized Controlled Trial'. *Family Practice* 23: 699–705.

Lewis, M., Hobday, J., and Hepburn, K. (2010). 'Internet-based Program for Dementia Caregivers'. *American Journal of Alzheimer's Disease & Other Dementias* 25: 674–679.

López, J., Crespo, M., and Zarit, S. H. (2007). 'Assessment of the Efficacy of a Stress Management Program for Informal Caregivers of Dependent Older Adults'. *Gerontologist* 47: 205–214.

López, J. and Crespo, M. (2008). 'Analysis of the Efficacy of a Psychotherapeutic Program to Improve the Emotional Status of Caregivers of Elderly Dependent Relatives'. *Aging & Mental Health* 12: 451–461.

Losada, B., Izal, F., Montorio, C., Marquez, G., and Perez, R. (2004). 'Differential Efficacy of two Psychoeducational Interventions for Dementia Family Caregivers'. *Revue Neurologique* 38: 701–708.

Losada, A., Márquez-González, M., Knight, B. G., Yanguas, J., Sayegh, P., et al. (2010). 'Psychosocial Factors and Caregivers' Distress: Effects of Familism and Dysfunctional Thoughts'. *Aging & Mental Health* 14: 193–202.

Losada, A., Márquez-González, M., and Romero-Moreno, R. (2011). 'Mechanisms of Action of a Psychological Intervention for Dementia Caregivers: Effects of Behavioural Activation and Modification of Dysfunctional Thoughts'. *International Journal of Geriatric Psychiatry* 26: 1119–1127.

Low, L.-F., Draper, B., Cheng, A., Cruysmans, B., Hayward-Wright, N., et al. (2009). 'Future Research on Dementia Relating to Culturally and Linguistically Diverse Communities'. *Australasian Journal on Ageing* 28: 144–148.

Low, L. and Anstey, K. (2009). 'Dementia Literacy: Recognition and Beliefs on Dementia of the Australian Public'. *Alzheimer's and Dementia* 5: 43–49.

Lubben, J. and Gironda, M. (1996). 'Assessing Social Support Networks among Older People in the United States'. In H. Litwin (ed.), *The Social Networks of Older People: A Cross-National Analysis* (pp. 143–162). Wesport, CT: Praeger.

Lugo Steidel, A. G. and Contreras, J. M. (2003). 'A New Familism Scale for Use with Latino Populations'. *Hispanic Journal of Behavioral Sciences* 25: 312–330.

McCurry, S., Gibbons, L., Logsdon, R., Vitiello, M., and Teri, L. (2005). 'Nighttime Insomnia Treatment and Education for Alzheimer's Disease: A Randomized, Controlled Trial'. *Journal of the American Geriatrics Society* 53: 793–802.

Magnusson, L., Hanson, E., and Borg, M. (2004). 'A Literature Review Study of Information and Communication Technology as a Support for Frail Older People Living at Home and their Family Carers'. *Technology and Disability* 16: 223–235.

Magnusson, L., Hanson, E., and Nolan, M. (2005). 'The Impact of Information and Communication Technology on Family Carers of Older People and Professionals in Sweden'. *Ageing Society* 25: 693–713.

Mahoney, D., Tarlow, B., and Jones, R. (2003). 'Effects of an Automated Telephone Support System on Caregiver Burden and Anxiety: Findings from the REACH for TLC Intervention Study'. *Gerontologist* 43: 556–567.

Majerovitz, S. (1995). 'Role of Family Adaptability in the Psychological Adjustment of Spouse Caregivers to Patients with Dementia'. *Psychology and Aging* 10: 447–457.

Marín, G. and Gamba, R. (1996). 'A New Measurement of Acculturation for Hispanics: The Bidimensional Acculturation Scale for Hispanics (BAS)'. *Hispanic Journal of Behavioral Sciences* 18: 297–316.

Markowitz, J., Gutterman, E., Sadik, K., and Papadopoulos, G. (2003). 'Health-related Quality of Life for Caregivers of Patients with Alzheimer Disease'. *Alzheimer Disease and Associated Disorders* 17: 209–214.

Márquez-González, M., Losada, A., Izal, M., Pérez-Rojo, G., and Montorio, I. (2007). 'Modification of Dysfunctional Thoughts about Caregiving in Dementia Family

Caregivers: Description and Outcomes of an Intervention Program'. *Aging & Mental Health* 11: 616–625.

Márquez-González, M., Romero-Moreno, R., and Losada, A. (2010). 'Caregiving Issues in a Therapeutic Context: New Insights from the Acceptance and Commitment Therapy Approach'. In N. Pachana, K. Laidlaw, and B. Knight (eds), *Casebook of Clinical Geropsychology: International Perspectives on Practice* (33–51). Oxford: Oxford University Press.

Marriott, A., Donaldson, C., Tarrier, N., and Burns, A. (2000). 'Effectiveness of Cognitive-behavioural Family Intervention in Reducing the Burden of Care in Carers of Patients with Alzheimer's Disease'. *British Journal of Psychiatry* 176: 557–562.

Martín-Carrasco, M., Martín, M., Valero, C., Millán, P., García, C., et al. (2009). 'Effectiveness of a Psychoeducational Intervention Program in the Reduction of Caregiver Burden in Alzheimer's Disease Patients' Caregivers'. *International Journal of Geriatric Psychiatry* 24: 489–499.

Marziali, E. and Garcia, L. (2011). 'Dementia Caregivers' Responses to 2 Internet-based Intervention Programs'. *American Journal of Alzheimer's Disease & Other Dementias* 26: 36–43.

MICINN (2011). 'Guía de Práctica Clínica sobre la Atención Integral a las Personas con Enfermedad de Alzheimer y otras Demencias' [Practical clinical guide about the integral attention to people with Alzheimer and other dementias]. In M. D. C. Innovación (ed.), Report by Ministerio de Ciencia e Innovación, Madrid, Spain. http://www.gencat.cat/salut/depsan/units/aatrm/pdf/gpc_alzheimer_demencias_pcsns_aiaqs_2011vc.pdf.

Miller, B. and Cafasso, L. (1992). 'Gender Differences in Caregiving: Fact or Artifact?' *Gerontologist* 32: 498–507.

Mittelman, M., Ferris, S., Steinberg, G., Schulman, E., Mackell, J., et al. (1993). 'An Intervention that Delays Institutionalization of Alzheimer's Disease Patients: Treatment of Spouse-caregivers'. *Gerontologist* 33: 730–740.

Mittelman, M., Ferris, S., Schulman, E., Steinberg, G., and Levin, B. (1996). 'A Family Intervention to Delay Nursing Home Placement of Patients with Alzheimer Disease: A Randomized Controlled Trial'. *Journal of the American Medical Association* 276: 1725–1731.

Mittelman, M., Roth, D., Coon, D., and Haley, W. (2004). 'Sustained Benefit of Supportive Intervention for Depressive Symptoms in Caregivers of Patients with Alzheimer's Disease'. *American Journal of Psychiatry* 161: 850–856.

Mittelman, M., Haley, W., Clay, O., and Roth, D. (2006). 'Improving Caregiver Well-being delays Nursing Home Placement of Patients with Alzheimer's Disease'. *Neurology* 67: 1592–1599.

Mittelman, M., Roth, D., Clay, O., and Haley, W. (2007). 'Preserving Health of Alzheimer Caregivers: Impact of a Spouse Caregiver Intervention'. *American Journal of Geriatric Psychiatry* 15: 780–789.

Mittelman, M., Brodaty, H., Wallen, A., and Burns, A. (2008). 'A 3 Country Randomized Controlled Trial of Psychosocial Intervention for Caregivers Combined with Pharmacological Treatment for Patients with Alzheimer's Disease: Effects on Caregiver Depression'. *American Journal of Geriatric Psychiatry* 16: 893–904.

Moniz-Cook, E., Vernooij-Dassen, M., Woods, R., Verhey, F., Chattat, R., et al. (2008). 'A European Consensus on Outcome Measures for Psychosocial Intervention Research in Dementia Care'. *Aging & Mental Health* 12: 14–29.

Montoro-Rodriguez, J. and Gallagher-Thompson, D. (2009). 'The Role of Resources and Appraisals in Predicting Burden among Latina and Non-Hispanic White Female

Caregivers: A Test of an Expanded Socio-cultural Model of Stress and Coping'. *Aging & Mental Health* 13: 648–658.

Moritz, D., Kasl, S., and Ostfeld, A. (1992). 'The Health Impact of Living with a Cognitively impaired Elderly Spouse: Blood Pressure, Self-rated Health, and Health Behaviors'. *Journal of Aging and Health* 4: 244–267.

Mukadam, N., Cooper, C., and Livingston, G. (2011). 'A Systematic Review of Ethnicity and Pathways to Care in Dementia'. *International Journal of Geriatric Psychiatry* 26: 12–20.

Neary, S. and Mahoney, D. (2005). 'Dementia Caregiving: The Experiences of Hispanic/Latino Caregivers'. *Journal of Transcultural Nursing* 16: 163–170.

Nielsen-Bohlman, L., Panzer, A., Hamlin, B., and Kindig, D. (2004). *Health Literacy: A Prescription to End Confusion*. Washington, DC: National Academies Press.

Nikmat, A., Hawthorne, G., and Ahmad Al-Mashoor, S. (2011). 'Dementia in Malaysia: Issues and Challenges'. *ASEAN Journal of Psychiatry* 12: 1–7.

Olazaran, J., Reisberg, B., Clare, L., Cruz, I. P.-C., J, Del Ser, T., et al. (2010). 'Nonpharmacological Therapies in Alzheimer's Disease: A Systematic Review of Efficacy'. *Dementia and Geriatric Cognitive Disorders* 30: 161–178.

Ory, M., Hoffman, R., III, Yee, J., Tennstedt, S. and Schulz, R. (1999). 'Prevalence and Impact of Caregiving: A Detailed Comparison between Dementia and Nondementia Caregivers'. *Gerontologist* 39: 177–186.

Ostwald, S., Hepburn, K., Caron, W., Burns, T., and Mantell, R. (1999). 'Reducing Caregiver Burden: A Randomized Psychoeducational Intervention for Caregivers of Persons with Dementia'. *Gerontologist* 39: 299–309.

Paasche-Orlow, M. K., Parker, R. M., Gazmararian, J. A., Nielsen-Bohlman, L. T., and Rudd, R. R. (2005). 'The Prevalence of Limited Health Literacy'. *Journal of General Internal Medicine* 20: 175–184.

Parry, J. and Weiyuan, C. (2011). 'Alzheimer's Disease International: Global Perspective'. *Alzheimer's Disease International* 21 (2). http://www.alz.co.uk/adi/pdf/gp201106.pdf.

Pearlin, L. and Schooler, C. (1978). 'The Structure of Coping'. *Journal of Health and Social Behavior* 19: 2–21.

Pearlin, L., Mullan, J., Semple, S., and Skaff, M. M. (1990). 'Caregiving and the Stress Process: An Overview of Concepts and their Measures'. *Gerontologist* 30: 583–594.

Perren, S., Schmid, R., and Wettstein, A. (2006). 'Caregivers' Adaptation to Change: The Impact of Increasing Impairment of Persons Suffering from Dementia on their Caregivers' Subjective Well-being'. *Aging & Mental Health* 10: 539–548.

Pinquart, M. and Sörensen, S. (2003). 'Differences between Caregivers and Noncaregivers in Psychological Health and Physical Health: A Meta-analysis'. *Psychology and Aging* 18: 250–267.

Pinquart, M. and Sörensen, S. (2005). 'Ethnic Differences in Stressors, Resources, and Psychological Outcomes of Family Caregiving: A Meta-analysis'. *Gerontologist* 45: 90–106.

Pinquart, M. and Sörensen, S. (2006). 'Helping Caregivers of Persons with Dementia: Which Interventions Work and How Large are their Effects?' *International Psychogeriatrics* 18: 577–595.

Plante, T. and Boccaccini, M. (1997). 'The Santa Clara Strength of Religious Faith Questionnaire'. *Pastoral Psychology* 45: 375–387.

Port, C., Zimmerman, S., Williams, C., Dobbs, D., Preisser, J., et al. (2005). 'Families Filling the Gap: Comparing Family Involvement for Assisted Living and Nursing Home Residents with Dementia'. *Gerontologist* 45: 87–95.

Powell, J., Chiu, T., and Eysenbach, G. (2008). 'A Systematic Review of Networked Technologies Supporting Carers of People with Dementia'. *Journal of Telemedicine and Telecare* 14: 154–156.

Prince, M. (2004). 'Care Arrangements for People with Dementia in Developing Countries'. *International Journal of Geriatric Psychiatry* 19: 170–177.

Prince, M., Acosta, D., Castro-Costa, E., Jackson, J., and Shaji, K. (2009). 'Packages of Care for Dementia in Low and Middle Income Countries'. *PLoS Medicine* 6: e1000176.

Prince, M., Brodaty, H., Uwakwe, R., Acosta, D., Ferri, C., et al. (2011). 'Strain and its Correlates among Carers of People with Dementia in Low and Middle Income Countries. A 10/66 Dementia Research Group Population-based Survey'. *International Journal of Geriatric Psychiatry* 27: 670–682.

Qualls, S. (1997). 'Transitions in Autonomy: The Essential Caregiving Challenge. An Essay for Practitioners'. *Family Relations* 46: 41–45.

Qualls, S. and Vair, C. (2013). 'Caregiver Family Therapy for Families Dealing with Dementia'. In P. Peluso, R. Vatts, and M. Parsons (eds), *Changing Aging, Changing Family Therapy: Practicing with 21st Century Realities*. New York: Routledge.

Rabinowitz, Y. G., Mausbach, B. T., Coon, D. W., Depp, C., Thompson, L. W., et al. (2006). 'The Moderating Effect of Self-efficacy on Intervention Response in Women Family Caregivers of Older Adults with Dementia'. *American Journal of Geriatric Psychiatry* 14: 642–649.

Rabinowitz, Y. G., Mausbach, B. T., Thompson, L. W., and Gallagher-Thompson, D. (2007). 'The Relationship between Self-efficacy and Cumulative Health Risk Associated with Health Behavior Patterns in Female Caregivers of Elderly Relatives with Alzheimer's Dementia'. *Journal of Aging and Health* 19: 946–964.

Rabinowitz, Y. G., Brent, M. T., and Gallagher-Thompson, D. (2009). 'Self-efficacy as a Moderator of the Relationship between Care Recipient Memory and Behavioral Problems and Caregiver Depression in Female Dementia Caregivers'. *Alzheimer Disease and Associated Disorders* 23: 389–394.

Radloff, L. (1977). 'The CES-D Scale: A Self-report Scale for Research in the General Population'. *Applied Psychological Measurement* 1: 385–401.

Roberts, J. and Connell, C. (2000). 'Illness Representations among First-degree Relatives of People with Alzheimer Disease'. *Alzheimer Disease and Associated Disorders* 14: 129–136.

Robinson-Whelen, S., Tada, Y., MacCallum, R., McGuire, L., and Kiecolt-Glaser, J. (2001). 'Long-term Caregiving: What Happens When It Ends?' *Journal of Abnormal Psychology* 110: 573–584.

Roff, L., Burgio, L., Gitlin, L., Nichols, L., Chaplin, W., et al. (2004). 'Positive Aspects of Alzheimer's Caregiving: The Role of Race'. *Journals of Gerontology, Series B: Social Sciences* 59: 185–190.

Sarasohn-Kahn, J. (2010). *How Smartphones are Changing Health Care for Consumers and Providers*. Oakland, CA: California Health Care Foundation. http://www.chcf.org/publications/2010/04/how-smartphones-are-changing-health-care-for-consumers-and-providers.

Scharlach, A., Li, W., and Dalvi, T. (2006). 'Family Conflict as a Mediator of Caregiver Strain'. *Family Relations* 55: 625–635.

Schneider, J., Murray, J., Banerjee, S., and Mann, A. (1999). 'EUROCARE: A Cross-national Study of Co-resident Spouse Carers for People with Alzheimer's Disease: I-Factors Associated with Carer Burden'. *International Journal of Geriatric Psychiatry* 14: 651–661.

Schulz, R., O'Brien, A., Bookwala, M., and Fleissner, K. (1995). 'Psychiatric and Physical Morbidity Effects of Dementia Caregiving: Prevalence, Correlates, and Causes'. *Gerontologist* 35: 771–791.

Schulz, R., Newsom, J., Mittelmark, M., Burton, L., Hirsch, C., et al. (1997). 'Health Effects of Caregiving. The Caregiver Health Effects Study: An Ancillary Study of the Cardiovascular Health Study'. *Annals of Behavioral Medicine* 19: 110–116.

Schulz, R. and Beach, S. (1999). 'Caregiving as a Risk Factor for Mortality: The Caregiver Health Effects Study'. *Journal of the American Medical Association* 282: 2215–2219.

Schulz, R. (ed.) (2000). *Handbook on Dementia Caregiving: Evidence-based Interventions for Family Caregivers*. New York: Springer.

Schulz, R., Burgio, L., Burns, R., Eisdorfer, C., Gallagher-Thompson, D., et al. (2003). 'Resources for Enhancing Alzheimer's Caregiver Health (REACH): Overview, Site-specific Outcomes, and Future Directions'. *Gerontologist* 43: 514–520.

Schulz, R., Belle, S., Czaja, S., McGinnis, K., Stevens, A., and Zhang, S. (2004). 'Long-term Care Placement of Dementia Patients and Caregiver Health and Well-being'. *Journal of the American Medical Association* 292: 961–967.

Schulz, R. and Martire, L. (2004). 'Family Caregiving of Persons with Dementia: Prevalence, Health Effects, and Support Strategies'. *American Journal of Geriatric Psychiatry* 12: 240–29.

Schulz, R., Martire, L., and Klinger, J. (2005). 'Evidence-based Caregiver Interventions in Geriatric Psychiatry'. *Psychiatric Clinics of North America* 28: 1007–1038.

Schulz, R., Boerner, K., Shear, K., Zhang, S., and Gitlin, L. (2006). 'Predictors of Complicated Grief among Dementia Caregivers: A Prospective Study of Bereavement'. *American Journal of Geriatric Psychiatry* 14: 650–658.

Shaji, K., Jotheeswaran, A., Girish, N., Bharath, S., Dias, A., et al. (2010). *The Dementia India Report 2010*. New Delhi: Alzheimer's and Related Disorders Society of India. http://www.alzheimer.org.in/assets/dementia.pdf.

Shaw, W., Patterson, T., Semple, S., Ho, S., Irwin, M., et al. (1997). 'Longitudinal Analysis of Multiple Indicators of Health Decline among Spousal Caregivers'. *Annals of Behavioral Medicine* 119: 101–109.

Sheikh, J. and Yesavage, J. (1986). 'Geriatric Depression Scale (GDS): Recent Evidence and Development of a Shorter Version'. *Clinical Gerontologist* 5: 165–173.

Smith, T. and Toseland, R. (2006). 'The Effectiveness of a Telephone Support Program for Caregivers of Frail Older Adults'. *Gerontologist* 46: 620–629.

Smits, C., De Lange, J., Dröes, R.-M., Meiland, F., Vernooij-Dassen, M., et al. (2007). 'Effects of Combined Intervention Programmes for People with Dementia Living at Home and their Caregivers: A Systematic Review'. *International Journal of Geriatric Psychiatry* 22: 1181–1193.

Sörensen, S., Pinquart, M., Habil, D., and Duberstein, P. (2002). 'How Effective are Interventions with Caregivers? An Updated Meta-analysis'. *Gerontologist* 42: 356–372.

Sörensen, S., Duberstein, P., Gill, D., and Pinquart, M. (2006). 'Dementia Care: Mental Health Effects, Intervention Strategies, and Clinical Implications'. *Lancet Neurology* 5: 961–973.

Spector, J. and Tampi, R. (2005). 'Caregiver Depression'. *Annals of Long-term Care: Clinical Care and Aging* 13: 177–185.

Spijker, A., Vernooij-Dassen, M., Vasse, E., Adang, E., Wollersheim, H., et al. (2008). 'Effectiveness of Nonpharmacological Interventions in Delaying the Institutionalization of Patients with Dementia: A Meta-analysis'. *Journal of the American Geriatrics Society* 56: 1116–1128.

Steadman, P., Tremont, G., and Davis, J. (2007). 'Premorbid Relationship Satisfaction and Caregiver Burden in Dementia Caregivers'. *Journal of Geriatric Psychiatry and Neurology* 20: 115–119.

Steffen, A. (2000). 'Anger Management for Dementia Caregivers: A Preliminary Study Using Video and Telephone Interventions'. *Behavior Therapy* 31: 281–299.

Steffen, A., McKibbin, C., Zeiss, A., Gallagher-Thompson, D., and Bandura, A. (2002). 'The Revised Scale for Caregiving Self Efficacy: Reliability and Validity Studies'. *Journals of Gerontology, Series B: Social Sciences* 57: P74–P86.

Suinn, R., Ahuna, C., and Khoo, G. (1992). 'The Suinn-Lew Asian Self-Identity Acculturation Scale: Concurrent and Factorial Validation'. *Educational and Psychological Measurement* 52: 1041–1046.

Tarlow, B., Wisniewski, S., Belle, S., Rubert, M., Ory, M., et al. (2004). 'Positive Aspects of Caregiving'. *Research on Aging* 26: 429–453.

Teri, L., Truax, P., Logsdon, R., Uomoto, J., Zarit, S., et al. (1992). 'Assessment of Behavioral Problems in Dementia: The Revised Memory and Behavior Problems Checklist'. *Psychology and Aging* 7: 622–631.

Teri, L., Logsdon, R., Uomoto, J., and McCurry, S. (1997). 'Behavioral Treatment of Depression in Dementia Patients: A Controlled Clinical Trial'. *Journals of Gerontology, Series B: Social Sciences* 52: P159–P166.

Teri, L., Gibbons, L., McCurry, S., Logsdon, R., Buchner, D., et al. (2003). 'Exercise plus Behavioral Management in Patients with Alzheimer Disease: A Randomized Controlled Trial'. *Journal of the American Medical Association* 290: 2015–2022.

Teri, L., McCurry, S., Logsdon, R., and Gibbons, L. (2005). 'Training Community Consultants to Help Family Members Improve Dementia Care: A Randomized Controlled Trial'. *Gerontologist* 45: 802–811.

Topo, P. (2009). 'Technology Studies to Meet the Needs of People with Dementia and their Caregivers: A Literature Review'. *Journal of Applied Gerontology* 28: 5–37.

Torti, F. J., Gwyther, L., Reed, S., Friedman, J., and Schulman, K. (2004). 'A Multinational Review of Recent Trends and Reports in Dementia Caregiver Burden'. *Alzheimer Disease and Associated Disorders* 18: 99–109.

Toseland, R., Rossiter, C., and Labrecque, M. (1989). 'The Effectiveness of Peer-led and Professionally Led Groups to Support Family Caregivers'. *Gerontologist* 29: 465–471.

Tremont, G., Davis, J., and Bishop, D. (2006). 'Unique Contribution of Family Functioning in Caregivers of Patients with Mild to Moderate Dementia'. *Dementia and Geriatric Cognitive Disorders* 21: 170–174.

Tsolaki, M., Papaliagkas, V., Anogianakis, G., Bernabei, R., Emre, M., et al. (2010). 'Consensus Statement on Dementia Education and Training in Europe'. *The Journal of Nutrition, Health and Aging* 14: 131–135.

Turner, R. M., Tran, C., Hinton, L., Gallagher-Thompson, D., Tzuang, M., Tran, C. H., and Valle, R. J. (under review). 'Coping with Dementia Behavior Problems: A Culturally-attuned Focus Group Study of Latino Caregivers'. *American Journal of Alzheimer's Disease and Other Dementias*.

Van Durme, T., Macq, J., Jeanmart, C., and Gobert, M. (2011). 'Tools for Measuring the Impact of Informal Caregiving of the Elderly: A Literature Review'. *International Journal of Nursing Studies* 49: 490–504.

Vitaliano, P. P., Zhang, J., and Scanlan, J. M. (2003). 'Is Caregiving Hazardous to One's Physical Health? A Meta-analysis'. *Psychological Bulletin* 129: 946–972.

Ware, J. (1998). 'The SF-36 Health Survey'. In M. Maruish (ed.), *The Use of Psychological Testing for Treatment Planning and Outcome Assessment* (2nd edn). Mahwah, NJ: Lawrence Erlbaum Associates.

Weiner, M. F., Rossetti, II. C., and Harrah, K. (2011). 'Videoconference Diagnosis and Management of Choctaw Indian Dementia Patients'. *Alzheimer's and Dementia* 7: 562–566.

Weingart, S., Rind, D., Tofias, Z., and Sands, D. (2006). 'Who Uses the Patient Internet Portal? The PatientSite Experience'. *Journal of the American Medical Informatics Association* 13: 91–95.

Wiglesworth, A., Mosqueda, L., Mulnard, R., Liao, S., Gibbs, L., et al. (2010). 'Screening for Abuse and Neglect of People with Dementia'. *Journal of the American Geriatrics Society* 58: 493–500.

Woods, B. (2010). 'Invited Commentary on: Non-pharmacological Interventions in Dementia'. *Advances in Psychiatric Treatment* 10: 178–179.

World Health Organization (2012). *WHO Quality of Life-BREF (WHOQOL-BREF)*. Geneva: World Health Organization. http://www.who.int/substance_abuse/research_tools/whoqolbref/en/.

World Health Organization and Alzheimer's Disease International (2012). *Dementia: A Public Health Priority*. http://www.who.int/mental_health/publications/dementia_report_(2012)/en/index.html (2012).

Wortmann, M., Andrieu, S., Mackell, J., and Knox, S. (2010). 'Evolving Attitudes to Alzheimer's Disease among the General Public and Caregivers in Europe: Findings from the IMPACT Survey'. *Journal of Nutrition, Health and Aging* 14: 531–536.

Yan, E. and Kwok, T. (2010). 'Abuse of Older Chinese with Dementia by Family Caregivers: An Inquiry into the Role of Caregiver Burden'. *International Journal of Geriatric Psychiatry* 26: 527–535.

Yee, J. and Schulz, R. (2000). 'Gender Differences in Psychiatric Morbidity among Family Caregivers: A Review and Analysis'. *Gerontologist* 40: 147–164.

Yeo, G. and Gallagher-Thompson, D. (eds) (2006). *Ethnicity and Dementias*. New York: Taylor and Francis.

Zarcadoolas, C., Pleasant, A., and Greer, D. (2005). 'Understanding Health Literacy: An Expanded Mode'. *Health Promotion International* 20: 195–203.

Zarit, S. H. and Femia, E. E. (2008). 'A Future for Family Care and Dementia Intervention Research? Challenges and Strategies'. *Aging & Mental Health* 12: 5–13.

Zeiss, L., Kwon, Y., Marquett, R., and Gallagher-Thompson, D. (eds) (2010). *Successful Interventions for Family Caregivers*. Chichester: Wiley.

Zhan, H. and Montgomery, R. (2003). 'Gender and Elder Care in China: The Influence of Filial Piety and Structural Constraints'. *Gender and Society* 17: 209–229.

Zhao, J., Zhang, Z., Guo, H., Li, Y., Xue, W., et al. (2010). 'E-health in China: Challenges, Initial Directions, and Experience'. *Telemedicine and e-Health* 16: 344–349.

CHAPTER 40

COGNITIVE GRIEF THERAPY

Coping with the Inevitability of Loss and Grief in Later Life

RUTH MALKINSON AND LIORA BAR-TUR

INTRODUCTION

Grief is the price we humans pay for our ability to form nurturing and rewarding attachment relationships. Our capacity to feel and understand loss and to adapt across a life-time reflects a mix of developmental and contextual influences, that result in considerable cultural and individual variability of outcome.

(Hansson and Stroebe 2007, p. 172)

Loss and grief in old age are inevitable and are embedded in a person's long life. We grieve for a variety of losses throughout our lives; a loss of relationship through death is one that is human, universal and normal yet one that reflects an attack on every aspect of our being. From the moment of birth and throughout our life relationships with significant others are being formed and transformed, at times being modified, at times, dissolved. The death of a loved one may be overwhelming, even traumatic, and may change us forever. Personal identity, the nature of our interpersonal fabric, and the quality of our relationships with the deceased undergo change and transform personal history and memory. Grief is the process of reorganizing one's relationship with the deceased and involves a variety of responses at the level of both internal and external functioning. It entails reorganizing our functioning, behaviour, thinking, and feeling in order to find a way of shaping the life that has changed, and the painful process of reworking the relationship with the deceased (Rubin, Malkinson, and Witztum 2012).

Traditionally, grief was seen as a healthy, normal, and universal process that aimed at decathexis—a term coined by Freud (1957/1917) to indicate relinquishing the bonds with the deceased, and investing the libidinal energy in new relationships. The idea that grief is a normal and universal process is still valid but the ideas concerning decathexis were not empirically supported (Wortman and Silver 1989). On the contrary, it was found that the relationship with the deceased often continues throughout life and is referred to as 'continuing bonds' (Klass, Silverman, and Nickman 1996; Malkinson and Bar-Tur 2004–2005; Rubin 1981, 1999). In most cases, grieving based on this conceptualization includes the act of reconstructing a world of meaning that was challenged by the loss. From this perspective, grief and mourning are regarded as a developmental process that serves to maintain a continuing bond with the deceased and involves grief for the individual lost, and the process of searching for and constructing meaning to life without the deceased.

In the common grieving process, reactions are known to be intense immediately following the loss and to decrease over time (Parkes and Prigerson 2010; Rando 1984). Their outcome is to find ways to balance between functioning and the inner relationship with the deceased's representation. When relationships with the deceased are balanced, there is no extreme and persisting denial, avoidance or flooding of the memory of the deceased's image (Niemeyer 2004; Rubin et al. 2012). As data have accumulated, a combination of several theoretical approaches has been proposed to better understand the multidimensional perspective of the bereavement process. Thus, the most salient are integrated models of stress and attachment such as Stroebe and Schut's Dual Process Model (DPM; 1999), which views bereavement as an oscillation between loss orientation and restoration orientation. Rubin's Two-Track Model of Bereavement (TTMoB) (1981, 1999) views intrapersonal and interpersonal aspects of loss as occurring on two parallel axes (functioning and relationship to the deceased) emphasizing the ongoing relationship with the deceased. In addition, Bonanno and Kaltman's (2001) socio-functional-integrative perspective includes cognitive stress, attachment, trauma and social-functional elements for an understanding of bereavement.

BEREAVEMENT IN OLD AGE

Old age is associated with expected losses. The terms 'natural' or 'anticipated' as opposed to sudden death best reflect this view (Fries 1980; Osterweis, Solomon, and Green 1984: 49). Moreover, old age is a stage when many changes associated with loss can be expected to occur in major life domains (see also the chapter on transitions in later life in this Handbook). Although expected, a loss through death involves a disruption to life, and in ageing it may in fact be an ongoing and continuous bereavement process as the individual approaches his or her own death.

Grief is a human, normal, and universal response to loss through death (Freud 1957/1917). The nature of bereavement experienced among older adults generally parallels that of younger persons, involving a mixture of affective, physical, cognitive, and behavioural symptoms, and social consequences. The course of bereavement reactions is also similar in that intense symptoms are to be expected in the first months post loss after which they begin to subside. Also relevant are individual differences that are related to interpersonal resources, personality, or disposition in the context of coping with bereavement, as well as nonpersonal resources such as cultural, religious, and social contexts, and the availability of support and care arrangements for bereaved persons.

A major difference however, is that bereavement following a loss through death in later life, in contrast to that in early life phases, is inseparable from the normative ageing process in which numerous changes associated with loss can be expected to occur in major life domains. Deterioration of one's health and the health of a spouse, retirement, relocation, occupational and financial loss, loss of social roles, loss of siblings and friends, and other losses pose an ongoing threat to everyday functioning, forcing the individual to adapt (Bar-Tur and Levi-Shiff 2000). One of the losses frequently studied is that of widowhood, and in particular, older widows in clinical settings (Parkes 1985; Parkes and Prigerson 2010). With additional studies conducted on nonclinical populations, the variability in adjusting to loss of a spouse was better understood. One such example is the study of Ott et al. (2007) who used the Complicated Grief Inventory (Prigerson et al. 1995b) and identified in a sample of 141 older spouses three distinct grief clusters that they termed common (49%), resilient (34%), and chronic (17%). Bereaved spouses in the common cluster experienced intense grief and depressive symptoms that decreased over time. Those in the resilient grief cluster experienced the lowest levels of grief and depression, and reported a high quality of life. The chronic cluster members experienced more sudden death, the highest levels of grief and depression, and the lowest levels of self-esteem, and highest marital dependency on the spouse. In addition, there are situations in later life when loss might be followed by relief if marital relationships are characterized by a high degree of conflict, or after care-giving for a chronically ill spouse (Bonanno, Wortman, and Nesse 2005; Schulz et al. 2003).

However, the experience of bereavement in later life extends well beyond the loss of a spouse. The longer one lives, the greater is the likelihood of also experiencing the death of children, even grandchildren, and these losses are associated with especially intense grief reactions. In old age it is likely that the number of deaths and losses experienced will increase; there may be multiple, concurrent losses and an accumulation of grief from losses that have occurred across the lifetime, possibly leading to bereavement overload (Kastenbaum 1969).

In contrast to younger adults' bereavement, the circumstances of bereavement vary substantially among older persons. As they face accumulated losses of significant others and the grief that follows, older persons as compared to younger ones are frequently left with fewer alternative resources, as a result of increased physical health problems, decreased energy, and less social and emotional support for comfort and companionship.

It is therefore critical to stress that the return to optimal health and becoming reintegrated following a loss through death may be harder to achieve when one is older, more frail, alone, or depleted of energy after caring for a chronically ill spouse for a long time. Physical and mental health deficits prior to the death together with multiple daily hassles and stressors and accumulated losses in old age can exacerbate the psychological, physical, and practical consequences of bereavement.

Poor outcome of bereavement in older adults, especially for the oldest-old, often results in greater dependency on family and community resources for basic needs and long-term care (Hansson and Stroebe 2007). Minor hassles or more major life events may interact with the process of bereavement and cause extreme suffering and distress.

Uncomplicated (Adaptive) and Complicated Grief

Experiences of intense yearning, pain, and intrusive thoughts are normal reactions immediately following loss through death. Despite the difficulties expected as a result of the ageing process, the majority of older bereaved adults appear to grieve resiliently, reorganize their life in an adaptive manner, and find remarkable resources to cope under the new life circumstances (Bonanno 2004; Rubin et al. 2012). Uncomplicated adaptation to previous losses is an important indication for the development of a robust self-concept that may enhance adaptation to subsequent bereavement.

Older adults may also present increased maturity, flexibility, and control in dealing with life events, as well as an emotional dampening, especially in respect to negative emotions (Carstensen et al. 2011). These emotional patterns may protect older adults from excessive bereavement-related trauma, and facilitate adjustment.

There may also be gender differences in bereavement; older widows may experience less trauma than younger ones, as death in old age is less unexpected and may relieve the surviving spouse of the burden of care-giving (Carr 2004; Hurd 1999; Keene and Prokos 2008; Stroebe, Stroebe, and Hansson 1994).

It has been suggested that one year after bereavement most widows start to rebuild their social lives and establish a new identity (Lieberman 1996). Carr (2004) found that older women who were dependent on their husbands had the lowest self-esteem prior to bereavement; these women had the highest self-esteem following bereavement, however. This suggests that the women's sense of independence increased on discovering that they were able to manage on their own.

Thus, widowhood can be a period of growth, development, and liberation, resulting in acquiring new friends and social activities in the remaining years of life (Chambers 2005; Davidson 2002; Hurd 1999) in contrast to the responsibility of providing care experienced by many older women (Davidson 2001; Graham 1985; Morgan and March 1992). Indeed, there is evidence to suggest that social participation and leisure time, such as activities with friends, actually increase for widows over the long term, around two to three years after loss, suggesting a compensatory effect and new-found freedom (Donnelly and Hinterlong 2010; Ferraro, Mutran, and Barresi 1984; Lopata 1973).

Yet for some widows and widowers, grief continues and for a prolonged period, and they find it difficult to accept the reality of the loss, displaying symptoms known as complicated grief. In most cases there is a gradual decrease in intensity of grief reactions, but for others this is not so. These individuals continue to experience intense yearning for the deceased, they have difficulties in accepting the reality of the loss and experience a loss in the meaning of life, and may develop complicated grief (MacCallum and Bryant 2010; Newson et al. 2011; Stroebe and Stroebe 1987).

Complicated grief is described as the intensification of grief which does not lead to assimilation of the loss, rather to repetitive stereotypic behaviour as well as impaired functioning (Boelen 2006; Malkinson 2007). Life has lost its meaning, there is a sense that life is over, there is preoccupation with the deceased, and there may be difficulties in sleeping, eating, and functioning. In complicated grief there are difficulties in organizing an inner relationship with the deceased, especially the oscillation between avoidance response and flooding, as well as dealing with the pain and yearning that follow the loss (Hansson and Stroebe 2007; Rubin and Malkinson 2001; Stroebe and Schut 1999).

Poor health, multiple losses and traumatic circumstances of death are known to increase the risk of complicated grief, and may result in additional reactions such as depression, anxiety states, and PTSD (Auster et al. 2008). Often, these coexist and overlap, stressing the importance of an assessment prior to applying treatment. Research studies have set the stage for differentiating complicated grief (obsessional preoccupation with the deceased, crying, persistent yearning and searching for the lost person or continuous avoidance) from depression (clinical signs of depression with preoccupation with self), and from anxiety or PTSD (Prigerson et al. 1995a; Shear et al. 2001; Shear et al. 2005). Moreover, complications in grief have been demonstrated as a separate condition from depression and anxiety in older adults as well, emphasizing the need for diagnostic criteria as a preventive measure in treatment (Newson et al. 2011).

Complicated grief may be part of older adults' bereavement process, especially those who experienced traumatic losses in their past and are now dealing with ageing-related losses. However there are major individual differences; while some older bereaved persons may demonstrate resilience and adequate functioning, others who exhibit risk may encounter exacerbation of repressed memories and delayed PTSD (Bonanno et al. 2004; Hansson and Stroebe 2007 Kahana and Kahana 1998).

Bereavement and Depression in Old Age

Depression-like symptoms are generally common in bereavement, especially during the acute phase, in contrast to the normal process in which they gradually diminish (Parkes and Prigerson 2010; Rubin et al. 2012). Most older bereaved people show resilience and remain active in coping with life events, but others respond by developing symptoms of depression or anxiety. In older people, sadness that at times resembles depressive symptoms is common, while psychological adjustment to ageing is complex, and is associated with chronic physical illness that limits the use of anti-depressants. Depression constitutes the most common emotional disorder found in older adults: although the estimate of the prevalence of major depression is 2–10%, milder forms of depression such as dysthymia affect 20–30% of older adults (Anderson 2002). Despite this drawback, older people are rarely offered psychological intervention (Serfaty et al. 2009). Many older patients with depression in primary care remain undetected, with somatization being one of the most important single problems associated with a missed diagnosis (Timonen and Liukkonen 2008).

Depression is not an inevitable outcome of ageing. Alterations in mood and behaviour as a result of depression are sometimes wrongly associated with the ageing process, overlooking the fact that they may be part of a bereavement process. Yet the older bereaved who suffered from depression prior to the loss may develop complicated grief as they continue to suffer from a chronic depression pattern long after the loss. In their study, Bonanno and associates (2004) examined the diversity of bereavement experience and depressive symptoms prior to the death of a spouse. Five bereavement patterns were identified: (1) common grief, an increase in depressive symptoms that receded within eighteen months (11%); (2) resilient pattern (46%), where depressive symptoms were low pre- and post-loss; (3) chronic grief pattern (16%), presenting low pre-loss symptoms that increased at six and eighteen months post-loss; (4) chronic depression (high symptoms of depression pre- and post-loss (8%); (5) depressed-improved: high pre-loss depression scores that abated at five and twenty-eight months (10%). Bereavement is an important predictor of depression among older adults; however, depressive symptoms decline within two years post-loss (Hansson and Stroebe 2007). It is therefore important to consider the timing of post-bereavement assessments, taking into account the non-linear course of symptomatology. Although the prevalence rate of complicated grief among older adults in the general population has not been clearly established, it is nevertheless notable as distinct from depression and anxiety, thus allowing its assessment and treatment as a separate condition or comorbidity (Newson et al. 2011).

INTERVENTIONS WITH THE OLD BEREAVED

Older bereaved individuals invariably experience difficulties in one or more areas in their life; thus, a careful and detailed assessment covering a broad range of factors influencing the bereaved individual's status is essential before formulating a therapy plan (Gallagher-Thompson and Thompson 2010a). Counselling older adults involves not only working with grief over a recent loss, including the behaviours and emotions surrounding it, but also working with accumulated past and present losses and the process of readjustment. Older clients bring into therapy their long-lasting past experiences and coping history, which affect present coping and are an integral part of the bereavement process.

Treatment of the older bereaved represents a challenge to mental health practitioners, who need specific knowledge and skills to work effectively with this subgroup of the bereaved. It incorporates several areas such as knowledge of the normal and pathological ageing processes, the process of uncomplicated and complicated grief, and assessment and suitable interventions for older adults in various settings.

Table 40.1 Elements for the comprehensive assessment of a bereaved person

(a) Physical and cognitive functions including a full record of medications and medical interventions prescribed now and prior to the loss

(b) A detailed account of the reactions and behaviours of the bereaved person since the death.

(c) Quality of relationship with the deceased as described by the bereaved.

(d) Assessment of changes and losses in role investment and in daily life since the loss.

(e) The reactions and expectations of family members and other significant people in the bereaved individual's life.

(f) Past experiences with losses, traumatic experiences, circumstances of the loss (prolonged illness or sudden death) and a history of adaptive or maladaptive functioning.

(g) Contextual and economic realities (i.e. location and neighbourhood, financial status).

(h) Social networks and social support (friends and professional) and especially family relationships and family care-givers who can provide support and enhance therapeutic involvement.

(i) Cohort and personal beliefs, generational issues and attitudes, spiritual and religious beliefs, cultural context, and values regarding old age, psychological intervention, widowhood, and illnesses.

(j) Sociocultural and religious context within which bereavement is experienced by the older adult.

Applying CBT in Normal and Complicated Grief in Older Bereaved

Cognitive-behavioural therapy (CBT) with older depressed has been reported as an effective time-limited intervention that focuses on changing negative thoughts and related emotions and behaviours as a way of minimizing the distress related to inflexible negative thinking (Gallagher-Thompson and Thompson 2010b; Gibson 2013; Laidlaw and MacAlpine 2008, 2010; Laidlaw et al. 2003; Pachana et al. 2010; Serfaty et al. 2009; Whitfield and Williams 2004). Similarly, a growing number of evidence-based studies indicate CBT as an effective treatment for complicated grief (Boelen and de Keijser 2007; Boelen et al. 2011; Shear et al. 2005). In their study, Shear et al. (2005) have modified standard IPT (interpersonal psychotherapy) for complicated grief and included elements of cognitive behaviour (Shear et al. 2001; Shear et al. 2005), which was later developed as complicated grief therapy (CGT) addressing both separate anxiety and traumatic anxiety elements (Shear 2010).

The ABC model of REBT

REBT (rational emotive behaviour therapy) is a CBT model reported to be an efficacious treatment in depression (Daniel, Lynn, and Ellis, 2010) and grief (Boelen et al. 2003; Boelen and Keijser 2007; Boelen et al. 2004). The ABC model (Adverse event—Beliefs—Consequences) is a cognitive theoretical model originated by Ellis (1994) that may be applied in cases of grief and bereavement in general and old age in particular. Like other cognitive models, the REBT model emphasizes the centrality of cognitive processes in understanding emotional disturbance following an adverse event. It views cognition as a mediator between the event and the emotional (and/or behavioural and somatic) response (see Table 40.2). The main feature of this model is the distinction between two sets of cognitions—rational and irrational ones—and their related emotional and behavioural consequences that differ in intensity, duration, and frequency, and mark the difference between healthy and unhealthy adaptation to adverse events (Malkinson 1996, 2001, 2007). This model emphasizes the distinction between healthy reactions to loss (sadness) and prolonged dysfunctional grief (depressive reaction). It provides guidelines for the assessment of bereaved individuals' interpretation of their experience of loss, and offers cognitive, emotional, and behavioural strategies for facilitating a healthier adaptive course of bereavement in cases of loss.

Assessment based on the ABC model, and cognitive therapy for complicated grief, is now outlined and clinical illustrations are provided.

What distinguishes rational from irrational thinking is the *interpretation* that is applied to events. Three main forms of distorted or irrational evaluations are self-downing, frustration intolerance (low frustration tolerance, LFT), and 'awfulizing' (evaluating events as extremely awful and unbearable). These are often followed at point C (Consequence) by emotional distress such as depressive response, anxiety, extreme shame, and guilt, as opposed to a rational evaluation of the event, which is followed by healthy negative emotions such as sadness, pain tolerance, or moderated anger. Frequently, the human tendency to think irrationally reaches a peak following a death event, especially when bereaved

Table 40.2 The ABC of loss and grief

	A Activating Event	
	Death of a significant other	
Irrational: Dysfunctional	**B Beliefs**	**Rational:** Functional
Devaluation of self, others and		Acceptance of self, others and the
the world		world
Unhealthy	**C Consequences**	**Healthy**
Depressive response, anxiety,	Emotional	Sorrow, concern, yearning, pain,
shame, guilt, anger	Behavioural	moderate anger
	Somatic	

individuals evaluate that the death should not have happened to them, or that it is too pain-ful for them to stand (Malkinson and Ellis 2000; Malkinson 2007; Rubin et al. 2012: 128).

Expressed differently, rational beliefs (B) are flexible realistic evaluations of adverse events over which one has no choice, and which stress acceptance of the self, high frustration tol-erance, and a realistic evaluation of the circumstances of the adverse event. The emotional consequences of these evaluations at point (C) are moderate negative and normative: sor-row, sadness, regret, frustration, and concern (Malkinson 2007). One's innate tendency of irrational thinking increases during crises such as a loss through death. Studies sup-port the notion that mental changes occur following a loss (Boelen et al. 2003; Boelen et al. 2004; Janoff-Bulman 1992; Niemeyer 2004). These changes are part of the normal process of bereavement and in most cases appear to be intense immediately following the loss and decrease with time. From the cognitive perspective, an adaptive healthy process of bereave-ment is the ability, even partially, to change one's evaluation of the new situation, to accom-modate to life without the loved one. Prolonged difficulties in doing so may suggest rigidity and inflexibility of irrational thinking that increases (along with other indications) the risk of complicated grief. Thus, treatment interventions should focus on identifying the patterns of irrational thinking and the emotional, non-adaptive consequences, and on adopting alterna-tive patterns of rational thinking, whose consequences are healthy negatives (see Table 40.3). Underlying cognitive-behavioural therapies is the assumption that people have a choice about interpreting events in their life including adverse ones (Ellis 1994; Malkinson 2007).

From this perspective, the grief process is a healthy form of thinking and emoting to help the bereaved person organize his or her disrupted belief system in a more acceptable, real-istic way. Thoughts about the death event are not avoided or ruminated (Nolen-Hoeksema 2002) rather they are rearranged in a balanced way of sadly deploring, and adaptively living, with the loss (see Table 40.3).

The major goals of the ABC of REBT in grief are: (1) to facilitate an adaptive process of grief that involves pronounced healthy negative emotions following the loss that will enable adjustment to the sad reality that no longer includes the deceased; (2) to change dysfunc-tional evaluations (irrational beliefs—irBs) into functional ones (rational beliefs—RBs) and minimize emotional distress; (3) to acquire and practise adaptive behaviours such as over-coming avoiding objects that remind the bereaved of their loved one.

Table 40.3 The ABC of functional and dysfunctional cognitions

Characteristics of grief-related beliefs

Rational (functional) beliefs	Irrational (dysfunctional) beliefs
Flexible evaluation of the event: 'We had a wonderful marriage, I miss her greatly and realize that life has changed forever.'	**Rigid and extreme evaluation of the event:** 'Since her death life is worthless.'
Consistent with reality: 'I get up in the morning feeling sad, thinking about him and realizing how difficult it is without him.'	**Inconsistent with reality:** 'I don't want to get up in the morning because it is another day without him and it is intolerable, awful.'
Acceptance of self and life without him or her: 'Whenever I think of her I cry, it's sad and painful, I miss her. I did all I could to save her.'	**Unacceptability of self and life without him or her:** 'I can't think that she is dead. It's too painful to think of her, I avoid it. I condemn myself for not taking her to the hospital.'
Continuing search for meaning to life: 'We talked a lot before he died and this gives me a lot of comfort in remembering the life we had together. I will always remember him. I think of additional ways to remember him.'	**Life is 'frozen' and lost its meaning:** 'To think that he will not be here means there is nothing left without him. Life is meaningless.'

In working with older bereaved this distinction has the potential for increasing one's inner acceptance or tolerance of uncontrollable events, as well as one's self-efficacy, and requires developing a therapeutic alliance wherein the patient learns the ABC connection and the distinction between rational and irrational beliefs. Cognitive strategies include coping statements, thought restructuring, alternative interpretations, and thought-stopping. Possible additional interventions can include rational emotive body imagery and rational letter writing (Rubin et al. 2012).

Two cases are given to illustrate the application of the ABC of REBT in grief.

Uncomplicated adaptive grief—Case 1

Sam, age 78, a retired engineer was referred to RM for consultation by his family physician. The family physician saw Sam together with his daughter who was worried about what she described as 'my father's depression'. Sam had lost his wife thirteen months earlier to cancer. At the first meeting Sam seemed energetic and a healthy person for his age, who introduced himself to RM with a big smile on his face describing himself and his reaction to his wife's death and his grief, adding that, according to his daughter, he was depressed and should be over his grief by now. Sam disagreed and said that he was sad over the death of his beloved wife, Rebecca. She was his best friend, companion, and confidante. Sam started crying in talking about his wife and described a very close, trusting relationship.

> She knew she was about to die. I realize she prepared me for her death, she showed me how to operate the washing machine; she taught me how to do the shopping and cook for myself.

I cherish every moment and I wasn't ready to hear her talking about it. Now I regret not being able to discuss it with her. We planned the last vacation exactly the way she wanted it and we had a wonderful time.' He looked very sad and in pain when he talked about his wife.

Sam said that although he is retired now, he continues his role as an engineer by going to work and advising his fellow workers on relevant issues. He is socially active and keeps up his daily physical activities.

The consultation included three sessions and was based on the elements of comprehensive assessment (Table 40.1). The following were assessed:

A Sam, age 78, physically healthy with above-average cognitive functioning. Although retired he continues to go to the office every day to consult his fellow workers. No history of medical problems and medications including high blood pressure treatment. Sam reported a routine of physical activity, mostly walking, and appeared fit.

B Sam's account of his reactions to the loss of his wife thirteen months earlier was very open and detailed. His description of his reactions to the loss was followed by spells of sadness and yearning for his beloved wife, recalling their last holiday together when she was ill. On the functioning level, Sam was active, looking after himself, doing shopping, exercises, seeing friends and going to his workplace as consultant. His eating and sleeping routine hadn't changed.

C Sam was very cooperative in recounting the relationship with his deceased wife. Moreover, he was grateful for having been given the opportunity to recall in detail their marital relationship, how they met and married and started their family life.

D Expectations of family members (in Sam's case, his daughter) were the reason for his referral for consultation. There was a discrepancy between Sam's grieving and his daughter's expectations. She was worried about his persistent crying and what she saw as depression. She expected him to resume 'normal' life and was anxious about his reaction. She felt that thirteen months after the loss of her mother Sam was expected to be over the loss. She assessed his ongoing sadness and continuing crying as symptoms of depression. She suggested considering medication.

Therapist's assessment: Despite his intense emotional reactions thirteen months after the death of his wife, his bereavement process is assessed as normative and adaptive. Crying when talking about how much he misses her, yearning for her, and experiencing the pain of the loss was his way of constructing continuing an inner relationship with his beloved wife ('continuing bonds') and reorganizing his memories and life without her.

Interventions included:

(a) Provision of information about grief and bereavement to Sam, his daughter and the family physician.

(b) Normalizing and legitimizing Sam's response to the loss of his wife.

(c) Applying psychoeducational elements of teaching the ABC of rational and irrational grief and the emotional consequences.

(d) Explaining to the daughter the difference between depressive response and grief as well as stressing the importance of providing support to the father's pace of grieving and his need to talk and cry about his beloved deceased wife.

(e) Additionally, strengthening his positive thinking about what had been lost, and enabling yearning to become an integrated part of his memories.

Commentary:

Provision of information to family members and care-givers about grief responses and its course is most important for two reasons: (1) reducing their anxiety regarding acute grief reactions, and (2) legitimizing and normalizing grief reactions.

Minimizing the pressure family members may impose on the older bereaved to terminate grief and return to 'normal' life.

Additionally, professionals need to be aware of, follow and accept the individual's idiosyncratic pace of grief in the older person.

Accumulated and complicated grief—Case 2

Edith, an 81-year-old widow, is a holocaust child survivor living in a nursing home. Edith's daughter referred her to LBR to help cope with her continuing grief and depression.

Edith's husband had died sixteen months prior to the consultation. Since then she had become detached from daily activities and social interactions and was spending most of the day at home or at her daughter's home feeling that she could not adjust to life without her husband. Additionally, six months prior to consultation, Edith's daughter was diagnosed with breast cancer. This was a real shock for Edith. She became very distressed and anxious, and more depressed. She stopped eating, could not sleep at night, lost a lot of weight and became very weak.

Edith's depression was treated by a psychiatrist who prescribed an anti-depressant.

Edith was married to David for almost sixty years and has two daughters and five grandchildren. She describes herself as very sensitive and insecure. She has suffered all her life from anxieties regarding her children and was very dependent on David, who was like a father to her. Edith still deeply grieves his death.

Edith and her sister are the only survivors of their family. She was saved by her sister, who lives overseas but still continues to play a significant role in her life. Her sister phones her every day to check her health and daily activities.

Assessment: complicated grief

Edith's grief over the loss of her husband is accompanied by accumulated past and present losses, some of which are traumatic losses of the holocaust. Unlike her sister and many survivors, she refuses to talk about her traumatic losses, giving the impression that they were never resolved. The loss of her husband, the relocation to a nursing home, deterioration in her health, and the unexpected diagnosis of her daughter's cancer have increased her vulnerability. Edith's bereavement is complicated and accompanied by depression.

Interventions

Treating Edith involved treatment of her anxieties, depression, and her complicated grief. Depleted of both physical and emotional resources at the early phases of the intervention, Edith needed a lot of encouragement and support from the therapist, her daughter, and the professional staff at the nursing home. This was a prerequisite for encouraging her to receive treatment. From the ABC of REBT perspective, Edith evaluated her accumulated losses (past and recent ones) in a very extreme way (in REBT terms: low frustration tolerance and self-downing and unfairness). The major target was:

(a) to provide information about grief and its components, along with
(b) normalizing and legitimizing her grief over past traumatic losses and recent losses,
(c) normalizing her grief over the loss of her husband, David, who was so important in her life, and
(d) teaching Edith the distinction between rational and irrational thinking and their related emotional consequences (i.e. sadness as adaptive response to loss, and the depressive response as a maladaptive one).

The intervention focused on helping Edith adapt to life without her husband as opposed to self–pity. 'It is normal to grieve for David; it is also painful to think that he is no longer available to support you. Having survived so many painful losses, what does it say about you? You are in spite of everything resilient.' Teaching her coping statements was important: 'It is so difficult to experience these losses but I can try and manage as best as I can.' 'Life is not fair but there is no point in ruminating.' 'I can recall nice memories to relieve my pain; David left me with ample supplies to keep on living.' 'There will be days that I feel depressed and there are days that I can cope.'

Commentary: In Edith's case and similar cases it is most important (a) to address the client's available resources to cooperate and be active in therapy which may require intense ongoing support and encouragement from the therapist, (b) to give active support, including reaching out, and frequent, short sessions, and (c) to provide a lot of emotional support to contain despair and agony.

Grief of a care-giver: ambiguous grief

So far we have been dealing with bereavement and grief over the death of loved ones, but significant losses are also experienced by older adults who act as primary care-givers for frail older adults. A change in relationship that occurs when one spouse is physically or cognitively impaired and requires continuous care can be experienced not only as a major strain but also as a major loss among couples, where a greater proportion of self and existence is intertwined with that of the other (Holtslander and Duggleby 2010). Care-giving is especially difficult when an older patient is cognitively impaired. Care-givers may experience symptoms of depression and grief reactions (Doka 1989, 2010; Hansson and Stroebe 2007; Marwit and Meuser 2002; Schulz et al. 2003). The care-giver's grief is about the 'person who was', who is physically alive but has 'died' cognitively and also perhaps emotionally.

In effect, the care-giver's grief is over an ambiguous loss that is unclear, has no resolution, and no closure (Boss 2011). The duality of a loved one's being absent and present at the same time is confusing, and finding a meaning or making sense of the situation becomes immensely challenging. For without meaning it is hard to cope. There is a lonely and often misunderstood mourning, a chronic sadness with an indefinite beginning and termination. Support for the difficulties experienced by widows who cared for their seriously ill husbands comes from a study on widowhood and depression conducted by Carnelley, Wortman, and Kessler (1999). They found that widows whose husbands had been seriously ill before dying did not express increased depression after two to three years, as opposed to widows whose husbands had not been seriously ill, thus suggesting that they had already begun to grieve before their spouse's death. Indeed Morgan and March (1992), in a study utilizing focus group interviews, found that in their sample of widows and care-givers, widowhood was associated with increased social interaction whereas care-giving was associated with increased social isolation.

The care-giver's grief can also be viewed as disenfranchised and, with no clear-cut grief, one that has no familiar rituals for guiding behaviour and bringing people together in support of this loss (Doka 1989, 2010). As time passes, there may be a diminished adaptive capacity among older care-givers, from whom intense, social support may be withdrawn after some time. The ensuing confusion and lack of support may lead to depression, anxiety, family fights, and rifts (Boss 2011). There may be oscillation between hope and despair, anger and intimacy, as well as fluctuations in functioning and changes in mood.

Ambiguous loss and anticipated grief—Case 3

Rachel is 68 years old and is a primary care-giver for her 80-year-old husband, Moses, diagnosed with Parkinson's disease. In the last two years he had two 'strokes' (CVAs) which left him unable to walk without help and unable to read. He has difficulties in talking and suffers from cognitive loss. Moses was a prominent lecturer in one of the leading academic institutions in Israel, and when he became sick Rachel's life changed dramatically. She retired from her successful job and devoted her entire life to taking care of him, managing their financial and professional affairs as well as continuing to help their five children and eleven grandchildren who kept in touch but rarely helped her to take care of their sick father.

Rachel has diabetes and suffers from arthritis. She requires regular medication and treatment but since Moses's illness, she hardly finds time to take care of her own health.

Her husband's deterioration and personality change have become the major source of pain and stress. Moses's frustration is expressed in temper tantrums, refusal to get help and restlessness, all directed against Rachel, which increases her frustration and helplessness. 'He behaves like a little child, screaming and shouting and insulting me in front of people. I do so much for him and instead of being appreciative and grateful he is hostile.' As she talks, Rachel cries a lot, oscillating from present to past as she describes to her therapist (LBR) what a brilliant and most respected person he was and still is when calm and clear-minded. Rachel cannot tolerate it when he starts abusing her and is unable to accept the fact that he has less control at times. Rachel often describes herself as a prisoner, trapped, as Moses wants her around him all the time.

Interventions: Rachel's grief over her husband's 'missing parts' is legitimized, as well as her present and anticipatory grief, as a way to increase her resilience under uncertain circumstances. An additional source of stress for Rachel is her guilt feelings over her thoughts, emotions, and behaviour towards her husband, and her low frustration tolerance over the uncertainty of the progress of his illness.

With the introduction of the ABC model, which distinguishes between the event and its evaluation and the emotional and physical consequences, Rachel is given information about alternative thinking as a way to reduce her emotional distress.

The goal of intervention is to listen to Rachel, provide her with a lot of support, assist her to recognize and legitimize her grief and express her pain and anger, as well teaching her how to accept ambiguity. Other goals include helping her to acquire a coping statement, increase her frustration tolerance while caring for her husband, and practise coping skills in a complex situation by focusing on the positive perceptions of herself and her role as a care-giver. These will decrease stress, and help her to accept herself and her grief as part of her life stage, and enable functioning alongside strengthening her support network. Thus, the experience of anticipated grieving for someone who is still alive but no longer the person that he used to be is a healthy response for well-being.

Commentary: Ambiguous loss challenges the care-giver's functioning and coping, and complicates the grieving process. To be a care-giver as in Rachel's case is an intensely emotional and complex role. Provision of support and legitimization of present and anticipatory grief for care-givers for their intense feelings and stress is of utmost importance. The aim is to assist them to accept their ambivalent and conflicting feelings without feeling guilty, and learn how to balance individuality and togetherness, to consider their own needs, to accept both what was and what remains, and adapt and cope with daily hassles and the uncertain reality that follows.

Summary

Old age is a phase in life where many expected as well as unexpected losses can occur in all life domains. Older bereaved persons may therefore need ongoing support as opposed to the younger bereaved who are more likely to need help earlier. Older bereaved persons are more likely also to experience more frequent oscillation between daily functioning requirements and loss-oriented issues as time goes on, and as bereavement-related symptoms, in some cases, become increasingly embedded in ageing and disablement. Additionally, with increased longevity, larger numbers of older spouses are likely to face ambiguous loss as care-givers for frail older adults and experience disenfranchised grief. Thus, interventions with older bereaved persons need to include strengthening both existing inner and external resources and focus on the choice one has of alternative evaluations of adverse events, assisting in managing the symptoms and maintaining optimal function rather than aiming at recovery or rehabilitation.

In their review of late-life bereavement Shah and Meeks (2012) conclude that although there is no clear boundary between complicated grief and uncomplicated grief, interventions targeted specifically at treating complicated grief have been found to be moderately effective. Although the majority of older bereaved persons will adapt well, some will likely experience complicated grief, at times with depression symptoms, and may need ongoing support as well as professional help.

Details of ways to assess the course of grief were presented in order to determine adaptive and/or maladaptive outcomes, stressing the importance of providing information, legitimizing anticipated grief, and increasing resilience together with applying cognitive-behavioural strategies.

The ABC model of REBT introduced in this chapter views grief as a normal, human, and universal response to loss of a significant person. From this perspective, the purpose of grief is to reorganize life without the deceased and cognitively and emotionally to adopt new evaluations of the bonds with the representation of the deceased. We have addressed normative adaptive grief following the loss of a loved one and the complications of grief in old age as well as grief of a care-giver for a frail older adult who experiences ambiguous loss. Complications from the cognitive perspective are viewed as a form of dysfunctional grief and defined as a persistence over time with no diminishing effect of dominant irrational evaluations regarding the loss event, the deceased, and the self (Malkinson 2007), a form of thought that delays or prevents adaptation to the reality that excludes the deceased. The therapeutic interventions described in the chapter are directed at facilitating the adaptive process to grief and the pain and yearning that are its components as ways to increase the well-being of the older bereaved.

> For everything there is a season and a time for every matter under heaven:
> A time to plant and a time to pluck up what is planted
> A time to be born and a time to die...
> A time to weep and a time to laugh
> A time to mourn and a time to dance...
> A time for war and a time for peace
>
> Ecclesiastes 3:1-9

Key References and Sources for Further Reading

Boss, P. (2011). *Loving Someone Who Has a Dementia: How to Find Hope while Coping with Stress and Grief*. San Francisco: Jossey-Bass.

Hansson, R. O. and Stroebe, M. S. (2007). *Bereavement in Later Life: Coping, Adaptation and Developmental Influences*. London: Tavistock.

Klass, D., Silverman, P. S. and Nickman, L. (1996). *Continuing Bonds*. Washington, DC: Taylor and Francis.

Malkinson, R. (2007). *Cognitive Grief Therapy: Constructing a Rational Meaning to Life Following Loss*. New York: W.W. Norton.

Rubin, S. S., Malkinson, R., and Witztum, E. (2012). *Working with the Bereaved: Multiple Lenses on Loss and Bereavement*. New York: Routledge.

References

Anderson, A. J. (2002). 'Treatment of Depression in Older Adults'. *International Journal of Psychosocial Rehabilitation* 6: 69–78.

Auster, T., Moutier, C., Lanouette, N., and Zisook, S. (2008). 'Bereavement and Depression: Implications for Diagnosis and Treatment'. *Psychiatric Annals* 38(10): 655–661.

Bar-Tur, L. and Levi-Shiff, R. (2000). 'Coping with Losses and Past Trauma in Old Age: The Separation-individuation Perspective'. *Journal of Personal and Interpersonal Loss* 5: 263–281.

Boelen, P. A., van den Bout, J., van den Hout, M. A. (2003). 'The Role of Cognitive Variables in Psychological Functioning after the Death of a First Degree Relation'. *Behaviour Research and Therapy* 41: 1123–1136.

Boelen, P. A., Kip, H. J., Voorsluijs, J. J., and van den Bout, J. (2004). 'Irrational Beliefs and Basic Assumptions in Bereaved University Students: A Comparison Study'. *Journal of Rational-emotive and Cognitive Behavior Therapy* 22(2): 111–129.

Boelen, P. A. (2006). 'Cognitive Behavior Therapy and Complicated Grief: Theoretical Underpinning and Case Description'. *Journal of Loss and Trauma* 11(1): 1–30.

Boelen, P. A. and de Keijser, J. (2007). 'Treatment of Complicated Grief: A Comparison between Cognitive Behavior Therapy and Supportive Counseling'. *Journal of Consulting and Clinical Psychology* 75(2): 277–284.

Boelen, P. A. and Prigerson, H. G. (2007). 'The Influence of Symptoms of Prolonged Grief Disorder, Depression, and Anxiety on Quality of Life among Bereaved Adults: A Prospective Study'. *European Archives of Psychiatry and Clinical Neuroscience* 257: 444–452.

Boelen, P. A., de Keijser, J., van den Hout, M. A., and van den Bout, J. (2011). 'Factors Associated with Outcome of Cognitive Behavioral Therapy for Complicated Grief: A Preliminary Study'. *Clinical Psychology & Psychotherapy* 18: 439–444.

Bonanno, G. A. and Kaltman, S. (2001). 'The Varieties of Grief Experience'. *Clinical Psychology Review* 21: 705–734.

Bonanno, G. A. (2004). 'Loss, Trauma and Human Resilience'. *American Psychologist* 59: 24–28.

Bonanno, G. A., Wortman, C. B., and Nesse, R. M. (2004). 'Prospective Patterns of Resilience and Maladjustment during Widowhood'. *Psychology & Aging* 19: 260–270.

Boss, P. (2011). *Loving Someone who has Dementia: How to find Hope while Coping with Stress and Grief*. San Francisco: Jossey-Bass.

Carnelley, K. B., Wortman, C. B., and Kessler, R. C. (1999). 'The Impact of Widowhood on Depression: Findings from a Prospective Survey'. *Psychological Medicine* 29: 1111–1123.

Carr, D. (2004). 'Gender, Pre Loss Marital Dependence, and Older Adults' Adjustment to Widowhood'. *Journal of Marriage and Family* 66(1): 220–236.

Chambers, P. (2005). *Older Widows and the Life Course: Multiple Narratives of Hidden Lives*. Farnham: Ashgate.

Carstensen, L. L., Turan, B., Scheibe, S., Ram, N., Ernser-Hershfield, H., et al. (2011). 'Emotional Experience Improves with Age: Evidence Based on over 10 Years of Experience Sampling'. *Psychology and Aging* 26(1): 21–33.

Daniel, D., Lynn, S. J, and Ellis, A. (2010). *Rational and Irrational Beliefs*. New York: Oxford University Press.

Davidson, K. (2001). 'Late Life Widowhood, Selfishness and New Partnership Choices: A Gendered Perspective'. *Ageing & Society* 21(3): 297–317.

Davidson, K. (2002). 'Gender Differences in New Partnership Choices and Constraints for Older Widows and Widowers'. *Ageing International* 27(4): 43–60.

Doka, K. J. (1989). 'Disenfranchised Grief'. In K. J. Doka (ed.), *Disenfranchised Grief: Recognizing Hidden Sorrow* (pp. 3–11). Lexington, MA: Lexington Books.

Doka, K.J. (2010). 'Grief, Multiple Loss and Dementia'. *Bereavement Care* 29: 20–35. http://dx.doi.org/10.1080/02682621.2010.255374

Donnelly, E. A. and Hinterlong, J. A. (2010). 'Changes in Social Participation and Volunteer Activity among Recently Widowed Older Adults'. *Gerontologist* 50(2): 158–169.

Ellis, A. (1994). *Reason and Emotion in Psychotherapy: A Comprehensive Method of Treating Human Disturbances* (rev. edn). New York: Birch Lane Press.

Ferraro, K., Mutran, E., and Barresi, C. (1984). 'Widowhood, Health, and Friendship Support in Later Life'. *Journal of Health and Social Behaviour* 25: 245–259.

Freud, S. (1957/1917). 'Mourning and Melancholia'. In J. Strachey (ed. and trans.), *Standard Edition of the Complete Psychological Works of Sigmund Freud* (vol. 14; pp. 237–258). London: Hogarth Press.

Fries, J. F. (1980). 'Aging, Natural Death and the Compression of Morbidity'. *New England Journal of Medicine* 303(3): 130–135.

Gallagher-Thompson, D. and Thompson, L. W. (2010a). *Treating Late-life Depression*. Oxford: Oxford University Press.

Gallagher-Thompson, D. and Thompson, L. W. (2010b). Effectively Using Cognitive Behavioral Therapy with the Oldest-old: Case Examples and Issues for Consideration. In N. A. Pachana, K. Laidlaw, and B. Knight (eds), *Casebook of Clinical Geropsychology* (pp. 275–282). Oxford: Oxford University Press.

Gibson, J. (2013). 'How Cognitive Behavior Therapy Can Alleviate Older People's Grief'. *Mental Health Practice* 15(6): 12–17.

Graham, H. (1985). 'Providers, Negotiators and Mediators: Women as the Hidden Carers'. In E. Lewin and V. Olesen (eds), *Women, Health and Healing: Toward a New Perspective*. London: Tavistock.

Hansson, R. O. and Stroebe, M. S. (2007). *Bereavement in Later Life: Coping, Adaptation, and Developmental Influences*. Washington, DC: American Psychological Association.

Holtslander, L. and Duggleby, W. (2010). 'The Psychosocial Context of Bereavement for Older Women who Were Caregivers for a Spouse with Advanced Cancer'. *Journal of Women and Aging* 22(2): 109–124.

Hurd, L. (1999). 'We're Not Old! Older Women's Negotiation of Aging and Oldness'. *Journal of Aging Studies* 13(4): 419–421.

Janoff-Bulman (1992). *Shattered Assumptions: towards a New Psychology of Trauma*. New York: Free Press.

Kahana, B. and Kahana, E. (1998). 'Toward a Temporal-spatial Model of Cumulative Life Stress: Placing Late-life Stress Effects in a Life-course Perspective'. In J. Lomranz (ed.), *Handbook of Aging and Mental Health: An Integrative Approach* (pp. 153–181). New York: Plenum.

Kastenbaum, R. (1969). 'Death and Bereavement in Later Life'. In A. H. Kutscher (ed.), *Death and Bereavement* (pp. 27–54). Springfield, IL: Charles Thomas.

Keene, J. and Prokos, A. (2008). 'Widowhood and the End of Spousal Care Giving: Relief or Wear and Tear?' *Ageing & Society* 28(4): 551–570.

Klass, D., Silverman, P. S., and Nickman, L. (eds) (1996). *Continuing Bonds*. Washington, DC: Taylor and Francis.

Laidlaw, K. and MacAlpine, S. (2008). 'Cognitive Behaviour Therapy: How Is It Different with Older People?' *Journal of Rational-Emotive and Cognitive-Behavior Therapy* 26(4): 250–262.

Laidlaw, K., Thompson, L. W., Dick-Siskin, L., and Gallagher-Thompson, D. (2003). *Cognitive Behavior Therapy with Older People*. Chichester: Wiley.

Laidlaw, K. (2010). 'Enhancing Cognitive Behaviour Therapy with Older People Using Gerontological Theories as Vehicles for Change'. In N. A. Pachana, K. Laidlaw, and B. G. Knight (eds), *Casebook of Clinical Geropsychology: International Perspectives on Practice*. Oxford: Oxford University Press, pp. 17–31.

Lieberman, M. (1996). *Doors Close, Doors Open: Widows Grieving and Growing*. New York: Grosset/Putnam.

Lopata, H. (1973). *Widowhood in an American City*. Cambridge, MA: Schenkman.

MacCallum, F. and Bryant, R. A. (2010). 'Attentional Bias in Complicated Grief'. *Journal of Affective Disorders* 125: 316–322.

Malkinson, R. (1996). 'Cognitive Behavioral Grief Therapy'. *Journal of Rational-Emotive and Cognitive-Behavior Therapy* 14(4): 156–165.

Malkinson, R. (2001). 'Cognitive Behavioral Therapy of Grief: A Review and Application'. *Research on Social Work Practice* 11(6): 671–698.

Malkinson, R. and Bar-Tur, L. (2004–2005). 'Long-term Bereavement Processes of Older Parents: The Three Phases of Grief'. *Omega* 50(2): 103–129.

Malkinson, R. (2007). *Cognitive Grief Therapy: Constructing a Rational Meaning to Life Following Loss*. New York: W.W. Norton.

Malkinson, R. and Ellis, A. (2000). 'The Application of Rational-emotive Behavior Therapy (REBT) in Traumatic and Non-traumatic Grief'. In R. Malkinson, S. Rubin, and E. Witztum (eds), *Traumatic and Non-traumatic Loss and Bereavement: Clinical Theory and Practice* (pp. 173–196). Madison, CT: Psychosocial Press.

Marwit, S. J. and Meuser, T. M. (2002). 'Development and Initial Validation of an Inventory to Assess Grief of Persons with Alzheimer Disease'. *Gerontologist* 42(6): 751–765.

Morgan, D. and March, S. (1992). 'The Impact of Life Events on Networks of Personal Relationships: A Comparison of Widowhood and Caring for a Spouse with Alzheimer's Disease'. *Journal of Social and Personal Relationships* 9(4): 563–584.

Newson, R. S., Boelen, P. A., Hek, K., Hofman, A., and Tiemeier, H. (2011). 'The Prevalence and Characteristics of Complicated Grief in Older Adults'. *Journal of Affective Disorders* 132: 231–238.

Niemeyer, R. A. (2004). 'Research on Grief and Bereavement: Evaluation and Revolution'. *Death Studies* 32: 489–490.

Nolen-Hoeksema, S. (2002). 'Ruminative Coping and Adjustment'. In M. S. Stroebe, R. O. Hansson, W. Stroebe, and H. Schut (eds), *Handbook of Bereavement Research: Consequences, Coping and Care* (pp. 545–562). Washington, DC: American Psychological Association.

Osterweis, M., Solomon, F., and Green, M. (eds) (1984). *Bereavement, Reactions, Consequences and Care*. Washington, DC: National Academy Press.

Ott, C. H., Lueger, R. J., Kelber, S. T., and Prigerson, H. G. (2007). 'Spousal Bereavement in Older Adults: Common, Resilient, and Chronic Grief with Defining Characteristics'. *Journal of Nervous and Mental Disease* 195(4): 332–341.

Pachana, A. N., Laidlaw, K., and Knight, B. G. (eds) (2010). *Casebook of Clinical Geropsychology: International Perspective on Practice*. Oxford: Oxford University Press.

Parkes, C. M. (1985). 'Bereavement'. *British Journal of Psychiatry* 146: 11–17.

Parkes, C. M. and Prigerson, H. G. (2010). *Bereavement: Studies of Grief in Adult Life* (4th edn). London: Routledge.

Prigerson, H. G., Frank, E., Kasl, S. V., Reynolds, C. F., III Anderson, B., et al. (1995a). 'Complicated Grief and Bereavement-related Depression as Distinct Disorders: Preliminary Empirical Validation in Elderly Bereaved Spouses'. *American Journal of Psychiatry* 152: 22–30.

Prigerson, H. G., Maceiejewski, P. K., Reynolds, C. F, III Bierhals, A. J., Newsom, J. T., et al. (1995b). 'Inventory of Grief: A Scale to Measure Maladaptive Symptoms of Loss'. *Psychiatry Research* 59: 65–79.

Rando, T. A. (1984). *Grief, Dying and Death: Clinical Interventions for Caregivers*. Champaign, IL: Research Press.

Rubin, S. S. (1981). 'A Two-track Model of Bereavement: Theory and Application in Research'. *American Journal of Orthopsychiatry* 51: 101–109.

Rubin, S. S. (1999). 'The Two-track Model of Bereavement: Prospects and Retrospect'. *Death Studies* 23: 681–714.

Rubin, S. S. and Malkinson, R. (2001). 'Parental Response of Child Loss across the Life Cycle: Clinical and Research Perspective'. In M. S. Stroebe, W. Stroebe, and R. O. Hansson (eds), *Handbook of Bereavement Research: Consequences, Coping and Caring* (pp. 219–240). Cambridge: Cambridge University Press.

Rubin, S. S., Malkinson, R., and Witztum, E. (2012). *Working with the Bereaved: Multiple Lenses on Loss and Mourning*. New York: Routledge.

Serfaty, M. A., Hawort, D., Blanchard, M., Buszewicz, M., Murad, S., et al. (2009). 'Clinical Effectiveness of Individual Cognitive Behavioral Therapy for Depressed Older People in Primary Care'. *Archive of General Psychiatry* 66(12): 1332–1340.

Schulz, R., Mendelson, A. B., Haley, W. E., Mahoney, D., Allen, R. S., et al. (2003). 'End-of-life Care and the Effects of Bereavement on Family Caregivers of Persons with Dementia'. *New England Journal of Medicine* 349: 1936–1942.

Shah, S. N. and Meeks, S. (2012). 'Late-life Bereavement and Complicated Grief: A Proposed Comprehensive Framework (Review)'. *Aging & Mental Health* 16(1): 39–56.

Shear, K. (2010). 'Complicated Grief Treatment: The Theory, Practice and Outcome'. *Bereavement Care* 29(3): 10–14. Also available: Bereavement Care http://www.informaworld.com/smpp/title~content=t901546305

Shear, K., Frank, E., Foa, E., Cherry, C., Reynolds, C. F. III, et al. (2001). 'Traumatic Grief Treatment: A Pilot Study'. *American Journal of Psychiatry* 158(9): 1506–1608.

Shear, K., Frank, E., Houck, P. R., and Reynolds, C. F. III (2005). 'Treatment of Complicated Grief: A Randomized Controlled Study'. *Journal of the American Medical Association* 293(21): 2601–2608.

Stroebe, W. and Stroebe, M. S. (1987). *Bereavement and Health: The Psychological and Physical Consequences of Partner Loss*. Cambridge: Cambridge University Press.

Stroebe, M., Stroebe, W., and Hansson, R. (1994). *Handbook of Bereavement: Theory, Research, and Intervention*. Cambridge: Cambridge University Press.

Stroebe, M. S. and Schut, H. (1999). 'The Dual Process Model of Coping with Loss'. *Death Studies* 23: 1–28.

Timonen, M. and Liukkonen, T. (2008). 'Management of Depression in Adults'. *Clinical Review* 336: 435–439.

Whitfield, G. and Williams, C. (2004). 'The Evidence Base for Cognitive-behavioral Therapy in Depression: Delivery in Busy Clinical Settings'. *Advances in Psychiatric Treatment* 9: 21–30.

Wortman, C. M. and Silver, R. (1989). 'The Myth of Coping with Loss'. *Journal of Consulting and Clinical Psychology* 57: 349–359.

CHAPTER 41

COMBINING MEDICATION AND PSYCHOTHERAPY FOR LATE-LIFE ANXIETY AND MOOD DISORDERS

JILL A. STODDARD, CHRISTOPHER BARMANN,
ERIC LENZE, AND JULIE L. WETHERELL

INTRODUCTION

OLDER adults are the fastest-growing segment of the population. It is estimated that two billion adults will be over the age of 60 by the year 2050 (United Nations 2010). Anxiety and mood disorders are common among older adults and result in significant impairment. In community samples, up to 19% meet criteria for at least one anxiety disorder (Flint 1994). In medically ill cohorts, rates may be even higher (De Beurs et al. 1999; Kennedy and Schwab 1997). Depression and dysthymic disorder are present in about 15% of older adults (Gareri et al. 2000) with recurrence rates of major depressive episodes ranging from 50–90% over the course of two to three years (Post, Benson, and Blumer 1998; Zis et al. 1980). Bipolar disorder, while less common in older adults (less than 1%), is associated with significantly higher rates of morbidity and mortality than in younger adults (Goodwin and Jamison 1990; Sajatovic, Popli, and Semple 1996) and significant utilization of healthcare resources (Bartels et al. 2000). In fact, all anxiety and mood disorders are associated with greater rates of mortality, high healthcare expenditures, and reduced quality of life (Beekman et al. 2000; Smit et al. 2006). If left untreated, anxiety and mood disorders tend to follow a chronic, unremitting course (Larkin, Copeland, and Dewney 1992).

While mental health issues in older adults have received increasing attention in recent years, a relative dearth of information remains. Currently, consensus is lacking as to the most appropriate treatment for anxiety and mood disorders in old age. This may in large part be due to conflicting evidence regarding the efficacy of many pharmacological and psychosocial treatments, as well as findings that many monotherapies (i.e. medication or therapy alone) fail to result in high-end-state functioning (Lenze et al. 2009).

Selective serotonin reuptake inhibitors (SSRIs) are generally considered first-line treatments for anxiety and depression in older adults because side-effects are manageable and the risk of overdose is low (Alexopoulos et al. 2001). Many studies have shown promising results with SSRI treatment; however, significant room for improvement exists. For example, one study of depressed older adults found that fewer than 50% achieved remission despite adequate dosing (Unutzer et al. 2002), and another found that SSRIs were only moderately efficacious in the treatment of generalized anxiety (Lenze et al. 2009). Benzodiazepines are commonly prescribed for anxiety. However, in late life, benzodiazepine use is associated with cognitive impairment, increased fall risk, and dependency (Benitez et al. 2008). In addition, many older adults are reluctant to take medications due to feared side-effects and potential issues associated with polypharmacy and multiple medical diagnoses (Gum et al. 2006). Thus, older patients often prefer psychosocial interventions (Wetherell et al. 2004).

For bipolar disorder, medications are considered an essential component of treatment. To our knowledge, only one double-blind, randomized efficacy trial addressing specific treatment recommendations for older adults with bipolar disorder has been conducted (Young, Gyulai, and Mulsant 2010). Apart from this study, pharmacological treatment of bipolar disorder in older adults has been derived from mixed-age and uncontrolled clinical studies of younger adults, stipulating the use of conventional mood stabilizers and anti-convulsants as a first-line treatment (Sajatovic et al. 2005a; Young et al. 2004). However, studies have shown that lithium tends to be poorly tolerated and possibly less effective in older patients, leading to increased side-effects and decreased rates of remission (Sajatovic, Madhusoodanan, and Coconea 2005a; Sajatovic, Calabrese, and Mullen 2008).

Nearly all randomized controlled trials investigating the efficacy of psychotherapy in older adults with mood and anxiety disorders have involved elements of cognitive-behavioural therapy (CBT), interpersonal therapy (IPT), or interpersonal and social rhythm therapy (IPSRT, a therapy that combines IPT with behavioural techniques aimed at mitigating circadian and sleep-wake vulnerabilities). While the majority of studies have shown these psychosocial treatments to be superior to wait-list and control conditions, many participants continue to have clinically elevated symptoms (Barrowclough et al. 2001; Thorp et al. 2009). For example, one study investigating group CBT for older adults with generalized anxiety disorder (GAD) found that only half of patients achieved a significant reliable change index at post-treatment. This increased to two-thirds at follow-up, but 30% were left with clinically significant symptoms six months following treatment termination (Wetherell et al. 2005).

While monotherapies may provide some benefit to older adults with anxiety and mood disorders, outcomes have been unimpressive and substantial room for improvement exists. Likewise treatment compliance may be influenced by patient preferences. In an effort to improve outcomes and retention, researchers have increasingly focused on optimizing treatment strategies by combining pharmacotherapy and psychosocial interventions. The remainder of this chapter will focus on a review of the treatment outcome literature investigating (1) combination treatment, (2) sequential treatment, and (3) augmentation treatment.

TREATMENT STRATEGIES DEFINED

Combination treatment involves starting two treatments simultaneously (i.e. medication and psychotherapy). The goal is to maximize the acute treatment response as quickly and effectively as possible. However, it may be argued that this strategy could expose some patients who would have otherwise responded to monotherapy to unnecessary interventions as well as avoidable costs and side-effects. In addition, combination treatment requires more of a patient when it comes to treatment compliance. Specifically, patients are obliged to adjust to a new daily medication and its side-effects, while simultaneously learning and practising novel therapy skills. Finally, combination treatment may not correspond to 'real-world' clinical practice.

In contrast, *sequential treatment* involves adding a second treatment after the acute period of an initial treatment has been completed. Some have suggested that sequential treatment may have several advantages over combination treatment. These include (1) allowing the provider and patient to focus sequentially on different aspects of treatment, rather than dividing focus among multiple treatments and components of illness at once; (2) offering treatment that is likely more reflective of real clinical practice, in which providers will examine a patient's response to one therapeutic option before adding another; and (3) allowing for one treatment to be a catalyst for the next (Fava, Park, and Sonino 2006). In GAD, for example, SSRI treatment can reduce acute distress and somatic symptoms, allowing CBT to address underlying worry control, engage cognitive distortions, and improve coping skills. Thus, with two interventions targeting different facets of the illness, treatment may be optimized leading to reductions in persistent residual features and relapse. The only potential disadvantage of sequential treatment is a possible slower time to response and recovery compared with combination treatment.

Augmentation treatment is a specific type of sequential strategy in which a second treatment is added only after an initial treatment has proven to be only partially effective. Augmentation treatment is cost-effective in that additional treatments are only added when definitively needed. However, there may be benefits to adding a second treatment even to those who are no longer symptomatic. For example, relapse prevention may be enhanced (Fava et al. 2006) or social functioning improved (Lenze et al. 2002).

COMBINATION TREATMENT

When monotherapies are inadequate, combined psychotherapy and medication may confer an advantage, particularly because the two treatments have different mechanisms of action and may be able to treat different aspects of the illness. In addition, combination treatment may work faster than monotherapies alone. While there have been numerous studies investigating combined medication and psychotherapy for mood and anxiety disorders in younger adults, far fewer studies have focused on an older population.

Mood disorders: depression

To our knowledge, only seven published studies have evaluated the impact of combined medication and psychotherapy on late-life depression; none have investigated treatment efficacy for dysthymia. The majority of studies have looked at IPT plus anti-depressant medication, with fewer investigating CBT plus anti-depressants and one examining dialectical behaviour therapy (DBT) and anti-depressant medication. Overall, the data suggest that, for certain samples, combined treatments are stronger than monotherapies for older adults with major depression.

In the earliest study investigating combined treatment for late-life depression (Reynolds et al. 1992), seventy-three adults aged 60 and older with nonbipolar, nonpsychotic depression were treated with open-label, simultaneous IPT and nortriptyline (80–120ng/ml). IPT was manualized and delivered weekly for fifty minutes. IPT focuses on four core problem areas thought to be particularly relevant for depressed older adults: grief/bereavement, role disputes, role transitions, and interpersonal deficits.

Participants received combined treatment until achieving response, at which point they were enrolled in sixteen weeks of continuation treatment. For those not achieving a full response after eight weeks, adjunctive medication (e.g. lithium or perphenazine) was added until response was achieved. To enter continuation, maintenance of response was required for three weeks after discontinuation of the adjunctive medication. During continuation, nortriptyline was continued at the same dose and IPT was reduced to every other week for eight weeks, then every three weeks for the final eight weeks. Following the sixteen-week continuation phase participants were randomized to one of four maintenance conditions: medication alone, placebo alone, medication plus monthly IPT, or placebo plus monthly IPT. Those in the non-IPT conditions met with a provider for thirty minutes in a medication clinic where they were asked about symptoms and side-effects but no therapy was provided. Participants were actively treated across conditions for three years or until recurrence of a major depressive episode, whichever occurred first.

Preliminary results from the acute and continuation phase of the study indicated that of sixty-one participants who completed acute treatment, forty-eight (78.7%) were full responders (defined as a score of 10 or less on the Hamilton Depression Rating Scale (Ham-D); Hamilton 1960), three were partial responders, and ten were non-responders. The mean reduction in Ham-D score was clinically significant at 71%. Overall, results were superior to past investigations of monotherapies for late-life depression (Georgotas et al. 1988; Gerson, Plotkin, and Jarvik 1988; Thompson, Gallagher, and Breckenridge 1987). However, these results were from the open-label phase and thus did not include random assignment, double blind conditions, or comparison groups. The results from the larger, full-scale study (Reynolds 1999a), which included these controls, will be reported below.

First, a follow-up report (Reynolds et al. 1994) described the thirty-two participants who were randomized to the two maintenance placebo conditions (placebo alone and placebo plus IPT) and experienced a return of symptoms during the transition phase. Upon relapse, participants were switched from placebo to active nortriptyline and IPT. Ninety percent of participants were re-stabilized and achieved remission. In addition, remission was achieved more quickly for the second episode compared with the first. Thus, in summary, combined IPT and nortriptyline successfully and rapidly treated recurrent episodes of depression in older adults. Again, this phase of the trial preceded the randomized, double blind portion which is described below.

In the final randomized controlled trial investigating nortriptyline and IPT as a maintenance strategy for late-life depression (Reynolds et al. 1999a), 180 depressed older adults were enrolled in the acute treatment phase. Of these, 107 participants fully recovered and were randomized to one of the four maintenance treatment conditions (described above). Fifty-nine experienced a recurrence at some point during the three-year maintenance phase, with most occurring during the first year. The combined treatment group had the least number of recurrences, with 80% remaining depression-free at the end of three years. Pair-wise analyses indicated that all three active treatment conditions significantly outperformed placebo with combined treatment performing best, followed by medication alone and IPT alone, which did not significantly differ from each other. In addition, social adjustment improved in the combined therapy group but declined in groups receiving monotherapy (Lenze et al. 2002).

Interestingly, when outcomes were split by age group (60–70 and 70 plus), older age was associated with higher and faster rates of relapse in all conditions except the combined IPT plus medication condition. In the younger age group, all three active treatments performed equally well.

Results from this study suggest that combined maintenance therapy is superior to monotherapy for preventing relapse of depression in older adults who have achieved remission. This is particularly important given the high rates of recurrence reported in the literature (Flint and Rifat 1998; Post, Benson, and Blumer 1998; Zis et al. 1980). While the focus of this study was relapse prevention, it is worth commenting on the efficacy of the acute, combined treatment as well. Of the 180 participants who began acute treatment, 159 completed the acute phase and 84% of those achieved full remission. In addition, of the 133 who entered the continuation phase, nearly 90% remained fully recovered (reasons for attrition are provided in the original article; Reynolds et al. 1999a). While these initial treatment phases did not include a comparison group, these rates of remission are higher than reported in many studies of monotherapies for older adults.

A related study investigating acute treatment with combined nortriptyline and IPT in older adults with a bereavement-related major depressive episode found similar results. Specifically, combined treatment resulted in the highest rates of remission compared to nortriptyline alone, placebo alone, and IPT plus placebo (Reynolds et al. 1999b). In both studies, the superior response associated with combined treatment may have, in part, been due to the ability of the two treatments to address both the biological and psychosocial elements associated with depression.

Currently, nortriptyline and other tricyclic anti-depressants, while clinically useful, are less commonly prescribed due to risk associated with overdose and greater side-effects. SSRIs are now favoured in contemporary clinical care settings. Thus, more recent studies have investigated combined psychotherapy and SSRI treatments.

In another placebo-controlled, double-blind, randomized controlled trial, Reynolds et al. (2006) investigated the efficacy of paroxetine and IPT in participants aged 70 and older with nonpsychotic, nonbipolar depression. All participants received an open trial of paroxetine (10-40mg/day) and weekly IPT until achieving response. This was followed by a sixteen-week continuation phase of continued paroxetine and IPT every other week. Those who achieved at least partial recovery were randomly assigned to one of four conditions: paroxetine plus monthly IPT, paroxetine alone, placebo plus monthly IPT, or placebo alone. Those in the paroxetine and placebo conditions also had monthly, thirty-minute clinical management sessions where they were asked about symptoms and side-effects but no therapy was provided. Participants received treatment for two years or until recurrence of a major depressive episode.

Of the 151 participants who began the continuation phase, 116 completed the phase and 100% of those were partially or fully recovered and were randomized into one of the four maintenance arms. Ninety participants completed the maintenance phase and fifty-one of those experienced a recurrence at some point during the two years. The combined treatment and paroxetine groups had the lowest rates of recurrence at 35% and 37%, respectively (after adjusting for censoring). Surprisingly, while 58% of the placebo only participants relapsed, the highest rate of recurrence was in the placebo plus IPT group (68%), suggesting that IPT does not protect against relapse when not combined with medication. Pair-wise analyses indicated that combined treatment and paroxetine alone significantly outperformed placebo plus IPT (p = .03). Combined treatment was also superior to placebo alone (p = .05). Paroxetine alone approached significance when compared to placebo alone (p = .06).

Interestingly, the highest recurrence rates (75%) occurred among participants who received additional pharmacotherapy (e.g. lithium). This is of particular importance given the common practice of physicians to augment treatment with additional medications if a single medication is not performing adequately. In addition, higher levels of anxiety, greater medical burden, and poorer sleep quality all predicted faster times to relapse. Thus, clinicians will want to pay particular attention to these variables when treating depressed older adults.

Results from this study suggest that paroxetine is effective for preventing relapse of depression in older adults who have achieved partial or full remission; the addition of IPT does not provide additional protective benefits. Moreover, IPT in the absence of active medication appears to be contraindicated as a maintenance strategy. This finding is inconsistent with the earlier studies reviewed (Reynolds et al. 1999a and 1999b) and may be due to the older age of the participants, greater medical burden, and greater cognitive impairment in the current sample. In addition, more participants in the current study were experiencing a first, late-onset episode of depression, compared with the former study which recruited only participants with recurrent depression. Late-onset depression may be different (e.g. related to dementia) and thus may respond differently to psychotherapy.

We found only one study that examined the efficacy of combined CBT and medication for late-life depression. In this randomized controlled trial, participants aged 60 and older with nonpsychotic, nonbipolar depression were randomized to one of three conditions: desipramine alone, CBT alone, or desipramine plus CBT (Thompson et al. 2001). Across conditions, participants were seen twice weekly for four weeks then once weekly for eight to twelve weeks. The mean level of desipramine was 90mg/day and the CBT intervention was manualized, based on Beck et al. (1979) with modifications for older adults (e.g. slower presentation, greater amount of practice). Generally speaking, CBT focuses on changing distorted beliefs and schemas (e.g. 'I'm a failure', 'Nothing ever goes right for me') as well as maladaptive behaviours (e.g. social isolation) that are thought to contribute to low mood.

Using growth-modelling analyses, results indicated significant per-session improvement across all three treatment conditions on the Ham-D, and significant improvement on the Beck Depression Inventory – short form (BDI-SF; Beck et al. 1961) in the CBT alone and CBT plus desipramine conditions, but not the desipramine alone condition. Rates of improvement differed across groups as well. On the Ham-D, the combined condition showed greater rates of change than the desipramine alone condition. There were no statistical differences between the combined and CBT alone groups, or the CBT alone and desipramine alone groups. On the BDI-SF, rates of improvement for the combined and CBT alone conditions were greater than the desipramine alone condition. The combined and CBT alone conditions did not differ from one another.

In intent-to-treat analyses, repeated measures analyses of variance revealed signifi-cant main effects for time, indicating that participants' scores on measures of depression improved over time across treatment groups. Significant time by group interactions were also found indicating that combined treatment outperformed desipramine alone on both measures, and CBT alone led to superior response compared to desipramine alone on the BDI-SF; improvement on the Ham-D was marginally significant (p = .053).

Findings from this study indicate that combining CBT and desipramine has clear advan-tages over drug therapy alone, and in some cases, CBT alone may also confer an advantage over drug therapy alone (e.g. on self-report measures of depression). The authors posited that subtherapeutic doses of desipramine may have accounted for these results; however, the findings held up even when medication dose and depression severity were controlled.

This study did not include a control group or placebo condition so it is impossible to state definitively that the active treatments were wholly responsible for improvement. In addi-tion, the sample was fairly young, white, healthy, educated, and high functioning; thus, results may not generalize to a more heterogeneous or impaired group.

One study investigated the impact of combined group DBT with standard medication management (SMM; Lynch et al. 2003). Thirty-four participants aged 60 and older with nonpsychotic, unipolar depression were randomly assigned to receive SMM alone or SMM plus group DBT. SMM consisted of visits with a psychiatrist approximately every thirteen weeks. Medication type, number, and dose were based on clinical expertise (as in 'treatment as usual' rather than a protocol devised for the study). DBT consisted of weekly, two-hour group sessions plus weekly thirty-minute telephone coaching sessions, all of which focused on attainment of skills via four treatment modules: emotion regulation, distress tolerance, interpersonal effectiveness, and mindfulness. The duration of the group was twenty-eight weeks; following the twenty-eight weeks, phone coaching continued for six months but was reduced to every other week for the first three months and monthly for the last three months.

Results indicated that both groups improved over time on clinician-rated measures of depression, but only the combined group improved on self-rated depression. In addi-tion, remission rates were better in the combined group (71%) compared to the SMM only group (47%) at post-treatment as well as at six-month follow-up (75% vs 31%, respectively). Finally, only those in the combined group showed significant improvements on measures of coping and sociotropy. This is particularly relevant as these constructs have been pro-posed to create vulnerability to depression. As shown in Table 41.1, the majority of current research demonstrates the efficacy of combined treatment as superior when compared to monotherapy for achieving and sustaining remission in older adults evidencing late-life depression.

Mood disorders: bipolar disorder

Contrary to the current notion that older adults with bipolar disorder are hospitalized less often due to a decreased likelihood of displaying disruptive manic features in late-life, research has shown that the utilization of mental health services by these individuals is on the rise (Broadhead and Jacob 1990).

Table 41.1 Combined treatment for late-life depression

Study author(s)	Treatment	Results
Reynolds et al. (1999a, 1999, 1992, 1994)	IPT plus nortriptyline	Combined maintenance therapy is superior to monotherapy for achieving remission and preventing relapse.
Reynolds et al. (2006)	IPT plus paroxetine	Combined treatment is significantly superior to placebo and medication alone for achieving and sustaining remission.
Thompson et al. (2001)	CBT plus desipramine	Combining CBT and desipramine is superior to medication monotherapy for achieving and sustaining remission.
Lynch et al. (2003)	DBT plus medication	Combining DBT plus medication led to increased remission rates and greater improvement on self-rated depression compared to medication alone.

In a study by Bartels et al. (2000), older adult patients with bipolar disorder used a significantly greater amount of total outpatient mental health services when compared with a unipolar major depression group ($p < 0.0001$). In addition, late-life bipolar patients were more likely to receive partial hospitalization care over the one-month study period and were three times more likely to have had acute psychiatric inpatient hospitalizations. Interestingly, older adults are continuing to experience a recurrence in symptoms leading to psychiatric hospitalizations despite the increased utilization of mental health services.

Unfortunately, a lack of scientific studies examining the efficacy of pharmacological treatments of bipolar disorder in late-life has consequently led to an increased recurrence of symptomatology when implementing a standard medication protocol (Sajatovic et al. 2005b; Young 2005). Despite the need for more serious inquiry into the issue of best practices in older patients with bipolar disorder, we were unable to find published studies evaluating the efficacy of medication plus simultaneous psychotherapy for the treatment of late-life bipolar disorder. However, consistent with the current trend in treating late-life bipolar disorder, mixed-age, randomized controlled studies have been conducted evaluating the efficacy of combining pharmacological and psychosocial treatment. In general, these findings have suggested that psychosocial treatments, like family-focused therapy (FFT) and IPSRT, play an important role in the management of bipolar disorder, predominantly decreasing the risk of relapse and re-hospitalization and increasing adherence to medication protocols (Miklowitz 2007; Miklowitz, Axelson, and Birmaher 2008; Rea et al. 2003).

Craighead and Miklowitz (2000) note that psychosocial interventions can be incorporated into treatment regimens to enhance the effects of pharmacological interventions. With late-life bipolar disorder, the combination of simultaneous medication and psychotherapy may result in a collaborative interaction, promoting medication compliance, symptom management, and decreased psychiatric hospitalizations. However, the efficacy of these findings in the treatment of older adults is unclear when taking into account medical comorbidities and age-related factors. As shown in Table 41.2, further research is needed to

Table 41.2 Combined treatment for late-life bipolar disorder

Study author(s)	Treatment	Results
Rea et al. (2003) Miklowitz (2007) Miklowitz et al. (2008)	FFT plus medication	Combined treatment led to a decrease in the risk for relapse and re-hospitalization, and an increase adherence to medication protocols.

determine the benefits of treatment protocols implementing simultaneous medication and psychosocial interventions for late-life bipolar disorder.

Anxiety disorders

To our knowledge, no studies have investigated the efficacy of combination treatment in older adults with anxiety disorders. The only study we were able to find focused on sequential treatment for GAD and will be discussed below.

SEQUENTIAL TREATMENT

While combined treatment may offer rapid rates of response, sequential treatment is likely more reflective of clinical practice, allows patients to focus on one treatment at a time, and may have a catalytic effect (Wetherell et al. 2010). Despite the strong arguments for sequential treatment, we came across no empirical studies of sequential treatments for depression, dysthymia, or bipolar disorder in older adults.

Anxiety disorders

We know of only one study that has investigated sequential treatment in older adults with anxiety. This recent multisite randomized controlled trial by Wetherell and colleagues (2013) investigated the impact of adding escitalopram to modular CBT in seventy-three adults aged 60 years and older with a principal diagnosis of GAD. Participants were excluded for evidence of psychosis or substance dependence in the past six months, current suicidal ideation, or cognitive impairment. All psychotropic medication was tapered prior to beginning the study.

Enrolled participants completed an acute treatment phase involving twelve weeks of open-label escitalopram (10–20mg depending on improvement and drug tolerance). Those improving by at least 20% during the acute treatment phase were randomized to one of four conditions (n = 73): (1) sequential phase of sixteen weeks of continued escitalopram plus sixteen CBT sessions, followed by twenty-eight weeks of maintenance escitalopram alone; (2) sixteen weeks of continued escitalopram without CBT, followed by twenty-eight weeks of maintenance escitalopram alone; (3) sixteen weeks of continued escitalopram plus sixteen sessions of CBT, followed by twenty-eight weeks of maintenance pill placebo; or (4) sixteen weeks of continued escitalopram without CBT, followed by twenty-eight weeks of maintenance pill placebo. For all participants, CBT was manualized and included psychoeducation, relaxation training, problem-solving, cognitive restructuring, and skills practice. For any participant with a supportive, local family member, treatment also included a family support module. For some participants, CBT included modules devoted to behavioural activation (for those who were identified as depressed according to assessments), exposure therapy (for those with other anxiety disorders), or sleep hygiene (for those with sleep complaints).

Results indicated that during the sequential phase, those receiving escitalopram alone did not differ from those receiving escitalopram plus CBT on the Ham-A, a measure of physiological anxiety. However, when looking at only the thirty-four participants who remained symptomatic at the end of the acute treatment phase, 53% who received medication plus CBT were classified as responders, compared with only 27% who were taking medication alone. Further, on the Penn State Worry Questionnaire (PSWQ; Meyer et al. 1990), a measure of worry, those receiving both medication and CBT were three times more likely to respond to treatment by the end of sixteen weeks compared to those receiving escitalopram alone. During the maintenance phase, both escitalopram groups (CBT and no CBT) resulted in significantly lower relapse rates than both placebo conditions. There were no differences in relapse rates for those receiving medication plus CBT compared with those receiving medication without CBT. Among the two placebo conditions, 65% relapsed without CBT compared with 25% who received CBT.

In summary, this study found support for sequential therapy for late-life GAD, which can be seen in Table 41.3. Escitalopram alone led to the greatest reductions in physiological anxiety, whereas escitalopram plus CBT led to better reductions in worry. Further, maintenance CBT protected against relapse relative to pill placebo. This suggests a few important things: (1) medication and CBT likely target different aspects of GAD (i.e. physiological symptoms vs worry, respectively), thus providing support for combining treatments and (2) patients may need to remain medicated or participate in CBT (if they wish to discontinue medication) in order to protect against relapse. The study was limited by its small sample size and lack of a psychotherapy comparison group; however, it is the first and only sophisticated multisite RCT investigating treatment sequencing for late-life anxiety.

Table 41.3 Sequential Treatment For Late–Life Anxiety Disorder

Study author(s)	Treatment	Results
Wetherell et al. (2013)	Escitalopram added to CBT	Escitalopram improved physiological anxiety; adding CBT led to greater reductions in worry; both protect against relapse.

Augmentation Treatment

A specific form of sequential treatment, augmentation involves adding a second treatment only when an initial treatment results in an inadequate response. Augmentation treatment may be more cost-effective than combination or traditional sequential treatment in that additional treatments are only added when definitively needed.

Mood disorders: depression

One study investigated the impact of augmenting combined treatment (paroxetine plus IPT) with additional medication (bupropion, nortriptyline, or lithium) for older adults with an inadequate response to acute treatment (Dew et al. 2007). One hundred and ninety-five participants aged 70 and older with nonpsychotic, unipolar depression were treated with paroxetine (10–40mg) and weekly IPT until response was achieved, followed by sixteen weeks of bi-weekly IPT and continued paroxetine. Non-responders and responders with early relapse received medication augmentation of either sustained-release bupropion (150–400mg), nortriptyline (120ng/L), or lithium carbonate (.5–.7 mEq/L; for details of the standardized protocol refer to Whyte et al. 2004 and Mulsant et al. 2001). If no clinical response was achieved via augmentation, the first augmentation medication was discontinued and another added.

Of the 195 initially enrolled in the combined IPT/paroxetine condition, seventy-seven (40%) were classified as non-responders and twenty-eight (14%) evidenced a loss of response; sixty-nine of the seventy-seven went on to receive augmentation treatment (see original article for reasons for attrition; Dew et al. 2007). Overall, those who never required augmentation were significantly more likely to recover than those who did require augmentation (87% of initial responders recovered vs 50% of non-responders vs 67% of early relapsers, x^2 = 21.8, p <.001). Additionally, participants requiring augmentation reported significantly greater side-effects than those who did not, irrespective of eventual responder status. Finally, non-responders requiring augmentation took longer to eventually recover (median of twenty-eight weeks) than responders and early relapsers (both with a median of twenty-four weeks). Both medical burden and anxiety at baseline were predictors of slower rates of recovery.

Results of this study provide some support for using medication augmentation in depressed older adults who either do not respond to acute treatment or evidence an early relapse. According to study authors, while participants who required augmentation were less likely to respond than those who did not, rates of eventual response in the augmentation group were still better than those in studies of younger depressed adults. However, many older adults may not be able to tolerate the added medication, especially given the finding that the non-responder augmentation group evidenced the highest levels of side-effects. In addition, thirty-six participants dropped out or refused augmentation, often for reasons related to medical burden. Among those who did receive augmentation, higher medical burden predicted slower time to recovery. Thus, augmentation may be a viable option for non-responding, depressed older adults; however, clinicians will need to be aware of the higher likelihood of side-effects and impact of baseline medical burden.

A more recent study investigated the impact of augmenting escitalopram with IPT in older adults with a partial response to medication alone (Reynolds et al. 2010). One hundred and twenty-four participants aged 60 and older taking 10mg of escitalopram for nonpsychotic, unipolar depression were randomized to receive augmentation treatment of sixteen weeks of IPT plus depression care management (DCM; sixty to seventy-five minutes per session) or DCM alone (forty-five to fifty minutes). In both conditions, participants continued treatment with escitalopram but the dose was raised from 10 to 20mg. DCM consisted of psychoeducation about late-life depression, anti-depressant medication, sleep hygiene, and suicidality. It also included review and management of symptoms and side-effects, encouragement to remain treatment compliant, and a reminder of a twenty-four-hour on-call service.

Results indicated that participants in both groups demonstrated similar response rates (58% in the IPT group vs 45% in the DCM group, p = .14) and similar median times to response (five weeks in the IPT group and six weeks in the DCM group), demonstrating that IPT offered no added benefit over DCM alone. However it should be noted that DCM added elements of a psychosocial treatment that went beyond a simple medication dose increase and this likely contributed to improved outcomes compared to past studies. Thus, while IPT was not superior to DCM, combining medication with some elements of psychosocial treatment still appeared to have advantages over monotherapy. Another consideration is that IPT augmentation was initiated after only six weeks at escitalopram 10mg. It is possible that many participants had a delayed response, or responded to the increase in escitalopram dose to 20mg, and therefore the augmentation phase included many people who were eventually going to respond to escitalopram alone.

Finally, this study was different in that very few exclusion criteria were imposed. Participants were included who had significant medical and psychiatric comorbidities, including current or past suicidal ideation and mild neurocognitive impairment. Thus, generalizability of results was improved over past studies. As seen in Table 41.4, further research is needed to demonstrate the efficacy of augmented treatment strategies for managing late-life depression.

Mood disorders: bipolar disorder

In the past decade, clinical outcome research has focused on augmentation treatment of bipolar disorder in mixed-age samples. Unfortunately, to our knowledge there are no

Table 41.4 Augmented treatment for late-life depression

Study author(s)	Treatment	Results
Dew et al. (2007)	Paroxetine with IPT augmented with additional medication	Medication augmentation was most effective for depressed older adults who either did not response to acute treatment or evidenced an early relapse.
Reynolds et al. (2010)	Escitalopram with IPT augmented with DCM	Psychosocial treatment augmentation appeared to have advantages over monotherapy.

known studies that have focused on the augmented use of psychosocial and pharmaco-logical treatments for bipolar disorder in older adults. Rather, there has been a focus, albeit minimal, on pharmacological augmentation for existing medication protocols in the treatment of late-life bipolar disorder. In this section, we will review the current lit-erature regarding pharmacological augmentation interventions specific to late-life bipolar disorder.

With the current preference to treat symptoms of late-life bipolar disorder through phar-macological modalities, scientific research has begun to focus on ways to further enhance existing medication protocols (Young et al. 2010). Various researchers have evaluated the effectiveness and safety of treating late-life bipolar disorder with traditional mood stabi-lizers in addition to anti-convulsants and atypical anti-psychotics (Gildengers et al. 2005; Sajatovic et al. 2008; Young et al. 2004). However, more controlled, double-blind studies of late-life bipolar disorder need to be conducted in order to elucidate efficacious treatments for older adults.

Young and colleagues (2010) have begun research into the conceptual and methodologi-cal issues in designing a randomized controlled treatment trial for geriatric bipolar disor-der. Their research gives evidence for the increased need to address high priority clinical concerns relevant to the routine pharmacological treatment of geriatric bipolar disorder. As a result, they have proposed a double-blind, randomized efficacy trial examining phar-macological treatment of late-life bipolar disorder. This study, better known as the Acute Pharmacotherapy of Late-life Mania (GERI-BD), plans to randomize adults aged 60 or older to treatment groups receiving: lithium carbonate prescribed in units of 150mg/cap-sule (range: 0.40–.99 mEq/L; target: 0.80–0.99 mEq/L) or divalproex sodium in units of 250 mg/capsule (range: 40–99 mcg/ml; target: 80–99 mcg/ml) twice daily for a period of three weeks to establish therapeutic levels. Lorazepam, then risperidone, respectively, will be added during the first three weeks in the event of excessive symptomatology consisting of agitation, aggression, anxiety, hyperactivity, or insomnia. If these symptoms persist follow-ing the three-week stabilization period, risperidone will be added as adjunctive, combined daily therapy to either lithium or divalproex. At the time of writing, the GERI-BD study is still in progress.

Sajatovic and colleagues (2005a) suggest that older adults may be more vulnerable to acute lithium toxicity with toxicity often occurring at lower doses than found in younger adults undergoing similar medication protocols. Due to the increase in adverse side-effects of lithium in older adults, clinical trials have been published examining the efficacy of first-line treatments for late-life bipolar disorder that attempt to account for pharmacoki-netic interactions seen within the older adult population. From these studies, the mood sta-bilizer lamotrigine and anti-convulsant divalproex have been shown to be beneficial in the treatment of older patients with bipolar disorder, particularly in adjunct with the traditional mood stabilizer lithium.

Schneider and Wilcox (1998) reviewed four case studies involving geriatric patients with rapid-cycling bipolar disorder. Their review concluded that when traditional lithium-based protocols were not effective in preventing symptom recurrence, augmentation of dival-proex sodium in combination with lithium carbonate appeared to increase the sensitiv-ity to lithium carbonate and prevent the recurrence of manic symptoms. These findings give clinicians the option to lower lithium concentrations to a tolerable and greater safety range, while enhancing treatment effectiveness with an anti-convulsant that produces fewer side-effects in older adults. Further investigation with double-blind, controlled studies would be required to explicate the efficacy of pharmacological treatment using divalproex augmentation.

Robillard and Conn (2002) conducted a small, open-label trial of adjunctive lamotrigine (an anti-convulsant) therapy involving five older adult women (mean age = 71.5) with bipolar disorder who had been hospitalized for symptom recurrence. The five participants had been on a lithium or valproate semisodium protocol for at least three months. Lamotrigine was started at a dosage of 25mg at bedtime, with weekly incremental increases of 12.5mg daily until a total dosage of either 75mg or 100mg was obtained. Improvement was measured by a clinical interview as well as by HAM-D scores. Participants were reassessed at six weeks and were considered improved if HAM-D scores had decreased by at least 50%.

Results from this study showed that three of the five participants had remission of symptoms as indicated by a 50% reduction in HAM-D scores and clinical interview. At the three-month follow-up, these three patients had not required re-hospitalization and maintained a decrease in symptoms. Additional double-blind, randomized controlled studies are needed to further support the efficacy of lamotrigine augmentation. For a more in-depth review of pharmacological treatment of bipolar disorder in older adults, please refer to Sajatovic et al. (2005b).

Augmenting minimally effective pharmacological interventions with psychosocial treatment may improve cognitive and interpersonal coping skills as well as medication compliance, resulting in increased quality of life and longer periods of symptom remission. Unfortunately, to our knowledge there are no known studies examining psychosocial augmentation strategies for the treatment of late-life bipolar disorder. Based on studies in mixed-age samples (Frank et al. 2005; Lam et al. 2003; Miklowitz 2008; Miklowitz et al. 2003; Rothbaum and Astin 2000;), it is possible that FFT and IPSRT are the best treatment strategies in older adults. However, as shown in Table 41.5, further research is needed to determine the efficacy of augmentation treatments for late-life bipolar disorder.

Table 41.5 Augmented pharmacological treatment for late–life bipolar disorder

Study author(s)	Treatment	Results
Young et al. (2010)	Lithium or divalproex sodium augmented with lorazepam followed by risperidone	Study still in progress.
Sajatovic et al. (2005a)	Lamotrigine augmented with divalproex in adjunct with lithium	Medication augmentation shown to be beneficial in reducing symptoms and preventing relapse.
Schneider and Wilcox (1998)	Lithium augmented with divalproex sodium	Medication augmentation increased sensitivity to lithium and prevented the recurrence of manic symptoms.
Robillard and Conn (2002)	Lithium or valproate augmented with lamotrigine	Medication augmentation decreased manic symptoms and occurrences of re-hospitalization.

Anxiety disorders

As mentioned above, we know of no studies that have investigated augmentation strategies for the treatment of anxiety disorders in older adults.

DIRECTIONS FOR FUTURE RESEARCH

Due to the paucity of research in the area of optimal treatment sequencing, a number of future research directions exist. Expansion is needed in terms of (1) the symptoms, disorders, and conditions being investigated, including the impact of medical and psychiatric comorbidity on treatment outcome, (2) better understanding the efficacy of different pharmacological treatments in combination with each other and with psychotherapy, (3) better understanding the efficacy of different psychosocial interventions and their components (e.g. cognitive vs behavioural strategies vs their combination; modifications for older age), and (4) comparing monotherapy vs combination vs sequential vs augmentation treatment strategies to fully understand their dynamics, advantages, and disadvantages.

Further, cognitive impairment is a common co-occurring condition in older adults with late-life anxiety. Yet, the most common combination treatment—SSRIs and CBT—combines two treatments that are each less efficacious in the context of cognitive impairment (Alexopoulos et al. 2001; Caudle et al. 2007). Thus, it remains unknown just how to manage anxiety disorders in older adults with co-occurring cognitive impairment. Given that this is a large and growing group, and given the enormous health and cost implications of this problem, research is urgently needed to develop, test, and implement novel or adapted treatments that target both anxiety and co-occurring cognitive impairment.

Unfortunately, despite the availability of effective treatments for anxiety and depression, many older adults do not receive the treatment they need (Swartz et al. 1998). This deficit requires a more thorough dissemination of research findings into clinical practice, especially within the domain of primary care. Older adults are more likely to present for treatment in primary care, and mental health problems are more likely to be identified by primary care providers. Thus, arming these providers with contemporary knowledge regarding optimal treatment options for older adults with mental health concerns should be a top priority.

IMPLICATIONS FOR PRACTICE

Despite a clear need for additional research, practitioners can still take away a number of valuable insights from what is already known. First, some combination of medication and psychotherapy appears to offer an advantage over medications or therapy alone for the treatment of anxiety and mood disorders in older adults. While the literature, as of yet, does not clearly support one specific strategy over another (i.e. combination vs sequencing vs augmentation), each has advantages and disadvantages (discussed in the Introduction) that can be considered depending on the individual patient. In addition, treatment planning in collaboration with the patient (i.e. attending to patient preferences and concerns) will likely result in lower attrition and greater adherence to medication and/or psychotherapy protocols. For example, a patient who is resistant to adding another medication to an already burdensome regimen may be willing to try psychotherapy first, only adding medication if s/he does not achieve adequate response. Alternatively, a patient who feels therapy requires too great a commitment may wish to try medication alone, agreeing to add therapy should remission not be achieved. Another patient may have a 'more is better' mentality, wanting to address symptoms using both medication and therapy from the beginning. If the clinician considers these viewpoints, knowing that the research supports each of these strategies, s/he may achieve the best compliance, and therefore increase the likelihood of successful treatment.

Summary

Despite the prevalence and burden of anxiety and mood disorders in late-life, a relative paucity of literature examining optimal treatment strategies exists. Evidence for the efficacy of monotherapies is mixed and consensus is lacking. However, contemporary researchers have attempted to devise novel protocols that allow for a thorough examination of the interplay between medications, psychotherapy, and stepped or collaborative care in the treatment of late-life anxiety and mood disorders.

Overall, the preponderance of evidence has lent support to the notion that combining psychosocial and medical treatments results in better outcomes for older adults with anxiety and mood disorders, even when taking older age and medical comorbidities into account. This is particularly important given that combined treatments in younger adults have not consistently proven to be superior to monotherapies. It should be noted, however, that this line of research is still in its infancy. The number of studies examining optimal treatment strategies for older adults is low, and while most of the studies reviewed in this chapter were scientifically rigorous, several limitations were noted (e.g. lack of placebo/control/comparison groups, limited sample size, lack of generalizability), and the majority focused on late-life depression. Thus, it is clear that additional well-controlled studies are needed to further elucidate these complex issues, especially in older adults with anxiety disorders and bipolar disorder.

Key References and Sources for Further Reading

Miklowitz, D. J., George, E. L., Richards, J. A., Simoneau, T. L., and Suddath, R. L. (2003). 'A Randomized Study of Family-focused Psychoeducation and Pharmacotherapy in the Outpatient Management of Bipolar Disorder'. *Archives of General Psychiatry* 60: 904–912.

Reynolds, C. F., Frank, E., Perel, J. M., Imber, S. D., Cornes, C., et al. (1999). 'Nortriptyline and Interpersonal Psychotherapy as Maintenance Therapies for Recurrent Major Depression: A Randomized Controlled Trial in Patients Older than 59 Years'. *Journal of the American Medical Association* 28: 39–45.

Reynolds, C. F., Dew, M. A., Pollock, B. G., Mulsant, B. H., Frank, E. et al. (2006). 'Maintenance Treatment of Major Depression in Old Age'. *New England Journal of Medicine* 354(11): 1130–1138.

Reynolds, C. F., Dew, M. A., Martire, L. M., Miller, M. D., Cyranowski, J. M., et al. (2010). 'Treating Depression to Remission in Older Adults: A Controlled Evaluation of Combined Escitalopram with Interpersonal Psychotherapy versus Escitalopram with Depression Care Management'. *International Journal of Geriatric Psychiatry* 25: 1134–1141.

Sajatovic, M., Madhusoodanan, S., and Coconcea, N. (2005). 'Managing Bipolar Disorder in the Elderly'. *Drugs and Aging* 22: 39–54.

Thompson, L. W., Coon, D. W., Gallagher-Thompson, D., Sommer, B. R., and Koin, D. (2001). 'Comparison of Desipramine and CBT in the Treatment of Elderly Outpatients with Mild-to-moderate Depression'. *American Journal of Geriatric Psychiatry* 9: 225–240.

Wetherell, J. L., Petkus A. J., White, K. S., Nguyen, H., Kornblith, S., et al. (2013). 'Antidepressant Medication Augmented with Cognitive-behavioral Therapy for Generalized Anxiety Disorder in Older Adults'. *American Journal of Psychiatry* 170: 782–789.

References

Alexopoulos, G. S., Katz, I. R., Reynolds, C. F., Carpenter, D., Docherty, J. P., et al. (2001). 'Pharmacotherapy of Depressive Disorders in Older Patients: A Summary of the Expert Consensus Guidelines'. *Journal of Psychiatric Practice* 7: 361–376.

Barrowclough, C., King, P., Colville, J., Russell, E., Burns, A., et al. (2001). 'A Randomized Trial of the Effectiveness of Cognitive-behavioral Therapy and Supportive Counseling for Anxiety Symptoms in Older Adults'. *Journal of Consulting and Clinical Psychology* 69(5): 756–762.

Bartels, S. J., Forester, B., Miles, K. M., and Joyce, T. (2000). 'Mental Health Service Use by Elderly Patients with Bipolar Disorder and Unipolar Major Depression'. *American Journal of Geriatric Psychiatry* 8: 160–166.

Beekman, A. F., De Beurs, E., Van Balkom, A. M., Deeg, D. H., Van Dyck, R., et al. (2000). 'Anxiety and Depression in Later Life: Co-occurrence and Communality of Risk Factors'. *American Journal of Psychiatry* 157: 89–95.

Beck. A. T., Rush, A. J., Shaw, B. F., and Emery, G. (1979). *Cognitive Therapy for Depression*. New York: Guilford Press.

Beck, A. T., Ward, C. H., Mendelson, M., Mock, J., and Erbaugh, J. (1961). 'An Inventory for Measuring Depression'. *Archives of General Psychiatry* 4: 561–571.

Benitez, C., Smith, K., Vasile, R. G., Rende, R., Edelem, M. O., et al. (2008). 'Use of Benzodiazepines and Selective Serotonin Reuptake Inhibitors in Middle-aged and Older Adults with Anxiety Disorders'. *American Journal of Geriatric Psychiatry* 16(1): 5–13.

Broadhead, J. and Jacoby, R. (1990). 'Mania in Old Age: A First Prospective Study'. *International Journal of Geriatric Psychiatry* 5: 215–222.

Caudle, D. D., Senior, A. C., Wetherell, J. L., Rhoades, H. M., Beck, J. G., et al. (2007). 'Cognitive Errors, Symptom Severity, and Response to Cognitive Behavior Therapy in Older Adults with Generalized Anxiety Disorder'. *American Journal of Geriatric Psychiatry* 15(8): 680–689.

Craighead, W. E. and Miklowitz, D. J. (2000). 'Psychosocial Interventions for Bipolar Disorder'. *Journal of Clinical Psychiatry* 61: 58–64.

De Beurs, E., Beekman, A. F., Van Balkom, A. M., Deeeb, D. H., Van Dyck, R., et al. (1999). 'Consequences of Anxiety in Older Persons: Its Effect on Disability, Well-being and Use of Health Services'. *Psychological Medicine* 29: 583–593.

Dew, M. A., Whyte, E. M., Lenze, F. J., Houck, B. R., Mulsant, B. H., et al. (2007). 'Recovery from Major Depression in Older Adults Receiving Augmentation of Antidepressant Pharmacotherapy'. *American Journal of Psychiatry* 164(6): 892–899.

Fava, G. A., Park, S. K., and Sonino, N. (2006). 'Treatment of Recurrent Depression'. *Expert Review of Neurotherapeutics* 6: 1735–1740.

Flint, A. J. (1994). 'Epidemiology and Comorbidity of Anxiety Disorders in the Elderly'. *American Journal of Psychiatry* 15: 640–649.

Flint, A. J. and Rifat, S. L. (1998). 'The Treatment of Psychotic Depression in Later Life: A Comparison of Pharmacotherapy and ECT'. *International Journal of Geriatric Psychiatry* 13: 23–28.

Frank, E., Kupfer, D. J., Thase, M. E. et al. (2005). 'Two-Year Outcomes for Interpersonal and Social Rhythm Therapy in Individuals with Bipolar I Disorder'. *Archives of General Psychiatry* 62: 995–1004.

Gareri, P., Falconi, U., De Fazio, P., and De Sarro, G. (2000). 'Conventional and New Antidepressant Drugs in the Elderly'. *Progress in Neurobiology* 61: 353–396.

Georgotas, A., McCue, R. E., Cooper, R. B., Nagachandran, N., and Chang, I. (1988). 'How Effective and Safe is Continuation Therapy in Elderly Depressed Patients? Factors Affecting Relapse Rate'. *Archives of General Psychiatry* 45: 929–932.

Gerson, S. C., Plotkin, D. A., and Jarvik, L. F. (1988). 'Antidepressant Drug Studies, 1964–1986: Empirical Evidence for Aging Patients'. *Journal of Clinical Psychopharmacology* 8: 311–322.

Gildengers, A. G., Mulsant, B. H., and Begley, A. E. (2005). 'A Pilot Study of Standardized Treatment in Geriatric Bipolar Disorder'. *American Journal of Geriatric Psychiatry* 13: 319–323.

Goodwin, F. K. and Jamison, K. R. (1990). *Manic Depressive Illness: Bipolar Disorders and Recurrent Depression*. Oxford University Press: New York.

Gum, A. M., Arean, P. A., Hunkeler, E., Tang, L., Katon, W., et al. (2006). 'Depression Treatment Preferences in Older Primary Care Patients'. *Gerontologist* 46(1): 14–22.

Hamilton, M. (1960). 'A Rating Scale for Depression'. *Journal of Neurology, Neurosurgery, and Psychiatry* 23: 56–62.

Kennedy, B. L. and Schwab J. J. (1997). 'Utilization of Medical Specialists by Anxiety Disorder Patients'. *Psychosomatics* 38: 109–112.

Lam, D. H., Watkins, E. R., Hayward, P., Bright, J., Wright, K., et al. (2003). 'A Randomized Controlled Study of Cognitive Therapy for Relapse Prevention for Bipolar Affective Disorder'. *Archives of General Psychiatry* 6: 145–152.

Larkin, B. A., Copeland, J. R., and Dewney, M. E. (1992). 'The Natural History of Neurotic Disorder in an Elderly Urban Population'. *British Journal of Psychiatry* 160: 681–686.

Lenze, E. J., Dew, M. A., Mazumdar, S., Begley, A. E., Comes, C., et al. (2002). 'Combined Pharmacotherapy and Psychotherapy as Maintenance Treatment for Late-life Depression: Effects on Social Adjustment'. *American Journal of Psychiatry* 159(3): 466–468.

Lenze, E. J., Rollman, B. L., Shear, M. K., Dew, M. A., Pollock, B. G., et al. (2009). 'Escitalopram for Older Adults with Generalized Anxiety Disorder'. *Journal of the American Medical Association* 31(3): 295–303.

Lynch, T. R., Morse, J. Q., Mendelson, T., and Robins, C. J. (2003). 'Dialectical Behaviour Therapy for Depressed Older Adults: A Randomized Pilot Study'. *American Journal of Geriatric Psychiatry* 11: 33–45.

Meyer, T. J., Miller, M. L., Metzger, R. L., and Borkovec, T. D. (1990). 'Development and Validation of the Penn State Worry Questionnaire'. *Behavior Research and Therapy* 28: 487–495.

Miklowitz, D. J., George, E. L., Richards, J. A., Simoneau, T. L., and Suddath, R. L. (2003). 'A Randomized Study of Family-focused Psychoeducation and Pharmacotherapy in the Outpatient Management of Bipolar Disorder'. *Archives of General Psychiatry* 60: 904–912.

Miklowitz, D. J. (2007). 'The Role of the Family in the Course and Treatment of Bipolar Disorder'. *Current Directions in Psychological Science* 16(4): 192–196.

Miklowitz, D. J. (2008). 'Adjunctive Psychotherapy for Bipolar Disorder: State of the Evidence'. *American Journal of Psychiatry* 165: 1408–1419.

Miklowitz, D. J., Axelson, D. A., and Birmaher, B. (2008). 'Family-focused Treatment for Adolescents with Bipolar Disorder: Results of a 2-year Randomized Trial'. *Archives of General Psychiatry* 65(9): 1053–1061.

Mulsant, B. H., Alexopoulos, G. S., Reynolds, C. F., III Katz, I. R., Abrams, R., et al. (2001). 'Pharmacological Treatment of Depression in Older Primary Care Patients: The PROSPECT Algorithm'. *International Journal of Geriatric Psychiatry* 16: 585–592.

Post, F., Benson, D. F., and Blumer D. (1998). *Psychiatric Aspects of Neurologic Disease*. New York: Grune and Stratton.

Rea, M. M, Thompson, M. C., Miklowitz, D. J., Goldstein, M. J., Hwang, S., et al. (2003). 'Family-focused Treatment versus Individual Treatment for Bipolar Disorder: Results of a Randomized Clinical Trial'. *Journal of Consulting and Clinical Psychology* 71(3): 482–492.

Reynolds, C. F., Frank. E., Perel, J. M., Imber, S. D., Comes, C., et al. (1992). 'Combined Pharmacotherapy and Psychotherapy in the Acute and Continuation Treatment of Elderly Patients with Recurrent Major Depression: A Preliminary Report'. *American Journal of Psychiatry* 149: 1687–1692.

Reynolds, C. F., Frank. E., Perel, J. M., Miller, M. D., Comes, C., et al. (1994). 'Treatment of Consecutive Episodes of Major Depression in the Elderly'. *American Journal of Psychiatry* 151: 1740–1743.

Reynolds, C. F., Frank, E., Perel, J. M., Imber, S. D., Comes, C., et al. (1999a). 'Nortriptyline and Interpersonal Psychotherapy as Maintenance Therapies for Recurrent Major Depression: A Randomized Controlled Trial in Patients Older than 59 Years'. *Journal of the American Medical Association* 281: 39–45.

Reynolds, C. F., Frank, E., and Dew. M. A., Houck, P. R., Miller, M., et al. (1999b). 'Treatment of 70+ year-olds with Recurrent Major Depression: Excellent Short-term but Brittle Long-term Response'. *American Journal of Geriatric Psychiatry* 7: 64–69.

Reynolds, C. F., Dew, M. A., Pollock, B. G., Mulsant, B. H., Frank, E., et al. (2006). 'Maintenance Treatment of Major Depression in Old Age'. *New England Journal of Medicine* 354(11): 1130–1138.

Reynolds, C. F., Dew, M. A., Martire, L. M., Miller, M. D., Cyranowsky, J. M., et al. (2010). 'Treating Depression to Remission in Older Adults: A Controlled Evaluation of Combined Escitalopram with Interpersonal Psychotherapy versus Escitalopram with Depression Care Management'. *International Journal of Geriatric Psychiatry* 25: 1134–1141.

Robillard, M. and Conn, D. K. (2002). 'Lamotrigine Use in Geriatric Patients with Bipolar Depression'. *Canadian Journal of Psychiatry* 47: 767–770.

Rothbaum, B. O. and Astin, M. C. (2000). 'Integration of Pharmacotherapy and Psychotherapy for Bipolar Disorder'. *Journal of Clinical Psychiatry* 61: 68–75.

Sajatovic, M., Calabrese J. R., and Mullen, J. (2008). 'Quetiapine for the Treatment of Bipolar Disorder in Older Adults'. *Bipolar Disorders* 10: 662–671.

Sajatovic, M., Gyulai, L., Calabrese, J. R., Thompson, T. R., Wilson, B. G., et al. (2005a). 'Maintenance Treatment Outcomes in Older Patients with Bipolar I Disorder'. *American Journal of Geriatric Psychiatry* 13: 305–311.

Sajatovic, M., Madhusoodanan, S., and Coconcea, N. (2005b). 'Managing Bipolar Disorder in the Elderly'. *Drugs and Aging* 22: 39–54.

Sajatovic, M., Popli, A., and Semple, W. (1996). 'Ten-year Use of Hospital-based Services by Geriatric Veterans with Schizophrenia and Bipolar Disorder'. *Psychiatry Services* 47: 961–965.

Schneider, A. L. and Wilcox, C. S. (1998). 'Divalproate Augmentation in Lithium-resistant Rapid Cycling Mania in Four Geriatric Patients'. *Journal of Affective Disorders* 47: 201–205.

Smit, F., Ederveen, A., Cuijpers, P., Deeg, D., and Beekman, A. (2006). 'Opportunities for Cost-effective Prevention of Late-life Depression'. *Archives of General Psychiatry* 63: 290–296.

Swartz, M. S., Wagner, H. R., Swanson, J. W., Burns, B. J., George, L. K., et al. (1998). 'Administrative Update: Utilization of Services I: Comparing Use of Public and Private Mental Health Services: The Enduring Barriers of Race and Age'. *Community Mental Health Journal* 34: 133–144.

Thompson, L. W., Gallagher, D. E., and Breckenridge, J. S. (1987). 'Comparative Effectiveness of Psychotherapies for Depressed Elders'. *Journal of Consulting and Clinical Psychology* 55: 385–390.

Thompson, L. W., Coon, D. W., Gallagher-Thompson, D., Sommer, B. R., and Koin, D. (2001). 'Comparison of Desipramine and CBT in the Treatment of Elderly Outpatients with Mild-to-moderate Depression'. *American Journal of Geriatric Psychiatry* 9: 225–240.

Thorp, S. R., Ayers, C. R., Nuevo, R., Stoddard, J. A., Sorrell, J. T., et al. (2009). 'Meta analysis Comparing Different Behavioral Treatments for Late-life Anxiety'. *American Journal of Geriatric Psychiatry* 17(2): 105–115.

United Nations, Department of Economic and Social Affairs (2010). *World Population Prospects, the 2010 Revision*. http://esa.un.org/unpd/wpp/Excel-Data/population.htm.

Unutzer, J., Katon, W., Callahan, C. M., Williams, J. W., Hunkeler, E., et al. (2002). 'Collaborative Care Management of Late-life Depression in the Primary Care Setting: A Randomized Controlled Trial'. *Journal of the American Medical Association* 288(22): 2836–2845.

Wetherell, J. L., Kaplan, R. M., Kallenberg, G., Dresselhaus, T. R., Sieber, W. J., et al. (2004). 'Mental Health Treatment Preferences of Older and Younger Primary Care Patients'. *International Journal of Psychiatry in Medicine* 34: 219–233.

Wetherell, J. L., Hopko, D. R., Diefenbach, G. J. et al. (2005). 'Cognitive-behavioral Therapy for Late-life Generalized Anxiety Disorder: Who Gets Better?' *Behavior Therapy* 36: 147–156.

Wetherell, J. L., Petkus, A. J., White, K. S., Nguyen, H., Kornblith, S., Andreescu, C., Zisook, S., and Lenze, E. J. (2013). 'Antidepressant Medication Augmented with Cognitive-behavioral Therapy for Generalized Anxiety Disorder in Older Adults'. *American Journal of Psychiatry* 170: 782–789.

Wetherell, J. L., Stoddard, J. A., White, K. S., Kornblith, S., Nguyen, H., et al. (2010). 'Augmenting Antidepressant Medication with Modular CBT for Geriatric Generalized Anxiety Disorder: A Pilot Study'. *International Journal of Geriatric Psychiatry* 26: 869–875.

Whyte, E. M., Basinski, J., Farhi, P., Dew, M. A., Begley, A., et al. (2004). 'Geriatric Depression Treatment in Nonresponders to Selective Serotonin Reuptake Inhibitors'. *Journal of Clinical Psychiatry* 65: 1634–1641.

Young, R. C. (2005). 'Bipolar Disorder in Older Persons: Perspectives and New Findings'. *American Journal of Geriatric Psychiatry* 13: 265-267.

Young, R. C., Gyulai, L., and Mulsant, B. H. (2004). 'Pharmacotherapy of Bipolar Disorder in Old Age: Review and Recommendations'. *American Journal of Geriatric Psychiatry* 12: 342–357.

Young, R. C., Schulberg, H. C., Gildengers, A. G., Sajatovic, M., Mulsant, B. H., et al. (2010). 'Conceptual and Methodological Issues in Designing a Randomized, Controlled Treatment Trial for Geriatric Bipolar Disorder: GERI-BD'. *Bipolar Disorders* 12: 56–67.

Zis, A. P., Grof, P., Webster, M., and Goodwin, F. K. (1980). 'Prediction of Relapse in Recurrent Affective Disorder'. *Psychopharmacology Bulletin* 16: 47–49.

CHAPTER 42

PAIN IN PERSONS WITH DEMENTIA AND COMMUNICATION IMPAIRMENT

A. LYNN SNOW AND M. LINDSEY JACOBS

PAIN IN DEMENTIA: WHY IT IS SPECIAL AND IMPORTANT

IT may seem surprising that an entire chapter is devoted to the apparently narrow topic of pain detection and treatment in persons with dementia. However, there are five compelling reasons why pain identification and management for persons with dementia is an especially challenging endeavour worthy of careful consideration. First, under-identification and subsequent under-treatment of pain are unfortunately common in this vulnerable population (Gibson 2007). Chart-documented rates of pain are one-third to one-half of the rates found when nursing home residents with mild to moderate dementia are interviewed verbally by researchers (Herman et al. 2009; Takai et al. 2010). Several studies report that only one-quarter or less of persons with dementia identified as being in pain by researchers were receiving analgesics in their clinical setting (Husebo et al. 2012; Hutt et al. 2006; Won et al. 2006). For example, in a study of hospital inpatients undergoing hip fracture surgery, persons with advanced dementia received only a third of the amount of opiate analgesic received by those without dementia (Morrison and Siu 2000), and in another study eleven years later other investigators again found opiate medication dosages to be lower in hip fracture inpatients with dementia (Sieber et al. 2011).

Second, the cognitive impairments that define dementia make it difficult for persons with dementia to understand and communicate about their pain (Snow et al. 2004). Third, because of these communication problems, poor detection of pain and under-treatment of pain are unfortunately the rule rather than the exception in this vulnerable population (Buffum et al. 2007). Fourth, self-report ability declines at uneven rates and in unpredictable patterns dependent both upon the type of dementia and unique characteristics of the individual, making it extremely difficult for clinicians finely to predict when self-report will no longer be accurate (Snow et al. 2004). This prediction difficulty is due to the fact that the

---

Box 42.1 Distress Messages

- Negative Facial Expressions: e.g., frowning; grimacing; squeezing eyes shut; looking sad, scared, anxious, angry, or worried*
- Negative Verbal Expressions: e.g., groaning; moaning; gasping; screaming; muttering; pain words like "ouch"; negative words like "no", "stop", "go away"
- Negative Body Language: e.g., bracing; rocking; freezing; flinching; guarding; pushing; hitting; pulling away

* For simplicity, affective words (sad, scared) are used here as a shorthand to describe facial expressions that most people interpret to indicate the presence of these affective states. A more accurate behavioural statement might be, for example, raising of eyebrows and widening of eyes rather than the phrase 'looking scared'. We refer the interested reader to the large body of research that has been conducted using the Facial Action Coding System to better understand the associations between facial muscle activity and internal experience of emotion (e.g., http://face-and-emotion.com/dataface/facs/description.jsp).

---

ability to self-report pain accurately is a higher-level complex cognitive skill relying upon a wide variety of other foundational cognitive skills including memory, expressive and receptive language, and abstract thought, such as being able to recognize one's distressing negative perceptual experiences as pain and understand the importance of communicating this pain to others.

Fifth, due to our decreased confidence in self-report, we must rely heavily upon observation of behaviours to determine when a person with dementia is in pain, and yet the behaviours that indicate pain are the same behaviours that indicate a wide variety of other causes of distress (Herr et al. 2011). These 'distress messages' (e.g. negative facial expressions, verbal expressions, and body language; see Box 42.1) are often misconstrued by others as being caused by conditions that do not require intervention (e.g. he just does that 'because of the dementia', he 'just' wants attention) and are then ignored (Buffum et al. 2007).

The Unmet Needs Conceptual Model

In this section we will explore a conceptual model that provides a critical foundation from which to build an understanding of how pain assessment and treatment should be approached in persons with dementia and communication impairment.

The Unmet Needs Model states that *all* distress behaviours (i.e. "problem behaviours" or "challenging behaviours", see section below (On Language: 'Distress' not 'Pain) for a discussion of this language choice) in persons with dementia are due to one or multiple unmet needs (Algase et al. 1996; Cohen, Mansfield, and Werner 1995). Unmet needs may be *physical, environmental, emotional*, or *social*. Unmet needs may thus be internal or external. The model also posits that *background factors* affect an individual's unique expression of distress behaviours (Algase 1996).

The Unmet Needs Model builds upon a rich history of theoretical work regarding the roles of needs and drives in motivating behaviour. Because the reach of influence and the evidence base of this preceding work is rich and thus lends support to the Unmet Needs Model, we briefly mention two of these approaches: Maslow's hierarchy of needs and self-determination theory. Maslow defined a 'need' as innate psychological as well as physical requirements for ongoing health and well-being, and posited that all humans possess a hierarchically organized collection of needs in which basic physiological needs (e.g. food, sleep) form the foundation upon which more complex needs layer, including safety, belongingness, and esteem (Maslow 1943, 1968, 1987). Although influential, Maslow's theory was not heavily based on evidence. Self-determination theory, however, is remarkably similar to Maslow's approach in terms of its conception of needs, and is based in and supported by a large body of experimental evidence (Deci 1980; Deci and Ryan 1980, 1985, 1991, 2013). Self-determination theory posits three basic needs: the needs for competence, relatedness, and autonomy.

Several excellent resources have built upon or complement the Unmet Needs Model, including the person-centred dementia care approach (Kitwood 1997), the whole person dementia assessment approach (Mast 2011), the detective approach (Camp 2012), the TREA approach (Treatment Routes for Exploring Agitation; Cohen-Mansfield 2011), and the Serial Trials Protocol (Kovach et al. 2006a; Kovach, Cashin, and Sauer 2006b). We will next briefly review each of the five main components of the Unmet Needs Model and two related categorizations.

Physical

'Start with the Physical!' exhorts Cameron Camp in a book that lays out his formula for responding to distress behaviours (Camp 2012). This is good advice and is echoed by Christine Kovach's Serial Trials Protocol, which directs nurses to begin with a *hands-on* physical assessment when distress behaviours are present (Kovach et al. 2006a, 2006b). Pain is of course one possible physical cause of distress behaviours. Failing to identify and/or adequately treat pain is the unmet need that is the primary focus of this chapter. If there is pain, where is it coming from?

A head-to-toe examination of the person with dementia is always a critical part of identifying clues to this question. Psychologists and other allied health professionals who are not trained in medical examination can still participate in this important activity in two ways. First, one does not have to be a nurse or a physician to gently and respectfully look over a person with dementia to note any obvious potential sources of discomfort. Observe the skin that is visible to you: do you see any areas of redness, swelling, flaking, constriction, discolouration? Do you see any body parts that appear to be positioned in potentially uncomfortable ways? Second, review the person's medical chart and/or interview the person and their closest care-givers to take a medical history. Does the person have any medical conditions that carry a high probability or potential for pain, such as arthritis, cancer, or a recent injury/fracture/surgery (see Box 42.2 for a partial listing of physical conditions with high potential for causing pain or discomfort)? Does the person have a history of pain? Does the person have a history of another condition that has a high probability of causing discomfort, thus leading to distress behaviours even if pain is not present, such as eczema (causing itching), urinary tract infections, constipation (causing gastrointestinal discomfort and potentially pain),

---

Box 42.2 Common physical causes of pain or discomfort

Physical conditions that are common causes of pain
  Musculoskeletal conditions: osteoporosis, slipped or bulging discs, spinal stenosis, compression fractures in the spine, fractures or sprains due to falls, soft tissue damage due to falls or accidents
  Nerve damage: diabetic neuropathy, other neuropathies, shingles, compressed nerves such as sciatica
  Joint conditions: arthritis, rheumatoid arthritis
  Cancer
  Fibromyalgia
  GI conditions: irritable bowel syndrome, ulcer, bowel impaction

Physical conditions that are common causes of physical discomfort*
  Urinary tract infections
  Bowel difficulties: gas, constipation
  Need to be helped to restroom to urinate or defecate
  Skin difficulties: rashes, hives, eczema, dry skin, itchy skin
  Discomfort due to irritation from clothing or furniture
  Too hot or too cold
  Lack of sleep
  Lack of physical movement leading to stiffness, soreness, limited range of motion
  Hunger
  Thirst
  Breathing difficulties due to a bad cold, asthma, bronchitis, pneumonia, COPD

  * Some people may experience these conditions as painful. Regardless of whether the condition causes discomfort or pain, these conditions can be highly distressing for people.

---

or ear infections (causing dizziness or vertigo)? Third, serve as an advocate for obtaining a thorough physical examination of the person. Even in a nursing home setting, one cannot assume a thorough physical examination has been recently conducted in a manner that would uncover potential physical causes of distress behaviour. During their randomized controlled trial of the Serial Trials approach in fourteen nursing homes, Kovach and colleagues reported that before intervention it was quite a common situation that licensed nurses did not regularly conduct physical examinations of nursing home residents (2006a). In a fascinating descriptive study, they document a high rate of new physical problems (143 in sixty-five residents over six weeks) and note that persons who received more frequent assessments had new problems identified and treated more quickly (Kovach et al. 2010). Further, subtle or even obvious signs of physical conditions that can cause pain and discomfort can be missed during strenuous activities like transferring or bathing individuals, so taking the time to conduct a physical examination with the express purpose of looking for potential physical causes of distress behaviours is an important assessment step.

Environmental

Kovach's Serial Trials Protocol directs the assessor to move next from physical to environmental factors. We typically think of environmental causes or contributors to distress behaviours as factors that overstimulate the person with dementia, such as an overly noisy, overly active, or overly cluttered environment. These are indeed important causal elements. The environmental press theory posits that dementia compromises the ability of a person to attend selectively to information (i.e. to be able to 'tune out' environmental information that is extraneous to what the person wishes to focus upon). As this ability to selectively attend becomes further compromised with the progression of dementia, the person becomes more and more sensitive to overstimulation, and more likely to react to overstimulation with distress behaviours (Lawton 1986; Lawton, Van Haitsma, and Klapper 1994). However, an understimulating environment can be equally problematic. Building upon Lawton's environmental press work, Kovach and colleagues proposed the Model of Imbalance in Sensoristasis (MIS), which states that distress behaviours may be 'initiated or exacerbated when there is an imbalance between sensory-stimulating and sensory-calming activity' (Kovach 2000; Kovach and Schlidt 2001; Kovach and Wells 2002). In support of the MIS, a randomized controlled trial of an intervention to balance periods of rest and individualized engaging activity resulted in significantly decreased agitation scores in seventy-eight nursing home residents with moderate to severe dementia (Kovach et al. 2004).

Emotional and Social

Regarding emotional and social needs, the person-centred approach developed by Thomas Kitwood (1997, 2008) and elaborated upon by many others since (Cheston and Bender 1999; Mast 2011; Power 2010) is an important companion to the Unmet Needs Model. Kitwood was among the first to write about the 'medicalization of dementia' and to promote a prioritization of the personhood of the person with dementia. Kitwood proposed that all people, including people with dementia, have needs for *comfort* (i.e. safety, security*), attachment, inclusion, occupation, and identity* (1997). These needs are often overlooked for people with dementia, particularly severely impaired people who have difficulty communicating. Yet, observational studies and observational measurement during non-pharmacological interventions such as those of Cohen-Mansfield and colleagues (Cohen-Mansfield and Werner 1995; Cohen-Mansfield et al. 2009; Cohen-Mansfield 2011), Kovach and colleagues (Kovach 2000; Kovach and Schlidt 2001; Kovach and Wells 2002; Kovach et al. 2004), Camp and colleagues (Camp and Skrajner 2004; Lee, Camp, & Malone, 2007), Meeks (Meeks et al. 2008), and others (Cahill and Diaz-Ponce 2011; Lawrence et al. 2012) provide evidence that persons with severe dementia need meaningful human contact and meaningful and pleasant activity (as well as appropriate balance between periods of rest and engagement). The Montessori intergenerational dementia programming approach developed by Camp and colleagues is a wonderful example of how even persons with severe dementia flower when their need for occupation (i.e. their need to feel that they are contributing and are valued) is met. Using spaced retrieval and rehabilitation scaffolding principles to allow these persons to serve as teachers of simple Montessori skills to toddlers, the authors report increased engagement and positive affect during the Montessori teaching activities (Skrajner and Camp 2007).

Regarding the need for identity, Kitwood wrote extensively about the negative effects of malignant social psychology on persons with dementia. Building upon this innovative framework, Cheston and Bender (1999) illustrated a 'vicious spiral' in which all social interactions of the person with dementia are impacted by the presence of the dementia label in ways that cause distress and disability in excess of the actual effects of the dementia itself. These include societal prejudice and altered interactions due to stigma and changed expectations based on disease status, leading then to low mood and internal devaluation, leading then to difficulties with concentration, energy, and self-efficacy, which in turn lead to lower mood and further difficulties (Cheston and Bender 1999: 117). The person-centred approach reminds the clinician of the importance of assessing carefully the emotional needs and social environment of the person with dementia to identify potential sources of excess disability, including assessing oneself for potential biases about what people with dementia can and cannot accomplish.

Engage!—optimal stimulation

Engagement is both a way to prevent distress behaviours stemming from unmet emotional and social needs and a way to respond to those unmet emotional needs. Optimal stimulation is a key to the success of engagement efforts. 'Engage!' is the second step in Cameron Camp's detective approach to responding to problematic behaviours (Camp,2012). In this second step, Camp emphasizes the power of engagement. As discussed in the previous section, the person with dementia will not have his or her needs met if the engagement activity is too hard, but will instead be subjected to a new form of environmental press (i.e. stress). Similarly, activities that are too easy will be experienced as a malignant social psychology message, telling the person with dementia that he is seen as too disabled to be of any real use and must be kept busy. Camp (2012) gives this anecdote of an assisted living resident's response to the question 'What's it like living here?' to describe how 'busy work' is experienced by people with dementia: 'They wake us up. They get us dressed. They bring us to breakfast. Then, they give us something to do to keep us busy...this is a beautiful prison.'

Individualization

Individualization is the key to providing engagement activities that are neither too hard nor too easy. Activities that are matched with the past and current preferences of persons with dementia are more engaging, as measured by an observational measure of engagement that took into account duration of engagement, quality of attention paid to the activity, and attitude towards the activity (Cohen-Mansfield et al. 2009). Gitlin and colleagues conducted a randomized trial of an eight-session, four-month structured occupational therapy intervention that assessed persons with dementia to determine their strengths, created 'activity prescriptions' that matched activities to the person's abilities, and educated family care-givers in the skills necessary for effective engagement. These included: cueing, relaxing the rules, not rushing, environmental set-up, simplifying communication, understanding the role of the environment and how to integrate activities in daily care routines, and stress reduction techniques so that the care-giver could provide activities in a calm manner (Gitlin et al., 2008; Gitlin et al., 2009). The investigators reported that the intervention resulted in significant reductions in the frequency of occurrences of problem behaviours, care-giver time providing instrumental care, and care-giver time in providing daily oversight, all with impressively large effect sizes (Cohen's d = .72, .88, 1.00, respectively). The intervention was also incrementally cost effective when the cost of providing the intervention (approximately $942/dyad) was compared to the cost savings represented by the resulting additional hour per day, on average, that care-givers reported gaining and maintaining over the four-month follow-up (Gitlin et al. 2010). Another helpful resource can be found in Cohen-Mansfield's excellent overview chapter on behaviour in persons with dementia (2008; see Table 11.3) in which she presents an example planning grid for matching activities to the needs of individuals based on five dimensions: current sense of identity; current sensory abilities; current motor abilities; current and past habits and preferences; and current needs (physical, emotional, social).

In conclusion, persons with dementia retain the same basic emotional and social needs of all humans, and meaningful and pleasant engagement in activity and individualization of engagement opportunities is critical for meeting these needs. Cohen-Mansfield has proposed an intervention she calls TREA (treatment routes for exploring agitation) that proposes a three-stage approach to developing treatment plans for unmet emotional and social needs (Cohen-Mansfield 2008). TREA elucidates several principles that are foundational for meeting the emotional and social needs of persons with dementia: first respond to distress behaviours by working to understand what need is communicated by the behaviour; psychosocial approaches should be used before pharmacological approaches are tried; psychosocial approaches should be individualized; organizations should prioritize provision of individualized treatments over group-based activities/care approaches,[1] a persistent detective approach to distress behaviours should be prioritized—avoid becoming resigned to the behaviour; and prioritize "prevention, accomodation, and flexibility" when responding to distress behaviours.

Background Factors

Finally, the Unmet Needs Model accounts for the uniqueness of each person with dementia by incorporating 'background factors' to explain inter-individual variation in the expression of distress behaviours. Algase identified four categories of background factors: neurological/cognitive abilities and impairments, physical/affective/functional abilities and impairments, premorbid personality, and premorbid interests and abilities (Algase 1996). Clinical professionals are well acquainted with the inconvenient truth that it is much easier to predict behaviour for a group of people than for an individual. The concept of background factors is a way of accounting for this difficult-to-predict individual variation. Ideally, the astute clinician can use knowledge of background factors to increase his or her prognostication accuracy. One's life story and operant learning history are additional tools for understanding distress behaviour that we would place in the category of background factors (Mast 2011: 84–85, 130, 136–145).

As an example of the importance of background factors, consider the following four persons, all with a diagnosis of vascular dementia of approximately five years duration: CJ, an 81-year-old white woman who was a schoolteacher in Savannah, Georgia for forty years, and has a lifelong history of taking overnight hikes in the woods for fun with her family; PH, a 65-year-old black man from inner city Chicago who became a physician and returned to Chicago to raise his sons; DK, a 90-year-old female from Poland who briefly lived in one of the infamous Auschwitz concentration camps before being sent to safety with a family friend but who left behind parents and siblings who died before the end of the war; and JD, a 70-year-old white male rancher from Texas who left the eighth grade to help out on the family farm. Even with the same diagnosis and approximate span of time since the first presentation of symptoms, CJ, PH, DK, and JD will likely have very different patterns of strengths and challenges in their cognitive and functional abilities, and very different patterns of needs due to their widely discrepant background factors. At a neurological/cognitive level, vascular dementia is an extremely broad category encompassing a wide range of neuropathologies that are only loosely related due to their relationship to the body's vascular systems. Thus, CJ may suffer from difficult-to-control hypertension such that the high intra-vessel pressures are progressively weakening and destroying the smallest vessel networks in the brain in a widely dispersed pattern that leads to cognitive symptoms much like Alzheimer's disease. In contrast, JD may have heavy plaque build-up in his large vessels that regularly break off and travel through his vessels until they become stuck, leading to death of that vessel and the area around it from lack of blood flow; such pathology might result in more focal cognitive symptoms depending upon the area of the brain where the occlusion occurred, and might lead to the hallmark 'stepwise' pattern of progression that is often associated with vascular disease. Level of education also strongly affects resulting cognitive and functional impairment because higher levels of educational attainment (such as PH's medical degree) provide a degree of 'cognitive reserve', such that a greater amount of neuropathology is accommodated before effects in behaviour can be observed. Similarly, individuals can benefit from 'physical reserve', so that a person with a healthy physique and a lifelong habit of exercise (such as CJ) may be able to accommodate a greater amount of neuropathology and continue to perform activities of daily living that require balance, dexterity, or strength (e.g., dressing, ambulating), than a person who was already somewhat deconditioned from years of sedentary living. Life story and operant learning are incredibly important because the rule of thumb regarding dementia progression is 'first in, last out'—that is, the longer an individual has possessed and used a unit of knowledge, the more opportunity that individual has had to create multiple, overlapping, and redundant neural pathways to access that information and thus the more neuropathology the person can accommodate before it becomes impossible to retrieve and use that information. For example, it is well known that language abilities acquired later in life, such as when DK emigrated from Poland to the US and learned English, are lost before native language abilities are affected. There is also increasing evidence that traumas (such as DK's forced emancipation) are a risk factor for the development of dementia (Burnes and Burnette 2013; Burri et al. 2013; Conn, Clarke, and Van Reekum 2000). It is further hypothesized that significant and severe traumas from earlier in life may be somewhat repressed and controlled by a healthy mind only to re-emerge as the inhibitory abilities of the frontal lobes are compromised by dementia (Mittal et al. 2001; Wolff 2012). It might be expected, therefore, that DK, due to her experiences in Auschwitz, may have a stronger need for security and safety than someone like CJ, who grew up in a safe and loving childhood and early adult environment.[2]

Internal vs External: Whose Problem is This?

A critically important contribution of the Unmet Needs Model is that it reminds us that causes of distress behaviours can be internal to the person with dementia, external to the person with dementia, or most likely a combination of the two. Camp's detective approach asks 'Who's *really* got the problem?' and he astutely observes: 'sometimes the problem, and therefore the focus of intervention, is not about the person with dementia. It could be in a caregiver or a staff member, or in the rules and regulations that were intended to lead to good care. Good intentions do not always translate into happiness' (Camp 2012: 80).

Fixed vs Mutable: Putting Effort in the Right Place

Finally, it is helpful to consider which causes of distress behaviours are fixed and which are mutable. For example, Alzheimer's disease itself is an incurable, progressive disease and is therefore fixed, but not mutable. It is obvious that this concept can aid one in deciding where to focus one's efforts when responding to distress behaviours. However, the more impactful contribution of this concept is likely the finding that care-givers tend to have significant difficulty distinguishing between fixed vs mutable causes, missing opportunities to respond to mutable causes and increasing frustration by focusing instead on fixed causes. Using seven focus groups and forty-one participants (persons with dementia, care-givers, nurse aides, physicians, and nurses), Kunik and colleagues developed a conceptual model of causes of disruptive behaviour (2003). When asked what caused disruptive behaviours, participants from all groups initially identified the disease process as the cause. Only upon further discussion did participants identify mutable causes of the behaviours. The final emergent model supported the Unmet Needs Model, identifying as primary causes unmet emotional, social, and physical needs as well as environmental factors.

Evidence Supporting the Unmet Needs Model: Bringing it Back to Pain

The astute reader may be wondering why so many words have been devoted to causes of distress behaviours when the focus of this chapter is on pain. The short answer is that for persons with dementia and impaired communication, the clinician or care-giver cannot know for sure that pain is present, only that distress is present. Pain is but one of the plethora of needs of a person with dementia that, if left unmet, can cause distress. Thus, pain cannot be approached, assessed, or addressed in a narrow specific way. Instead, it is necessary for the clinician or care-giver to approach all distress behaviours with an open, hypothesis-testing attitude and only to conclude that pain is the cause of the distress based upon evidence gathered from assessment and from observations of response to intervention efforts.

Several intervention trials provide evidence supporting the Unmet Needs Model and evidence supporting our assertion that one cannot 'assess specifically for pain' in this vulnerable population. A clinical trial of a psychiatric consultation intervention recruited nursing home residents with moderate to severe dementia who were exhibiting one or more distress behaviours as listed on the Cohen-Mansfield Agitation Inventory and engaging in those behaviours several times each day (Opie et al. 2002). A consultation team including a psychiatrist, psychologist, and nurse assessed the participants and, based upon their findings, recommended individualized interventions. All interventions fit within the categories of the Unmet Needs Model. Interestingly, eighteen of the ninety-nine participants received interventions to address pain. Overall, the consultation programme resulted in significant decreases in aggression and verbal and physical agitation. In conclusion, pain was a frequent cause of distress behaviour and was effectively identified and treated through a protocol that focused on broadly assessing for all distress behaviours, but also note that 81 of the participants had distress *not* deemed to be due to pain. Supporting a similar conclusion, Kovach and colleagues conducted a double-blind randomized controlled trial of the Serial Trials Protocol (STP) in fourteen nursing homes with 114 participants, all of whom suffered from moderate to severe dementia (Kovach et al. 2006a, 2006b). The purpose of the STP as stated by the investigators was to 'address problems of pain and other unmet needs'. The STP directs the nurse to respond to distress behaviours identified by the Discomfort–Dementia of the Alzheimer's Type (Discomfort–DAT) and/or the BEHAVE-Alzheimer's Disease (AD) scales by first conducting a physical assessment (with response if a potential behaviour cause is found), then an affective/environmental assessment if behaviours continue (with response if a potential behaviour cause is found). If the behaviours continue, the next steps, in order, are a trial of a non-pharmacological intervention, then a trial of an analgesic intervention, then a consultation with a mental health expert, and possibly a psychotropic trial. The treatment group had significantly less discomfort than the control group at post-testing and more frequently had behavioural symptoms return to baseline. The group of nurses using the STP also showed more persistence in assessing and intervening than the control group. The STP clearly illustrates our assertion that there is no such thing as pain assessment in persons with dementia and impaired communication—pain assessment *is* distress assessment. One can only conclude that pain was indeed the culprit causing a behaviour *after* the behaviour has been reduced or eliminated through a pain intervention trial.

Having now grounded ourselves within the larger context of distress, we are ready to move on to consider the evidence regarding pain interventions more specifically. In the next section we will consider the evidence regarding efficacy and effectiveness of pharmacological and non-pharmacological pain interventions. We shall then return to the distress concept and discuss how the language of distress has a foundational role in an integrative clinical approach to assessing and treating causes of distress, including pain, in persons with dementia.

Pain Interventions

There is an abundance of research dedicated to evaluating the efficacy of pain interventions. Pain interventions are broadly defined as methods of treatment that aim to decrease patients' pain. In research and practice, pain interventions are separated into pharmacological and non-pharmacological treatments at the individual level. Although the efficacy of these interventions is an important factor to consider when deciding which treatment to recommend, the fidelity of treatment delivery also plays a substantial role in the overall success of the intervention. In complex healthcare systems, there are many factors that can interfere with intervention fidelity such as staff knowledge and attitudes about pain, assessments, and interventions. Interventions at the systems level, which we discuss below within the non-pharmacological section, target the organization's care practices to improve the effectiveness of pain intervention access, delivery, and quality. Fortunately, there is an important body of work that is focused on investigating the effectiveness of systemic interventions. Below, we provide an overview of the evidence regarding pharmacological (individual) and non-pharmacological (individual and systemic) pain interventions.

Pharmacological Interventions

Pharmacological therapy is typically the first class of intervention used for treatment of pain. For example, most practice guidelines for pain interventions either heavily emphasize or exclusively address pharmacological interventions (American Pain Society 2003; American Medical Directors Association 2012; Australian Pain Society Expert Panel on Older Persons 2005; Gibson 2007; Horgas et al. 2012; McConigley et al. 2008; National Opioid Use Guideline Group 2010). However, medication poses a higher risk in older adults compared to younger adults due to factors such as polypharmacy, slower metabolism, thinner skin, and higher likelihood of having compromised renal and liver function (Weiner and Hanlon 2001). These factors have implications for the type of analgesic that can be prescribed as well as the method of medication administration. Because of the major focus on pharmacological interventions in practice and the higher risk posed to older adults, the most recent practice guidelines published by the American Geriatrics Society Panel on the Pharmacological Management of Persistent Pain in Older Persons (AGS) focus solely on research and recommendations for medication therapy (2009; the assessment guidance and the non-pharmacological guidance from the 2002 guideline was determined still to be up to date and was therefore not addressed in the 2009 guideline).

The World Health Organization (WHO 1996, 2009) has outlined a three-step analgesic ladder that provides a general guide to pharmacological pain management. Although it was developed over two decades ago for use with persons with cancer pain, it is still used today and is consistently referenced in reviews and practice guidelines for pain management in older adults. The motto for pharmacological pain management that has been endorsed in multiple practice guidelines is known as 'start low, and go slow' (AGS 2009; AMDA 2012). This concept is illustrated in the three-step analgesic ladder as a stepwise process that is based on the pain intensity experienced by the individual. As mentioned previously, persons with dementia may be unable to voice their pain. Therefore, observations of frequency, number, and duration of distress behaviours become an important determining factor in pharmacological trials.

Acetaminophen and NSAIDs

Acetaminophen and non-steroidal anti-inflammatory drugs (NSAIDs) are the pharmacological therapies on the lowest step of the analgesic ladder. Because acetaminophen is effective for the management of musculoskeletal pain (a common type of pain in older adults) and poses relatively little risk to older adults, it can be used as an assessment method to determine the cause of distress behaviours in persons with dementia when clinicians are uncertain of the presence of pain. Chibnall and colleagues (2005) illustrated the use of acetaminophen as an assessment method in their study of nursing home residents with moderate to severe dementia. Regular administration of 1000 mg of acetaminophen at each mealtime resulted in increased engagement and decreased distress among the study participants, supporting the researchers' hypothesis that pain was the cause of the residents' distress behaviours.

Patients respond best to acetaminophen when the medication is given every four to six hours, when the person is not already taking a stronger pain analgesic, and when the pain intensity is *mild*. A study by Buffum and colleagues (2004) found regularly scheduled and as-needed (i.e. PRN) low-dose administration of acetaminophen to be ineffective for treating discomfort. Nursing home residents with severe dementia and medical conditions known to be associated with pain were prescribed 650mg of acetaminophen. Participants' pain levels, as measured by distress behaviours, did not vary between the regularly scheduled and PRN groups. Further analysis revealed that most participants had moderate or greater pain. Thus, results of the study indicated that low-dose acetaminophen is not a successful treatment for persons with greater pain intensity. In fact, low-dose opioids may be a more appropriate start point for persons with probable moderate to severe pain as indicated by the analgesic ladder (see next section, Opioids).

Although NSAIDs are listed as a starting point for an analgesic trial in persons with mild pain, they are associated with a number of adverse events in older adults including gastrointestinal toxicity, gastrointestinal bleeding, renal impairment, hypertension, and other vascular and cardiac adverse events including heart failure (AGS 2009). Therefore, AGS (2009) recommends that NSAIDs be used rarely and with caution in people with stomach disease, cardiovascular disease, congestive heart failure, or renal disease. Because of the high risk associated with NSAIDs, cyclooxygenase-2 selective inhibitor NSAID (COX-2) was created as a substitute. However, results of clinical trials have provided indication that negative events are associated with COX-2 (AGS 2009; Dahlberg et al. 2009). Due to the complications that can occur with the use of NSAIDs and COX-2, especially among people in high-risk groups, the AGS (2009) recommends that acetaminophen be used as the first form of pharmacotherapy, especially for persons with musculoskeletal pain. Moreover, low-dose opioids are less likely to cause health complications that have been observed with NSAIDs and COX-2, and they may be a better alternative when prescribed at a very low dosage.

Opioids

Opioids have gained attention since research has highlighted the adverse events associated with NSAID use. Opioids are classified as weak or strong, with the former representing step 2 and the latter representing step 3 on the WHO analgesic ladder (http://www.who.int/cancer/palliative/painladder/en/). Research has shown that opioids are effective for pain management for musculoskeletal and neuropathic pain conditions (AGS 2009). However, clinicians are less likely to prescribe opioids for chronic pain in persons with cognitive impairment (Closs, Barr, and Briggs 2004; Pickering, Jourdan, and Dubray, 2006). Compared to medications recommended at the first level of the analgesic ladder, opioids are stronger and the effects last longer in older adults (Mitchell 2001). Short-term side-effects, such as confusion, drowsiness, and itching, can occur with opioid use (Mitchell 2001). Some risk is also associated with long-term use, such as constipation, sedation, nausea, and respiratory depression; however, these events are more likely to occur when a person is given excessive doses of the medication (AGS 2009; Mitchell 2001). In fact, at very low doses, weak opioids produce fewer side-effects than some of the medications on the first level of the three-step analgesic ladder. Moreover, when weak opioids are started at a low dosage and titrated slowly, individuals are better able to adjust to the medication, and side-effects such as drowsiness subside.

Strong opioids, which are indicated on the last level of the analgesic ladder and are recommended for severe pain, are associated with more side-effects and higher risk compared to weak opioids. Physicians may be hesitant to prescribe potent opioids, especially on a long-term basis, due to the fear of their sedating effects. However, these side-effects can be managed with careful planning and continual reassessment by a clinician. Iatrogenic effects of strong opioids should always be weighed against the negative effects associated with severe, persistent pain. Furthermore, when pain is not appropriately managed, older adults have an increased risk of developing confusion and delirium (Schreier 2010). Jamison and colleagues (2003) investigated the neuropsychological effects of long-term opioid use in persons with chronic pain aged 18 to 70, and found that oxycodone and transdermal fentanyl increased performance on two neuropsychological tests. Therefore, the use of strong opioids may allow the person with severe pain to function at a more optimal level, nullifying the concerns of possible medication side-effects. Rather than withholding opioid treatment due to the potential ramifications, physicians should monitor the presence of side-effects and treat them as needed.

Similar to the use of acetaminophen as an assessment tool for pain, careful use of opioids is beneficial for assessing possible pain when the cause of distress behaviours in persons with dementia is unknown. A study by Manfredi and colleagues (2003) provided evidence that opioids, such as long-acting oxycodone and morphine, can reduce agitation in nursing home residents. After adjusting for sedation in their analyses, the investigators (2003) found that opioids significantly reduced agitation in a group of nursing home residents with severe dementia; however, this effect was only observed in residents above the age of 85. Husebo and colleagues (2011) demonstrated the feasibility and effectiveness of a trial stepwise approach to pharmacological interventions in their study of nursing home residents with moderate to severe dementia in eighteen nursing homes. They started residents on acetaminophen and increased the dose and type of medication (e.g. weak and strong opioids) based on observations made during consistent monitoring. Agitation in residents that completed the trial significantly decreased, and the pain intervention also resulted in a significant reduction in overall severity of neuropsychiatric symptoms. The study by Husebo et al. (2011) illustrates the necessary consideration of pain when developing treatments for agitation and other distress behaviours in persons with cognitive impairment.

The use of opioids in persons with dementia, and indeed the use of opioids in general, is the subject of much controversy. The past twenty years have seen a complete swinging of the pendulum of public and medical opinion from a perhaps overly conservative stance to a perhaps overly liberal stance, and we can only hope that now the pendulum is settling into a middle ground that more accurately reflects reality. There are good reasons to be very cautious in the use of opioids in persons with dementia (Chau et al. 2008). They have the highest frequency of side-effects, particularly in the early stages of use when dosage is being titrated (Lin, Heacock, and Fogel 2010). Common side-effects of opioids include nausea, constipation, sedation, and thinking difficulties. Falls are significantly more common in older persons taking opioids than those taking other types of analgesics (Cooper et al. 2007; Hanlon et al. 2009).

However, there are also good reasons to consider opioids for use in persons with dementia, in some cases even as first-line treatments (Auret and Schug 2005; Brown 2010). Opioids do not carry the toxicity risks to kidneys and liver that NSAIDS do. Opioids have a higher potency, which is important for treating chronic pain. Finally, lower doses of strong opioids may be a better choice than doses of weak opioids when codeine and tramadol (the weak opioids on the WHO analgesic stepladder) are contraindicated. Codeine is ineffective for pain in approximately 30% of the population due to a genetic mutation that is relatively common. Tramadol is contraindicated in persons with a history of seizures and may be contraindicated in those taking SSRI medications due to increased risk of serotonergic syndrome (Dworkin et al. 2007). Finally, there is growing evidence that anti-psychotics and benzodiazapines are more responsible for falls than opioids (Hartikainen, Lönnroos, and Louhivuori 2007; Lavsa et al. 2010), and that cumulative anticholinergic burden is a more powerful predictor of fall risk than the use of opioids per se (Fox et al. 2011). Given the large number of anticholinergic medications that are commonly prescribed to older adults, it is much more important to focus on reducing polypharmacy and cumulative anticholinergic burden than avoiding opioids at all costs (Kelly, Frich, and Hale 2011; Langballe 2011). An anticholinergic cumulative burden tool was developed by Fox and colleagues, and is available at http://www.indydiscoverynetwork.com.

There is also growing evidence that failures to 'start low and go slow' are more likely to be responsible for falls than opioids per se. This may be due in part to confusion about what 'low' is for persons with dementia, particularly very old individuals (over age 80) or individuals with advanced dementia. Indeed, what is considered a 'low' dose in a healthy older adult may be a high dose in frail persons with dementia (Ito and Kanemoto 2013). Three studies have found that weak opioids are responsible for more falls than strong opioids; investigators speculate that this is due to dosage titration being less likely to be carefully approached at sufficiently low starting levels because the opioids are considered 'weak' (Buckeridge et al. 2010; Miller et al. 2011; Wolff et al. 2012). Similarly, there is evidence that opioid-naïve nursing home residents with advanced dementia are more likely be placed on long-acting strong opioids (i.e. fentanyl patch) compared to those without dementia; presumably because providers were attracted by the the advantages of using a patch (rather than oral administration for persons with advanced dementia who often have swallowing difficulties) and subsequently overlooked the risks of starting the opioid-naïve person with a strong opioid at a relatively high fixed dose (due to patches only coming in certain dosages) (Bell et al. 2011; Dosa et al. 2009). During our recent study of the tolerability and efficacy of low-dose opiates (Lortab) to treat discomfort in persons with advanced dementia, we found that even doses so low as to be considered to be subtherapeutic in normal persons were sedating for two of our participants. Finally, there is evidence that side-effects are more common in the very old, perhaps another indicator that lower starting doses are needed in this population (Petre et al. 2012).

Individual Non-pharmacological Interventions

Compared to pharmacological interventions, non-pharmacological therapies have been under-researched, undervalued, and underused. For example, Cramer and colleagues

(2000) found that out of all patients receiving analgesic medications in four long-term care organizations, only 31% had received a non-pharmacological intervention in the past three months. Another study (Allcock, McGarry, and Elkan 2002) surveyed sixty-eight nursing homes and found that non-pharmacological physical therapies were prescribed less often compared to medication, and complementary therapies were rarely or never used. The underuse of non-pharmacological interventions is likely a result of the lack of research and the increased staff time required to implement non-pharmacological therapy compared to pharmacological treatment. The bounty of pharmacological research is attributed to the funding from pharmacological companies and necessity of research due to known risks involved in medication use. In contrast, non-pharmacological intervention research is funded by fewer companies, and it is more costly and difficult to control standardization in non-pharmacological pain management research.

Cohen-Mansfield and colleagues (2012) conducted a study to identify the barriers of implementation of non-pharmacological interventions targeted at decreasing distressing behaviours. They found that there were three types of barrier: resident barriers (e.g. unwillingness to participate, unresponsiveness), availability barriers (e.g. resident unavailable due to other activities or sleeping), and external barriers (e.g. physician did not indicate the presence of pain, materials for intervention were not available). Cohen-Mansfield et al. (2012) suggested that some barriers could be improved while care-givers should respond to others with accommodation. For example, better education on detecting and reporting pain could be provided for physicians. However, resident-related barriers can be difficult to change and should be accommodated. Non-pharmacological interventions should be tailored to the patient's level of functioning to maximize the likelihood of engagement and success.

Non-pharmacological pain interventions can be described as psychosocial and physical/functional therapies aimed at managing persistent pain. The purpose of psychosocial interventions is to provide distraction from pain or to help the patient cope with pain and minimize the negative effects on emotional well-being. Psychosocial interventions indirectly target pain and include relaxation therapy, cognitive-behavioural therapy, and music therapy. In contrast, physical/functional therapies aim to decrease pain and improve physical function by directly targeting pain areas. Physical/functional pain interventions include strategies that require passive participation (e.g. repositioning, hot/cold compresses, massage, transcutaneous electrical nerve stimulation (TENS), tactile simulation, and reflexology) and active participation (e.g. physical therapy and exercise). Each intervention requires assistance from clinicians, yet, due to the deficiency of non-pharmacological research, clinicians may be uncertain about the optimal duration of each therapy.

Psychosocial Interventions

Psychosocial interventions are the least commonly used pain management strategies in nursing homes (Cohen-Mansfield et al. 2012). The most well-documented psychosocial intervention used for management of pain in community-dwelling individuals is cognitive-behavioural therapy (CBT). Because CBT inherently has a cognitive component to treatment, it is not suitable for persons with severe cognitive impairment. However, with proper modifications to treatment delivery, CBT can be an effective intervention in long-term care facilities with persons with mild to moderate dementia. For example a two-part study investigated the effectiveness of a multimodal cognitive-behavioural therapy (MCBT) in nursing home residents with mild to moderate cognitive impairment (Cipher, Clifford, and Roper 2007). The investigators found that eight sessions of MCBT resulted in significant reductions in pain and other factors related to pain, such as emotional stress and activity interference. Furthermore, the nursing home residents had fewer, shorter, less intense distress behaviours at the end of the study. A comparison of matched controls revealed that the study participants had fewer physician visits compared to controls. Several CBT manuals and books offer helpful modifications that can be used for administering CBT to older adults, and a few sources provide recommendations on how to adjust therapy based on level of cognitive abilities (Snow, Powers, and Liles 2006). As Cipher and colleagues (2006) observed, modifications, such as working collaboratively with family members and nursing home staff, addressing problems relevant and valued by the residents, developing structured treatment plans in collaboration with an interdisciplinary team, and using a variety of techniques to identify successful methods of therapy, can result in favourable outcomes.

Relaxation therapy is typically a component of CBT, but it can be used as a standalone treatment for chronic pain in older adults. When used alone, relaxation therapy is conceptualized as a mind-body intervention. Relaxation techniques include progressive muscle relaxation, meditation, yoga, tai chi, and qi gong. A review by Morone and Greco (2007) summarizes the literature on mind-body interventions used for pain management in older adults. They found twenty controlled trials, though only one was conducted in a nursing home setting. The authors concluded that mind-body interventions are well suited for older adults and can be effective at managing pain. However, research is lacking in this area, especially concerning older adults with dementia in long-term care settings.

Physical/Functional Interventions

Physically focused non-pharmacological interventions are diverse in the symptoms and causes they treat. For example, an ice pack could be used to treat the symptom of pain in the lower back, though this intervention would not treat the cause of pain. Physical therapy could be used to increase strength which would directly treat the cause of back pain. In general, physically focused therapies are more often used in nursing home settings compared to psychosocial interventions, though the length of time between therapies is typically long and the therapy schedules are not as structured compared to pharmacological interventions.

Basic non-pharmacological pain management strategies target the site of pain and include repositioning the resident to a more aligned, relaxed position, using pillows to provide cushion and comfort, and applying hot and/or cold compresses. Often, these basic strategies are overlooked because of the simplistic nature of the techniques and the major focus on analgesics for pain relief. Out of the 31% of nursing home residents who received non-pharmacological interventions in the study by Cramer et al. (2000), only 6.6% of those patients received application of hot/cold compresses. Similarly, Reynolds and colleagues (2008) found that 7.1% of nursing home residents in their study were prescribed hot/cold compresses for pain management. Interestingly, basic pain management techniques may be used more often in hospitals compared to nursing homes. A study by Titler et al. (2009) investigated pain management strategies used in hospitals for the treatment of pain associated with hip fractures in older adults. The most frequent non-pharmacological intervention was repositioning (76%), followed by use of a pressure relief device (21.4%), and cold applications (14.3%).

Physical therapy is often used as a pain management strategy and involves passive and active participation. Therapy that is passive (i.e. does not require active participation or movement from the patient) includes massage and TENS. Massage alleviates pain by reducing the muscle tension and stiffness that accompany pain. Not only does massage offer one-on-one contact, it can also block or interfere with pain signals to the brain by sending different sensations to nerve cells. Tactile stimulation (i.e. touching) and reflexology (i.e. application of pressure to small targeted areas or pressure points) have the benefit of one-on-one contact without the strong applied pressure typically used for massages. These techniques have not received as much attention in the literature compared to other therapies, but the evidence is suggestive of reduced pain. The use of TENS for pain management has received mixed reviews, but the basic mechanism for alleviating pain is similar to that of massage therapy. TENS produces an electric current that stimulates nerve cells and interferes with pain signals. Active physical therapy, such as exercise, requires the patient to move and can increase the pain threshold. In addition, active physical therapy decreases functional impairment that is associated with pain. However, the use of exercise as a pain management strategy for older persons with frailty or dementia has received mixed reviews in the literature, so it is important to consider the individual's needs and abilities as well as potential contraindications related to existing conditions.

Systemic Non-pharmacological Interventions

The ultimate outcome of a pain intervention is not only determined by its efficacy but also by the *fidelity* with which it is delivered. Systemic interventions are unique compared to individual pain treatments in that they aim to improve an entire organization's overall approach to care rather than just that of the individual clinician. The need for systemic pain interventions was guided by research findings that older adults with cognitive impairment who live in long-term care facilities receive substandard care for pain management, and that the inadequate care was often a result of multiple systemic factors including staff attitudes and knowledge about pain in persons with dementia, lack of a standard observational assessment instrument and pain assessment protocol, and poor coordination among clinical team members.

Swafford and colleagues (2009) conducted a literature synthesis of systemic pain management interventions in nursing homes and identified ten studies that focused on nursing homes and described evaluations of either quality improvement programmes or process interventions targeting pain assessment, pain management, or both (Alexander et al. 2005; Baier et al. 2004; Buhr and White 2006; Hanson et al. 2008; Horner et al. 2005; Jones et al. 2004; Kovach et al. 2006a; Resnick et al. 2004; Stevenson et al. 2006; Weissman et al. 2000). Overall, the aggregated findings of these studies strongly indicate that pain management practices can improve with the adoption of systematic assessment and/or management practices. Although the interventions described in these studies varied widely, the authors were able to identify several key components of these systems that were consistent across many of the reports. Based upon the synthesis, the authors developed a set of recommendations for systemic pain management interventions, indicating the level of evidence for each recommendation. These recommendations are summarized in Box 42.3.

Box 42.3 Recommendations for systemic pain management approaches

---

1 Conduct audit of current pain care practices, critical elements for success include: formation of a QI pain team using a systematic implementation process model, clear quality indicators, ongoing education system
2 Use evidenced-based clinical decision-making algorithms to assess and treat pain
3 Engage all care team members (include residents, families, front-line staff, nurses, nurse managers, nurse leaders, allied health clinicians, prescribing clinicians, medical directors, pharmacists, activity, and chaplaincy) when considering pain care process changes
4 Target team building to facilitate communication improvement between care team members, particularly between prescribers and nurses
5 Implement a plan for regular evaluation of pain management processes and resident outcomes
6 Consult with experts in pain management and process improvement strategies; be sure to include on-site consultation/bedside training

Reproduced from Kristen Lynne Swafford, Lois Lachmann Miller, Pao-Feng Tsai, Keela Ann Herr, and Mary Ersek, Improving the Process of Pain Care in Nursing Homes: A Literature Synthesis, *Journal of the American Geriatrics Society*, 57(6), pp. 1080–1087 © 2009, Copyright the Authors. Journal compilation © 2009, The American Geriatrics Society.

CLINICAL IMPLICATIONS. DISTRESS FIRST— AN INTEGRATIVE CLINICAL INTERVENTION APPROACH

In this section we present a clinical intervention approach that clinicians from any discipline can use to guide their work. This approach integrates assessment and treatment. It also includes guidelines for integrating paraprofessionals and family members as critical members of the intervention team. This approach is described in terms of persons with dementia severe enough to cause communication impairment, but the astute reader will notice that the approach is also applicable to persons with milder dementia and cognitive impairments. Indeed, because the approach is based upon identifying and responding to universal human needs, the approach is arguably applicable to anyone by modifying the assessment to focus more heavily on verbal interchange with cognitively intact persons.

On Language: 'Distress' Not 'Pain'

The real voyage of discovery consists not in seeking new landscapes but in having new eyes.

Marcel Proust

We urge clinicians to use the word 'distress' rather than 'pain' when engaging in assessment and treatment efforts for persons with dementia severe enough to cause communication impairment. There is compelling evidence that language use actually affects cognition (Bowman, Ronch, and Madjaroff 2010: 31–32). By using the word 'distress' to describe a behaviour rather than 'pain' the clinician takes the cognitive position of 'discovery', (to use Proust's language), and is thus open to a variety of hypotheses regarding the possible causes and possible clinical responses to the behaviour. This open-minded cognitive stance is extremely important because the behaviours that indicate pain in persons with dementia severe enough to cause communication impairment are exactly the same group of behaviours that indicate a variety of other types of distress, including boredom, fright, and physical discomforts that are not pain (i.e. itching, uncomfortable positioning, rough clothing). By using the word 'pain' before a proper assessment is completed, the clinician is setting him or herself up to forget that the cause of the behaviour may not be pain at all. A second reason to use the word 'distress' is that the inappropriately early use of the word 'pain' narrows the clinician's sense of purpose to one of relieving only pain rather than relieving all forms of distress. More importantly, use of the word 'pain' inadvertently communicates this narrower sense of purpose to treatment team and family members, and even to the person with dementia (in the case of less cognitively impaired persons). In contrast, we emphatically state that our shared purpose should be to address *all* forms of distress, no matter what their cause. One final consideration regarding treatment teams, family members, and persons with dementia is that the word 'pain' is an emotionally charged word that means different things to different people. For some people, 'pain' brings up associations of past experiences in which a person was over-medicated or inappropriately medicated for pain, with disastrous results. For others, 'pain' brings up associations of past experiences in which someone complained of pain as part of drug-seeking or attention-seeking behaviour. For some people with dementia, complaining of 'pain' is seen as a sign of weakness. Thus, another excellent reason to use the word 'distress' is the avoidance of the baggage that often accompanies the use of the word 'pain'.

Experiences in four different studies of pain and dementia have convinced us of the importance of using the word 'distress' rather than 'pain'. In a study of the tolerability of opiates for persons with severe dementia we often encountered pain screening (PAINAD) scores of 0 (meaning no behavioural indicators of pain present), and yet a member of the clinical team had referred the person to the study and furthermore our team of trained assessors would report positive pain screening scores on observation. Conversations with nursing staff yielded the explanations such as 'yes, I have also heard the veteran muttering to himself under his breath,' (a behaviour that is described as 'negative vocalization' by the PAINAD) 'but that's just something he always does, it's not because he is in pain'. Qualitative interviews with nurses yielded similar sentiments during an implementation study of a pain screening system for persons with dementia. The nurses were tasked with coaching nursing assistants who were asked to complete a pain screening measure (NOPPAIN) after providing morning care to residents. Unfortunately, the nurses also needed some coaching. The nurses often reported during these interviews that they had to 'correct' the nursing assistants for endorsing behaviours 'incorrectly'; in fact the behaviours (such as negative vocalizations and facial expressions) were present, but the nurses interpreted these behaviours as not indicative of pain and therefore coached the nursing assistants that the behaviours should be marked 'absent' on the screening form.

We believe the word 'pain' on these screening forms is what led the staff astray. Nursing home staff have typically been trained in the medical model to complete charting information in a narrow and focused way. This habit is adaptive when deciding what to write in the medical chart so that formal documentation can communicate important information quickly and reduce opportunities for liability by not documenting too much information, but this habit is not helpful for promoting a broader critical thinking approach to understanding cause and effect. In support of this contention, we found in a recent series of cognitive interviews with nurses and nursing assistants for a pain instrumentation study that when staff were asked to reflect about the causes of distress behaviours, they were likely to dismiss the behaviours as not worthy of attention if they believed the behaviours were not caused by pain. Finally, we learned a lot about the language of pain during a study in which we provided dyadic psychoeducation to care-givers and persons with pain and mild to moderate dementia. On several occasions the therapist would be surprised on her first visit to hear denials of pain from the care-giver and/or person with dementia, despite having endorsed pain during a phone assessment just days beforehand. Once the therapist pulled out her notes and reviewed the conditions that had been explored as causes of pain, the participants would inevitably issue exclamations of agreement and explanations such as 'oh yes, we forgot about that!', or 'yes, he does complain a lot about his knee but we think it's just the depression'. For example, one person with mild dementia and his wife stridently denied any pain when the therapist asked for a description of his pain. The therapist then pulled out the intake notes and said, 'It says here that during the phone assessment you mentioned that Mr. Smith has pain in his foot from an old combat injury, is this incorrect?' The care-giver and person with dementia immediately laughed and enthusiastically agreed that there was indeed a foot problem, saying, 'Oh yes! That old foot! We had forgotten about that!' Later in the conversation, it turned out that the pain from the foot injury was so intense that the person with dementia often could not sleep at night and had in fact been up half the previous night because of the pain. We now regularly use the word 'distress' and make sure that clinicians inquiring about potentially painful experiences persevere in describing the potential experience in multiple ways so they can be assured of hearing about experiences that participants label with different words than 'pain'.

Ancient Japanese Zen masters often used odd or nonsensical language as a tool to shock the mind, thus helping their students to 'wake up' to important truths. In more modern times, we greatly enjoyed the movie Fight Club, starring Brad Pitt and Edward Norton, and found the 'rules of fight club' (espoused by Brad Pitt's character) to sound much like a Zen koan. Thus, influenced by both the ancient and the modern, we humbly offer the following poem to sum up our approach to pain in persons with dementia and communication impairment.

The first rule of treating pain is you do not assess for pain.
The second rule of treating pain is you do not assess for pain.
Instead you assess for distress.
The final rule of treating pain is you treat the distress, regardless of if it is caused by pain or
    caused by something else.

THE PROCESS: LOOK• LISTEN• GUESS• RESPOND• REPEAT

Look•Listen•Guess•Respond•Repeat (LLGRR) is our moniker for a recommended approach that builds upon the evidence-supported successes of the interventions reviewed in the previous sections, particularly the Serial Trials Protocol. The LLGRR process is concordant with the most recent guidelines regarding assessment in persons with dementia and is summarized in Box 42.4 (Hadjistavropolous et al. 2007; Herr et al. 2011; Royal College of Physicians, British Geriatrics Society, and British Pain Society 2007). LLGRR is grounded in

---

Box 42.4 Look • Listen • Guess • Respond • Repeat (LLGRR)

(1) Look and Listen For Distress Messages and Their Causes: *Assessment*
  a) Assessment Dimensions
    i. Internal: Physical & Emotional
    ii. External: Social & Environmental
      a. Background:
        a. Neurologic/Cognitive abilities and impairments
          1. Neurologic: specific regional brain involvement, neurotransmitter imbalance, circadian rhythm deterioration, motor ability
          2. Cognitive: attention, memory, visual-spatial ability, language skills
        b. Physical/affective/functional abilities and impairments
          1. General health
          2. Functional ability
          3. Affective state
          4. Psychosocial characteristics: gender, education, occupation, history of psychosocial stressors and responses to stress
        c. Premorbid and current personality
        d. Premorbid and current interests and abilities
        e. Life story, self-identity
  b) Assessment Sources of Information
    i. Person with Dementia
      a. Interview the person with dementia
      b. Observe the person with dementia, note appearance and behaviour
      c. Advocate for a physical examination of the person with dementia
    ii. Medical chart
      a. Review current conditions and status
      b. Review medical/psychosocial history
    iii. Collateral sources (family, care-givers)
      a. Interview collateral sources
      b. Observe collateral sources interact with the person with dementia
    iv. Environment
      a. Observe the environment
      b. Observe interactions between environment and person with dementia

(Continued)

Box 42.4 (Continued)

---

    c) Assessment Questions

        i. Is there optimal stimulation? Is there engagement? Is the engagement individualized and meaningful?

        ii. Where should I concentrate my efforts?

           a. Which causes are fixed?

           b. Which of the identified potential causes are most mutable?

           c. Who's the Problem?

        iii. Might operant learning play a role? Are there unintended reinforcers of distress behaviours?

(2) Guess: *Clinical Hypothesis Testing*

(3) Respond: *Treatment Planning and Intervention*

    i. Non-pharmacologic interventions first

    ii. With exception of Pharmacologic intervention first when clinical confidence is high regarding cause

(4) Repeat: *Re-assess, Revise, Reach Out to Others/Refer (Consultation)*

    i. Analgesic trial

    ii. Consultation

    iii. Psychotropic trial last if indicated

---

the Unmet Needs Model. The clinician's first step in LLGRR is to carefully assess the person with dementia to identify distress messages when they are present and to identify potential causes of those distress messages. Guided by the Unmet Needs Model, the clinician assesses for unmet physical, emotional, social, and environmental unmet needs/causes of distress messages as well as contributory background factors. The clinician gathers information from the person with dementia, collaterals, the medical record, and the environment through interview, observation, and record review. In evaluating and synthesizing the assessment data, the clinician is guided by three critical questions informed by the rich theoretical and evidence base that has grown around the Unmet Needs Model (as discussed in the Unmet Needs Conceptual Model section): 1) is there optimal stimulation; 2) where should I concentrate my efforts; and 3) is operant learning playing a role in the development or maintenance of distress messages? The clinician then develops hypotheses about the causes of the identified distress behaviours as informed by the assessment. Next, the clinician works with other members of the clinical team, the person with dementia, and staff and family members as appropriate to develop an action plan for addressing the hypothesized causes. Non-pharmacological interventions should always be tried first. The exception to this rule are cases in which the clinician has high confidence in a cause hypothesis and a pharmacological response is clearly indicated for that cause (e.g. arthritis is causing pain, there is subsequent resistance to care during transfers and bathing, and therefore an anti-inflammatory analgesic is indicated prior to transfers and baths). Finally, the LLGRR cycle is repeated. Reassessment for the presence of distress behaviours is conducted. If distress behaviours are still present, potential causes are evaluated and clinical hypotheses are revised based upon those data. If the assessment data indicate additional potential causes, non-pharmacological treatments should again be preferred for initially addressing any newly hypothesized causes, and again the LLGRR cycle is repeated. If distress behaviours persist and non-pharmacological treatment of all reasonable hypothesized causes has been explored, the clinician should consider an *analgesic trial*. Kovach reports excellent success in using analgesic trials (i.e. scheduled doses of a non-opioid analgesic such as acetaminophen) to explore the possibility that pain due to an unidentified cause is driving the distress behaviour. The analgesic trial is an important step because pain is so prevalent in this population and because the multiple comorbidities typically represented in these individuals can easily result in pain while masking the cause. Finally, consultation with other experts, such as a geropsychiatrist or a pain management expert, would be indicated if the analgesic trial is a failure. A psychotropic trial, such as an anti-depressant or anti-psychotic, should be explored at this time. The most important ingredients in the LLGRR protocol are tenacity and diligence on the part of the clinician. As the Serial Trials Protocol studies demonstrate, clinical persistence is necessary when responding to distress messages in persons with dementia and communication impairment. Indeed, Kovach and colleagues found that an average of nine cycles of the Serial Trials Protocol were required to achieve significant decreases in distress behaviours.

The Eight ('-ate') Action Principles: Enculturate, Educate, Communicate, Advocate, Activate, Participate, Evaluate, and Reformulate

Now that we have addressed the LLGRR process that is recommended for the clinician, the last component of the Distress First intervention approach is how the clinician interfaces with his or her own organizational environment in pursuing quality care for the person with dementia. As we discussed earlier, there is evidence that healthcare organizations are most effective in providing quality pain care for their patients when they include these critical elements: having a quality improvement (QI) process for pain management, using evidence-based algorithms, engaging all members of the care team, providing ongoing education to the care team members (including access to consultants), and engaging in periodic evaluation and improvement of these processes. Although the individual clinician cannot change an entire organization, the clinician can approach her or his individual clinical work with an attitude and commitment to action that is concordant with and supportive of these critical elements. Thus, we strongly recommend that the clinician work to support these action principles: *educate, communicate, enculturate, advocate, activate, evaluate, and reformulate*. A mnemonic to assist in remembering these principles is that there are eight of them and they all end in '-ate', thus the eight ('-ate') actions.

Regarding *educate, communicate, enculturate, and advocate*, the clinician should work to share and recommend the alternative language of 'Distress First' with fellow clinical team members as well as family members and friends of the person with dementia. By educating about and communicating the importance of using a 'Distress First' approach to language and behaviour cause conceptualization, the clinician can promote improved quality of care. Consistently guiding others to discuss 'distress messages' and engage in 'distress assessment' can, over time, have a strong effect on the thought processes and actions of others, thus changing the culture. We recommend LLGRR as a process rather than its closest inspiration, the Serial Trials Protocol, specifically because of its educational value. The language of Look •Listen•Guess•Respond•Repeat is understandable to individuals regardless of clinical background or lack thereof, and avoids potentially confusing jargon such as 'clinical hypothesis testing' and 'treatment planning'. Gently exploring the pain (and distress) beliefs, attitudes, and experiences of fellow clinical team members, persons with dementia, and their families and friends will provide opportunities for further education and communication. Fears about pain medications are common not just in lay people but also among fellow clinical professionals who have suffered through past experiences of seeing patients over-medicated, resulting in sedation, confusion, deconditioning, and falls. Fears of addiction to pain medication are common, particularly amongst family members and people with dementia. By openly discussing past experiences, the clinician can help facilitate improved treatment planning among clinical team members and improved treatment compliance among people with dementia and their families and friends.

Regarding *activate, evaluate, and reformulate*, the clinician can work personally to model a QI approach to change as well as to collaborate with others to put QI elements in place in the organization. Choosing a pain assessment tool and using it regularly with one's own case load is a small way to begin. The clinician can identify best practice guidelines and request that the clinical team develop assessment and treatment algorithms based upon those guidelines, if the organization does not already have such in place. Conducting a review of one's own case load on a regular basis to attempt to identify opportunities for improvement is yet another way to model a commitment to evaluation and reformulation principles.

Implications for Practice

In summary, the clinician is encouraged always to consider pain as a potential condition when working with persons with dementia and communication impairment. Assessing for distress messages through observations of behaviour should be a continual process with this vulnerable population. All clinicians should include in their responsibilities the education of members of the treatment team of the person with dementia, including family members and front-line care providers such as nursing assistants and home health aides, about the unmet needs model and the importance of being alert for distress messages. LLGRR should be used by clinicians and taught to all team members (including families and front-line care partners) as the systematic approach of choice for detecting and responding to distress messages. Clinicians should serve as advocates for the communicatively impaired person with dementia, gently but persistently persuading the clinical team to assure that thorough assessments of physical, emotional, social, and environmental dimensions are conducted, including all possible information sources (chart, proxies, observation) and taking into account background factors. Clinicians should also advocate for pharmacological interventions to be delayed until non-pharmacological alternatives can be tried. Knowing that persistence is the key to success, clinicians should continue to advocate for multiple cycles of

LLGRR, not accepting 'it's just the dementia' as an explanation for distress behaviours. With regards to consideration of analgesic treatment, clinicians are encouraged to consider the risks of polypharmacy, psychotropic use, and cumulative anticholinergic burden. Informed pharmacological treatment decision-making is recommended: a) start slow and go slow; b) take into account the risks of opioid analgesic treatment, compared to the risks of NSAID or weak opioid/NSAID combination treatment and benefits; c) remember that there are significant risks associated both with the under-treatment of pain as well as the pharmaceutical over-treatment, so persist in treatment titration until an ideal balance is achieved.

SUMMARY

Pain assessment and management in persons with dementia and communication impairment are especially challenging and important topics because: under-identification and under-treatment is unfortunately common in this vulnerable population; the cognitive impairments that define dementia make it difficult for persons with dementia to understand and report their pain; difficulty in predicting when self-report in persons with dementia will become inaccurate makes it difficult for clinicians accurately to assess pain and requires increased reliance on observational assessment; and yet distress behaviours in persons with dementia are often misunderstood and, while sensitive, behavioural indicators of pain are not *specific* pain indicators. This chapter recommended the Unmet Needs conceptual model as an important paradigm for understanding causes of pain in persons with dementia. Pharmacological and non-pharmacological pain interventions are described. An integrative clinical assessment and intervention approach, 'Distress First', was presented. Clinicians are encouraged to use the term 'distress' rather than 'pain' for this population. An assessment and treatment approach, 'Look•Listen•Guess•Respond•Repeat', was recommended. Finally, a set of eight '-ate' action principles, 'Enculturate, Educate, Communicate, Advocate, Activate, Participate, Evaluate, Reformulate', is presented to guide clinicians toward action at both individual and systemic levels to improve pain assessment and management for this population

NOTES

1. This is not to denigrate the value of group-based activities, but to acknowledge that the current culture of dementia care is overly skewed toward group-based solutions, and a rebalancing is needed.
2. The film *Ex Memoria* offers a portrait of life as seen through the eyes of a woman with dementia, loosely based upon the life history of the director's Jewish grandmother from Poland. This excellent film was made with support from the Bradford Dementia Group, which provides an excellent discussion of issues including the effect of the Holocaust on Jewish people in Poland and how such effects may manifest in persons with dementia. For more information please see: (1) Bradford Dementia Group. 'Handouts on Issues Raised by the Film *Ex Memoria*'. http://www.bradford.ac.uk/health/career-areas/bradford-dementia-group/resources/ex-memoria-a-short-film/; (2) Appignanesi, J.

(director and writer), and Bays, M. (Producer). (2006). *Ex Memoria* (DVD). http://www.exmemoriafilm.co.uk/; (3) Appignanesi, J., and Baum, D. (2006). 'Ex Memoria: Filming the Face'. *Third Text* 20(1): 85–97. doi:10.1080/09528820500472530.

Key References and Sources for Further Reading

American Geriatrics Society Panel on the Pharmacological Management of Persistent Pain in Older Persons (2009). 'Pharmacological Management of Persistent Pain in Older Persons'. *Journal of the American Geriatrics Society* 57(8):1331–1346. doi:10.1111/j.1532-5415.2009.02376.x. For pharmacological treatment guidance.

American Geriatrics Society Panel on Persistent Pain in Older Persons (2002). 'Clinical Practice Guidelines: The Management of Persistent Pain in Older Persons'. *Journal of the American Geriatrics Society* 50: S205–S224 (2002). For nonpharmacological treatment guidance.

Camp, C. (2012). *Hiding the Stranger in the Mirror: A Detective's Manual for Solving Problems Related to Alzheimer's Disease and Related Disorders*. Cleveland, OH: Center for Applied Research in Dementia.

Cohen-Mansfield, J. (2011). 'The Language of Behavior'. In B. Bowers and M. Downs (eds), *Excellence in Dementia Care: Research into Practice*. New York: McGraw Hill.

Herr, K., Coyne, P. J., McCaffery, M., Manworren, R., and Merkel, S. (2011). 'Pain Assessment in the Patient Unable to Self-report: Position Statement with Clinical Practice Recommendations'. *Pain Management Nursing* 12(4): 230–250. doi:10.1016/j.pmn.2011.10.002.

Kovach, C. R., Logan, B. R., Noonan, P. E., Schlidt, A. M., Smerz, J., et al. (2006a). 'Effects of the Serial Trial Intervention on Discomfort and Behavior of Nursing Home Residents with Dementia'. *American Journal of Alzheimer's Disease and Other Dementias* 21(3): 147–155. doi:10.1177/1533317506288949.

Kovach, C. R., Cashin, J. R., and Sauer, L. (2006b). 'Deconstruction of a Complex Tailored Intervention to Assess and Treat Discomfort of People with Advanced Dementia'. *Journal of Advanced Nursing* 55(6): 678–688. doi:10.1111/j.1365-2648.2006.03968.x.

Mast, B. (2011). *Whole Person Dementia Assessment*. Baltimore, MD: Health Professions Press.

Swafford, K. L., Miller, L. L., Tsai, P.-F., Herr, K. A., and Ersek, M. (2009). 'Improving the Process of Pain Care in Nursing Homes: A Literature Synthesis'. *Journal of the American Geriatrics Society* 57(6): 1080–1087. doi:10.1111/j.1532-5415.2009.02274.x.

References

Alexander, B. J., Plank, P., Carlson, M. B., Hanson, B., Picken, K., et al. (2005). 'Methods of Pain Assessment in Residents of Long-term Care Facilities: A Pilot Study'. *Journal of the American Medical Directors Association* 6: 137–143.

Algase, D. L., Beck, C., Kolanowski, A., Whall, A., Berent, S., et al. (1996). 'Need-driven Dementia-compromised Behavior: An Alternative View of Disruptive Behavior'. *American Journal of Alzheimer's Disease and Other Dementias* 11(6): 10–19. doi:10.1177/153331759601100603.

Allcock, N., McGarry, J., and Elkan, R. (2002). 'Management of Pain in Older People within the Nursing Home: A Preliminary Study'. *Health and Social Care in the Community* 10(6): 464–471. http://www.ncbi.nlm.nih.gov/pubmed/12485133.

American Geriatrics Society Panel on the Pharmacological Management of Persistent Pain in Older Persons (2009). 'Pharmacological Management of Persistent Pain in Older Persons'. Journal of the American Geriatrics Society 57(8):1331–1346. doi:10.1111/j.1532-5415.2009.02376.x.

American Geriatrics Society Panel on Persistent Pain in Older Persons (2002). 'Clinical Practice Guidelines: The Management of Persistent Pain in Older Persons'. Journal of the American Geriatrics Society 50: S205–S224 (2002). For nonpharmacological treatment guidance.

American Medical Directors Association (2012). Pain Management in the Long-term Care Setting. Baltimore, MD: American Medical Directors Association.

American Pain Society (2003). Principles of Analgesic Use in the Treatment of Acute Pain and Chronic Cancer Pain (5th edn). Chicago: American Pain Society.

Appignanesi, J. and Bays, M. (2006). Ex Memoria (DVD). http://www.exmemoriafilm.co.uk/.

Auret, K. and Schug, S. (2005). 'Underutilisation of Opioids in Elderly Patients with Chronic Pain: Approaches to Correcting the Problem'. Drugs & Aging 22(8): 641–654. http://www.ncbi.nlm.nih.gov/pubmed/16060715.

Australian Pain Society Expert Panel on Older Persons (2005). Pain in Residential Aged Care Facilities: Management Strategies (pp. 1–85). Sydney: Australian Pain Society.

Baier, R. R., Gifford, D. R., Patry, G, et al. (2004). 'Ameliorating Pain in Nursing Homes: A Collaborative Quality-improvement Project'. Journal of the American Geriatrics Society 52: 1988–1995.

Bell, J. S., Laitinen, M.-L., Lavikainen, P., Lönnroos, E., Uosukainen, H., et al. (2011). 'Use of Strong Opioids among Community-dwelling Persons with and without Alzheimer's Disease in Finland'. Pain 152(3): 543–547. doi:10.1016/j.pain.2010.11.003.

Bowman, C., Ronch, J., and Madjaroff, G. (2010). The Power of Language to Create Culture. Chicago: Hulda B. and Maurice L. Rothschild Foundation. http://www.pioneernetwork.net/CultureChange/PowerOfLanguage/.

Brown, R. (2010). 'Broadening the Search for Safe Treatments in Dementia Agitation: A Possible Role for Low-dose Opioids? International Journal of Geriatric Psychiatry 25(10): 1085–1086. doi:10.1002/gps.2423.

Buckeridge, D., Huang, A., Hanley, J., Kelome, A., Reidel, K., et al. (2010). 'Risk of Injury Associated with Opioid Use in Older Adults'. Journal of the American Geriatrics Society 58(9): 1664–1670. doi:10.1111/j.1532-5415.2010.03015.x.

Buffum, M. D., Sands, L., Miaskowski, C., Brod, M., Washburn, A., et al. (2004). 'A Clinical Trial of the Effectiveness of Regularly Scheduled versus As-needed Administration of Acetaminophen in the Management of Discomfort in Older Adults with Dementia'. Journal of the American Geriatrics Society 52(7): 1093–1097. http://search.ebscohost.com/login.aspx?direct=trueanddb=psyhandAN=2004-15349-007andsite=ehost-live.

Buffum, M. D., Hutt, E., Chang, V. T., Craine, M. H., and Snow, A. L. (2007). 'Cognitive Impairment and Pain Management: Review of Issues and Challenges'. Journal of Rehabilitation Research and Development 44(2): 315. doi:10.1682/JRRD.2006.06.0064.

Buhr, G. T. and White, H. K. (2006). 'Quality Improvement Initiative for Chronic Pain Assessment and Management in the Nursing Home: A Pilot Study. Journal of the American Medical Directors Association 7: 246–253.

Burnes, D. P. R. and Burnette, D. (2013). 'Broadening the Etiological Discourse on Alzheimer's Disease to include Trauma and Posttraumatic Stress Disorder as Psychosocial Risk Factors'. Journal of Aging Studies 27(3): 218–224. doi:10.1016/j.jaging.2013.03.002.

Burri, A., Maercker, A., Krammer, S., and Simmen-Janevska, K. (2013). 'Childhood Trauma and PTSD Symptoms Increase the Risk of Cognitive Impairment in a Sample of Former Indentured Child Laborers in Old Age'. PLoS One 8(2): e57826. doi:10.1371/journal.pone.0057826.

Cahill, S. and Diaz-Ponce, A. M. (2011). ' "I Hate Having Nobody Here. I'd Like to Know Where They All Are": Can Qualitative Research Detect Differences in Quality of Life among Nursing Home Residents with Different Levels of Cognitive Impairment?' *Aging & Mental Health* 15(5): 562–572. doi:10.1080/13607863.2010.551342.

Camp, C. J. and Skrajner, M. J. (2004). 'Resident-assisted Montessori Programming (RAMP): Training Persons with Dementia to Serve as Group Activity Leaders'. *Gerontologist* 44(3): 426–431. http://www.ncbi.nlm.nih.gov/pubmed/15197297.

Camp, C. (2012). *Hiding the Stranger in the Mirror: A Detective's Manual for Solving Problems Related to Alzheimer's Disease and Related Disorders*. Cleveland, OH: Center for Applied Research in Dementia.

Chau, D. L., Walker, V., Pai, L., and Cho, L. M. (2008). 'Opiates and Elderly: Use and Side Effects'. *Clinical Interventions in Aging* 3(2): 273–278. http://www.pubmedcentral.nih.gov/articlerender.fcgi?artid=2546472andtool=pmcentrezandrendertype=abstract.

Cheston, R. and Bender, M. (1999). *Understanding Dementia: The Man with the Worried Eyes*. London: Jessica Kingsley.

Chibnall, J. T., Tait, R. C., Harman, B., and Luebbert, R. A. (2005). 'Effect of Acetaminophen on Behavior, Well-being, and Psychotropic Medication Use in Nursing Home Residents with Moderate-to-severe Dementia'. *Journal of the American Geriatrics Society* 53(11): 1921–1929. doi:10.1111/j.1532-5415.2005.53572.x.

Cipher, D. J., Clifford, P. A., and Roper, K. D. (2006). 'Behavioral Manifestations of Pain in the Demented Elderly'. *Journal of the American Medical Directors Association* 7(6): 355–365. doi:10.1016/j.jamda.2005.11.012.

Cipher, D. J., Clifford, P. A., and Roper, K. D. (2007). 'The Effectiveness of Geropsychological Treatment in Improving Pain, Depression, Behavioral Disturbances, Functional Disability, and Health Care Utilization in Long-term Care'. *Clinical Gerontologist* 30(3): 23–40.

Closs, S. J., Barr, B., and Briggs, M. (2004). 'Cognitive Status and Analgesic Provision in Nursing Home Residents'. *The British Journal of General Practice* 54(509): 919–921. http://www.pubmedcentral.nih.gov/articlerender.fcgi?artid=1326110andtool=pmcentrezandrendertype=abstract.

Cohen-Mansfield, J. and Werner, P. (1995). 'Environmental Influences on Agitation: An Integrative Summary of an Observational Study'. *American Journal of Alzheimer's Care and Related Disorders and Research* 10(1): 32–39.

Cohen-Mansfield, J., Marx, M. S., Regier, N. G., and Dakheel-Ali, M. (2009). 'The Impact of Personal Characteristics on Engagement in Nursing Home Residents with Dementia'. *International Journal of Geriatric Psychiatry* 24(7): 755–763. doi:10.1002/gps.2192.

Cohen-Mansfield, J. (2011). 'The Language of Behavior'. In B. Bowers and M. Downs (eds), *Excellence In Dementia Care: Research into Practice*. New York: McGraw Hill.

Cohen-Mansfield, J., Thein, K., Marx, M. S., and Dakheel-Ali, M. (2012). 'What are the Barriers to Performing Nonpharmacological Interventions for Behavioral Symptoms in the Nursing Home?' *Journal of the American Medical Directors Association* 13(4): 400–405. doi:10.1016/j.jamda.2011.07.006.

Cooper, J. W., Freeman, M. H., Cook, C. L., Burfield, A. H. (2007). 'Assessment of Psychotropic and Psychoactive Loads and Falls in Nursing Facility Residents'. *Consultant Pharmacist* 22: 483–489.

Conn, D. K., Clarke, D., and Van Reekum, R. (2000). 'Depression in Holocaust Survivors: Profile and Treatment Outcome in a Geriatric Day Hospital Program'. *International Journal of Geriatric Psychiatry* 15(4): 331–337. http://www.ncbi.nlm.nih.gov/pubmed/10767733.

Cramer, G. W., Galer, B. S., Mendelson, M. A., and Thompson, G. D. (2000). 'A Drug Use Evaluation of Selected Opioid and Nonopioid Analgesics in the Nursing Facility Setting'. *Journal of the American Geriatrics Society* 48(4): 398–404.

Dahlberg, L. E., Holme, I., Høye, K., and Ringertz, B. (2009). 'A Randomized, Multicentre, Double-blind, Parallel-Group study to Assess the Adverse Event-related Discontinuation Rate with Celecoxib and Diclofenac in Elderly Patients with Osteoarthritis'. *Scandinavian Journal of Rheumatology* 38(2): 133–143.

Deci, E. L. (1980). *The Psychology of Self-determination.* Lexington, MA: Heath.

Deci, E. L. and Ryan, R. M. (1980). 'The Empirical Exploration of Intrinsic Motivational Processes'. In L. Berkowitz (ed.), *Advances in Experimental Social Psychology* (vol. 13, pp. 39–80). New York: Academic Press.

Deci, E. L. and Ryan, R. M. (1985). *Intrinsic Motivation and Self-determination in Human Behavior.* New York: Plenum.

Deci, E. L. and Ryan, R. M. (1991). 'A Motivational Approach to Self: Integration in Personality'. In R. Dienstbier (ed.), *Nebraska Symposium on Motivation. Vol. 38. Perspectives on Motivation* (pp. 237–288). Lincoln: University of Nebraska Press.

Deci, E. L. and Ryan, R. M. (2013). 'The "What" and "Why" of Goal Pursuits: Human Needs and the Self-determination of Behavior'. *Psychological Inquiry* 11(4): 227–268.

Dosa, D. M., Dore, D. D., Mor, V., and Teno, J. M. (2009). 'Frequency of Long-acting Opioid Analgesic Initiation in Opioid-naïve Nursing Home Residents'. *Journal of Pain and Symptom Management* 38(4): 515–521. doi:10.1016/j.jpainsymman.2008.11.008/

Dworkin, R. H., O'Connor, A. B., Backonja, M., Farrar, J. T., Finnerup, N. B., et al. (2007). 'Pharmacologic Management of Neuropathic Pain: Evidence-based Recommendations'. *Pain* 132(3): 237–251. doi:10.1016/j.pain.2007.08.033.

Fox, C., Richardson, K., Maidment, I. D., Savva, G. M., Matthews, F. E., et al. (2011). 'Anticholinergic Medication Use and Cognitive Impairment in the Older Population: The Medical Research Council Cognitive Function and Ageing Study'. *Journal of the American Geriatrics Society* 59(8): 1477–1483. doi:10.1111/j.1532-5415.2011.03491.x.

Gibson, S. J. (2007). 'IASP Global Year against Pain in Older Persons: Highlighting the Current Status and Future Perspectives in Geriatric Pain'. *Expert Review of Neurotherapeutics* 7(6): 627–635. doi:10.1586/14737175.7.6.627.

Gitlin, L. N., Winter, L., Burke, J., et al. (2008). 'Tailored Activities to Manage Neuropsychiatry Behavior in Persons with Dementia and Reduce Caregiver Burden: A Randomized Pilot Study'. *American Journal of Geriatric Psychiatry* 16: 229–239.

Gitlin, L. N., Winter, L., Earland, T. V., et al. (2009). 'The Tailored Activity Program (TAP): A Nonpharmacologic Approach to Improving Quality of Life at Home for Persons with Dementia and their Family Caregivers'. *Gerontologist* 49: 428–439.

Gitlin, L. N., Hodgson, N., Jutkowitz, E., and Pizzi, L. (2010). 'The Cost-effectiveness of a Nonpharmacologic Intervention for Individuals with Dementia and Family Caregivers: The Tailored Activity Program'. *American Journal of Geriatric Psychiatry* 18(6): 510–519. doi:10.1097/JGP.0b013e3181c37d13.

Hadjistavropoulos, T., Herr, K., Turk, D. C., Fine, P. G., Dworkin, R. H., et al. (2007). 'An Interdisciplinary Expert Consensus Statement on Assessment of Pain in Older Persons'. *Clinical Journal of Pain* 23(suppl. 1): S1–S43. doi:10.1097/AJP.0b013e31802be869.

Hanlon, J. T., Boudreau, R. M., Roumani, Y. F., Newman, A. B., Ruby, C. M., et al. (2009). 'Number and Dosage of Central Nervous System Medications on Recurrent Falls in Community Elders: The Health, Aging and Body Composition Study'. *Journals of Gerontology, Series A: Biological Sciences and Medical Sciences* 64(4): 492–498. doi:10.1093/gerona/gln043.

Hanson, L. C., Reynolds, K. S., Henderson, M., and Pickard, C. G. (2008). 'A Quality Improvement Intervention to Increase Palliative Care in Nursing Homes'. *Journal of Palliative Medicine* 8: 576–584.

Hartikainen, S., Lönnroos, E., and Louhivuori, K. (2007). 'Medication as a Risk Factor for Falls: Critical Systematic Review'. *Journals of Gerontology, Series A: Biological Sciences and Medical Sciences* 62(10): 1172–1181. http://www.ncbi.nlm.nih.gov/pubmed/17921433.

Herman, A. D., Johnson, T. M., Ritchie, C. S., and Parmelee, P. A. (2009). 'Pain Management Interventions in the Nursing Home: A Structured Review of the Literature'. *Journal of the American Geriatrics Society* 57(7): 1258–1267. doi:10.1111/j.1532-5415.2009.02315.x.

Herr, K., Coyne, P. J., McCaffery, M., Manworren, R., and Merkel, S. (2011). 'Pain Assessment in the Patient Unable to Self-report: Position Statement with Clinical Practice Recommendations'. *Pain Management Nursing* 12(4): 230–250. doi:10.1016/j.pmn.2011.10.002.

Horgas, A. L., Yoon, S. L., and Grall, M. (2012). 'Nursing Standard of Practice Protocol: Pain Management in Older Adults'. In *Evidence-Based Geriatric Nursing Protocols for Best Practice* (4th edn; p. 7). Springer Publishing Company.

Horner, J. K., Hanson, L. C., Wood, D., Silver, A. G., and Reynolds, K. S. (2005). 'Using Quality Improvement to Address Pain Management Practices in Nursing Homes'. *Journal of Pain and Symptom Management* 30: 271–277.

Husebo, B. S., Ballard, C., Sandvik, R., Nilsen, O. B., and Aarsland, D. (2011). 'Efficacy of Treating Pain to Reduce Behavioural Disturbances in Residents of Nursing Homes with Dementia: Cluster Randomised Clinical Trial'. *British Medical Journal* 343(7816): 1–10.

Husebo, B. S., Achterberg, W. P., Lobbezoo, F., Kunz, M., Lautenbacher, S., et al. (2012). 'A Review of Pain Assessment and Treatment Challenges; Pain in Patients with Dementia'. *Norsk Epidemiologi/Norwegian Journal of Epidemiology* 22(2): 243–251.

Hutt, E., Pepper, G. A., Vojir, C., Fink, R., and Jones, K. R. (2006). 'Assessing the Appropriateness of Pain Medication Prescribing Practices in Nursing Homes'. *Journal of the American Geriatrics Society* 54(2): 231–239. doi:10.1111/j.1532-5415.2005.00582.x.

Ito, G. and Kanemoto, K. (2013). 'A Case of Topical Opioid-induced Delirium Mistaken as Behavioural and Psychological Symptoms of Dementia in Demented State'. *Psychogeriatrics* 13(2): 118–123. doi:10.1111/psyg.12007.

Jamison, R. N., Schein, J. R., Vallow, S., Ascher, S., Vorsanger, G. J., et al. (2003). 'Neuropsychological Effects of Long-Term Opioid Use in Chronic Pain Patients'. *Journal of Pain and Symptom Management* 26(4): 913–921. doi:10.1016/S0885-3924(03)00310-5.

Jones, K. R., Fink, R., Vojir, C., Pepper, G., Hutt, E., et al. (2004). 'Translation Research in Long-term care: Improving Pain Management in Nursing Homes'. *Worldviews on Evidence-based Nursing* 1(suppl. 1): S13–S20.

Kelly, D. M., Frick, E. M., and Hale, L. S. (2011). 'How the Medication Review Can Help to Reduce Risk of Falls in Older Patients'. *Journal of the American Academy of Physician Assistants* 24(4): 30–34 55. http://www.ncbi.nlm.nih.gov/pubmed/21534380.

Kitwood T. (1997). *Dementia Reconsidered: The Person Comes First*. New York: McGraw-Hill.

Kitwood, T. (2008). 'Towards a Theory of Dementia Care: The Interpersonal Process'. *Ageing and Society* 13(1): 51. doi:10.1017/S0144686X00000647.

Kovach, C. R. (2000). 'Sensoristasis and Imbalance in Persons with Dementia'. *Journal of Nursing Scholarship* 32: 379–384.

Kovach, C. R. and Schlidt, A. M. (2001). 'The Activity-agitation Interface of People with Dementia in Long-term Care'. *Journal of Alzheimer's Disease* 16: 1–7.

Kovach, C. R. and Wells, T. (2002). 'Pacing of Activity as a Predictor of Agitation for People with Dementia in Acute Care'. *Journal of Gerontological Nursing* 28: 28–35.

Kovach, C. R., Taneli, Y., Dohearty, P., Schlidt, A. M., Cashin, S., et al. (2004). 'Effect of the BACE Intervention on Agitation of People with Dementia'. *Gerontologist* 44(6): 797–806. http://www.ncbi.nlm.nih.gov/pubmed/15611216.

Kovach, C. R., Logan, B. R., Noonan, P. E., Schlidt, A. M., Smerz, J., et al. (2006a). 'Effects of the Serial Trial Intervention on Discomfort and Behavior of Nursing Home Residents With Dementia'. *American Journal of Alzheimer's Disease and Other Dementias* 21(3): 147–155. doi:10.1177/1533317506288949.

Kovach, C. R., Cashin, J. R., and Sauer, L. (2006b). "Deconstruction of a Complex Tailored Intervention to Assess and Treat Discomfort of People with Advanced Dementia'. *Journal of Advanced Nursing* 55(6): 678–688. doi:10.1111/j.1365-2648.2006.03968.x

Kovach, C. R., Logan, B. R., Simpson, M. R., and Reynolds, S. (2010). 'Factors Associated with Time to Identify Physical Problems of Nursing Home Residents with Dementia'. *American Journal of Alzheimer's Disease and Other Dementias* 25(4): 317–323. doi:10.1177/1533317510363471.

Kunik, M. E., Lees, E., Snow, A. L., Cody, M., Rapp, C. G., et al. (2003). 'Disruptive Behavior in Dementia: A Qualitative Study to Promote Understanding and Improve Treatment'. *Alzheimer's Care Quarterly* 2(4): 125–136.

Langballe, E. M., Engdahl, B., Selbaek, G., and Nordeng, H. (2011). 'Concomitant Use of Anti-dementia Drugs with Psychotropic Drugs in Norway: A Population-based Study'. *Pharmacoepidemiology and Drug Safety* 20(12): 1319–1326. doi:10.1002/pds.2211.

Lavsa, S. M., Fabian, T. J., Saul, M. I., Corman, S. L., and Coley, K. C. (2010). 'Influence of Medications and Diagnoses on Fall Risk in Psychiatric Inpatients'. *American Journal of Health-system Pharmacy* 67(15): 1274–1280. doi:10.2146/ajhp090611.

Lawrence, V., Fossey, J., Ballard, C., Moniz-Cook, E., and Murray, J. (2012). 'Improving Quality of Life for People with Dementia in Care Homes: Making Psychosocial Interventions Work'. *British Journal of Psychiatry* 201(5): 344–351. doi:10.1192/bjp.bp.111.101402.

Lawton, M. P. (1986). *Environment and Aging*. Albany, NY: Center for the Study of Aging.

Lawton, M. P., Van Haitsma, K., and Klapper, J. (1994). 'A Balanced Stimulation and Retreat Program for a Special Care Dementia Unit'. *Alzheimer Disease and Associated Disorders* 8(suppl. 1): S133–S138.

Lee, M. M., Camp, C. J., and Malone, M. L. (2007). 'Effects of Intergenerational Montessori-based Activities Programming on Engagement of Nursing Home Residents with Dementia'. *Clinical Interventions in Aging* 2(3): 477–83.

Lin, R. Y., Heacock, L. C., and Fogel, J. F. (2010). 'Drug-induced, Dementia-associated and Non-dementia, Non-drug Delirium Hospitalizations in the United States 1998–2005: An Analysis of The National Inpatient Sample'. *Drugs and Aging* 27(1): 51–61. doi:10.2165/11531060-000000000-00000.

Lee, M. M., Camp, C. J., and Malone, M. L. (2007). 'Effects of Intergenerational Montessori-based Activities Programming on Engagement of Nursing Home Residents with Dementia'. *Clinical Interventions in Aging* 2(3): 477–483. http://www.pubmedcentral.nih.gov/articlerender.fcgi?artid=2685273andtool=pmcentrezandrendertype=abstract.

McConigley, R., Toye, C., Goucke, R., and Kristjanson, L. J. (2008). 'Developing Recommendations for Implementing the Australian Pain Society's Pain Management Strategies in Residential Aged Care'. *Australasian Journal on Ageing* 27(1): 45–49. doi:10.1111/j.1741-6612.2007.00266.x.

Manfredi, P. L., Breuer, B., Wallenstein, S., Stegmann, M., Bottomley, G., et al. (2003). 'Opioid Treatment for Agitation in Patients with Advanced Dementia'. *International Journal of Geriatric Psychiatry* 18(8): 700–705. doi:10.1002/gps.906.

Maslow, A. H. (1943). 'A Theory of Human Motivation'. *Psychological Review* 50: 370–396.

Maslow, A. H. (1968). *Toward a Psychology of Being*. New York: D. Van Nostrand Co.

Maslow, A. H. (1987). *Motivation and Personality* (3rd edn). New York: Harper and Row.

Mast, B. (2011). *Whole Person Dementia Assessment*. Baltimore, MD: Health Professions Press.

Meeks, S., Looney, S. W., Van Haitsma, K., and Teri, L. (2008). 'BE-ACTIV: A Staff-assisted Behavioral Intervention for Depression in Nursing Homes'. *Gerontologist* 48:105–114.

Miller, M., Stürmer, T., Azrael, D., Levin, R., and Solomon, D. H. (2011). 'Opioid Analgesics and the Risk of Fractures in Older Adults with Arthritis'. *Journal of the American Geriatrics Society* 59(3): 430–438. doi:10.1111/j.1532-5415.2011.03318.x.

Mitchell, C. (2001). 'Assessment and Management of Chronic Pain in Elderly People'. *British Journal of Nursing* 10(5): 296–304. http://www.ncbi.nlm.nih.gov/pubmed/12170672.

Mittal, D., Torres, R., Abashidze, A., and Jimerson, N. (2001). 'Worsening of Post-traumatic Stress Disorder Symptoms with Cognitive Decline: Case Series'. *Journal of Geriatric Psychiatry and Neurology* 14(1): 17–20. http://www.ncbi.nlm.nih.gov/pubmed/11281311.

Morone, N. E. and Greco, C. M. (2007). 'Mind-body Interventions for Chronic Pain in Older Adults: A Structured Review'. *Pain Medicine* 8(4): 359–375. doi:10.1111/j.1526-4637.2007.00312.x.

Morrison, R. S. and Siu, A. L. (2000). 'A Comparison of Pain and its Treatment in Advanced Dementia and Cognitively Intact Patients with Hip Fracture'. *Journal of Pain and Symptom Management* 19(4): 240–248. http://www.ncbi.nlm.nih.gov/pubmed/10799790.

National Opioid Use Guideline Group (2010). *Canadian Guideline for Safe and Effective Use of Opioids for Chronic Non-Cancer Pain: Part B—Recommendations for Practice*. Hamilton, ON: National Opioid Use Guideline Group.

Opie, J., Doyle, C., and Connor, D. W. O. (2002). 'Challenging Behaviours in Nursing Home Residents with Dementia: A Randomized Controlled Trial of Multidisciplinary Interventions'. *International Journal of Geriatric Psychiatry* 17(1): 6–13. doi:10.1002/gps.493

Petre, B. M., Roxbury, C. R., McCallum, J. R., Defontes, K. W., Belkoff, S. M., et al. (2012). 'Pain Reporting, Opiate Dosing, and the Adverse Effects of Opiates after Hip or Knee Replacement in Patients 60 Years Old or Older'. *Geriatric Orthopaedic Surgery and Rehabilitation* 3(1): 3–7. doi:10.1177/2151458511432758.

Pickering, G., Jourdan, D., and Dubray, C. (2006). 'Acute versus Chronic Pain Treatment in Alzheimer's Disease'. *European Journal of Pain* 10(4): 379–84. doi:10.1016/j.ejpain.2005.06.010.

Power, G. A. (2010). *Dementia Beyond Drugs: Changing the Culture of Care*. Baltimore, MD: Health Professions Press.

Resnick, B., Quinn, C., and Baxter, S. (2004). 'Testing the Feasibility of Implementation of Clinical Practice Guidelines in Long-term Care Facilities'. *Journal of the American Medical Directors Association* 5: 1–8.

Reynolds, K. S., Hanson, L. C., Devellis, R. F., Henderson, M., and Steinhauser, K. E. (2008). 'Disparities in Pain Management Between Cognitively Intact and Cognitively Impaired Nursing Home Residents'. *Journal of Pain and Symptom Management* 35(4): 388–396. doi:10.1016/j.jpainsymman.2008.01.001.

Royal College of Physicians, British Geriatrics Society and British Pain Society (2007). *The Assessment of Pain in Older People: National Guidelines. Concise Guidance to Good Practice Series, No 8*. London: RCP.

Schreier, A. M. (2010). 'Nursing Care, Delirium, And Pain Management for the Hospitalized Older Adult'. *Pain Management Nursing* 11(3): 177–185. doi:10.1016/j.pmn.2009.07.002.

Sieber, F. E., Mears, S., Lee, H., and Gottschalk, A. (2011). 'Postoperative Opioid Consumption and its Relationship to Cognitive Function in Older Adults with Hip Fracture'. *Journal of the American Geriatrics Society* 59(12): 2256–2262. doi:10.1111/j.1532-5415.2011.03729.x.

Skrajner, M. J. and Camp, C. J. (2007). 'Resident-Assisted Montessori Programming (RAMP): Use of a Small Group Reading Activity Run by Persons with Dementia in Adult

Day Health Care and Long-term Care Settings'. *American Journal of Alzheimer's Disease and Other Dementias* 22(1): 27–36. http://www.ncbi.nlm.nih.gov/pubmed/17533999.

Snow, A. L., O'Malley, K. J., Cody, M., Kunik, M. E., Ashton, C. M., et al. (2004). 'A Conceptual Model of Pain Assessment for Noncommunicative Persons with Dementia'. *Gerontologist* 44(6): 807–817. http://www.ncbi.nlm.nih.gov/pubmed/15611217.

Snow, A. L., Powers D., and Liles, D. (2006). 'Cognitive-Behavioral Therapy for Long-Term Care Patients with Dementia'. In L. Hyer and R. Intrieri (eds), *Clinical Applied Gerontological Interventions in Long-term Care* (pp. 265–293). New York: Springer.

Stevenson, K. M., Dahl, J. L., Berry, P. H., Beck, S. L., and Griffie, J. (2006). 'Institutionalizing Effective Pain Management Practices: Practice Change Programs to Improve the Quality of pain Management in Small Health Care Organizations'. *Journal of Pain and Symptom Management* 31: 248–261.

Swafford, K. L., Miller, L. L., Tsai, P.-F., Herr, K. A., and Ersek, M. (2009). 'Improving the Process of Pain Care in Nursing Homes: A Literature Synthesis'. *Journal of the American Geriatrics Society* 57(6): 1080–1087. doi:10.1111/j.1532-5415.2009.02274.x.

Takai, Y., Yamamoto-Mitani, N., Okamoto, Y., Koyama, K., and Honda, A. (2010). 'Literature Review of Pain Prevalence among Older Residents of Nursing Homes'. *Pain Management Nursing* 11(4): 209–223. doi:10.1016/j.pmn.2010.08.006.

Titler, M. G., Herr, K., Brooks, J. M., Xie, X.-J., Ardery, G., et al. (2009). 'Translating Research into Practice Intervention Improves Management of Acute Pain in Older Hip Fracture Patients'. *Health Services Research* 44(1): 264–287. doi:10.1111/j.1475-6773.2008.00913.x,

Weiner, D. K. and Hanlon, J. T. (2001). 'Pain in Nursing Home Residents: Management Strategies'. *Drugs and Aging* 18(1): 13–29. http://www.ncbi.nlm.nih.gov/pubmed/11232736.

Weissman, D. E., Griffie, J, Muchka, S., et al. (2000). 'Building an Institutional Commitment to Pain Management in Long-term Care Facilities'. *Journal of Pain and Symptom Management* 20: 35–43.

Wolff, M. L. (2012). 'Case report: Post-traumatic Memories Triggered by Donepezil in a Dose-dependent Pattern'. *American Journal of Geriatric Pharmacotherapy* 10(3): 219–222. doi:10.1016/j.amjopharm.2012.03.001.

Wolff, M. L., Kewley, R., Hassett, M., Collins, J., Brodeur, M. R., et al. (2012). 'Falls in Skilled Nursing Facilities Associated with Opioid Use'. *Journal of the American Geriatrics Society* 60(5): 987. doi:10.1111/j.1532-5415.2012.03913.x.

World Health Organization (1996). *Cancer Pain Relief with a Guide to Opioid Availability* (2nd edn). Geneva: World Health Organization.

World Health Organization (2009). 'WHO's Pain Relief Ladder'. http://www.who.int/cancer/palliative/painladder/en/.

Won, A., Lapane, K. L., Vallow, S., Schein, J., Morris, J. N., et al. (2006). 'Long-term Effects of Analgesics in a Population of Elderly Nursing Home Residents with Persistent Nonmalignant Pain'. *Journals of Gerontology, Series A: Biological Sciences and Medical Sciences* 61(2): 165–169.

PART V

NEW HORIZONS

CHAPTER 43

PSYCHOLOGICAL INTERVENTIONS IN NON-MENTAL HEALTH SETTINGS

MARIA E. A. ARMENTO AND
MELINDA A. STANLEY

INTRODUCTION

MOOD and anxiety disorders are the two most prevalent groups of mental disorders treated in primary care (Ansseau et al. 2004; Kroenke et al. 2007). Prevalence estimates among older adults range from 3–11.9% for mood disorders and from 7.6–15.3% for anxiety disorders (Beattie, Pachana, and Franklin 2010; Byers et al. 2010; Kessler et al. 2005).

When seeking treatment, older adults generally present to a non-mental health medical care setting (Blazer, Geroge, and Hughes 1991; Wittchen et al. 2002), most often their primary care clinic, making diagnosis and treatment in this setting important. In primary care in the US, for example, the most prevalent mood and pervasive anxiety disorders in late life are Major Depressive Disorder (MDD) and Generalized Anxiety Disorder (GAD) (Kroenke et al. 2007; Stanley et al. 2003). However, only a minority of patients with anxiety or depression (15–36%) are recognized in this setting; and most of these patients go untreated (Kroenke et al. 2007). Older adults with mood and/or anxiety disorders are two to three times less likely to seek treatment than their middle-aged counterparts (Mackenzie et al. 2011); and when they do seek treatment, they often present with symptoms that overlap with coexistent medical disorders, making diagnosis difficult (Byers et al. 2010; Stanley et al. 2003). Other age-related factors such as differences in emotional expression and symptomology, high rates of depression and anxiety comorbidity, and treatment stigma may also contribute to the lack of treatment use in up to 70% of community-dwelling older adults with mood and anxiety disorders (Byers, Areán, and Yaffe 2012; Byers et al. 2010; Kroenke et al. 2007; Wolitzky-Taylor et al. 2010).

Mood and anxiety disorders in older adults are generally treated with pharmacotherapy, individual psychotherapy, or a combination of the two (see 'Interventions' below). Although medication for anxiety and depression may be useful, any positive gains must be weighed against risks for older adults taking psychotropic medications (Pinquart and

Duberstein 2007). A recent meta-analytic review (Pinquart, Duberstein, and Lyness 2006) reported comparable effect sizes for psychotherapy and pharmacotherapy targeting major depression among older adults. Older people with dysthymia or subthreshold symptoms, however, were more likely to benefit from psychotherapy than from medication. Pharmacological and psychotherapeutic interventions for anxiety are also both effective, with review studies suggesting equivalent effects relative to control conditions (Gonçalves and Byrne 2012; Pinquart and Duberstein 2007), and studies targeting older adults with panic disorder and/or mixed groups of anxiety disorders suggesting preferential outcomes following pharmacotherapy (Hendriks et al. 2010; Schuurmans et al. 2009). Research points to four evidence-based psychotherapeutic interventions for anxiety in older adults: cognitive-behaviour therapy (CBT), cognitive therapy, relaxation training, and supportive therapy (Ayers et al. 2007). Several psychotherapies also are effective with older adults with depression: CBT, interpersonal psychotherapy, problem-solving therapy, and brief psychodynamic psychotherapy (Ellison, Kyomen, and Harper 2012).

Since the preponderance of outcome data has been collected in academic mental health clinics despite the small number of patients who actually seek treatment in these settings, there is a need to focus on treatment delivery and outcomes in non-mental health settings, where the most frequent patient visits take place. Better understanding of diagnosis and treatment in these settings may help advance reach and accessibility of treatment, as well as patient engagement for the older-adult community.

BROADENING TREATMENT BEYOND THE TRADITIONAL MENTAL HEALTH SETTING

A number of studies have begun to look at the effectiveness of treatment for late-life depression and anxiety in non-mental health settings where older adults receive services, in particular primary care and community-based service settings. Most of this work has focused on depression, but recent studies have begun to address the treatment of anxiety and comorbid mental and physical illnesses in non-mental health settings.

Primary care-based treatments

Primary care has been the most common setting in which older adults are screened and treated for depression and anxiety (Gitlin et al. 2012; Stanley et al. 2003). However, numerous barriers exist to proper diagnosis and treatment in these settings, including patient concern about stigma, discomfort talking about personal problems with a healthcare provider, and lack of treatment engagement. These barriers are especially problematic for racial-ethnic minority groups, who tend more than majority populations to be under-diagnosed in primary care, under-represented in clinical trials, and inadequately treated (Areán et al. 2003; Byers et al. 2012; Cooper et al. 2003).

Models have been developed for integrating mental healthcare into primary care in real-world practice throughout the world. A number of countries, including Australia,

Brazil, South Africa, and the UK, have developed models for integrating mental health-care into primary care. Australia and Brazil have integrated care with consultation from mental health specialists as needed, South Africa has several working models for integration, and the UK has a holistic care model to conceptualize integration (WHO-Wonca 2008). In the US, integration includes collaborative care, care management, and blended models (Zeiss and Karlin 2008). Each model relies on a continuum of care providers. Collaborative care generally includes a mental health provider (e.g. psychologist or social worker) who actively works on issues of patient care with other medical providers. Care management involves 'care managers' (e.g. registered nurses with mental health training), who may assess and provide regular follow-up for patients referred by primary care physicians. The Depression Care Model, in particular, includes a care manager that uses a systematic team approach grounded in a chronic disease care model (Snowden, Steinman, and Frederick 2008). The blended model generally involves a combination of both collaborative care and care management, including early access to mental health providers and regular patient follow-up (Jameson and Cully 2011). Several interventions, including those tested in the PROSPECT (Bruce et al. 2004) and IMPACT (Unützer et al. 2002) trials, have investigated use of these care models. The PROSPECT intervention consists of two core components: a clinical algorithm used to increase physician knowledge, and care management by depression care managers. The algorithm initially suggests a trial of a selective serotonin reuptake inhibitor. If the patient declines the selective serotonin reuptake inhibitor, the physician then recommends interpersonal psychotherapy with a care manager. Care managers, including social workers, nurses, and psychologists, provided physicians with recommendations for treatment, clinical monitoring, and follow-up, but, ultimately, the responsibility for clinical care remained with the physician. Care managers received regular supervision from psychiatrists and met in person or on the phone with patients at scheduled intervals and other times as clinically warranted (Alexopoulos et al. 2005; Bruce et al. 2004). In the IMPACT model, care managers and primary care physicians worked together to create and implement treatment. Patients were initially provided educational materials, including a videotape and booklet about depression, and offered a chance to meet with a depression clinical specialist (DCS). The DCS (nurse or psychologist care managers trained for the study) conducted clinical histories and discussed patient preferences for treatment. The DCS worked with the primary care provider and the patient to establish a treatment plan matching a treatment algorithm (generally, a choice of anti-depressant medication or problem-solving therapy), but, ultimately, care choice was up to the patient and his/her physician. The DCS also provided follow-up to patients and consulted with psychiatrists about patients who did not improve. Results from both the PROSPECT and IMPACT trials illustrated the utility of these care models that were superior to usual care for older primary care patients suffering with depressive symptoms.

The first large randomized controlled trial (RCT) of late-life anxiety treatment in primary care examined the effects of CBT relative to enhanced usual care (EUC) for GAD (Stanley et al. 2009). CBT consisted of ten individual sessions in which patients learned skills (e.g. cognitive therapy, relaxation training, sleep management, exposure, and problem-solving), followed by four brief telephone booster sessions every three months over one year. Patients in EUC received bi-weekly calls for three months, which provided support and assessed for safety issues. Compared with EUC, patients treated with CBT reported more improvement in worry severity, depressive symptoms, sleep disturbance, and general mental health (Bush et al. 2012; Stanley et al. 2009). Gains were maintained or improved over one-year follow-up.

In the move to investigate treatment outcomes in non-mental health settings, research in mental healthcare has shifted from efficacy to effectiveness trials and, more recently, to hybrid trials that also consider implementation (Cully et al. 2012; Curran et al. 2012). Although some evidence-based interventions for depression in primary care have been widely replicated (http://impact-uw.org), many intervention trials have used delivery models that do not translate smoothly into real-world care (Stanley et al. 2009) because of the use of expert providers, relatively long and frequent sessions, and academic clinic settings. Translating treatment models into real-world care is difficult not only in the US but also in other countries throughout Europe and elsewhere, where widespread implementation of these models may be hindered by lack of infrastructure, dearth of trained personnel, lack of consensus in practice, and, in the US in particular, Medicare payment policies (Ell 2006; Karel, Gatz, and Smyer 2012; Muijen 2012; Snowden et al. 2008). These difficulties may be even greater in countries with underdeveloped mental health services.

Recent primary care work in late-life anxiety in the US has begun to address real-world practice concerns by training non-expert providers to deliver care, incorporating telephone-based care to reduce barriers, and using electronic medical records to identify patients and communicate with providers (Brenes, Ingram, and Danhauer 2011; Calleo et al. 2013; Stanley et al. 2014). Innovative developments with respect to primary care 'real-world' delivery are also occurring in other parts of the world, particularly to serve more geographically isolated populations. For example, one-third of Australia's population lives in non-metropolitan areas (Australian Institute of Health and Welfare 2005); of this population, nearly 20% reside in rural and remote communities with fewer than 5000 residents. Many such communities are composed of a largely indigenous population. Innovative models of primary care in such communities tend to strive for comprehensive and integrated service delivery. The Aboriginal Community Controlled Health Service model has been well studied and generally viewed as a successful example of such a model, emphasizing improved health outcomes by addressing underlying social determinants of health (e.g. Robinson et al. 2003). Here primary care is integrated with preventative and health promotion activity, as well as governance and community capacity building, working with key Aboriginal community stakeholders.

A more complex constellation of symptoms occurs when older adults present with comorbid physical and mental health concerns. Novel treatments are being developed to address concurrently the management of chronic illness and anxiety/depressive symptoms. Studies in this domain have looked at treatment programmes for depression and anxiety targeting patients with comorbid arthritis, diabetes, gastrointestinal disorders, and heart and lung diseases (Blanchard et al. 1992; Gellis, Kenaley, and Ten Have 2014; Huffman et al. 2014; Kunik et al. 2008; Lustman et al. 1998; Sharpe et al. 2001).

In general, there is modest support for the effectiveness of psychotherapy for depression and anxiety comorbid with chronic physical illness; but few psychological interventions have been accepted and adopted in medical care settings (Jameson and Cully 2011). CBT is widely accepted in mental health contexts and is beginning to be used more frequently in non-mental health settings (Roy-Byrne et al. 2010; Stanley et al. 2009, 2014; Wetherell et al. 2011). CBT-based treatments for depression and/or anxiety for patients with chronic obstructive pulmonary disease (COPD), arthritis, diabetes mellitus, and Parkinson's disease have demonstrated decreases in depression (Armento et al. 2012; Dobkin et al. 2011; Kunik et al. 2008; Lin et al. 2003; Lustman et al. 1998; Sharpe et al. 2001; Williams et al. 2004), decreased anxiety, and increased quality of life (Kunik et al. 2008). Some improvement in physical functioning has also been reported; for example, improvement in disease marker CRP (C-reactive protein—aids in evaluating severity) for arthritis (Sharpe et al. 2001), decreased pain and improved functional status (Lin et al. 2003), and improved glycaemic control for patients with diabetes (Lustman et al. 1998). Unfortunately, implementation of these treatments still involves limitations. Educational interventions to change clinical practice require a multilevel approach to address barriers that arise in the care setting (Sullivan, Blevins, and Kauth 2008), and external facilitation at all levels (facility, clinic, clinician) remains critical. Research continues to examine outcomes of facilitation efforts and potential implementation barriers, including time, communication, and cost (Kauth et al. 2010).

Community-based treatments

Older community-dwelling adults generally do not receive mental healthcare in equal proportion to need, and this reflects a global phenomenon. For example, US epidemiological data suggest that approximately 70% of respondents meeting diagnostic criteria for MDD and 72% of those meeting criteria for an anxiety disorder in the past year had not received care in the past twelve months (Garrido et al. 2011). In a small study in the Netherlands using data from the second Dutch National Survey of General Practice (Volkers et al. 2004), only just over 20% of patients aged over 55 with a diagnosis of major depression in the last twelve months were classified as depressed by their GP, with 32% of the patients with major depression classified as having a psychological problem other than depression and 13% as having 'social problems'. The authors stressed the continuing need for clinical education and guideline implementation in primary care settings and the need for GPs to be able correctly to differentiate depression from other psychiatric conditions, as well as social issues in later life. Attitudes related to mental healthcare, including low symptom severity self-perception, desire to resolve difficulties independently, and fear about treatment, appeared to delay or cause them to avoid seeking treatment. Attitudes of mental health providers may also be a barrier in the US (Montano 1999) and other countries (Burroughs et al. 2006; Koder and Ferguson 1998).

In the US, access to mental health services is generally even lower among minority older adults (Agency for Healthcare Research and Quality 2009), who are less likely to be identified and receive or use mental health services (Brenes et al. 2008; Joo et al. 2010). African Americans, in particular, consistently receive poorer-quality depression care than white patients because of barriers at the patient (e.g. stigma), environment (e.g. geography, transportation), provider (e.g. lack of training), and system levels (e.g. lack of care coordination) (Gitlin et al. 2012). In other countries, access may be limited by geography, transportation, stigma, cost, and coordination of care (Mucic 2011; Kronfol 2012; Woodward and Pachana 2009).

Community-based treatments may increase accessibility and utilization of treatment in older adults. Several studies have tested psychosocial interventions and collaborative care in community settings, including community-based service agencies, faith-based organizations, and patient homes, to facilitate provision of mental healthcare in more comfortable and 'preferable' locations (Casado et al. 2008; Ciechanowski et al. 2004; Frederick et al. 2007; Gitlin et al. 2012; Shrestha et al. 2012), thereby increasing accessibility and reach.

Studies of psychosocial and collaborative-care, community-based treatments for depression in older adults have produced positive results (Areán et al. 2010; Frederick et al. 2007; Steinman et al. 2007). For example, Healthy IDEAS (Quijano et al. 2007), an intervention that integrates depression identification, linkage referral, and behavioural activation and is delivered by non-specialty providers (case managers), has been implemented successfully in several community-based social service organizations. Another community-based programme, PEARLS (Ciechanowski et al. 2004), provides in-home problem-solving treatment for older adults and has led to a significant reduction in depressive symptoms and improved health status in older adults also suffering from comorbid chronic illness. Other groups have emphasized the important role of case management in community-delivered depression interventions (Areán et al. 2005; Miranda et al. 2006). Gitlin et al. (2012, 2014) tested a community-integrated, home-based depression intervention in the US for older African Americans (Beat the Blues) in a randomized trial. Outcomes demonstrated improvement in depression, anxiety, and quality of life relative to a wait-list control.

Treatments for anxiety in older adults are less well developed but have integrated content and delivery options to meet personal client needs. Individualized, modular treatment for anxiety used in community settings is flexible, allowing patients to choose what kinds of skills they learn, how many sessions of treatment to receive, and whether to incorporate telephone sessions and cultural adaptations, including optional integration of religious/spiritual beliefs into therapy. Modular-based treatments for late-life anxiety have positive preliminary outcomes (Calleo et al. 2013; Shrestha et al. 2012; Wetherell et al. 2009).

Developing community partnerships

An important part of bringing mental healthcare into primary care or a community setting is developing partnerships. Many primary care physicians experience barriers in treating older adults with mental health concerns, including lack of time and referral sources (Van Etten 2006). Integration of mental health treatment into the primary care setting can provide physicians with a direct referral source for their patients. Development of a relationship with positive rapport between mental health providers, other healthcare providers, and clinic administrative staff is important (Stanley et al. 2003).

Building partnerships in the community also involves building positive rapport, but it is necessary to consider other unique issues in community settings. The Clinical and Translational Science Award (CTSA) Consortium's Community Engagement Key Function Committee and CTSA Community Engagement Workshop Planning Committee (2008) provide a comprehensive summary of best practices in community engagement, including how to interact with partners, successfully customize clinical care in a way that works for the community, and integrate community involvement into decision-making.

Dobransky-Fasiska et al. (2009) developed a community-based partnership to facilitate treatment of depression in under-served populations and identified six stages of building a community partnership: collaborating to secure funding, building a communications platform, fostering enduring relationships, assessing needs, initiating specific collaborative projects, and maintaining a 'sustainable and productive partnership'. The Calmer Life Program (CL Program; Jameson et al. 2012; Shrestha et al. 2012) provides another example of building an effective community partnership in the process of providing community-based anxiety treatment to older adults. The CL Program is anchored in an academic-community partnership with faith-based and social service agency leaders, who provided guidance in the development of a treatment approach, participant referral, and community outreach.

IMPLICATIONS FOR PRACTICE

Once partnerships are developed within a non-mental healthcare setting, a number of important barriers still impact practice. Among primary care patients, nearly 60% report at least one barrier to psychotherapy that is significant enough to make treatment very difficult to impossible (Mohr et al. 2006). Given current data suggesting that nearly three-quarters of community-dwelling older adults who need mental health treatment do not receive care (Garrido et al. 2011), barriers to mental healthcare in non-traditional settings are an important concern for mental health practice.

Practical barriers patients may encounter include lack of time (convenience/accessibility), lack of transportation, or other financial issues; while personal barriers may include low perceived need of mental health services or having to deal with comorbid physical conditions (Brown et al. 2010; Jameson and Cully 2011; Karlin, Duffy, and Gleaves 2008; Unützer et al. 1999; Van Etten 2006; Woodall et al. 2010; Woodward and Pachana 2009).

Practical barriers appear to be easier to overcome than personal barriers (Woodall et al. 2010). Non-mental healthcare settings are ideal for addressing these kinds of barriers by allowing flexibility in treatment, including in-person meetings in settings where patients already come for services, creating a less fragmented treatment-delivery system, telephone delivery options, and treatments tailored to fit a patient's schedule. The following case example illustrates effective resolution of practical barriers in a non-mental healthcare setting.

> Ms S (60 years old) had difficulty with mobility due to increased symptoms of multiple sclerosis. She had become concerned about her financial future and her ability to care for herself and reported feeling 'down and blue'. She saw a brochure in her doctor's office about a treatment for anxiety and/or depression in older adults. When she called to inquire about the programme, she mentioned her mobility issues and was informed that a staff member could set up a meeting in her home or doctor's office, and that telephone sessions would also be an option. Ms S was happy to have the opportunity to participate in a programme from which she would otherwise not have been able to benefit.

Personal barriers to treatment are more complex to resolve. Issues such as low perceived need of care and comorbid chronic illness can complicate receipt of mental health treatment. Older adults are as likely as younger adults to seek treatment for serious mental health concerns (e.g. schizophrenia symptoms, suicidal ideation) but not as likely to seek treatment for less severe symptomology such as anxiety and depression (Robb et al. 2003). Lack of treatment for even subthreshold symptoms of anxiety and depression is related to other difficulties in older adults, including cognitive and physical health decline (Ellison et al. 2012; Grenier et al. 2011; Pietrzak et al. 2012), making adequate care for all mental health concerns important. Chronic physical illness can also interfere with receipt of mental healthcare in older adults because of a focus on physical rather than mental illness, limited resources, and overlap of symptomatology, leading to difficulties in both initial diagnosis and further treatment of anxiety and depression. Once they begin receiving care, these patients require some kind of integration of care to ensure that both mental and physical healthcare needs will be met (Jameson and Cully 2011). The following are two case examples illustrating how personal barriers to care were overcome in a non-mental health setting, illustrating how even complex difficulties may be overcome through flexibility and accessibility of treatment:

> Ms R (67) had become increasingly anxious over the last several years. Three years after her husband passed away, finances became extremely tight. Then one year ago, Ms R's daughter and three-year-old grandson moved in with her and she quickly became the main care-giver for her grandson. Ms R was also worried about her health, as the stress in her life led to significant decline in her physical well-being. Ms R was an active member of her church and had heard a guest speaker talking about a treatment programme for anxious older adults. She wanted to participate, but she was concerned about spending time in the programme since her symptoms 'are not that bad'. Ms R was concerned about taking away even more time from caring for her grandson for her own doctor appointments and felt she should just 'try to handle this myself'. Her friends encouraged her to contact a staff member from the programme for more information. The staff member discussed barriers with Ms R about receiving treatment and let Ms R know that the schedule of treatment could be flexible and delivery could be in person or on the phone. Ms R was also informed that she could do as many or as few sessions as she chose and that treatment would be tailored to her needs. Given this flexibility, Ms R decided that she would be able to participate and receive important care for herself while still fulfilling other important life obligations.
>
> Mr H was diagnosed with COPD and had many questions and concerns for his doctors. About one year after diagnosis, his anxiety and depressive symptoms became noticeable and began interfering with his quality of life. Mr H expressed his negative emotions to his doctor and told him that these symptoms, combined with his struggle with COPD, were keeping him from being able to enjoy life the way he used to. His doctor suggested he participate in a programme being offered in the clinic for older adults with depression and/or anxiety. Mr H called the treatment team to get more information about the programme. He expressed his concern about finding someone who would understand how his physical health affected his feelings of anxiety and depression, and concern about his trouble separating out his experiences. The staff member from the treatment team talked with Mr H about the interconnectedness of physical and mental health. Mr H was informed that his treatment would take into account his COPD diagnosis, in regard to a meeting schedule conducive to his COPD healthcare and through communication with his primary care physician and structured skill-building focused on relief of anxiety and depression symptoms, his physical health condition and overall quality of life. Mr H was very happy to be involved in a programme that respected his unique condition, combined consideration of physical and mental health issues, and provided care within the same system through which he was receiving his other medical care.

Future Directions

Providing access to mental healthcare in non-traditional settings may provide some older adults increased access to treatment. Because depression and anxiety in older adults are associated with other healthcare risks (e.g. cognitive decline and vascular disease), it is important to approach treatment of these mental health concerns when trying to modify overall quality of life for this age group (Ellison et al. 2012; Pietrzak et al. 2012). Even subthreshold anxiety is related to significant physical health difficulties in older adults (Grenier et al. 2011; Stillman et al. 2011), pointing to the importance of early diagnosis and treatment availability and flexibility to meet the needs of older-adult clients. There are a number of potential future directions for treatment of anxiety and depression in non-mental health settings. The following are two important future areas of growth for care: implementation of prevention efforts and utilization of technology in delivery of services.

Developing and implementing prevention efforts is an important future direction for research and clinical care. Prevention of mental health symptoms can be thought of as 'pre-emptive' and 'protective' (Reynolds 2009) and could lead to decreases in the significant economic burden associated with mental healthcare for older adults (Vasiliadis et al. 2012). Community-dwelling older adults with depression/anxiety have significantly higher healthcare costs (Vasiliadis et al. 2012), with ambulatory costs up to 52% higher for depressed older adults (Katon et al. 2003). Psychotherapy-based interventions with older adults have the potential to decrease incidence and remission rates of depression (Lee et al. 2012), and the possibility of screening for subthreshold symptoms of anxiety (Grenier et al. 2011) may provide an opportunity for early treatment, contributing to increased overall quality of life while decreasing national mental health expenditure. Preventive techniques for older adults may include loosening inclusion criteria, developing partnerships to serve those who most need public health services, using outcomes beyond symptom ratings, instituting longer follow-up periods, and using a modular-based approach to treatment.

Another potential future direction for mental health treatment in older adults is telemental healthcare and incorporation of technology in treatment. Although there are various approaches and methods to telemental health and internet-based psychotherapeutic treatment, the literature shows a generally positive trend for effectiveness (Barak et al. 2008; Brenes et al. 2011).

Telemental health can increase reach of treatment for patients who may otherwise have difficulty accessing services by providing mental healthcare across geographical distance (Brenes et al. 2011). Telehealth services are in use in a wide range of countries, including Australia, where a research team recently received a grant to develop telehealthcare to residential aged-care facilities (Mucic 2011; UQ News 2012). The American Telemedicine Association (2009) has provided guidelines for best practice in evidence-based telemental health. These guidelines suggest that telehealth, including interactive television, teleconferencing and consultation, and telepsychotherapy, may improve access to treatment for geriatric patients who face barriers related to transportation, cost, and mobility.

Internet-assisted treatment, on the other hand, consists of various internet applications of treatment. Differing amounts of human communication and type of delivery (delayed or real-time) are just two potential areas of variation in internet-assisted treatment (Barak et al. 2008). Internet-based delivery has a number of advantages, including decreased cost, increased reach and access, the availability to personalize treatment through use of complex algorithms, and continuous monitoring of treatment progress. Internet-assisted treatment has improved reach and decreased barriers for mental health treatment among younger adults in both US populations and other countries such as Australia (Bennett et al. 2010; Kaltenthaler and Cavanagh 2010), and participants and providers have embraced it (MacGregor et al. 2009).

Barriers specific to older adults include lack of access and knowledge about technology, as well as sensory and cognitive changes that accompany ageing. These barriers also vary between the developed and the developing world. For example, data from the 2009 US National Health Interview Survey suggest that over half of people age 55 to 64 and 34% of those aged 65 to 74 use the internet to locate general health information (Choi 2011). Technology skills and knowledge in older adults have been increased through e-health literacy programmes in some countries (Xie 2011). Other countries are indirectly facilitating such work, such as Australia's strategic plan to have a national broadband system in place in the near future. Further research in this area may include investigating the usefulness of education and training about technology as part of the treatment programme and ongoing provider contact to facilitate skill use. Interventions will also need to include personalized and culturally sensitive approaches to facilitate use among not only those groups generally using the internet but also among other low-income, disadvantaged groups.

SUMMARY

Mental healthcare in non-traditional settings has the possibility of increasing reach and accessibility of treatment for older adults. Flexibility and the opportunity to meet individual patient needs through modular-based treatment may make treatment more appealing to this age group, creating opportunities for participation in treatment that might not otherwise exist. Continued research is needed to expand this care through continued implementation in primary care and community settings, and, potentially, beyond, through telemental health and internet-based psychotherapy. As this area continues to broaden, so does the possibility of reaching many older adults who are experiencing anxiety and depression, thereby increasing their overall quality of life.

KEY REFERENCES AND SOURCES FOR FURTHER READING

American Telemedicine Association (2009). *Evidence-based Practice for Telemental Health.* http://www.americantelemed.org/practice/standards/ata-standards-guidelines/evidence-based-practice-for-telemental-health.

Jameson, J. P., Shrestha, S., Escamilla, M., Clark, S., Wilson, N., et al. (2012). 'Establishing Community Partnerships to Support Late-life Anxiety Research: Lessons Learned from the Calmer Life Project'. *Aging & Mental Health* 16(7): 874–883.

Shrestha, S., Robertson, S., and Stanley, M. A. (2011). 'Innovations in Research for Treatment of Late-life Anxiety'. *Aging & Mental Health* 15(7): 811–821

WHO-Wonca (2008). *Integrating Mental Health into Primary Care: A Global Perpective.* Geneva and London: WHO and Wonca. http://www.who.int/mental_health/policy/services/mentalhealthintoprimarycare/en/.

REFERENCES

Agency for Healthcare Research and Quality (2009). *National Healthcare Quality and Disparities Reports* (2009). Rockville, MD: Agency for Healthcare Research and Quality. http://www.ahrq.gove/qual/qrdr09.htm.

Alexopoulos, G. S., Katz, I. R., Bruce, M. L., Heo, M., Ten Have, T., et al. (2005). 'Remission in Depressed Geriatric Primary Care Patients: A Report from the PROSPECT Study'. *American Journal of Psychiatry* 162: 718–724.

American Telemedicine Association (2009). *Evidence-based Practice for Telemental Health*. http://www.americantelemed.org/practice/standards/ata-standards-guidelines/evidence-based-practice-for-telemental-health.

Ansseau, M., Dierick, M., Buntinkx, F., Cnockaert, P., De Smedt, J., et al. (2004). 'High Prevalence of Mental Disorders in Primary Care'. *Journal of Affective Disorders* 78: 49–55.

Areán, P. A., Alvidrez, J., Nery, R., Estes, C., and Linkins, K. (2003). 'Recruitment and Retention of Older Minorities in Mental Health Services Research'. *Gerontologist* 43: 36–44.

Areán, P. A., Gum, A., McCulloch, C. E., Bostrom, A., Gallagher-Thompson, D., and Thompson, L. (2005). 'Treatment of Depression in Low-income Older Adults'. *Psychology and Aging* 20: 601–609.

Areán, P. A., Mackin, S., Vargas-Dwyer, E., Raue, P., Sirey, J. A., et al. (2010). 'Treatment of Depression in Disabled Low-income Elderly: A Conceptual Model and Recommendations for Care'. *International Journal of Geriatric Psychiatry* 25: 765–769.

Armento, M. E. A., Stanley, M. A., Marsh, L., Kunik, M. E., York, M., et al. (2012). 'Cognitive Behavioral Therapy (CBT) for Depression and Anxiety in Parkinson's Disease: A Clinical Review'. *Journal of Parkinson's Disease* 2(2): 135–151. doi: 10.3233/JPD-2012–12080.

Australian Institute of Health and Welfare (2005). *Rural, Regional and Remote Health: Indicators of Health*. Catalogue No. PHE 59. Canberra: Australian Institute of Health and Welfare .

Ayers, C. R., Sorrell, J. T., Thorp, S. R., and Wetherell, J. L. (2007). 'Evidence-based Psychological Treatments for Late-life Anxiety'. *Psychology and Aging* 22: 8–17.

Barak, A., Hen, L., Boniel-Nissim, M., and Shapira, N. (2008). 'A Comprehensive Review and a Meta-analysis of the Effectiveness of Internet-based Psychotherapeutic Interventions'. *Journal of Technology in Human Services* 26: 109–159.

Beattie, E., Pachana, N. A., and Franklin, S. J. (2010). 'Double Jeopardy: Comorbid Anxiety and Depression in Late Life'. *Research in Gerontological Nursing* 3: 209–220.

Bennett, K., Reynolds, J., Christensen, H., and Griffiths, K. M. (2010). 'e-hub: An Online Self-help Mental Health Service in the Community'. *Medical Journal of Australia* 192(11): S48–S52.

Blanchard, E. B., Schwarz, S. P., Suls, J. M., Gerardi, M. A., Scharff, L., et al. (1992). 'Two Controlled Evaluations of Multicomponent Psychological Treatment of Irritable Bowel Syndrome'. *Behaviour Research & Therapy* 30: 175–189.

Blazer, D., George, L. K., and Hughes, D. (1991). 'The Epidemiology of Anxiety Disorders: An Age Comparison'. In: C. Salzman and B. D. Lebowitz (eds), *Anxiety in the Elderly: Treatment and Research* (pp. 17–30). New York: Springer.

Brenes, G. A., Knudson, M., McCall, W. V., Williamson, J. D., Miller, M. E., et al. (2008). 'Age and Racial Differences in the Presentation and Treatment of Generalized Anxiety Disorder in Primary Care'. *Journal of Anxiety Disorder* 22: 1128–1136.

Brenes, G. A., Ingram, C. W., and Danhauer, S. C. (2011). 'Benefits and Challenges of Conducting Psychotherapy by Telephone'. *Professional Psychology: Research and Practice* 42: 543–549.

Brown, C., Conner, K. O., Copeland, V. C., Grote, N., Beach, S., et al. (2010). 'Depression Stigma, Race, and Treatment Seeking Behavior and Attitudes'. *Journal of Community Psychology* 38: 350–368.

Bruce, M. L., Ten Have, T. R., Reynolds, C. F., III, Katz, I. I., Schulberg, H. C., et al. (2004). 'Reducing Suicidal Ideation and Depressive Symptoms in Depressed Older Primary Care Patients'. *Journal of the American Medical Association* 291: 1081–1091.

Burroughs, H., Lovell, K., Morley, M,. Baldwin, R., and Burns, A. (2006). '"Justifiable Depression": How Primary Care Professionals and Patients View Late Life Depression? A Qualitative Study'. *Family Practice* 23: 369–377.

Bush, A. L., Kunik, M. E., Novy, D. M., Rhoades, H. M., Weiss, B. J., et al. (2012). 'The Pittsburgh Sleep Quality Index in Older Primary Care Patients with Generalized Anxiety Disorder: Psychometrics and Outcomes Following Cognitive Behavioral Therapy'. *Psychiatry Research* 199(1): 24–30.

Byers, A. L., Yaffe, K., Covinsky, K. E., Friedman, M. B., and Bruce, M. L. (2010). 'High Occurrence of Mood and Anxiety Disorders among Older Adults: The National Comorbidity Survey Replication'. *Archives of General Psychiatry* 67: 489–496.

Byers, A. L., Areán, P. A., and Yaffe, K. (2012). 'Low Use of Mental Health Services among Older Americans with Mood and Anxiety Disorders'. *Psychiatric Services* 63: 66–72.

Calleo, J., Bush, A. L., Cully, J. A., Wilson, N. L., Kraus-Schumann, C., et al. (2013). 'Treating Late-life Generalized Anxiety Disorder in Primary Care: An Effectiveness Pilot Study'. *Journal of Nervous and Mental Disease* 201(5): 414–420.

Casado, B. L., Quijano, L. M., Stanley, M. A., Cully, J. A., Steinberg, E. H., et al. (2008). 'Healthy IDEAS: Implementation of a Depression Program through Community-based Case Management'. *Gerontologist* 48: 828–838.

Choi, N. (2011). 'Relationship between Health Service Use and Health Information Technology Use among Older Adults: Analysis of the US National Health Interview Survey'. *Journal of Medical Internet Research* 13: E33.

Ciechanowski, P., Wagner, E., Schmaling, K., Schwartz, S., Williams, B., et al. (2004). 'Community-integrated Home-based Depression Treatment in Older Adults'. *Journal of the American Medical Association* 291: 1569–1577.

Cooper, L. A., Gonzales, J. J., Gallo, J. J., Rost, K. M., Meredith, L. S., et al. (2003). 'The Acceptability of Treatment for Depression among African-American, Hispanic and White Primary Care Patients'. *Medical Care* 41: 479–489.

CTSA Consortium's Community Engagement Key Function Committee and the CTSA Community Engagement Workshop Planning Committee (2008). *Researchers and Their Communities: The Challenge of Meaningful Community Engagement: A Summary of the Best Practices Emerging from a Series of National and Regional Workshops on Community Engagement.* https://www.dtmi.duke.edu/about-us/organization/duke-center-for-community-research/Researchers%20and%20Their%20Communities.pdf/view.

Cully, J. A., Armento, M. E. A., Mott, J., Nadorff, M. R., Naik, A. D., et al. (2012). 'Brief Cognitive Behavioral Therapy in Primary Care: A Hybrid Type 2 Patient Randomized Effectiveness-implementation Design'. *Implementation Science* 7:64. doi:10.1186/1748-5908-7-64.

Curran, G. M., Bauer, M., Mittman, B., Pyne, J. M., and Stetler, C. (2012). 'Effectiveness-implementation Hybrid Designs: Combining Elements of Clinical Effectiveness and Implementation Research to Enhance Public Health Impact'. *Medical Care* 50: 217–226.

Dobkin, R. D., Menza, M., Allen, L. A., Gara, M. A., Mark, M. H., et al. (2011). Cognitive Behavior Therapy for Depression in Parkinson's Disease: A Randomized Controlled Trial'. *American Journal of Psychiatry* 168(10): 1066–1074.

Dobransky-Fasiska, D., Brown, C., Pincus, H. A., Nowalk, M. P., Wieland, M., et al. (2009). 'Developing a Community-academic Partnership to Improve Recognition and Treatment of Depression in Underserved African American and White Elders'. *American Journal of Geriatric Psychiatry* 17(11): 953–964.

Ell, K. (2006). 'Depression Care for the Elderly: Reducing Barriers to Evidence Based Practice'. *Home Health Care Services Quarterly* 25: 115–148.

Ellison, J. M., Kyomen, H. H., and Harper, D. G. (2012). 'Depression in Later Life: An Overview with Treatment Recommendations'. *Psychiatric Clinics of North America* 35: 203–229.

Frederick, J. T., Steinman, L. E., Prohaska, T., Satariano, W. A., Bruce, M., et al. (2007). 'Community-based Treatment of Late Life Depression: An Expert Panel-informed Literature Review'. *American Journal of Preventive Medicine* 33: 222–249.

Garrido, M. M., Kane, R. L., Kaas, M., and Kane, R. A. (2011). 'Use of Mental Health Care by Community-dwelling Older Adults'. *Journal of the American Geriatrics Society* 59: 50–56.

Gellis, Z. D., Kenaley, B. L., and Ten Have, T. (2014). 'Integrated Telehealth Care for Chronic Illness and Depression in Geriatric Home Care Patients: The Integrated Telehealth Education and Activation of Mood (I-TEAM) Study'. *Journal of the American Geriatrics Society* 62: 889–895.

Gitlin, L. N., Harris, L. F., McCoy, M., Chernett, N. L., Jutkowitz, E., et al. (2012). 'A Community-integrated Home Based Depression Intervention for Older African Americans: Description of the Beat the Blues Randomized Trial and Intervention Costs'. *BMC Geriatrics* 12: 1–11.

Gitlin, N. L., Harris, L. F., McCoy M. C., Chernett N. L., Pizzi, L. T., Jutkowitz, E., Hess, E., and Hauck, W. W. (2013). 'A Home-based Intervention to Reduce Depressive Symptoms and Improve Quality of Life in Older African Americans: A Randomized Trial'. *Annals of Internal Medicine* 159: 243–252.

Gonçalves, D. C. and Byrne, G. J. (2012). 'Interventions for Generalized Anxiety Disorder in Older Adults: Systematic Review and Meta-analysis'. *Journal of Anxiety Disorders* 26: 1–11.

Grenier, S., Potvin, O., Hudon, C., Boyer, R., Préville, M. et al. (2011). 'Twelve-month Prevalence and Correlates of Subthreshold and Threshold Anxiety in Community-dwelling Older Adults with Cardiovascular Diseases'. *Journal of Affective Disorders* 136: 724–732.

Hendriks, G. J., Keijsers, G. P. J, Kampman, M., Oude Voshaar, R. C., Verbraak, M. J. P. M., et al. (2010). 'A Randomized Controlled Study of Paroxetine and Cognitive-behavioural Therapy for Late-life Panic Disorder'. *Acta Psychiatrica Scandinavica* 122(1): 11–19.

Huffman, J. C., Mastromauro, C. A., Beach, S. R., Celano, C. M., DuBois, C. M., Healy, B. C., Suarez, L., Rollman, B. L., and Januzzi, J. L. (2014). 'Collaborative Care for Depression and Anxiety Disorders in Patients with Recent Cardiac Events: The Management of Sadness and Anxiety in Cardiology (MOSAIC) Randomized Clinical Trial'. *JAMA Internal Medicine*, published on-line 24 April 2014.

Jameson, J. P. and Cully, J. A. (2011). 'Cognitive Behavioral Therapy for Older Adults in the Primary Care Setting'. In K. Sorocco and S. Lauderdale (eds), *Anxiety in the Elderly: Treatment and Research* (pp. 291–316). New York: Springer.

Jameson, J. P., Shrestha, S., Escamilla, M., Clark, S., Wilson, N., et al. (2012). 'Establishing Community Partnerships to Support Late-life Anxiety Research: Lessons Learned from the Calmer Life Project'. *Aging & Mental Health* 16(7): 874–883.

Joo, J. H., Morales, K. H., De Vries, H. F., and Gallo, J. J. (2010). 'Disparity in Use of Psychotherapy Offered in Primary Care between Older African American and White Adults: Results from a Practice-based Depression Intervention Trial'. *Journal of the American Geriatrics Society* 58: 154–160.

Kaltenthaler, E. and Cavanagh, K. (2010). 'Computerised Cognitive Behavioural Therapy and its Uses'. *Progress in Neurology and Psychiatry* 14: 22–29.

Karel, M. J., Gatz, M., and Smyer, M. A. (2012). 'Aging and Mental Health in the Decade Ahead: What Psychologists Need to Know'. *American Psychologist* 67: 184–198.

Karlin, B. E., Duffy, M., and Gleaves, D. H. (2008). 'Patterns and Predictors of Mental Health Service Use and Mental Illness among Older and Younger Adults in the United States'. *Psychological Services* 5: 275–294.

Katon, W. J., Lin, E., Russo, J., and Unutzer, J. (2003). 'Increased Medical Costs of a Population-based Sample of Depressed Elderly Patients'. *Archives of General Psychiatry* 60: 897–903.

Kauth, M. R., Sullivan, G., and Blevins, D., Cully, J. A., Landes, R. D., et al. (2010). 'Employing External Facilitation to Implement Cognitive Behavioral Therapy in VA Clinics: A Pilot Study'. *Implementation Science* 5: 1–11.

Kessler, R. C., Berglund, P., Demler, O., Jin, R., Merikangas, K. R., et al. (2005). 'Lifetime Prevalence and Age-of-onset Distributions of DSM-IV Disorders in the National Comorbidity Survey Replication'. *Archives of General Psychiatry* 62: 593–602.

Koder, D. A. and Ferguson, S. J. (1998). 'The Status of Geropsychology in Australia: Exploring why Australian Psychologists are not Working with Elderly Clients'. *Australian Psychologist* 33: 96–100.

Kroenke, K., Spitzer, R. L., Williams, J. B. W., Monahan, P. O., and Löwe, B. (2007). 'Anxiety Disorders in Primary Care: Prevalence, Impairment, Comorbidity, and Detection'. *Annals of Internal Medicine* 146: 317–325.

Kronfol, N. M. (2012). 'Health Services to Groups with Special Needs in the Arab World: A Review'. *East Mediterranean Health Journal* 18(12): 1247–1253.

Kunik, M. E., Veazey, C., Cully, J. A., Souchek, J., Graham, D. P., et al. (2008). 'COPD Education and Cognitive Behavioral Therapy Group Treatment for Clinically Significant Symptoms of Depression and Anxiety in COPD Patients: A Randomized Controlled Trial'. *Psychological Medicine* 38: 385–396.

Lee, S. Y., Franchetti, M. K., Imanbayev, A., Gallo, J. J., Spira, A. P., et al. (2012). 'Non-pharmacological Prevention of Major Depression among Community-dwelling Older Adults: A Systematic Review of the Efficacy of Psychotherapy Interventions'. *Archives of Gerontology and Geriatrics* 55(3): 522–529. doi: 10.1016/j.archger.2012.03.003.

Lin, E. H. B., Katon, W., Von Korff, M., Tang, L, Williams, J. W., Jr, et al. (2003). 'Effect of Improving Depression Care on Pain and Function among Older Adults with Arthritis'. *Journal of the American Medical Association* 290: 2428–2803.

Lustman, P. J., Griffith, L. S., Freedland, K. E., Kissel, S. S., and Clouse, R. E. (1998). 'Cognitive Behavior Therapy for Depression in Type 2 Diabetes Mellitus. A Randomized, Controlled Trial'. *Annals of Internal Medicine* 129: 613–621.

MacGregor, A. D., Hayward, L., Peck, D. F., and Wilkes, P. (2009). 'Empirically Grounded Clinical Interventions'. *Behavioural and Cognitive Psychotherapy* 37: 1–9.

Mackenzie, C. S., Reynolds, K., Cairney, J., Striner, D. L., and Sareen, J. (2011). 'Disorder-specific Mental Health Service Use for Mood and Anxiety Disorders: Associations with Age, Sex, and Psychiatric Comorbidity'. *Depression and Anxiety* 29(3): 234–242.

Miranda, J., Green, B. L., Krupnick, J. L., Chung, J., Siddique, J., et al. (2006). 'One-year Outcomes of a Randomized Clinical Trial Treating Depression in Low-income Minority Women'. *Journal of Consulting and Clinical Psychology* 74: 99–111.

Mohr, D. C., Hart, S. L., Howard, I., Julian, L., Vella, L., et al. (2006). 'Barriers to Psychotherapy among Depressed and Nondepressed Primary Care Patients'. *Annals of Behavioral Medicine* 32: 254–258.

Montano, C B. (1999). 'Primary Care Issues Related to the Treatment of Depression in Elderly Patients'. *Journal of Clinical Psychiatry* 60: 45–51.

Mucic, D. (2011). 'Telemental Health in Treatment of Ethnic Minorities in EU'. *European Psychiatry* 26(1): 2194.

Muijen, M. (2012). 'The State of Psychiatry in Europe: Facing The Challenges, Developing Consensus'. *International Review of Psychiatry* 24(4): 274–277.

Pietrzak, R. H., Maruff, P., Woodward, M., Fredrickson, J., Fredrickson, A., et al. (2012). 'Mild Worry Symptoms Predict Decline in Learning and Memory in Healthy Older Adults: A 2-year Prospective Cohort Study'. *American Journal of Geriatric Psychiatry* 20: 266–275.

Pinquart, M. and Duberstein, P. R. (2007). 'Treatment of Anxiety Disorders in Older Adults: A Meta-analytic Comparison of Behavioral and Pharmacological Interventions'. *American Journal of Geriatric Psychiatry* 15: 639–651.

Pinquart, M., Duberstein, P. R., and Lyness, J. M. (2006). 'Treatments for Later-life Depressive Conditions: A Meta-analytic Comparison of Pharmacotherapy and Psychotherapy'. *American Journal of Psychiatry* 169: 1493–1501.

Quijano, L. M., Stanley, M. A., Petersen, N. J., Casado, B. L, Steinberg, E. H., et al. (2007). 'Healthy IDEAS: A Depression Intervention Delivered by Community-based Case Managers Serving Older Adults'. *Journal of Applied Gerontology* 26(2): 139–157.

Reynolds, C. F., III (2009). 'Prevention of Depressive Disorders: A Brave New World'. *Depression and Anxiety* 26: 1062–1065.

Robb, C., Haley, W. E., Becker, M. A., Polivka, L. A., and Chwa, H. J. (2003). 'Attitudes towards Mental Health Care in Younger and Older Adults: Similarities and Differences'. *Aging & Mental Health* 7: 142–152.

Robinson, G., d'Abbs, P., Togni, S., and Bailie, R. (2003). 'Aboriginal Participation in Health Service Delivery: Coordinated Care Trials in the Northern Territory of Australia'. *International Journal of Healthcare Technology and Management* 5: 45–62.

Roy-Byrne, P., Craske, M. G., Sullivan, G., Rose, R. D., Edlund, M. J., et al. (2010). 'Delivery of Evidence-based Treatment for Multiple Anxiety Disorders in Primary Care: A Randomized Controlled Trial'. *Journal of the American Medical Association* 303: 1921–1928.

Schuurmans, J., Comijs, H., Emmelkamp, P. M., Weijnen, I. J., van den Hout, M., et al. (2009). 'Long-term Effectiveness and Prediction of Treatment Outcome in Cognitive Behavioral Therapy and Sertraline for Late-life Anxiety Disorders'. *International Psychogeriatrics* 6: 1148–1159.

Sharpe, L., Sensky, T., Timberlake, N., Ryan, B., Brewin, C. R., et al. (2001). 'A Blind, Randomized, Controlled Trial of Cognitive-behavioural Intervention for Patients with Recent Onset Rheumatoid Arthritis: Preventing Psychological and Physical Morbidity'. *Pain* 89: 275–283.

Shrestha, S., Armento, M. E. A., Bush, A. L., Huddleston, C., Zeno, D., et al. (2012). 'Pilot Findings from a Community-based Treatment Program for Late-life Anxiety'. *International Journal of Person Centered Medicine* 2(3): 400–409.

Snowden, M., Steinman, L., and Frederick, J. (2008). 'Treating Depression in Older Adults: Challenges to Implementing the Recommendations of an Expert Panel'. *Preventing Chronic Disease* 5: 1–7.

Stanley, M. A., Diefenbach, G. J., Hopko, D. R., Novy, D., Kunik, M. E., et al. (2003). 'The Nature of Generalized Anxiety in Older Primary Care Patients: Preliminary Findings'. *Journal of Psychopathology and Behavioral Assessment* 25: 273–280.

Stanley, M. A., Wilson, N., Novy, D. M., Rhoades, H. M., Wagener, P. D., et al. (2009). 'Cognitive Behavior Therapy for Older Adults with Generalized Anxiety Disorder in Primary Care: A Randomized Clinical Trial'. *Journal of the American Medical Association* 301: 1460–1467.

Stanley, M.A., Wilson, N.L., Amspoker, A. B., Kraus-Schuman, C., Wagener, P. D., Calleo, J. S. Cully, J. A. et al. (2014). 'Lay Providers Can Deliver Effective Cognitive Behavioral Therapy for Older Adults With Generalized Anxiety Disorder: A Randomized Trial'. *Depression and Anxiety* 31: 391–401.

Steinman, L. E., Frederick, J. T., Prohaska, T., Satariano, W. A., Dornberg-Lee, S., et al. (2007). 'Recommendations for Treating Depression in Community-based Older Adults'. *American Journal of Preventive Medicine* 33: 175–181.

Stillman, A. N., Rowe, K. C., Arndt, S., and Moser, D. J. (2011). 'Anxious Symptoms and Cognitive Function in Non-demented Older Adults: An Inverse Relationship'. *International Journal of Geriatric Psychiatry* 27(8): 792–798. doi:10.1002/gps.2785.

Sullivan, G., Blevins, D., and Kauth, M. R. (2008). 'Translating Clinical Training into Practice in Complex Mental Health Systems: Towards Opening the "Black Box" of Implementation'. *Implementation Science* 3: 1–7.

Unützer, J., Katon, W., Sullivan, M., and Miranda, J. (1999). 'Treating Depressed Older Adults in Primary Care: Narrowing the Gap between Efficacy and Effectiveness'. *Milbank Quarterly* 77: 225–256.

Unützer, J., Katon, W., Callahan, C. M., Williams, J. W., Jr, Hunkeler, E., et al. (2002). 'Collaborative Care Management of Late-life Depression in the Primary Care Setting'. *Journal of the American Medical Association* 288: 2836–2845.

UQ News (2012). 'Telehealth Grant Awarded for Residential Aged Care Facilities'. http://www.uq.edu.au/news/index.html?article=25458.

Van Etten, D. (2006). 'Psychotherapy with Older Adults: Benefits and Barriers'. *Journal of Psychosocial Nursing* 44: 28–33.

Vasiliadis, H. M., Dionne, P. A., Préville, M., Gentil, L., Berbiche, D., et al. (2012). 'The Excess Healthcare Costs Associated with Depression and Anxiety in Elderly Living in the Community'. *American Journal of Geriatric Psychiatry* 21(6): 536–548.

Volkers, A. C., Nuyen, J., Verhaak, P. F., Schellevis, F. G. (2004). 'The Problem of Diagnosing Major Depression in Elderly Primary Care Patients. *Journal of Affective Disorders* 82(2): 259–263.

Wetherell, J. L., Ayers, C. R., Sorrell, J. T., Thorp, S. R., Nuevo, R., et al. (2009). 'Modular Psychotherapy for Anxiety in Older Primary Care Patients'. *American Journal of Geriatric Psychiatry* 17: 483–492.

Wetherell, J. L., Afari, N., Rutledge, T., Sorrell, J. T., Stoddard, J. A., et al. (2011). 'A Randomized, Controlled Trial of Acceptance and Commitment Therapy and Cognitive-behavioral Therapy for Chronic Pain'. *Pain* 152: 2098–2107.

WHO-Wonca (2008). *Integrating Mental Health into Primary Care: A Global Perspective*. Geneva and London: WHO and Wonca. http://www.who.int/mental_health/policy/services/mentalhealthintoprimarycare/en/.

Williams, J., Jr, Katon, W., Lin, E. H. B., Nöel, P. H., Worchel, J., et al. (2004). 'The Effectiveness of Depression Care Management on Diabetes-related Outcomes in Older Patients'. *Annals of Internal Medicine* 140: 1015–1024.

Wittchen, H. U., Kessler, R. C., Beesdo, K., Krause, P., Hofler, M., and Hoyer, J. (2002). 'Generalized Anxiety and Depression in Primary Care: Prevalence, Recognition, and Management'. *Journal of Clinical Psychiatry* 63(suppl. 8): 24–34.

Wolitzky-Taylor, K. B., Castriotta, N., Lenze, E. J., Stanley, M. A., and Craske, M. G. (2010). 'Anxiety Disorders in Older Adults: A Comprehensive Review'. *Depression and Anxiety* 27: 190–211.

Woodall, A., Morgan, C., Sloan, C., and Howard, L. (2010). 'Barriers to Participation in Mental Health Research: Are There Specific Gender, Ethnicity and Age Related Barriers?' *BMC Psychiatry* 10(103): 1–31.

Woodward, R. and Pachana, N. A. (2009). 'Attitudes Toward Psychological Treatment Among Older Australians'. *Australian Psychologist* 44(2): 86–93.

Xie, B. (2011). 'Effects of an eHealth Literacy Intervention for Older Adults'. *Journal of Medical Internet Research* 13: e90.

Zeiss, A. M. and Karlin, B. E. (2008). 'Integrating Mental Health and Primary Care Services in the Department of Veterans Affairs Health Care System'. *Journal of Clinical Psychology in Medical Settings* 15: 73–78.

CHAPTER 44

POSITIVE AGEING

New Horizons for Older Adults

LIORA BAR-TUR AND RUTH MALKINSON

The illiterate of the 21st century will not be those who cannot read and write, but those who cannot learn, unlearn, and relearn.

Herbert Gerjuoy in Alvin Toffler (1970 p. 367)

INTRODUCTION

POSITIVE psychology is the scientific study of positive experiences, positive individual traits, and the institutions that facilitate their development. The scientific and professional movement concerned with well-being and optimal functioning was established in 1998 by Martin Seligman (Seligman 2000). Positive psychology encompasses studies on well-being, happiness, positive emotions, character strengths, virtues, excellence, thriving, flourishing, resilience, optimal functioning, and the like. The new focus on the science of thriving or optimal functioning proposes new ways to address some of the most pressing issues facing modern societies. In the applied sphere, it underlies numerous viewpoints, including that one can learn optimism (Seligman 1991), increase positive emotions (Fredrikson 2009), find flow (Csikszentmihalyi 1997), apply strategies of gratitude, forgiveness, and altruism (Hill 2011), and, put more broadly, work towards a better life (Lyubomirsky 2008; Seligman 2011). The science of positive psychology has recently also been applied to educational systems, workplaces, leadership, and the well-being and welfare of society at large (Donaldson 2011).

Positive psychology is especially relevant in the twenty-first century, as societies are more affluent in many ways. Longevity is increasing, and quality of life for a majority of older adults is improving, with better health due to advances in medicine and a more widespread knowledge of healthy living. Interest in how to live a good and fulfilling long life is a natural concern once society's basic needs are met and threats have been relatively contained. Compared to the past, there is more freedom today to pursue different life styles and to acquire knowledge of more choices. This is even more the case for older adults who, as they age, may encounter the freedom to experience a fulfilling existence for the first time in their lives.

Positive psychology emphasizes not only the individual's actualization, but also the development of positive environments, such as families, workplaces, schools, senior clubs, and communities, within the framework of their contribution to society. When given the opportunity, large numbers of seniors are active in their communities through volunteer work and frequently even by taking low-paid part-time jobs. Many also provide care to family members. While older adults often contribute a great deal to society (Williamson and Christie 2009), there are still vast differences in the ageing experience, which can be accompanied by an increase in disability (Jacobzine, Cambois, and Robine 2002). How to age successfully, despite age-related losses, is therefore the focus of much concern and a great challenge to positive psychology studies. The major concepts of positive psychology being investigated in ageing populations include mental health, well-being, successful ageing, and positive health.

PSYCHOLOGICAL WELL-BEING

In the 2000s' research has led to a major change in understanding that mental health is not merely the absence of mental illness, but rather the presence of 'a state of well-being in which the individual realizes his or her own abilities, can cope with normal stresses of life, can work productively and fruitfully, and is able to make a contribution to his or her community' (World Health Organization 2004: 12). Complete mental health is thus a state in which the individuals are flourishing (Keyes 2009). Psychological well-being is now understood as comprising positive psychological resources, such as positively affecting satisfaction with life (Diener 1984), autonomy, competence, relatedness (Ryan and Deci 2001), self-acceptance, purpose, personal growth (Ryff 1989a; Ryff and Singer 2008), personal resilience (Doyle, McKee, and Sherriff 2010; Windle, Woods, and Markland 2010), and flourishing (Seligman 2011).

Diener and Biswas-Diener (2008) introduced the concept of psychological wealth as the experience of well-being and high quality of life. It includes life satisfaction, the feeling that life is full of meaning, a sense of engagement in interesting activities, the pursuit of important goals, the experience of positive emotional feelings, and a sense of spirituality that connects people to things. Seligman (2011) delineated five measurable elements of well-being—Positive emotion, including happiness and life satisfaction; Engagement; positive Relationships; Meaning; and Accomplishment—which he referred to as PERMA. Some aspects of these five elements are measured subjectively by self-report while other aspects are measured objectively (for more on this see Box 44.1).

According to the well-being concept, the goal of positive psychology is to increase the amount of flourishing in the individual's own life and beyond. Positive psychologists argue that well-being can be improved, and their research focuses on testing interventions and special positive psychology exercises that can increase happiness and life satisfaction thereby encouraging individuals to engage in interesting and meaningful activities (Lopez and Snyder 2003; Lyubomirsky 2008).

Box 44.1 Well-being (PERMA)

Positive emotion: The pleasant life (of which happiness and life satisfaction are all aspects). It is assessed subjectively and the subjective state is in the present.

  Engagement: Something that one is absorbed with, in a state of flow. It is assessed only subjectively. The subjective state for engagement is only retrospective.

  Positive relationships: Positive relationships or their absence have profound influences on well-being. They contribute to well-being and can bring about positive emotion, engagement, meaning, or accomplishment. Other people are the best antidote to the downs of life and the single most reliable up.

  Meaning: Belonging to and serving something that one believes is bigger than the self. It is both subjective and objective. Meaning is defined and measured independently of the other components of well-being.

  Accomplishment: Achievement or achieving life, what people choose to do, is often pursued for its own sake, even when it does not contribute to the other components of well-being.

  Data from Seligman, M. E. P., Flourish: A Visionary New Understanding of Happiness and Well-being, 2011, Free Press.

WELL-BEING AND OLD AGE

In contrast to the stereotypic associations in the literature between old age and declining functional capacities, recent studies have focused more on the possibilities of continued growth and development in the later years. An increased awareness of the richness and rewards of long life has led to such concepts as successful ageing, optimal ageing, and positive health. It is well recognized that there are vast individual differences in the subjective well-being and functioning of older adults. Whereas some individuals age successfully, experiencing rewarding time and maintaining their competence, independence, interests, and good mental and physical health, others experience decline early and live out their final years in poor health, often without social supports, The aim of positive psychology is thus to promote common knowledge of how to age well and to suggest effective strategies for moderating the hassles and stressors of old age.

  The contribution of positive psychology to the study of ageing lies in identifying the psychological components that facilitate positive ageing. Positive psychology seeks to understand the concepts of recovery, adaptation, and resilience, rather than focusing on dysfunction and psychopathology. It examines how older adults recover and maintain their health and well-being in the face of cumulative adversities and how people sustain a positive outlook and functional capacity as life challenges multiply. Potential protective factors are investigated on multiple levels (biological, psychological, social, and cultural), and the ways in which people can deal effectively with losses in various domains of the ageing process are explored. There is increasing interest in the importance of later-life resilience to an understanding of how we can reduce older individuals' dependency and the future costs of caring for the older population (Ryff and Singer 2000a; Seligman 2008, 2011). This in fact is one of the pivotal questions that gerontologists ask in their quest for an integrated model of successful ageing as a means of proving that there are alternatives to deterioration, and that positive mental health is not only desirable but also an achievable goal (Gilleard and Higgs 2008). For example, taking an active role to promote mental and physical health using proactive adaptation can help to maintain well-being despite illness. Proactive adaptation includes operating the individual's internal and external resources, such as health promotion (exercise), planning ahead, and marshalling support (Kahana, Kelley-Moore, and Kahana 2011b). In fact, many older adults nowadays are active, vital, self-reliant, socially active, and creatively involved with their communities (Ranzijn 2002; Williamson and Christie 2009).

Positive Ageing: From Negative to Positive Models of Ageing Well

Positive ageing can be viewed as a scientific multidimensional concept that combines various terms describing ageing well: optimal, successful, productive, and healthy ageing. Positive ageing consists of five independent factors: health, cognition, activity, affect, and physical fitness. It is described in practice by a broad set of biopsychosocial factors and is assessed through both objective and subjective indicators (Fernandez-Ballesteros 2011). The terms dealing with positive ageing aim to combat the negative images of ageing. One of the most popular and controversial terms in use is 'successful aging'. While this concept has been discussed and studied for almost fifty years (Havighurst 1963), there is still an on-going debate about what defines success and how it is measured (Bowling and Dieppe 2005; Pruchno, Wilson-Genderson, and Cartwright, 2010). Various models of successful ageing (Baltes and Baltes 1990; Rowe and Kahn 1987; Ryff 1989a; Ryff and Singer 2008) have explored the components and dimensions of well-being and positive function in older adults. Rowe and Kahn (1998) have listed three objective criteria for characterizing successful ageing: the ability to maintain a low risk of disease and disease-related disability; high mental and physical function; and active engagement with life. Although their model stimulated significant research, there remains no precise definition of successful ageing or specific ways of measuring it (Kahn 2003) (for more on this see Box 44.2).

In attempting to define successful ageing, some studies have focused on objective measures of disability or physical function, while others have defined it in relative terms as a process of

---

Box 44.2 What constitutes successful ageing?

Rowe and Kahn (1987, 1998): The ability to maintain a low risk of disease and disease-related disability; high mental and physical function; and active engagement with life.

Ryff (1989a; Ryff and Singer, 2008): Six components of subjective experience of psychological well-being: self-acceptance, positive relationships, autonomy, environmental mastery, purpose in life, personal growth.

Baltes and Baltes (1990; Baltes and Castensen 1996; Baltes and Lang 1997): Successful adaptation using strategies of selection, optimization, and compensation: 'the attainment of goals which can differ widely among people and can be measured against diverse standards and norms' (Baltes and Castensen 1996: 399).

Pruchno, Wilson-Genderson, and Cartwright (2010): A two-factor model of objective components of health conditions and functional ability, and subjective components: the evaluation that individuals make of their own ageing experience at one point in time, e.g. positive, successful ageing.

successful adaptation to age-related changes (Baltes and Baltes 1990; Baltes, Lindenberger, and Staudinger 1998; Kling, Seltzer, and Ryff 1997; Myers and Diener 1995; Strongman and Overton 1999). Baltes and Baltes' (1990) selective optimization with compensation (SOC) model suggested a series of strategies for ageing successfully, providing a framework for the understanding of developmental changes and resilience across the lifespan. The three elements, selection, optimization, and compensation, interplay with one another so that a person may suffer from a reduced general capacity and losses in specific functions, but still create a transformed and effective life through the process of SOC (Freund and Baltes 1998).

Not only have definitions of successful ageing varied among studies, the term 'successful' also has several meanings. Alternative terms employed include 'healthy ageing', 'ageing well', 'effective ageing', 'optimal ageing', and 'productive ageing'. Depp and Jeste (2006) found twenty-nine definitions in their examination of empirical studies of successful ageing and an equal number of measures that operationalized them. Another difficulty in reaching an accepted term for successful ageing is attributable to the significant differences found in studies comparing the term's objective and subjective definitions (Montross et al. 2006; Strawbridge, Wallhagen, and Cohen 2002).

However, the term 'successful ageing' emphasizes that in adulthood it is possible to engage in behaviours that will impact on how a person ages. In other words, at any age, including old and very old, people are to some extent in charge of and responsible for their own quality of life (Hill 2005), a point that is well presented in Ryff and Singer's (2008) six dimensions of well-being model. This integrated model (originally called 'successful ageing' and later 'well-being and positive functioning'), first presented by Ryff (1989a) and Ryff and Essex (1991) and later by Ryff and Singer (1996, 2008), incorporates lifespan developmental theories, clinical theories of personal growth, and mental health perspectives. It comprises six dimensions of positive functioning: self-acceptance; positive relations with others; autonomy; environmental mastery; purpose in life; and personal growth (for more on this see Box 44.3).

Box 44.3 Dimensions of well-being

Self-acceptance: Long-term self-evaluation that involves awareness, and acceptance, of both personal strengths and weaknesses.

Positive relations with others: Warm, satisfying, trusting, and intimate relationships with others. The ability to love and to feel empathy. This dimension is critical to the promotion of health-related processes.

Autonomy: Self-determination, independence, having an internal locus of evaluation, whereby one does not look to others for approval, but evaluates oneself by personal standards.

Environmental mastery: A sense of mastery and competence. The individual's ability to choose or create environments suitable to his or her psychic conditions

Personal growth: A feeling of continued development, openness to new experiences, the feeling that the self is growing and expanding, and that there is a development in self-knowledge and effectiveness.

Purpose in life: A feeling that there is purpose in and meaning to present and past life. The individual has goals in life and a sense of directedness.

Data from Ryff, C. D., & Singer, B., Psychological well-being: Meaning, measurement, and implications for psychotherapy research, *Psychotherapy and Psychosomatics*, 65, pp. 14–23 1996, S. Karger A. G., Basel, Ryff, C. D., & Singer, B., Interpersonal flourishing: A positive health agenda for the new millennium, *Personality and Social Psychology Review*, 4(1), pp. 30–44, 2000, Society for Personality and Social Psychology, Inc., and Ryff, C. D., & Singer, B., Know thyself what you are: A eudaimonic approach to psychological well-being, *Journal of Happiness Studies*, 9, pp. 13–39, 2008, Springer Science and Business Media.

Further research revealed that these dimensions of well-being and healthy mental functioning are shaped by socio-demographic characteristics (e.g. age, gender, socio-demographic status, ethnicity, and culture), as well as by individual experiences, including both unexpected life stresses and planned, normative transitions (Ryff and Essex 1991; Ryff and Singer 1996). Hedonic well-being generally shows gains with age, that is, older adults tend to show increments in positive affect and decrements in negative affect, at least until very old age. In contrast, eudemonic well-being, reflecting a sense of purpose, is more inclined to reflect decrements in the later years, especially in terms of assessment of purpose in life and personal growth (Ryff and Singer 2008).

How Older Adults Define Well-being and Optimal Ageing

The vast increases in the older population's longevity, health, and quality of life in recent years, together with substantial technological, social, political, and life-style changes, have led to an understanding that the concepts of well-being and successful ageing need constant re-evaluation and refinement as new generations of ageing individuals bring different standards and ideals for evaluation of themselves and others. It is also essential that older adults provide their own definitions of positive or ideal functioning at their respective stages in life and their different cultures, as there is a wide variation in individual experiences of ageing.

Interviews with middle-aged and older adults, exploring how older adults define positive functioning and well-being, revealed that acceptance of change was considered to be an important quality of positive functioning (Montross et al. 2006; Ryff 1989b). Such acceptance pertains to changes within the self, such as biological ageing, as well as changes in the surrounding world. It also involves developing the capacity to accept life's twists and turns, which may be progressively beyond one's control. The emphasis on accepting change was expressed together with a concern for continued growth by both middle-aged and older adults. Thus, positive functioning was defined in terms of adapting to as well as initiating change. Moreover, reference to positive relations with others was a focal point for both age groups and for both sexes.

In another study (Tate, Leedine, and Cuddy 2003), the most frequently cited definitions of successful ageing related to physical and mental health, high cognitive and physical functioning, and active engagement with life, including positive relationships with family and friends. These findings agreed with those of Ryff (1989a), Baltes and Baltes' SOC model (1990), and Rowe and Kahn's (1998) concept of successful ageing. An interesting point is that the second most frequently reported description of successful ageing after 'health' was 'happiness, enjoying life, having a satisfying life style, "no worries, be happy"'. A study by Reichstadt et al. (2010) confirmed these components of successful ageing, reporting that older adults viewed successful ageing as a balance between self-acceptance and self-contentedness on the one hand, and engagement with life and self-growth in later life on the other.

The term 'successful ageing' or 'positive ageing' is regarded today as an 'umbrella' for various aspects of well-being and positive functioning (Fernandez-Ballesteros 2011; Ryff 2012). It is suggested to be a multidimensional model that includes both objective criteria and subjective perceptions. Psychological well-being, social engagements, and physical activities are significant factors that contribute to ageing well. More studies are needed to understand the precursors and different aspects of successful ageing from the young to the 'old-old' (Doyle et al. 2010; Pruchno et al. 2010; Strawbridge et al. 2002).

Whereas early models of successful ageing dealt with positive functioning and strategies for ageing well, there is a growing literature that links attitudes and states of mind to physical well-being in older adults. Physical activity, social interaction, cognitive function, and physical and mental health are inextricably linked in very complex ways. Researchers in positive psychology investigating the nature of the reciprocal influences have revealed some telling indicators of the nature of these relationships. For example, it was found that subjective self-ratings of health (e.g. 'What would you say your health is like these days?') are better predictors of morbidity and mortality than are physical health assessments by physicians or laboratory tests (Helmer et al. 1999; Menec, Chipperfield, and Perry 1999).

Furthermore, having a positive mood and engaging in enjoyable activities were found to be more strongly related to self-rated health than were functional ability and medical indicators (Benyamini et al. 2000). Indeed, the overriding theme that emerges from the past decade of positive psychology research is that mental health and subjective well-being can protect one from physical illness, and that the reverse is also true: good health is a significant factor contributing to happiness in older age, together with positive qualities of mind such as altruism and a good sense of humour (Scottish Executive 2006; Vaillant 2000). Altruistic attitudes refer to other-oriented concerns or compassion that is motivated by generativity, as suggested by Erikson (1968), by concern for the welfare of others (Dovidio et al. 2006), and by the need for meaningful connectedness (Kahana et al. 2011a). The important role of prosocial behaviour for well-being in late life is well evident in the literature (Coalman 2007; Greenfield and Marks 2004; Kahana et al. 2011a, 2013; Li and Ferraro 2005; Musick and Wilson 2008; Morrow-Howell et al. 2003; Thoits and Hewitt 2001).

In summary, the term 'positive ageing' describes an individual acting on resources available to her or him to optimize the ageing experience, with the assumption that it is possible to modify one's own ageing experience (for more on this see Box 44.4).

Box 44.4 Characteristics of positive ageing

1. Mobilizing resources to cope with age-related decline: Using assimilative coping and accommodative coping in accordance with age-related decline.
2. Making life-style choices to preserve well-being: Maintaining and implementing preventive health behaviours to preserve the person's health. Accommodating life style to one's health condition.
3. Cultivating flexibility across the lifespan: So that the person can adjust goals and priorities when necessary, can regulate emotions, and create meaning and optimism in the presence of age-related decline.
4. Focusing on the positive vs the negative aspects of growing old: Cultivating a sense of well-being by focusing selectively on the meaningful aspects of one's old age.

Data from Hill, R.D., Positive aging: A guide for mental health professionals and consumers, 2005, W. W. Norton & Co.

POSITIVE HEALTH

The term positive health, as proposed by Ryff and Singer (1998; Ryff and Singer 2000b; Ryff, Singer, and Love 2004; Ryff et al. 2006) and Seligman (Seligman et al. 2005; Seligman 2008, 2011), is an integrated concept concerned with the connections between subjective and physical well-being. Positive health is defined as the neurophysiological substance of flourishing (Ryff and Singer 1998). Human flourishing, whether in the form of deeply engaged life purposes or richly experienced love relationships, is likely to affect multiple biological systems. The key issue is how psychological well-being is linked with biology. Do such things as high-quality relationships and purpose in life provide protection against adverse health outcomes, and, if so, what are the intermediate mechanisms?

Assuming that positive health provides a buffer against physical and mental illness, Seligman (2008) proposed that the field of positive health has direct parallels to the field of positive psychology. These parallels suggest that the focus on health rather than illness will lead to cost savings in terms of increased longevity, decreased health expenditure, better mental health, and improved prognosis. According to Seligman (2008), positive health consists of three independent quantifiable variables: subjective characteristics, such as optimism, hope, zest, a sense of good health, vitality, and life satisfaction; biological indicators; and functional aspects, such as a satisfying marriage, rich friendships, engaging pastimes, and a flourishing work life (Seligman 2011). The combination of these three assets can be used to predict health targets of interest, such as longevity, mental health, disease prognosis, and ageing. The definition of positive health is currently being tested empirically by Seligman and his colleagues (see Seligman 2011: 210), who are re-analysing six large long-term studies of predictors of illness, which originally focused on risk factors rather than on health assets. Thus, the purpose of longitudinal studies made by Seligman and others on positive health is the conceptualization and measurement of positive health and its effects on longevity, health costs, mental health, and prognosis. Resilience is a prominent component of well-being (Huppert and So 2009) and older adults' 'flourishing' (Windle et al. 2010). Psychological resilience in older adults is defined as 'the capacities of some ageing persons to stay well, recover, or even improve, in the face of cumulating challenge' (Ryff et al. 1998: 69). Ryff and her colleagues distinguish between resilience as a set of outcome criteria (Bonanno et al. 2006; O'Rourke 2004) and as an internal and dynamic process (Navarro et al. 2006; Windle, Markland, and Woods 2008).

The intervening influence of psychological resources on health and subjective well-being has emerged from various studies. In a cohort study of 7000 people, known as MIDS (the Mid-Life in the US National Study of Americans, conducted from 2004 through 2009), Ryff and colleagues (Ryff and Lachman 2006; Ryff and Davidson 2009) found that people with a high level of eudemonic well-being, which derives from living with a sense of purpose, had a lower risk of developing cardiovascular disease or Alzheimer's disease. Other recent studies have linked eudemonic well-being and the role of a resilient self (the inner capacity to adapt to negative changes) in moderating the negative effects of ill-health in later life on subjective well-being (Boyle et al. 2010; Windle et al. 2010). These findings suggest that people with a sense of purpose are more able to take care of their health, appraise their surroundings, and see the positive side of things.

Several studies have confirmed the significant positive effects of personality traits (Turiano et al. 2012), and the impact of optimism and positive health on physical health (Rasmussen, Scheier, and Greenhouse 2009), on cardiovascular disease, and on mortality (e.g. Buchanan 1995; Giltay et al. 2004; Kubzansky et al. 2001; Leedham et al. 1995; Seligman 2008). These studies suggest that optimism is robustly associated with cardiovascular health and pessimism with cardiovascular risk, since optimists take care of themselves and have healthier life styles.

Diener and Biswas-Diener (2008) claim that happy people tend to have not only better cardiovascular health but also stronger immune systems. Research clearly points to a mechanism that links social support to health outcomes via neural regulation of stress reactivity. Accordingly, the active attempt to manage one's environment so that it is relatively low in stress, and high in social support is another means of guarding against the adverse effects of stress.

Keyes (2005) investigated the association of mental health with chronic physical conditions related to age, and concluded with two important findings. First, adults who were completely mentally healthy had the lowest number of chronic physical conditions at all ages. Second, the youngest adults who were languishing had the same number of chronic physical ailments as older flourishing adults. In another study, Keyes and Grzywacz (2005) found the utilization of healthcare services to be the lowest among flourishing adults.

The outcome of these studies is that flourishing is a desirable, central component of complete mental health and should be protected or promoted.

In a series of conversations with Mr B, a 90-year-old widower, published in a book entitled *Life in a Second Thought* (Bar-Tur 2009), Mr B describes how consulting with his therapist (Liora Bar-Tur: LB) on adjustment to widowhood and preparing himself for old age was 'my insurance policy for aging well'. Despite his advanced age, Mr B is fully involved, plays active professional and social roles, and carefully focuses his energy on important and meaningful activities. His 'motto' is clear regarding what old people need to do to preserve their dignity and positive self-image: manage their health, regulate their activities effectively, plan their future, invest in their families, be involved socially, and contribute to their families or communities. He argues that old people are responsible for their old age and should learn how to plan it carefully, while maintaining their independence for as long as possible.

As Seligman (2008) argues, bringing about well-being through engagement, purpose, accomplishments, positive emotions, and positive relationships is one of the best weapons against mental disorder. Healthy people who have good psychological well-being, social support, and love in their life are at less risk for illness and early death. The lesson to be learned is that building supportive social networks for older adults (especially for the very old who may be isolated and lonely) and encouraging active participation in them are of the utmost importance. This is the major task of positive psychology researchers and professionals today.

IMPLICATIONS FOR PRACTICE

Positive psychology, as a body of theory, research, and practical tools, can be added to any intervention or coaching practice regardless of theoretical or professional orientation

(Biswas-Diener and Dean 2007). Given the accumulated research on positive health and positive functioning, positive psychology interventions follow the model of primary prevention, which is concerned with preventing predictable problems, protecting existing states of health, and promoting desired goals for older adults. These interventions are designed to help the older adults improve their well-being and acquire the necessary skills and strategies to adjust to their changing reality, and effectively draw on proactive adaptation to deal with possible future unpreventable adversities. They provide professionals and non-professional adults with evidence-based tools that can be easily taught and applied.

The aim of these interventions is to reach as many older adults as possible, especially those who avoid psychological support because of their negative beliefs and attitudes towards psychotherapy or mental health professionals. Our experience with older adults suggests that short-term intervention or coaching, which focuses on personal strengths and promotion of health, is more appealing than traditional therapy, and generates less negativism (Bar-Tur 2005). The focus is on proactive coping, defined as 'an effort to build up general resources that facilitate promotion towards challenging goals and personal growth' (Schwarzer 2000: 349). These include internal resources such as optimism and self-efficacy and external resources such as time, knowledge, money, planning skills, and social and/or practical support (Begovic 2005; Greenglass 2002; Kahana et al. 2011b). Support for this approach was reported in a study conducted on community-dwelling Australian adults (Sougleris and Ranzijn 2011), suggesting the effects of proactive coping on personal growth and purpose in life, with a weaker but still marked effect on satisfaction with life.

Suggested Positive Psychology Interventions for Older Adults

Comprehensive Assessment of the Older Person's Mental and Physical Health in the Sociocultural and Historical Context

This is one of the prominent features of positive psychology interventions with older clients and represents a major departure from traditional medical assessment and intervention. Many practitioners in complex specialties overlook the fundamental unity of the whole person in the context of his/her physical, social, and mental environment. The focus should be on understanding the person's needs and expectations and evaluating his/her resources, limitations, or problems. A comprehensive assessment should take into consideration not only mental and physical health, including cognitive functioning and personality, but also the full context of the person's present life and past history, including social, cultural, and spiritual factors.

Positive Assessment of the Client' Strengths and Reserve Capacities

We suggest that practitioners and therapists working with older clients move away from the traditional medical assessment model. Instead of focusing on the older person's weaknesses (a broken bone, a broken heart, or a broken community situation), helping professionals should assess and activate client strengths and reserve capacities, as well as the strengths of relevant primary groups (family, friends, close associates, etc.) and secondary groups (large-scale organizations, communities, cultural groups, etc.) to achieve desired goals and prevent predictable problems (Kivnick and Murray 2001; Klein and Bloom 1997). Thus, rather than asking 'What is wrong?' (the typical question asked when visiting the physician), the aim is to find out 'What is good about me? What is still working? What is my reserve capacity?' (Bar-Tur 2005).

Promoting Positive Health

The purpose of psychological intervention should be to help older adults become fully aware of and value their personal resources and their positive health in all its psychological, physical, and social aspects. Psychological intervention should be carried out as part of a multidisciplinary team effort aimed at the promotion of optimal health behaviours involving life-style changes in diet, smoking, and drinking, and physical and cognitive exercises, including stress management and relaxation. By promoting positive health the older person can be helped to deal more effectively with possible ageing losses including memory loss and mood decline.

Promoting Optimal Ageing

Promoting and protecting individual physical, mental, and psychosocial strengths can be achieved by using key elements of the ABC (Activating events-adversities, Beliefs-Consequences) model of optimal ageing such as unconditional self-acceptance and frustration tolerance, which focus on one's ability to accept ageing-related aggravations (Ellis and Velten 1998). In addition, re-establishing meaning and purpose can be applied by using the six 'keys' for positive functioning (Ryff and Singer 1998, 2008). They can practise self-acceptance by learning how to maintain a positive attitude towards oneself and one's past. They can invest more in positive relations with significant others. They can practise autonomy by increasing their independent functioning, express their personal voices, and strengthen their ability to make their own decisions on how to live their lives, while resisting social pressure from family, friends, and others to think or act in certain ways. Another 'key' is aimed at achieving environmental mastery, or the capacity to manage everyday life and create a surrounding context that fits one's personal needs and values. Finding purpose in life, by having a sense of direction, finding meaning in one's present and past, and setting goals to stay active and engaged form another significant dimension of increasing positive functioning which can be achieved through engagements in satisfying social activities. Volunteering is a recommended engagement that can activate and benefit from a person's resources. Older people who volunteered reported feeling more cheerful, more peaceful, more satisfied, and more full of life (Greenfield and Marks 2004).

By having all the five 'keys', older adults thus preserve a sense of personal growth (the sixth key), that is, a feeling of continued development and openness to new experiences. In addition, practising the six keys for positive functioning can enhance the ability to adapt to changing reality and to achieve development of optimal potential (Ryff and Singer 1998, 2008).

Promoting Older Adults' Community Connectedness

One of the major tasks of helping professionals should be to assist older adults in protecting and promoting their social and emotional support, to provide strategies for maintaining community attachment, and to facilitate better use of their neighbourhoods, communities, and sociocultural systems for dealing with stress and loneliness. This can be achieved through proactive interactions and attempts to reach out to older lonely people in the community, by offering regular contacts to 'touch base', inviting them to participate in social events and join programmes designed for older adults, and providing them with psychoeducation and support. A network of 'gatekeepers' made up of people in the community who are trained to identify depressed or at-risk older adults can also be developed.

Positive Psychology Intervention for Depression

Positive psychotherapy may be especially helpful for adults who experience depressive symptoms as a result of accumulated losses in ageing and who need professional support. A substantial body of research suggests that interventions, such as using strengths, writing down three good things or blessings every evening, gratitude exercises, and savouring, can build positive states and alleviate depressive symptoms caused by a lack of well-being, positive emotion, engagement, and meaning in life (Rashid and Seligman 2011; Seligman, Rashid, and Parks 2006; Seligman et al. 2005). For older individuals who suffer from emotional problems or mental disorders, positive psychology interventions can be incorporated into more traditional psychotherapy approaches, such as CBT-REBT or IPT (interpersonal psychotherapy) for depression in older adults (Ellis and Velten 1998; Malkinson 2007; Miller 2009)—see also chapters 30 and 40 in this Handbook on IPT for older adults and the CBT-REBT model applied to grief.

Assimilating Positive Psychology Strategies

Helping professionals in clinical and medical settings should play an important role in conveying information about positive psychology ideas, research, and suggested strategies to increase well-being, and in teaching new skills for positive functioning to the non-clinical community of older adults in general. Professionals should aim to recruit and train leaders from the community to help assimilate positive psychology strategies. They should also provide referral services to clients, particularly primary prevention services, by helping them to help themselves. By promoting clients' prevention-protection-promotion behaviour, the number of consultations with treatment and rehabilitation professionals may be reduced.

Expanding Professionals' Horizons

Positive psychology interventions have the potential to be successful if helping professionals working with older adults are themselves optimistic and in good health. Many professionals still need to overcome their own ageist attitudes if they are effectively to assist what will be an increasingly larger proportion of their clientele (Bar-Tur 2010; Eyal and Bar-Tur 2002; Helmes and Gee 2000). Helping professionals, especially psychologists, should also engage in strategic advocacy for the extension of medical insurance for psychological services, mainly in the areas of prevention, screening, and early intervention (Karlin and Humphreys 2007) (for more on this see Box 44.5).

Box 44.5 Positive psychology interventions for older adults

1. Comprehensive assessment of the older person's mental and physical health in the sociocultural and historical context
2. Positive assessment of the client' strengths and reserve capacities
3. Promoting positive health
4. Promoting optimal ageing
5. Promoting older adults' community connectedness
6. Assimilating positive psychology strategies
7. Positive psychology intervention for depression
8. Expanding professionals' horizons

In sum, positive psychology interventions are better delivered away from health clinics and private practice to reach the non-clinical population at large in their own surroundings, such as senior citizens' clubs and retirement communities. Moreover, open communication channels, such as radio, television, and internet, should be used to contact older adults. Teaching basic skills to increase optimism, develop positive thinking, and learn how to set goals for more involvement and meaningful participation in the community will also contribute to older adults' quality of life.

Wellness and Mental Fitness Kit for Positive Ageing?

This is an example of a group intervention designed by LB to help older adults enhance their positive functioning and well-being (Bar-Tur 2003, 2005). It can be applied in different communities and settings among older adults to assist them explore and activate personal and social resources and reserve capacities. It has been applied by LB in retirement programmes in various communities and with young and old clients individually.

The Wellness and Mental Fitness Kit for Positive Ageing is designed as a psychological journey with eight or twelve stations, each of which offers a two-hour session on a different topic. The journey begins with an introductory lecture by the group leader, which reviews the latest studies and suggested models for positive psychology and positive ageing (Baltes and Baltes 1990; Baltes and Carstensen 1996; Diener and Biswas-Diener 2008; Ellis and Velten 1998; Fredrikson, 2009; Lyubomirsky 2008; Ryff and Singer 2008; Seligman 2011). The mental fitness kit includes a 'personal map, compass, sail and oars' to help older adults decide what they want to go and see, do, and experience along their way (Ellis and Velten 1998). Together they provide participants with tools for achieving positive ageing by assisting them to review their past accomplishments and successful coping as well as present resources and strengths.

Positive psychology strategies are introduced in each session, such as exploring personal strengths and practising new ways to use them, learning how to invest in significant relationships, visualising one's best self, keeping a gratitude diary or a list of good things that happened during the day, seeking out activities that produce flow, practising mindfulness and acts of kindness, and learning components of hope and accessing stories from their own lives to hone their sense of hope (Kauffman 2011; Lyubomirsky 2013). Homework assignments are included to practise these strategies together with other assignments following the topic of each session.

The journey begins by addressing the issue of 'Who am I?', i.e. identity and the ageing self. The first task deals with identity, self-acceptance, and positive self-regard. This is the older person's 'visiting card' in the ageing phase, and is significant in affecting motivation, beliefs, and attitudes towards engagement and an active life.

Maintaining positive self-regard is often associated with the quality of relations with others, as well as a sense of autonomy and environmental mastery, self-realization, and personal growth, with the latter serving to enhance the pursuit of life's goals. Possessing a sense of purpose is a key feature in maintaining coherence. As purposeful living can be expressed in many contexts, older adults who were fully engaged in work or social roles, as well as widows and widowers who were assuming the role of care-giver, may need guidance in finding suitable contexts for gaining a sense of control and purpose in their lives.

'Wellness and Positive Ageing' encourages older adults to examine their present reality, as well as their past. The second issue deals with ' Where do I come from?', i.e. significant milestones in my life. Reviewing past achievements and accomplishments provides a road map of the individual's talents and skills and the domains in which self-efficacy has been cultivated. In gaining a sense of direction and a realistic view of identity and self-image, older adults are enabled to plan and set goals that maintain or increase their well-being. The programme teaches them to identify positive, realistic goals and to use the adaptive mechanisms of selection, optimization, and compensation (SOC) (Baltes and Baltes 1990). This allows the older adults to continue maximizing their chosen activities in life, especially as they grow older and their resources decline (Jopp and Smith 2006).

Participants then focus on their purpose in life through the process of goal attainment. 'What are my short term goals and what would I consider my long-term goals?' Goals provide order and structure to life, helping to orient people to a more valuable, meaningful, and purposeful life. Setting clear, realistic, measurable, and significant goals and structuring how time is spent are important elements as people age and find that they have increased free time and declining commitments (e.g. work and family obligations) (Emmons 2003).

Thereafter, participants identify and increase their health-promoting behaviours. This process fosters the individual's self-acceptance, self-esteem, and integrated identity. By learning the ABC (Activating events-adversities, Beliefs-Consequences) for optimal ageing (Ellis and Velten 1998), older adults are better able to cope with the adversities encountered in growing old. They learn to identify and replace their irrational beliefs and attitudes with rational and more realistic ones, as unrealistic expectations, beliefs, and attitudes regarding old age affect well-being and impede goal attainment. With the group's help, they also seek and create emotional and social support (for more on this see Box 44.6). The mental fitness kit is in fact an intervention that may be used in group and individual therapy or coaching for use with older and younger adults. It is also an effective screening tool where the counsellor can clearly point out to the older client which 'key' needs to be 'fixed'.

Box 44.6 Wellness and Mental Fitness Kit for Positive Ageing

A. Introductory lecture
B. Applying the well-being keys—personal identity, personal map, reviewing significant milestones, past accomplishment, present resources, and strengths, setting short- and long-term goals
C. Teaching and practising the ABC-REBT for optimal aging...
D. Practising positive psychology strategies, new skills and behaviour for healthy life style, and flourishing
E. Creating emotional and social support in the immediate environment
F. Planning an 'emergency kit' for possible 'bad days'

SUMMARY AND FUTURE DIRECTIONS

Positive psychology is a scientific and professional movement concerned with well-being and optimal functioning. Given the increase in longevity and the quality of life of older adults, a major shift in psychological research and in the approach to interventions for the older population is necessary. Traditionally, old people were viewed as 'irrelevant' and as a financial drain on society, whereas recent research is demonstrating that many older adults are relatively healthy, active, and independent. Nowadays, they have many more resources for ageing successfully and maintaining high levels of well-being, and being socially active and creatively involved with their communities.

Growing old in the twenty-first century is still a great challenge nonetheless, and entails high risk, especially for the 'old-old' and the 'oldest-old'. Thus, ageing successfully depends to a large extent on coping effectively with age-related life events. The challenge for older adults is to maintain their independence, and even more so to increase their personal resources so as not to overwhelm societal resources with their needs. Thus, older adults should bear some responsibility for making sure that they maintain a healthy life style and engage in challenging activities within their communities. Interventions that incorporate practising positive psychology strategies can help older adults to increase their autonomy, environmental mastery, and purpose in life by identifying manageable activities and available resources that increase their well-being. As for the oldest-old and/or disabled and sick older adults, their main challenge is to adjust to their changing reality, and to come to terms with their dependence while keeping their psychological autonomy and mastery.

But this is not enough. The surroundings in which older adults live exert a powerful influence on their well-being, and their opportunities to flourish may be restricted. Although findings indicate that the majority of the older population has a resourceful interpersonal milieu and varied social networks (Litwin and Shiovitz-Ezra 2011), there is also the risk of future disability and limitations in mobility which can increase loneliness and reduce well-being. Surroundings are thought to affect successful ageing (Lomranz and Bar-Tur 1998; Nussbaum et al. 2000). A prime point of intervention is to identify the resources and facilitate the social network cooperation that will keep older adults socially and physically active and involved in their communities. More research is needed on the positive aspects of ageing in order to maintain a more realistic and broader vision of ageing, and the aged, as well as to reduce negative images and their consequences on individuals and society at large. Professionals can also help if they recruit and train leaders from the community who will help incorporate strategies and tools for optimal functioning into their treatment approach.

More than that, it is important to understand that positive ageing does not begin in the sixties age group. The foundations are laid early in life by adopting a healthy life style. The development of healthy habits depends to a great extent on social and cultural contexts along the lifespan. Therefore, from a very early age, it is imperative to use educational programmes and media channels in the community to promote public strategies for positive functioning and well-being in general, and for retirement and old age in particular. In fact, the creation of positive institutions, including families, schools, businesses, communities, and society at large, is one of the present and future pillars of positive psychology. Thus, future research on post-retirement society should focus on the adaptive competence of the individual and society as each is affected by the other. Further, the challenge of present and future societies is to provide older persons with meaningful roles and opportunities for self-realization, continued personal growth and social engagements through appropriate positive institutions and suitable surrounding contexts.

As Featherman, Smith, and Peterson (1990) suggested in the early 1990s, 'Successful aging is individuals' learning to plan and society's planning to learn' (84).

KEY REFERENCES AND SOURCES FOR FURTHER READING

Ellis, A. and Velten, E. (1998). *Optimal Aging: Get Over Getting Older*. New York: Open Court.
Hill, R. D. (2005). *Positive Aging: A Guide for Mental Health Professionals and Consumers*. New York: W. W. Norton.
Lyubomirsky, S. (2008). *The How of Happiness: A Scientific Approach to Getting the Life You Want*. New York: Penguin Press.
Lyubomirsky, S. (2013). *The Myths of Happiness: What Should Make You Happy, but Doesn't. What Shouldn't Make You Happy, but Does*. New York: Penguin.
Seligman, M. E. P. (2011). *Flourish: A Visionary New Understanding of Happiness and Well-being*. New York: Free Press.

WEBSITE RESOURCES

Authentic Happiness. http://www.authentichappiness.sas.upenn.edu.
Centre for Confidence and Well-being. http://www.centreforconfidence.co.uk/pp.
University of Pennsylvania, Positive Psychology Center. http://www.ppc.sas.upenn.edu.

REFERENCES

Baltes, P. B. and Baltes, M. M. (1990). 'Psychological Perspectives on Successful Aging: The Model of Selective Optimization with Compensation'. In P. B. Baltes and M. M. Baltes (eds),

Successful Aging: Perspectives from the Behavioral Sciences (pp. 1–34). Cambridge: Cambridge University Press.

Baltes, P. B. and Carstensen, L. L. (1996). 'The Process of Successful Aging'. *Aging and Society* 16: 397–422.

Baltes, P. B. and Lang, F. R (1997). 'Everyday Functioning and Successful Aging: The Impact of Resources'. *Psychology and Aging* 3: 433–443.

Baltes, P. B., Lindenberger, U., and Staudinger, U. M. (1998). 'Life-span Theory in Developmental Psychology'. In R. M. Lerner (ed.), *Handbook of Child Psychology, vol. 1: Theoretical Models of Human Development* (5th edn; pp. 1029–1143). New York: Wiley.

Bar-Tur, L. (2003). *The Mental Fitness Kit for Optimal Aging.* Paper presented at the World Federation for Mental Health Biennial Congress, Melbourne, Australia (February).

Bar-Tur, L. (2005). *The Challenge of Aging: Mental Health, Assessment and Therapy.* Jerusalem: Eshel. (In Hebrew.)

Bar-Tur, L. (2009). *Life in a Second Thought: Conversations with Naftali.* Haifa: Ach Publishing. (In Hebrew.)

Bar-Tur, L. (2010). 'Who Cares for the Caretaker? Professional and Emotional Skills of Practitioners Working with the Elderly'. Gerontology: *Journal of Aging Studies*, 37(2–3), 69-85 (Journal of the Israel Gerontological Society). (In Hebrew.)

Begovic, A. (2005). *Older Adults' Residential Moves, Coping, and Adaptation.* Unpublished Doctoral Dissertation, University of Akron, Ohio.

Benyamini, Y., Idler, E. L., Leventhal, H., and Leventhal, E. A. (2000). 'Positive Affect and Function as Influences on Self-assessments of Health: Expanding our View beyond Illness and Disability'. *Journal of Gerontology, Series B: Psychological Sciences* 55B(2): 107–116.

Biswas-Diener, R. and Dean, B. (2007). *Positive Psychology Coaching: Putting the Science of Happiness to Work for your Clients.* New Jersey: Wiley.

Bonanno, G. A., Galea, S., Bucciarelli, A., and Vlahov, D. (2006). 'Psychological Resilience after a Disaster: New York City in the Aftermath of the September 11th Terrorist Attack'. *Psychological Science* 17: 181–186.

Bowling, A. and Dieppe, P. (2005). 'What Is Successful Ageing and Who Should Define It?' *British Medical Journal* 331: 24–31.

Boyle, P. A., Buchman, A. S., Barnes, L. L., and Bennett, D. A. (2010). 'Effect of a Purpose in Life on Risk of Incident Alzheimer Disease and Mild Cognitive Impairment in Community-dwelling Older Persons'. *Archives of General Psychiatry* 67(3): 301–310.

Buchanan, G. M. (1995). 'Explanatory Style and Coronary Heart Disease'. In G. M. Buchanan and M. E. P. Seligman (eds), *Explanatory Style* (pp. 225–232). Hillsdale, NJ: Erlbaum.

Coalman, M. (2007). 'Positive Psychology: A New Way to Support Wellness in Older Adults?' *Journal on Active Aging* 6(4): 51–54.

Csikszentmihalyi, M. (1997). *Finding Flow.* New York: Basic Books.

Depp, A. C. and Jeste, D. V. (2006). 'Definitions and Predictors of Successful Aging: A Comprehensive Review of Larger Quantitative Studies'. *Journal of Geriatric Psychiatry* 14(1): 6–20.

Diener, E. (1984). 'Subjective Well-being'. *Psychological Bulletin* 95: 542–575.

Diener, E. and Biswas-Diener, R. (2008). *Happiness: Unlocking the Mysteries of Psychological Wealth.* New York: Wiley.

Donaldson, S. I. (2011). 'Determining What Works, if Anything, in Positive Psychology'. In S. I. Donaldson, M. Csikszentmihalyi, and J. Nakamura (eds), *Applied Positive Psychology: Improving Everyday Life, Health, Schools, Work, and Society* (pp. 3–11). New York: Routledge.

Dovidio, J. F., Piliavin, J. A., Schroeder, D. A., and Penner, L. A. (2006). *The Social Psychology of Prosocial Behavior*. Mahwah, NJ: Lawrence Erlbaum.

Doyle, Y. G., McKee, M., and Sherriff, M. (2010). 'A Model of Successful Aging in British Populations'. *European Journal of Public Health* 22(1): 71–76.

Ellis, A. and Velten, E. (1998). *Optimal Aging: Get Over Getting Older*. New York: Open Court.

Emmons, R. A. (2003). 'Personal Goals, Life Meaning, and Virtue: Wellsprings of a Positive Life'. In C. L. M. Keyes and J. Haidt (eds), *Flourishing* (pp. 105–128). Washington, DC: American Psychological Association.

Erikson, E. H. (1968). 'Generativity and Ego Integrity'. In B. L. Neugarten (ed.), *Middle Age and Aging* (pp. 85–87). Chicago: University of Chicago Press.

Eyal, N. and Bar-Tur, L. (2002). 'A Light on the Psychology of Aging: The Missed Dance, the Therapist's Refusal and the Patient's Refusal'. *Psycho-Actualia* April: 24–28. (In Hebrew.)

Featherman, D. L., Smith, J., and Peterson, J. G. (1990). 'Successful Aging in a Post-retired Society'. In P. B. Baltes and M. M. Baltes (eds), *Successful Aging: Perspectives from the Behavioral Sciences* (pp. 50–91). Cambridge: Cambridge University Press.

Fernandez-Ballesteros, R. (2011). 'Positive Ageing: Objective, Subjective, and Combined Outcomes'. *Electronic Journal of Applied Psychology* 7(1): 22–30.

Fredrikson, B. L. (2009). *Positivity: Groundbreaking Research Reveals How to Embrace the Hidden Strengths of Positive Emotions, Overcome Negativity, and Thrive*. New York: Crown.

Freund, A. M. and Baltes, P. B. (1998). 'Selection, Optimization and Compensation as Strategies of Life Management. Correlations with Subjective Indicators of Successful Aging'. *Psychology and Aging* 13(4): 531–543.

Gilleard, C. and Higgs, P. (2008). 'Editorial: Promoting Mental Health in Later Life'. *Aging & Mental Health* 12(3): 283–284.

Giltay, E., Geleijnse, J., Zitman, F., Hoekstra, T., and Schouten, E. (2004). 'Dispositional Optimism and All-cause and Cardiovascular Mortality in a Prospective Cohort of Elderly Dutch Men and Women'. *Archives of General Psychiatry* 61: 1126–1135.

Greenfield, E. A. and Marks, N. (2004). 'Formal Volunteering as a Protective Factor for Older Adults' Psychological Well-being'. *Journals of Gerontology, Series B: Psychological Sciences and Social Sciences* 59B(5): S258–S264.

Greenglass, E. R. (2002). 'Proactive Coping and Quality of Life Management'. In E. Frydenberg (ed.), *Beyond Coping: Meeting Goals, Visions, and Challenges* (pp. 37–62). New York: Oxford University Press.

Havighurst, R. J. (1963). 'Successful Aging'. In R. H. Williams, C. Tibbitts, and W. Donahue (eds), *Process of Aging* (vol. 1, pp. 299–320). New York: Atherton Press.

Helmer, C., Barberger-Gateau, P., Letenneur, L., and Dartigues, J.-F. (1999). 'Subjective Health and Mortality in French Elderly Women and Men'. *Journal of Gerontology, Series B: Social Sciences* 54B(2): S84–S92.

Helmes, E. and Gee, S. (2000). 'Development of a Training Program in Clinical Geropsychology'. *Australasian Journal on Ageing* 19(3): 113–117.

Hill, R. D. (2005). *Positive Aging: A Guide for Mental Health Professionals and Consumers*. New York: W. W. Norton.

Hill, R. D. (2011). 'A Positive Aging Framework for Guiding Geropsychology Interventions'. *Behavior Therapy* 42: 66–77.

Huppert, F. and So, T. (2009). 'What Percentage of People in Europe Are Flourishing and What Characterizes Them' http://www.isquols2009/institutodeglinnocent.itqContent_en/Huppert.pdf.

Jacobzine, S., Cambois, E., and Robine, J. (2002). *Is the Health of Older People in the OECD Countries Improving Fast Enough to Compensate for Population Ageing?* OECD Economic Studies 30. Paris: OECD.

Jopp, D. and Smith, J. (2006). 'Resources and Life-management Strategies as Determinants of Successful Aging: On the Protective Effect of Selection, Optimization, and Compensation'. *Psychology and Aging* 21(2): 253–265.

Kahana, E., Kahana, B., Lovegreen, L., Kahana, J., Brown, J., et al. (2011a). 'Health-care Consumerism and Access to Health Care: Educating Elders to Improve both Preventive and End-of-life Care'. *Research in the Sociology of Health Care* 29: 173–193. doi: 10.1108/S0275-4959(2011)0000029010

Kahana, E., Kelley-Moore, J., and Kahana, B. (2011b). 'Proactive Aging: A Longitudinal Study of Stress, Resources, Agency, and Well-being in Late Life'. *Aging & Mental Health* 16(4): 438–451.

Kahana, E., Bhatta, M. M., Lovegreen, L. D., Kahana, B., and Midlarsky, E. (2013). 'Altruism, Helping, and Volunteering: Pathways to Well-being in Later Life'. *Journal of Aging and Health* 25(1): 159–187.

Kahn, R. L. (2003). 'Successful Lagging: Intended and Unintended Consequences of a Concept'. In L. W. Poon, S. H. Gueldner, and B. M. Sprouse (eds), *Successful Aging and Adaptation with Chronic Diseases* (pp. 55–69). New York: Springer.

Karlin, B. E. and Humphreys, K. (2007). 'Improving Medicare Coverage of Psychological Services for Older Americans'. *American Psychologist* 62(7): 637–649.

Kauffman, C. (2011). 'Applied Positive Psychology in Action: New Developments for Coaching, Consulting or Therapy'. Workshop presented at the International Positive Psychology Conference, Philadephia, PA.

Keyes, C. L. M. (2005). 'Mental Illness and/or Mental Health? Investigating Axiom of the Complete State Model Health'. *Journal of Consulting and Clinical Psychology* 73: 539–548.

Keyes, C. L. M. (2009). 'Towards a Science of Mental Health'. In C. R. Snyder and S. J. Lopez (eds), *Oxford Handbook of Positive Psychology* (pp. 89–95). Oxford: Oxford University Press.

Keyes, C. L. M. and Grzywacz, J. G. (2005). 'Health as a Complete State: The Added Value in Work Performance and Healthcare Costs'. *Journal of Occupational and Environmental Medicine* 47: 523–532.

Kivnick, H. Q. and Murray, S. V. (2001). 'Life Strengths Interview Guide: Assessing Elder Clients' Strengths'. *Journal of Gerontological Social Work* 34(4): 7–31.

Klein, W. C. and Bloom, M. (1997). *Successful Aging: Strategies for Healthy Living.* New York: Plenum.

Kling, K. C., Seltzer, M. M., and Ryff, C. D. (1997). 'Distinctive Late-life Challenges: Implications for Coping and Well-being'. *Psychology and Aging* 12(2): 288–295.

Kubzansky, L., Sparrow, D., Vokonas, P., and Kawachi, I. (2001). 'Is the Glass Half Empty or Half Full? A Prospective Study of Optimism and Coronary Heart Disease in the Normative Aging Study'. *Psychosomatic Medicine* 63: 910–916.

Leedham, B., Meyerowitz, B. E., Muirhead, J., and Frist, W. H. (1995). 'Positive Expectations Predict Health after Heart Transplantation'. *Health Psychology* 14: 74–79.

Li, Y. and Ferraro, K. F. (2005). 'Volunteering and Depression in Later Life: Social Benefit or Selection Processes?' *Journal of Health and Social Behavior* 46(1): 68–84. doi: 10.1177/002214650504600106.

Litwin, H. and Shiovitz-Ezra, S. (2011). 'Social Network Type and Subjective Well-being in a National Sample of Older Americans'. *Gerontologist* 51: 379–388.

Lomranz, J. and Bar-Tur, L. (1998). 'Mental Health in Nursing Homes'. In A. S. Bellack and M. Hersen (eds), *Handbook of Clinical Geropsychology* (vol. 7, pp. 1–21). New York: Elsevier Science.

Lopez, S. J. and Snyder, C. R. (eds) (2003). *Positve Psychological Assessment: A Handbook of Models and Measures.* Washington, DC: American Psychological Association.

Lyubomirsky, S. (2008). *The How of Happiness: A Scientific Approach to Getting the Life You Want.* New York: Penguin.

Malkinson, R. (2007). *Cognitive Grief Therapy: Constructing a Rational Meaning To Life Following Loss.* New York: W. W. Norton.

Menec, V. H., Chipperfield, J. G., and Perry, R. P. (1999). 'Self-perceptions of Health: A Prospective Analysis of Mortality, Control, and Health'. *Journal of Gerontology, Series B: Psychological Sciences* 54B(3): P85–P93.

Miller, M. D. (2009). *Clinical Guide to Interpersonal Psychotherapy in Later life.* New York: Oxford University Press.

Montross, L. P., Depp, C. A., Daly, J., Reichstadt, J., Golshan, S., et al. (2006). 'Correlates of Self-rated Successful Aging among Community Dwelling Older Adults'. *American Journal of Geriatric Psychiatry* 14: 43–51.

Morrow-Howell, N., Hinterlong, J., Rozario, P. A., and Tang, F. (2003). 'Effects of Volunteering on the Well-being of Older Adults'. *Journals of Gerontology, Series B: Psychological Sciences and Social Sciences* 58: S137–S145. doi: 10.1093/geronb/58.3.S137

Musick, M. A. and Wilson, J. (2008). *Volunteers: A Social Profile.* Bloomington, IN: Indiana University Press.

Myers, D. G. and E. Diener (1995). 'Who Is Happy?' *Psychological Science* 6: 10–19.

Navarro, A. B., Bueno, B., Buz, J., and Mayoral, P. (2006). 'Perceptió n de autoeficacia en el afrontamiento de los problemas y su contributió n en la satisfactió n vital de las personas muy mayores' [Perception of self-efficacy in coping with problems and its contribution to life satisfaction in very old people]. *Revista Espanola de Geriatria y Gerontologia* 41(4): 222–227.

Nussbaum, J. F., Pecchioni, L. L., Robinson, J. D., and Thompson, T. L. (2000). *Communication and Aging* (2nd edn). Mahwah, NJ: Erlbaum.

O'Rourke, N. (2004). 'Psychological Resilience and the Well-being of Widowed Women'. *Ageing International* 29(3): 267–280.

Pruchno, R. A., Wilson-Genderson, M., and Cartwright, F. (2010). 'A Two-factor Model of Successful Aging'. *Journal of Gerontology, Series B: Psychological Sciences* 65B: 671–679.

Ranzijn, R. (2002). 'Towards a Positive Psychology of Ageing: Potentials and Barriers'. *Australian Psychologist* 37(2): 79–85.

Rashid, T. and Seligman, M. E. P. (2011). 'An Overview of Fourteen Sessions of PPT'. In M. E. P. Seligman (ed.), *Flourish: A Visionary New Understanding of Happiness and Well-being* (pp. 41–43). New York: Free Press.

Rasmussen, H., Scheier, M., and Greenhouse, J. (2009). 'Optimism and Physical Health: A Meta-analytic Review. *Annals of Behavioral Medicine* 37: 239–256.

Reichstadt, J., Geetika, M. S., Sengupta, M. D, Palinkas, L. A., and Jeste, D. V. (2010). 'Older Adults' Perspectives on Successful Aging: Qualitative Interviews'. *American Journal of Geriatric Psychiatry* 18(7): 567–575.

Rowe, J. W. and Kahn, R. L. (1987). 'Human Aging: Usual and Successful'. *Science* 237: 143–149.

Rowe, J. W. and Kahn, R. L. (1998). *Successful Aging.* New York: Pantheon Books.

Ryan, R. M. and Deci, E. L. (2001). 'On Happiness and Human Potentials: A Review Of Research on Hedonic and Eudaimonic Well-being'. *Annual Review of Psycholology* 52: 141–166.

Ryff, C. D. (1989a). 'Beyond Ponce de Leon and Life Satisfaction: New Directions in Quest of Successful Aging'. *International Journal of Behavioral Development* 12: 35–55.

Ryff, C. D. (1989b). 'In the Eye of the Beholder: Views of Psychological Well-being among Middle-aged'. *Psychology and Aging* 4(2): 195–210.

Ryff, C. D. and Essex, M. (1991). 'Psychological Well-being in Adulthood and Old Age: Descriptive Markers and Explanatory Processes'. In W. Schaie and M. P. Lawton (eds), *Annual Review of Gerontology and Geriatrics,* vol. 11 (pp. 144–171). New York: Springer.

Ryff, C. D. and Singer, B. (1996). 'Psychological Well-being: Meaning, Measurement, and Implications for Psychotherapy Research'. *Psychotherapy and Psychosomatics* 65: 14–23.

Ryff, C. D. and Singer, B. (1998). 'The Contours of Positive Health'. *Psychological Inquiry* 9: 1–28.

Ryff, C. D., Singer, B., Love, G. D., and Essex, M. J. (1998). 'Resilience in Adulthood and Later Life: Defining Features and Dynamic Processes'. In J. Lomranz (ed.), *Handbook of Aging and Mental Health: Integrative Approach* (pp. 69–96). New York: Plenum.

Ryff, C. D. and Singer, B. (2000a). 'Biopsychosocial Challenge of the New Millennium'. *Psychotherapy and Psychosomatics* 69: 170–177.

Ryff, C. D. and Singer, B. (2000b). 'Interpersonal Flourishing: A Positive Health Agenda for the New Millennium'. *Personality and Social Psychology Review* 4(1): 30–44.

Ryff, C. D., Singer, B. H., and Love, G. D. (2004). 'Positive Health: Connecting Well-being with Biology'. *Philosophical Transactions of the Royal Society of London B* 359: 1383–1394.

Ryff, C. D. and Lachman, M. E. (2006). 'National Survey of Midlife Development in the United States (MIDUS II): Cognitive project, 2004–2006'. MIDUS—Midlife in the United States: A National Longitudinal Study of Health & Well-Being. http://www.icpsr.umich.edu/icpsrweb/ICPSR/series/203/studies/25281.

Ryff, C. D., Love, G. D., Urry, H. L., Muller, D., Rosenkranz, M. A., et al. (2006). 'Psychological Well-being and Ill-being: Do They Have Distinct or Mirrored Biological Correlates?' *Psychotherapy & Psychosomatics* 75: 85–95.

Ryff, C. D. and Singer, B. (2008). 'Know Thyself What You Are: A Eudaimonic Approach to Psychological Well-being'. *Journal of Happiness Studies* 9: 13–39.

Ryff, C. D. and Davidson, R. (2009). 'National Survey of Midlife Development in the United States (MIDUS II): Neuroscience Project'. MIDUS—Midlife in the United States: A National Longitudinal Study of Health & Well-Being. http://www.icpsr.umich.edu/icpsrweb/ICPSR/series/203/studies/28683.

Ryff, C. D. (2012). 'Understanding Positive Aging as an Integrated Biopsychosocial Process'. Institute on Aging, University of Wisconsin-Madison. http://aging.wisc.edu/research/affil.php?Ident=55.

Schwarzer, R. (2000). 'Manage Stress at Work through Preventive and Proactive Coping'. In E. A. Locke (ed.), *The Blackwell Handbook of Principles of Organizational Behavior* (pp. 342–355). Oxford: Blackwell.

Scottish Executive (2006). *Research Governance Framework for Health and Community Care* (2nd edn). Scottish Excecutive Health Department: n.p. http://www.cso.scot.nhs.uk/Publications/ResGov/Framework/RGFEdTwo.pdf.

Seligman, M. E. P. (1991). *Learned Optimism*. New York: Knopf.

Seligman, M. E. P. (2000). 'Positive Psychology: An Introduction'. *American Psychologist* 55(1): 5–14.

Seligman, M. E. P., Steen, T. A., Park, N., and Peterson, C. (2005). 'Positive Psychology Progress: Empirical Validation of Interventions'. *American Psychologist* 60: 410–421.

Seligman, M. E. P., Rashid, T., and Parks, A. C. (2006). 'Positive Psychotherapy'. *American Psychologist* 61: 774–788.

Seligman, M. E. P. (2008). 'Positive Health'. *Applied Psychology* 75: 3–18.

Seligman, M. E. P. (2011). *Flourish: A Visionary New Understanding of Happiness and Well-being*. New York: Free Press.

Sougleris, C. and Ranzijn, R. (2011). 'Proactive Coping in Community Dwelling Older Australians'. *International Journal of Aging and Human Development* 72(2): 155–168.

Strawbridge, W. J., Wallhagen, M. I., and Cohen, R. D. (2002). 'Successful Aging and Well Being: Who Can Be Characterized as Successfully Aged?' *Gerontologist* 42: 272–733.

Strongman, K. T. and Overston, A. E. (1999). 'Emotion in Late Adulthood'. *Australian Psychologist* 34(2): 104–110.

Tate, R. B., Leedine, L., and Cuddy, T. E. (2003). 'Definition of Successful Aging by Elderly Canadian Males: The Manitoba Follow-up Study'. *Gerontologist* 43: 735–744.

Thoits, P. A. and Hewitt, L. N. (2001). 'Volunteer Work and Well-being'. *Journal of Health and Social Behavior* 42(2): 115–131. doi: 10.2307/3090173.

Toffler, A. (1970). *Future Shock*. New York: Random House.

Turiano, N. A., Pitzer, L., Armour, C., Karlamangla, A., Ryff, C. D., et al. (2012). 'Personality Trait Level and Change as Predictors of Health Outcomes: Findings from a National Study of Americans (MIDUS)'. *The Journals of Gerontology Series B: Psychological Sciences and Social Science* 67(1): 4–12.

Vaillant, G. E. (2000). 'Adaptive Mental Mechanisms: Their Role in a Positive Psychology'. *American Psychologist* 55(1): 89–98.

Williamson, G. M. and Christie, J. (2009). 'Aging Well in the 21st Century: Challenges and Opportunities'. In C. R. Snyder and S. J. Lopez (eds), *Oxford Handbook of Positive Psychology* (pp. 65–170). New York: Oxford University Press.

Windle, G., Markland, D. A., and Woods, B. (2008). 'Examination of a Theoretical Model of Psychological Resilience in Older Age'. *Aging & Mental Health* 12(3): 285–292.

Windle, G., Woods, R. T., and Markland, D. A. (2010). 'Living with Ill-health in Older Age: The Role of a Resilient Personality'. *Journal of Happiness Studies* 11: 763–777.

World Health Organization (2004). *Promoting Mental Health: Concepts, Emerging Evidence, Practice* (Summary report). Geneva: World Health Organization.

CHAPTER 45

BARRIERS TO MENTAL HEALTHCARE UTILIZATION

CANDACE KONNERT AND
ANA PETROVIC-POLJAK

INTRODUCTION

I (CK) read a chapter that reviewed psychological service barriers when I was a budding geropsychologist (Gatz et al. 1985). It influenced me greatly. Now over twenty-five years have passed. Some barriers have been reduced (e.g. attitudes towards mental health utilization), but others have been woefully neglected (e.g. rural populations). Few studies have examined the broad range of psychological service barriers applicable to older adults. The purpose of this chapter is to evaluate progress towards reducing these barriers. Our goal with respect to barriers to mental healthcare utilization in older persons is to provide an overview of the current literature, highlight gaps in that literature, and highlight unique and innovative programmes for which there is empirical support.

CLIENT VARIABLES

Stigma

Do older adults hold more negative views of mental illness compared to younger adults? To date, findings have been inconsistent. Angermeyer and Dietrich (2006: 170) reviewed research between 1990 and 2004, examining age differences in attitudes towards people with mental illness. This comprehensive literature review included studies from a broad range of primarily European countries and included thirty-three national and twenty-nine local and regional samples. Studies focused on both mental illness in general and specific mental health problems, including severe and persistent disorders. They reported that negative attitudes were positively associated with age in thirty-two studies, negatively associated with age in one study, with no relationship found in ten studies. Other research from

North America failed to find age differences in stigma (Cook and Wang 2010; Pepin, Segal, and Coolidge 2009; Segal et al. 2005). Yet, as part of the Changing Minds campaign in Great Britain, a population survey of 1725 individuals was conducted in 1998 and again in 2003. In both surveys, the most negative views were held by those between the ages of 16 and 19 for six of the seven mental health problems that were included (Crisp et al. 2005). In part, these inconsistent results may have to do with the multidimensional nature of stigma and different methods of assessment. For example, Segal et al. (2005: 365) found that older adults believed that those with mental illness had poorer social and interpersonal skills (e.g. were more embarrassing or untrustworthy), yet did not differ from younger respondents regarding beliefs about incurability or dangerousness.

As Angermeyer and Dietrich (2006: 170) indicated, the extent to which age differences in stigma represent an ageing or cohort effect remains unknown. If they are due to a cohort effect, one might hope that future generations would hold less stigmatizing views due to clinical, research, and policy initiatives on stigma reduction. Pescosolido et al. (2010: 1321–1330) analysed data from the 1996 and 2006 General Social Survey to determine whether attitudes towards those with schizophrenia, depression, and alcohol dependence had changed over time. They found that, although respondents were more likely to endorse neurobiological explanations for these disorders, this did not lead to decreases in stigma. Levels of stigma remained high and, in fact, increased for some stigma indicators for schizophrenia and alcohol dependence (Pescosolido et al. 2010: 1323). Moreover, stigma against persons with Alzheimer's disease and their family members has been reported in numerous studies by Werner and colleagues (Werner and Giveon 2008; Werner and Heinik 2008) and is a significant predictor of care-giver burden (Werner et al. 2012). Thus, the 1990s Decade of the Brain, with its increased emphasis on neurobiological and genetic aetiologies, does not appear to have had an impact on stigmatizing attitudes. These data attest to the pervasiveness, stability, and negative consequences of these attitudes and suggest the continued importance of stigma reduction campaigns for future cohorts of older adults.

Ideally, stigma reduction efforts should involve inter-agency collaborations. In the Canadian context, the Canadian Coalition for Seniors' Mental Health is partnering with the Mental Health Commission of Canada (MMCC) to better understand the unique needs and experiences of stigma in the older population. Building on the Technical Consensus Statement produced by the Old Age Psychiatry section of the World Psychiatric Association and the World Health Organization (Graham et al. 2003), and the conceptual model of Link and Phelan (2001), Canadian researchers are engaged in a programme of research investigating the unique needs and experience of stigma among older adults. Recognizing that anti-stigma efforts must target multiple stakeholders, initial work has focused on surveying health providers in the ageing sector. Preliminary data suggest that more than half of respondents did not have anti-stigma programmes in place, and over one-third indicated that they simply had not thought of it. Thus, there is much to be done in the area of stigma reduction among healthcare professionals working with older adults (Wilson 2012). Although stigma continues to be prevalent in society in general, research suggests that it is not the most significant barrier to help-seeking among older adults and that other factors may more strongly account for patterns of under-utilization (Mackenzie, Pagura, and Sareen 2010; Mackenzie et al. 2008; Pepin et al. 2009).

Perception of need and attitudes towards mental health treatment

What are the strongest predictors of mental heath service use among older adults? There is considerable support in the literature for perceived need as the strongest predictor of mental health service use among older adults (Karlin, Duffy, and Gleaves 2008), including those with anxiety disorders and symptoms (Scott et al. 2010). There is also compelling evidence from two studies with large, nationally representative samples that older adults have lower levels of perceived need compared to their younger counterparts (Karlin et al. 2008; Mackenzie et al. 2010). Similarly, Garrido et al. (2009: 707) reported that, in their sample of adults 65 years and older, perceived need was lower among those of advanced age. Even among older adults who had a psychiatric diagnosis (mood, anxiety, or substance-related disorder), only 47% perceived a need for treatment, with the majority of these (69.2%) citing a preference for 'handling problems themselves' (Mackenzie et al. 2010). This tendency was also observed by Garrido et al. (2011: 53), who reported that, of those who indicated a perceived need for care but delayed seeking that care for at least a month, 75.4% wanted to handle the problem on their own. However, results are preliminary because, although both studies involved large datasets of older adults, these findings are based on small sub-samples of thirty-six (Mackenzie et al. 2010) and forty-three (Garrido et al. 2011) who met the inclusionary diagnostic criteria and perceived a need for care.

In one of the largest studies to date, Garrido et al. (2009: 704–712) used the Collaborative Psychiatric Epidemiology Survey to assess the correlates of perceived need among 1339 adults, 65 years of age and older (mean age of 74.6 years), residing in the community. Consistent with the findings of Mackenzie et al. (2010: 1103–1115), only half of the respondents who met diagnostic criteria for major depressive disorder (MDD) or generalized anxiety disorder (GAD) within the past year perceived a need for care. Overall, perceived need was highest among those who met criteria for MDD or GAD; however, subthreshold GAD and the number of symptoms of depression and anxiety were also significantly related to greater perceived need. Alcohol abuse and/or dependence was associated with greater perceived need among those with a diagnosis of GAD but not MDD within the past year. Lifetime occurrence of chronic health problems was associated with greater perceived need but measures of general health were not, suggesting that those who have a history of interacting with health systems are more likely to perceive a need for mental healthcare.

How do older adults view mental health services? A growing body of literature suggests that older adults have generally favourable views (James and Buttle 2008; Mackenzie, Gekoski, and Knox 2006; Woodward and Pachana 2009) and that there are no age differences in the willingness to seek out professional psychological help (Segal et al. 2005). Using the National Comorbidity Survey Replication, Mackenzie et al. (2008: 1014) found that over 80% of adults 55 and older held positive help-seeking attitudes. The most positive views were held by the first wave of the baby boom generation (ages 55 to 64), who were almost three times as likely to endorse positive views compared to young adults (ages 18 to 24). However, for the total sample, those with a diagnosed mood or anxiety disorder held the most negative views within the past year. Mackenzie et al. (2006: 577) found that never-married older adults were most likely to be open to seeking help. In addition, Mackenzie et al. (2010: 1110) found that, in their sample of older adults, advanced age was related to help seeking. Among those who were 75 years and older, very few who perceived a need did not seek help for it, indicating a significant age difference between the young-old and old-old. Further research is needed to better understand the relationship between perception of need and help seeking, and why this may be stronger among the very old.

While these results are encouraging, it is important to emphasize that these samples of older adults tend to be better educated, healthier, and ethnically homogeneous. Furthermore, these data suggest that many older adults with mental health problems do not perceive a need for care and may have more negative attitudes towards psychological services. This is consistent with the findings of Crabb and Hunsley (2006: 306), who reported that depressed older adults under-utilize mental health services.

Mental health literacy

Can those who work with older adults recognize a mental health problem? An important initiative that is vital to overcoming barriers to mental health utilization is the training of those individuals who interact with older adults in the course of their daily activities, for example, those working in the continuum of medical and supportive services that are available to older adults. Australia is the leader in mental health literacy, defined as 'knowledge and beliefs about mental disorders which aid in their recognition, management, or prevention' (Jorm et al. 1997: 182). The Mental Health First Aid Training (MHFA) and Research Program was developed in Australia to promote mental health literacy, and has been adapted for implementation in fifteen other countries (Jorm and Kitchener 2011). Jorm (2012: 238), in his review of evaluated programmes, states 'there is good evidence that the mental health literacy of a whole community can be improved'. However, these programmes typically involve community campaigns (e.g. *beyondblue* in Australia), or outreach to younger adults, cultural minorities, or people in developing countries. There is tremendous potential for extending mental health literacy programmes to older adults, their family members, and those who work with seniors. For example, direct care workers are in a pivotal position to benefit from mental health literacy training, as they are important gatekeepers in the detection of mental health problems among frail and isolated seniors, a particularly vulnerable group. To the best of our knowledge, Singapore is the only country to offer Mental Health First Aid with a specific focus on the older person (http://www.mhfa. com.sg/mhfa-op.html). The ability to recognize the signs and symptoms of a mental health problem is the first step in getting appropriate assessment and treatment for older adults.

THERAPIST VARIABLES

Attitudes towards older adults

To what extent are attitudes towards older adults significant barriers to mental health treatment? There are two broad categories of barriers. First, mental health professionals who begin working with older adults may be concerned about how much specialized knowledge is needed. Concerns about competency may lead to a general reluctance to engage older adults in clinical practice. Competency tools such as the Pikes Peak measure and the recognition of geropsychology as a proficiency area of practice by the American Psychological Association in 2010 are positive steps towards overcoming this barrier. Furthermore, there are a variety of ways of integrating geropsychology content into pre-doctoral training programmes in clinical psychology (Qualls et al. 2010).

Second, therapists' and societal attitudes about older adults' prognosis and worthiness have been viewed as significant barriers, particularly in light of the severe scarcity of mental health resources and many competing at-risk groups, including children. In 2002, a review by Robb, Chen, and Haley (1–12) indicated that older adults are treated differently by the medical system, for example, in terms of screening and access to treatment. However it was unclear whether this was due to an age bias or other factors. There have been surprisingly few studies of age bias among mental health professionals, and those that have been carried out primarily utilize vignette methodologies. Collectively, these studies suggest that age bias does not appear to influence the diagnostic process, at least in the case of depression, but that it does contribute to more negative attitudes towards treatment and perceptions of poorer prognosis among US psychologists and trainees and Australian psychologists and counsellors (Helmes and Gee 2003; Meeks 1990). Interestingly, when asked directly about barriers to mental healthcare, both younger and older adults ranked ageism as the least influential barrier (Pepin et al. 2009).

Although age biases are often thought of as negative, equally important are positive biases. Knight (2010: 109–110) discussed the role of positive ageing stereotypes among supervisees and suggested that therapists in training (and even more experienced therapists) may have difficulty identifying substance abuse or cognitive impairment in a client. These biases may prevent older adults from getting the help that they need and are potentially just as serious as negative biases. More generally, students are attracted to clinical geropsychology because they truly like and care about older adults and this may contribute to 'blind spots', whereby they tend to view their clients through the lens of positive stereotypes of ageing. Knight (2010: 113–114) also noted that older trainees or therapists that feel negatively about their own ageing may convey an inappropriately positive view of age-related losses, minimizing the impact they have on older clients.

Training issues

Are we making progress towards addressing the well-documented lack of trained professionals in geriatric mental health (Institute of Medicine 2012)? There have been significant developments in the area of education and training, most notably the development of the Pikes Peak model of training in geropsychology (Knight et al. 2009) and the associated measure of competency, the Pikes Peak Geropsychology Knowledge and Skill Assessment Tool (Karel et al. 2012a). This tool was recently used in an online survey of 764 clinical and counselling graduate students in the US, Canada, Australia, and New Zealand (Woodhead et al. 2013). Approximately 80% of respondents indicated that they anticipated working with older adults in the future; self-rated competencies were positively and significantly related to ageing-related course work, practicum hours with older clients, and greater faculty with ageing-related interests. Exposure to course work and clinical practica in ageing have consistently been found to predict interest in working with this population in both psychology (Koder and Helmes 2008; Pachana et al. 2010) and social work trainees (Cummings and Galambos 2002). The barriers that were most often cited to providing additional training were an inability to recruit staff and difficulties in finding appropriate practicum experiences.

Not only is there a marked lack of mental health professionals trained to work with older adults, the training that they do receive appears to reflect the broader trend towards the assessment and diagnosis of cognitive disorders to the neglect of treatment, in spite of the demonstrated efficacy of many psychological interventions. For example, geropsychology training in accredited clinical and counselling internship programmes in Canada provides more training on diagnosis and assessment and less on individual psychotherapy with older adults (Konnert, Dobson, and Watt 2009). Of those internships with geropsychology rotations, only 47.6% of US and 63.6% of Canadian sites offered individual psychotherapy training experiences (Pachana et al. 2010). Opportunities for this type of experience were significantly higher in Australia, with 85.7% of training sites reporting that they offered this training.

One of the exciting training developments has been the growth of doctoral programmes that offer training in primary care settings, for example, at the University of Colorado at Colorado Springs (Novotney 2012) and Yeshiva University (Zweig, Siegel, and Snyder 2006). In the US, the federally sponsored Graduate Psychology Education programme provides funds to train geropsychology doctoral students in primary care, and preliminary data are very promising. In short, 'geropsychology training in primary care represents a win-win opportunity for doctoral psychology programmes, physicians and healthcare systems, and older adults in need of services' (Zweig et al. 2006: 27). These programmes are particularly effective at targeting older adults of minority status, a group that experiences significant barriers to mental healthcare. Increasingly, psychologists and other mental health providers will work in diverse settings that serve older adults, each with their own unique organizational structures. Currently, setting-specific competencies are considered a core aspect of training in geropsychology competencies (Knight et al. 2009).

Mental Health System Variables

Knight and Sayegh (2011: 228–243) described the fragmented, multisystem network of mental healthcare for older adults in the US and the historical factors that influenced its development. The various systems of care include specialty mental health, acute medical, long-term, dementia, and substance abuse. Often these systems have conflicting cultures, policies, and procedures, and compete for limited funding. Moreover, services are delivered as if one size fits all, with no recognition that older adults have diverse mental health needs. For example, those with chronic mental illness have very different needs from those with late-onset disorders.

Concerns about access

Can older people find a therapist? In the spring of 2006, the Committee on Aging of the Group for the Advancement of Psychiatry collaborated with Jeanne Phillips, the author of the daily column 'Dear Abby', the most widely syndicated in the world with more than

10 000 letters and e-mails per week (Koh et al. 2010). In her column, she solicited information about, 'how older people feel about mental health problems, where you seek help for them, what you feel needs to be done to improve services, and whether you'd like more mental health services than you are getting now' (Koh et al. 2010: 1146). Of the over eight hundred replies received, the overwhelming concern was access to a mental health professional. While this was not a particularly scientific study, the results reflect those of Pepin et al. (2009: 774), who reported that on the Barriers to Mental Health Services Scale, the subscale 'belief about inability to find a psychotherapist' was the highest and second to highest ranked barrier for older and younger adults respectively. Also ranked highly were concerns about a psychotherapist's qualifications, a very realistic perception given the shortage of mental health providers with specialized training. Similarly, among older adults with a perceived need for mental healthcare, concerns about where to go or who to see were ranked as the first (Karlin et al. 2008) and second (Mackenzie et al. 2010) most significant barriers.

Knight and Shurgot (2008: 454) made the case that future cohorts of older adults will be more likely to seek psychological services and Mackenzie et al. (2008: 1016) reported that the first wave of baby boomers (ages 55–64) held the most favourable attitudes towards mental health seeking. In addition, the baby boom cohort may be more sophisticated in terms of their understanding of the efficaciousness of psychological treatments. Therefore, concerns about access will not only include finding competent and trained providers, but also obtaining evidence-based treatments. Gatz (2007: 52–53) described evidence hurdles, those issues that research has failed to address well. These include an absence of literature but also issues that are relevant to the efficacy–effectiveness continuum, that is, moving from the lab to the real-world delivery of interventions (e.g. sampling, comorbidity, fidelity) where contextual factors play an important role in the delivery of psychological interventions to older adults.

There is also a pressing need to disseminate evidence-based interventions more widely to older adults, and, globally, health agencies have a strong commitment (both at the policy level and with dedicated funding) to supporting knowledge uptake and translational activities. The World Health Organization's (WHO) recent publication provides a framework for knowledge translation in ageing and health, including 'push' and 'pull' strategies for promoting evidence-based practice (WHO 2012). Many of these strategies have great potential for overcoming barriers to the uptake of evidence-based psychological interventions with older adults. Eli (2006: 121–125) provides a comprehensive review of the barriers depressed older adults face in seeking evidence-based care, and provides useful strategies for translating research into practice.

Recently, Ward et al. (2012: 298) argued that conceptualizations of knowledge translation need to go beyond simply examining barriers and enablers in the relationship between research and practice. Their qualitative data examined how knowledge exchange unfolded in real time within three service delivery teams in a mental health organization in the UK. Ward et al. (2012: 302) make the important point that knowledge uptake is a process that is highly contextual and that 'context' has typically been narrowly defined. More broadly, knowledge uptake is a social and political process that involves, among other things, a good understanding of norms, professional identities, and individual beliefs. As clinical geropsychologists continue to deliver services in a variety of contexts, it will become important to better understand these contexts in order to facilitate the knowledge uptake of evidence-based psychological treatments. For example, long-term care residents are among the most underserved older adults in terms of their mental health needs. If depression is viewed as normative in these environments and if those who work in long-term care do not see themselves as mental health providers, then the probability that evidence-based mental health treatments will be provided is low.

Integrated models of care

It is now widely recognized that integrated models of care are the wave of the future, as outlined in the document *Blueprint for Change: Achieving Integrated Health Care for an Aging Population* (American Psychological Association 2008). Mackenzie et al. (2006: 579) and James and Buttle (2008: 38) reported that older adults were more likely to seek psychological help from a primary care physician than a mental health professional. Unfortunately, the mental healthcare they receive in primary care settings is often inadequate (Moak 2011). As noted by Karel et al. (2012b: 189–190) and Moak (2011: 278–280), mental healthcare is particularly effective when integrated into primary and community care, and they provide examples of evaluated programmes designed to treat a range of mental health problems in these contexts. (See also Armento and Stanley on psychological interventions in primary care settings in this Handbook.)

In a randomized trial, Bartels et al. (2004: 1455–1462) compared integrated mental healthcare with enhanced referral to specialty mental health clinics among 2022 patients (mean age 73.5 years) with depression, anxiety, or at-risk alcohol use, across ten sites. Various indices of treatment engagement clearly indicated the superiority of integrated care. Comparing integrated to specialized care respectively, 71% vs 49% of clients made at least one visit, and mean number of visits was 3.04 vs 1.91. In addition, two particularly important findings emerged from the data. First, the integrated model appeared to function particularly well for individuals with at-risk alcohol use and those with active suicidal ideation. Second, treatment engagement was positively related to closer proximity of mental health/substance use services to primary care. Bartels et al. (2004: 1460) suggested that integration should be viewed along a continuum across multiple dimensions that involve not only physical proximity but also temporal proximity, communication, and collaboration across health and mental health providers, range of mental health services, and the degree to which billing for physical and mental health services can be coordinated and streamlined.

The first step in integrated care involves enhanced outreach and referral capacity. In Singapore, the Community-based Early Psychiatric Interventional Strategy (CEPIS) utilized community outreach strategies at seventy-six sites, including active screening programmes, psychoeducation, and case manager support to enhance access and primary care referrals for depression among seniors (Nyunt et al. 2009). Of the 4633 participants (mean age 73.7), 370 screened positive for depression. Of these, fewer than a quarter perceived a need for help and, in the past year, only 10.3% sought treatment. The CEPIS outreach strategies improved the rate of referral for further assessment and treatment to 73.8%. The majority of the referrals were for older adults with subsyndromal depression, a group that is at high risk for major depressive disorder. Notably, the study sample was comprised of older individuals (aged 70+) who were of lower socio-economic status and in poor health, a group that is at greater risk of mental health problems and an important target group for preventive interventions.

On a cautionary note, Moak (2011: 279–280) suggests that integrated care is not suitable for all mental health problems and some older adults with more severe problems may need more intensive services. In addition, integrating mental healthcare into primary care will only be successful if staffed by mental health professionals with geriatric training. The workforce shortage and acute funding deficits in primary care limit the potential for new and innovative programmes such as integrated care. In the US, recent changes to reimbursement plans increased payment to some primary care providers while at the same time reduced fees for specialized providers, in particular those with geriatric mental health training. As stated by Moak (2011:281), 'the detrimental impact of this on the development of geriatric mental health services cannot be underestimated'.

Often overlooked in this discussion is the fact that many older adults with serious mobility problems or lack of transportation are unable to benefit from mental health treatment in primary care or specialized programmes. Davitt and Gellis (2011: 314–315) discussed the complexities of providing mental health services through Medicare home care benefits in the US, identifying two specific barriers. First, mental health is assessed in the context of a much longer and more burdensome evaluation protocol (i.e. the Outcome and Assessment Information Set–C) and the mental health items lack sensitivity and specificity. Furthermore, those administering the items may lack sufficient training in mental health screening. Second, Medicare policy restricts the provision of mental health services to psychiatrically trained nurses, effectively reducing access to other potential mental health providers, such as social workers. This policy essentially serves to curtail costs and ultimately restricts the availability of mental health services to homebound older adults. Davitt and Gellis (2011: 317–320) provide recommendations in the practice, policy, and research arenas that have the potential to improve access to care. For example, social workers (or other mental health professionals) could train those doing home care assessments in detecting mental health problems and making appropriate referrals. They could also be more involved in providing treatment to home care clients, a particularly important initiative given that many home health agencies do not have psychiatric nurses on staff, especially in rural areas.

SPECIAL POPULATIONS

Older populations in rural areas

The proportion of older adults living in rural areas is growing due to the global increase of persons reaching old age and the increasing urban migration of younger people from rural areas (Kaufman et al. 2007). Jameson and Blank (2007: 284–287) provide an excellent overview of the problems facing rural residents of all ages who need mental healthcare. These problems are particularly acute among older rural residents. Barriers to care can be broadly grouped into poor availability, limited accessibility, and acceptability of mental health services (see Figure 45.1, Fox, Merwin, and Blank 1995).

In addition to these barriers, the heterogeneity of rural older persons is rarely addressed. Characteristics such as race, ethnicity, religion, socio-economic status, distance from urban centres, and population density differ significantly between, and even within, rural communities, which create subgroups of individuals that experience unique challenges (Kaufman

ACCESSIBILITY
Geographic location
Transportation
Inability to afford services
AVAILABILITY
Services
Trained professionals
Funding
ACCEPTABILITY
Stigma
Cultural values
Issues of confidentiality and multiple relationships

FIGURE 45.1 The three As of barriers to mental healthcare for older populations in rural areas.

et al. 2007). Focus groups conducted in Canadian rural communities revealed four types of rural older persons: community active, stoic, frail, and marginalized, and each had different perceptions of and needs for services (Keating and Eales 2012). This type of information offers essential and practical strategies for the development of effective mental health services to meet diverse needs in rural communities. All too often, programmes that work in urban settings are assumed to be equally effective in rural settings; however, this top-down approach fails to appreciate the distinct social and cultural milieux within rural environments. In contrast, bottom-up approaches have greater potential to create programmes that are more palatable to older adults living in rural areas and may be more sustainable in these environments (Bull et al. 2001).

An innovative approach was employed by the ElderLynk programme, which served to link existing mental health and social services with primary care providers and provided geriatric mental health education to professionals and the general public (McGovern et al. 2008). The researchers employed a community-based participatory research process that included community partners and stakeholders (e.g. local practitioners, community members) in the development, implementation, and evaluation of the programme. Although not without its challenges, this approach assisted in bringing together mental health providers, enhanced cooperation and increased community involvement, and may serve as a useful model for creating culturally sensitive, community-specific services (Blevins, Morton, and McGovern 2008).

Furthermore, there is a strong need for the evaluation of innovative service delivery among rural older cohorts in order to inform practice and research, as presently outcome evaluations of programmes in place fail to be conducted or appropriately disseminated. Kaufman and colleagues (2007: 355–361) employed a helpful strategy by sharing the challenges their team encountered in recruitment (e.g. irregular referrals, suspicious attitudes) and provision of services (e.g. travel time, illiteracy, stigma, poverty) as part of the Project to Enhance Aged Rural Living that examined the effectiveness of providing cognitive-behaviour therapy (CBT) to older adults living in such areas. By sharing the challenges they encountered, and how they accommodated for them, the authors effectively disseminated implications for practice and research. Within a limited population of researchers and service providers that specialize in geriatric rural mental health, such open and active discourse is particularly essential to allow for significant progress in the design, evaluation, and provision of mental health services to rural older adults.

Telehealth and rural older adults

Technology-based service delivery methods (e.g. telephone, email, videoconferencing, website access), referred to as telehealth, have increased access to cost-effective, high-quality mental healthcare for older persons living in rural areas, and have provided many creative possibilities for providing care (Buckwalter et al. 2002). Most notably, assessment and treatment via telehealth have proven comparable to face-to-face approaches among older adults, with similar patient satisfaction (Mitka 2003).

What types of telehealth programmes are available for rural older adults and/or their care-givers? The University of California Davis Medical Center eMental Health Consultation Service serves as a comprehensive 'virtual mental health clinic' that successfully provides psychiatric (i.e. medication consultation) and psychological (e.g. brief solution-focused therapy and CBT) clinical services, as well as consultations and education to rural primary care clinics through telehealth, secure email, and telephone (Neufeld et al. 2007). Moreover, telepsychiatry consultations for depression and dementia-related behaviour problems have been employed in a rural nursing facility (Johnston and Jones 2001), with the ability to respond promptly to residents' clinical needs, efficient use of consultants' time, greater follow-through of recommendations, and high levels of family and resident satisfaction with the quality of care provided. Computerized therapy programmes, whereby therapy interventions are presented on a computer in place of face-to-face contact with a therapist, are also being evaluated. A four-year prospective randomized controlled trial is currently underway comparing the effectiveness of evidence-based treatments for depression in older persons delivered via in-home videophone or traditional face-to-face services in such rural areas (Egede et al. 2009). Furthermore, use of telehealth in long-term care (LTC) facilities may have an even greater role than in community settings, as the LTC sector is generally disconnected from specialist services, including mental health services. Notably, many of the services that are provided on site in urban LTC facilities can be provided via telehealth to rural LTC facilities (Gray et al. 2012: 145). The use of telehealth in such settings would also be more economically viable as multiple residents, staff, and family members could use the same equipment (Gray et al. 2012).

In addition to providing services to older adults, telehealth interventions have the potential to assist rural family care-givers, for example the Telehelp Line for Caregivers, which provides supportive services and resources through a call-in helpline and structured telephone counselling sessions (Dollinger and Chwalisz 2011). In addition, there is great potential for the use of internet-based intervention programmes for care-givers, which have yielded outcomes similar to those of face-to-face support groups (Marziali and Garcia 2011). Although use of technology with older persons raises concerns about technological skills, recent programmes have incorporated simplified computer training manuals and regular support, in addition to simplifying technology (e.g. using remote control devices), as well as making accommodations for individuals with cognitive, intellectual, and sensory deficits (Buckwalter et al. 2002). In addition to providing greater access to services, videoconferencing via the internet has also proven useful in enhancing professional development for isolated rural professionals by increasing access to clinical supervision, improved consultation, and training programmes to front-line staff (Troisi 2001).

Some challenges remain with the use of telehealth, such as inconsistent reimbursement and compensation by third-party payers, initial direct costs of technology equipment and software, perceived 'emotional distance' between consumers and providers, nervousness about using new technologies, problems with licensure, and weaker technological infrastructure of rural communities (Jameson and Blank 2007; Whitten 2001). A recent review of Medicare expenditure in Australia for psychiatric consultations showed that consultations delivered via videoconference are currently being under-utilized given the level of funding provided for such consultations (Smith et al. 2012:170). It is important to further examine the barriers to using telehealth as part of regular care. These include the infrastructure for using telehealth, such as equipment and software, as well as clinical and administrative support systems required to support telehealth in the clinical environment (Smith et al. 2012: 170). Furthermore, the quality of research examining the clinical effectiveness of use of telehealth with older adults has been limited and there is a great need for more robust studies and randomized controlled trials (Brignell, Wootton, and Gray 2007). Much of this research has addressed a limited number of questions and is frequently focused on user acceptance and reliability (Edirippulige et al. 2013). Future studies should examine telehealth interventions more broadly and avoid focusing on a single aspect of care provided by a given specialty. For example, many studies examining telehealth in LTC focus generally on the reliability of dementia diagnoses provided by psychiatry (Edirippulige et al. 2013).

Overall, with the proliferation of technology in our society, and the increasing familiarity with technology among baby boomers, it is likely that telehealth will receive increased acceptance and use among providers and consumers. Although further evaluation of the efficacy and effectiveness of telehealth in service provision for older persons in rural areas is needed, this service modality holds significant promise.

Ethnic minority groups

Surveys that address barriers to mental healthcare utilization among older adults often do not include ethnic minorities, but report on samples that are almost exclusively Caucasian,

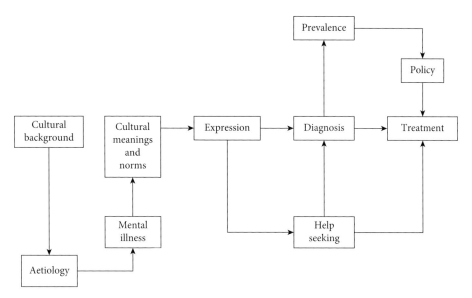

FIGURE 45.2 The Cultural Influences on Mental Health (CIMH) model.

in spite of the fact that older persons from minority backgrounds are at greater risk for mental health problems and are less likely to utilize mental health services (Sorkin, Pham, and Ngo-Metzger 2009). Reasons for under-utilization are complex and varied, and must be understood in the context of conceptual frameworks, such as the Cultural Influences on Mental Health Model (see Figure 45.2; Hwang et al. 2008). These authors provide an excellent overview of the multiple pathways and barriers to help seeking among culturally diverse groups, recognizing the unique influences of immigration background (e.g. refugees), acculturation and enculturation, racism and discrimination, socio-economic status, stigma, and attitudes/beliefs that are unique to specific groups. In general, the literature on barriers to mental healthcare among older ethnic minority groups is very sparse.

Much of the research has focused on older Asian populations, reflecting the increased numbers of Asian immigrants in many countries. For example, in Canada from 1981 to 2006, the percentage of visible minorities grew from 4.7% to 16.2% of Canada's total population, with Asians and South Asians comprising the two largest groups (Natural Resources Canada 2009). By 2017, this percentage is expected to increase from 19% to 23%, depending on the growth scenario utilized (Statistics Canada 2005). This, coupled with an ageing population, has led to a significant increase in the number of older Asians living in Canada. Moreover, the prevalence of depressive symptoms among older Chinese-Canadians is twice as high as estimates in the general older Canadian population (Lai 2000), a finding that is consistent with US data (Mui and Kang 2006).

The literature on barriers to mental healthcare among Asian older adults has focused on mental health literacy, the expression of psychological distress, acculturation and enculturation, and cultural attitudes and beliefs. Using a case vignette methodology, depression literacy was found to be poorer among older (mean age = 70) Chinese immigrants compared to a population-based survey of Canadian-born older adults, with 11.3% and 74% respectively correctly identifying depression (Tieu, Konnert, and Wang 2010). In addition, the majority (52.8%) of Chinese older persons believed that the person depicted in the vignette would fully or partially recover from depression without receiving professional help, in contrast to 9.4% of Canadian-born older adults. General practitioners were viewed as helpful by 43.4% of Chinese participants and 89.3% of Canadian-born participants. There is some evidence that Chinese people express distress somatically; however, not all research supports this finding (Ryder et al. 2008). Cultural differences in the expression of depression may account, in part, for the low recognition of depression in the vignette. In addition, significantly more Chinese older adults endorsed the views that full or partial recovery from depression would occur without professional intervention and that general practitioners were not particularly helpful (Tieu et al. 2010). These beliefs may act as significant barriers to help seeking among older Chinese persons. This is particularly true given that general practitioners are the major treatment providers for mental health problems and act as gatekeepers to the mental health system in Canada.

In a study specifically designed to assess attitudes towards seeking mental health services, 150 Chinese-Canadian immigrants, mean age 74 years (range = 55 to 95 years), were interviewed in either Mandarin or Cantonese using the Inventory of Attitudes toward Seeking Mental Health Services (IASMHS) scale (Mackenzie et al. 2004; Tieu and Konnert 2012). Participants who were younger, married, and proficient in English reported significantly more positive attitudes towards seeking mental health services, as did those with more perceived social support. The results of this study clearly indicate the importance of English literacy in attitudes towards mental health services, and the need for providing mental health services in multiple languages. The results also reinforce the challenges associated with changing attitudinal barriers among older Chinese adults with less perceived support who are not married, as these individuals may be most vulnerable to mental health problems.

Other factors that may act as barriers to mental health services include acculturation/enculturation and attitudes and beliefs. Models of acculturation have become more complex, recognizing the dual processes of acculturation (i.e. adopting the cultural norms of the dominant society) and enculturation (i.e. retaining the norms of the indigenous culture) (Ryder, Alden, and Paulus 2000). Where older adults fall on these two dimensions may have significant implications for their attitudes about mental healthcare utilization and their willingness to access these resources. Moreover, because family members are often pivotal in helping older adults access the mental health system, their acculturation/enculturation may also play a role, with a potential for conflict if, for example, the younger generation is more accepting of mental health services but these attitudes are not shared by older generations.

Beliefs and values of the indigenous culture also play a significant role. For example, traditional Chinese medicine takes a holistic view, integrating mind, body, and spirit with an emphasis on balance in life and harmony with nature (Lai and Surood 2009). Psychiatric illnesses have been attributed to ghosts, evil spirits, infection, injuries, intoxication, nutritional deficiency, somatic illness, and congenital factors. As a result, there may be different pathways to seeking help among older Chinese persons, for example alternative and complementary approaches. Confucianism, Taoism, and Buddhism heavily influence Chinese beliefs, and cultural values such as *filial piety* and the *preservation of face* may play a significant role in accessing mental health services. To date, research in this area has focused on younger Chinese adults (e.g. Yang, Phelan, and Link 2008), with virtually no attention paid to how these factors may influence access to mental healthcare among older adults across a variety of ethnic backgrounds.

Implications for Practice

What do practitioners need to know? Perceiving a need for mental healthcare is the best determinant of accessing care. Mental health literacy initiatives are important because they aid in the detection and recognition of mental health problems, potentially increasing perceptions of need. For those who are reluctant to seek help, providing information that many mental health disorders are very treatable with time-limited and focused interventions may also increase the likelihood of seeking help. In addition, older adults have generally favourable views of mental health services. However, they are concerned about how to find a therapist who is qualified and familiar with issues that are relevant to them. It is not uncommon for mental health professionals to advertise specific areas of expertise and populations of interest (depression, children and adolescence) within their practice domains. If mental health professionals have an interest in and familiarity with working with older adults, this information should be advertised and broadly disseminated to venues and in ways that are most likely to reach older adults (e.g. seniors' magazines, seniors' centres, primary care physicians, etc.). Most importantly, a consistent theme in the geropsychology literature is the need to embed mental health services into places where older adults are. Thus, practitioners need to think creatively about how to work within the continuum of services for older adults, and increase their visibility in settings where older adults live, work or volunteer, and engage in recreation.

Summary

One of the exciting, yet challenging aspects of being a gerontologist is thinking about how what we know today will translate to future cohorts of older persons. How can we overcome barriers to mental healthcare both now and in the future? Several findings from this review suggest some promising avenues of research. First, the literature strongly suggests that perceived need is the best predictor of mental health service use (Karlin et al. 2008; Scott et al. 2010) and that younger adults have greater levels of perceived need than older adults (Mackenzie et al. 2010). Although these findings are cross-sectional, it is likely that future cohorts will perceive a need for mental health services. Educational campaigns are promising. There is strong evidence that mental health literacy campaigns are effective for whole communities and countries, such as Australia, Germany, and Norway (Jorm 2012). Recognition of need is the first step but mental health literacy also encompasses knowledge of evidence-based treatments, the qualifications and skills to look for in a mental health therapist, and effective self-help strategies. It also has clear links to universal and/or targeted prevention strategies. The question remains how best to capitalize on the success of mental health literacy efforts to overcome barriers to mental healthcare among older adults, both now and in the future.

Second, what can we do to meet the growing demand for mental health treatment among future cohorts, particularly those older adults who are most vulnerable? Training initiatives focusing on core competencies in clinical geropsychology and assessment measures, such as the Pikes Peak tool, are welcome additions to the training landscape. The move towards setting-specific competencies is also laudable, and hopefully will extend to a wider variety of settings, with a greater availability of practicum and internship experiences in these settings. For example, Knight and Sayegh (2011: 238) suggest that religious institutions and prisons are emerging areas of practice for psychologists who are interested in working with older adults with serious mental health problems. Canadian researchers have begun developing interventions for homeless or marginally housed older people, many of whom have long-standing mental health issues (Ploeg et al. 2008). It is these groups that often experience the greatest barriers to mental healthcare.

In addition to broadening the range of training settings, attracting trainees who are multilingual would enhance the provision of mental health services to ethnic minority older persons. Training in telehealth interventions has tremendous potential to reach future cohorts of increasingly technologically sophisticated older adults, including those living in rural environments and isolated seniors. Perhaps most importantly, there needs to be an increased emphasis on how to address systemic barriers to mental healthcare for older adults and how to advocate for them. Karel et al. (2012b) provide several good examples of ageing policy and practice areas where psychologists have simply not been at the table. Learning how to be at the table and have a voice to affect broader change is an important skill that should be integrated into training curricula in clinical geropsychology.

Finally, overcoming barriers to implementing evidence-based treatments with older adults is an ongoing challenge. Evidence-based assessments and treatments are not uniformly embraced by all individuals and professions that work within systems of care for older adults. Even in environments that support evidence-based practice, there remains the question of how best to maintain fidelity while, at the same time, being flexible and adapting it to the context in which it is being delivered. Psychologists have been at the forefront of developing evidence-based practices, but less active in the area of knowledge translation. On a hopeful note, as psychologists become increasingly integrated into a variety of settings that serve older adults, their familiarity with these contexts will be highly beneficial in facilitating and promoting knowledge uptake of evidence-based practice.

KEY REFERENCES AND SOURCES FOR FURTHER READING

Bartels, S. J., Coakley, E. H., Zubritsky, C., Ware, J. H., Miles, K. M., et al. (2004). 'Improving Access to Geriatric Mental Health Services: A Randomized Trial Comparing Treatment Engagement with Integrated versus Enhanced Referral Care for Depression, Anxiety, and At-risk Alcohol Use'. *American Journal of Psychiatry* 161(8): 1455–1462.

Eli, K. (2006). 'Depression Care for the Elderly: Reducing Barriers to Evidence-based Practice'. *Home Health Care Services Quarterly* 25(1–2): 115–148.

Hwang, W., Myers, H. F., Abe-Kim, J., and Ting, J. Y. (2008). 'A Conceptual Paradigm for Understanding Culture's Impact on Mental Health: The Cultural Influences on Mental Health (CIMH) Model'. *Clinical Psychology Review* 28: 211–227.

Jameson, J. P. and Blank, M. B. (2007). 'The Role of Clinical Psychology In Rural Mental Health Services: Defining Problems and Developing Solutions'. *Clinical Psychology: Science and Practice* 14(3): 283–283.

Jorm, A. J. (2012). 'Mental Health Literacy: Empowering the Community to Take Action for Better Mental Health'. *American Psychologist* 67(3): 231–243.

Moak, G. S. (2011). 'Treatment of Late-life Mental Disorders in Primary Care: We Can Do a Better Job'. *Journal of Aging and Social Policy* 23(3): 274–285.

Nyunt, M. S. Z., Ko, S. M., Kumar, R., Fones, C., and Ng, T. P. (2009). 'Improving Treatment Access and Primary Care Referrals for Depression in a National Community-based Outreach Programme for the Elderly'. *International Journal of Geriatric Psychiatry* 24(11): 1267–1276.

References

American Psychological Association (2008). *Blueprint For Change: Achieving Integrated Health Care for an Aging Population.* http://www.apa.org/pi/aging/resources/guides/exec-summary. aspx.

Angermeyer, M. C. and Dietrich, S. (2006). 'Public Beliefs about and Attitudes towards People with Mental Illness: A Review of Population Studies'. *Acta Psychiatrica Scandinavica* 113(3): 163–179.

Bartels, S. J., Coakley, E. H., Zubritsky, C., Ware, J. H., Miles, K. M., et al. (2004). 'Improving Access to Geriatric Mental Health Services: A Randomized Trial Comparing Treatment Engagement with Integrated versus Enhanced Referral Care for Depression, Anxiety, and At-risk Alcohol Use'. *American Journal of Psychiatry* 161(8): 1455–1462.

Blevins, D., Morton, B., and McGovern, R. (2008). 'Evaluating a Community-based Participatory Research Project for Elderly Mental Healthcare in Rural America'. *Clinical Interventions in Aging* 3: 535–545.

Brignell, M., Wootton, R., and Gray, L (2007). 'The Application of Telemedicine to Geriatric Medicine'. *Age and Ageing* 36(4): 369–374.

Buckwalter, K. C., Davis, L. L., Wakefield, B. J., Kienzle, M. G., and Murray, M. A. (2002). 'Telehealth for Elders and their Caregivers in Rural Communities'. *Family and Community Health* 25: 31–40.

Bull, C. N., Krout, J. A., Rathbone-McCuan, E., and Shreffler, J. (2001). 'Access and Issues of Equity in Remote/Rural Areas'. *Journal of Rural Health* 17: 356–359.

Cook, T. M. and Wang, J. (2010). 'Descriptive Epidemiology of Stigma against Depression in a General Population Sample in Alberta'. *BMC Psychiatry* 10: 29–39.

Crabb, R. and Hunsley, J. (2006). 'Utilization of Mental Health Care Services among Older Adults with Depression'. *Journal of Clinical Psychology* 62(3): 299–312.

Crisp, A., Gelder, M., Goddard, E., and Meltzer, H. (2005). 'Stigmatization of People with Mental Illnesses: A Follow-up Study within the Changing Minds Campaign of the Royal College of Psychiatrists'. *World Psychiatry* 4(2): 106–113.

Cummings, S. M. and Galambos, C. (2002). 'Predictors of Graduate Social Work Students' Interest in Age-related Work'. *Journal of Gerontological Social Work* 39: 77–94.

Davitt, J. K. and Gellis, Z. D. (2011). 'Integrating Mental Health Parity for Homebound Older Adults under the Medicare Home Health Care Benefit'. *Journal of Gerontological Social Work* 54(3): 309–324.

Dollinger, S. C. and Chwalisz, K. (2011). 'Reaching Rural Caregivers with a Multicomponent Telehealth Intervention: The Telehelp Line for Caregivers'. *Professional Psychology: Research and Practice* 42: 528–534.

Edirippulige, S., Martin-Kahn, M., Beattie, E., Smith, A. C., and Gray, L. C. (2013). 'A Systematic Review of Telemedicine Services for Residents in Long Term Care Facilities'. *Journal of Telemedicine and Telecare.* (e-pub ahead of print).

Egede, L. E., Frueh, C. B., Richardson, L. K., Acierno, R., Mauldin, P. D., et al. (2009). 'Rationale and Design: Telepsychology Service Delivery for Depressed Elderly Veterans'. *Trials* 10(1): 22–35.

Eli, K. (2006). 'Depression Care for the Elderly: Reducing Barriers to Evidence-based Practice'. *Home Health Care Services Quarterly* 25(1–2): 115–148.

Fox, J., Merwin, E., and Blank, M. (1995). 'Defacto Mental Health Services in the Rural South'. *Journal of Health Care for the Poor and Underserved* 6: 434–468.

Garrido, M. M., Kane, R. L., Kaas, M., and Kane, R. A. (2009). 'Perceived Need for Mental Health Care among Community-dwelling Older Adults'. *Journal of Gerontology, Series B: Psychological Sciences* 64B(6): 704–712.

Garrido, M. M., Kane, R. L., Kaas, M., and Kane, R. A. (2011). 'Use of Mental Health Care by Community-dwelling Older Adults'. *Journal of the American Geriatrics Society* 59(1): 50–56.

Gatz, M., Popkin, S. J., Pino, C., and VandenBos, G. R. (1985). 'Psychological Interventions with Older Adults'. In J. E. Birren and K. W. Schaie (eds), *Handbook of the Psychology of Aging* (2nd edn; pp. 755–785). New York: Van Nostrand Reinhold.

Gatz, M. (2007). 'Commentary on Evidence-based Psychological Treatments for Older Adults'. *Psychology and Aging* 22(1): 52–55.

Graham, N., Lindesay, J., Katona, C., Bertolote, J. M., Camus, V., et al., (2003). 'Reducing Stigma and Discrimination against Older People with Mental Disorders: A Technical Consensus Statement'. *International Journal of Geriatric Psychiatry* 18: 670–678.

Gray, L., Edirippulige, S., Smith, A. C., Beattie, E., Theodoros, D., et al. (2012). 'Telehealth for Nursing Homes: The Utilisation of Specialist Services for Residential Care'. *Journal of Telemedicine and Telecare* 18(3): 142–146.

Helmes, E. and Gee, S. (2003). 'Attitudes of Therapists toward Older Clients: Educational and Training Imperatives'. *Educational Gerontology* 29(8): 657–670.

Hwang, W., Myers, H. F., Abe-Kim, J., and Ting, J. Y. (2008). 'A Conceptual Paradigm for Understanding Culture's Impact on Mental Health: The Cultural Influences on Mental Health (CIMH) Model'. *Clinical Psychology Review* 28: 211–227.

Institute of Medicine (2012). *The Mental Health and Substance Use Workforce for Older Adults: In Whose Hands?* http://www.iom.edu/Reports/2012/The-Mental-Health-and-Substance-Use-Workforce-for-Older-Adults.aspx.

James, S. A. and Buttle, H. (2008). 'Attitudinal Differences towards Mental Health Services between Younger and Older New Zealand Adults'. *New Zealand Journal of Psychology* 37(3): 33–43.

Jameson, J. P. and Blank, M. B. (2007). 'The Role of Clinical Psychology in Rural Mental Health Services: Defining Problems and Developing Solutions'. *Clinical Psychology: Science and Practice* 14(3): 283–283.

Johnston, D. and Jones, B. N. (2001). 'Telepsychiatry Consultations to a Rural Nursing Facility: A 2-year Experience'. *Journal of Geriatric Psychiatry and Neurology* 14: 72–75.

Jorm, A. F., Korten, A. E., Jacomb, P. A., Christensen, H., Rodgers, B., et al. (1997). '"Mental Health Literacy": A Survey of the Public's Ability to Recognise Mental Disorders and their Beliefs about the Effectiveness of Treatment'. *Medical Journal of Australia* 166: 182–186.

Jorm, A. F. and Kitchener, B. A. (2011). 'Noting a Landmark Achievement: Mental Health First Aid Training Reaches 1% of Australian Adults'. *Australian and New Zealand Journal of Psychiatry* 45: 808–813.

Jorm, A. J. (2012). 'Mental Health Literacy: Empowering the Community to Take Action for Better Mental Health'. *American Psychologist* 67(3): 231–243.

Karel, M. J., Holley, C., Whitbourne, S. K., Segal, D. L., Tazeau, Y. N., et al. (2012a). 'Preliminary Validation of Tool to Assess Competencies for Professional Geropsychology Practice'. *Professional Psychology: Research and Practice* 43(2): 110–117.

Karel, M. J., Gatz, M., and Smyer, M. A. (2012b). 'Aging and Mental Health in the Decade Ahead: What Psychologists Need to Know'. *American Psychologist* 67(3): 184–198.

Karlin, B. E., Duffy, M., and Gleaves, D. H. (2008). 'Patterns and Predictors of Mental Health Service Use and Mental Illness among Older and Younger Adults in the United States'. *Psychological Services* 5(3): 275–294.

Kaufman, A. V., Scogin, F. R., Burgio, L. D., Morthland, M. P., and Ford, B. K. (2007). 'Providing Mental Health Services to Older People Living in Rural Communities'. *Journal of Gerontological Social Work* 48(3–4): 349.

Keating, N. and Eales, J. (2012). 'Diversity among Older Adults in Rural Canada: Health in Context'. In J. C. Kulig and A. M. Williams (eds), *Health in Rural Canada* (pp. 427–446). Vancouver, BC: UBC Press.

Knight, B. G. and Shurgot, G. R. (2008). 'Psychological Assessment and Treatment with Older Adults: Past Trends and Future Directions'. In K. Laidlaw and B. Knight (eds), *Handbook of Emotional Disorders in Later Life: Assessment and Treatment* (pp. 453–464). Oxford: Oxford University Press.

Knight, B. G., Karel, M. J., Hinrichsen, G. A., Qualls, S. H., and Duffy, M. (2009). 'Pikes Peak Model for Training in Professional Geropsychology'. *American Psychologist* 64: 205–214.

Knight, B. G. (2010). 'Clinical Supervision for Psychotherapy with Older Adults'. In N. A. Pachana, K. Laidlaw, and B. G. Knight (eds), *Casebook of Clinical Geropsychology* (pp. 107–117). Oxford: Oxford University Press.

Knight, B. G. and Sayegh, P. (2011). 'Mental Health and Aging in the 21st Century'. *Journal of Aging and Social Policy* 23: 228–243.

Koder, D. A. and Helmes, E. (2008). 'The Current Status of Clinical Geropsychology in Australia: A Survey of Practicing Psychologists'. *Australian Psychologist* 43: 22–26.

Koh, S., Blank, K., Cohen, C. I., Cohen, G., Faison, W., et al. (2010). 'Public's View of Mental Health Services for the Elderly: Responses to Dear Abby'. *Psychiatric Services* 61(11): 1146–1149.

Konnert, C., Dobson, K. S., and Watt, A. (2009). 'Geropsychology Training in Canada: A Survey of Doctoral and Internship Programs'. *Canadian Psychology* 50(4): 255–260.

Lai, D. (2000). 'Prevalence of Depression among the Elderly Chinese in Canada'. *Canadian Journal of Public Health* 91(1): 64–66.

Lai, D. W. L. and Surood, S. (2009). 'Chinese Health Beliefs of Older Chinese in Canada'. *Journal of Aging and Health* 21(1): 38–62.

Link, B. G. and Phelan, J. C. (2001). 'Conceptualizing Stigma'. *Annual Review of Sociology* 47: 363–385.

McGovern, R. J., Lee, M. M., Johnson, J. C., and Morton, B. (2008). 'ElderLynk: A Community Outreach Model for the Integrated Treatment of Mental Health Problems in the Rural Elderly'. *Ageing International* 32(1): 43–53.

Mackenzie, C. S., Knox, V. J., Gekoski, W. L., and Macaulay, H. L. (2004). 'An Adaptation and Extension of the Attitudes Toward Seeking Professional Psychological Help Scale'. *Journal of Applied Social Psychology* 34: 2410–2435.

Mackenzie, C. S., Gekoski, W. L., and Knox, V. J. (2006). 'Age, Gender, and the Underutilization of Mental Health Services: The Influence of Help-seeking Attitudes'. *Aging & Mental Health* 10(6): 574–582.

Mackenzie, C. S., Scott, T., Mather, A., and Sareen, J. (2008). 'Older Adults' Help-seeking Attitudes and Treatment Beliefs Concerning Mental Health Problems'. *American Journal of Geriatric Psychiatry* 16(12): 1010–1019.

Mackenzie, C. S., Pagura, J., and Sareen, J. (2010). 'Correlates of Perceived Need for and Use of Mental Health Services by Older Adults in the Collaborative Psychiatric Epidemiology Surveys'. *American Journal of Geriatric Psychiatry* 18(12): 1103–1115.

Marziali, E. and Garcia, L. J. (2011). 'Dementia Caregivers' Responses to 2 Internet-based Intervention Programs'. *American Journal of Alzheimer's Disease and Other Dementias* 26: 36–43.

Meeks, S. (1990). 'Age Bias in the Diagnostic Decision-making Behavior of Clinicians'. *Professional Psychology: Research and Practice* 21(4): 279–284.

Mitka, M. (2003). 'Telemedicine Eyed for Mental Health Services: Approach Could Widen Access for Older Patients'. *Journal of the American Medical Association* 290(14): 1842–1843.

Moak, G. S. (2011). 'Treatment of Late-life Mental Disorders in Primary Care: We Can Do a Better Job'. *Journal of Aging and Social Policy* 23(3): 274–285.

Mui, A. C. and Kang, S. (2006). 'Acculturation Stress and Depression among Asian Immigrant Elders'. *Social Work* 51(3): 243–255.

Natural Resources Canada (2009). *The Atlas of Canada: Visible Minority Population*. http://atlas.nrcan.gc.ca/site/english/maps/peopleandsociety/population/visible_minority.

Neufeld, J. D., Yellowlees, P. M., Hilty, D. M., Cobb, H., and Bourgeois, J. A. (2007). 'The E-mental Health Consultation Service: Providing Enhanced Primary-care Mental Health Services through Telemedicine'. *Psychosomatics* 48(2): 135–141.

Novotney, A. (2012). 'A Boost for Integrated Care'. *APA Monitor* 43(4): 20–21.

Nyunt, M. S. Z., Ko, S. M., Kumar, R., Fones, C., and Ng, T. P. (2009). 'Improving Treatment Access and Primary Care Referrals for Depression in a National Community-based Outreach Programme for the Elderly'. *International Journal of Geriatric Psychiatry* 24(11): 1267–1276.

Pachana, N. A., Emery, E., Konnert, C. A., Woodhead, E., and Edelstein, B. A. (2010). 'Geropsychology Content in Clinical Training Programs: A Comparison of Australian, Canadian, and U.S. Data'. *International Psychogeriatrics* 22(6): 909–918.

Pepin, R., Segal, D. L., and Coolidge, F. L. (2009). 'Intrinsic and Extrinsic Barriers to Mental Health Care among Community-dwelling Younger and Older Adults'. *Aging & Mental Health* 13(5): 769–777.

Pescosolido, B. A., Martin, J. K., Long, J. S., Medina, T. R., Phelan, et al. (2010). 'A Disease Like any Other? A Decade of Change in Public Reactions to Schizophrenia, Depression, and Alcohol Dependence'. *American Journal of Psychiatry* 167: 1321–1330.

Ploeg, J., Hayward, L., Woodward, C., and Johnston, R. (2008). 'A Case Study of a Canadian Homelessness Intervention Programme for Elderly People'. *Health and Social Care in the Community* 16(6): 593–605.

Qualls, S. H., Scogin, F., Zweig, R., and Whitbourne, S. K. (2010). 'Predoctoral Training Models in Professional Geropsychology'. *Training and Education in Professional Psychology* 4(2): 85–90.

Robb, C., Chen, H., and Haley, W. E. (2002). 'Ageism in Mental Health and Health Care: A Critical Review'. *Journal of Clinical Geropsychology* 8(1): 1–12.

Ryder, A. G., Alden, L. E., and Paulus, D. L. (2000). 'Is Acculturation Unidimensional or Bidimensional? A Head-to-head Comparison in the Prediction of Personality, Self-identity, and Adjustment'. *Journal of Personality and Social Psychology* 79: 49–65.

Ryder, A. G., Yang, J., Zhu, X., Yao, S., Yi, J., et al. (2008). 'The Cultural Shaping of Depression: Somatic Symptoms in China, Psychological Symptoms in North America? *Journal of Abnormal Psychology* 117(2): 300–313.

Scott, T., Mackenzie, C. S., Chipperfield, J. G., and Sareen, J. (2010). 'Mental Health Service Use among Canadian Older Adults with Anxiety Disorders and Clinically Significant Anxiety Symptoms'. *Aging & Mental Health* 14(7): 790–800.

Segal, D. L., Coolidge, F. L., Mincic, M. S., and O'Riley, A. (2005). 'Beliefs About Mental Illness and Willingness to Seek Help: A Cross-sectional Study'. *Aging & Mental Health* 9(4): 363–367.

Smith, A. C., Armfield, N. R., Croll, J., and Gray, L. C. (2012). 'A Review of Medicare Expenditure in Australia for Psychiatric Consultations Delivered in Person and via Videoconference'. *Journal of Telemedicine and Telecare* 18(3): 169–171

Sorkin, D. H., Pham, E., and Ngo-Metzger, Q, (2009). 'Racial and Ethnic Differences in the Mental Health Needs and Access to Care of Older Adults in California'. *Journal of the American Geriatrics Society* 57(12): 2311–2317.

Statistics Canada (2005). *Population Projections of Visible Minority Groups, Canada, Provinces and Regions 2001–2017*. Catalogue no. 91-541-XIE, Statistics Canada, Ottawa.

Tieu, Y., Konnert, C., and Wang, J. (2010). 'Depression Literacy among Older Chinese Immigrants in Canada: A Comparison with a Population-based Survey'. *International Psychogeriatrics* 22(8): 1318–1326.

Tieu, Y. and Konnert, C. (2012). 'Chinese Older Adults' Attitudes toward Seeking Mental Health Services'. Paper presented to the Scientific Meeting of the Canadian Psychological Association, Halifax 13–15 June.

Troisi, J. (2001). 'Training to Provide for Healthy Rural Aging'. *Journal of Rural Health* 17: 336–340.

Ward, V., Smith, S., House, A., and Hamer, S. (2012). 'Exploring Knowledge Exchange: A Useful Framework for Practice and Policy'. *Social Science and Medicine* 74: 297–304.

Werner, P. and Giveon, S. M. (2008). 'Discriminatory Behavior of Family Physicians toward a Person with Alzheimer's Disease'. *International Psychogeriatrics* 20(4): 824–839.

Werner, P. and Heinik, J. (2008). 'Stigma by Association and Alzheimer's Disease'. *Aging & Mental Health* 12(1): 92–99.

Werner, P., Mittelman, M. S., Goldstein, D., and Heinik, J. (2012). 'Family Stigma and Caregiver Burden in Alzheimer's Disease'. *Gerontologist* 52(1): 89–97.

Whitten, P. (2001). 'E-health Holds Promise and Many Questions'. *Aging Today* 22: 9–11.

Wilson, K. (2012). 'Eliminating Stigma: A Focus on Seniors' Mental Health'. Paper presented at the 5th International Stigma Conference, Ottawa, 4–6 June.

Woodhead, E., Emery, E., Pachana, N., Konnert, C., Scott, T., et al. (2013). 'Geropsychology Content in Graduate Training: Student Competencies And Career Decision-making'. *Professional Psychology: Research and Practice* 44(5): 355–362.

Woodward, R. and Pachana, N. A. (2009). 'Attitudes toward Psychological Treatment among Older Australians'. *Australian Psychologist* 44(2): 86–93.

World Health Organization (2012). *Knowledge Translation on Ageing and Health*. http://www.who.int/ageing/publications/knowledge_translation/en/index.html.

Yang, L. H., Phelan, J. C., and Link, B. G. (2008). 'Stigma and Beliefs of Efficacy towards Traditional Chinese Medicine and Western Psychiatric Treatment among Chinese-Americans'. *Cultural Diversity and Ethnic Minority Psychology* 14(1): 10–18.

Zweig, R. A., Siegel, L., and Snyder, R. (2006). 'Doctoral Gero-psychology Training in Primary Care: Preliminary Findings from a Clinical Training Project'. *Journal of Clinical Psychology in Medical Settings* 13(1): 21–30.

CHAPTER 46

....

SENIORS' ONLINE COMMUNITIES AND WELL-BEING IN LATER LIFE

....

GALIT NIMROD

INTRODUCTION

THE advancement of computer technologies and the cybernetic revolution provide older adults with many new opportunities. One of them is the opportunity to participate in seniors' online communities, namely, groups of older adults who interact online through diverse applications such as chat rooms and forums. Such communities seem to be very welcome by their target audiences. The number of seniors' online communities is growing, and some of them have hundreds and even thousands of members. Moreover, a recent study (Nimrod 2010), which followed a full year's activity in leading seniors' communities, indicated that during the research period there was a constant increase in the daily activity level. The number of threads (i.e. discussions, stream of posts concerning the same topic and with the same opening post) has doubled, and the number of authors and posts (i.e. messages) has tripled. Hence, participating in seniors' online communities may be described as a significant trend in older adults' use of information and communication technology (ICT).

Based on a series of studies that utilized various methods (including content analysis, virtual ethnography, and online survey with community members), this chapter aims to explain why these communities became so popular. It demonstrates that all the utilities of ICT for older adults identified in previous research (e.g. Opalinski 2001; Xie 2007) are offered by seniors' online communities. Accordingly, as these functions were found to have a significant contribution to seniors' well-being (e.g. Dickenson and Hill 2007; Fokkema and Knipscherr 2007), the main argument of this chapter is that seniors' online communities have significant potential to enhance psychological well-being in later life. Preliminary empirical support for this argument is provided.

OLDER ADULTS AND ICT

The cybernetic revolution did not bypass the senior population. According to a recent report by the Organisation for Economic Co-operation and Development (OECD), the percentage of internet users among people who are 65 years old and over is still much lower than among younger age groups. This 'age divide' is present in all OECD countries, but differs from one country to another, with Poland, Slovenia, and Greece demonstrating the widest 'age divide'. However, the number of older internet users grows rapidly every year. On average, older adults have increased their use of the internet by 44% since 2007, and in some countries (e.g. Norway, Iceland, Luxembourg, and Japan), the rate of internet users in this age group is higher than 60% (OECD 2011).

The 'age divide' is reflected not only in terms of percentage of internet users, but also in the usages people make of the internet. Whereas younger users are involved in a large variety of online activities, including advanced online entertainment (e.g. downloading videos) and social media use, the online activities of older adults are typically limited to using email and search engines, conducting online research and information gathering, and involvement in e-commerce (Pew Internet and American Life Project (PIALP) 2009). Nevertheless, older adults stand to benefit from ICT in various ways.

Previous research has identified a host of utilities of ICT for older adults. The main functions described are: (1) communication medium—ICT is used for maintenance of social networks with family and friends, as well as a tool for making new friends, and helps to remove geographic and transportation limits; (2) information source—increased access to current affairs, health and medical information, consumer information, online courses, etc.; (3) task-oriented tool (e.g. shopping, financial management, and travel planning); and (4) leisure activity—older adults use many leisure activities offered by the web, such as researching family trees, making photo albums, playing games, and participating in other virtual hobbies (Cody et al. 1999; Iyer and Eastman 2006; Kiger 2006; Loges and Jung 2001; Opalinski 2001; PIALP 2004, 2009; White et al. 1999; White and Weatherall 2000; Xie 2007).

In addition to the practical benefits of using the internet, its use seems to have a strong impact on older adults' psychological well-being. Learning computer and internet skills enhances a sense of independence (Henke 1999), and creates a process of empowerment (transition from helplessness to control, and from passiveness to activeness) as a result of the power of change and the power of knowledge (Fuglsang 2005; McMellon and Schiffman 2002; Shapira, Barak, and Gal 2007). In addition, involvement in the virtual world, according to Furlong (1989), is likely to strengthen the self-image and self-confidence of older people.

Internet use also seems to have a role in maintaining older users' social networks, which enhance their psychological well-being. It is associated with higher levels of social connectivity, higher levels of perceived social support, decreased feelings of loneliness, lower levels of depression, and generally more positive attitudes toward ageing (Cody et al. 1999; Dickenson and Hill 2007; Fokkema and Knipscherr 2007; Nahm and Resnick 2001; Van De Watering 2005; White et al. 2002). Moreover, older persons involved in the virtual world relate to their computer as an independent presence in their homes, and tend to attribute human qualities to it, as if it is a component in their social network (Blit-Cohen and Litwin 2004; Kadlec 2007).

Seniors' Online Communities

The study of online communities has been a predominant theme in the social scientific examination of the internet. The concept was first used by Rheingold (1994), following his experiences in an early online community called the WELL (Whole Earth Lectronic Link). He defined online communities as 'a group of people who may or may not meet one another face to face, and who exchange words and ideas through the mediation of computer...networks' (Rheingold 1994: 57). Lazar and Preece (1998) complemented this definition by outlining four components of an online community: people, purpose, policies, and system. The people are community members, who interact online in order to satisfy a certain need and/or perform a specific role. These people have a shared purpose, such as an interest, a need, or a service. In order to achieve that purpose, the community develops formal and informal policies in the form of implied assumptions, rituals, rules, or guides, and it relies on computer systems to support the online interaction.

Online communities may operate through diverse applications such as email distribution lists, newsgroups, interactive sites, chat rooms, or forums/message boards. They may also use the technological platform of social network sites (SNSs) such as Facebook or Google Plus, but there is a significant distinction between online communities and social networks. Although one can establish new relationships via SNSs (Tufekci 2010), the available research suggests that most SNSs primarily support pre-established interpersonal relationships between individuals. SNS users construct a public or semi-public profile, define a list of other users with whom they share a connection, and view and traverse their list of connections. Connection between users is direct and built one at a time, and people typically have only one social network. Similar to SNS users, members in online communities may create a personal profile and form relationships that are not visible to others. However, online communities are held together by the common interests of a large group of people. Although community members may have a pre-existing interpersonal relationship, it is not required, and typically new members do not know most of the people in the community. Individuals may participate in multiple communities, and thus communities may overlap. In addition, communities are nested, so that one community may contain another (Boyd and Ellison 2007; Wu 2011).

Compared with face-to-face groups, online communities have several advantages, including accessibility, anonymity, invisibility and status neutralization, greater individual control over the time and pace of interactions, opportunity for multi-conversing, and opportunities for archival searches (Barak 2007; Barak, Boniel-Nissim, and Suler 2008; McKenna and Bargh 2000; Meier 2004). These characteristics, along with availability and simplicity of use, may explain the popularity of online communities among internet users. Some of these qualities, especially the anonymity and the invisibility, may also be considered as advantages when comparing online communities with SNSs.

This chapter discusses the specific qualities of seniors' online communities. Due to the multiple technological platforms of online communities, it focuses on the most dominant type of communities, namely, forums/message boards. A simple Google search identifies dozens of forums dedicated to older adults. Some of them are hosted by forum sites (e.g. Yahoo! Groups), while others are provided by portals for seniors (e.g. 'My Senior Portal') that have, in addition to the forums, many sections providing useful information for seniors, as well as newsletters, webcasts, and so forth. Most communities, however, are available on independent websites that contain forums only.

Seniors' online communities are usually recognizable by their names, which suggest a focus on older adults (e.g. 'Fifty Plus Forum' or 'Third Age'). Others have more neutral names, but they explicitly state their target audience on their home pages. For example, an

Australian community named 'Your Life Choices' is presented as 'for fun in your 50s, 60s and beyond'. Like any other forum, each forum-based community for seniors is made up of various sections (e.g. Health and Wellbeing, Politics or Hobbies). Users can simply choose a topic, then browse the various threads within that topic and join one of the online discussions. Alternatively, they can open a new thread. The following part of this chapter provides examples of the various discussions that take place in seniors' online communities, and demonstrates the various uses seniors make of these communities.

THE USES THAT OLDER ADULTS MAKE OF SENIORS' ONLINE COMMUNITIES

Communication medium

Online communities are predominantly a medium for interpersonal communication. They provide a virtual public sphere (Papacharissi 2002), in which individuals can communicate with other community members, or simply follow others' communication exchanges ('lurk'). This is similar to any other offline multi-participant conversation, in which some participants take a more active role than others. The main differences are that the communication is written instead of oral, and that the non-active participants are invisible.

In addition to participating in public conversations, members can communicate via private messages, which are similar to emails. In some communities, they can also open a private online chat. The latter enables synchronous communication, whereas communication in the public forum and via private messages is asynchronous. As the communication in the private messages and chats is concealed, there is no way to explore its contents.

The contents of the *public* online conversations in seniors' online communities were examined in several studies which aimed to explore the social support exchanged in the communities. Wright (2000), for example, analysed 360 pages of messages posted in SeniorNet (an American community). Analysis revealed that the online discussions were characterized by a high level of self-disclosure and that community members deeply appreciated the social support they received from their online peers. Pfeil (2007) explored 1200 messages posted in the same community to develop a code scheme for analysing empathy and social support in online communities for older people. Six categories were identified, including: light support, deep support, information, community building, self-disclosure, and off-topic. These categories were later used to examine the associations between the communication content and the social network patterns (Pfeil and Zaphiris 2010).

To explore the *subjects* discussed in the communities, one study examined a full year's data from fourteen English-language-based leading communities from the US, Canada, the UK, and Australia (Nimrod 2010). The overall database included 19 963 threads and 686 283 posts. The number of authors was 79 665. Using a novel computerized system for content analysis, the study identified thirteen main subjects discussed in the communities, including (in descending order) 'Fun on line' (i.e. games, jokes, riddles, etc.), 'Retirement', 'Family', 'Health', 'Work and Study', 'Recreation', 'Finance', 'Religion and Spirituality', 'Technology', 'Aging', 'Civic and Social issues', 'Shopping', and 'Travels'.

Surprisingly, the volume of posts relating to each topic does not accurately reflect community members' reported interests. In a recently completed online survey with 218 members of sixteen English-language-based seniors' online communities, respondents were presented with a list of the thirteen most-discussed subjects, and asked to rate their interest in these subjects using a four-point scale ranging from 'have no interest' to 'very interested'. All subjects discussed in the communities were of high interest, and relatively few reported having no interest in one of the subjects. Yet there was only a little consistency between subjects' volume and appeal (see Table 46.1). The most significant gaps were evident with regard to 'Fun on line', which had the highest volume but relatively little reported interest, and with regard to 'Technology', 'Civic and Social issues', and 'Travel', which had relatively little volume but very high reported interest.

There are several explanations for these gaps, including social desirability, as some subjects may be perceived as more legitimate or appreciated than others. Another explanation is the fact that the communities examined in the survey only partially overlapped with the communities examined in the content analysis (as some community administrators refused to collaborate with the research team). In addition, the survey was conducted three years after the content analysis, and thus members' characteristics could have changed with the many newcomers to the communities. Moreover, the indicator for volume in the content analysis could have been misleading. There are differences in the length of posts relating to

Table 46.1 The most discussed subjects: volume and members' reported interest

Subject	Volume		Interested members			Ranking gap
	# of posts	Ranking	% of sample	(N)	Ranking	
'Fun on line'	133878	1	36	211	10	−9
Retirement	94200	2	63	213	4	−2
Family	77252	3	62	210	5	−2
Health	55888	4	75	215	1	3
Work and studies	50834	5	51	211	8	−3
Leisure	48572	6	57	213	7	−1
Finances	29220	7	60	212	6	1
Religion and spirituality	28824	8	33	212	12	−4
Technology	27235	9	71	213	2	7
Aging	19039	10	60	214	6	4
Civic and social issues	17740	11	66	211	3	8
Shopping	9671	12	43	212	9	3
Travel	3425	13	60	214	6	7

Note: The data regarding volume is adapted from Nimrod (2010) and based on content analysis of messages posted in fourteen communities between 1 April 2007 and 31 March 2008. The data regarding members' interests is based on an online survey conducted between July and October 2011. Survey participants that reported being 'very interested' or 'quite interested' were defined as interested members.

the various topics. Posts in the 'Fun on line' category are typically very short, whereas posts in more informed intellectual discussions may be rather long. The content analysis related to the number of posts, but not to the total amount of text. Lastly, it is possible that there is no correlation between the number of authors and number of posts for each topic (e.g. in the 'Fun on line' a small number of community members post a very large number of messages).

Regardless of this incongruity, the findings of the content analysis suggest that the communities serve as a platform for discussing every possible subject, ranging from very *private* subjects, such as problematic relationships or fear of death, to *public* subjects such as global warming or politics. Subjects range from very *serious* (e.g. employees' exploitation) to very *casual* (e.g. jokes), and while some of them are *exclusive* to seniors (e.g. ageing, retirement rights), many of them are *general*. Moreover, it seems that the communities also enable the expression of a wide range of emotions, ranging from very *negative* (e.g. sadness, anger, grief) to very *positive* (e.g. happiness and playfulness). Tone analysis, which was based on the frequency and the intensity of more than 2000 defined expressions, suggested that the overall tone of the discussions was somewhat more positive than negative, but overall there seemed to be a balance (Nimrod 2010). The terminology in the online discussions featured significant usage of general positive expressions (e.g. good, great), but also words expressing difficulties and pain (e.g. problem, loss).

The fact that the public conversations include, among others, discussions of private and problematic personal issues, supports previous notions (e.g. Pfeil 2007; Wright 2000) that online communities provide immediate, intensive, and heartfelt support for seniors in need. In addition, they offer more casual social interaction as well as intellectual stimulation. Therefore joining online communities may provide an expansion of existing real-life social networks and/or compensation for lost friendships as a result of various constraints (e.g. poorer health or friends' disability or death). Participating in seniors' online communities can keep seniors socially engaged, provide meaningful interaction and, to a certain extent, a sense of belonging. This may explain why one of the most salient benefits of participation in seniors' online communities is companionship (Kanayama 2003; Nimrod 2014; Pfeil and Zaphiris 2010). Such relations probably cannot replace real relationships and/or significantly help seniors who suffer from loneliness. Still, some community members report making new offline friends and even meeting new spouses through the communities (Nimrod 2014). Therefore the socio-emotional benefits of the communities may extend beyond the online communication.

Information source

A study that aimed to assess the information needs of older adults among prospective Korean senior portal users over 50 years of age, found that users have a high preference for seeing the following content on senior portals: health/medical issues, banking, travel, current terminology, and real estate (Yoon, Yoon, and George 2011). These findings echoed earlier analyses in an American context which demonstrated that older adults use the internet as a tool for research, shopping, and banking (PIALP 2009).

The aforementioned results of the content analysis (Nimrod 2010) suggest that seniors' online communities may answer many of the information needs of their members. Generally, this information may be divided into two types: 'practical information' and 'content'. 'Practical information' can be used in members' daily lives. For example, a discussion found in one of the forums was entitled 'Flu shot, best time to get it?' This discussion included various pieces of advice concerning flu shots, as well as links to scientific articles and medical websites. The accumulated information provided in this discussion could support community members' decision-making about getting flu shots.

'Content' includes articles, information, and news about a topic of interest to community members. These mainly expand one's horizons rather than support practical tasks. Examples of such content may easily be found in discussions of social issues (e.g. discussions dealing with elections, economic policy, or conflicts in the Middle East) and spirituality (e.g. discussions on selected chapters from the Bible, mindfulness, or atheism). The existence of this type of discussion may explain why one of the most salient benefits of participation in seniors' online communities is intellectual stimulation (Nimrod 2014).

Task-orientated tool

The 'practical information' shared in senior's online communities may be very useful and serve as a task-oriented tool. To support this argument we use the findings of two studies. The first is a study that examined tourism-related contents (Nimrod 2012). This study was based on the same dataset used in the aforementioned content analysis (Nimrod 2010), but while the former study used a quantitative approach, the current investigation was qualitative and applied an online ethnography approach (Kozinets 2002, 2006; Langer and Beckman 2005; Sade-Beck 2004). Key tourism-related words (e.g. 'tour', 'travel', and 'trip') were used to select appropriate posts, and the overall database included 3425 posts.

Analysis led to identifying three categories: 'practical information exchange', 'search for contacts', and 'travel stories'. The majority of posts belonged to the first category, and provided practical information to community members who were planning a trip or vacation. The scope of discussed issues in this category was broad, and included 'Destinations' (e.g. tourist attractions), 'Accommodation' (e.g. hotels), 'Travels' (e.g. transportation options), and 'Preparations' (e.g. health insurance). All this information could be usefully applied by community members planning to travel. In addition, some members used the online communities as a platform for establishing contacts which would contribute to their planned travels. Some were looking for *travel companions*, and others were looking for *home exchange*. Furthermore, although many posts that included recommendations also included descriptions of personal experiences, there were also many posts by people who shared their travel stories just for the sake of sharing. These findings suggest that members of seniors' online communities use them as a valuable resource both before and after travelling.

A study by Xie (2008) examined an online community of older Chinese individuals. Based on in-depth interviews with thirty-three community members, this study indicated that the online forum in this community was primarily used for informational support about technology and computer use. This finding may be explained by the fact that the community was formed to serve the alumni of a computer training programme for older adults. Therefore it was perceived by community members as an extension of the programme. Still, as technology is one of main subjects discussed in seniors' online communities (Nimrod 2010), it seems that many use the information provided by their peers to face technology-related challenges.

The various instrumental contributions of seniors' online communities may be divided into two types: age-related and general contributions (Nimrod 2014). The information provided by their peers may help community members to deal with challenges associated with later life (e.g. retirement and widowhood) and as a means to learning about seniors' rights and services (e.g. senior centres). However, many instrumental contributions are not age-related. These often include using the communities as a means to finding a job or promoting members' businesses (e.g. financial consultancy or legacy books publishing), and as a useful tool for coping with various daily challenges, from cooking a special Thanksgiving dinner to purchasing a new car.

Leisure activity

Leisure is the 'quality of activity defined by relative freedom and intrinsic satisfaction' (Kelly 1996: 22). The leisure literature distinguishes between *serious leisure* and *casual leisure* (for a review, see Stebbins 2007). Casual leisure serves mainly to clarify the meaning of serious leisure, which is characterized by considerable commitment, effort, and perseverance. However, it is in itself an important form of leisure, and far more people participate in it than in serious leisure (Hutchinson and Kleiber 2005). It is defined as 'an immediately, intrinsically rewarding, relatively short-lived pleasurable core activity, requiring little or no special training to enjoy it' (Stebbins 1997: 18).

Casual leisure includes eight types of activity: play (e.g. dabbling, dilettantism), relaxation, passive entertainment (e.g. watching TV), active entertainment (e.g. party games), sociable conversation, sensory stimulation, casual volunteering, and pleasurable aerobic activity (e.g. walking). These eight types of casual leisure all share a hedonic nature, and may be pursued in combinations of two and three at least as often as they are pursued separately (Stebbins 2007). Participating in an online community is a free-time activity that may involve various types of casual leisure. First and foremost, it involves *sociable conversation*, but for members participating in sections dedicated to 'fun' (such as Games, Quizzes, Jokes, Humour, or Other), it also involves *play* and *active entertainment*.

A recent study (Nimrod 2011) explored these fun sections using an online ethnography approach. The study analysed a full year's data from six out of the fourteen communities examined in the content analysis (Nimrod 2010). The final database included about 50 000 posts. Results indicated that in a reality of limited alternatives for digital games that meet older adults' needs and interests (Griffiths et al. 2004; Ijsselsteijn et al. 2007; De Schutter and Abeele 2008), seniors found an independent system to satisfy their need for play. The majority of posts were part of online social games, including cognitive, associative, and creative games. Cognitive games mainly included *trivia games* that challenged participants' general knowledge, and *alphabetical games*, which tested their vocabulary. The associative games were somewhat similar to the cognitive games in their mechanisms, but in these cases, the previous participant's post triggered the next one based on free associations. Creative games required more imagination, and their outcome was a story, a limerick, or a poem. Hence, the games provided both cognitive stimulation and a creative outlet for the participants.

Most of the texts in the fun sections were written by the 'regulars', who visited the communities quite often and posted on a regular basis. Most of the members, however, seemed to be 'lurkers'. Examination of data from the archives' numerators regarding popular threads showed that the number of views was sometimes dozens and even hundreds of times greater than the number of replies. For the 'lurkers', the type of casual leisure may be best described as *passive entertainment*, which is similar to watching TV. It is possible that they enjoy following real people and dynamics, an activity that is similar to watching reality or talk shows on TV. Assuming that the 'lurkers' are older adults as well, it is also likely that they enjoy following people their age, as they can identify with them. In addition, as the 'regulars' usually have 'group humour', and they tend to exhibit self-humour, it is likely that it is the humoristic atmosphere in the communities that attracts the 'lurkers'.

Casual leisure is associated with five benefits: creativity or serendipitous discovery, 'edutainment' (i.e. entertaining education), regeneration or re-creation, development and maintenance of interpersonal relationships, and enhanced well-being (Stebbins 2001). As the communities provide various types of casual leisure, which may be pursued in combinations of two and three (as in the case of the 'fun' sections), they may provide, at least to some extent, the various benefits associated with casual leisure. This may explain why one of the most salient benefits of participation in senior's online communities is joyfulness (Nimrod 2014). Moreover, the communities also serve as a resource in seniors' offline leisure, as many posts deal with recommendations relating to recreation, shopping, and travel. In fact, members report that they use the information provided by other community members to promote their existing and new interests and hobbies (Nimrod 2014). Therefore, as leisure has a key role in the well-being of older adults (e.g. Fernandez-Ballesteros, Zamarron, and Ruiz 2001; Kelly 1987; Nimrod 2007), seniors' online communities may have both direct and indirect impact on seniors' leisure and well-being.

SENIORS' ONLINE COMMUNITIES
AND WELL-BEING

The discussion above leads to the conclusion that all the uses of ICT for older adults identified in previous research (e.g. Opalinski 2001; Xie 2007) are offered by seniors' online communities. The communities serve (1) as a communication medium for both public and private communication. They are used as a tool for making new friends, and provide social interaction, intellectual stimulation, and emotional support for those in need. In addition, they are used (2) as an information source for both 'content' (articles, information, and news about topics of interest) and 'practical information', and the latter serves (3) as a task-oriented tool that helps community members to deal with challenges associated with later life as well as various daily challenges. Lastly, in parallel to serving as a resource in seniors' offline leisure, participation in the communities is also (4) a leisure activity in itself, which involves various forms of casual leisure. As these four utilities were found to make a significant contribution to the psychological well-being of seniors (e.g. Dickenson and Hill 2007; Fokkema and Knipscherr 2007), seniors' online communities have a great potential to enhance psychological well-being in later life.

Several exploratory studies have tried to delineate the benefits of participation in seniors' online communities. These studies demonstrated the communities' potential to provide instrumental information (Camarinha-Matos and Afsarmanesh 2004; Pfeil 2007; Xie 2008), emotional support (Furlong 1989; Ito et al. 2001; Pfeil 2007; Pfeil and Zaphiris 2010; Wright 2000), companionship (Kanayama 2003; Nimrod 2014; Pfeil and Zaphiris 2010), a sense of belonging (Burmeister 2012), intellectual stimulation and joyfulness (Nimrod 2014). Without de-emphasizing the contribution of these studies, it should be noted that they portrayed a rather limited picture. This resulted from various reasons. First, most were based on qualitative methods (e.g. qualitative content analysis, focus groups, and in-depth interviews with members), while quantitative studies were rather scarce. Second, in most studies, interviewees and/or contents were sampled from one online community only. Third, most previous studies tended to regard the communities as online support groups. Any lay review of the contents posted in such communities would reveal that most of them are not defined as support groups. On the contrary, the communities' positioning tends to emphasize the recreational aspects of participation. Moreover, while some discussions in the communities may indeed be described as supportive, others are intellectual or very casual in nature. Lastly, none of the previous studies used measures of psychological well-being.

Although only a trial study that would use a single-component intervention and control for non-community components may prove the potential of seniors' online communities to enhance psychological well-being in later life, preliminary empirical support may be provided by the aforementioned online survey with members of seniors' online communities. In that survey, respondents were asked to answer mostly closed and some open-ended questions regarding their participation patterns, demographic and socio-demographic background, interest in issues discussed in the communities, and benefits of participation (measured by the Paragraphs About Leisure—Form E (PAL-E), developed by Tinsley and Kass 1980a, 1980b). In addition, they were presented with the short version of Ryff's Psychological Well Being Scale (Ryff and Keyes 1995).

Sample size was 218. Most respondents were 55 to 75 years old, and the mean was 64.7 years. Fifty-six percent were female, 64% were married and most of the rest (18%) were divorced. The average number of years of education was 15.1. Fifty-four percent of the respondents reported having an average income and 26% reported income higher than average. Forty-eight percent were from the USA, 33% were from the British Isles, 13% from Australia and 4 % from Canada. Relatively few (2%) resided in non-English-speaking countries. Seventy-three percent perceived their health to be good or excellent, and only 6 % perceived their health to be poor. These sample characteristics suggest that the current users of seniors' online communities are rather young, healthy, educated, and well-to-do seniors.

Heavy users were defined as members that visited the community from which they were referred to the survey and/or other seniors' communities every day or almost every day. They comprised 40.2% of the sample. The rest of the sample (59.8%) was comprised of light users, who visited the community and/or other seniors' communities fewer than three times a week. There was a significant association (p = 0.001) between the frequency of the visits and the duration of respondents' typical visit in the communities. Far more heavy users (42% vs 16%) reported that their typical visit lasted more than thirty minutes, whereas most light users (60% vs 30%) reported that their typical visit lasted up to fifteen minutes.

Analysis indicated significant differences between the two segments in their perceived benefits of participation and background characteristics (see Table 46.2). The heavy users reported a higher level of agreement with eleven out of the twenty-seven paragraphs describing the psychological benefits of participation in seniors' online communities. These included companionship (e.g. a chance to make friends, as well as a chance to express

Table 46.2 Differences between heavy and light users

	Sig.	T	Light users (N = 122)		Heavy users (N = 82)	
			SD	Mean	SD	Mean
Benefits of participation						
Making a creative contribution	.000	3.952	1.125	2.67	1.157	3.32
A chance to help, to be of service, or to do things for other people	.001	3.534	1.092	2.78	1.211	3.35
A feeling of accomplishment	.001	3.281	1.124	2.43	1.270	2.99
Having an easy-going, humorous attitude towards life	.001	3.435	1.082	3.35	1.041	3.88
A chance to improve skills	.001	3.293	1.110	2.56	1.232	3.11
Being considerate of others and going out of the way to help them	.002	3.163	1.042	3.16	1.092	3.65
A chance to make friends	.004	2.880	1.118	2.33	1.226	2.81
Useful information and emotional support	.007	2.736	1.085	2.96	1.067	3.38
A chance to be active	.010	2.610	1.132	2.45	1.151	2.88
Getting something in return for the effort	.012	2.539	1.044	2.63	1.136	3.03
A chance to express bottled up feelings	.039	2.075	1.071	2.05	1.281	2.40
Socio-demographics						
Age	.026	2.239	9.385	63.32	7.826	66.26
Education	.027	-2.231	2.967	15.69	3.922	14.54
Self-rated health	.037	1.997	.797	1.97	.888	2.32

Note: Benefits were measured using a five-point scale ranging from 1 = 'not true' to 5 = 'definitely true'. Education was measured by total years of education. Health was measured on a four-point scale ranging from 1 = excellent to 4 = poor. Hence, light users reported better health.

bottled-up feelings), self-expression and growth (e.g. a chance to be active, to improve skills, and to be of service to others), as well as a sense of achievement (e.g. a feeling of accomplishment and of getting something in return for one's efforts).

Findings also indicated differences between the two segments in their background characteristics. Heavy users were significantly older than the light users (mean age = 66.26 vs 63.32), which may explain why they reported poorer health (2.32 vs 1.97 on a four-point scale ranging from 1 = excellent to 4 = poor). In addition, while both groups reported a high level of education, the heavy users were significantly less educated than the light users (14.54 vs 15.69 years of education). These findings suggest that the communities may be particularly beneficial for older and frailer seniors, whose participation in offline social activities is more constrained. Unfortunately, this is exactly the population which, according to the various statistical reports (e.g. OECD 2011), is less involved with the internet.

Based on the differences between the groups in their background characteristics, one might expect that the heavy users would report lower well-being than the light users. However, a comparison of the mean well-being scores showed no significant difference. To explore possible explanations for this finding, all differentiating variables

Table 46.3 Step-wise regression analysis of variables differentiating between heavy and light users (benefits and socio-demographics) with members' psychological well-being

Variable	Un-standardized coefficient		Standardized coefficient
	B	SE B	β
(constant)	78.725	2.508	
Self-rated health	−3.528	.656	−.318*
Having an easy-going, humorous attitude towards life	2.246	.503	.272*
A chance to express bottled-up feelings	−1.626	.476	−.209**
A chance to help, to be of service or to do things for other people	1.292	.475	.170**

$R\ square = 0.281$, $F\ score = 20.832$.

$^* p < .001$, $^{**} p < 0.01$.

(socio-demographics and benefits) were used as independent variables in a stepwise regression with the level of well-being as the dependent variable (see Table 46.3). The overall regression model accounted for 28.1% of the variance in well-being. Hence, there are probably other variables, not included in the model, which may explain members' well-being. Nevertheless, results indicated that poor health and the benefit of expressing bottled-up feelings (which may indicate a high level of loneliness) were negatively associated with well-being ($p < 0.01$), whereas two benefits, namely, 'having an easy-going, humorous attitude towards life' and 'a chance to help others', were positively associated with well-being ($p < 0.01$). Hence, it is possible that these two benefits enhanced the well-being of the heavy users, *in spite* of their being frailer, bringing it to the level of well-being enjoyed by the light users.

Conclusions

Seniors' online communities are, to an extent, a cybernetic social club. They provide a virtual sphere where older adults can meet new friends with whom they can chat, play, and exchange ideas, information, and emotional support. As such, the communities may enhance seniors' well-being in three ways, the first being *psychological*. Just as in offline seniors' clubs, the relationships created in the communities do not replace existing social networks, but they may expand members' social networks and somewhat compensate for the loss of friends and relatives as a result of retirement, relocation, physical or mental disability, or death. This is particularly true when members develop meaningful relationships through the private communication channels offered by the communities (i.e. private messages and chats), which turn into offline friendships and even conjugal relationships. Yet this may be valid even if the social interaction remains online and does not permeate into daily offline reality.

The literature on older adults' social networks suggests a positive association between various parameters of the social network and different dimensions of emotional well-being such as happiness, life satisfaction, morale, mood, depression, and so forth (e.g. Lang and Baltes 1997; McLaughlin et al. 2010). This association may be explained by the social support provided by the social network. Such social support helps people to cope effectively with stressful life events by influencing coping processes (Antonucci and Akiyama 1991), strengthening personal control and self-worth (Atchley 1991), and fostering hope and optimism (Nunn 1996).

It should be noted that the communities discussed here are not *intended* to provide social support. It would be more accurate to say that the social support exchanged by community members is an *outcome* of the relationships formed in the communities. There are numerous communities specifically designed to provide social support for older adults in need, such as persons with emotional disorders (e.g. depression), people coping with specific health conditions (e.g. dementia), care-givers and so forth. Such communities are not defined as seniors' online communities but rather as online support groups, and there is a significant body of scientific literature examining them (cf. Glueckauf et al. 2004; Griffiths et al. 2009).

The seniors' online communities are more social and recreational in their nature. In fact, the only shared 'purpose' (Lazar and Preece 1998) community members have is the desire to interact with others of a similar age. However, as the communities enable anonymity and invisibility, members tend to consult their peers with regard to personal and sensitive issues. The opportunity to receive and provide emotional support may have an empowering effect. The immediate social support offered by community members may help individuals in coping with stressful life events and losses. At the same time, being able to support others may provide members with a sense of meaning and purpose. The latter, as well as the easygoing, humorous, and playful atmosphere in the communities, seem to be particularly important factors in their well-being, as suggested by the results presented above.

The potential contribution of the communities to their members' psychological well-being is not limited to emotional aspects only. Participating in online communities may also contribute to members' cognitive health, as many of the discussions and games require activating cognitive abilities. Even if one is just 'lurking' in the online communication and does not take an active part in it, these abilities are still triggered. In addition, participation in seniors' online communities enables older adults to maintain a high level of social involvement, which is associated with better cognitive performances (e.g. Stoykova et al. 2011) and may even help to reduce cognitive decline in older adults (Béland et al. 2005; Holtzman et al. 2004; Seeman et al. 2001).

In addition to their psychological impact, the communities may have *instrumental* and *physical* contributions. The information provided by community members may serve as a practical tool, which helps seniors in processes of decision-making and managing age-related and general daily tasks, from handling their pensions to shopping and leisure planning. In addition, the contents of the many discussions of health may contribute to health management. Moreover, the literature on seniors' social networks provided evidence for their positive impact on exercise behaviour (Resnick et al. 2002), self-rated health (Zunzunegui et al. 2004), physical functioning (Unger et al. 1999), disability (Walter-Ginzburg, Blumstein, and Guralnik 2004), and even mortality (Rasulo,

Christensen, and Tomassini 2005). Therefore the social networks created in the communities may affect members' health.

At the same time, however, excessive use of the communities may lead to negative effects, such as limited physical activity, as found among older American adults embedded in family network types (Litwin 2012), as well as neck–shoulder and low back pain as a result of spending many hours in front of the computer (Hakala, Rimpelä, and Saarni 2006). Additional (non-physical) risks may be reduced involvement in offline relationships and internet addiction (Shaw and Black 2008). Hence, just like any other positive activity, some balance is required to keep participation in seniors' online communities beneficial.

As may be expected, heavy users of seniors' online communities report more perceived benefits from participation than light users. These benefits may be both an outcome of participation and a motivating factor that encourages continuous participation (Kleiber, Walker, and Mannell 2011). Nevertheless, the fact that heavy users of the communities are somewhat older than light users, and report lower education and poorer health, suggests that the communities may be particularly beneficial for frail older adults who face physical constraints that limit their abilities to participate in various outdoor activities. The communities offer such people an enjoyable and varied social activity that may replace and somewhat compensate for lost opportunities. Such mechanisms of optimization and compensation fit the Selective Optimization and Compensation (SOC) model of successful ageing, advanced by Baltes and colleagues (Baltes and Baltes 1990; Baltes and Carstensen 1999). They help older adults make the best of what is possible.

IMPLICATIONS FOR PRACTICE

Although a trial study that uses a single-component intervention and controls for non-community components is still required, the existing body of knowledge already suggests implications for practice. Because the communities have significant potential to enhance psychological well-being in later life, older adults should be informed about such communities and encouraged to participate in them. This is relevant to all seniors, but is specifically important with regard to frail, older people, including homebound seniors, people in nursing homes, and the oldest old.

Due to the aforementioned 'age divide', this task is not easy, but it may be achieved in various ways. First, more effort should be invested in providing training programmes that would enable seniors to acquire computer and internet skills. Instructors of computer and internet classes for older adults should address the subject of seniors' online communities. They should teach class participants how to locate such seniors' communities on the internet using search engines, and how to use them. Second, in order to create awareness among seniors who already use the internet, community administrators should use various promotion tactics including public relations and advertising (both online and offline).

In addition, designers of seniors' online communities should use the various insights provided by the literature on gerontechnology (cf. Chou, Lai, and Liu 2012; Cornejo, Favela, and Tentori 2010; Gibson et al. 2010) to make the communities' interface more senior-friendly. This includes, for example, designing aesthetically pleasing displays of information which support the monitoring of information without distracting or burdening the user, meeting seniors' visual requirements (e.g. by enlarging the bottom size and identification), providing accessibility assistance (e.g. by offering parent–child account number applications to enable younger family members to assist with registration processes), and reducing users' anxiety by offering a more tentative, incremental approach to revealing their identity. Lastly, practitioners working with older adults, such as psychologists, psychiatrists, geriatric nurses, social workers, and recreation therapists, should be informed about the communities' potential to enhance psychological well-being in later life, so that they may consider the communities in their professional interventions. Hopefully, this chapter will play a role in reaching that goal.

Summary

This chapter demonstrated how all the utilities of ICT for older adults that were identified in previous research, namely, a communication medium, an information source, a task-oriented tool, and a leisure activity, are offered by seniors' online communities. As these functions were found to make significant contribution to seniors' well-being, the main argument of this chapter was that seniors' online communities have significant potential to enhance psychological well-being in later life. Preliminary support for this argument was provided by original findings from a survey study comparing light and heavy users of the communities. Although additional research is still required, the existing body of knowledge already suggests implications for practice.

Acknowledgements

The author wishes to express her appreciation to Prof. Howard E. A. (Tony) Tinsley, who graciously provided her with information about his research and a copy of the PAL-E questionnaire for use in the study presented in this chapter. The author also wholeheartedly thanks Prof. Carol Ryff for providing her with a copy of the Psychological Well Being scale and for the permission to use it.

Key References and Sources for Further Reading

Bennett, J. (2011). *Online Communities and the Activation, Motivation and Integration of Persons Aged 60 and Older: A Literature Review*. Bern: Third Age Online (TAO). http://www.thirda geonline.eu/wp-content/uploads/2011/11/tao_preliminary_study_60_plus_literature_ review_20111103.pdf.
Burmeister, O. K., Foskey, R., Hazzlewood J., and Lewis, R. (2012). 'Sustaining Online Communities Involving Seniors'. *Journal of Community Informatics* 8(1). http://ci-journal. net/index.php/ciej/article/view/554/902.
Lampe, C., Wash, R., Velasquez, A., and Ozkaya, E. (2010). 'Motivations to Participate in Online Communities'. *CHI* 4: 10–15. Available at: http://rickwash.org/papers/pap1604_lampe.pdf.

Wellman, B. and Gulia, M. (1999). 'Net Surfers Don't Ride Alone: Virtual Community as Community'. In B. Wellman (ed.), *Networks in the Global Village* (pp. 331–367). Boulder, CO: Westview Press.

Xie, B., Huang, M., and Watkins, I. (2012). 'Technology and Retirement Life: A Systematic Review of the Literature on Older Adults and Social Media'. In M. Wang (ed.), *The Oxford Handbook of Retirement* (pp. 493–509). New York: Oxford University Press.

Websites: Examples of Seniors' Online Communities

Age Concern. http://www.ageuk.org.uk/.

Age Net. http://www.age-net.co.uk/.

Circles of Friends. http://www.circlesoffriends.net/.

Fifty Plus Forum. http://www.fiftyplusforum.co.uk/.

My Senior Portal. http://www.myseniorportal.com/.

Pensioners Forum. http://www.pensionersforum.co.uk/.

The Over 50 Golden Group. http://www.theover50goldengroup.com/.

Third Age. http://www.thirdage.com/.

Your Life Choices. http://www.yourlife-yourchoices.com/.

50 Plus Forum. http://www.50plusforum.co.uk/.

References

Antonucci, T. C. and Akiyama, H. (1991). 'Social Relationships and Aging Well'. *Generations* 15: 39–44.

Atchley, R. (1991). 'The Influence of Aging and Frailty on Perception and Expression of the Self: Theoretical and Methodological Issues'. In J. E. Birren, J. Lubben, J. Rowe, and D. Deutchman (eds), *The Concept and Measurement of Quality of Life in the Frail Elderly* (pp. 207–225). San Diego, CA: Academic Press.

Baltes, P. B. and Baltes, M. M. (1990). *Successful Aging: Perspectives from the Behavioral Sciences*. New York: Cambridge University Press.

Baltes, M. M. and Carstensen, L. L. (1999). 'Social-psychological Theories and their Applications to Aging: From Individual to Collective'. In V. L. Bengston and K. W. Schaie (eds), *Handbook of Theories of Aging* (pp. 209–226). New York: Springer.

Barak, A. (2007). 'Emotional Support and Suicide Prevention through the Internet: A Field Project Report'. *Computers in Human Behavior* 23: 971–84.

Barak, A., Boniel-Nissim, M., and Suler, J. (2008). 'Fostering Empowerment in Online Support Groups'. *Computers in Human Behavior* 24: 1867–1883.

Béland, F., Zunzunegui, M. V., Alvarado, B., Otero, A., and Del Ser, T. (2005). 'Trajectories of Cognitive Decline and Social Relations'. *Journals of Gerontology, Series B: Social Sciences* 60: 320–330.

Blit-Cohen, E. and Litwin, H. (2004). 'Elder Participation in Cyberspace: A Qualitative Analysis of Israeli Retirees'. *Journal of Aging Studies* 18(4): 385–398.

Boyd, D. M. and Ellison, N. B. (2007). 'Social Network Sites: Definition, History, and Scholarship'. *Journal of Computer-mediated Communication* 13: 210–230.

Burmeister, O. K. (2012). 'What Seniors Value about Online Community'. *Journal of Community Informatics* 8(1). http://ci-journal.net/index.php/ciej/article/view/545/880.

Camarinha-Matos, L. M. and Afsarmanesh, H. (2004). 'TeleCARE: Collaborative virtual Elderly Support Communities', in *Proceedings of the 1st Workshop on Tele-Care and Collaborative Virtual Communities in Elderly Care, TELECARE 2004* (pp. 1–12). Porto, Portugal: TELECARE 2004 in conjunction with ICEIS 2004.

Chou, W. H., Lai, Y. T., and Liu, K. H. (2012). 'User Requirements of Social Media for the Elderly: A Case Study in Taiwan'. *Behaviour & Information Technology*. Available at: http://www.tandfonline.com/doi/abs/10.1080/0144929X.2012.681068.

Cody, M. J., Dunn, D., Hoppin, S., and Wendt, P. (1999). 'Silver Surfers: Training and Evaluating Internet Use among Older Adult Learners'. *Communication Education* 48(4): 269–286.

Cornejo, R., Favela, J., and Tentori, M. (2010). 'Ambient Displays for Integrating Older Adults into Social Networking Sites'. *Collaboration and Technology* 6257: 321–36.

De Schutter, B. and Abeele, V. (2008). 'Meaningful Play in Elderly Life'. Paper presented at the *58th Annual Conference of the International Communication Association*, Montreal, Canada.

Dickenson, A. and Hill, R. L. (2007). 'Keeping in Touch: Talking to Older People about Computers and Communication'. *Educational Gerontology* 33(8): 613–30.

Fernandez-Ballesteros, R., Zamarron, M., and Ruiz, M. (2001). 'The Contribution of Socio-demographic and Psychosocial Factors to Life Satisfaction'. *Aging & Society* 21(1): 25–43.

Fokkema, T. and Knipscheer, K. (2007). 'Escape Loneliness by Going Digital: A Quantitative and Qualitative Evaluation of a Dutch Experiment in Using ECT to Overcome Loneliness among Older Adults'. *Aging & Mental Health* 11(5): 496–504.

Fuglsang, L. (2005). 'IT and Senior Citizens: Using the Internet for Empowering Active Citizenship'. *Science, Technology & Human Values* 30(4): 468–495.

Furlong, M. (1989). 'An Electronic Community for Older Adults: The Seniornet Network'. *Journal of Communication* 39: 145–153.

Gibson, L., Moncur, W., Forbes, P., Arnott, J., Martin, C., et al. (2010). 'Designing Social Networking Sites for Older Adults'. In *Proceedings of the 2010 British Computer Society Conference on Human-Computer Interaction, BCS-HCI 2010* (pp. 186–194). Dundee (Scotland): BCS.

Glueckauf, R. L., Ketterson, T. U., Loomis, J. S., and Dages, P. (2004). 'Online Support and Education for Dementia Caregivers: Overview, Utilization, and Initial Program Evaluation'. *Telemedicine Journal & e-Health* 10: 223–232.

Griffiths, M. D., Davies, M. O. N., and Chappell, D. (2004). 'Online Computer Gaming: A Comparison of Adolescent and Adult Gamers'. *Journal of Adolescence* 27(1): 87–96.

Griffiths, K. M., Calear, A. L., Banfield, M., and Tam, A. (2009). 'Systematic Review on Internet Support Groups (ISGs) and Depression: What is Known about Depression ISGs?' *Journal of Medical Internet Research* 11(3): e41. http://www.jmir.org/2009/3/e40/.

Hakala, P. T., Rimpelä, A. H., and Saarni, L. A. (2006). 'Frequent Computer-related Activities Increase the Risk of Neck-shoulder and Low Back Pain in Adolescents'. *European Journal of Public Health* 16: 536–541.

Henke, M. (1999). 'Promoting Independence in Older Persons through the Internet'. *CyberPsychology & Behavior* 2(6): 521–527.

Holtzman, R. E., Rebok, G. W., Saczynski, J. S., Kouzis, A. C., Doyle, K. W., et al. (2004). 'Social Network Characteristics and Cognition in Middle-aged and Older Adults'. *Journals of Gerontology, Series B: Psychological Sciences and Social Sciences* 59: 278–284.

Hutchinson, S. L. and Kleiber, D. A. (2005). 'Gifts of the Ordinary: Casual Leisure's Contribution to Health and Well Being'. *World Leisure* 47(3): 2–16.

Ijsselsteijn, W. A., Nap, H. H., de Kort, Y. A. W., and Poels, K. (2007). 'Digital Game Design for Elderly Users'. *In Proceedings of 2007 Conference on Future Play* (pp. 17–22). Toronto, Canada: The Game Developers Conference® Canada.

Ito, M., O'Day, V., Adler, A., Linde, C., and Maynatt, E. (2001). 'Making a Place for Seniors on the Net: Seniornet, Senior Identity, and the Digital Divide'. *Computers and Society* 31(3): 15–21.

Iyer, R. and Eastman, J. K. (2006). 'The Elderly and their Attitude toward the Internet: The Impact on Internet Use, Purchase, and Comparison Shopping'. *Journal of Marketing Theory and Practice* 14(1): 57–67.

Kanayama, T. (2003). 'Ethnographic Research on the Experience of Japanese Elderly People Online'. *New Media & Society* 5(2): 267–288.

Kadlec, D. (2007). 'Senior Netizens'. *Time* 169(7): 94.

Kelly, J. R. (1987). *Peoria Winter: Styles and Resources in Later Life*. Lanham, MD: Lexington Books.

Kelly, J. R. (1996). *Leisure* (3rd edn). Boston: Allyn & Bacon.

Kiger, P. J. (2006). 'Generation Xboxers'. *AARP Bulletin* 47(2): 3–4.

Kleiber, D. A., Walker, G. J., and Mannell, R. C. (2011). *A Social Psychology of Leisure* (2nd edn). State College, PA: Venture.

Kozinets, R. V. (2002). 'The Field behind the Screen: Using Netnography for Marketing Research in Online Communities'. *Journal of Marketing Research* 39: 61–72.

Kozinets, R. V. (2006). 'Netnography 2.0'. In R.W. Belk (ed.), *Handbook of Qualitative Research Methods in Marketing* (pp. 129–42). Cheltenham, UK and Northampton, MA: Edward Elgar.

Lang, F. R. and Baltes, M. M. (1997). 'Being with People and Being Alone in Late Life: Costs and Benefits for Everyday Functioning'. *International Journal of Behavioral Development* 21(4): 729–746.

Langer, R. and Beckman, S. C. (2005). 'Sensitive Research Topics: Netnography Revisited'. *Qualitative Market Research* 8(2): 189–203.

Lazar, J. and Preece, J. (1998). 'Classification Schema for Online Communities'. In *Proceedings of the 1998 Association for Information Systems Americas Conference* (pp. 84–86). Baltimore, MD: Association for Information Systems.

Litwin, H. (2012). 'Physical Activity, Social Network Type, and Depressive Symptoms in Late Life: An Analysis of Data from the National Social Life, Health and Aging Project'. *Aging & Mental Health* 16: 608–616.

Loges, W. and Jung, J. (2001). 'Exploring the Digital Divide: Internet Connectedness and Age'. *Communication Research* 28(4): 536–562.

McKenna, K. Y. A. and Bargh, J. A. (2000). 'Plan 9 from Cyberspace: The Implications of the Internet for Personality and Social Psychology'. *Personality and Social Psychology Review* 4: 57–75.

McLaughlin, D., Vagenas, D., Pachana, N. A., Begum, N., and Dobson, A. (2010). 'Gender Differences in Social Network Size and Satisfaction in Adults in their 70s'. *Journal of Health Psychology* 15: 671–679.

McMellon, C. A. and Schiffman, L. G. (2002). 'Cybersenior Empowerment: How Some Older Individuals are Taking Control of their Lives'. *Journal of Applied Gerontology* 21: 157–75.

Meier, A. (2004). 'Technology-mediated Groups'. In C. D. Garvin, L. M. Gutiérrez, and M. J. Galinsky (eds), *Handbook of Social Work with Groups* (pp. 497–503). New York: Guilford Press.

Nahm, E. and Resnick, B. (2001). 'Homebound Older Adults' Experiences with the Internet and E-mail'. *Computers in Nursing* 19(6): 257–263.

Nimrod, G. (2007). 'Retirees' Leisure: Activities, Benefits, and their Contribution to Life Satisfaction'. *Leisure Studies* 26(1): 65–80.

Nimrod, G. (2010). 'Seniors' Online Communities: A Quantitative Content Analysis'. *Gerontologist* 50(3): 382–392.

Nimrod, G. (2011). 'The Fun Culture in Seniors' Online Communities'. *Gerontologist* 51(2): 226–237.

Nimrod, G. (2012). 'Online Communities as a Resource in Older Adults' Tourism'. *Journal of Community Informatics* 8(1). http://ci-journal.net/index.php/ciej/article/view/757/857.

Nimrod, G. (2014). 'The Benefits of and Constraints to Participation in Seniors' Online Communities'. *Leisure Studies* 33(3): 247–266.

Nunn, K. P. (1996). 'Personal Hopefulness: A Conceptual Review of the Relevance of the Perceived Future to Psychiatry'. *British Journal of Medical Psychology* 69(3): 227–245.

Opalinski, L. (2001). 'Older Adults and the Digital Divide: Assessing Results of a Web-based Survey'. *Journal of Technology in Human Services* 18(3/4): 203–221.

Organisation for Economic Co-operation and Development (2011). *The Future of the Internet Economy: A Statistical Profile*. http://www.oecd.org/dataoecd/24/5/48255770.pdf.

Papacharissi, Z. (2002). 'The Virtual Sphere: The Internet as a Public Sphere'. *New Media & Society* 4(1): 9–27.

Pew Internet and American Life Project (2004). *Older Americans and the Internet*. http://www.pewinternet.org/pdfs/PIP_Seniors_Online_2004.pdf.

Pew Internet and American Life Project (2009). *Generational Differences in Online Activities*. http://www.pewinternet.org/Reports/2009/Generations-Online-in-2009.aspx.

Pfeil, U. (2007). 'Online Social Support for Older People'. *SIGACCESS Newsletter* 88: 3–8.

Pfeil, U. and Zaphiris, P. (2010). 'Investigating Social Network Patterns within an Empathic Online Community for Older People'. *Computers in Human Behavior* 25(5): 1139–1155.

Rasulo, D., Christensen, K., and Tomassini, C. (2005). 'The Influence of Social Relations on Mortality in Later Life: A Study on Elderly Danish Twins'. *Gerontologist* 45(5): 601–8.

Resnick, B., Orwig, D., Magaziner, J., and Wynne, C. (2002). 'The Effect of Social Support on Exercise Behavior in Older Adults'. *Clinical Nursing Research* 11(1): 52–70.

Rheingold, H. (1994). 'A Slice of Life in my Virtual Community'. In L. M. Harasim (ed.), *Global Networks: Computers and International Communication* (pp. 57–80). Cambridge, MA: MIT.

Ryff, C. D. and Keyes, C. L. M. (1995). 'The Structure of Psychological Well-being Revisited'. *Journal of Personality and Social Psychology* 69(4): 719–727.

Sade-Beck, L. (2004). 'Internet Ethnography: Online and Offline'. *International Journal of Qualitative Methods* 3(2): 1–14.

Seeman, T. E., Lusignolo, T. M., Albert, M., and Berkman, L. (2001). 'Social Relationships, Social Support, and Patterns of Cognitive Aging in Healthy, High-functioning Older Adults: Macarthur Studies of Successful Aging'. *Health Psychology* 20: 243–255.

Shapira, N., Barak, A., and Gal, I. (2007). 'Promoting Older Adults' Well Being through Internet Training and Use'. *Aging & Mental Health* 11(5): 477–84.

Shaw, M. and Black, D. W. (2008). 'Internet Addiction: Definition, Assessment, Epidemiology and Clinical Management'. *CNS Drugs* 22(5): 353–365.

Stebbins, R. A. (1997). 'Casual Leisure: A Conceptual Statement'. *Leisure Studies* 16: 17–25.

Stebbins, R. A. (2001). 'The Costs and Benefits of Hedonism: Some Consequences of Taking Casual Leisure Seriously'. *Leisure Studies* 20: 305–309.

Stebbins, R. A. (2007). *Serious Leisure: A Perspective for our Time*. New Brunswick, NJ: Transaction.

Stoykova, R., Matharan, F., Dartigues, J. F., and Amieva, H. (2011). 'Impact of Social Network on Cognitive Performances and Age-related Cognitive Decline across a 20-year Follow-up'. *International Psychogeriatrics* 1: 1–8.

Tinsley, H. E. A. and Kass, R. A. (1980a). 'The Construct Validity of the Leisure Activities Questionnaire and of the Paragraphs about Leisure'. *Educational and Psychological Measurement* 40: 219–226.

Tinsley, H. E. A. and Kass, R. A. (1980b). 'Discriminant Validity of the Leisure Activities Questionnaire and the Paragraphs about Leisure'. *Educational and Psychological Measurement* 40: 227–233.

Tufekci, Z. (2010). 'Who Acquires Friends through Social Media and Why? "Rich Get Richer" versus "Seek and Ye Shall Find"'. In *Proceedings of the 4th International AAAI Conference on Weblogs and Social Media (ICWSM, 2010)* (pp. 170–177). Palo Alto, CA: AAAI Press.

Unger, J. B., McAvay, G., Bruce, M. L., Berkman, L., and Seeman, T. (1999). 'Variation in the Impact of Social Network Characteristics on Physical Functioning in Elderly Persons: MacArthur Studies of Successful Aging'. *Journals of Gerontology, Series B: Psychological Sciences and Social Sciences* 54B(5): 245–251.

Van De Watering, M. (2005). *The Impact of Computer Technology on the Elderly*. http://www.few.vu.nl/~rvdwate/HCI_Essay_Marek_van_de_Watering.pdf.

Walter-Ginzburg, A., Blumstein, T., and Guralnik, J. M. (2004). 'The Israeli Kibbutz as a Venue for Reduced Disability in Old Age: Lessons from the Cross-sectional and Longitudinal Aging Study (CALAS)'. *Social Science & Medicine* 59(2): 389–403.

White, H., McConnell, E., Clipp, E., Bynum, L., Teague, C., et al. (1999). 'Surfing the Net in Later Life: A Review of the Literature and Pilot Study of Computer Use and Quality of Life'. *Journal of Applied Gerontology* 18(3): 358–78.

White, J. and Weatherall, A. (2000). 'A Grounded Theory Analysis of Older Adults and Information Technology'. *Educational Gerontology* 26(4): 371–386.

White, H., McConnell, E., Clipp, E., Branch, L. G., Sloane, R., et al. (2002). 'A Randomized Controlled Trial of the Psychosocial Impact of Providing Internet Training and Access to Older Adults'. *Aging & Mental Health* 6(3): 213–221.

Wright, K. B. (2000). 'The Communication of Social Support within an On-line Community for Older Adults: A Qualitative Analysis of the SeniorNet Community'. *Qualitative Research Reports in Communication* 1(2): 33–43.

Wu, M. (2011). *Social Networks vs. Online Communities: The Important Distinctions to Know*. http://www.mycustomer.com/topic/social-crm/social-networks-vs-online-communities-important-distinctions/126967.

Xie, B. (2007). 'Information Technology Education for Older Adults as a Continuing Peer Learning Process: A Chinese Case Study'. *Educational Gerontology* 33(5): 429–450.

Xie, B. (2008). 'Multimodal Computer-mediated Communication and Social Support among Older Chinese Internet Users'. *Journal of Computer-mediated Communication* 13(3): 728–750.

Yoon, J., Yoon, T. E., and George, J. F. (2011). 'Anticipating Information Needs for Senior Portal Contents'. *Computers in Human Behavior* 27(2): 1012–1020.

Zunzunegui, M. V., Koné, A., Johri, M., Béland, F., Wolfson, C., et al. (2004). 'Social Networks and Self-rated Health in Two French-speaking Canadian Community Dwelling Populations over 65'. *Social Science & Medicine* 58(10): 2069–2081.

CHAPTER 47

....

MOBILE COMPUTING TECHNOLOGY IN REHABILITATION SERVICES

....

DUNCAN R. BABBAGE

INTRODUCTION

....

THE coming decades usher in a marked shift in the age profile of the world population, with a higher proportion of older adults than ever seen previously, and a substantial increase in people over 85. There will be proportionally fewer younger adults to assist senior members of their communities. More developed countries anticipate dramatic change, but a demographic shift is projected in almost every country. (See Pollack 2005, for a discussion of these issues.) Professional and community carers will still play an important role, but their time will be divided across a greater number of older adults. Assistive technology for cognition has the potential to support older adults to remain more functionally independent, compensating for disability and increasing participation for people with cognitive impairment (Gartland 2004). While older adults do not want technology to replace human interactions in healthcare (Walsh and Callan 2011), technology offers one avenue to ameliorate the negative effects of carer scarcity, assisting independent living in the community for longer (Jorge 2001; Pollack 2005).

Pollack (2005) outlined three uses for assistive technology in supporting older adults: to ensure older adults are safe and performing necessary daily activities, to help older adults compensate for impairments, and to assess cognitive status. All three are worthwhile applications of assistive technology, but the second is the primary focus of this chapter—assisting older adults to maximize functioning by compensating for cognitive impairment with portable assistive technology. For a discussion of other areas, see Bharucha et al. (2009) and Pollack (2005).

KEY CONCEPTS AND PRINCIPLES

....

In thinking about the use of mobile computing technology with older adults, clinicians and researchers are likely to have a number of questions. Will older adults adapt to the use of mobile technology if they are not already familiar with it? Are our clinical teams sufficiently familiar with the technology to support older adults in this? Does the use of this technology lead to better outcomes for older adults with cognitive difficulties? If so, what kind of technology should we pursue in our research and practice for best outcomes?

CURRENT KNOWLEDGE

Older adults will utilize useful technology

Pre-existing familiarity with similar technology is often cited as a factor in the success or failure to implement the use of assistive technology, and there is some support for this notion (e.g. see Walsh and Callan 2011). Some technologies may be under-utilized by older adults (Mann et al. 2007). However, research does not bear out the fairly widespread misconception that older adults may be less *willing* to use technology or may even actively resist such use (Olson et al. 2011). Older adults are frequently open to and actively interested in technologies—when they see clearly demonstrable and current benefits to them to use them (Wilkowska et al. 2009). For instance, older adults are at least as likely as younger adults to persist with computerized approaches to cognitive-behavioural therapy, though they may require more technical support (Crabb et al. 2012). The usability of the technology itself may be a substantial contributing factor—both in terms of its generic usability for any person (anyone would find this device hard to use), and also the match with a particular person's cognitive abilities and difficulties (people with particular cognitive impairments would find this device hard to use; De Joode et al. 2010; LoPresti, Mihailidis, and Kirsch 2004). Carers are likewise supportive of the use of assistive technology when it is well matched with the needs of a person (Rosenberg, Kottorp, and Nygård 2011).

In 1989, when even many younger adults still had little experience with portable electronic devices, Giles and Shore (1989) suggested that paper diaries were likely to be easier to use for people with severe memory impairments due to their prior familiarity. The current generation of people in their 70s and 80s will likewise have variable familiarity with current mobile technology. In particular the touchscreen smartphones that have the most promise for this kind of work were only introduced as a product category in 2007, after the majority of these people had retired. The experience levels of older adults with mobile technology will clearly change in the near future. Jorge (2001), discussing the use of technology to support cognitively impaired older adults, stated that at that time, 'current mobile and ubiquitous technologies typically exert a high cognitive load on users and are targeted for highly trained subsets of the population' (p. 4). In contrast, our research with more recent technology indicated that younger to middle-aged adults with traumatic brain injuries were able fairly successfully to use a smartphone to complete a range of everyday tasks, having never used one previously, without training, and after only ten to fifteen minutes of self-directed familiarization (i.e. playing) with the device (Howard and Babbage 2009a). This kind of research is yet to be replicated in older adults, although there is data indicating that older adults are able to comfortably learn and use the gestural interfaces of touchscreen devices (Stößel et al. 2010), and examining how best to design interface elements like icons for older adults (Leung, McGrenere, and Graf 2011). Smartphones appear to be reaching the point where people are able to spontaneously (and correctly) use these devices without training. This gives much greater hope that people with cognitive impairments will be able to make successful use of such devices, with relatively limited (and thus cost-effective) training, and even if they do not subsequently recall any training they have had. Given anecdotal observation of many healthy older adults adopting such technology, smartphones clearly warrant investigation even in clinical samples without prior familiarity with this technology.

Clinicians are capable of supporting mobile technology

Gillespie, Best, and O'Neill (2012) defined assistive technologies for cognition as 'any technology which assists cognitive functioning during task performance', and observed that 'historically, it is high functioning people who have used [assistive technologies for cognition] to extend their ability' (Gillespie et al. 2012, p. 1). However, in the past these devices were more commonplace in corporate settings than healthcare settings, and many clinicians have not utilized technology such as PDAs and smartphones until recently. Gartland (2004) notes the significant commitment of time and effort necessary for rehabilitation professionals to keep abreast of the latest developments in technology in order to utilize it with their clients. Only by personally using mobile computing aids themselves will rehabilitation professionals have the intimate familiarity with the technology necessary to train a person with neurodisability to use them successfully. Clinicians are open to the use of assistive technologies for cognition, but only a minority are actually doing so (De Joode et al. 2012). Smartphones are now in many pockets that never held a PDA, and perhaps finally this may facilitate implementation of this technology with clients too. However, clinicians need to personally use these devices for more than just making phone calls and sending text messages if they are to become truly conversant with the technology. If a rehabilitation professional cannot use a smartphone to record information about their own contacts, organize their own appointments, and record important information they encounter in their day, what hope can they have of training their clients with cognitive difficulties to do so?

Mobile assistive technology for cognition looks useful—but hard evidence is needed

We know surprisingly little about mobile assistive technology for cognition in older adults. Even with younger adults, the majority of evidence in this field is based on individual case studies, case series, or small group studies. Such studies are weak if not carefully controlled, and the usefulness of assistive technology for cognition for people with dementia, and other older adults, is thus not well demonstrated (Van de Roest et al. 2012). Despite this, it is a fairly widely held view that assistive technology holds significant promise in assisting people with dementia with memory difficulties and in other areas (Cahill et al. 2007). People with mild dementia themselves report the potential value of such technological assistance (Nugent et al. 2007).

Casting a wider net across all age ranges and health populations, Gillespie et al.'s (2012) systematic review examined assistive technology for cognition. Sixty-one studies (67%) reported a positive treatment effect, with just four single-subject experiments (4%)

reporting mixed effects. (Again, this review covered all age groups, not just older adults.) The remaining twenty-six studies were usability studies or in two cases simply did not measure treatment effects. Therefore, 94% of the studies examining treatment effects reported a positive effect. This is a surprisingly high proportion, raising questions about the effects of design weaknesses (e.g. the lack of a robust control group in group studies) and the falsifiability of studies. Nevertheless, the weight of current evidence supports the general efficacy of assistive technology for cognition. The focus of the vast majority of these studies was younger adults (i.e. in this context 18–64-year-olds), typically with non-progressive cognitive impairment (Bharucha et al. 2009). However, some studies have been conducted with older adults, and these are outlined below.

Focusing attention

O'Neill and McMillan (2004) described a simple device that emits an audible alarm that signals when a neglected body part has not moved for a period. Examined in a series of studies after cerebrovascular accident (CVA), including a single-blind randomized controlled trial (RCT), improvements were maintained in motor functioning twenty-four months after treatment (Robertson, North, and Geggie 1992; Robertson, Hogg, and McMillan 1998; Robertson et al. 2002; mean age of the thirty-nine RCT participants was 69 years). This study is distinctive both for being one of just two RCTs of assistive technology including older adults, and also for novel use of quite simple and inexpensive technology that demonstrated a positive long-term outcome.

Older adults with mild or more serious cognitive impairment may have difficulty orienting to internal goal states ('What am I supposed to be doing?' and 'Am I actually achieving my goal?'). In just a few cases with older adults, assistive technology has been utilized to cue users to review internal goal states through 'content-free' cueing, resulting in improved task completion. Manly et al. (2004) used an auditory tone for this effect in participants with CVAs, with three of their seven participants being in their 70s. While such a small sample leaves this evidence fairly weak, it is relevant to note that this kind of approach using other forms of content-free cueing has likewise been found to be useful in younger adult samples, including those with cognitive impairment—for example, sending a text message saying 'stop' to somewhat paradoxically prompt task initiation (Fish et al. 2007; twenty adults with traumatic brain injury; TBI), or using content-free tactile cues (Rich 2009; three students aged 12–14). Given that these content-free cues have been shown to be effective (Gillespie et al. 2012) across a range of populations and contexts, and they can be delivered using even extremely basic technology, they would be a worthwhile target for more systematic research in older adults. Meanwhile, no studies to date have focused on older adults receiving messages that direct attention to specific points of focus. Such research has been conducted with younger adults, such as using cues provided through text prompts (Culley and Evans 2010; eleven adults with TBI) and auditory prompts (Hart, Hawley, and Whyte 2002; ten adults with TBI)—both of which resulted in increased goal-directed behaviour and improved recall of therapeutic goals. However, a particular research question for the use of cueing for older adults would be whether the older adults still saw content-free cues as applicable to their needs, given the particular importance older adults place on immediate usability. On the one hand, the simple technology that delivers content-free cues would be likely to be appealing (e.g. a device in your pocket that beeps from time to time). However, content-free cues might inherently be seen, particularly by older adults, as more abstract than something that draws attention to particular tasks that need to be completed (e.g. 'Remember to pay the power bill').

Memory and remembering

Inglis et al. (2004) described a (younger adult) participant who carried a bulky lever-arch file around with him, who expressed a desire to store all of this information in an electronic memory device. Inglis et al. described this as 'ultimately unrealistic'. Today this client's request would be easily met: a smartphone can now hold in local storage a full copy of a cloud-based database designed for just such a purpose. While no studies have yet been conducted in this area with older adults, there is no reason why older adults cannot access such services. Moreover, if they are provided with interfaces to these services that have been designed to compensate for sensory or cognitive disabilities (e.g. providing larger text sizes—which can often be achieved on a smartphone or tablet device through operating system level preferences; customizing interfaces to reduce the number of interface elements displayed on a screen at one time and thus reduce cognitive complexity), so much the better. Even in advance of formal research on such services, it is perfectly reasonable for clinicians to be trialling such interventions with their clients. Indeed, the most likely source of information on the effectiveness of such interventions will come from clinician-led evaluations based on a single case or a small series of cases, which can provide high-quality evidence—as discussed further in the later part of this chapter.

While the approaches above examine helping a person to access information and knowledge more generally, a number of approaches have trialled interventions to stimulate recall of personal autobiographical experiences and information. Alm et al. (2004) trialled digital versions of paper reminiscence books with six people with dementia, while Berry et al. (2007), working with a younger (63-year-old) man with limbic encephalitis, examined a device that made a photographic record of his day for later review. While these are interesting approaches, support for these interventions is at this stage limited—they have simply not been adequately examined (Gillespie et al. 2012). See Jamieson et al. (2013) for a more extensive review.

Self-management

Across all age groups, higher-level cognitive functions are the most frequently examined domain for assistive technology intervention, with 36% of studies examining interventions for time management, and 27% focusing on organization and planning (Gillespie et al. 2012). Most notable among these studies is the only RCT of scale in the area of assistive technology for cognition, conducted by Wilson et al. (2001, 2005). Their study examined people with memory complaints from 8 to 83 years of age, and provided strong evidence for interventions for everyday task completion and for completion of tasks at a scheduled time by presenting text-based reminders sent to pagers. Disappointingly, Fish et al. (2008) examined the subgroup of thirty-six people with CVA from that study, and concluded they had failed to maintain gains at follow-up. However, other smaller studies have supported such interventions as effective (e.g. Inglis et al. 2003; ten older and seven memory-impaired people). Reminders have also been found to be effective using voice messages from others (Leirer et al. 1991; sixteen older adults), using digital recorders enabling a person to listen to time-triggered verbal prompts in their own voice (Yasuda et al. 2002; nine older adults with dementia), or viewing and hearing video reminders recorded and scheduled by carers and presented on a mobile phone (O'Neill, Moran, and Gillespie 2010; seven older adults with mild cognitive impairment and two with Alzheimer's disease). Pollack (2005) argued that many current assistive technology devices 'function like glorified alarm clocks', noting, 'older adults...do not live their lives according to unchanging schedules' (p. 16). She suggested that schedule-management systems needed to be significantly more flexible, and discussed just such a system being developed by her research team. Pollack (2005) noted it would be straightforward to schedule and present reminders if the only criterion was to ensure the user was aware of planned activities. She outlined three other goals in reminder presentations that should also be balanced with that first goal: 'achieving a high level of user and caregiver satisfaction...avoiding introducing inefficiency into the user activities; and...avoiding making the user overly reliant on the reminder system, which would have the detrimental effect of decreasing, rather than increasing user independence' (Pollack 2005, p. 17).

The final point is debatable. One does not set a goal that an amputee will make decreasing use of their prosthetic limb over time. Likewise, neuropsychological rehabilitation focuses on functional outcomes, not the means of achieving them. 'User independence' is a function of the person plus the reminder system, not the person in isolation. If full function is achieved with the aid of a cognitive prosthetic, a person is not considered disabled in the social model of disability (World Health Organization 2002). Ongoing reliance on a reminder system should not in itself be seen as a negative outcome. Rather, factors that might limit continued use of the reminder system (e.g. high recurring cost, other resource constraints) should be identified as environmental barriers. Ensuring a person does not become *overly* reliant has merit. An artificial intelligence approach as discussed by Pollack (2005) is complex and thus has concomitant difficulties, so whether this is the best approach remains to be seen. The chief drawback to the system developed by Pollack et al. is that while the first research on it was published over a decade ago, the system remains a research project and is still not available commercially—so this proposed intervention approach has still had no impact on the lives of people outside the group's research trials. This criticism can similarly be levelled at other complex technology interventions.

In the area of supporting task organization and planning, there has been moderate support for interventions (Gillespie et al. 2012) that have ranged from providing verbal prompts on task steps that are responsive to verbal feedback from the user (O'Neill et al. 2010; six people with peripheral vascular disease, two with diabetes mellitus, with six over 65) to a more complex (though not portable) system that uses video cameras to monitor steps towards completion of handwashing, moderating auditory cues as appropriate to guide progress (Mihailidis, Barbenel, and Fernis 2004; Mihailidis et al. 2008; ten and six people with dementia). The use of video cameras comes with privacy and ethical concerns that need to be carefully weighed up (see Niemeijer et al. 2010). Such interventions also remain out of reach of most clinical settings, and are likely to remain so until sophisticated ambient technology is ubiquitous. Less complex interventions to assist self-management are, however, more feasible with current consumer technology. For example, it would be straightforward to present to a person with dementia a series of photos on a smartphone with associated audio instructions for each image in order to assist with task sequencing. This is simply a technology-based extension of work that many therapists have done with printed photographs and written instructions in the past. However, the technology offers multiple alternatives: photos can be quickly taken, immediately used, and replaced, with the cost of this mostly limited to the one-off cost of the smartphone itself. With the right system, such task sequences could even be updated remotely, and their use could also be monitored. Evaluation of such interventions in mainstream practice is now practical and appropriate.

Language

There is at least some degree of evidence for the use of electronic aids for enhancing conversational skills in Alzheimer's disease (Bourgeois 1990), though this small study (n = 3) examined improved outcomes only over a six-week period. (Other studies have found similar results for paper-based memory aids; e.g. Bourgeois 1993; Hoerster, Hickey, and Bourgeois 2001; six and four people with dementia, respectively.) Bharucha et al. (2009) reviewed two cognitive aids designed to assist people with aphasia with cooking tasks by providing visual or video-based prompts, with some tentative support found for such interventions in people with more severe aphasia. There are of course a myriad of areas in which aphasia would affect the ability to follow written step-by-step instructions beyond just cooking (Bharucha et al. 2009). Future research could examine the efficacy of a more generic tool for presenting step-by-step visual instructions to an end user, which could be quickly programmed for new tasks by a carer or clinician. As with the task sequencing example above, such a tool would not be difficult to develop for a modern camera-equipped smartphone or tablet device, and would provide a much more generalizable intervention for assisting people with aphasia. (For a review of the wider field of augmentative and alternative communication, see Fried-Oken, Beukelman, and Hux (2012).)

Wayfinding

Studies have examined technologies that provide information to users about their location using either GPS technology, or for indoor wayfinding, using electronic tags or environmental cues that a device could use to identify its own location. Evidence in this area is limited (Gillespie et al. 2012), with much of the related research being designed for people with sensory impairments or mobility difficulties rather than cognitive impairments (Pollack 2005). Despite this, for outdoor wayfinding, current technology seems highly promising for users who can manage their own basic safety on the roads. Some research with specialist devices has been reported (Liao et al. 2007; single experimental case; Kautz et al. 2002) though custom devices would appear unnecessary in most cases today. GPS navigation is now widely used by people in the general population, using both dedicated GPS devices and smartphones, when navigating by vehicle and on foot. For wandering patients with dementia, there are also passive technologies like GPS monitors embedded in the heels of shoes (Mahoney and Mahoney 2010). Clinical experience of the author and anecdotal reports from others indicates that some people with significant brain injuries are now successfully using GPS devices to drive between predefined locations. (These are otherwise safe drivers who have marked difficulty following a route to a destination without assistance. Clearly there are always more complex considerations regarding driving in older adults with progressive dementias; Ott and Daiello 2010.) Both this and the use of GPS devices for navigating while walking warrant formal documentation in single-case experimental designs or larger studies. Indoor wayfinding remains more complex due to the unreliability of GPS signals inside buildings, though there are small-scale trials of interest (e.g. Liu et al. 2008; seven adults with a range of disabilities). It seems likely that successful widespread adoption of indoor location-based supports will only be possible following global availability of submetre accuracy location data indoors, whether through improved GPS or complementary technology. (For a wider discussion of location-based services, see Raper et al. 2007a, 2007b.)

Emotional functioning

Various uses of assistive technology in relation to emotional functioning have been examined (e.g. the use of personal music devices to distract from hallucinations in schizophrenia, and using biofeedback to moderate symptoms of anxiety; see Gillespie et al. 2012, for an overview). Mobile devices have also been used to support various psychotherapeutic interventions, and the use of mobile assistive technology for cognitive domains may itself have positive effects on mood for people with cognitive impairment (Lancioni et al. 2009) and may reduce carer strain (Teasdale et al. 2009). There is also a burgeoning literature on the use of mobile devices in psychotherapies, such as for people with mood and anxiety disorders, and these interventions may well also be relevant to older adults. However, such applications are beyond the scope of the current chapter.

Other cognitive functions

To date, there has been no research examining assistive technology for cognition focused on psychomotor functions, perceptual functions, thought functions, or mental functions of sequencing complex movements in either older adults or more generally, and also no research examining calculation functions in older adults (Gillespie et al. 2012). These areas are characterized by the intimate relationships between a person's body position and movement, their environment, their internal experience, and control of all of these. As such, a plausible assistive technology device would require substantially more information about the current state of the person and environment than is required for more simple tasks such as directing attention to a predefined stimulus, providing orientation to current time and place, providing cues about task sequencing, or providing prompts to assist memory recall. Assistance with all of these other domains can rely on predefined information—such as a schedule—and objective external data—such as the current time, or the device's location determined by GPS positioning. However, mobile devices like smartphones are increasingly gaining sophisticated sensors to collect information about their environment and, in some cases (usually with additional peripherals), about the state of their user (e.g. a heart-rate monitor). It may be that in the future, these other domains will become more amenable to assistive technology intervention, particularly, as Gillespie et al. (2012) suggest, with some assistance elicited from the user such as through monitoring thoughts expressed verbally.

Adaptive assistants

Jorge (2001) outlined a vision of 'social assistants', ubiquitous machine-learning systems that could take the place of carers in supporting many of the needs of moderately cognitively impaired older adults. Whether implemented via personal robots in healthcare settings (Pollack et al. 2002; 2003), or in handheld devices, we are yet to see such a comprehensive vision played out. However, initial stages of such technology are now entering the mainstream with smartphones combining relatively well-established voice recognition software with a breadth and depth of natural language processing not seen before on a mobile device (or arguably, on any mainstream device). Some of the roles that Jorge ascribed to an intelligent assistant can also already be fulfilled with less sophisticated, now well-established cloud-based services. (That is, services provided through lightweight client software on a mobile device supported by powerful, often distributed, back-end servers on the internet that underpin the bulk of the intelligence and information processing required to provide the service.) For instance, Jorge's description of an assistant providing turn-by-turn walking directions to enable a person to navigate across a city, even with a degree of route-finding difficulty, is now embodied in the navigation apps available on all smartphones. In hindsight, it is interesting to note that Jorge (2001) argued custom technology developments to support wayfinding for people with disabilities might be applicable to a mainstream audience. In contrast, it has been development of services for a mainstream audience that has now brought such hoped-for services to the cognitively disabled population as well. It is mainstream software and hardware platforms with ubiquitous internet access, interfaces for easy data synchronization through cloud-based services, and sophisticated tools for rapid software development that will enable a myriad of additional assistive technologies to be deployed in coming years.

LIMITATIONS OF OUR KNOWLEDGE

In assistive technology for cognition, there is a surprising preponderance of peer-reviewed papers that offer opinions and recommendations, apparently divorced from actual data or any literature review (Babbage 2011). Measures of research quality indicate there are few well-controlled studies, and even fewer with substantial numbers of participants (Gillespie et al. 2012). The proportion of better-controlled studies has remained low over time, which may be a function of rapid technological development (Gillespie et al. 2012)—there is insufficient time to build on earlier exploratory studies with large-scale clinical trials as technology has changed. Research funding bodies may also be less motivated to support clinical trials based on compensatory technology, if they perceive the value of the findings to be eroding before the initial results have even been published. (In contrast, the framework outlined later in this chapter indicates that such research can have important relevance beyond the lifespan of the particular technology or device being examined.) There are difficulties with blinding; while research participants can usually be kept blind to the treatment conditions that other participants are receiving, it is clearly not possible for them to remain blind to treatment *they* receive. Meanwhile, the most robust assessment of functional performance would be in situ behavioural observation, which cannot be blinded to the use of assistive technology. (Perhaps at some point in the future, some assistive technologies may become unobtrusive enough that blinding of assessors may become feasible—devices providing in-ear audio prompts for example, or a heads-up display projected on standard glasses.) In any case, direct behavioural assessment is frequently impractical in functional contexts, and therefore most research in this field relies on self- and care-giver-reports of behaviour (e.g. task completion logs) that are unreliable. Due to these difficulties, at times research focuses on proxies for the desired behaviour, which arguably may not be adequate (e.g. recording memory for goals after goal prompts, rather than measuring goal completion). Finally, ethical considerations in this field of research could usefully receive greater and more nuanced attention (Zwijsen, Niemeijer, and Hertogh 2011). These issues all constrain our knowledge.

IMPLICATIONS FOR PRACTICE

Rate of technological change

Smartphones have achieved mainstream use, have substantially greater capacity than the mobile devices that preceded them and are also touted as being easier to use. They are ubiquitous, flexible, and far more cost effective than specialized assistive technology devices. However, while there has been a large shift towards mobile devices in assistive technology for cognition (Gillespie et al. 2012), the virtual absence of touchscreen smartphones in research published to date underscores a temporal disconnect. Compared to progress in technology, academic research is glacial. We have studies demonstrating the value of earlier assistive technologies for cognition, but current technology that is obviously superior has not been subjected to empirical evaluation for use in rehabilitation. There is reason to believe that this state of affairs will *always* be true. By the time one generation of technology has been scrutinized in clinical trials through to publication, superior alternatives have been released to market. At least three factors contribute to this: it takes too long to obtain grant funds. We design RCTs that require large numbers of participants to have sufficient power to answer simple *intervention works/does not work* questions. Finally, once we have actually collected data, it takes far too long to write papers about the work and even longer before they successfully complete peer review and are published. None of this even addresses the potential divide that separates most approaches examined in research trials from interventions that might plausibly be put into practice. There are many dilemmas for researchers examining assistive technology, and for clinicians who seek empirical guidance.

Testing abstract solutions

An evidence-based practice purist might hold back from utilizing new compensatory technology until it had been established by empirical research to lead to rehabilitation outcomes that were as robust as preceding devices, even when the newer devices are essentially presenting the same functional tasks in a new format and/or package. With an energetic

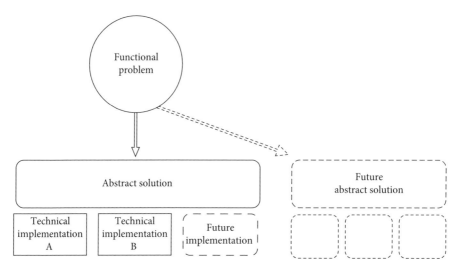

FIGURE 47.1 Relationship between functional problems, abstract solutions, and technical implementations.

and well-funded international research effort, it seems we could confidently make such pronouncements of efficacy about each technology around the time it was superseded by something newer—a recipe for full employment of assistive technology researchers, but not particularly effective rehabilitation.

I therefore argue (Babbage 2011, this chapter) that rather than focusing on *technological implementations*, research should be primarily concerned with testing *abstract solutions* to *functional problems*. Figure 47.1 outlines these relationships. For any particular functional problem, there should be a number of potential abstract solutions, and for each abstract solution, a number (perhaps an unlimited number) of possible technical implementations. A researcher may examine assisting people with dementia with task sequencing (the functional problem), by providing step-by-step prompts (an abstract solution) using a smartphone app (a technical implementation). Evaluating a successful outcome, a traditional researcher would conclude there is evidence you can assist with task sequencing if you use that particular app, and that attributes of the specific smartphone model may also have contributed to the outcome. The researcher might reasonably state that other similar interventions might also assist with impaired task sequencing, a hypothesis that would need examination in further studies. In contrast, the interpretative framework recommended here is that for relatively low-risk compensatory aids for cognition, technical implementations should be seen as exemplars of abstract solutions. By default, we should accrue the evidence to the abstract solution, rather than solely the one technical implementation tested. The study outlined above would thus be seen as providing evidence for the efficacy of providing step-by-step prompts in order to assist with impaired task sequencing, rather than evidence of efficacy of just that app. This framework essentially reverses the usual burden of proof in the case of technical implementations—it argues that by default all technical implementations of a particular abstract solution should be treated as equally supported. This would include future technical implementations of the same solution, which could be argued already to have empirical support from existing research. A technical implementation would then only be treated as more or less effective than another when there is specific evidence *against* equivalence—for instance, a well-designed study demonstrating that a particular app is indeed more effective for task sequencing than the default task sequencing approach. Of course, not all technical implementations are solving a problem in the same way, and the model in Figure 47.1 provides for the possibility of future abstract solutions that differ from those that have already been examined. In such cases, research specifically examining that particular abstract solution would be needed—as usual, through examining one or more technical implementations of that solution.

This model and this line of reasoning seems consistent with the approach of Gillespie et al. (2012), who concluded that they 'see the efficacy of prospective memory aids (reminding devices) established in principle...the established efficacy of Neuropage-like devices generalizes to the basic idea of *using reminding devices to assist prospective memory*' (p. 14, emphasis added). Some thought needs to be given regarding how broadly one can abstract a solution. One approach to weighing up a proposed definition of an abstract solution would be to consider whether other abstract solutions can be imagined—if the definition appears to encapsulate every possible solution to the functional problem, this may be an indication that it is merely restating the simple negation of the problem and is too broad a definition. (For example, simply 'a way of assisting with remembering events' would be too broad, whereas 'assisting with remembering by recording notes about events in writing' might be an appropriate abstract solution.) Again, this model is proposed as a way of handling a problem in an unusual research context: assistive technology for cognition is a relatively low-risk intervention, and one where the pace of development of one of the treatment components (the technology) vastly outstrips our ability to examine new developments in a timely fashion.

Observation of current practice suggests that many clinicians are already implementing much of the outlined approach, either consciously or intuitively. It is common to encounter clinicians making attempts to use the latest technology, extrapolating from previous research, supported by careful thinking and a dose of clinical intuition. For clinicians who have felt qualms about the empirical basis of this, the framework discussed here may resolve cognitive dissonance—such an approach seems justified in the assistive technology area. It is now important for health and disability funders also to recognize the practical necessity of extrapolating from past technologies to their logical descendants—refusing funding for an assistive technology because there is not yet peer-reviewed evidence for that particular brand/model/generation of technical implementation is short-sighted and is unlikely to be acting in the best interests of a client.

Use mainstream technology

Gillespie et al. (2012) outlined a range of ways in which assistive technology has the potential to maximize functioning for people with cognitive impairment, to improve relationships between people with cognitive impairment and their carers, and to reduce carer burden. They also noted, however, that assistive technology devices 'have yet to achieve this potential' (p. 2). There is a range of possible explanations for this discrepancy. Mihailidis, Fernie, and Barbenel (2001) asserted, 'Previous researchers have maintained that, for a cognitive device to be effective for a particular user, it must be developed as a one-of-a-kind device...Typically, up to 1,000 different parameters need to be customized for each user for a cognitive device to be effective' (pp. 26–27). If this is true, it is no wonder that we do not see an abundance of assistive technology for cognition in use in clinical settings. For example, Mihailidis et al. (2001) discussed three cognitive orthotic devices that were commercially available at that time; none of them had been subjected to clinical trials in older adults, and only one of them had been formally trialled in younger populations. Meanwhile, devices developed in research contexts rarely seem to become widely commercially available, if available at all. More importantly, however, it appears that while devices developed in research contexts may be well ahead of mainstream technology at their inception, they are rarely able to keep pace with the rate of development in mainstream technology. There are good reasons, therefore, to question the approach of designing specialized assistive devices and then highly customizing them to a user.

Where off-the-shelf products and services are not sufficient out of the box, these should be minimally modified, primarily focusing on customizations at the user application layer. For instance, this might involve creating a custom app for a standard smartphone, which provides a less cognitively complex interface to an existing service, but still storing all data with that service so that it remains accessible via the service's other interfaces. Where the standard physical sensors and interfaces to a mainstream device are insufficient, we should strive wherever possible to create additional sensors and input devices for the original mainstream device rather than creating an entirely new device. In this way, the specialized assistive device is responsible for only one layer of the overall service being provided, and there is a much greater chance that the specialized component will continue to evolve and remain relevant as new technologies become mainstream. Alongside this, the ideal is a universal design approach that begins in the product design stage (Sanford 2012). Clinicians and even most researchers in this field may feel some distance from being able to influence such processes, but a focus on the use of mainstream devices in healthcare settings will provide additional impetus for manufacturers to create mainstream devices that are accessible for all.

It seems likely that specialist devices will increasingly give way to superior mainstream alternatives, or at least to specialized apps running on mainstream hardware and software platforms. For instance, in discussing technology to alleviate social isolation for older adults, Pollack (2005) described the Dude's Magic Box (Siio, Rowan, and Mynatt 2002, cited in Pollack 2005), 'an innovative system that allows children to interact with grandparents who are far away by placing their toys or other objects of interest into a box that projects a picture onto a touch-sensitive screen at the grandparents' home' (p. 11). Today, you would simply buy the grandparent a mainstream tablet or smartphone with a built-in camera and simple-to-operate video chat, providing virtually unlimited communication over a wireless broadband connection for a basic monthly fee. This illustrates an important principle: most valuable technologies will be independently implemented for the mainstream before researchers have perfected it in the assistive technology sphere, and the mainstream alternative will be more advanced and be sold at a more competitive price.

A focus on currently available technology may also lead to more realistic solutions. For instance, in discussing the 'surprising' (p. 10) lack of assistive technology for assisting recognition or perceptual interpretation, Gillespie et al. (2012) proposed the possibility of a device that might verbally prompt the names of people in their environment via an unobtrusive earpiece, after recognition by the device via camera or voice recognition. Such technology remains well beyond current device capabilities, however. Pollack (2005) suggested that it is essential that any assistive technology system for cognition 'be able to observe and reason about the elder's performance of daily activities' and that 'the ability to recognize the performance of routine activities is also essential for compensation systems, so that they can provide useful assistance that is tailored to the current needs of the user' (Pollack 2005, both p. 12). Bharucha et al. (2009) presumably agree, because they eliminated entirely from their review 'cognitive aids that lack the ability to determine the user's current activity context and necessity or appropriateness of an intervention, such as simple reminder systems' (Bharucha et al. 2009, p. 3).

These requirements continue to present technological challenges, but their necessity for a cognitive aid to be useful is questionable. Less complex approaches have been shown to be viable utilizing users' areas of intact functioning to provide input. For instance, our research team is examining the ability of people with brain injuries to improve their functional capacity in the area of face-name recognition simply by the person with brain injury visually comparing the person in front of them to photographic or illustrated representations of those people on their smartphone (Howard and Babbage 2009b; Howard, Babbage, and Leathem 2011). This face-name recognition app, coded by Howard and Babbage, is currently being trialled using a single-case experimental design approach with six people with TBI. Rather than the smartphone providing face-recognition algorithms—a complex technology that relies on the user to engage in the socially awkward act of taking a photo of a person in their vicinity—the system uses GPS location information and other criteria to present the user with the most likely options for consideration first, and also provides for user input quickly to narrow the potential choices down to a manageable set. A simple interface is designed to reduce cognitive complexity. Initial results are encouraging (Howard et al. 2011). Other examples were reviewed earlier in this chapter across a range of domains, and no doubt other research taking this kind of approach is also currently being conducted. Rather than envisaging technologies not yet available, these kinds of intervention make novel use of current technology platforms and so have the potential for more immediate benefits in rehabilitation practice.

Closing the feedback loop

Feedback loops play a fundamental role in human performance (e.g. Yates 1963), yet we are often flying blind in rehabilitation practice regarding the extent to which clients use the compensatory interventions they are provided with and whether they are effective or not, and what the long-term outcome is (Babbage 2014). With some customization at the application level, compensatory mobile apps can be designed to log a person's use and automatically send this information back to a remote researcher or clinician. Clients who are struggling with the technology can then be identified and supported proactively, instead of relying on retrospective reports from clients and their families about compensatory aids. Such facilities also enable accurate analyses of dose-response relationships in compensatory aids. Given the substantial error in such analyses that is otherwise associated with being uncertain whether compensatory aids are even being used, this is a fundamental advantage of mobile-technology-mediated interventions over alternative approaches.

Single-case research

Given the inherent difficulty in accumulating evidence through large-scale studies in this area, there is high value in clinicians and researchers pursuing single-case experimental designs to evaluate their interventions. It appears this may already have been recognized, as these represent 74% of studies in the field (Gillespie et al. 2012). There are concrete steps that can be taken to ensure that such studies provide high-quality evidence that can reliably inform future practice. A single-case experimental design approach is ideally suited to examining treatment outcomes in heterogeneous populations such as older adults (Perdices and Tate 2009). It provides robust evidence as to whether the actual treatment was the cause of any effect observed, and each participant acts as their own control. This methodology is increasingly being recognized as providing Class I evidence that rivals RCTs and is highly practice-relevant. Meanwhile, it is a methodology that a clinician can embed within their clinical practice and utilize without devoting significant time to research as a separate activity; it can produce robust data about change in a single case or a small series of cases. Perdices and Tate (2009) and Mateer (2009) discuss these issues further, and Tate et al. (2008) present a single-case experimental design evaluation tool that can also be productively used as a checklist to learn about this approach to research and to guide the research planning process from the outset of a study.

Weighing risks and benefits

Clearly, the risks of any intervention must be considered. For instance, Bharucha et al. (2009) state, 'The accuracy of context-awareness when delivering a prompt is important since distraction at the wrong time (e.g. crossing a street or driving a car) could be life-threatening' (p. 3). There is some merit in this consideration, though it should be noted that one implication of this line of reasoning would also be to ensure no person with dementia ever carried a mobile phone, lest someone call them at an inopportune time. (There are, of course, a number of obvious counter-arguments as to why carrying a mobile phone would increase the overall safety of a person with dementia.) The risk of over-weighting such safety considerations is that developing additional complexity in systems will defer progress in actually delivering compensatory aids en masse to people who would benefit from them. Indeed, the substantial majority of devices and systems reviewed by Bharucha et al. (2009) were noted to be undergoing (mostly small-scale) research and were not yet commercially available—a situation essentially unchanged today. Actual delivery of interventions that can be utilized on a large scale and at reasonable cost should be a highly prized outcome of research.

SUMMARY

This chapter outlines that there is good evidence for the rehabilitative effectiveness of mobile devices as compensatory aids, particularly in some key domains. However, frequently weak methodological design limits the conclusions that can be drawn from small sample sizes. The vast majority of this research has been conducted with younger adults or children. While it is reasonable to be hopeful about applicability to older adults, research formally establishing this is clearly a priority. To this end, this chapter laid out a framework for the generalization of research findings, exhorted researchers and also clinicians to embrace solutions based on mainstream services and devices to protect longevity in the usefulness of interventions, and recommended intervention evaluation using robust single-case experimental design methodology. In concert, these approaches have the greatest probability of leading to improvements in the interventions delivered in front-line rehabilitation services for older adults with cognitive impairment.

DISCLOSURE

The author is a shareholder in Apple Inc. The views expressed in this chapter were not influenced by that investment, and were largely formed prior to that investment.

KEY REFERENCES AND SOURCES FOR FURTHER READING

Armstrong, N., Nugent, C., Moore, G., and Finlay, D. (2010). 'Using Smartphones to Address the Needs of Persons with Alzheimer's Disease'. *Annals of Telecommunications–Annales des Télécommunications* 65: 485–495.

Bharucha, A. J., Anand, V., Forlizzi, J., Dew, M. A., Reynolds, C. F., et al. (2009). 'Intelligent Assistive Technology Applications to Dementia Care: Current Capabilities, Limitations, and Future Challenges'. *American Journal of Geriatric Psychiatry* 17: 88–104.

Gillespie, A., Best, C., and O'Neill, B. (2012). 'Cognitive Function and Assistive Technology for Cognition: A Systematic Review'. *Journal of the International Neuropsychological Society* 18: 1–19.

Kurz, A. F., Leucht, S., and Lautenschlager, N. T. (2011). 'The Clinical Significance Of Cognition-focused Interventions for Cognitively Impaired Older Adults: A Systematic Review of Randomized Controlled Trials'. *International Psychogeriatrics* 23: 1364–1375.

Jamieson, M., Cullen, B., McGee-Lennon, M., Brewster, S., and Evans, J. J. (2013). 'The Efficacy of Cognitive Prosthetic Technology for People with Memory Impairments: A Systematic Review and Meta-analysis'. *Neuropsychological Rehabilitation* (epub ahead of print).

Reijnders, J., Van Heugten, C., and Van Boxtel, M. (2013). 'Cognitive Interventions in Healthy Older Adults and People with Mild Cognitive Impairment: A Systematic Review'. *Ageing Research Reviews* 12: 263–275.

Sanford, J. A. (2012). *Universal Design as a Rehabilitation Strategy: Design for the Ages*. New York: Springer.

WEBSITES AND OTHER RESOURCES

Center for Aging Services Technology: http://ww.leadingage.org/cast.aspx.

Center for Technology and Aging. http://ww.techandaging.org.

Centre for Excellence in Universal Design: www.universaldesign.ie.

RESNA Standards Committee on Cognitive Technologies. http://www.resna.org/atStandards/standards.dot.

REFERENCES

Alm, N., Astell, A., Ellis, M., Dye, R., Gowans, G., et al. (2004). 'A Cognitive Prosthesis and Communication Support for People with Dementia'. *Neuropsychological Rehabilitation* 14: 117–134.

Babbage, D. R. (2011). 'Systematic Review of the Use of Mobile Computing Technology in Neurorehabilitation'. Paper presented at the New Zealand Rehabilitation Association Conference, Auckland, New Zealand.

Babbage, D. R. (2014). 'Open and Abundant Data Is the Future of Rehabilitation and Research'. *Archives of Physical Medicine and Rehabilitation* 95: 795–798. doi:10.1016/j.apmr.2013.12.014.

Berry, S. M., Kapur, N., Williams, L., Hodges, S., Watson, P., et al. (2007). 'The Use of a Wearable Camera, SenseCam, as a Pictorial Diary to Improve Autobiographical Memory in a Patient with Limbic Encephalitis: A Preliminary Report'. *Neuropsychological Rehabilitation* 17: 582–601.

Bharucha, A. J., Anand, V., Forlizzi, J., Dew, M. A., Reynolds, C. F., et al. (2009). 'Intelligent Assistive Technology Applications to Dementia Care: Current Capabilities, Limitations, and Future Challenges'. *American Journal of Geriatric Psychiatry* 17: 88–104.

Bourgeois, M. S. (1990). 'Enhancing Conversation Skills in Patients with Alzheimer's Disease Using a Prosthetic Memory Aid'. *Journal of Applied Behavior Analysis* 23: 29–42.

Bourgeois, M. S. (1993). 'Effects of Memory Aids on the Dyadic Conversations of Individuals with Dementia'. *Applied Behavior Analysis* 26: 77–87.

Cahill, S., Macijauskiene, J., Nygård, A.-M., Faulkner, J.-P., and Hagen, I. (2007). 'Technology in Dementia Care'. *Technology and Disability* 19: 55–60.

Crabb, R. M., Cavanagh, K., Proudfoot, J., Learmonth, D., Rafie, S., et al. (2012). 'Is Computerized Cognitive-behavioural Therapy a Treatment Option for Depression in Late-life? A Systematic Review'. *British Journal of Clinical Psychology* 51: 459–464.

Culley, C. and Evans, J. J. (2010). 'SMS Text Messaging as a Means of Increasing Recall of Therapy Goals in Brain Injury Rehabilitation: A Single-blind Within-subjects Trial'. *Neuropsychological Rehabilitation* 20: 103–119.

De Joode, E., Van Heugten, C., Verhey, F., and Van Boxtel, M. (2010). 'Efficacy and Usability of Assistive Technology for Patients with Cognitive Deficits: A Systematic Review'. *Clinical Rehabilitation* 24: 701–714.

De Joode, E. A., Van Boxtel, M. P. J., Verhey, F. R., and Van Heugten, C. M. (2012). 'Use of Assistive Technology in Cognitive Rehabilitation: Exploratory Studies of the Opinions and Expectations of Healthcare Professionals and Potential Users'. *Brain Injury* 26: 1257–1266.

Fish, J., Evans, J. J., Nimmo, M., Martin, E., Kersel, D., et al. (2007). 'Rehabilitation of Executive Dysfunction Following Brain Injury: "Content-free" Cueing Improves Everyday Prospective Memory Performance'. *Neuropsychologia* 45: 1318–1330.

Fish, J., Manly, T., Emslie, H., Evans, J. J., and Wilson, B. A. (2008). 'Compensatory Strategies for Acquired Disorders of Memory and Planning: Differential Effects of a Paging System for Patients with Brain Injury of Traumatic versus Cerebrovascular Aetiology'. *Journal of Neurology, Neurosurgery and Psychiatry* 79: 930–935.

Fried-Oken, M., Beukelman, D. R., and Hux, K. (2012). 'Current and Future AAC Research Considerations for Adults with Acquired Cognitive and Communication Impairments'. *Assistive Technology* 24: 56–66.

Gartland, D. (2004). 'Considerations in the Selection and Use of Technology with People who Have Cognitive Deficits Following Acquired Brain Injury'. *Neuropsychological Rehabilitation* 14: 61–75.

Giles, G. M. and Shore, M. (1989). 'The Effectiveness of an Electronic Memory Aid for a Memory-impaired Adult of Normal Intelligence'. *American Journal of Occupational Therapy* 43: 409–411.

Gillespie, A., Best, C., and O'Neill, B. (2012). 'Cognitive Function and Assistive Technology for Cognition: A Systematic Review'. *Journal of the International Neuropsychological Society* 18: 1–19.

Hart, T., Hawkey, K., and Whyte, J. (2002). 'Use of a Portable Voice Organizer to Remember Therapy Goals in Traumatic Brain Injury Rehabilitation: A Within-subjects Trial'. *Journal of Head Trauma Rehabilitation* 17: 556–570.

Hoerster, L., Hickey, E. M., and Bourgeois, M. S. (2001). 'Effects of Memory Aids on Conversations between Nursing Home Residents with Dementia and Nursing Assistants'. *Neuropsychological Rehabilitation* 11: 399–427.

Howard, P. and Babbage, D. R. (2009a). 'Cognitive and Physical Demands of Multi-touch Interfaces after Traumatic Brain Injury'. Paper presented at the AFRM/NIRR/NZRA conference, incorporating the 17th Annual Scientific Meeting of the Australasian Faculty of Rehabilitation Medicine, Queenstown, New Zealand.

Howard, P. and Babbage, D. R. (2009b). 'Multi-touch interface trial after traumatic brain injury'. Paper presented at the m-health conference, Auckland, New Zealand.

Howard, P., Babbage, D. R., and Leathem, J. M. (2011). 'Smartphone-based Compensation for Face Naming Difficulties after Brain Injury'. *Brain Impairment* 12: 77.

Inglis, E. A., Szymkowiak, A., Gregor, P., Newell, A., Hine, N., et al. (2003). 'Issues Surrounding the User-centred Development of a New Interactive Memory Aid'. *Universal Access in the Information Society* 2: 226–234.

Inglis, E. A., Szymkowiak, A., Gregor, P., Newell, A. F., Hine, N., et al. (2004). 'Usable technology? Challenges in Designing a Memory Aid with Current Electronic Devices'. *Neuropsychological Rehabilitation* 14: 77–87.

Jamieson, M., Cullen, B., McGee-Lennon, M., Brewster, S., and Evans, J. J. (2013). 'The Efficacy of Cognitive Prosthetic Technology for People with Memory Impairments: A Systematic Review and Meta-analysis'. *Neuropsychological Rehabilitation* (epub ahead of print).

Jorge, J. A. (2001). 'Adaptive Tools for the Elderly: New Devices to Cope with Age-induced Cognitive Disabilities'. In *WUAUC'01 Proceedings of the 2001 EC/NSF workshop on Universal Accessibility of Ubiquitous Computing: Providing for the Elderly* (pp. 66–70). New York: ACM.

Kautz, H., Fox, D., Etzioni, O., Borriello, G., and Arnstein, L. (2002). 'An Overview of the Assisted Cognition Project'. Paper presented at the AAAI-2002 Workshop on Automation as Caregiver: The Role of Intelligent Technology in Elder Care, Edmonton, Alberta.

Lancioni, G., Singh, N., O'Reilly, M., Zonno, N., Flora, A., et al. (2009). 'Persons with Mild and Moderate Alzheimer's Disease Use Verbal-instruction Technology to Manage Daily Activities: Effects on Performance and Mood'. *Developmental Neurorehabilitation* 12: 181–190.

Leirer, V. O., Morrow, D. G., Tanke, E. D., and Pariante, G. M. (1991). 'Elder's Nonadherence: Its Assessment and Medication Reminding by Voice Mail'. *Gerontologist* 31: 514–520.

Leung, R., McGrenere, J., and Graf, P. (2011). 'Age-related Differences in the Initial Usability of Mobile Device Icons'. *Behaviour and Information Technology* 30: 629–642.

Liao, L., Patterson, D. J., Fox, D., and Kautz, H. (2007). 'Learning and Inferring Transportation Routines'. *Artificial Intelligence* 171: 311–331.

Liu, A. L., Hile, H., Kautz, H., Borriello, G., Brown, P. A., et al. (2008). 'Indoor Wayfinding: Developing a Functional Interface for Individuals with Cognitive Impairments'. *Disability and Rehabilitation: Assistive Technology* 3: 69–81.

LoPresti, E. F., Mihailidis, A., and Kirsch, N. (2004). 'Assistive Technology for Cognitive Rehabilitation: State of the Art'. *Neuropsychological Rehabilitation* 14: 5–39.

Mahoney, E. L. and Mahoney, D. F. (2010). 'Acceptance of Wearable Technology by People with Alzheimer's Disease: Issues and Accommodations'. *American Journal of Alzheimer's Disease and Other Dementias* 25: 527–531.

Manly, T., Heutink, J., Davidson, B., Gaynord, B., Greenfield, E., et al. (2004). 'An Electronic Knot in the Handkerchief: "Content Free Cueing" and the Maintenance of Attentive Control'. *Neuropsychological Rehabilitation* 14: 89–116.

Mann, W. C., Belchior, P., Tomita, M. R., and Kemp, B. J. (2007). 'Older Adults' Perception and Use of PDAs, Home Automation System, and Home Health Monitoring System'. *Topics in Geriatric Rehabilitation* 23: 35–46.

Mateer, C. A. (2009). 'Neuropsychological Interventions for Memory Impairment and the Role of Single-case Design Methodologies'. *Journal of the International Neuropsychological Society* 15: 623–628.

Mihailidis, A., Barbenel, J. C., and Fernie, G. (2004). 'The Efficacy of an Intelligent Cognitive Orthosis to Facilitate Handwashing by Persons with Moderate to Severe Dementia'. *Neuropsychological Rehabilitation* 14: 135–171.

Mihailidis, A., Boger, J., Craig, T., and Hoey, J. (2008). 'The COACH Prompting System to Assist Older Adults with Dementia through Handwashing: An Efficacy Study'. *BMC Geriatrics* 8: 28.

Mihailidis, A., Fernie, G. R., and Barbenel, J. C. (2001). 'The Use of Artificial Intelligence in the Design of an Intelligent Cognitive Orthosis for People with Dementia'. *Assistive Technology* 13: 23–39.

Niemeijer, A. R., Frederiks, B. J. M., Riphagen, I. I., Legemaate, J., and Eefsting, J. A. (2010). 'Ethical and Practical Concerns of Surveillance Technologies in Residential Care for People with Dementia or Intellectual Disabilities: An Overview of the Literature'. *International Psychogeriatrics* 22: 1129–1142.

Nugent, C., Mulvenna, M., Moelaert, F., Bergvall-Kåreborn, B., Meiland, F., et al. (2007). 'Home Based Assistive Technologies for People with Mild Dementia'. *Pervasive Computing for Quality of Life Enhancement* 4541: 63–69.

O'Neill, B. and McMillan, T. M. (2004). 'The Efficacy of Contralesional Limb Activation in Rehabilitation of Unilateral Hemiplegia and Visual Neglect: A Baseline-intervention Study'. *Neuropsychological Rehabilitation* 14: 437–447.

O'Neill, B., Moran, K., and Gillespie, A. (2010). 'Scaffolding Rehabilitation Behaviour Using a Voice-mediated Assistive Technology for Cognition'. *Neuropsychological Rehabilitation* 20: 509–527.

Olson, K., O'Brien, M., Rogers, W., and Charness, N. (2011). 'Diffusion of Technology: Frequency of Use for Younger and Older Adults'. *Ageing International* 36: 123–145.

Ott, B. R. and Daiello, L. A. (2010). 'How Does Dementia Affect Driving in Older Patients?' *Aging Health* 6: 77–85.

Perdices, M. and Tate, R. L. (2009). 'Single-subject Designs as a Tool for Evidence-based Clinical Practice: Are they Unrecognised and Undervalued?' *Neuropsychological Rehabilitation* 19: 904–927.

Pollack, M. E. (2005). 'Intelligent Technology for an Aging Population: The Use of AI to Assist Elders with Cognitive Impairment'. *AI Magazine* 26: 9.

Pollack, M. E., Brown, L., Colbry, D., McCarthy, C. E., Orosz, C., Peintner, B., Ramakrishnan, S., and Tsamardinos, I. (2003). Autominder: An Intelligent Cognitive Orthotic System for People with Memory Impairment. *Robotics and Autonomous Systems* 44: 273–282.

Pollack, M. E., McCarthy, C. E., Ramakrishnan, S., Tsamardinos, I., Brown, L., et al. (2002). 'Autominder: A Planning, Monitoring, and Reminding Assistive Agent'. International Conference on Intelligent Autonomous Systems.

Raper, J., Gartner, G., Karimi, H., and Rizos, C. (2007a). 'Applications of Location-based Services: A Selected Review'. *Journal of Location Based Services* 1: 89–111.

Raper, J., Gartner, G., Karimi, H., and Rizos, C. (2007b). 'A Critical Evaluation of Location Based Services and their Potential'. *Journal of Location Based Services* 1: 5–45.

Rich, L. P. (2009). 'Prompting Self-monitoring with Assistive Technology to Increase Academic Engagement in Students with Attention-deficit/Hyperactivity Disorder Symptoms'. Dissertation, Hofstra University.

Robertson, I. H., Hogg, K., and McMillan, T. M. (1998). 'Rehabilitation of Visual Neglect: Improving Function by Contralesional Limb Activation'. *Neuropsychological Rehabilitation* 8: 19–29.

Robertson, I. H., McMillan, T. M., MacLeod, E., Edgeworth, J., and Brock, D. (2002). 'Rehabilitation by Limb Activation Training Reduces Left-sided Motor Impairment in Unilateral Neglect Patients: A Single-blind Randomised Control Trial'. *Neuropsychological Rehabilitation* 12: 439–454.

Robertson, I. H., North, N. T., and Geggie, C. (1992). 'Spatiomotor Cueing in Unilateral Neglect: Three Cases of Its Therapeutic Effects'. *Journal of Neurology, Neurosurgery & Psychiatry* 55: 799–805.

Rosenberg, L., Kottorp, A., and Louise, N. R. (2011). 'Readiness for Technology Use with People with Dementia: The Perspectives of Significant Others'. *Journal of Applied Gerontology* 28 January. doi:10.1177/0733464810396873.

Sanford, J. A. (2012). *Universal Design as a Rehabilitation Strategy: Design for the Ages*. New York: Springer.

Stößel, C., Wandke, H., Blessing, L., Kopp, S., and Wachsmuth, I. (2010). *Gestural Interfaces for Elderly Users: Help or Hindrance? Gesture in Embodied Communication and Human-Computer Interaction*. Berlin/Heidelberg: Springer.

Tate, R. L., McDonald, S., Perdices, M., Togher, L., Schultz, R., et al. (2008). 'Rating the Methodological Quality of Single-subject Designs and n-of-1 trials: Introducing the Single-Case Experimental Design (SCED) Scale'. *Neuropsychological Rehabilitation* 18: 385–401.

Teasdale, T. W., Emslie, H., Quirk, K., Evans, J., Fish, J., et al. (2009). 'Alleviation of Carer Strain during the Use of the NeuroPage Device by People with Acquired Brain Injury'. *Journal of Neurology, Neurosurgery and Psychiatry* 80: 781–783.

Van de Roest, H. G., Wenborn, J., Dröes, R. M., and Orrell, M. (2012). 'Assistive Technology for Memory Support in Dementia'. *Cochrane Database of Systematic Reviews*: CD009627.

Walsh, K. and Callan, A. (2011). 'Perceptions, Preferences, and Acceptance of Information and Communication Technologies in Older-adult Community Care Settings in Ireland: A Case-Study and Ranked-Care Program Analysis'. *Ageing International* 36: 102–122.

Wilkowska, W., Ziefle, M., Holzinger, A., and Miesenberger, K. (2009). *Which Factors Form Older Adults' Acceptance of Mobile Information and Communication Technologies? HCI and Usability for e-inclusion*. Berlin/Heidelberg: Springer.

Wilson, B. A., Emslie, H., Quirk, K., Evans, J., and Watson, P. (2005). 'A Randomized Control Trial to Evaluate a Paging System for People with Traumatic Brain Injury'. *Brain Injury* 19: 891–894.

Wilson, B. A., Emslie, H. C., Quirk, K., and Evans, J. J. (2001). 'Reducing Everyday Memory and Planning Problems by means of a Paging System: A Randomised Control Crossover Study'. *Journal of Neurology, Neurosurgery & Psychiatry* 70: 477–482.

World Health Organization (2002). *Towards a Common Language for Functioning, Disability and Health (ICF)*. Geneva: World Health Organization.

Yasuda, K., Misu, T., Beckman, B., Wantanabe, O., Ozawa, Y., and Nakamura, T. (2002). 'Use of an IC-Recorder as a Voice Output Memory Aid for Patients with Prospective Memory Impairment'. *Neuropsychological Rehabilitation* 12: 155.

Yates, A. J. (1963). 'Delayed Auditory Feedback'. *Psychological Bulletin* 60: 213–232.

Zwijsen, S. A., Niemeijer, A. R., and Hertogh, C. M. (2011). 'Ethics of Using Assistive Technology in the Care for Community-dwelling Elderly People: An Overview of the Literature'. *Aging & Mental Health* 15: 419–427.

CHAPTER 48

VIRTUAL REALITY TECHNIQUES IN OLDER ADULTS

Exposure Therapy, Memory Training, and Training of Motor Balance

KATHARINA MEYERBRÖKER AND
PAUL M. G. EMMELKAMP

INTRODUCTION

VIRTUAL reality (VR) integrates real-time computer graphics, body tracking devices, visual displays, and other sensory inputs to immerse individuals in a computer-generated virtual environment. First, we will discuss whether virtual reality exposure therapy (VRET) is applicable to older anxious patients. Although age-dependent information processing or controlling posture may affect the feasibility and usefulness of virtual reality techniques, there is a growing body of evidence that virtual reality can be a useful tool in assessment and rehabilitation of patients with neurodegenerative disorders of ageing such as Alzheimer's disease or patients who have suffered from stroke (Farrow and Reid 2004; McGee et al. 2000) or Parkinson's disease (Arias et al. 2012). Additionally, there are indications that virtual reality can be a beneficial component in treating memory impairment in older adults (Optale et al. 2010). Research will be discussed with respect to the use of virtual reality in preventing or delaying cognitive decline. In addition, research into controlling posture and balance in virtual reality in older patients will be discussed in terms of assessment and the type of interventions used. Finally, we will briefly discuss research into the increased risk of cybersickness in older patients.

VIRTUAL REALITY EXPOSURE THERAPY IN LATE-LIFE ANXIETY DISORDERS

In geriatric psychiatry it is often held that mood disorders are more prevalent in older adults than anxiety disorders, but epidemiological studies have shown that anxiety disorders are in fact more common in older adults than major depression and dysthymia, and usually persist over years when untreated (Schuurmans et al. 2005). There is some evidence that cognitive-behaviour therapy (CBT) for anxiety disorders in older persons is less effective when compared to treatment with anti-depressants (Pinquart and Duberstein 2007). Data comparing the short-term effectiveness of CBT and sertraline for late-life anxiety, described in a study by Schuurmans et al. (2006), revealed higher effect sizes for sertraline. Dropouts were present in both treatment groups, with a total attrition rate of 32%. No significant differences between treatment groups were found in treatment response and end-state functioning. In addition, at one-year follow-up effect sizes of older patients who completed treatment for sertraline remained in the moderate to large range (Cohen's d = 0.60–1.62), while effect sizes for CBT were small to moderate (Cohen's d = 0.22–0.70) (Schuurmans et al. 2009).

Given the relatively small effects of CBT in anxious older persons and given that there are often contraindications for prescribing anti-depressants in such persons (French et al. 2006), it would be an important development if VRET was shown to be effective in such patients with an anxiety disorder. VRET is a modern alternative to classical exposure in vivo therapy. The rationale of exposure therapy is to confront patients with their anxiety-provoking stimuli to enhance habituation (Emmelkamp 2013). During VRET the patient is not exposed to real threatening stimuli, but guided by a therapist through a virtual environment with anxiety-provoking cues to elicit specific fears in the patient. In a recent study with patients with panic disorder and agoraphobia, synchrony of temporal processes involved in VRET and exposure in vivo on weekly avoidance measures and cognitive measures was demonstrated (Meyerbroeker et al. 2013). It has been demonstrated that VRET can be as effective in specific phobias (i.e. acrophobia and fear of flying) as the state-of-the-art treatment exposure in vivo (Opris et al. 2012; Powers and Emmelkamp 2008). In more complex anxiety disorders such as panic disorder with agoraphobia, results with exposure in vivo were slightly better than with VRET (Meyerbroeker et al. 2013), but in post-traumatic stress disorder (PTSD) the results of VRET have been less convincing (Goncalves et al. 2012; Meyerbröker and Emmelkamp 2010; Meyerbröker 2014), something that will be discussed later in this chapter.

However, while in most trials the efficacy of VRET in specific phobias has been demonstrated (Meyerbröker and Emmelkamp 2010), to our knowledge there has been almost no research into the factor of age. This is especially important given the increase in the use of technology in daily life. If in future therapy is increasingly to be delivered digitally, either by e-health, mobile health (or m-health) or virtual reality technologies, it is important to evaluate whether these newer therapeutic instruments are viable alternatives in older populations, in order to prevent exclusion of older adults because of the complexity of hardware/ software or other considerations.

As noted above, although there is robust evidence that VRET is as effective as the gold standard exposure in vivo in acrophobia and fear of flying, and nearly as effective in agoraphobia, most studies excluded older persons (above the age of 65). Most research concerning VRET in older adults has been done in war veterans suffering from PTSD. The essential feature of PTSD is the development of persistent and recurrent re-experiencing of trauma, avoiding situations, thoughts, and emotions associated with trauma, and experiencing increased arousal after having been exposed to a traumatic event involving direct personal threat, death, or serious injury (APA 2000). To our knowledge there are not many randomized controlled trials (RCTs) published in patients with PTSD and VRET, which might be due to the complexity of the disorder. We will limit our review to war veterans and exclude studies with active duty members, given the difference in age.

One of the first studies with older war veterans (but see discussion below) was an open clinical trial, wherein Vietnam combat veterans with a diagnosis of PTSD (APA 2000) underwent sixteen sessions of VRET (Rothbaum et al. 2001). From the sixteen patients who started treatment, ten completed all therapy sessions. PTSD symptoms were rated on clinician-rated and self-report measures including the Clinician Administered PTSD Scale (CAPS; Blake et al. 1995; Weathers, Keane, and Davidson 2001), the Combat Exposure Scale (CES; Foy et al. 1984), and the Impact of Event Scale (IES; (Horowitz, Wilner, and Alvarez 1979). Patients were exposed to two virtual environments: a virtual Huey helicopter flying over a virtual Vietnam and a clearing surrounded by jungle. On the CAPS at six-month follow-up an overall statistically significant decrease of PTSD symptoms from baseline was measured. Significant decreases were measured in all three symptom clusters. However, patient self-reported intrusion symptoms as measured by the IES were significantly lower at three-month follow-up but not at six months. One major limitation of this study is that it concerns an open trial with no randomization to either treatment or a control group. Additionally, it concerned a small group of patients with a substantial dropout rate (28%). In this patient population high dropout rates were expected given the complex symptoms from which patients were suffering. No indications were mentioned by the authors that dropout of patients was related to age. Finally, the mean age of patients was 51 years (SD = 3.16), which means that generalizability to older populations is limited.

In a more recent study with Portuguese war veterans, VRET was compared to exposure in imagination (EI) and a waiting list (WL) condition (Gamito et al. 2010). In this rather small study ten patients were randomly assigned to receive twelve exposure sessions either in virtual reality or imagination, or to WL. Patients in the VRET condition were exposed to a virtual footpath surrounded by dense vegetation, where patients had to follow a column of virtual soldiers. Intensity of sessions was manipulated by increasing the frequency of the following cues: ambush, sounds of gun firing and tracing bullets, mortar, sound of blasting amidst black smoke and spraying particles, waiting for an evacuation, waiting near an injured soldier for a helicopter to fly in and to evacuate him. The mean age of patients was 63 (SD = 4.43) years and from the ten patients who started treatment one dropped out from the VRET condition. PTSD symptoms were assessed with the CAPS and the IES. Unfortunately, no statistically significant effects of treatment were found at the post-test on the CAPS. Further, non-significant similar symptom reduction was found in the WL group as in both active treatment groups, indicating that the small symptom changes could possibly be explained by time. Given the small numbers per group, no group comparisons were made.

In another small study eleven Vietnam War veterans were randomly assigned to receive either ten sessions of VRET or present-centred therapy (PCT), which avoided traumatic content and was based on a problem-solving approach (Ready et al. 2010). Patients were recruited with flyers and presentations at the Atlanta VA Medical Centre for Mental Health Clinic, where they had been under treatment for their PTSD for the preceding three months. They were assessed at pre- and post-treatment, and at six-month follow-up. The mean age of patients was 57.5 (SD = 3.03) years. Two virtual Vietnam environments were used. One environment was a 'landing-zone' with rolling hills that included a swampy rice-paddy area surrounded by jungle that was experienced to be about two acres wide. Effects included muzzle flashes from the jungle, the sound of a land mine exploding, helicopters flying overhead, helicopters landing and taking off, darkness and fog. Additionally, auditory effects included jungle sounds such as crickets, distant gun-fire and explosions, enemy machine gun-fire, mortars being launched, sloshing sounds in the swampy area, screaming and male voices yelling, 'Move out! Move out!' The other environment consisted of a ride with a Huey helicopter, which included different Vietnam-like terrains and touching down in a 'hot' landing zone. Combining the groups, significant treatment effects were found from pre- to post-treatment and from pre-treatment to follow-up. No statistically significant effects were found when individual treatment conditions were compared—neither on PTSD symptoms as assessed with the CAPS nor on general depressive symptoms as assessed on the Beck Depression Inventory (BDI; Beck et al. 1988). However, a high variability in CAPS scores and the small sample size did not allow for more explicit interpretation of the data.

The reviewed VRET studies with older adults with PTSD, however, are minimal. None of the studies demonstrated stable effects of VRET in treating older adults with PTSD. It is difficult to conclude that age-related aspects affected therapy given that this was not investigated in these studies. The fact that VRET was not found to be effective may be attributed to other factors, including that the number of sessions were too few for such a complex disorder. Additionally, evidence-based protocols in treating PTSD consist usually of more components than pure exposure to the traumatic event (Kulkarni, Barrad, and Cloitre, 2014). It might therefore be possible, that trauma memory might have been triggered by VRET (which would explain the high variability in CAPS scores in some of the studies) but could not adequately be processed in all individuals to cure trauma memory.

In summary, to our knowledge there is no evidence yet that VRET is effective in older adults with PTSD. More research into human variables (e.g. age, culture) is needed to investigate whether or not VRET is a viable alternative in older adults for the state-of-the-art CBT for PTSD. Until now there has been no reason to recommend VRET for older adults with PTSD. This conclusion is not only based on the studies into VRET in older adults discussed here but also on the few efficacy trials into VRET and PTSD in adults which have been published (e.g. Difede et al. 2007; McLay et al. 2011; Ready et Gerardi et al. 2010). In these trials only very small effects were found. Although VRET showed some promising effects, it still cannot be presented as an empirically supported treatment for PTSD. Given the complexity of PTSD and the existence of evidence-based treatments for PTSD (Kulkarni, Barrad, and Cloitre 2014), it is recommended that older adults receive state-of-the-art treatment rather than VRET.

THE EFFECTS OF VIRTUAL REALITY ON COGNITIVE DECLINE

Although there are arguments that older adults cannot benefit sufficiently from virtual reality techniques due to declining cognitive abilities (e.g. Salthouse 2004), these arguments lack empirical support. On the contrary, there is a growing body of evidence that virtual reality can be a beneficial technique to improve memory deficiencies in older adults. In older adults it was found that decline in mental and physical activity is paralleled by decline in cognitive functioning (Mackinnon et al. 2003). To improve memory deficits or prevent memory from declining in older adults, different strategies are used. Based on research that suggests physical exercise may prevent or delay dementia in older adults who are at risk for Alzheimer's disease (see chapter 26 in this Handbook, and also Larson 2008), one approach combines physical activity with enhanced virtual reality in cybercycling (Anderson-Hanley et al. 2012) to prevent cognitive decline. Cybercycling involves the use of a static exercise bike in an enhanced virtual environment that provides a changing 'landscape' as the user rides the bike, and may modify the cycling difficulty for the user as terrain changes (i.e. as in the real world, it is harder to ride up a hill than down the other side). Meanwhile, in a more traditional approach, memory training activities for older adults have been 'translated' into virtual reality to treat memory deficits (e.g. Man, Chung, and Lee 2012; Optale et al. 2010). Research into both approaches will be discussed below.

Physical activity and cybercycling

In a cluster RCT, the effects on cognitive functioning of cybercycling were compared to the effects of traditional exercise in older adults (Anderson-Hanley et al. 2012). The intervention consisted of a three-month training either in cybercycling (mean age = 75.7, SD = 9.9) or a comparable intervention on a traditional stationary bike (mean age = 81.6, SD = 6.2) viewing the same biofeedback information as was provided to the cybercycle group. The cybercycle group participants experienced 3D tours and competed with their own 'ghost' rider (their last best ride). During the third month participants were instructed to outpace on-screen riders. Main outcome measures were executive functioning (measured by Colour Trails Difference, Stroop C, and Digits Backward), clinical status (cognitive impairment), and exercise effort/fitness. Intent-to-treat analyses showed a significant group by time interaction for cognitive functioning. Cybercycling yielded a medium effect over traditional exercise and resulted in a 23% relative risk reduction in the progression of their clinical status. Thus, virtual reality in combination with physical exercise (cybercycling) has a positive impact on cognitive functioning in older adults, suggesting some potential for preventing cognitive decline.

In another study done by the same group, competitiveness moderated the exercise efforts in older adults when cybercycling (Anderson-Hanley et al. 2011). In a small trial (n = 14) it was shown that in cybercycling virtual social facilitation (increased exercise effort induced by competing avatars) increased exercise effort among more competitive exercising older adults as compared to less competitive older persons.

Virtual reality based cognitive training

Given that the success of motor rehabilitation may relate to varying degrees of cognitive processing, it is worthwhile considering whether virtual reality based cognitive training could improve cognitive functioning in older adults. In earlier studies older healthy adults benefited significantly from computer-based memory training (Mahncke, Bronstone, and Merzenich 2006a; Mahncke et al. 2006b; Smith et al. 2009). These benefits could not be demonstrated in the active control group and remained stable at three-month follow-up.

In a group of older adults with chronic schizophrenia (n = 27), a virtual reality cognitive training programme was compared to treatment as usual (Chan et al. 2010). The mean age of participants was 66.2 years. The intervention group received ten sessions of a virtual reality program consisting of two activities: 'Ball and bird' and 'Shark bait'. In the first scenario, the users see themselves standing in a pastoral setting where balls of different colours emerge from peripheral locations flying towards them. The participants can use any part of their body to contact the ball. Different intensity of ball contact will either make the ball 'burst' or 'transform' into doves and fly away. In the other scenario, 'Shark bait', the participant sees a video reflection of himself beneath the sea. The participant can navigate in the sea by leaning from side to side or by squatting. They have to follow a yellow star to avoid sharks and eels. The level of difficulty can be adjusted by the number of distractors. The group receiving the virtual reality intervention performed significantly better than the control condition on overall cognitive functioning and on the subscales of Repetition and Memory. Engaging in a virtual reality cognitive training programme would appear to offer potential for gains in cognitive functioning in older adults with schizophrenia.

In more traditional approaches memory training programmes for older adults have been developed in virtual reality to treat memory decline. In an RCT thirty-six older adults were assigned to receive either a six-month virtual reality memory training, which involved auditory stimulation and VR experiences in path finding (Optale et al. 2010), or equivalent face-to-face training sessions using music therapy. The mean age of participants in the virtual reality memory training condition was 78.5 (SD = 10.9) and in the control condition the mean age was 81.6 (SD = 5.0). The effects of treatment on memory functioning were measured on general cognitive abilities (Mini Mental State Examination and Mental Status in Neurology), verbal memory (Digit Span test), executive functions (Phonemic Verbal Fluency Test, the Dual Task Performance Test, and the Cognitive Estimation Test), and visuospatial processing (Clock Drawing Test). Neuropsychological and functional measurements were performed at baseline, after the initial training phase (after three months) and after the booster training phase (after six months). On General Cognitive Abilities a non-significant effect for time was found, but a significant between-group effect favouring virtual reality memory training was found (Cohen's d = 0.26–0.48). The virtual reality memory training condition showed significant improvements on memory tests. In contrast, the control condition showed progressive decline in memory functions. The beneficial results of the virtual reality memory training were not only limited to the trained functions but also extended to other cognitive abilities (e.g. verbal memory). The changes in executive function abilities, however, were non-significant.

In another RCT forty-four older adults with questionable dementia (being at risk of progressing to dementia) were assigned to receive either a virtual reality based or a therapist-led memory training programme (Man et al. 2012). The virtual reality based memory training consisted of different tasks ranging from simple to more complex in terms of the number and similarity of objects to be remembered as well as the duration of distraction. Two virtual environments were used as a memory training surrounding. Participants received instructions by verbal and written messages displayed by the computer (e.g. a list of items which had to be memorized and after a distraction phase had to be taken out of the refrigerator). The therapist-led training consisted of a psychoeducational approach and was similar to the virtual approach. Treatment sessions consisted of ten individual sessions of thirty minutes. Mean age of the participants was 80.3 (SD = 1.25). Participants were assessed pre- and post-intervention with measures of dementia severity (CDR scale; Hughes et al. 1982), the Mini Mental State Examination (MMSE; Folstein, Folstein, and McHugh 1975), the Geriatric Depression Scale (Yesavage et al. 1983), the Multifactorial Memory Questionnaire (MMQ; Troyer and Rich 2002), and the Fuld Object–Memory Evaluation (FOME; Fuld 1977). The virtual reality based memory training demonstrated significant improvement in all three FOME scores (total encoding, total recall, delayed recall) and on the MMQ scale strategy, whereas the therapist-led group showed significant improvement on two of the three sub-scales of the FOME (total recall, delayed recall) and on the MMQ scale Contentment. These results suggest that the virtual reality based memory training was slightly superior to the therapist-led control group; however, no effect sizes were reported by the authors.

Taken together, results of the studies discussed here show that virtual reality can provide active tools for older adults to improve their memory performance.

Controlling Posture during Virtual Reality

Older adults often require more time to reweight sensory information for maintaining bal-ance, which is especially demanding in changing virtual environments. In a study comparing younger (mean age = 22.8, SD = 3.3 years) and older adults (mean age = 71.5, SD = 4.9 years) in engaging in the reweighting of sensory information, the visual surround information during a collision avoidance task was manipulated (Eikema et al. 2011). Participants stood for 240 seconds on a force platform under two experimental conditions: quiet standing and standing while anticipating randomly approaching virtual objects which had to be avoided. In the quiet standing condition the older persons showed greater sway variability and were more severely affected by changing the visual surrounding information when compared to young adults. During visual anticipation no differences between groups were found. These findings are in line with earlier findings (Bugnariu and Fung 2007) and suggest that there are no differences in sensory reweighting in dynamic virtual environments between young and older adults. However, older adults show less efficient sensory reweighting in quiet standing due to greater visual field dependence.

A few studies have investigated whether older persons may profit from virtual reality training of motor balance. Buccello-Stout and colleagues investigated whether prolonged exposure to perceptual-motor mismatch increased the adaptability and retention of balance in older adults (mean age = 72.2, SD = 5.3) (Buccello-Stout et al. 2008). In the experimental group participants walked on a treadmill for twenty minutes while viewing a rotating visual scene that provided a perceptual-motor mismatch. In the control group participants like-wise walked on a treadmill for twenty minutes, but did so while viewing a static visual scene. Training occurred twice a week for a four-week period. Effects were measured by a scoring system in an obstacle course, where participants had to avoid the obstacles. If participants hit an obstacle penalty scores were given and time was registered to complete the obstacle course. It was demonstrated that older adults benefit from sensorimotor adaptation training by improving their balance and control; the experimental group moved faster through the obstacle course with fewer penalties.

In another study (Bisson et al. 2007) the training programme to improve functional balance and mobility consisted of virtual reality training, which required participants to lean sideways to juggle a virtual ball. The other group received biofeedback training viewing a red dot representing their centre of gravity on a screen, and were required to move that dot to the four corners of the monitor. Both groups completed a ten-week training programme consisting of two thirty-minute sessions per week. Mean age was 74.4 years. Both groups showed significant improvement in functional balance and mobility and decreased reaction times. No differences were found for sway in quiet stance.

In summary, older adults show less efficient sensory reweighting in quiet standing conditions due to greater visual field dependence. Research indicates that older adults benefit from sensorimotor training as well as dynamic training, and are able to improve their balance and control in a virtual environment. However, further research is required to clarify whether such training is superior, inferior, or equally as effective as non-virtual alternatives in this population.

Cybersickness

Cybersickness is a complicating factor in treatment with virtual reality techniques across all ages. Cybersickness is a condition in which a disagreement exists between visually perceived movement and the vestibular system's sense of movement, often caused by a very slight delay in the tracking system. Dizziness, fatigue, headache, and nausea are the most common symptoms of cybersickness. While it was first assumed that motion sickness and cybersickness overlap because of the similarity of symptoms (Wiederhold and Wiederhold 2005), now there is some evidence that motion sickness declines with age; this is not true for cybersickness, which may increase with age (Arns and Cerney 2005).

In an earlier study on the effects of age and simulator sickness, 148 participants completed a driving assessment in a virtual driving environment (Liu, Watson, and Miyazaki 1999). Participants were categorized according to their age (13–35; 36–55; 56+ years). Simulator sickness increased significantly with age; this was especially the case for women. However, symptoms reported by the older group (56+) were no more severe than those reported by the mid-aged group (36–55). Nevertheless, a significant relationship between increasing age and complaints about the Head Mounted Display (HMD) used for presentation of the virtual worlds was found. Given that cybersickness increases with age but not more significantly after a certain age, it may be concluded that virtual reality is a feasible instrument to treat older adults, but that the choice of the hardware can be crucial given the significantly increasing complaints about the HMD.

In another study, participants (n = 387) were visitors to a virtual reality tour day (Arns and Cerney 2005). No overall effect between cybersickness severity and age was found, but mean scores for those participants aged 40–60 years were higher than the mean scores reported for participants until the age of 26 years. In a study with patients with chronic schizophrenia (Chan et al. 2010), a virtual reality intervention for cognitive training was completed. Within the first session a significant improvement in cybersickness symptoms was found. One limitation concerning this study is the 2D nature of the virtual environments and the use of a single-screen projection system. This could explain the relatively low severity of experienced cybersickness. The results suggest that virtual reality might be a suitable intervention for older persons as long as they have an adequate amount of time to become accustomed to the virtual reality system. Additionally, the use of a single-screen projection system might help to reduce the amount of experienced cybersickness.

In line with the results above, in another study potential factors influencing cybersickness in older persons were investigated. Participants (n = 32) were exposed to a classroom that contained tables, chairs, bookcases, and other objects (Liu 2009). Participants were asked to search for objects, which were listed in a checkbox on the screen. Navigational rotating speed and duration of exposure were assessed. Cybersickness severity was low after five minutes of exposure, but increased significantly after ten minutes and continued to increase for fifteen to twenty minutes. Additionally, cybersickness increased significantly with an increase in rotating speed. Thus, it can be concluded that not only age is a risk factor for cybersickness: duration of exposure and an increase in navigational rotating speed can account for increases in experienced cybersickness.

In summary, results concerning cybersickness in older adults are less clear than assumed. Although it was found in an early study (Liu et al. 1999) that cybersickness increases with age, in a more recent study only a trend towards the expected effect was found (Arns and Cerney 2005). However, there is some evidence that older adults are more vulnerable to factors such as the weight and comfort of the HMD. Additionally, it was found that in particular the length of duration of exposure and navigational rotation speed influenced the level of experienced cybersickness (Liu 2009).

Summary

The main aim of this chapter was to review the existing literature on the use of virtual reality techniques in older adults, in both healthy and clinical samples. Relatively few studies have investigated these newer techniques in the elderly. The few controlled studies that involved older adults with PTSD did not provide robust evidence that VRET is an effective treatment for older persons with PTSD, indicating that other treatments might be more feasible for this group of patients (e.g. trauma-focused CBT or Eye Movement Desensitization and Reprocessing; Kulkarni et al. 2014). Although no RCTs have been reported on the use of VRET in older persons with specific phobias, a number of RCTs in adults indicate that VRET is highly effective in adults with acrophobia and fear of flying (Meyerbröker and Emmelkamp 2010; Powers and Emmelkamp 2008). We assume that VRET will also be effective in older persons with specific phobias when special measures are taken as discussed below.

Furthermore, research shows that virtual reality techniques may potentially be a beneficial tool to prevent cognitive decline. Promising results were achieved via cybercycling (Anderson-Hanley et al. 2011; Anderson-Hanley et al. 2012) as well as via classical memory training in virtual reality (Chan et al. 2010; Man et al. 2012; Optale et al. 2010). This indicates that even patients suffering from dementia or Alzheimer's disease are able to follow virtual reality trainings and therapies.

This is important in the treatment of anxiety disorders with VRET because it implies that older adults can benefit from virtual reality training. Cybercycling and its positive effects on older adults are particularly interesting. Given the limited mobility of older adults, cybercycling could be an interesting instrument to encourage older patients to retain their mobility as well as enhance social interaction. Meanwhile, no clinical evidence has been found to suggest that declines in cognitive processing are a contraindication for the treatment of older adults with VRET. On the contrary, it has been found that with a sufficient amount of training, older adults can benefit from virtual reality treatment and even improve their cognitive performances.

A few studies have investigated whether older persons may profit from virtual reality training of motor balance, and the results are largely positive. Results indicate that although older persons show less efficient sensory reweighting in quiet standing, they can benefit from sensorimotor training or dynamic training and are able to improve their balance and control in a virtual environment. We conclude that it is possible for older adults to adapt to changes in virtual environments and recover their balance.

This is an important finding given that in most anxiety disorders (e.g. specific phobias and agoraphobia) anxiety comes along with bodily sensations (e.g. feeling dizzy, nauseous, or unsure in maintaining balance). In older persons these symptoms can be even more serious because normal ageing slows down the processing of sensory information and therefore lengthens the postural adaptation phase (Eikema et al. 2011). This is an important point when patients are treated with VRET because sensory information in the virtual environment has to be processed at the same time as anxiety symptoms. For example, in the treatment of fear of heights it is necessary for patients to lean over a railing and look into the depth to habituate to heights and depths; thus patients need constantly to reweight sensory information. Therefore it might be more difficult for older adults to adapt to VRET in fear of heights (acrophobia) given the more demanding virtual environments. We recommend in the treatment of specific phobias to slow down virtual exposure to give older adults a better chance to adapt to the changing circumstances. However, in regards to fear of flying, where treatment consists of virtual flights sitting in an aircraft chair, no difficulties for older adults are expected. In the treatment of fear of flying to our knowledge there are no indications that increasing age can be a complicating factor.

Results concerning cybersickness in older adults are less clear than assumed. Effects of age on cybersickness were found in only one study (Liu et al. 1999) while in another study only a trend was found (Arns and Cerney 2005). It was found that older adults are more vulnerable to such factors as the weight and comfort of the HMD. Furthermore, the length of duration of exposure and navigational rotation speed also influence cybersickness (Liu 2009). Given the mixed results, it is recommended that older persons are provided with an adequate amount of time to become accustomed to the system. In addition, using lightweight hardware to prevent symptoms related to cybersickness is recommended.

The research on virtual reality techniques in older adults is promising. Especially in memory training these developments may prove beneficial in the future for helping in preventing cognitive decline in older adults via either the benefits of exercise in virtual environments (e.g. cybercycling) or direct interventions for cognition such as memory retraining. In the treatment of anxiety disorders with VRET results are less clear. While there was no evidence found in support of treating older war veterans with PTSD using virtual environments, some findings indicate that older adults with other anxiety disorders (e.g. specific phobias) can be treated with VRET—as long as a sufficient amount of time is provided for them to adapt to the virtual environment.

Key References and Sources for Further Reading

Meyerbröker, K. and Emmelkamp, P. M. G. (2010). 'Virtual Reality Exposure Therapy in Anxiety Disorders: A Systematic Review of Process-and-outcome Studies'. *Depression & Anxiety* 27(10): 933–944.

Meyerbröker, K. (2014). 'Virtual Reality Exposure'. In P. M. G. Emmelkamp and T. Ehring (eds), *The Wiley Handbook of Anxiety Disorders*, vol. II. Oxford: Wiley-Blackwell.

References

Anderson-Hanley, C., Snyder, A. L., Nimon, J. P., and Arciero, P. J. (2011). 'Social Facilitation in Virtual Reality-enhanced Exercise: Competitiveness Moderates Exercise Effort of Older Adults'. *Clinical Interventions in Aging* 6: 275–280.

Anderson-Hanley, C., Arciero, P. J., Brickman, A. M., Nimon, J. P., Okuma, N., et al. (2012). 'Exergaming and Older Adult Cognition: A Cluster Randomized Clinical Trial'. *American Journal of Preventive Medicine* 42: 109–119.

APA (2000): Diagnostic and Statistical Manual of Mental Disorders, Text Revision, ed 4. Washington DC: American Psychiatric Association.

Arias, P., Robles-Garcia, V., Sanmartin, G., Flores, J., and Cudeiro, J. (2012). 'Virtual Reality as a Tool for the Evaluation of Repetitive Rhythmic Movements in the Elderly and Parkinson's Disease Patients'. *PLoS One* 7(1): 1–8.

Arns, L. L. and Cerney, M. M. (2005). 'The Relationship between Age and Incidence of Cybersickness among Immersive Environment Users'. *Proceedings IEEE Virtual Reality* 5: 267–268.

Beck, A., Brown, G., Epstein, N., and Steer, R. (1988). 'An Inventory for Measuring Clinical Anxiety: Psychometric Properties'. *Journal of Consulting and Clinical Psychology* 56(6): 893–897.

Bisson, E., Contant, B., Sveistrup, H., and Lajoie, Y. (2007). 'Functional Balance and dual-task Reaction Times in Older Adults Are Improved by Virtual Reality and Biofeedback Training'. *Cyberpsychology & Behavior* 10: 16–23.

Blake, D. D., Weathers, F. W., Nagy, L. M., Kaloupek, D. G., Gusman, F. D., et al. (1995). 'The Development of a Clinician-administered PTSD Scale'. *Journal of Traumatic Stress* 8: 75–90.

Buccello-Stout, R. R., Bloomberg, J. J., Cohen, H. S., Whorton, E. B., Weaver, G. D., et al. (2008). 'Effects of Sensorimotor Adaptation Training on Functional Mobility in Older Adults'. *Journal of Gerontology* 63: 295–300.

Bugnariu, N. and Fung, J. (2007). 'Aging and Selective Sensorimotor Strategies in the Regulation of Upright Balance'. *Journal of Neuroengineering and Rehabilitation* 4: 19–25.

Chan, C. L. F., Ngai, E. K. Y., Leung, P. K. H., and Wong, S. (2010). 'Effect of the Adapted Virtual Reality Cognitive Training Program among Chinese Older Adults with Chronic Schizophrenia: A Pilot Study'. *International Journal of Geriatric Psychiatry* 25: 643–649.

Difede, J., Cukor, J., Jayasinghe, N., Patt, I., Jedel, S., et al. (2007). 'Virtual Reality Exposure Therapy for the Treatment of Posttraumatic Stress Disorder Following September 11, 2001'. *Journal of Clinical Psychiatry* 68(11): 1639–1647.

Eikema, D. J. A., Hatzitaki, V., Tzovaras, D., and Papaxanthis, C. (2011). 'Age-dependent Modulation of Sensory Reweighting for Controlling Posture in a Dynamic Virtual Environment'. *Age* 34(6): 1381–1392.

Emmelkamp, P. M. G. 2013. 'Behavior Therapy with Adults'. In M. J. Lambert (ed.), *Bergin and Garfield's Handbook of Psychotherapy and Behavior Change* (6th edn). New York: Wiley.

Farrow, S. and Reid, D. (2004). 'Stroke Survivors' Perceptions of a Leisure-based Virtual Reality Program'. *Technology and Disability* 16: 69–81.

Folstein, M. F., Folstein, S. E., and McHugh, P. R. (1975). 'Mini-mental State: A Practical Method for Grading the Cognitive State of Patients for Clinicians'. *Journal of Psychiatric Research* 12: 189–198.

Foy, D. W., Rueger, D. B., Sipprelle, R. C., and Carroll, E. M. (1984). 'Etiology of Posttraumatic Stress Disorder in Vietnam Veterans—Analysis of Premilitary, Military, and Combat Exposure Influences'. *Journal of Consulting and Clinical Psychology* 52(1): 79–87.

French, D. D., Campbell, R., Spehar, A., Cunningham, F., Bulat, T., et al. (2006). 'Drugs and Falls in Community-dwelling Older People: A National Veterans Study'. *Clinical Therapeutics* 28: 619–630.

Fuld, P. A. (1977). *Fuld Object-memory Evaluation: Instruction Manual*. Wood Dale, IL: Stoelting.

Gamito, P., Oliveira, J., Rosa, P., Morais, D., Duarte, N., et al. (2010). 'PTSD Elderly War Veterans: A Clinical Controlled Pilot Study'. *Cyberpsychology Behavior and Social Networking* 13(1): 43–48.

Goncalves, R., Pedrozo, A. L., Coutinho, E. S. F., Figueira, I., and Ventura, P. (2012). 'Efficacy of Virtual Reality Exposure Therapy in the Treatment of PTSD: A Systematic Review'. *PLoS One* 7(12): e48469–e48469.

Horowitz, M. J., Wilner, N., and Alvarez, W. (1979). 'Impact of Event Scale: A Measure of Subjective Distress'. *Psychosomatic Medicine* 41: 207–218.

Hughes, C. P., Berg, L., Danziger, W. L., Coben, L. A., and Martin, R. L. (1982). 'A New Clinical Scale for the Staging of Dementia'. *British Journal of Psychiatry* 140: 566–572.

Kulkarni M., Barrad A., and Cloitre M. (2014). 'Posttraumatic Stress Disorder: Assessment and Intervention'. In P. M. G. Emmelkamp, and T. Ehring (eds), *The Wiley Handbook of Anxiety Disorders*, vol. I. Oxford: Wiley-Blackwell.

Kulkarni, M., Barrad, A., and Cloitre, M. (2014). 'Posttraumatic Stress Disorder: Assessment and Intervention'. In P. M. G. Emmelkamp and T. Ehring (eds), *The Wiley Handbook of Anxiety Disorders*, vol. II. Oxford: Wiley-Blackwell.

Larson, E. (2008). 'Physical Activity for Older Adults at Risk for Alzheimer Disease'. *Journal of the American Medical Association* 300: 1077–1079.

Liu, C. L. (2009). 'A Neuro-fuzzy Warning System for Combating Cybersickness in the Elderly Caused by the Virtual Environment on a TFT-LCD'. *Applied Ergonomics* 40: 316–324.

Liu, L., Watson, B., and Miyazaki, M. (1999). 'VR for the Elderly: Quantitative and Qualitative Differences in Performance with a Driving Simulator'. *Journal of Cybertherapy & Rehabilitation* 2: 567–576.

McGee, J. S., Van der Zaag, C., Buckwalter, J. G., Thiebaux, M., Van Rooyen, A., et al. (2000). 'Issues for the Assessment of Visuospatial Skills in Older Adults Using Virtual Environment Technology'. *Cyberpsychology & Behavior* 3(3): 469–482.

Mackinnon, A., Christensen, J., Hofer, S. M., Korten, A. E., and Jorm, A. F. (2003). 'Use It and Still Lose It? The Association between Activity and Cognitive Performance Established Using Latent Growth Techniques in a Community Sample'. *Aging, Neuropsychology and Cognition* 10(3): 215–229.

McLay, R. N., Wood, D. P., Webb-Murphy, J. A., Spira, J. L., Wiederhold, M. D., et al. (2011). 'A Randomized, Controlled Trial of Virtual Reality-Graded Exposure Therapy for Post-Traumatic Stress Disorder in Active Duty Service Members with Combat-Related

Post-Traumatic Stress Disorder'. *Cyberpsychology Behavior and Social Networking* 14(4): 223–229.

Mahncke, H. W., Bronstone, A., and Merzenich, M. M. (2006a). 'Brain Plasticity and Functional Losses in the Aged: Scientific Bases for a Novel Intervention'. *Progress in Brain Research* 157: 81–109.

Mahncke, H. W., Connor, B. B., Appelman, J., Ahsanuddin, O. N., Hardy, J. L., et al. (2006b). 'Memory Enhancement in Healthy Older Adults Using a Brain Plasticity-Based Training Program: A Randomized Controlled Study'. *Proceedings of the National Academy of Sciences of the United States of America* 103(33): 12523–12528.

Man, D. W. K., Chung, J. C. C., and Lee, G. Y. Y. (2012). 'Evaluation of a Virtual Reality-Based Memory Training Programme for Hong Kong Chinese Older Adults with Questionable Dementia: A Pilot Study'. *International Journal of Geriatric Psychiatry* 27: 513–520.

Meyerbroeker, K., Morina, N., Kerkhof, G. A., and Emmelkamp, P. M. G. (2013). 'Virtual Reality Exposure Therapy Does Not Provide Any Additional Value in Agoraphobic Patients: A Randomized Controlled Trial'. *Psychotherapy and Psychosomatics* 82(3): 170–176.

Meyerbröker, K. and Emmelkamp, P. M. G. (2010). 'Virtual Reality Exposure Therapy in Anxiety Disorders: A Systematic Review of Process-and-outcome Studies'. *Depression & Anxiety (1091–4269)* 27(10): 933–944.

Meyerbröker, K. (2014). 'Virtual Reality Exposure'. In P. M. G. Emmelkamp and T. Ehring (eds), *The Wiley Handbook of Anxiety Disorders*, vol. II. Oxford: Wiley-Blackwell.

Opris, D., Pintea, S., Garcia-Palacios, A., Botella, C., Szamoskoezi, S., et al. (2012). 'Virtual Reality Exposure Therapy in Anxiety Disorders: A Quantitative Meta-analysis'. *Depression and Anxiety* 29(2): 85–93.

Optale, G., Urgesi, C., Busato, V., Marin, S., Piron, L., et al. (2010). 'Controlling Memory Impairment in Elderly Adults Using Virtual Reality Memory Training: A Randomized Controlled Pilot Study'. *Neurorehabilitation and Neural Repair* 24(4): 348–357.

Pinquart, M. and Duberstein, P. R. (2007). 'Treatment of Anxiety Disorders in Older Adults: A Meta-analytic Comparison of Behavioral and Pharmacological Interventions'. *American Jouranl of Geriatric Psychiatry* 15: 639–651.

Powers, M. B. and Emmelkamp, P. M. G. (2008). 'Virtual Reality Exposure Therapy for Anxiety Disorders: A Meta-analysis'. *Journal Of Anxiety Disorders* 22(3): 561–569.

Ready, D. J., Gerardi, R. J., Backscheider, A. G., Mascaro, N., and Rothbaum, B. O. (2010). 'Comparing Virtual Reality Exposure Therapy to Present-Centered Therapy with 11 US Vietnam Veterans with PTSD'. *Cyberpsychology Behavior and Social Networking* 13(1): 49–54.

Rothbaum, B., Hodges, L., Ready, D., Graap, K., and Alarcon, R. (2001). 'Virtual Reality Exposure Therapy for Vietnam Veterans with Posttraumatic Stress Disorder'. *Journal of Clinical Psychiatry* 62(8): 617–622.

Salthouse, T. (2004). 'What and When of Cognitive Aging'. *Current Directions in Psychological Science* 13(4): 140–144.

Schuurmans, J., Comijs, H., Beekman, A., De Beurs, E., Deeg, D., et al. (2005). 'The Outcome of Anxiety Disorders in Older People at 6-year Follow-up: Results from the Longitudinal Aging Study Amsterdam'. *Acta Psychiatrica Scandinavica* 111(6): 420–428.

Schuurmans, J., Comijs, H., Emmelkamp, P., Gundy, C., Weijnen, I., et al. (2006). 'A Randomized, Controlled Trial of the Effectiveness of Cognitive-behavioral Therapy and Sertraline versus a Waitlist Control Group for Anxiety Disorders in Older Adults'. *American Journal of Geriatric Psychiatry* 14(3): 255–263.

Schuurmans, J., Comijs, H., Emmelkamp, P. M. G., Weijnen, I. J. C., Van Den Hout, M., et al. (2009). 'Long-term Effectiveness and Prediction of Treatment Outcome in Cognitive

Behavioral Therapy and Sertraline for Late-life Anxiety Disorders'. *International Psychogeriatrics* 21(6): 1148–1159.

Smith, G. E., Housen, P., Yaffe, K., Ruff, R., Kennison, R. F., Mahncke, H. W., et al. (2009). 'A Cognitive Training Program Based on Principles of Brain Plasticity: Results from the Improvement in Memory with Plasticity-based Adaptive Cognitive Training (IMPACT) Study'. *Journal of the American Geriatrics Society* 57: 594–603.

Troyer, A. K. and Rich, J. B. (2002). 'Psychometric Properties of a New Metamemory Questionnaire for Older Adults'. *Journal of Gerontological Behaviour Psychological Science Social Science* 57(1): 19–27.

Weathers, F. W., Keane, T. M., and Davidson, J. R. T. (2001). 'Clinician-administered PTSD Scale: A Review of the First Ten Years of Research'. *Depression and Anxiety* 13(3): 132–156.

Wiederhold, B. K. and Wiederhold, M. D. (2005). *Virtual Reality Therapy For Anxiety Disorders: Advances in Evaluation and Treatment*. Washington, DC: American Psychological Association.

Yesavage, J. A., Brink, T. L., Rose, T. L., Lum, O., Huang, V., et al. (1983). 'Development and Validation of a Geriatric Depression Rating Scale: A Preliminary Report'. *Journal of Psychological Research* 17: 27.

CHAPTER 49

EXERCISE AND HEALTH PROMOTION FOR OLDER ADULTS WITH COGNITIVE IMPAIRMENT

LINDA TERI, SUSAN M. MCCURRY, REBECCA G. LOGSDON, AND ELLEN L. MCGOUGH

INTRODUCTION

FOR the rapidly ageing population, protection of cognitive health as a means of maintaining quality of life has become a paramount concern. Ageing is associated with changes in cognitive function, and the rate of dementia throughout the world is predicted to double every twenty years to 81.1 million by 2040 (Ferri et al. 2005). Thus, identification of intervention strategies or life-style changes that may prevent or slow dementia onset and progression is critically important. There is a growing body of evidence from epidemiological studies that a history of exercise or physical activity may delay onset and progression of dementia in older adults (Abbott et al. 2004; Andel et al. 2008; Colcombe and Kramer 2003; Larson et al. 2006; Laurin et al. 2001). Increased exercise may also ameliorate some of the negative physical sequelae associated with dementing illnesses, such as risk for falls and fractures, reduced neuromuscular function, and decreased cardiopulmonary function (Rolland et al. 2007), as well as improve functioning in daily activities and mood (Kwak et al. 2008; Williams and Tappen 2007). In this chapter, we will briefly review the literature supporting the value of exercise for older adults across the continuum of cognitive function, and then describe how our own work at the University of Washington in the US fits with this larger body of research.

Physical performance in older adults with cognitive impairment

A temporal relationship exists between declining cognitive and physical performance in older adults (Buchman et al. 2011; Wittwer, Webster, and Menz 2010). Reduced function in problem-solving and executive function tasks (Rosenberg et al. 2011; Rozzini et al. 2007), instrumental activities of daily living (IADL) (Mariani et al. 2008; Perneczky et al. 2006), and physical performance tasks (Liu-Ambrose et al. 2008) are common in older adults with mild cognitive impairment (MCI). This relationship between cognitive and physical function is evident through positive associations between cardiopulmonary fitness and cognitive function in older adults without dementia (Erickson et al. 2009) and those with early Alzheimer's disease (Burns et al. 2008). In addition, reduced functional mobility often precedes the onset of dementia (Aggarwal et al. 2006; Kluger et al. 1997, 2008) and progressively worsens with advancing stages of dementia (O'Keeffe et al. 1996). Performance of complex tasks such as IADLs decline in prodromal and early stages of dementia (Mariani et al. 2008), followed by a progressive decline in basic activities of daily living (ADLs) such as walking, eating, toileting, and bathing in later stages of dementia (Hauer and Oster 2008). Slowed gait speed alone is associated with reduced cognitive function in non-demented older adults (Beauchet et al. 2008; O'Keeffe et al. 1996), and increased severity of cognitive impairment and associated disability in those with dementia (Beauchet et al. 2008; Espeland et al. 2007). Gait and balance impairments as well as fall-related complications frequently result in hospitalization and transitions from independent or assisted living to skilled nursing care (Kenny et al. 2008; Morris, Rubin, and Buchner 1987; Tinetti and Kumar 2010) where increased assistance is needed for basic ADLs (Tornatore et al. 2003). Taken together, cognitive impairment and reduced fitness negatively impact participation in exercise routines necessary to maintain optimal fitness and functional mobility. Thus, effective exercise interventions for improving fitness and functional mobility should be individualized to address physical, cognitive, and environmental barriers. There is strong evidence that older adults with cognitive impairment demonstrate improved function in response to individualized exercise interventions of sufficient intensity, frequency, and duration (Chodzko-Zajko et al. 2009). Thus, effective strategies are needed to enhance exercise interventions for improving fitness and functional mobility in older adults with cognitive impairment.

Observational exercise studies

Positive associations between regular exercise and cognitive functions, including processing speed, memory, executive function, and global cognitive function, have been reported in observational studies of healthy older adults (Angevaren et al. 2008; Bixby et al. 2007; Clarkson-Smith and Hartley 1989; Hillman et al. 2006). Exercise intensity is also positively associated with cognitive function (Angevaren et al. 2007), with higher levels of exercise in mid- and late-life associated with less global cognitive decline (Van Gelder et al. 2004; Yaffe et al. 2001), less incident MCI (Geda et al. 2010; Middleton, Kirk, and Rockwood 2008), and less incident dementia (Larson et al. 2006; Rovio et al. 2005). A retrospective study of older women has reported cognitive health benefits associated with physical activity throughout the lifespan. Older women who were more active as teenagers had the highest cognitive function and the lowest rates of cognitive impairment, but those who were physically active at any age were less likely to have cognitive impairment compared to women who remained inactive (Middleton et al. 2008). However, the strength of associations between exercise and cognitive function in observational studies suggests that the protective effects may be stronger in women (Laurin et al. 2001; Middleton et al. 2008).

Exercise intervention studies with older adults

A number of recent reviews and meta-analyses have examined the impact of exercise on cognitive function in clinical trials. A Cochrane Review (Angevaren et al. 2008) reported evidence for improvements in motor function, cognitive speed, and auditory and visual attention resulting from aerobic exercise in randomized controlled trials (RCTs). Both aerobic exercise and resistance training have been reported to be effective in improving cognitive function, especially performance on executive function tasks (Colcombe and Kramer 2003; Van Uffelen et al. 2008a), and these beneficial effects have been observed in studies of older adults with and without cognitive decline. Randomized trials of resistance exercise alone have also demonstrated improved cognitive function, especially executive functions, in cognitively healthy older adults (Cassilhas et al. 2007; Liu-Ambrose et al. 2010; Perrig-Chiello et al. 1998).

Other studies, however, have reported little to no positive effect of exercise on cognitive function (Van Uffelen et al. 2008a). Several aerobic exercise trials in healthy older adults have resulted in little to no improvement in cognitive function following interventions ranging from two months (Madden et al. 1989) to ten months (Smiley-Oyen et al. 2008). One recent study with women ages 65 to 75 found that progressive resistance training and weight-bearing exercise practice either once or twice a week produced improvements in performance on executive function tasks compared to training in balance and toning exercises, but differences between groups were not observed until the twelve-month follow-up, suggesting that sustained exercise may be important for treatment effects to emerge (Liu-Ambrose et al. 2010). A preservative effect on cognitive function may also be a factor influencing interpretation of mixed study results. For instance, in one six-month aerobic exercise RCT in older adults (ages 60 to 73) the intervention group had no significant improvement, but the control group had a significant decline in cognitive function (Hill, Storandt, and Malley 1993). This provides support for the notion that aerobic exercise may help older adults maintain cognitive function and slow age-related cognitive decline even if it does not improve cognitive test performance from baseline (Hill et al. 1993).

Exercise studies in older adults with mild cognitive impairment

Among individuals with MCI, randomized controlled trials examining the impact of exercise on cognitive function have shown mixed results. In their recent review, Ahlskog and colleagues (2011) reported modest improvement in cognitive function after six to eighteen months of exercise, compared to usual activity or low-intensity-activity control groups. A twenty-four-week RCT comparing a home-based walking programme to usual care with 170 community-dwelling adults with MCI (ages $\geq$ 50 years) resulted in a modest gain in performance on the Alzheimer's Disease Assessment Scale—Cognitive Subscale (1.3; SD 2.38–0.03) in the walking group at six and eighteen months follow-up, compared to the control group (Lautenschlager et al. 2008). A six-month RCT of high-intensity aerobic exercise compared to a stretching control group in older adults with amnestic MCI (aMCI) (n = 33, ages 55–85) reported improved performance on the Trail Making, part B in the aerobic exercise group (Baker et al. 2010). However, a twelve-month RCT with 152 older adults (ages

70–80) with MCI comparing moderate-intensity walking plus non-aerobic exercise, plus vitamin B supplementation, to a placebo pill control group demonstrated no difference in cognitive function between the groups at twelve months (Van Uffelen et al. 2008b).

Exercise studies in older adults with dementia

Several meta-analyses and reviews of exercise interventions in individuals with dementia have reported positive effects of exercise, including improved physical performance (walking speed, balance, and endurance), fitness, cognitive function, ADLs, and behaviour (Blankevoort et al. 2010; Heyn, Abreu, and Rottenbacher 2004; Kwak et al. 2008). There is notable evidence that cognitively impaired individuals can improve physical function through participation in a regular exercise programme (Hauer et al. 2012; Heyn et al. 2004; Littbrand et al. 2011a). In particular, activity-specific and functional weight-bearing exercises improve balance and the ability to move from sitting to standing (transfers) in people with dementia (Littbrand, Stenvall, and Rosendahl 2011b; Roach et al. 2011). Another study reported improved postural control, dynamic balance, transfer ability, and walking after three months of participation in a group strength and functional training programme in older adults with mild to moderate dementia (mean age = 82.6 years) (Hauer et al. 2011). These physical gains in response to exercise training despite cognitive impairment are important, considering the additional disability burden that physical and functional mobility limitations place on persons with dementia and their care-givers (Rovio et al. 2005).

THE SEATTLE PROTOCOLS

For the past decade, our research group in Seattle has been exploring the use of exercise as part of a systematic body of research using targeted behavioural interventions to improve the mood, function, and behaviour of community-dwelling persons with cognitive impairment. These programmes, part of a collective referred to as the Seattle Protocols (Teri, Logsdon, and McCurry 2005), were designed to decrease physical disability as well as delay disease progression using a standardized approach to care that focuses on: (1) identifying, initiating, and maintaining participation in enjoyable physical exercise; (2) teaching behavioural strategies and problem-solving skills for overcoming obstacles to such exercise; (3) engaging interpersonal supports to maintain exercise regimens; and (4) encouraging walking and other easy-to-achieve, accessible, and available physical activities in the community.

Theoretical rationale

The Seattle Protocols are based on social learning and gerontology theories, and grounded in an understanding of the neuropsychological and behavioural changes that occur in individuals with dementia. The Protocols that include physical activity incorporate findings from evidence-based research on exercise training in older adults with clinical expertise regarding how best to incorporate such training into programmes for individuals with cognitive impairment. We use strategies that have been shown to facilitate learning and behaviour change without relying heavily on cognitive skills. Exercise is conceptualized as an observable and modifiable chain of behaviours that can be initiated and maintained using principles of goal setting, self-monitoring, provision of feedback, problem-solving, and reinforcement. Complex behaviours are broken into small steps, and, as each step is mastered, the next one is added. Visual cues, reminders, and other tools are used to help individuals with MCI maintain their exercise programme on their own between individual or group sessions and after treatment concludes. For persons with more significant cognitive impairment (who are unable to initiate or maintain the programme on their own), training includes a care-giving family member, friend, or staff person who can assist them with identifying and remembering how to perform the exercises safely and consistently.

Key components

Each Protocol begins with an orientation that provides participants with a rationale for training and establishes mutually agreed-upon goals. Each concludes with specific recommendations and plans for maintaining and generalizing gains achieved during treatment. The central phase of each protocol focuses on training skills addressing the target behaviour of interest, in this case, exercise or increased physical activity. In addition to exercise training, skills that are critical to the successful implementation and maintenance of the exercise programme are covered. For example, each protocol addresses systematic ways to increase pleasant events (ideally making physical activity one of these pleasant events). Participants are assisted in setting appropriate and achievable activity goals, problem-solving potential obstacles and setbacks to continued physical activity, and identifying strategies to maintain motivation and measure progress. Safety is emphasized, and participants are coached about how to choose appropriate walking shoes, identify safe walking routes, and plan exercise during safe weather conditions. Additional health promotion topics may be included as warranted, such as maintaining good nutrition and using relaxation techniques to improve mood and sleep. When care-givers are involved, problem-solving training also focuses on ensuring that they understand how cognitive limitations can impact a participant's understanding and cooperation with the exercise programme, and helping them learn to use effective communication, pleasant events, and behavioural strategies to guide and motivate the person with dementia.

Exercise training

Exercises included in the Seattle Protocols were developed based upon national recommendations for maintaining strength and mobility in older adults (ACSM 1998; Cress et al. 2005). They include activities to promote gentle stretching, strength training, balance, and endurance. Gentle stretching provides a warm-up and cool down for other exercises, and increases participants' awareness of their muscles and muscle tension. Strength training is designed to help individuals maintain mobility and muscle strength safely to perform daily activities such as standing up from a chair, getting in and out of a car, carrying groceries, and walking. Balance exercises help individuals perform movements necessary for safe mobility, including weight shifting and body awareness. Last but not least, endurance activities help to maintain or improve overall cardiovascular health, physical status, and mood. All exercise activities focus on ease, availability, and accommodating individual preferences. For example, walking is the most commonly employed endurance activity—it has the advantage of being a well-learned activity, it is relatively easy to vary intensity based on the participant's current level of fitness, and walking routes can be planned that incorporate pleasant events into the outing.

Pleasant events

Exercise that is not enjoyed will not be sustained. Consequently, we endeavour to help participants select activities that they will enjoy and to modify what they do to maximize their enjoyment. We also provide creative and fun instructions that participants can enjoy and incorporate into their own plans. For example, in a quadriceps strengthening exercise, we instruct participants to stand and sit very slowly, like a mother hen sitting on her eggs, urging everyone to be careful not to break the eggs. Balance training incorporates simple dance steps that shift weight from side to side, or tandem walking on an imaginary tightrope. For endurance, exercises may vary depending on the individual's preference: some participants walk, others ride a stationary bike; some walk indoors, others outdoors. In any case, the object is for the person to identify an activity or activities that they can enjoy at their present level of cognitive and physical function and that can be adapted as changes occur. Finally, and importantly, we strive to identify what would make a given exercise more fun for each individual, and therefore more likely to be maintained.

Problem-solving

Engaging in exercise takes effort and planning. Obstacles to initiating a new programme and maintaining it when illness, family issues, or travel occurs must be identified and overcome. Using our well-established A-B-C approach to behaviour management (Teri et al. 2002) we teach participants and their care-givers to problem-solve their way around obstacles to ensure they can engage in exercise in a regular and productive manner. In brief, participants are asked to identify and gather information about the behaviour (B) that is causing them distress, and to observe and modify the antecedents (A)—actions which precede the behaviour and may, therefore be triggering it—and consequences (C)—actions that follow the behaviour, and may, therefore be sustaining it.

Since most participants in our studies are sedentary upon enrolment, we work with them to establish reasonable exercise goals, and provide clear instructions to both participants and their exercise partners about how to monitor progress and problem-solve obstacles that arise. Throughout the process, we emphasize the importance of rewarding successes and having fun. An example of this problem-solving process might be the case of an individual who needs to increase his daily walking (the B—Behaviour). The information-gathering stage would include identifying how often and how long he walked in the past week, and examining whether he is more or less likely to walk with certain individuals, at certain times of day, in certain locations or weather conditions, or after certain activities (these are the A—or triggering antecedents). In addition, it is helpful to know what happens when he does not want to walk: does the exercise partner acquiesce to the refusal, argue, matter-of-factly gather up their coats and head out the door, or offer to buy a favourite ice-cream treat on the way home? Each of these responses (the C—or Consequence) may increase or decrease the likelihood that a walk will be pleasant, and will occur. Helping participants find a way to incorporate exercise into a daily routine that is enjoyable and that makes them feel success-ful is the key to long-term maintenance.

EMPIRICAL BASIS OF THE SEATTLE PROTOCOLS FOR INCREASING PHYSICAL ACTIVITY IN INDIVIDUALS WITH COGNITIVE IMPAIRMENT

RDAD: Reducing Disability in Alzheimer's Disease (Teri et al. 2003)

The RDAD study was a randomized controlled clinical trial involving 153 Alzheimer's patients and their family care-givers randomized to an exercise and behaviour man-agement protocol or to routine medical care. During a twelve-week treatment period, care-givers receiving the Protocol were taught to guide their demented care recipient in an individualized programme of endurance activities (primarily walking), strength-training, balance, and flexibility exercises. In addition, care-givers were taught behavioural and problem-solving strategies to increase exercise behaviour and decrease undesirable agi-tated or depressed behaviours in their care recipients (Logsdon, McCurry, and Teri 2005; Teri et al. 1998). Subjects were evaluated at baseline, post-treatment, and at six-, twelve-, eighteen-, and twenty-four-month follow-up. Patient health status was measured with the Medical Outcomes Study Short Form (SF-36), the Sickness Impact Profile (SIP), the Cornell Depression Scale for Dementia, and care-giver reports of patients' restricted activity days, bed disability days, falls, and exercise participation.

Study findings indicated that care-givers were able to learn and direct patients to follow scheduled exercise activities. Eighty-one percent of active treatment patients attempted exercise recommendations. Significant differences between active and control conditions were obtained. At post-test, active treatment subjects exercised more (odds ratio (95% CI) 2.82 (1.22, 6.49)), had fewer restricted activity days (odds ratio 3.10 (1.08, 8.95)), and improved significantly more than controls on primary outcomes of physical activity (mean SF-36 Physical Role Functioning difference score 19.29 (8.75, 29.83)) and depression (mean Cornell Depression Scale difference score 1.03 (−0.17, −1.91)). Over twenty-four months of follow-up, changes in physical activity were maintained and improvements in SIP mobil-ity occurred. For patients entering the study with higher levels of depression, significant improvements in depression were maintained at twenty-four months. There was also a trend among active treatment patients to have less institutionalization due to behavioural disturbance throughout the twenty-four-month follow-up period (Teri et al. 2003).

NITE-AD: Nighttime Insomnia Treatment and Education in Alzheimer Disease (McCurry et al. 2005, McCurry et al. 2011)

NITE-AD focused on the use of exercise to reduce sleep disturbances in persons with dementia. In an early pilot study, thirty-six participants were randomly assigned to either a combination intervention which included walking, light exposure, and training in behavioural problem-solving (NITE-AD) or to an educational contact control. Exercise instructions included asking NITE-AD subjects to set a goal of walking daily for thirty continuous minutes. In cases where the Alzheimer's disease (AD) patient was too frail to walk that duration, he or she started with a shorter time goal, and worked with the interventionist to increase daily walking time gradually over the two-month treatment period (McCurry et al. 2003). At the two-month post-treatment and six-month follow-ups, sleep (as measured by wrist actigraphy) in NITE-AD subjects had improved significantly, while in contact control subjects it had declined. NITE-AD subjects' average time awake at night decreased by thirty-six minutes (p = .030) and they had fewer nightly awakenings (p = .012). NITE-AD patients also exercised significantly more days per week (p = .010), and had significantly lower levels of depression (p = .007) than controls (McCurry et al. 2005).

A subsequent randomized trial assigned 132 community-dwelling AD patients and care-givers into one of four treatment conditions (walking only, light exposure only, combination NITE-AD, and education contact control) (McCurry et al. 2011). Patients assigned to each of the three active treatment conditions showed post-treatment improvements in actigraphically measured total wake time (p <.05; effect size 0.51–0.63) and sleep percent (walking, light p = .07; NITE-AD p = .02; effect size 0.45–0.63) compared to control subjects. However, unlike the earlier study, significant group differences were not observed for any outcome at six months. One reason hypothesized for the lack of sustained treatment impact was the observation that the frequency and duration of both walking and light box used declined over the six-month period. Patients with greater adherence (4+ days/ week) to walking and light exposure recommendations had significantly (p <.05) less total wake time and better sleep efficiency than those with lesser adherence. Examination of factors associated with better walking adherence showed that AD participants who walked more had lower levels of behavioural disturbance and were less depressed; the care-givers of walking participants tended to be spouses and reported less perceived stress (McCurry et al. 2010). Feedback from participants in follow-up evaluations also indicated that dyads faced a variety of obstacles to daily walking, including dealing with inclement weather, neighbourhood walkability, care-giver or participant physical limitations, care-giver competing family or work-time demands, and participant resistance. Some participants and care-givers enthusiastically embraced the walking programme, but others (who, in some cases, had never enjoyed exercising) did not. Since many persons with dementia will be unable to implement and maintain an exercise programme safely without care-giver oversight, these results indicate the importance of tailoring exercise recommendations to the unique circumstances and preferences of the dyad to increase the likelihood of long-term success.

RALLI: Resources and Activities for Life Long Independence (Logsdon et al. 2007)

RALLI is geared to enhancing the cognitive supports that individuals with MCI may need when engaging in an exercise programme. Exercises are taught in a series of easy-to-remember steps that are repeated several times during training sessions in order to help participants' initial learning and facilitate subsequent recall. Each week, participants receive handouts and tracking forms to help them remember what was covered that week. Written instructions for all exercises are laminated and have small magnets attached to the back of the page, so participants can put them on their refrigerator doors. This provides a visual cue for participants to remember to do the exercises each day, as well as providing a handy reminder of how to do them. These memory aids and cues are incorporated throughout training.

RALLI was developed as a group intervention for residents living in retirement communities. In a pilot study (n = 37), attendance and compliance with the intervention was excellent, with participants attending 90% of scheduled classes. All subjects completed their six-month follow-up assessment, with no dropouts or attrition. At post-test (twelve weeks), 82% of participants had exercised at least once during the prior week, compared with 59% who had exercised at least once during the week prior to baseline (p <.0001), and mean exercise time increased by 172 minutes per week (p <.0001). On the SF-36, the Physical Components Scale and General Health Perceptions Subscale significantly improved (p <.0001 and p <.05, respectively); HDL cholesterol improved by 2.4 points (p <.05); and MMSE scores improved by 1.2 points at post test (p <.06). Participants' overall ratings of change indicate improvement in perceived physical health and emotional well-being as a result of the intervention. Anonymous ratings of class materials and instructor effectiveness also indicated a very high level of satisfaction. Thus, RALLI is a promising intervention to promote exercise in individuals with MCI, and it is currently being evaluated in a larger randomized controlled clinical trial.

EnhanceMobility in Assisted Living Memory Care Units

EnhanceMobility (EM) is an individualized, small-group exercise programme designed specifically for individuals with mild to moderate dementia, based on a combination of two evidence-based exercise interventions, EnhanceFitness (EF) and Reducing Disability in Alzheimer's Disease (RDAD). EF is nationally recognized as an effective group exercise programme for older adults without cognitive impairment, and RDAD is an evidence-based exercise programme for people with dementia who live at home with a family care-giver. EM has been pilot tested in the memory care units of four residential care facilities: twelve staff members and thirty-one residents (average age of 84 (range 67–96) and MMSE of 12 (range 2–26)). Exercise classes were conducted three times a week and lasted about thirty minutes per session. Direct assessments of participants were conducted by a trained interviewer before they began attending the EM Exercise Program (baseline) and four months after the baseline. As expected, cognitive functioning declined in participants over the four months of the study, with an average 1.88 point decline on the MMSE (p <.01). Despite this, participants' functional mobility improved significantly, with a 2.28 improvement on a Physical Functioning Scale (p <.05). Participants also exhibited significantly fewer behaviour problems following EM on the RMBPC (p <.001), including fewer depressive behaviours (p >.01). Current efforts are underway to develop and test this programme via a larger RCT.

RDAD Translation

RDAD has subsequently been implemented and evaluated in the US in a state-wide programme involving the Ohio Department of Aging, Alzheimer's Association chapters in Ohio and the Benjamin Rose Institute on Aging. Initially, the Alzheimer's Association, Northwest Ohio Chapter, served as the core implementation site; subsequent to the success achieved at that site, staff throughout the state of Ohio have been trained and implemented RDAD.

RDAD was selected because of its 'fit' with other programmes already provided in Ohio, as well as its unique focus on both the person with dementia and their family care-giver. The care-giver education and behavioural training aspects of RDAD were compatible with groups already offered at the Alzheimer's Association, but RDAD included additional skills to help staff extend services to family care-givers living with various stages of dementia and their concomitant behavioural problems. The exercise component of RDAD was novel and enabled the chapters to offer a new service, therefore increasing the scope of their support services. Staff members are bachelor's and master's prepared clinicians (primarily nurses, social workers and gerontologists) with an average eighteen years' experience in the field (range 5–36 years). To preserve treatment fidelity, all RDAD-Ohio staff participated in a two-day training programme conducted by University of Washington (UW) trainers followed by regular group supervision sessions to discuss and problem-solve implementation strategies and challenges in offering the programme. Thus far, 405 families have participated in RDAD-Ohio and preliminary results indicate strong positive responses from care-givers, care recipients, and staff.

More recently, our UW research group has received funding to translate RDAD throughout Washington and Oregon States in partnership with eight Area Agencies on Aging (AAAs) (1R01AG041716-01; L. Teri, PI). Two hundred and eight older adults (65+ years) with dementia who are living in the community and their family care-givers will be recruited from existing and future caseloads of collaborating AAAs. Case managers from each AAA attend a three-day workshop that provides training in both the RDAD exercises and the ABC problem-solving, communication, and pleasant events components of the intervention. Both persons in the participating dyads (care-givers and care-recipients) are instructed to practise the daily exercise routine, and repeated telephone assessments are being conducted over a one-year period to examine the impact on their mood, physical function, and independence. UW is working closely with AAA agency directors at every stage of implementation to ensure that any issues that arise with regard to case ascertainment, treatment delivery, outcome evaluation, and ongoing sustainability are addressed in a timely fashion. Although this latest translation of the RDAD programme has just recently begun, it has been enthusiastically received by the AAAs as a valuable addition to the portfolio of services they have available to offer persons with dementia and care-givers in their regions.

Need for Future Research

While the studies described here strongly support the effectiveness of exercise training for older adults, with and without cognitive impairment, the exact relationship between cognitive and physical health is still a topic with many contributing factors and complex associations. Significant questions remain about the causal mechanisms that may underlie the relationship between physical activity and cognitive status. Regular exercise may impact multiple modifiable risk factors that in turn impact brain health and cognitive function in older adults (Fotuhi, Do, and Jack 2012). Neuroprotective and neuroplastic effects have been reported in cognitive function as well as specific cortical regions of the brain in older adults who have participated in moderate levels of aerobic exercise (Erickson et al. 2009, 2011). Increases in volume in the temporal and prefrontal cortical regions of the brain have been found following a six-month moderate-intensity walking programme, compared to a stretching and toning programme, in previously sedentary community-dwelling older adults (ages 60–79) (Colcombe et al. 2004; Erickson et al. 2009; Erickson et al. 2011) and additional research involving physical activity and brain imaging is needed further to explore this evidence of neuroplasticity.

Furthermore, despite the positive successes of RDAD, NITE-AD, and EM, these programmes have not yet been conducted in large multisite trials. The diversity of those with intact cognition, MCI, and dementia, as well as their care-givers, requires large numbers of individuals of various cultural and ethnic groups, varied socio-economic status, and geographical distribution in order to better identify who is most (or least) likely to benefit, as well as to investigate the types of programmes most amenable to community-based translation.

Implications for Practice

Exercise Recommendations for All Older Adults (Chodzko-Zajko et al. 2009):

1. Given the high prevalence of comorbid medical conditions in older adults, evaluation by a healthcare professional is advised prior to initiating a moderate to vigorous exercise programme in older adults with cognitive impairment.
2. In cases of moderate to severe dementia and/or comorbid medical conditions, appropriate levels of supervision and exercise-response monitoring should be determined by a trained professional.
3. Exercise for older adults should include aerobic exercise, muscle-strengthening exercises, and flexibility exercises.
4. Individuals who are prone to falling or mobility impairment should perform specific exercises to improve balance, with oversight by a physical therapist or other health professional.

5. A combination of aerobic and resistive exercise training seems to be more effective than either form of training alone in counteracting the detrimental effects of a sedentary life style on health and functioning of the cardiovascular system and skeletal muscles.

6. Although there are clear benefits associated with higher-intensity exercise training programmes in healthy older adults, moderate intensity exercise is effective in reducing chronic cardiovascular and metabolic disease.

7. Exercise programmes should be individualized to meet the preferences and abilities of older adults.

8. Minimum exercise recommendations (Chodzko-Zajko et al. 2009; Garber et al. 2011) for all older adults include:

   (a) 150 minutes per week (thirty minutes, five days/week) of moderate-intensity aerobic exercise *or* twenty minutes, three days/week of vigorous-intensity. For individuals with limited exercise capacity, aerobic exercise can be accrued in 10-minute bouts.

   (b) resistance exercises for major muscle groups two days/week,

   (c) neuromuscular fitness (balance, agility, and coordination) two days/week, and

   (d) flexibility exercises two days/week.

Incorporating Exercise into Interventions for Cognitively Impaired Individuals

The Seattle Protocols clinical trials involving exercise have demonstrated that exercise can be effectively delivered by a variety of care-givers (including family members, home healthcare providers, and retirement community staff) in a variety of settings (private homes, congregate care, and retirement communities). Positive objective and subjective health and emotional status outcomes have been observed for both care-givers and care recipients. What follows is an overview of observations and lessons we have learned while conducting these interventions, along with recommendations for maximizing the impact of the exercise programme (Logsdon et al. 2005).

Care-giver characteristics

The success of any exercise intervention depends on paid or family care-givers' abilities to follow through outside the actual training sessions. When care-givers are unavailable or too frail or burdened to participate, an alternative 'exercise partner' may need to be found. The care-giver or exercise partner should be available to exercise with the participant on a regular basis (preferably daily, but at least three days a week), familiar with the exercises, and physically able to assist the participant as needed to ensure that exercises are done correctly and safely. The care-giver or exercise partner may also need assistance in motivating the participant to exercise, and training to deal with any behaviour problems that arise during exercise practice.

Participant characteristics

Individuals at all levels of cognitive impairment can benefit from exercise, but degree of impairment must be taken into consideration in developing a specific programme. Some individuals can follow written instructions, some can imitate movements demonstrated by the trainer, and others may require physical guidance. If walking is incorporated into the exercise routine, the participant's ability to walk alone safely (without getting lost, confused, or injured) must be considered. If the participant walks outdoors, a companion will usually be required. It is important to adjust the difficulty of the programme and not assign exercises that are beyond the capability of the participant. If an exercise is too difficult, the participant may become frustrated and refuse to do it, or may do it incorrectly and risk injury.

Many individuals with AD have co-existing chronic illnesses or physical limitations. The care-giver should consult with the participant's primary physician before initiating a new exercise programme, to ensure that there are no contraindications or safety concerns. Exercises must be monitored frequently, to insure that they are physically safe and appropriate for each participant. If a family care-giver is assisting the participant, care should be taken to assure that the care-giver is also physically capable of the activity. Participants and care-givers should be instructed to discontinue any activity that is painful, and to consult with their physician or the trainer about persistent discomfort.

Trainer qualifications

Exercise can be encouraged, taught, and monitored by a variety of home health providers, as long as they are knowledgeable about dementia symptoms, behaviour management techniques, and exercise. Many providers may have expertise in one area, but not in another. Resources for skill acquisition and consultation will vary across different communities, but potential sources of information include physical therapists, nurses, counsellors, and exercise specialists. Access to ongoing consultation regarding individualized care and issues that arise during treatment, as well as clinical flexibility and problem-solving skills will help to ensure the success of the programme.

Introducing the exercise programme

Before beginning an exercise programme, it is essential to provide an introduction and rationale for the programme, including the importance and potential benefits of exercise for the participant. The rationale should be specific to the individual participant to maximize 'buy in' and improve compliance with the programme. It is also useful to discuss immediate vs long-term benefits. For example, an individual who complains of feeling tired all the time may feel more energetic a few weeks after starting to exercise regularly. It is also useful to identify the participant's past exercise patterns and active hobbies. Often these past experiences form the basis for the current programme. For example, if the individual never enjoyed being outdoors but loved shopping, mall walking would be a better activity choice than outdoor hiking.

Record keeping

An exercise log or diary is a useful tool to remind participants and care-givers to complete assigned exercises throughout the week. A simple one-page checklist that can be posted on the refrigerator or in another conspicuous location is often the most effective tool, because it serves as a visual reminder when the participant sees it, and it provides immediate rein-forcement each time the participant checks off completing the exercise.

Summary

Identification of life-style factors and intervention strategies that may prevent or slow cog-nitive decline is critically important in our ageing society. Equally important is to motivate individuals to incorporate these changes into their lives and to maintain a healthy life style throughout the developmental, occupational, physical, and cognitive changes that accom-pany ageing. There is a growing body of evidence that exercise or daily physical activity delays onset and progression of cognitive impairment, reduces risk for falls and fractures, improves neuromuscular and cardiopulmonary function, improves functioning in daily activities, improves sleep, and elevates mood in older adults. Despite these promising find-ings, results of RCTs of exercise are mixed, with some studies demonstrating improve-ment in cognitive function and others demonstrating no significant differences between treatment and control groups. In general, better outcomes are seen in studies of moder-ate or greater intensity aerobic and resistance exercises, performed several times a week, for a long-term period. Additional research regarding behavioural strategies to encourage long-term maintenance of physical activity and to incorporate long-term follow-up assess-ment is needed to evaluate preservation of cognitive and physical function in older adults.

Key References and Sources for Further Reading

Ahlskog, J. E., Geda, Y. E., Graff-Radford, N. R., and Petersen, R. C. (2011). 'Physical Exercise as a Preventive or Disease-modifying Treatment of Dementia and Brain Aging'. *Mayo Clinic Proceedings* 89: 876–884.

Angevaren, M., Aufdemkampe, G., Verhaar, H. J., Aleman, A., and Vanhees, L. (2008). 'Physical Activity and Enhanced Fitness to Improve Cognitive Function in Older People without Known Cognitive Impairment'. *Cochrane Database of Systematic Reviews*, July 16, CD005381.

Teri, L., McCurry, S. M., Buchner, D., Logsdon, R. G., Lacroix, A., et al. (1998). 'Exercise and Activity Level in Alzheimer's Disease: A Potential Treatment Focus'. *Journal of Rehabilitation Research and Development* 35: 411–419.

Teri, L., Gibbons, L. E., McCurry, S. M., Logsdon, R. G., Buchner, D. M., et al. (2003). 'Exercise plus Behavior Management in Patients with Alzheimer Disease: A Randomized Controlled Trial'. *Journal of the American Medical Association* 290: 2015–2022.

Teri, L., Logsdon, R. G., and McCurry, S. M. (2008). 'Exercise Interventions for Dementia and Cognitive Impairment: The Seattle Protocols'. *Journal of Nutrition and Aging* 12: 391–394.

Teri, L., McKenzie, G., Logsdon, R. G., McCurry, S. M., Bollin, S., et al. (2012). 'Translation of Two Evidence-based Programs for Training Families to Improve Care of Persons with Dementia'. *Gerontologist* 52: 352–459.

WEBSITES AND OTHER RESOURCES

NIH Senior Health: Benefits of Exercise. http://nihseniorhealth.gov/exerciseforolderadults/healthbenefits/01.html.

Administration on Aging Alzheimer's Disease Supportive Services Program/Current Projects. http://www.aoa.gov/AoARoot/AoA_Programs/HPW/Alz_Grants/index.aspx.

Alzheimer's Association. http://www.alz.org/index.asp.

University of Washington Northwest Roybal Center. http://nursing.uw.edu/centers/northwest-roybal-center/northwest-roybal-center.html.

Faculty author websites (contact for information on exercise treatment protocols)

Linda Teri. http://www.son.washington.edu/faculty/faculty_bio.asp?id=104.

Susan McCurry. http://www.son.washington.edu/faculty/faculty_bio.asp?id=73.

Rebecca Logsdon. http://www.son.washington.edu/faculty/faculty_bio.asp?id=67.

Ellen McGough. http://www.rehab.washington.edu/education/faculty/nonproviderbios/mcgough.asp.

REFERENCES

Abbott, R. D., White, L. R., Ross, G. W., Masaki, K. H., Curb, J. D., et al. (2004). 'Walking and Dementia in Physically Capable Elderly Men'. *Journal of the American Medical Association* 292: 1447–1453.

ACSM (1998). 'ACSM Position Stand: The Recommended Quantity and Quality of Exercise for Developing and Maintaining Cardiorespiratory and Muscular Fitness, and Flexibility in Healthy Adults'. *Medicine & Science in Sports & Exercise* 30: 975–991.

Aggarwal, N. T., Wilson, R. S., Beck, T. L., Bienias, J. L., and Bennett, D. A. (2006). 'Motor Dysfunction in Mild Cognitive Impairment and the Risk of Incident Alzheimer Disease'. *Archives of Neurology* 63: 1763–1769.

Ahlskog, J. E., Geda, Y. E., Graff-Radford, N. R., and Petersen, R. C. (2011). 'Physical Exercise as a Preventive or Disease-modifying Treatment of Dementia and Brain Aging'. *Mayo Clinic Proceedings* 89: 876–884.

Andel, R., Crowe, M., Pedersen, N. L., Fratiglioni, L., Johansson, B., et al. (2008). 'Physical Exercise at Midlife and Risk of Dementia Three Decades Later: A Population-based Study of Swedish Twins'. *Journals of Gerontology, Series A: Biological Sciences and Medical Sciences* 63: 62–66.

Angevaren, M., Vanhees, L., Wendel-Vos, W., Verhaar, H. J., Aufdemkampe, G., et al. (2007). 'Intensity, but not Duration, of Physical Activities is Related to Cognitive Function'. *European Journal of Cardiovascular Prevention and Rehabilitation* 14: 825–830.

Angevaren, M., Aufdemkampe, G., Verhaar, H. J., Aleman, A., and Vanhees, L. (2008). 'Physical Activity and Enhanced Fitness to Improve Cognitive Function in Older People without Known Cognitive Impairment'. *Cochrane Database of Systematic Reviews*, July 16, CD005381.

Baker, L. D., Frank, L. L., Foster-Schubert, K., Green, P. S., Wilkinson, C. W., et al. (2010). 'Effects of Aerobic Exercise on Mild Cognitive Impairment: A Controlled Trial'. *Archives of Neurology* 67: 71–79.

Beauchet, O., Allali, G., Berrut, G., Hommet, C., Dubost, V., et al. (2008). 'Gait Analysis in Demented Subjects: Interests and Perspectives'. *Neuropsychiatric Disease and Treatment* 4: 155–160.

Bixby, W. R., Spalding, T. W., Haufler, A. J., Deeny, S. P., Mahlow, P. T., et al. (2007). 'The Unique Relation of Physical Activity to Executive Function in Older Men and Women'. *Medicine and Science in Sports and Exercise* 39: 1408–1416.

Blankevoort, C. G., Van Heuvelen, M. J., Boersma, F., Luning, H., De Jong, J., et al. (2010). 'Review of Effects of Physical Activity on Strength, Balance, Mobility and ADL Performance in Elderly Subjects with Dementia'. *Dementia and Geriatric Cognitive Disorders* 30: 392–402.

Buchman, A. S., Boyle, P. A., Leurgans, S. E., Barnes, L. L., and Bennett, D. (2011). 'Cognitive Function is Associated with the Development of Mobility Impairments in Community-dwelling Elders'. *American Journal of Geriatric Psychiatry* 19: 571–580.

Burns, J. M., Anderson, H. S., Smith, H. J., and Donnelly, J. E. (2008). 'Cardiorespiratory Fitness in Early-stage Alzheimer Disease'. *Alzheimer Disease and Associated Disorders* 22: 39–46.

Cassilhas, R. C., Viana, V. A., Grassmann, V., Santos, R. T., Santos, R. F., et al. (2007). 'The Impact of Resistance Exercise on the Cognitive Function of the Elderly'. *Medicine & Science in Sports & Exercise* 39: 1401–1407.

Chodzko-Zajko, W. J., Proctor, D. N., Fiatarone Singh, M. A., Minson, C. T., Nigg, C. R., et al. (2009). 'American College of Sports Medicine Position Stand. Exercise and Physical Activity for Older Adults'. *Medicine & Science in Sports & Exercise* 41: 1510–1530.

Clarkson-Smith, L. and Hartley, A. A. (1989). 'Relationships between Physical Exercise and Cognitive Abilities in Older Adults'. *Psychology and Aging* 4: 183–189.

Colcombe, S. and Kramer, A. F. (2003). 'Fitness Effects on the Cognitive Function of Older Adults: A Meta-analytic Study'. *Psychological Science* 14: 125–130.

Colcombe, S. J., Kramer, A. F., Erickson, K. I., Scalf, P., McAuley, E., et al. (2004). 'Cardiovascular Fitness, Cortical Plasticity, and Aging'. *Proceedings of the National Academy of Sciences of the United States of America* 101: 3316–3321.

Cress, M. E., Buchner, D. M., Prohaska, T., Rimmer, J., Brown, M., et al. (2005). 'Best Practices for Physical Activity Programs and Behavior Counseling in Older Adult Populations'. *Journal of Aging and Physical Activity* 13: 61–74.

Erickson, K. I., Prakash, R. S., Voss, M. W., Chaddock, L., Hu, L., et al. (2009). 'Aerobic Fitness is Associated with Hippocampal Volume in Elderly Humans'. *Hippocampus* 19: 1030–1039.

Erickson, K. I., Voss, M. W., Prakash, R. S., Basak, C., Szabo, A., et al. (2011). 'Exercise Training Increases Size of Hippocampus and Improves Memory'. *Proceedings of the National Academy of Sciences of the United States of America* 108: 3017–3022.

Espeland, M. A., Gill, T. M., Guralnik, J., Miller, M. E., Fielding, R., et al. (2007). 'Designing Clinical Trials of Interventions for Mobility Disability: Results from the Lifestyle Interventions and Independence for Elders Pilot (LIFE-P) Trial'. *Journals of Gerontology, Series A: Biological Sciences, and Medical Sciences* 62: 1237–1243.

Ferri, C. P., Prince, M., Brayne, C., Brodaty, H., Fratiglioni, L., et al. (2005). 'Global Prevalence of Dementia: A Delphi Consensus Study'. *Lancet* 366: 2112–2117.

Fotuhi, M., Do, D., and Jack, C. (2012). 'Modifiable Factors that Alter the Size of the Hippocampus with Ageing'. *Nature Reviews Neurology* 8: 189–202.

Garber, C. E., Blissmer, B., Deschenes, M. R., Franklin, B. A., Lamonte, M. J., et al. (2011). 'American College of Sports Medicine Position Stand. Quantity and Quality of Exercise for Developing and Maintaining Cardiorespiratory, Musculoskeletal, and Neuromotor Fitness in Apparently Healthy Adults: Guidance for Prescribing Exercise'. *Medicine & Science in Sports & Exercise* 43: 1334–1359.

Geda, Y. E., Roberts, R. O., Knopman, D. S., Christianson, T. J., Pankratz, V. S., et al. (2010). 'Physical Exercise, Aging, and Mild Cognitive Impairment: A Population-based Study'. *Archives of Neurology* 67: 80–86.

Hauer, K. and Oster, P. (2008). 'Measuring Functional Performance in Persons with Dementia'. *Journal of the American Geriatrics Society* 56: 949–950.

Hauer, K., Lord, S. R., Lindemann, U., Lamb, S. E., Aminian, K., et al. (2011). 'Assessment of Physical Activity in Older People with and without Cognitive Impairment'. *Journal of Aging and Physical Activity* 19: 347–372.

Hauer, K., Schwenk, M., Zieschang, T., Essig, M., Becker, C., et al. (2012). 'Physical Training Improves Motor Performance in People with Dementia: A Randomized Controlled Trial'. *Journal of the American Geriatrics Society* 60: 8–15.

Heyn, P., Abreu, B., and Ottenbacher, K. (2004). 'The Effects of Exercise Training on Elderly Persons with Cognitive Impairment and Dementia: A Meta-analysis'. *Archives of Physical Medical Rehabilitation* 85: 1694–1704.

Hill, R. D., Storandt, M., and Malley, M. (1993). 'The Impact of Long-term Exercise Training on Psychological Function in Older Adults'. *Journals of Gerontology, Series B: Psychological Sciences and Social Sciences* 48: P12–P17.

Hillman, C. H., Motl, R. W., Pontifex, M. B., Posthuma, D., Stubbe, et al. (2006). 'Physical Activity and Cognitive Function in a Cross-section of Younger and Older Community-Dwelling Individuals'. *Health Psychology* 25: 678–687.

Kenny, A. M., Bellantonio, S., Fortinsky, R. H., Dauser, D., Kleppinger, A., et al. (2008). 'Factors Associated with Skilled Nursing Facility Transfers in Dementia-specific Assisted Living'. *Alzheimer Disease and Associated Disorders* 22: 255–260.

Kluger, A., Gianutsos, J. G., Golomb, J., Ferris, S. H., George, A. E., et al. (1997). 'Patterns of Motor Impairment in Normal Aging, Mild Cognitive Decline, and Early Alzheimer's Disease'. *Journals of Gerontology, Series B: Psychological Sciences and Social Sciences* 52: P28–P39.

Kluger, A., Gianutsos, J. G., Golomb, J., Wagner, A., Jr, Wagner, D., et al. (2008). 'Clinical Features of MCI: Motor Changes'. *International Psychogeriatrics* 20: 32–39.

Kwak, Y. S., Um, S. Y., Son, T. G., and Kim, D. J. (2008). 'Effect of Regular Exercise on Senile Dementia Patients'. *International Journal of Sports Medicine* 29: 471–474.

Larson, E. B., Wang, L., Bowen, J. D., McCormick, W. C., Teri, L., et al. (2006). 'Exercise is Associated with Reduced Risk for Incident Dementia among Persons 65 Years of Age and Older'. *Annals of Internal Medicine* 144: 73–81.

Laurin, D., Verreault, R., Lindsay, J., MacPherson, K., and Rockwood, K. (2001). 'Physical Activity and Risk of Cognitive Impairment and Dementia in Elderly Persons'. *Archives of Neurology* 58: 498–504.

Lautenschlager, N. T., Cox, K. L., Flicker, L., Foster, J. K., Van Bockxmeer, F. M., et al. (2008). 'Effect of Physical Activity on Cognitive Function in Older Adults at Risk for Alzheimer Disease: A Randomized Trial'. *Journal of the American Medical Association* 300: 1027–1037.

Littbrand, H., Carlsson, M., Lundin-Olsson, L., Lindelöf, N., Håglin, L., et al. (2011a). 'Effect of a High-intensity Functional Exercise Program on Functional Balance: Preplanned Subgroup Analyses of a Randomized Controlled Trial in Residential Care Facilities'. *Journal of the American Geriatrics Society* 59: 1274–1282.

Littbrand, H., Stenvall, M., and Rosendahl, E. (2011b). 'Applicability and Effects of Physical Exercise on Physical and Cognitive Functions and Activities of Daily Living among People with Dementia: A Systematic Review'. *American Journal of Physical Medicine, and Rehabilitation* 90: 495–518.

Liu-Ambrose, T. Y., Ashe, M. C., Graf, P., Beattie, B. L., and Khan, K. M. (2008). 'Increased Risk of Falling in Older Community-dwelling Women with Mild Cognitive Impairment'. *Physical Therapy* 88: 1482–1491.

Liu-Ambrose, T., Nagamatsu, L. S., Graf, P., Beattie, B. L., Ashe, M. C., et al. (2010). 'Resistance Training and Executive Functions: A 12-month Randomized Controlled Trial'. *Archives of Internal Medicine* 170: 170–178.

Logsdon, R. G., McCurry, S. M., and Teri, L. (2005). 'A Home Health Care Approach to Exercise for Persons with Alzheimer's Disease'. *Care Management Journals* 6: 90–97.

Logsdon, R. G., McCurry, S. M., and Teri, L. (2007). 'Evidence-based Interventions to Improve Quality of Life for Individuals with Dementia'. *Alzheimer's Care Today* 8: 309–318.

McCurry, S. M., Gibbons, L. E., Logsdon, R. G., Vitiello, M. V., and Teri, L. (2003). 'Training Caregivers to Change the Sleep Hygiene Practices of Patients with Dementia: The NITE-AD Project'. *Journal of the American Geriatrics Society* 10: 1455–1460.

McCurry, S. M., Gibbons, L. E., Logsdon, R. G., Vitiello, M. V., and Teri, L. (2005). 'Nighttime Insomnia Treatment and Education for Alzheimer's Disease: A Randomized Controlled Trial'. *Journal of the American Geriatrics Society* 53: 793–802.

McCurry, S. M., Pike, K. C., Logsdon, R. G., Vitiello, M. V., Larson, E. B., et al. (2010). 'Predictors of Short and Long-term Adherence to a Daily Walking Program in Persons with Alzheimer's Disease'. *American Journal of Alzheimer's Disease and Other Dementias* 25: 505–512.

McCurry, S. M., Pike, K. C., Vitiello, M. V., Logsdon, R. G., Larson, E. B., et al. (2011). 'Increasing Walking and Bright Light Exposure to Improve Sleep in Community-dwelling Persons with Alzheimer's Disease: Results of a Randomized, Controlled Trial'. *Journal of the American Geriatrics Society* 59: 1393–1402.

Madden, D. J., Blumenthal, J. A., Allen, P. A., and Emery, C. F. (1989). 'Improving Aerobic Capacity in Healthy Older Adults Does not Necessarily Lead to Improved Cognitive Performance'. *Psychology and Aging* 4: 307–320.

Mariani, E., Monastero, R., Ercolani, S., Rinaldi, P., Mangialasche, F., et al. (2008). 'Influence of Comorbidity and Cognitive Status on Instrumental Activities of Daily Living in Amnestic Mild Cognitive Impairment: Results from the ReGAl Project'. *International Journal of Geriatric Psychiatry* 23: 523–530.

Middleton, L., Kirkland, S., and Rockwood, K. (2008). 'Prevention of CIND by Physical Activity: Different Impact on VCI-ND Compared with MCI'. *Journal of the Neurological Sciences* 269: 80–84.

Morris, J. C., Rubin, E. H., and Buchner, D. M. (1987). 'Senile Dementia of the Alzheimer's Type: An Important Risk Factor for Serious Falls'. *Journal of Gerontology* 42: 412–427.

O'Keeffe, S. T., Kazeem, H., Philpott, R. M., Playfer, J. R., Gosney, M., et al. (1996). 'Gait Disturbance in Alzheimer's Disease: A Clinical Study'. *Age and Ageing* 25: 313–316.

Perneczky, R., Pohl, C., Sorg, C., Hartmann, J., Komossa, K., et al. (2006). 'Complex Activities of Daily Living in Mild Cognitive Impairment: Conceptual and Diagnostic Issues'. *Age and Ageing* 35: 240–245.

Perrig-Chiello, P., Perrig, W. J., Ehrsam, R., Staehelin, H. B., and Krings, F. (1998). 'The Effects of Resistance Training on Well-being and Memory in Elderly Volunteers'. *Age and Ageing* 27: 469–475.

Roach, K. E., Tappen, R. M., Kirk-Sanchez, N., Williams, C. L., and Loewenstein, D. (2011). 'A Randomized Controlled Trial of an Activity Specific Exercise Program for Individuals with Alzheimer Disease in Long-term Care Settings'. *Journal of Geriatric Physical Therapy* 34: 50–56.

Rolland, Y., Pillard, F., Klapouszczak, A., Reynish, E., Thomas, D., et al. (2007). 'Exercise Program for Nursing Home Residents with Alzheimer's Disease: A 1-year Randomized, Controlled Trial'. *Journal of the American Geriatrics Society* 55: 158–165.

Rosenberg, P. B., Mielke, M. M., Appleby, B., Oh, E., Leoutsakos, J. M., et al. (2011). 'Neuropsychiatric Symptoms in MCI Subtypes: The Importance of Executive Dysfunction'. *International Journal of Geriatric Psychiatry* 26: 364–372.

Rovio, S., Kåreholt, I., Helkala, E. L., Viitanen, M., Winblad, B., et al. (2005). 'Leisure-time Physical Activity at Midlife and the Risk of Dementia and Alzheimer's Disease'. *Lancet Neurology* 4: 705–711.

Rozzini, L., Chilovi, B. V., Conti, M., Bertoletti, E., Delrio, I., et al. (2007). 'Conversion of Amnestic Mild Cognitive Impairment to Dementia of Alzheimer Type is Independent to Memory Deterioration'. *International Journal of Geriatrics Psychiatry* 22: 1217–1222.

Smiley-Oyen, A. L., Lowry, K. A., Francois, S. J., Kohut, M. L., and Ekkekakis, P. (2008). 'Exercise, Fitness, and Neurocognitive Function in Older Adults: The 'Selective Improvement' and 'Cardiovascular Fitness' Hypotheses'. *Annals of Behavioral Medicine* 36: 280–291.

Teri, L., McCurry, S. M., Buchner, D., Logsdon, R. G., Lacroix, A., et al. (1998). 'Exercise and Activity Level in Alzheimer's Disease: A Potential Treatment Focus'. *Journal of Rehabilitation Research and Development* 35: 411–419.

Teri, L., Logsdon, R. G., and McCurry, S. M. (2002). 'Nonpharmacologic Treatment of Behavioral Disturbance in Dementia'. *Medical Clinics of North America* 86: 641–656.

Teri, L., Gibbons, L. E., McCurry, S. M., Logsdon, R. G., Buchner, D. M., et al. (2003). 'Exercise plus Behavior Management in Patients with Alzheimer Disease: A Randomized Controlled Trial'. *Journal of the American Medical Association* 290: 2015–2022.

Teri, L., Logsdon, R. G., and McCurry, S. M. (2005). 'The Seattle Protocols: Advances in Behavioral Treatment of Alzheimer's Disease'. In B. Vellas, L. J. Fitten, B. Winblad, H. Feldman, M. Grundman, et al. (eds), *Research and Practice in Alzheimer's Disease and Cognitive Decline*. Paris: Serdi Publisher.

Teri, L., Logsdon, R. G., and McCurry, S. M. (2008). 'Exercise Interventions for Dementia and Cognitive Impairment: The Seattle Protocols'. *Journal of Nutrition and Aging* 12: 391–394.

Teri, L., McKenzie, G., Logsdon, R. G., McCurry, S. M., Bollin, S., et al. (2012). 'Translation of Two Evidence-based Programs for Training Families to Improve Care of Persons with Dementia'. *Gerontologist* 52: 352–459.

Tinetti, M. E. and Kumar, C. (2010). 'The Patient Who Falls: "It's Always a Trade-off"'. *Journal of the American Medical Association* 303: 258–266.

Tornatore, J. B., Hedrick, S. C., Sullivan, J. H., Gray, S. L., Sales, A., et al. (2003). 'Community Residential Care: Comparison of Cognitively Impaired and Noncognitively Impaired Residents'. *American Journal of Alzheimer's Disease and Other Dementias* 18: 240–246.

Van Gelder, B. M., Tijhuis, M. A., Kalmijn, S., Giampaoli, S., Nissinen, A., et al. (2004). 'Physical Activity in Relation to Cognitive Decline in Elderly Men: The FINE Study'. *Neurology* 63: 2316–2321.

Van Uffelen, J. G., Chin, A. P. M. J., Hopman-Rock, M., and Van Mechelen, W. (2008a). 'The Effects of Exercise on Cognition in Older Adults with and without Cognitive Decline: A Systematic Review'. *Clinical Journal of Sports Medicine* 18: 486–500.

Van Uffelen, J. G., Chinapaw, M. J., Van Mechelen, W., and Hopman-Rock, M. (2008b). 'Walking or Vitamin B for Cognition in Older Adults with Mild Cognitive Impairment? A Randomised Controlled Trial'. *British Journal of Sports Medicine* 42: 344–351.

Williams, C. L. and Tappen, R. M. (2007). 'Effect of Exercise on Mood in Nursing Home Residents with Alzheimer's Disease'. *American Journal of Alzheimer's Disease and Other Dementias* 22: 389–397.

Wittwer, J. E., Webster, K. E., and Menz, H. B. (2010). 'A Longitudinal Study of Measures of Walking in People with Alzheimer's Disease'. *Gait & Posture* 32: 113–117.

Yaffe, K., Barnes, D., Nevitt, M., Lui, L. Y., and Covinsky, K. (2001). 'A Prospective Study of Physical Activity and Cognitive Decline in Elderly Women: Women who Walk'. *Archives of Internal Medicine* 161: 1703–1708.

CHAPTER 50

GEROPSYCHOLOGICAL RESEARCH AND PRACTICE IN MENTAL HEALTH IN MAINLAND CHINA

DAHUA WANG AND XIANMIN GONG

BACKGROUND

'AGEING and health', as the topic of World Health Day in 2012, demonstrates the imperative of focusing on ageing issues around the world. The World Health Organization (WHO) predicts that the world will soon have more older people than children, as life expectancy has increased significantly over the past century. In China, the challenges brought by the rapid pace of ageing and the huge older population seem more severe than anywhere else. The data from the Sixth Chinese National Population Census, released by the National Bureau of Statistics of China (NBSC), show that the population of people aged over 60 and 65 had reached 178 million (13.3% of the total population) and 120 million (8.9% of the total population) respectively by 2010 (more details can be found on the website http://www.stats.gov.cn). According to projections, the number of Chinese people over 60 years old will reach its peak of 430 million around the year 2050; this means that there will be one older person for every three persons in China (Zhang 2011). In addition, the drastic transition of economy and culture in Chinese society, begun about thirty years ago, has increased the challenges coming with the 'silver tides'.

Undoubtedly, it calls for efforts from the whole of society to solve the problems associated with ageing. The contribution of geropsychology is an indispensable part of these efforts. On the fiftieth anniversary of its foundation, celebrated in December 2000 in Italy, the International Association of Gerontology (IAG) explicitly proposed that gerontological research should aim at improving quality of life (QoL) for older people. Unfortunately, little agreement has been achieved so far even on the definition of QoL per se, as it is a complicated concept (Hunt 1997). In early literature on the subject, QoL was often defined in terms of objective aspects of living conditions, such as physical health, personal circumstances, and so forth (Morris 1979). In more recent years, more and more researchers have argued that the subjective or psychological aspects of an individual's life, including satisfaction, happiness, etc., should not be neglected and need to be taken into account as well (Diener and Suh 1997).

As a major branch of gerontology, geropsychology plays an essential role in the subjective domain of older adults' QoL. However, having started very late at the end of the last century, geropsychology in China is still at a very young age. And its influence, either in terms of academic research or practical application, has so far been quite limited, though it indicates great potential as well. In order to outline the current progress of geropsychological research and practice in China, we have carried out some reviews of research in China. We used two web resources: one is the China National Knowledge Infrastructure (CNKI), the most comprehensive and influential scholar database in China which includes nearly all Chinese academic publications; the other is the ISI Web of Knowledge, used to search English-language articles. Using 'across life OR life-span OR lifespan OR late life OR later life OR gerontism OR gerontology OR gerontal OR gerontic OR geriatric OR senile OR senium OR senility OR senior OR age OR aging OR ageing OR old OR older OR elder OR elderly' and 'Chinese OR China' as keywords in title, and 'psychology', 'geriatrics', 'gerontology', and 'psychiatry' as key words in field, in the end we only discovered a little more than seven hundred articles in the Chinese language and three hundred in the English language literature. These are all about geropsychological research in mainland China and were published between 1981 and 2010. Further, looking into these articles reveals that the majority concern the mental health of older adults, and are dominated in number by survey or epidemiological studies.

Accordingly, in this chapter, we first focus on the epidemiology of several kinds of mental health problems and related risk factors (mainly social-demographical factors), among which some unique cultural factors are addressed specifically. Then we shift to research and practice on prevention of or intervention in older people's mental health concerns from the standpoint of both formal social support and family support.

THE MENTAL HEALTH OF OLDER PEOPLE IN MAINLAND CHINA FROM THE PERSPECTIVE OF EPIDEMIOLOGY

Depression

Epidemiological characteristics of depression in the older population

Depression is one of the most common mental health problems among older adults. Though there has been no longitudinal investigation with population-based samples, the trend of rapid increase in the prevalence rate of depression among the older population turns out to be apparent when analysing publications from the last three decades. A meta-analysis of ten surveys conducted between 1983 and 1993 showed that the prevalence rates of depressive illness and depressive symptoms were 3.9% and 14.8%, respectively, among older people in mainland China (Chen, Copeland, and Wei 1999). Nonetheless, surprisingly, the prevalence rate of depressive symptoms climbed to 64.1% for rural older people and 44.5% for urban older people in 2006, according to a nationwide investigation, the Sampling Survey of the Aged Population in Urban/Rural China 2006, sponsored by the China National Committee on Ageing (CNCA)

(Zhang and Guo 2009). Similarly, the rate for the older population as a whole was 39.9%, according to another nationwide investigation conducted between 2007 and 2008 (Yu et al. 2012). Another meta-analysis (Zhang, Xu, and Nie 2011), of twenty-five surveys published between 2000 and 2010, reported it as 22.6%. Some other research listed in Table 50.1 found this rate to be over 30.0% as well. From Table 50.1, we can also see that the changing pattern of prevalence rates of depressive illness resembles rates of depressive symptoms.

Influential patterns of social-demographical risk factors of depression

Some previous research has found that the prevalence of depression in China was lower than that in Western countries (Parker, Cheah, and Roy 2001). However, the gap seems to have been diminishing in recent years. With regard to the underlying reasons, some argue that the sharply increasing prevalence of depression among older Chinese people is partly due to the gradual loss of some protective factors, including a lower level of urbanization, traditional values of filial piety, strong social support, etc. (Bromet et al. 2011; Parker et al. 2001; Yu et al. 2012).

However, much research targeting the Chinese older population turned back on the view that less industrialization and urbanization arrests the prevalence of depression, which has been widely verified and recognized in Western societies. Here in China, older people living in less industrialized and urbanized areas, such as the rural and western regions (Chinese western regions are generally less developed than eastern regions), tend to have higher depression rates (e.g. Ma et al. 2008; Ma et al. 2010; Zhang and Guo 2009). Another distinct pattern reflects the close relationship between depression rate and family support. Family support is a strong predictor of depressive symptoms, and better family support is usually tied to fewer health problems and better QoL (Leung et al. 2007; Yu et al. 2012). Later in this chapter, we will concentrate on the topic of family support as a specific section.

As shown in Table 50.1, other risk factors frequently examined include: (1) advanced age, though several researchers reported that the correlation between age and depression rate was not significant after controlling other confounding variables (Yu et al. 2012); (2) low educational level, though a recent large-sample study called CONVERGE suggested that females with more years of education are surprisingly more likely to have major depressive disorder in mainland China (Flint et al. 2011); and (3) being female, poor health conditions, low social-economic status, having an unhappy relationship, etc., which are commonly accepted as risk factors without much controversy.

Dementia

Dementia is another frequently occurring mental disorder which can greatly impact on the life of older adults. To our knowledge, there has been no nationwide investigation on the epidemiology of dementia in mainland China. By piecing together the results of several recent surveys (Rodriguez et al. 2008; Yan, Li, and Huang 2008; Zhang et al. 2005; Zhou et al. 2006), we tentatively conclude that the dementia rate in the Chinese older population may currently fluctuate at approximately 5.0%. Alzheimer's disease (AD) and vascular dementia (VaD) are the two major subtypes of dementia in mainland China (Dong et al.

Table 50.1 Prevalence of depressive illness and depressive symptoms in older people in mainland China

First author and year published	Survey date	Location	Urban/rural	Age (y) and subject number	Tools	Prevalence (CI) (%)		Risk factors
						Depressive illness	Depressive mood/symptom	
Chen et al. 1999[a]	1983–1993	Multiple	U/R	≥ 60; 13656	Multiple	3.9 (2.6–4.0)	14.8 (14.2–15.6)	Advanced age, retirement, poor physical health, poor social support, low income, mental stress, negative life events
Zhang et al. 2011[b]	2000–2010	Multiple	U/R	≥ 60; 28922	Multiple	–	22.6 (18.9–26.7)	Female, living in rural or less developed regions
Li et al. 1999	1997	Beijing	U	≥ 60; 1593	GDS, HAMD, ICD-10	1.8 (–)	–	Female, poor physical health, advanced age, lower educational level
Meng et al. 2000	1993	Beijing	U/R	≥ 60; 2299	CES-D	–	13.4 (–)	Advanced age, female, living in rural area
Chen et al. 2004	2001	Anhui	U	≥ 65; 1736	GMS-AGECAT	2.2 (1.5–2.9)	–	Low income
Chen et al. 2005	2003	Anhui	R	≥ 60; 1600	GMS-AGECAT	6.0 (4.8–7.3)	–	Female, poor physical health, low income, poor social support, bad relationship, negative life events
Ma et al. 2006	2004	Anhui	R	≥ 60; 1236	GMS-AGECAT	7.2[c] (–)	–	Negative life events
Chen et al. 2007	–	Hubei	U	≥ 60; 898	GDS	–	6.4	Low income, lower educational level, bad housing conditions and family relationship
Pan et al. 2008	2005	Beijing, Shanghai	U	50–70; 3289	CES-D	–	9.5 (–)	Female, poor physical health, low income, lower educational level, living alone, without spouse, poor medical insurance, few social activities
Chen et al. 2008	2006	Beijing	U	≥ 60; 1542	GDS-15	–	10.6	Advanced age, chronic disease, low ADL, without spouse, lonely, lower educational level, poor economic insurance

Study	Year	Region	U/R	Age; N	Instrument	Prevalence	First-incidence	Risk factors
Ma et al. 2008	2006	Beijing	U/R	≥ 60; 1601	CIDI 1.0	7.8 (-)	-	Female, low income, lower educational level, living in rural area, poor major medical conditions
Ma et al. 2010	2008	Anhui	U/R	≥ 65; 1757	GMS -AGECAT	Urban: 3.6 (1.6–5.8) Rural: 6.2 (4.7–7.8)	-	Living alone, worrying about children, less communication, negative life events, living in rural area
Yuan et al. 2010	-	Hunan	U	≥60; 460	GDS	-	33.5 (-)	Female, poor physical health, lower educational level, low income, bad marital status, bad housing conditions
Li et al. 2011	-	Hunan	-	≥60; 896	PHQ-9	MDD: 15.0 (-)	-	Female, low income, unmarried
Yu et al. 2012	2007-2008	Nationwide	U	≥55; 4945	CES-D	-	39.9 (-)	Poor family support, poor health status, bad marital status, lower educational level, in less developed region

Notes: a: This meta-analysis includes ten research surveys conducted through 1983 to 1993, which surveyed the prevalence of depressive illness or depressive symptoms among the elderly in different regions in mainland China;

b: This meta-analysis contains twenty-five research surveys published between 2000 and 2010, including one survey from Hong Kong and one from Macao. The rest of the surveys are not included in the two meta-analyses;

c: This datum refers to the first-incidence rate of depressive illness in the past year, while all other data in the same and the next column refer to the prevalence rate; U: urban; R: rural; GDS: Geriatric Depression Scale; HAMD: Hamilton Depression Scale; ICD-10: *The International Statistical Classification of Diseases and Related Health Problems* (10th revision); CES-D: Center for Epidemiologic Studies Depression Scale; GMS: Geriatric Mental State; AGECAT: Automated Geriatric Examination for Computer Assisted Taxonomy; CIDI: Composite International Diagnostic Interview; PHQ-9: Patient Health Questionnaire-9; CI: confidence interval; MDD: major depression disorder; –: not investigated or unmentioned.

2007; Zhang et al. 2005). In a systematic analysis of 1980–2004 studies about dementia in mainland China, Dong et al. (2007) reported that, among all kinds of dementia, the proportions of AD and VaD were 54.3% and 25.5%, respectively.

In addition, Dong et al. (2007) also argued that the pooled average dementia rate in China for older people above 60 years was 2.8% (95%, CI = 2.5–3.1%), and that the rates of both dementia and AD have increased while the rates of VaD have been stable for the past twenty-four years. Given the salient gap between 2.8% and 5.0%, we might intuitively suppose that the rate has increased during the last few years. However, this assumption could not be robust enough when generalized to the whole population of older people in China, considering the heterogeneity of samples from different researchers. In different studies, subjects might come from different regions with different cultural and socio-economic backgrounds, and gender and age ratios often differed as well. As a result, these differences could make findings less comparable, especially when considering that in China these factors are tightly related to the epidemiology of dementia.

With respect to risk factors, advanced age, female gender, lower education, physical disease, and motor-sensory disability have been consistently recognized to be associated with dementia (Chen et al. 2011; Li et al. 1999; Shen et al. 1994; Yan et al. 2008).

Anxiety and loneliness

A cross-culture study showed that in China fewer than 0.4% of urban and rural older people suffered from anxiety disorder, far lower than in other developing countries such as Latin America and India (Prina et al. 2011). However, the rate of anxiety symptoms may be remarkably high in Chinese older people. For example, one study showed that as many as 21.6% of home-dwelling healthy older adults suffer from anxiety symptoms (Zhang, Zeng, and Yang 2010). So far, no studies with larger samples have been developed to investigate the situation of anxiety in mainland China; more effort needs to be invested in future research. As to risk factors, being female, disease, a lower level of socio-economic status, and lower level of education have frequently been found to be closely related to anxiety in older adults (Prina et al. 2011; Zhang, Zeng, and Yang 2010).

Several large-sample or nationwide investigations looked into the loneliness of older adults in mainland China. About 15.6% of the older people reported feeling lonely in 1992, and 29.6% in 2000 (Yang and Victor 2008). In 2006, this rate was reported as 20.8% for urban and 34.4% for rural older Chinese according to the Sampling Survey of the Aged Population in Urban/Rural China 2006 (Guo and Chen 2009). Another study reported that the rate of loneliness among old people in rural Anhui province reached a rate of 78.1%. The author suggested that the remarkably high rate of loneliness may arise from lack of social support and family function (Wang et al. 2011). More specifically, in rural areas, lower levels of social resources and sociability limit older people's social activities. The limitation in social activities, in turn, leads older people to rely more on family function, and makes them more vulnerable to the ongoing social and family transitions in mainland China. In sum, all these data suggest that a great number of Chinese older people are living with loneliness.

Suicide

Though suicide per se is not a specific kind of mental disorder, it is closely associated with individuals' mental health. Suicide is a principal cause of death in China and its rate is higher in older populations than in other age groups, according to the China Health Statistic Yearbook 2010 released by the Ministry of Health of the People's Republic of China (MOH, for more information please refer to the website: http://www.moh.gov.cn) and the study by Zhang and colleagues (2002). In line with Durkheim's theories of suicide, a set of influential theories in Western countries, researchers argue that urbanization, industrialization, and modernization may relate to an increasing suicide rate (Lester 2001). However, it appears to be another story in China. The MOH's annual reports and quite a few studies have demonstrated a downward trend in the suicide rate in mainland China during the last thirty years, against a background of fast economic growth and rapid urbanization and industrialization (Qin and Mortensen 2001; Yang et al. 2004; Zhang et al. 2010).

Research has also found that the distribution of suicide rates among the older population in mainland China is distinct from that in Western countries. First, the suicide rate among older people in rural areas is higher, and the downward trend of suicide over time in rural areas is less remarkable than that in urban areas (Li, Xiao, and Xiao 2009). The discrepancy between rural and urban populations may be due to the shortage of social welfare services in rural areas, including economic security, medical insurance, and so on (Li et al. 2009). Again, the research runs counter to the argument that urbanization and industrialization may be contributing to the suicide rate in China. Second, early studies found a higher suicide rate among females than among males in China, which was contrary to the findings in Western countries. Some researchers ascribed the gender difference to cultural factors, i.e. the unequal treatment of women (Qin and Mortensen 2001). As the idea of equality between men and women is now becoming widely accepted, the gap is expected to diminish soon (Yip et al. 2005). Data released by the MOH (2010, see website above) has confirmed Yip et al's (2005) prediction that the suicide rate among females is no longer significantly higher, and is sometimes even lower, than that of males.

It may be quite surprising that the exacerbation of some mental health problems, such as depression and dementia, is combined with a decreasing suicide rate among the older population in mainland China. This paradoxical phenomenon may be the result of several causes. First, despite an increasing rate of certain mental health problems (i.e. depression and dementia), the situation of mental health and well-being as a whole may be improving in the older Chinese population. Another possibility is that the suicide rate may not be as closely associated with mental health as is widely imagined. Some studies supported this counter-intuitive point of view and suggested a low correlation between mental health and suicide in China. They found a low level of mental health illness in suicide victims; in other words, mental health did not strongly predict suicidal behaviour (Law and Liu 2008; Li et al. 2009). So what makes the pattern of suicide rate unique in China, and what are the major risk factors for suicide if a mental health condition is not among them? At present, few researchers have provided convincing answers.

Summary of mental health problems

According to a study conducted during 2001–2002, using *DSM-IV* as the diagnostic criteria, 8.2% people over 65 years of age in mainland China suffered from at least one kind of mental disorder (Lee et al. 2007). Given the large number of older persons with mental illness, the research investment and the findings in the past three decades have been relatively insufficient. First, measuring techniques are still immature. Almost all the commonly used tools, such as questionnaires, inventories, scales, and diagnostic criteria, were introduced from Western countries. Some of these were not rigorously examined for reliability, validity, or the appropriateness of cut-off points. This might be one source of evident divergence among different studies. Second, the samples in most published articles lacked representativeness. One of the most common shortcomings was that the sampling was usually limited to only one or a few regions. China is a huge country with a vast territory and great diversity of nationalities and subcultures, which makes it extremely difficult to draw any general conclusions about older adults' mental health from regional samples. Given the complicated components of the older population in this country, it is difficult and improbable to imagine that an individual project or study could adequately manage a comprehensive nationwide investigation. Thus it is time to call for government investment to support this kind of work. Fortunately, central government has realized the urgency and importance of promoting the life quality and mental health of older people. In the near future, we can expect more accurate figures specifically about the mental health of the older population from reliable sources.

With respect to the risk factors, we have discussed in detail the specific mental health problems of depression, dementia, and suicide. In general, poor physical health, low income, a lack of social support, a lower educational level, and being female are predictors of worse mental health for older people.

Social Support as an Important Protective Factor of Older People's Mental Health

As we can see from the above, social support is a critical factor influencing older people's QoL. There are two types of social support: formal support and informal support. The latter mainly refers to family support, such as support from spouses and children. The former is non-family support and can include support from governments, communities, and social organizations.

Family as the informal source of social support

Social support from children

To emphasize family values is a core tradition in China: supporting older people is presented as the basic obligation of family members. Much research has confirmed the positive effects of family support on older adults in mainland China. For example, better family support is demonstrated to have a close relationship with lower depression, less anxiety, higher self-esteem, and greater well-being (Chen and Silverstein 2000; Leung et al. 2007;

Silverstein, Cong, and Li 2006; Wang et al. 2004; Wang, Wang, and Shen 2006). In mainland China, support from children is one main source of family support for older adults. According to data from the 2000 Chinese National Population Census, 43.8% of older people's financial income came from the aid of their family members, though this percentage is lower than 57.1% in 1994 (Du 2003). In addition to financial support, descendants are also important care-givers for older adults. A survey (Zhang, Liu, and Tang 2004) focusing on care-givers reported that 96% of older patients with dementia were taken care of at home. Among the primary care-givers, 44% of them were sons and daughters-in-law, 15% were daughters and sons-in-law, 6% were grandchildren, and 31% were spouses (Zhang et al. 2004). With regard to practical help, children are usually the first to assist their older parents. Take shopping for example: 90.1% of older people in urban areas and 89.8% in rural areas received assistance from their adult children. And in another example, 89.7% of older people in urban areas and 90.6% of older people in rural areas were accompanied by their children when they went to visit doctors (Zhang and Guo 2009). Children also provide older parents with emotional support, one of the most important types of support for older people. A recent study targeting older females in rural Anhui, a province located in central mainland China, showed that 81.3% of the participants would like to seek emotional support from their sons, 54.5% from daughters, and 44.9% from their spouses (Huang, Lin, and Xu 2012).

However, family support from descendants, formerly the main source of support for older people, is now being undermined. The changes may result from two aspects of social transition. On the one hand, the family structure in mainland China is undergoing drastic transformation. First, the only-child policy, started in 1979 to slow down population growth in mainland China, will result in the '4-2-1' family structure becoming the dominant type if the policy continues without any adjustment. The '4-2-1' structure means a young/middle-aged couple have to look after four old parents (i.e. their own parents and parents-in-law), and have one child. Although the only-child policy has been adjusted to a so-called 'two only children' policy, which means that each couple can have two children if the wife and husband are both only children, the total fertility rate is still very low. For example, it was estimated as 1.22 in 2000 and 1.18 in 2010 by the sixth census (Fu, Zhang, and Li 2013). The total number of children is falling dramatically and this trend might continue for generations in China. It is not difficult to predict that children's support for older parents will inevitably decrease (Zimmer and Kwong 2003).

Second, changes in life style have contributed to changes in family structure. The pressure to find an ideal job as well as better opportunities for career development is taking young generations away from their parents and home towns, in a serious violation of the traditional value of filial piety in which taking care of one's parents is regarded as the fundamental responsibility of children. It was estimated that there would be 159 million peasant workers living away from their homes in mainland China in 2011 (see more information on the NBSC website: http://www.stats.gov.cn). In fact, the subjective willingness of older people to live with their children is dropping as well, as data show that 58.7% (43.0% in urban areas, 62.6% in rural areas) of older people were willing to live with children in 2000, while the rate dropped to less than 50.0% (37.1% in urban areas, 54.5% in rural areas) in 2006 (Zhang and Guo 2009). The population mobility of younger generations as well as the increasing preference of the older generation to live alone is prompting the boom of 'empty nests', especially in rural areas. According to CNCA, 38.3% of the 108 million rural older people were in an 'empty-nest' situation in 2006, and in some regions the rate might exceed 60%. For those 'empty-nest' seniors, lacking local support from children is likely to bring more challenges, especially if dysfunction, illness, or disability make it difficult for them to look after themselves. A number of studies (e.g. Liu and Guo 2007, 2008; Silverstein et al. 2006; Wang and Shi 2008) have also shown that seniors in 'empty nests' may be more at risk for mental health disorders. Compared to older adults who are not in the 'empty-nest' situation, they may be subject to more mental stresses, more frequent loneliness, a higher level of depressive symptoms, less family support, less subjective well-being, and lower life satisfaction.

The shift in social ideology may also drive the change in family support from descendants. It is necessary to think back to the concept of patrimonialism in Chinese traditional culture. In ancient China, as in some other earlier cultures, the father's role reflected his superior position in the family, and family members had to obey their eldest living forefather—the father, grandfather, or great-grandfather (Hamilton 1990). As they had the power of absolute authority in the family, the older adults never needed to worry about failing support from descendants. However, this utter superiority has become a legend that only existed in olden times. The absolute patrimonialism that prevailed in China for thousands of years is collapsing, and has been replaced by a more democratic, or even an inverse, power pattern between forefathers and their descendants. The downgrading of patriarchy has led to changes in intergenerational relationships, which in turn have led to a decline in the values of filial piety. Nowadays, whether the children will support their parents and grandparents depends more on their own willingness and less on compulsory obligation than at any previous time. Though this reflects a kind of ideological emancipation from the standpoint of individual development, it may simultaneously cause the undesired consequence that some younger adults will use it as an excuse to fail in fulfilling their duty to take care of the older adults in the family. It is not surprising that quite a number of older people worry about their children's dereliction of the duty to look after them (Guo and Chen 2009). Nevertheless, it is worth noting that the transition of filial piety does not always bring negative consequences to the stability of family support. It can also have some positive effects. For instance, modern filial piety may consist less of an imposed sense of obligation and more of a feeling of humanity and emotional support, which may sometimes be more important to boost older people's mental health and life satisfaction (Leung et al. 2007).

In summary, the change in family structure and the transition in ideology about intergenerational relationships may be combining to relax the central role of family support from children to parents in the care of older Chinese people.

Social support from spouse

In addition to children, the spouse is another significant other and another main source of family support for older people. A myriad of studies have illustrated the critical positive effect of satisfying marital status on the mental health and well-being of older adults (Wade and Pevalin 2004). Marital attachment is one of the important indicators of marital quality in older adults. In our study we found that marital attachment in mainland China could be classified into three types: secure, anxious, and avoidant attachment (Zhai et al. 2010). We also found that a majority (56.2%) of older people in our study could be categorized into the secure type, similar to a study from Taiwan (Liu 2000) in which 69.6% of older people reported secure attachment to their spouse. In contrast, insecure attachment is the most common type in Western countries (Diehl et al. 1998; Magai et al. 2001). This cultural discrepancy, including social support as an influential component, might strongly indicate that Chinese older people may enjoy more satisfying marital relationships.

In light of the findings about marital attachment, Chinese older couples seem to have a healthier marriage quality compared to their Western counterparts. However, problems should not be overlooked. According to CNCA, 23.0% of older people lived without a spouse in 2006, and the rate increased in older age groups. From another perspective, the highly skewed sex ratio of the population might worsen marriage status in mainland China. In 2010, the male to female ratio was 1.05:1, which means the number of surplus men was as high as 34 million. What's more, the boy to girl ratio at birth will stay above 1.1:1 before 2050, so the effect of this unbalanced sex ratio will last for a long time (Porter 2010). It is highly likely that these problems will affect social support from the spouse, which in turn will influence the older people's mental health and quality of life.

Summary of family support

Social ties are important for human beings, and interventions targeting social ties have been demonstrated by some studies to be effective in improving mental health (Kawachi and Berkman 2001). In China, family support may be the most important aspect of social ties, especially for older people. Older people receive support from other family members, and become more dependent on their children and spouse during the ageing process. This kind of traditional old-age support pattern has been delivered from generation to generation for thousands of years until recent decades, when drastic changes to family structure and ideologies took place which may threaten the integrity of family support. Given this background, family support cannot fulfil older people's needs in all cases. Thus, formal support, as supplementary help from outside the family, is becoming a necessity for older people to guarantee their mental health and well-being.

Formal social support

Government as the fundamental source of formal support

Given the greatly increased population of older people, both the central and regional governments in mainland China have realized the coming pressures of social and economic consequences and recognized that it is urgent and important to work out effective policies and coping strategies as soon as possible. However, not all the provincial governments are investing the same amount of effort into this issue, as the social and economic levels are obviously different among the various regions. Generally, the better developed regions display stronger support for their older residents. Undoubtedly, Beijing, the capital city and national centre of politics, culture, and economy, possesses optimal sources of social support for older people. Though the case of Beijing is not necessarily representative, it is helpful to understand the government's aim and direction here, as the efforts of Beijing play a leading role in the country as a whole. In this section, we talk more about the government's investment in the capital city.

First of all, to work out and enact supporting policies to enhance the QoL of older people is the core function of the government. Recently, several important strategies have been carried out to guarantee the benefits of older residents in Beijing. Since 2009, all residents above the age of 60 have rights to special care (http://zhengwu.beijing.gov.cn/zwzt/lnr/t999886.htm) in the following aspects of social life.

Medicare

Large- and medium-sized medical institutes provide 'six privileges' for older patients regardless of their in- or outpatient status. These privileges include registration, visiting a doctor, medical tests, examination, paying fees, and receiving medicine. Given the costs in time and fatigue for an older patient to queue for each of the steps that are part of the normal procedure for a hospital visit, the 'six privileges' are a careful and useful consideration. With respect to community medical institutes, they also provide some benefits for older residents. For instance, they offer free physical examinations once a year for those older adults who have no social insurance.

Social life service

Older people who are 65 years or older can apply for a special Identification Card for Senior Residents (ICSR) from the local government department, such as the residents' committee. An ICSR gives access to free bus transport in the city. Residents who are 90 years old or older will receive a sum of money (RMB100 Yuan if below 100 years old and RMB200 Yuan if 100 years old or above) every month as an advanced age allowance. Older people who are in disadvantaged circumstances, such as being disabled or living alone, will be provided with appropriate subsidies from the government.

Entertainment and cultural life

Access to most public parks and natural places of interest sponsored by the government is free to residents of advanced age. An ICSR is effectively an entrance ticket. For people aged between 60 and 65 there are concessionary entrance fees. All the museums, libraries, memorial places, etc. funded by the government are free to anyone aged 60 or above. In addition, many of the communities in the city have established senior clubs or recreational centres to offer various kinds of entertainment for older residents. A free hotline (96156) has been set up specifically to offer psychological counselling for older people.

Legal rights service

Law firms, notary offices, and other legal service offices are required to provide free or discounted legal services to older residents. Older people who have no source of income or social insurance should have their application for legal aid attended to as a priority.

In addition to the beneficial policies listed above, another main initiative of the government to improve older people's well-being has been to initiate better social ideology. For example, the government has recently proposed the concept of mental care, to be regarded as a counterpart to the medical care of older people. To take care of older people's mental health is the core principle of this concept. In 2011, command No. 113, announced by the Beijing Civil Affairs Bureau, addressed the work of enhancing mental care for older people. In the command, the government's aim of mental care is described as a five-year plan. The main goal of mental care is to establish a four-grade mental health service: city, county (district), subdistrict, and community (village). A service group comprised of professional psychological counsellors, volunteers, and community psychological assistants will be raised to make the system develop effectively.

Social organization as an important formal source of support: the case of an NGO

The government has put older people's mental care on its agenda and devised a sound framework and goal. However, it is unlikely that the government will be able to implement each of these initiatives (e.g. the hotline service mentioned above) by itself. Thus, it is necessary to recruit other sources of support, such as private and social forces. In recent years, non-profitable NGOs have begun to play an important role in assisting the government with public social affairs. In 2006, an NGO named Cun Cao Chun Hui (CCCH), with the specialty of providing services for the psychological well-being of older people, was registered at the Beijing Civil Affairs Bureau. This is the first NGO in China devoted to psychological practice and its aim is to promote older people's mental health. In the years after its birth, CCCH gradually developed a mode of working that fits both the needs of the government and its target population. In this section, we introduce the framework of CCCH's services to make sense of their role in relationship to the government and older people's mental health.

As depicted in Figure 50.1, the mental care service offered by CCCH can be divided into five parts. First, they provide psychological counselling via the hotline 96156. From October 2010 to October 2011, there were a total of 4371 case calls on this line (Guo, Liu, and Zhang, unpublished manuscript). However, only about 16% of calls were from people older than 60. Most of the calls from older people were associated with family problems in which 'empty-nest' and family relationships were the most frequently mentioned difficulties.

Second, CCCH provides home visits for older people, especially those in disadvantaged conditions, such as being disabled and living alone. In this case, CCCH organizes volunteers, mainly university students, into small groups (of three to four people) to make home

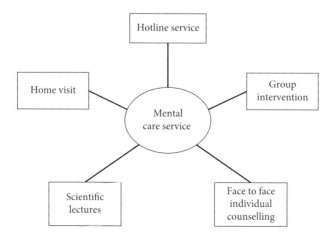

FIGURE 50.1 Contents of CCCH's mental care service.

visits. They visit their target older family once every two weeks. The main job of home visitors is to communicate with their host and to give emotional support. So far, CCCH has maintained constant home visits for about a hundred older families in the past few years.

Third, CCCH provides psychological awareness through giving public talks to older residents in communities. So far, their talks have been delivered to all sixteen administrative districts (counties) of Beijing, and the topics have been very popular as they are so close to older people's daily lives. For instance, the themes have included how to prevent memory decline, adapting to retirement, marriage in later life, relationship between daughters-in-law and mothers-in-law, grandparenting, art and health, filial piety and the mental care of older parents, learning in old age, and so on.

Fourth, CCCH recruits a group of licensed counsellors to provide voluntary individual psychological counselling for those who are in need. Recently, CCCH has tentatively established psychotherapeutic rooms in some communities in order to fulfil the needs of older people who would like to receive face-to-face counselling.

Fifth, CCCH provides group training to improve older people's mental health. For example, a group activity named the 'Old People's Intellectual Game', organized jointly by CCCH and our research team, has been favoured by older residents in communities in recent years. Typically, the game takes the form of an intelligence competition among groups, with each group consisting of five to eight older residents. The games were designed by our team based on paradigms and findings from the domains of cognitive psychology and cognitive ageing. The main purpose of the 'Old People's Intellectual Game' is to improve the social involvement of older residents, and to provide them with knowledge of cognitive ageing and possible ways to ameliorate their cognitive decline.

The latter two activities began only recently, but the former three activities have been the routine occupation of CCCH, whose contribution to enhancing the mental health of older people is widely accepted and cited by the government.

Summary of formal source of social support

Although there are other sources of non-family social support, the government joining together with NGOs has undoubtedly been the major source. Within the social and political system of China, government always plays a critical role in social life. Even NGOs must seek support from the government, which results in close cooperation between the two. In the case of CCCH, the government purchased the hotline counselling service from it to benefit older residents (Guo et al., manuscript). In this way, NGOs and other enterprises are encouraged to develop products for older adults that the government will buy for its people.

However, formal support for older people has not been as effective as it is hoped to be, especially with respect to mental health. For one thing, to seek psychological help from outside the family—on a hotline, for example—is still considered shameful or a threat to their self-esteem for many older people. Thus it is not surprising to find that less than 20% of calls on the mental care line 96156 were from older people, even though this line was specifically set up for them. So far, we have not found any direct empirical data from older people, but findings from the reports of college students suggest that about 15% of young people believe it to be shameful (Chen et al. 2010) and are unwilling to seek professional psychological help (Zhao, Jiang, and Wang 2011).The effect is that, compared with family, government and social organizations are comparatively impotent in their attempts to provide emotional support that is immediately related to mental health.

Summary

Nowadays the number of people aged 65 or above accounts for nearly 10% of the total population in China. The huge number of older adults in the population raises the problem of ageing for the entire country. The issues of older people's QoL have become a concern for society as a whole. Geropsychological research and practice play indispensible roles in coping with the issues. Epidemiological studies demonstrate a passive situation with respect to the older population's mental health, for example in the aspects of depression, dementia, anxiety, loneliness, and suicide. Social support is a critical protective factor for the mental health of older adults. In mainland China, informal support (i.e. family support from children and spouse), and formal support (i.e. from government and society) are the two main pillars of social support for older people. However, the transitions that Chinese society is undergoing are undermining the function of family support, and this increases the relative importance of support from government and society. Fortunately, government and society are paying increasing attention to the mental health of the older population. It could be forecasted that older people will receive better care in the near future.

Key References and Sources for Further Reading

Dong, M., Peng, B., Lin, X., Zhao, J., Zhou, Y. R., et al. (2007). 'The Prevalence of Dementia in the People's Republic of China: A Systematic Analysis of 1980–2004 Studies'. *Age and Ageing* 36: 619–624.

Lee, S., Tsang, A., Zhang, M., Huang, Y., Shen, Y., et al. (2007). 'Lifetime Prevalence and Inter-cohort Variation in DSM-IV Disorders in Metropolitan China'. *Psychological Medicine* 37: 61–72.

Yu, J., Li, J., Cuijpers, P., Wu, S., and Wu, Z. (2012). 'Prevalence and Correlates of Depressive Symptoms in Chinese Older Adults: A Population-based Study'. *International Journal of Geriatric Psychiatry* 27(3): 305–312.

Websites

China National Committee on Ageing (CNCA). http://www.cncaprc.gov.cn/en

Website of National Bureau of Statistics of China (NBSC):http://www.stats.gov.cn.

Ministry of Health of the People's Republic of China (MOH): http://www.moh.gov.cn.

References

Note: [C] indicates that the article or book is published in the Chinese language.

Bromet, E., Andrade, L. H., Hwang, I., Sampson, N., Alonso, J., and de Girolamo, G., et al. (2011). 'Cross-national Epidemiology of DSM-IV Major Depressive Episode'. *BMC Medicine* 9: 90–105.

Chen, J., Zhang, L., and Gao, L. (2007). 'Prevalence of Elderly's Depressive Mood and its Influencing Factors in Wuhan City'. *Chinese Journal of Gerontology* 27: 275–276.[C]

Chen, L., Chen, G., and Zheng, X. (2008). 'Analysis of Depression Symptoms and their Related Factors in Urban Widowed Elderly in Beijing'. *Chinese Journal of Gerontology* 28: 696–698.[C]

Chen, R., Copeland, J., and Wei, L. (1999). 'A Meta-analysis of Epidemiological Studies in Depression of Older People in the People's Republic of China'. *International Journal of Geriatric Psychiatry* 14: 821–830.

Chen, R., Hu, Z., Qin, X., Xu, X., and Copeland, J. R. (2004). 'A Community-based Study of Depression in Older People in Hefei, China—The GMS-AGECAT Prevalence, Case Validation and Socio-economic Correlates'. *International Journal of Geriatric Psychiatry* 19: 407–413.

Chen, R., Wei, L., Hu, Z, Qin, X., Copeland, J. R., et al. (2005). 'Depression in Older People in Rural China'. *Archives of Internal Medicine* 165: 2019.

Chen, R., Hu, Z., Wei, L., Ma, Y., Liu, Z., et al. (2011). 'Incident Dementia in a Defined Older Chinese Population'. *PLoS One* 6: e24817.

Chen, X. and Silverstein, M. (2000). 'Intergenerational Social Support and the Psychological Well-being of Older Parents in China'. *Research on Aging* 22: 43–65.

Chen, Y., Wu, D., Zhao, Y., and Ma, L. (2010). 'The Research on the Students' Attitude towards Psychological Counseling'. *Medicine and Society* 23: 83–85.[C]

Diehl, M., Elnick, A. B., Bourbeau, L. S., and Labouvie-Vief, G. (1998). 'Adult Attachment Styles: Their Relations to Family Context and Personality'. *Journal of Personality and Social Psychology* 74: 1656–1669.

Diener, E. and Suh, E. (1997). 'Measuring Quality of Life: Economic, Social, and Subjective Indicators'. *Social Indicators Research* 40: 189–216.

Dong, M., Peng, B., Lin, X., Zhao, J., Zhou, Y. R., et al. (2007). 'The Prevalence of Dementia in the People's Republic of China: A Systematic Analysis of 1980–2004 Studies'. *Age and Ageing* 36: 619–624.

Du, P. (2003). 'Current Situation and Changes of Main Economic Resources of Chinese Elderly'. *Population Research* 27: 37–43.[C]

Flint, J., Chen, Y., Shi, S., and Kendler, K. S. (2011). 'Epilogue: Lessons from the CONVERGE Study of Major Depressive Disorder in China'. *Journal of Affective Disorders* 140: 1–5.

Fu, C., Zhang, L., and Li Y. (2013). 'Characteristics of the Changes of Population Fertility in China Based on the Sixth Census'. *Statistical Research* 30: 68–75.

Guo, P. and Chen, G. (2009). *Data Analysis of the Follow-up Investigation on the Situation of the Old Population in Urban and Rural China in the Year 2006.* Beijing: China Social Press.[C]

Guo, P., Liu, H., and Zhang, Y. (n.d.). 'Management Mode and Service Efficacy of Non-government Organizations in Beijing'.

Hamilton, G. G. (1990). 'Patriarchy, Patrimonialism, and Filial Piety: A Comparison of China and Western Europe'. *British Journal of Sociology* 41: 77–104.

Huang, L., Lin, X., and Xu, X. (2012). 'On Rural Elder Women's SWB Relating to their Choices for their Offspring's Emotional Support: Based on a Questionnaire Survey in Anhui Province'. *Journal of Nanjing College for Population Programme Management* 28: 3–8.[C]

Hunt, S. M. (1997). 'The Problem of Quality of Life'. *Quality of Life Research* 6: 205–212.

Kawachi, I. and Berkman, L. F. (2001). 'Social Ties and Mental Health'. *Journal of Urban Health* 78: 458–467.

Law, S. and Liu, P. (2008). 'Suicide in China: Unique Demographic Patterns and Relationship to Depressive Disorder'. *Current Psychiatry Reports* 10: 80–86.

Lee, S., Tsang, A., Zhang, M., Huang, Y., Shen, Y., et al. (2007). 'Lifetime Prevalence and Inter-cohort Variation in DSM-IV Disorders in Metropolitan China'. *Psychological Medicine* 37: 61–72.

Lester, B. Y. (2001). 'Learning from Durkheim and Beyond: The Economy and Suicide'. *Suicide and Life-threatening Behavior* 31: 15–31.

Leung, K. K., Chen, C., Lue, B. H., and Hsu, S. T. (2007). 'Social Support and Family Functioning on Psychological Symptoms in Elderly Chinese'. *Archives of Gerontology and Geriatrics* 44: 203–213.

Li, S., Chen, C., Zhang, W., Jia, X., Liu, M., et al. (1999). 'The Prevalence of Dementia and Depression of the Elderly in the Urban Community in Beijing'. *Chinese Mental Health Journal* 13: 266–268.[C]

Li, X., Xiao, Z., and Xiao, S. (2009). 'Suicide among the Elderly in Mainland China'. *Psychogeriatrics* 9: 62–66.

Li, Z., Xiao, Y., Xie, Z., Chen, L., Xiao, S., et al. (2011). 'Use of Patient Health Questionnaire-9(PHQ-9) among Chinese Rural Elderly'. *Chinese Journal of Clinical Psychology* 19: 171–174. [C]

Liu, L. and Guo, Q. (2007). 'Loneliness and Health-related Quality of Life for the Empty Nest Elderly in the Rural Area of a Mountainous County in China'. *Quality of Life Research* 16: 1275–1280.

Liu, L. and Guo, Q. (2008). 'Life Satisfaction in a Sample of Empty-nest Elderly: A Survey in the Rural Area of a Mountainous County in China'. *Quality of Life Research* 17: 823–830.

Liu, M. (2000). 'Relation between Interpersonal Relationship, Attachment and Wellbeing in Old Adults'. Unpublished Master Thesis, National Kaohslung Normal University.[C]

Ma, S., Qin, X., Chen, R., and Hu, Z. (2006). 'Relationship of Life Events and the Incidence of Geriatric Depression'. *Chinese Mental Health Journal* 20: 157–159.[C]

Ma, X., Xiang, Y., Li, S., Xiang, Y., Guo, H. L., et al. (2008). 'Prevalence and Sociodemographic Correlates of Depression in an Elderly Population Living with Family Members in Beijing, China'. *Psychological Medicine* 38: 1723–1730.

Ma, Y., Chen, R., Qin, X., Li, L., Ren, Y., et al. (2010). 'Prevalence and Related Factors of Depression among Old People Living in Rural and Urban Community in Anhui Province'. *Chinese Mental Health Journal* 24: 752–756.[C]

Magai, C., Cohen, C., Milburn, N., Thorpe, B., McPherson, R., et al. (2001). 'Attachment Styles in Older European American and African American Adults'. *Journals of Gerontology, Series B: Psychological Sciences and Social Sciences* 56: S28–S35.

Meng, C. and Tang, Z. (2000). 'Analysis and Comparison of Elderly's Depression Symptom in Urban and Rural Beijing'. *Chinese Journal of Gerontology* 20: 196–199.[C]

Morris, M. D. (1979). *Measuring the Conditions of the World's Poor: The Physical Quality of Life.* NY: Pergamon Press. 17.

Pan, A., Franco, O. H., Wang, Y., Yu, Z., Ye, X. W., et al. (2008). 'Prevalence and Geographic Disparity of Depressive Symptoms among Middle-aged and Elderly in China'. *Journal of Affective Disorders* 105: 167–175.

Parker, G., Cheah, Y. C., and Roy, K. (2001). 'Do the Chinese Somatize Depression? A Cross-cultural Study'. *Social Psychiatry and Psychiatric Epidemiology* 36: 287–293.

Porter, M. (2010). 'Marriage and the Elderly in China'. In K. Eggleston and S. Tuljapurkar (eds), *Aging Asia*. Stanford, CA: Walter H. Shorenstein Asia-Pacific Research Center, 80.

Prina, A. M., Ferri, C. P., Guerra, M., Brayne, C., and Prince. M. (2011). 'Prevalence of Anxiety and its Correlates among Older Adults in Latin America, India and China: Cross-cultural Study'. *British Journal of Psychiatry* 199: 485–491.

Qin, P. and Mortensen, P. B. (2001). 'Specific Characteristics of Suicide in China'. *Acta Psychiatrica Scandinavica* 103: 117–121.

Rodriguez, J. J. L., Ferri, C. P., Acosta, D., Guerra, M., Huang, Y., et al. (2008). 'Prevalence of Dementia in Latin America, India, and China: A Population-based Cross-sectional Survey'. *Lancet* 372: 464–474.

Shen, Y., Li, G., Li, S., Chen, H., Li, S. R., et al. (1994). 'Three-year Follow-up Study of Age-related Dementia in an Older Population of Beijing Urban Area'. *Chinese Mental Health Journal* 8: 165–166.[C]

Silverstein, M., Cong, Z., and Li, S. (2006). 'Intergenerational Transfers and Living Arrangements of Older People in Rural China: Consequences for Psychological Well-being'. *Journals of Gerontology, Series B: Psychological Sciences and Social Sciences* 61: S256–S266.

Wade, T. J. and Pevalin, D. J. (2004). 'Marital Transitions and Mental Health'. *Journal of Health and Social Behavior* 45: 155–170.

Wang, D., Tong, Y., Zhou, L., and Shen, J. (2004). 'Inner-mechanisms between Intergenerational Social Support and Subjective Well-being of the Elderly'. *Acta Psychologica Sinica* 36: 78–82.[C]

Wang, G., Zhang, X., Wang, K., Li, Y., Shen, Q., et al. (2011). 'Loneliness among the Rural Older People in Anhui, China: Prevalence and Associated Factors'. *International Journal of Geriatric Psychiatry* 26: 1162–1168.

Wang, L. and Shi, Y. (2008). 'Social Support and Mental Health of the Empty-nest Elderly People in Urban Areas'. *Chinese Mental Health Journal* 22: 118–122.[C]

Wang, X., Wang, D., and Shen, J. (2006). 'The Effects of Social Support on Depression in the Aged'. *Chinese Journal of Clinical Psychology* 14: 73–74.[C]

Yan, F., Li, S., and Huang, Y. (2008). 'Longitudinal Study on Dementia in an Urban Community of Beijing City in Two Decades'. *Chinese Mental Health Journal* 22: 110–113.[C]

Yang, G. H., Zhou, L. N., Huang, Z. J., and Chen, A. P. (2004). 'The Trend and Geographic Distribution of Suicide in the Chinese Population'. *Chinese Journal of Epidemiology* 25: 280–284.[C]

Yang, K. and Victor, C. R. (2008). 'The Prevalence of and Risk Factors for Loneliness among Older People in China'. *Ageing and Society* 28: 305–328.

Yip, P. S. F., Liu, K., Hu, J., and Song, X. (2005). 'Suicide Rates in China during a Decade of Rapid Social Changes'. *Social Psychiatry and Psychiatric Epidemiology* 40: 792–798.

Yu, J., Li, J., Cuijpers, P., Wu, S., and Wu, Z. (2012). 'Prevalence and Correlates of Depressive Symptoms in Chinese Older Adults: A Population-based Study'. *International Journal of Geriatric Psychiatry* 27(3): 305–312.

Yuan, Q., He, G., Feng, H., and Gao, J. (2010). 'Analysis of Factors Influencing Community Elderly's Depression Symptom in Changsha City'. *Chinese Journal of Gerontology* 30: 746–748.[C]

Zhai, X., Li, C., Wei, H., and Wang, D. (2010). 'The Development of the Questionnaire of Marital Attachment for Older Adults'. *Psychological Development and Education*: 26: 197–203.[C]

Zhang, A., Zeng, X., and Yang, D. (2010). 'Investigation of the Influential Factors of Anxiety State in the Elderly Rooming House'. *Chinese Journal of Gerontology* 30: 672–674.[C]

Zhang, J., Jia, S., Wieczorek, W. F., and Jiang, C. (2002). 'An Overview of Suicide Research in China'. *Archives of Suicide Research* 6: 167–184.

Zhang, J., Ma, J., Jia, C., Sun, J., Guo, X., et al. (2010). 'Economic Growth and Suicide Rate Changes: A Case in China from 1982 to 2005'. *European Psychiatry* 25: 159–163.

Zhang, K. and Guo, P. (2009). *Blue Book of Population Ageing and the Situation of Old Population in China*. Beijing: China Social Press. 215[C]

Zhang, L., Xu, Y., and Nie, H. (2011). 'A Meta-analysis of the Elderly's Depression Rate in China from 2000 to 2010'. *Chinese Journal of Gerontology* 31: 3349–3352.[C]

Zhang, X. (2011). 'Analysing the Changes Related to the Types of Old People Issues against the Background of the Ageing Problem'. *Journal of Guizhou University (Social Science)* 29: 73–77. [C]

Zhang, Z., Liu, X., and Tang, M. (2004). 'A Caregiver Survey in Beijing, Xian, Shanghai and Chengdu: Health Service Status for the Elderly with Dementia'. *Acta Academiae Medicinae Sinicae*: 26: 116–121. [C]

Zhang, Z., Zahner, G. E. P., Roman, G. C., Liu, J., et al. (2005). 'Dementia Subtypes in China: Prevalence in Beijing, Xian, Shanghai, and Chengdu'. *Archives of Neurology* 62: 447–453.

Zhao, L., Jiang, G., and Wang, Y. (2011). 'Correlation between Trust of Counseling and Professional Help Seeking in College Students'. *Chinese Mental Health Journal* 25: 249–253. [C]

Zhou, D., Wu, C., Qi, H., Fan, J., Sun, X. D., et al. (2006). 'Prevalence of Dementia in Rural China: Impact of Age, Gender and Education'. *Acta Neurologica Scandinavica* 114: 273–280.

Zimmer, Z. and Kwong, J. (2003). 'Family Size and Support of Older Adults in Urban and Rural China: Current Effects and Future Implications'. *Demography* 40: 23–44.

CHAPTER 51

WHY WE NEED AN INTERNATIONAL CLINICAL GEROPSYCHOLOGY

NANCY A. PACHANA

INTRODUCTION

IT is perhaps a truism that the world is getting smaller. So many advances in technology and communications have shrunk all sorts of putative distances—between people, between places, and even one might say, conceptual distances. The internet has increased the ease of access to information, and combined with increased ease of travel to even remote corners of the world, all parts of the globe are more interconnected than ever before. But in truth, networks between peoples through trade, migration, and exploration have existed for hundreds of years. Food, customs, ideas, and, at a basic level, the people themselves have been shared across cultures, with at times tensions but more often innovation and creativity resulting.

Sharing innovations and knowledge in a wide range of areas has benefit—for example, in the areas of technological advances and healthcare. Increasingly, coordinated responses on a global scale are required in the area of disease control—the recent coordinated global efforts on severe acute respiratory system (SARS) outbreaks are an example (Quammen 2012). But there are also worldwide efforts to improve and enhance quality of life. For example, the WHO age-friendly environments programme is aimed at positively impacting the health and well-being of older adults by ensuring the physical and social aspects of their living environments support their needs (WHO 2007). In order to foster and share information gained by participation in the programme, the WHO Global Network of Age-friendly Cities and Communities (GNAFCC) was established, allowing easy communication of innovations worldwide.

Global interconnectedness can have positive implications for the science and practice of clinical geropsychology. These consequences in our discipline are across the areas of the spread of ideas and approaches, sharing of datasets, the development and testing of tools and interventions, and the training of new clinical geropsychologists and enhancing the career paths of those already working. The implications of the global ageing of the population in the developed as well as the developing world flow through and in turn influence clinical geropsychology internationally.

Clinical geropsychology as a discipline as well as clinical geropsychologists themselves benefit from a global outlook in a variety of ways. Advances and ideas are proposed in one quarter, and then tested, refined, and expanded by other individuals, who may also comment on the cross-cultural and societal implications of the ideas. Areas of the world where geropsychology is not so strong can access both the extant literature and collegial assistance in enhancing geropsychology in their local area. Clinical geropsychologists working in academia often require evidence of an international profile to apply for promotion; students can take advantage of international conferences to find expertise and mentorship in areas of scholarship unavailable in their own university.

In this chapter, some of the ways in which clinical geropsychology has matured into an international field are explored, with reference to the chapters in this *Oxford Handbook of Clinical Geropsychology* where appropriate.

SHARING IDEAS AND APPROACHES IN GEROPSYCHOLOGY

We have illustrated in this Handbook a variety of clinical ideas and concepts that have migrated internationally, and been enriched by that peregrination; there are also examples in the Handbook of constructs which may be less well known internationally, but should be better known. Two main illustrations of the benefits of cross-cultural exposure involve theories of ageing and clinical assessment and intervention techniques.

Theories of ageing

It is important to gauge how well theories of ageing apply cross-culturally and cross-nationally. For example, Carstensen's Socioemotional Selectivity Theory (Charles and Carstensen 2010), and particularly the aspect of that theory known as the positivity effect (Carstensen and Mikels 2005), whereby older adults appear to avoid attention to and memory of negative information, are well known. This theory is discussed in Kessler and colleagues' chapter on 'Clinical Geropsychology: A Lifespan Perspective', as well as elsewhere in this text. But how does the positivity effect play out internationally?

Fung and colleagues (2008) have looked at the positivity effect in an Asian population. In a series of studies this group has shown that older adults in Hong Kong do not demonstrate preferential cognitive processing of positively valenced stimuli relative to negatively valenced stimuli, in contrast to findings in Western samples. Fung and colleagues had hypothesized that persons operating in cultural contexts that attach less importance to positive emotions might not show the same effects. They posit that in cultures such as Japan and China, the desire to fit into social contexts motivates individuals to be attuned to negative emotions to avoid social faux pas (Kitayama and Karasawa 1995). Such international research efforts bring geropsychology theories a broader, more nuanced, and frankly more interesting view. This is demonstrated well in the chapter on 'Social Capital and Gender', with many cross-national studies on Antonucci's Social Convoy Model (Antonucci 1985) cited.

Kessler and colleagues' chapter also introduces several theories which have had less exposure internationally than Carstensen's theories. One is the Dual-Process Model of Assimilative and Accommodative Coping (Brandtstädter and Rothermund 2002), which helps make sense of two key means to achieving one's objectives in the face of ageing: striving to pursue goals (assimilative strategies) and adjusting goals to suit constraints (accommodative strategies). This theory includes such concepts as rescaling personal expectations and letting go of self-images that do not fit the actual self anymore. Likewise, in the chapter in this Handbook on 'Successful Development and Ageing', the Self-Management of Well-being Theory (Steverink, Lindenberg, and Slaets 2005), an extension of the Social Production Functions (SPF)–Successful Aging theory (Steverink and Lindenberg 2006; Steverink, Lindenberg, and Ormel 1998), is discussed. The SPF theory encompasses a hierarchy of universal human needs, instrumental goals, and resources, such as maintaining friendships in later life; the better an individual's needs are fulfilled, the higher their subjective well-being. Many of the theories presented in this Handbook, whether established or relatively new, would profit from greater exposure internationally. Steverink's Self-Management of Well-being theory relies on hierarchies presented as universal, and so testing the theory across the widest possible cultural contexts would be useful.

Clinical assessment and intervention approaches

More efficacious and age-sensitive assessment of cognitive decline is of interest internationally. In the chapter on 'Assessing Changes of Cognitive Trajectories over Time', what can be expected of normal and abnormal cognitive changes with increasing age are outlined. The value of assessing such changes over multiple occasions is explored. Careful calculation of clinically relevant changes in scores (i.e. reliable change index methods) offer compelling data, as individual trajectories for decline are unique and informative, superior to a simple individual assessment with regard to both diagnosis and recommendations for care. The value of broadening out cognitive assessment to encompass emotional functioning, activities of daily living, social functioning, and the environment is discussed in the 'Geropsychological Assessment' chapter. These approaches are supplemented by careful attention to how the results of such tests are relayed back to referral sources and patients in the chapter on 'Evaluation and Treatment of Geriatric Neurocognitive Disorders'. Involving older persons collaboratively in both the investigation of assessment goals and the feedback of assessment results has value, as they may be concerned about the consequences of such an evaluation. This is particularly true in parts of the world where educational attainment of older cohorts is low, and contact with psychologists infrequent.

Finally, recommendations for how rehabilitation strategies might move forward, given a holistic approach to assessment, are nicely captured by the Functional Integrative Approach to rehabilitation described in the chapter on 'Cognitive Development in Ageing'. In this approach an individualized intervention that targets resources, environmental demands, and change expectations of the patient is stressed. This ensures an intervention approach which is effective as well as personally relevant for patients' satisfaction with their cognitive health. What each of these chapters stresses is the value of trying to ascertain how an individual is functioning over time, in their unique context, and relaying assessment information back to the person while addressing their specific concerns and designing a tailored strategy to address these. Such approaches benefit the practice of clinical geropsychology internationally by offering alternatives to a largely medical approach to assessment, particularly of dementia, and providing a detailed evidence base to support these more age-friendly and ageing-sensitive assessment approaches.

In a similar manner, many forms of psychotherapy and psychotherapeutic intervention strategies have been developed either for older persons specifically or applied to older persons, and these are being tested more frequently across cultural contexts. Perhaps the most widely practised and researched of these, cognitive-behavioural therapy (CBT; Beck et al. 1979), was developed in the US by Aaron Beck and proliferated widely. Research on the use of CBT with older adults quickly became a strong and vibrant topic within geropsychology. In this Handbook, the chapters on 'Interpersonal Psychotherapy for the Treatment of Late-life Depression', 'Neuropsychiatric Approaches to Working with Depressed Older People', and 'The Use of CBT for Behaviours that Challenge in Dementia' illustrate the breadth of current use of CBT in older populations. The practice of CBT with older persons has been explored by many writers but particularly Laidlaw and colleagues in the UK (Laidlaw and McAlpine 2008) and the US, who have discussed more precisely the ways in which the processes inherent within the practice of CBT both remain the same as practice with young and mid-aged adults, and how they might differ when treating older adults. The chapter on 'Cognitive-Behaviour Therapy with Older People' in this Handbook explores these ideas in more depth. Here is an illustration of a productive cross-national conversation that has increased our understanding of how CBT works with older people.

Interpersonal therapy (IPT) has proved to have great utility in treating depression in older persons (Hinrichsen 1997), and its efficacy is recognized by its support and dissemination within the US Department of Veterans Affairs, as described in the 'Interpersonal Therapy for the Treatment of Late-life Depression' chapter. Cognitive Analytic Therapy (CAT; Hepple and Sutton 2004) is also gaining in popularity as an approach with older adults, as described in the 'Cognitive Analytic Therapy and Later Life' chapter. Yet both the largely US-focused IPT and the largely British CAT have been slower to disseminate elsewhere. Future areas of research on these two therapeutic approaches might be to ascertain how they are impacting the health-service systems in which they are utilized, and how they might usefully be adapted for other settings and contexts.

Acceptance and commitment therapy (Luoma, Hayes, and Walser 2007) is also being increasingly used with older populations, as described in the chapters on 'ACT and CBT in Older Age' chapter and 'Acceptance and Commitment Therapy with Dementia Care-givers' chapter. For example, Wetherell and colleagues (2011) examined the utility of ACT versus CBT for generalized anxiety disorder in older adults; they found high levels of satisfaction with treatment in both approaches, and patients received benefits from both treatment approaches. The goal may be to ascertain better fits between patients and approaches so as to minimize dropout, as more CBT than ACT patients discontinued treatment in their trial.

Further work with each of these intervention methods is warranted across cultures and also with particular patient populations, such as those with comorbid medical illnesses (as described in the chapter on 'Physical Comorbidity with Mood Disorders'). More work is also needed to look at these various interventions in combination with pharmacological treatments (as detailed in the chapter on 'Combining Medication and Psychotherapy for Late Life Anxiety and Mood Disorders'). In light of *DSM-5* changes as well as renewed interest in the topic, the issues explored in the chapter on 'Disorders of Personality in Late-life' warrant further intervention research in older persons.

Innovations in therapeutic interventions also may involve the direct use of technology in therapy to forward treatment aims. The potential uses of 'Virtual Reality Techniques in Older Adults' and 'Mobile Computing Technology in Rehabilitation Services' are topics of chapters in this volume, as well as fertile areas for future research efforts, particularly given that the size and cost of such devices continues to decline, while potential uses continue to increase. For example, touch-screen technologies are helping older persons with dementia by enhancing communication with care-givers. The CIRCA system is an interactive, multimedia touch-screen system containing stimuli to prompt reminiscing; results suggest the device can assist communication and enhance engagement in persons with dementia (Astell et al. 2010). The development of assistive technologies for persons with dementia is a burgeoning field (Peterson and Prasad 2012).

In the chapter on 'Positive Ageing: New Horizons for Older Adults', how older persons meet their needs through social engagement is discussed. One new means of older adults engaging with friends, family, and the world is through social media; in the chapter in this Handbook on 'Seniors' Online Communities and Well-being in Later Life', research on how older adults use the internet and social media, and the potential of such use to influence well-being and social connectedness in a positive manner, is explored. Social networks and their consequences, particularly at advanced ages (McLaughlin et al. 2010), are deserving of greater research attention. How social networks grow and change in later life with the use of social media is another fruitful area for attention.

Finally, the increasing importance of meta-analyses to inform the interventions used with older adults also impacts the importing of interventions across national boundaries. The chapter on 'Meta-analyses in Clinical Geropsychology' makes the point that varying levels of evidence exist for interventions, and such research also points to gaps in the literature in need of further research. This can both guide research efforts and prevent multiple inventions of the proverbial wheel, particularly a less than useful wheel, important in these times of constrained research and healthcare funding.

Sharing Large Datasets, Including Longitudinal Studies

Cross-national sharing of data, particularly large datasets, is another area of increasing activity in the geropsychology field. Research is expensive, and some of the most expensive research involves longitudinal research. As was discussed in the chapter in this Handbook on 'Longitudinal Studies and Clinical Geropsychology', many of the questions in the field of gerontology can be best answered via longitudinal research. Many longstanding longitudinal studies, such as the Seattle Longitudinal Study (Schaie 1993) or the Berlin Aging Studies (Baltes et al. 1993), have served as an important foundation for research worldwide.

Issues with cross-national datasets

However, even with such large studies, not all questions can be answered. First, a nationally based large ageing study may have limited generalizability to other countries. Even within relatively contained geographical regions such as Europe, or where countries can appear much more similar than different (e.g. perhaps, the US and Canada), differences remain, and these can be significant for issues regarding ageing. For example, in the chapter on 'Loneliness and Health in Later Life' in this Handbook, differences between Northern and Southern Europe in terms of loneliness and social connectedness are mentioned. Similarly, the implications of the recognition of same-sex marriage in Canada (and the until recent and still uneven recognition of this social institution in the US) loom large with respect to claiming benefits and inheritance for older LGBT individuals, as discussed in the chapter on 'Lesbian, Gay, Bisexual, and Transgender Ageing'.

Even within a country, individual longitudinal studies can offer more powerful data when combined. Anstey and colleagues have taken on the challenge of harmonizing the nine longitudinal studies on ageing in Australia (Anstey et al. 2010). Each of these longitudinal studies on its own offered unique contributions, whether it was the focus on gender and health (Brown et al. 1999; McLaughlin et al. 2011), or a particular health condition, typified by the Blue Mountain Eye Study (Hong et al. 2013), or whether it attempted to strike a core balance between data collection by post and face to face, allowing the maximization of subjective and objective observations (Graham, Ryan, and Luszcz 2011; Luszcz et al. 2007). However, combining these studies has led to key insights into ageing and older adults in Australia, particularly with respect to mental health and dementia (Anstey et al. 2010).

Now there is a growing interest in replicating versions of longitudinal studies cross-nationally to answer questions of a comparative nature. Interest in this for ageing studies and particularly centenarian studies has grown (Poon et al. 2007; see also the link for the International Centenarian Consortium at the end of this chapter). Using similar questions allows, of course, for direct comparisons of data, but more important is the thinking through of such questions in an international context. For example, even collecting demographic data can be challenging across countries. In the US, many studies ask for income or income brackets; this data is harder to access in cultures where disclosing this data is not part of the cultural norm (Brown et al. 1998). Similarly, if a particular demographic categorization predicts an outcome, but that categorization differs by country, then cross-national comparisons are made more difficult. For example, if marital status predicts health outcomes, but marital status is conceived differently in two countries (e.g. emphasis on married vs unmarried persons within the culture, or a lack of distinction between married and long-term partner in that society), then this fact has implications for collecting and interpreting data. Moreover, often these differences in categorization reflect the different sociopolitical structures in countries. For example, in a country where marriage is not required to collect benefits or claim inheritance, the population datasets (such as census data) may not contain the same data as countries where these variables have more legal and social implications.

The importance of social connections, or conceptions about the importance of mental health interventions and how these are best delivered, will differ even more widely cross-nationally perhaps than socio-demographic constructions. In the chapter on 'Social

Capital and Gender', the implications of how social connections play out in other cultures is cited as critical in influencing well-being in later life. Similarly, in the chapter on 'Geropsychological Research and Practice in Mental Health in Mainland China', the recent increase in interest in providing geropsychological services to older adults, and the changing role of the government in the provision of mental health services (now being augmented with NGO providers) is highlighted.

The impact of culture on cross-national research

Cultural influences on diagnosis, for example, are fairly well known (e.g. the ways in which culture can influence how people explain or define their symptoms, whom they approach for help, and how likely they are to access mental health services, as described in the chapter on 'Psychosis in Older Adults'). However, cross-national definitions of *individual words themselves* can differ widely, and can affect research into the issues around them.

The term dementia, like many illnesses, carries social and cultural weight, and is associated with stigma (e.g. Graham et al. 2003). For example, in China, dementia is often seen as the result of 'worrying too much', 'wrongdoing', or 'fate' and described as 'craziness' or 'contagious' (Hinton, Franz, and Friend 2004). Being affected by dementia, whether as one diagnosed with the illness or by being related to a person with dementia, thus has a negative connotation and suggests an attitude that the person with dementia or his/her family is at least partly responsible for developing the disease (Liu et al. 2008; Low et al. 2011).

The idea that dementia may be the result of a normal ageing process as well as a mental illness process which is stigmatizing are apparently contradictory and yet often co-exist in Chinese care-givers (Guo et al. 2000). Such opposing attitudes may contribute to care-giver stress by discouraging help-seeking and service engagement, and they may also affect care-givers' willingness to participate in care-giving research studies (Hinton et al. 2000; Sun, Ong, and Burnette 2012; Yeo and Gallagher-Thompson 2006). The consequences of the meanings of dementia in the Chinese context have reverberated internationally, as highlighted in the chapter on 'Caring for Care-givers of a Person with Dementia', where the difficulties in engaging care-givers are expanded upon.

There are many gains to be had from pursuing cross-national research, both in terms of the data itself and how we think about instigating, collecting, and interpreting such data. The pursuit of cross-national collaborations goes beyond identical datasets; indeed, seeking to import or impose a set of questions onto another country can appear to be a form of imperialism. This is especially true in cultures and countries seeking to understand what might be termed 'the other'. For example, seeking to set up a longitudinal study in an Asian country certainly goes beyond offering a set of questions or even offering money to pursue a research agenda; understanding how Asian countries pursue health and social research, particularly the close ties between research and the government, are key. In many Asian countries translational research is a given because there is a close (and possibly enviable alignment) of research agendas and the implementation of assessment and intervention strategies on a regional or national level. This situation affects everything from gaining ethical clearances to how fieldwork is implemented and, finally, to how and in what manner research findings are disseminated. This has resulted in exciting translational research opportunities (e.g. Coopmans, Graham, and Hamzah 2012). The importance of the nurturance of close, collaborative, and long-term partnerships in this region, and perhaps more broadly with respect to cross-national research, cannot be overstated.

DEVELOPMENT OF TOOLS AND INTERVENTIONS

A moment of personal reflection: as a clinical geriatric neuropsychologist trained in the US, but now living in the Southern Hemisphere, I went through three distinct phases of professional acculturation as a geropsychologist living in a different country and a different culture. First, there was the realization that even in so-called 'English-speaking' countries, language varies. Holding up a pen and having to decide whether 'Biro' (a brand of pen) was the correct answer on the MMSE, while an amused group of trainee clinicians looked on, was an interesting moment. And so the first hurdle in cross-national assessment, language, was made salient to me. Language does matter, particularly in testing. Tests (and indeed clinical interviews) are standardized, and moving these across cultures can be no easy feat, even when all care has been taken with back translations. (For information about this see the excellent articles by Sousa and Rojjanasrrirat 2011 and Van de Vijver and Hambleton 1996).

The second phase of my acculturation involved the perils of test development. Although frustrated for many years at the uncanny resemblance of a beaver to a platypus when administering the Boston Naming Test in Australia, when designing the Geriatric Anxiety Inventory (Pachana et al. 2007; Byrne and Pachana 2011), my colleagues and I blithely put in many culturally specific idiomatic expressions (e.g. 'I feel as though I have butterflies in my stomach'). This was justified (post hoc, of course) in that using the common vernacular is important in interviewing and testing older persons in the mental health context, a point well-made in the chapter on 'Interviewing Older Adults' in this Handbook. However, it still caused havoc with translations for countries where this expression was unknown. A flexible strategy was adopted; the phrase became 'I feel as though I have ants in my stomach' (Spain) and 'I feel tight like the strings of a violin' (Italian, and very poetic too). The need for specific translations for national populations (individualized Portuguese versions for both Portugal and Brazil, for example; Martiny et al. 2011) have led me to an increased awareness of what is required to make a test available internationally (Pachana and Byrne 2012).

The value of making tests, particularly tests designed specifically for older adult populations, and available to a wider audience, have great implications for both research and clinical practice in geropsychology. Several chapters in this Handbook have made the point about the utility of measures for various cultural and language groups (e.g. Caring for Care-givers chapter; 'Barriers to Mental HealthCare Utilization' chapter). The need for careful 'translations' of constructs, be they what is a standard drink ('Substance Use, Misuse, and Abuse' chapter) to how capacity is defined ('International Perspectives on Capacity Assessment' chapter) to what is valued at the end of life ('Transitions in Later Life' chapter), is apparent. Even the apparently ubiquitous notion of sleep (or at least, the significance of sleeping patterns, as described in the chapter on 'Late-life Insomnia') varies across nations, as anyone who has attempted to eat dinner in Madrid before 9pm can attest...

The third stage of my acculturation is the one I currently occupy. It involves being a practitioner who administers tests for a living in a multicultural society, and is struggling to do so in a changing multicultural landscape. My clients in a large Australian city come from various nations, but have come to Australia at different points in their own history, and their family's history. So issues of degree of acculturation crop up in terms of test administration and interpretation. Immigration laws are still relatively favourable in Australia for bringing ageing parents to live with relocated children; I see increasing numbers of persons with dementia only recently arrived from abroad. My last assessment client seen in an aged care facility arrived from Switzerland *and was taken directly to a nursing home from the airport.* The need for translators is dwarfed by the pressing need to understand the implications for such global migrations on care staff, families, and individuals themselves, in this case an individual with moderate dementia. Never mind what tool to choose; how can I make sense of the changing world I am seeing?

Tests used across populations

With respect to tests, one is guided by overarching assessment principles, including the excellent guidance given in the two chapters on 'Geropsychological Assessment' chapter as well as 'Clinical Evaluation and Assessment Methods' chapter offered in this Handbook. The need to be attuned keenly to culture in the clinical practice of geropsychology has been an important part of the CALTAP model of clinical interventions with older adults offered by Knight and Poon (2008).

Many tests mentioned in these chapters are deserving of further research, particularly cross-national validation. These include the useful Geriatric Suicide Ideation Scale (GSIS; Heisel and Flett 2006) mentioned in the chapter on 'Suicidal Ideation in Late-life', and the Everyday Problems Test (EPT; Diehl, Willis, and Schaie 1995; Willis and Marsiske 1993), an objective (i.e. performance-based) objective measure of a patient's ability to solve IADL problems relevant to everyday life, as described in the chapter on 'Functional Sequelae of Cognitive Decline in Later Life'.

Interventions tested across populations

Some intervention strategies have taken shape from particular healthcare niches (such as primary care; see the chapter on 'Psychological Interventions in Non-mental Health Settings'). While the specifics of primary care, or care by a general practitioner (GP), vary between countries, the recent explosion of research into providing psychological interventions in the realm of general practice across a variety of countries speaks to the global interest in this area (Kroenke et al. 2007; Stanley, Diefenback, and Hopko 2003; Verhaak, Bensing, and Brink-Muinen 2007).

Other interventions spring from looming healthcare issues, such as the growing number of persons globally that suffer from cognitive decline and dementia, as described in the chapters on 'Exercise and Health Promotion for Older Adults with Cognitive Impairment' chapter and 'Lifestyle Risks and Cognitive Health' chapter. Prince et al. (2013) estimated that globally, 35.6 million people lived with dementia in 2010, with numbers expected to nearly double every twenty years, to 65.7 million in 2030 and 115.4 million in 2050. This growing population of patients with dementia increases the risk for elder abuse; just as dementia is of growing concern internationally, ways to treat and in particular prevent elder abuse are being developed in many parts of the globe (see the chapter on 'Elder Abuse'). It also increases the need for interventions at the family level, as described in the chapter on 'Family Therapy with Ageing Families'.

Nearly every intervention chapter in this Handbook has mentioned important intervention approaches that could usefully be studied and adapted for use cross-culturally. For example, two types of reminiscence therapy—life review and life review therapy—have compelling support as efficacious treatments for improving well-being and for reducing depression in older persons, as detailed in the chapter on 'Reminiscence Therapy'. The chapter on 'Pain in Persons with Dementia and Communication Impairment' describes a systematic hypothesis-testing method that integrates assessment and treatment of pain, which is required to identify, assess, and treat pain appropriately in older persons.

Training and Practice in Geropsychology Internationally

The world is becoming older, and the training of health professionals, and particularly mental health professionals, to cope with increasing numbers of geriatric patients, is lagging (Karel et al. 2010; Kneebone 1996). However, in thinking about expanding the workforce to cope with increasing numbers of older clients, the idea of 'training' must expand to encompass 're-skilling' and the branching into geriatrics of health professionals who have mainly practised with adults (or even children). Finally, we must consider what is a minimum competency to practise as a clinical psychologist in an ageing world; increasingly, older clients will turn up everywhere (for example, as primary carers of grandchildren).

Training strategies and resources

Training in geropsychology varies internationally (Karel et al. 2010; Pinquart 2007). Cross-national comparative studies of geropsychology training (Pachana et al. 2010) and more recently competencies (Woodhead et al. 2013) have begun to appear in the literature. In the US, there has been a consolidation of training programmes in clinical geropsychology (Knight et al. 2009) and the development of an excellent resource in geropsychology (see link to GeroCentral website below); both of these initiatives have a nascent international component. (See also relevant sections of the chapter on 'Interprofessional Geriatric Healthcare: Competencies and Resources for Teamwork.') Peak psychology bodies internationally often have interest groups or divisions focusing on ageing. Most of these societies or organizations have practice, teaching, and research resources, tip sheets and other materials for clients, and information on mentoring and consultation outreach programmes. In many cases these resources are freely available online. (For interest, please see Appendix 1 for an undoubtedly incomplete list of such geropsychology organizations and peak bodies, internationally.) In general, Europe, North America, and Australia and New Zealand have well-developed networks of peak bodies and training programmes in geriatrics across health and mental health disciplines. This is a growing area in Asia and South America, but due to demographic realities geriatric subspecialties and training are probably least developed in Africa.

In the US, a set of clinical geropsychology competencies has been developed, and these are beginning to be known outside the US context. The Pikes Peak Model for Training in Professional Geropsychology details competencies important for psychological practice with older adults (Karel et al 2010; Knight et al. 2009). These geropsychology competencies have now been transformed into an online tool which serves to assess competencies, as well as point a new or re-skilling practitioner to areas for which they may need to do either further reading or seek supervision and guidance (again, see the GeroCentral website link at the end of this chapter). Outside the US, there are often already existing national and/or regional guides for practice and, by extension, training for work with older adults (e.g. Pachana, Helmes, and Koder 2006; Fernández-Ballesteros 2007). Now the challenge will be in more coordinated, systematic training efforts in geropsychology, hopefully guided by empirical research.

Training in geropsychology for work with particular populations within geriatrics is also of concern. One such population is older persons living in nursing homes. There are not enough clinical psychologists with particular training and expertise in working in long-term care settings, as described in the chapter on 'Older Adults and Long Term Care'.

Finally, introducing a more international perspective into training will equip geropsychology trainees with a bigger toolkit and a broader appreciation of cross-cultural and cross-national issues in ageing. A laudable internationalized training model in gerontology is the European Masters programme in Gerontology (EuMaG), which until recently was funded by the European Commission (Heijke 2004). Developed and delivered by a network of twenty European universities, EuMaG helped to train dozens of young European gerontologists. Its strong emphasis on cross-national comparisons of data, and its policy of various European universities hosting modules of content meant its graduates truly had an international view of ageing research, practice, and policy.

Potential hurdles and resources in geropsychology training

What might be some potential barriers or concerns with respect to increasing or improving our geriatric mental health workforce? Ageism among both mental health practitioners in general, and psychology trainee practitioners in particular (Gonçalves et al. 2011) may be one such barrier. Attempts to systematically address ageism in healthcare delivery systems and those who work in them are growing (Huang, Larente, and Morais 2011; Liu et al. 2012). Research efforts themselves are not free of ageism and age biases (Cherubini et al. 2010). Of course, psychology itself is not immune (e.g. Helmes and Gee 2003), and certainly addressing ageism and its consequences is deserving of more research in general clinical psychology as well as geropsychology training contexts. Again, contact with older persons is important if we are to stimulate students to work with older adults, and also potentially to stem negative attitudes towards older people (Gonçalves et al. 2011).

What resources are out there to help young clinicians gain the necessary skills and attitudes to work successfully with older adults? Careful explications of how to do therapy with older adults are important. Manualized approaches to therapy, such as those described in many chapters in this Handbook, as well as explanations of how particular components of therapy work with older adults, such as homework (Kazantzis, Pachana, and Secker 2003), are important. Many authors in this text make a point about the need for increasing dissemination of strategies to work with older people in training programmes. Similarly, the need for improved training in interdisciplinary approaches is highlighted in the chapter 'Interprofessional Geriatric Healthcare: Competencies and Resources for Teamwork' in this Handbook.

Finally, there remain many areas of research that remain under-developed, such as 'Late-life Anxiety', which are discussed in this Handbook. If we are ever to close the research gap in such important areas, we need to train young clinical psychology investigators, and to do that, we must encourage more of them to choose later life as a specialty area. The demographics of the world are changing at an increasing rate (see chapter on 'The Demography and Epidemiology of Population Ageing'); young researchers and clinicians both have to be across this data, and be armed with appropriate tools and knowledge with which to help older cohorts. This is especially true for practitioners, who may face a gap of many decades in age and several cohorts in lived experience when seeing their clients (Laidlaw and Pachana 2009).

Summary

We live in an ageing world. Older adults are a heterogeneous and growing population. Moreover, they migrate as well as stay rooted in their home (sometimes literally) of origin. They speak one or a dozen languages. They offer challenges to us with respect to ageing well and ageing with disorders of both a physical and psychological nature.

We currently have too few people trained to serve the needs of this diverse population of older persons. Our instruments and interventions proliferate, but would a more holistic view of their potential for cross-national application, as well as the limits to their application in particular regions or populations, help reduce inefficiencies and make stretched research and healthcare dollars go further?

I think the future of geropsychology lies in the international arena, and I think that future is a bright one.

Appendix 1: Peak Geropsychology Groups and Organizations

Internationally

Austria

Austrian Psychological Association, Geropsychology section. http://www.boep.or.at/Geron topsychologie.241.0.html.

Austrian Psychotherapeutic Association, Geropsychology section. http://www.psycho therapie.at/gerontopsychotherapie.

Australia

Psychology and Aging Interest Group (PAIG). http://www.groups.psychology.org.au/paig/.

Canada

Canadian Psychological Association: Adult Development and Aging. http://www.cpa.ca/aboutcpa/cpasections/adultdevelopmentandaging/.

China

Division of Aging Psychology, Gerontological Society of China (no webpage available).

Europe

European Federation of Psychologists' Associations: Geropsychology Information. http://geropsychology.efpa.eu/introduction/.

Netherlands

Netherlands Institute of Psychologists (NIP), Elderly Psychology Section. http://www.psynip.nl/sectoren-en-secties/sector-gezondheidszorg/ouderenpsychologie.html.

New Zealand

New Zealand Psychologists of Older Persons (NZPOPs). http://nzpops.co.nz/.

Sweden

Swedish Psychological Association, Geropsychologists Association. http://www.psykolog forbundet.se/Yrkesforeningar/Geropsykologer/.

UK

British Psychological Society (BPS), Division of Clinical Psychology. http://dcp.bps.org.uk/.
    Faculty of Psychologists of Older People (FPOP, a faculty of the Division of Clinical Psychology, BPS). http://www.psige.org/info/about+psige

USA

American Psychological Association, Society of Clinical Geropsychology (Division 12/II): http://www.geropsychology.org/.

Adult Development and Aging (Division 20). http://www.apadivisions.org/division-20/.

APA Office on Aging. http://www.apa.org/pi/aging/.

Council of Professional Geropsychology Training Programs (CoPGTP). http://www.copgtp.org/.

GeroCentral. http://gerocentral.org/.

Psychologists in Long Term Care (PLTC). http://www.pltcweb.org/index.php.

Websites

Age Platform Europe—Towards an Age-Friendly EU. http://www.age-platform.org/.

Australian Longitudinal Study on Aging. http://www.flinders.edu.au/sabs/fcas/alsa/.

Australian Longitudinal Study of Women's Health. http://www.alswh.org.au.

Dynamic Analyses to Optimize Aging (DYNOPTA) study. http://dynopta.anu.edu.au/.

GeroCentral. http://gerocentral.org/.

Gerontological Society of America: http://www.geron.org.

International Association of Gerontology and Geriatrics (IAGG): http://www.iagg.info.

International Centenarian Consortium. https://www.publichealth.uga.edu/geron/research/intl-centenarian-study.

International Centenarian Consortium. https://www.publichealth.uga.edu/geron/research/intl-centenarian-study.

International Federation on Aging. http://www.ifa-fiv.org.

International Psychogeriatric Association (IPA). http://www.ipa-online.net.

Survey of Health, Aging and Retirement in Europe. http://www.share-project.org/.

Sydney Blue Mountains Eye Study. http://www.cvr.org.au/bmes.htm.

United Nations Department of Economic and Social Affairs—Aging Social Policy and Development Division. http://undesadspd.org/Aging.aspx.

United Nations Principles for Older Persons (A/RES/46/91). http://www.un.org/Docs/asp/ws.asp?m=A/RES/46/91.

US Department of Health and Human Services—National Institute on Aging. http://www.nia.nih.gov/.

US Health and Retirement Study (HRS). http://hrsonline.isr.umich.edu/.

World Health Organization Study on Global Aging and Adult Health (SAGE). http://www.who.int/healthinfo/systems/sage/en.

References

Anstey, K. J., Burns, R. A., Birrell, C. L., Steel, D., Kiely, K. M., et al. (2010). 'Estimates of Probable Dementia Prevalence from Population-based Surveys Compared with Dementia Prevalence Estimates Based on Meta-analyses'. *BMC Neurology* 10(62). doi:10.1186/1471-2377-10-62.

Anstey, K. J., Byles, J. E., Luszcz, M. A., Mitchell, P., Steel, D., et al. (2010). 'Cohort Profile: The Dynamic Analyses to Optimize Aging (DYNOPTA) Project'. *International Journal of Epidemiology* 39(1): 44–51. doi:10.1093/Ije/Dyn276.

Antonucci, T. C. (1985). 'Personal Characteristics, Social Support, and Social Behavior'. In E. Shanas and R. H. Binstock (eds), *Handbook of Aging and the Social Sciences* (pp. 94–128). New York: Academic Press.

Astell, A. J., Ellis, M. P., Bernardi, L., Alm, N., Dye, R., et al. (2010). 'Using a Touch Screen Computer to Support Relationships between People with Dementia and Caregivers'. *Interacting with Computers* 22: 267–275.

Baltes, P. B., Mayer, K. U., Helmchen, H., and Steinhagen-Thiessen, E. (1993). 'The Berlin Aging Study (BASE): Overview and Design'. *Aging & Society* 13(4): 483–515. doi:10.1017/S0144686X00001343.

Beck, A. T., Rush, A. J., Shaw, B. F., and Emery, G. (1979). *Cognitive Therapy of Depression*. New York: Guilford Press.

Brandtstädter, J. and Rothermund, K. (2002). 'The Life-course Dynamics of Goal Pursuit and Goal Adjustment: A Two-process Framework'. *Developmental Review* 22(1): 117–150. doi:http://dx.doi.org/10.1006/drev.2001.0539.

Brown, W. J., Bryson, L., Byles, J. E., Dobson, A. J., Lee, C., et al. (1998). 'Women's Health Australia: Recruitment for a National Longitudinal Cohort Study'. *Women and Health* 28(1): 23–40.

Brown, W. J., Dobson, A. J., Bryson, L., and Byles, J. E. (1999). 'Women's Health Australia: On the Progress of the Main Cohort Studies'. *Journal of Women's Health and Gender-based Medicine* 8(5): 681–688.

Byrne, G. J. A. and Pachana, N. A. (2011). 'Development and Validation of a Short Form of the Geriatric Anxiety Inventory—the GAI-SF'. *International Psychogeriatrics* 23(1): 125–131.

Carstensen, L. L. and Mikels, J. A. (2005). 'At the Intersection of Emotion and Cognition: Aging and the Positivity Effect'. *Current Directions in Psychological Science* 14: 117–121.

Charles, S. T. and Carstensen, L. L. (2010). 'Social and Emotional Aging'. *Annual Review of Psychology* 61: 383–409. doi:10.1146/annurev.psych.093008.100448.

Cherubini, A., Del Signore, S., Ouslander, J., Semla, T., and Michel, J.-P. (2010). 'Fighting against Age Discrimination in Clinical Trials'. *Journal of the American Geriatrics Society* 58(9): 1791–1796.

Coopmans, C., Graham, C., and Hamzah, H. (2012). 'The Lab, the Clinic, and the Image: Working on Translational Research in Singapore's Eye Care Realm'. *Science, Technology, and Society* 17(1): 57–77.

Diehl, M., Willis, S. L., and Schaie, K. W. (1995). 'Everyday Problem Solving in Older Adults: Observational Assessment and Cognitive Correlates'. *Psychology and Aging* 10: 478.

Fernández-Ballesteros, R. (2007). *Geropsychology: European Perspectives for an Aging World*. Göttingen, Germany: Hogrefe and Huber.

Fung, H. H., Isaacowitz, D. M., Lu, A. Y., Wadlinger, H. A., Gooren, D., et al. (2008). 'Age-related Positivity Enhancement is not Universal: Older Hong Kong Chinese Look away from Positive Stimuli'. *Psychology and Aging* 23: 440–446.

Gonçalves, D. C., Guedes, J., Foneca, A. M., Cabral Pinto, F., Martin, I., et al. (2011). 'Attitudes, Knowledge and Interest: Preparing University Students to Work in an Aging World'. *International Psychogeriatrics* 23(2): 315–321.

Graham, N., Gray, J., Jacobsson, L., Kingma, M., Kuhne, N., et al. (2003). 'Reducing Stigma and Discrimination against Older People with Mental Disorders: A Technical Consensus Statement'. *International Journal of Geriatric Psychiatry* 18(8): 670–678. doi:10.1002/gps.876.

Graham, P. L., Ryan, L. M., and Luszcz, M. A. (2011). 'Joint Modelling of Survival and Cognitive Decline in the Australian Longitudinal Study of Aging'. *Journal of the Royal Statistical Society: Series C (Applied Statistics)* 60: 221–238. doi:10.1111/j.1467-9876.2010.00737.x

Guo, Z., Levy, B. R., Hinton, W. L., Witzman, P. F., and Levkoff, S. E. (2000). 'The Power of Labels: Recruiting Dementia-affected Chinese American Elders and their Caregivers'. In S. E. Levkoff, T. R. Prohaska, P. F. Weitzman, and M. G. Ory (eds), *Recruitment and Retention in Minority Populations: Lessons Learned in Conducting Research on Health Promotion and Minority Aging* (pp. 103–112). New York: Springer.

Heijke, L. (2004). 'The European Masters Programme in Gerontology'. *European Journal of Aging* 1: 106–108.

Heisel, M. J. and Flett, G. L. (2006). 'The Development and Initial Validation of the Geriatric Suicide Ideation Scale'. *American Journal of Geriatric Psychiatry* 14(9): 742–751.

Helmes, E. and Gee, S. (2003). 'Attitudes of Australian Therapists toward Older Clients: Educational and Training Imperatives'. *Educational Gerontology* 29(8): 657–670.

Hepple, J. and Sutton, L. (eds) (2004). *Cognitive Analytic Therapy and Later Life*. Hove and New York: Brunner Routledge.

Hinrichsen, G. A. (1997). 'Interpersonal Psychotherapy for Depressed Older Adults'. *Journal of Geriatric Psychiatry* 30: 239–257.

Hinton, L., Franz, C., and Friend, J. (2004). 'Pathways to Dementia Diagnosis: Evidence for Cross-ethnic Differences'. *Alzheimer Disease and Associated Disorders* 18: 134–144.

Hinton, L., Guo, Z., Hillygus, J., and Levkoff, S. (2000). 'Working with Culture: A Qualitative Analysis of Barriers to the Recruitment of Chinese–American Family Caregivers for Dementia Research'. *Journal of Cross-cultural Gerontology* 15: 119–137.

Hong, T., Mitchell, P., Rochtchina, E., Fong, C., Chia, E. M., et al. (2013). 'Long-term Changes in Visual Acuity in an Older Population over a 15-year Period: The Blue Mountains Eye Study'. *Ophthalmology* 120(10): 2091–2099.

Huang, A. R., Larente, N., and Morais, J. A. (2011). 'Moving towards the Age-friendly Hospital: A Paradigm Shift for the Hospital-based Care of the Elderly'. *Canadian Geriatrics Journal* 14(4): 100–103.

Karel, M. J., Knight, B. G., Duffy, M., Hinrichsen, G. A., and Zeiss, A. M. (2010). 'Attitude, Knowledge, and Skill Competencies for Practice in Professional Geropsychology: Implications for Training and Building a Geropsychology Workforce'. *Training and Education in Professional Psychology* 4(2): 75–84.

Kazantzis, N., Pachana, N. A., and Secker, D. L. (2003). 'Cognitive-behavioral Therapy for Older Adults: Practical Guidelines for the Use of Homework Assignments'. *Cognitive and Behavioral Practice* 10: 324–332.

Kitayama, S. and Karasawa, M. (1995). 'Self: A Cultural Psychological Perspective'. *Japanese Journal of Experimental Social Psychology* 35: 133–163.

Kneebone, I. I. (1996). 'Teaching about Aging: The New Challenge for Australian Clinical Psychology'. *Australian Psychologist* 31(2): 124–126. doi:10.1080/00050069608260191.

Knight, B. G. and Poon, C. Y. M. (2008). 'Contextual Adult Life Span Theory for Adapting Psychotherapy with Older Adults'. *Journal of Rational-emotive and Cognitive Behavior Therapy* 26: 232–249.

Knight, B. G., Karel, M. J., Hinrichsen, G. A., Qualls, S. H., and Duffy, M. (2009). 'Pikes Peak Model for Training in Professional Geropsychology'. *American Psychologist* 64(3): 205–214.

Kroenke, K., Spitzer, R. L., Williams, J. B. W., Monahan, P. O., and Löwe, B. (2007). 'Anxiety Disorders in Primary Care: Prevalence, Impairment, Comorbidity, and Detection'. *Annals of Internal Medicine* 146: 317–325.

Laidlaw, K., McAlpine, S. (2008). 'Cognitive Behaviour Therapy: How is it Different with Older People?' *Journal of Rational-emotive and Cognitive-behaviour Therapy* 26(4): 250–262.

Laidlaw, K. and Pachana, N. A. (2009). 'Aging, Mental Health, and Demographic Change'. *Professional Psychology: Research and Practice* 40(6): 601–608.

Liu, D., Hinton, L., Tran, C., Hinton, D., and Barker, J. C. (2008). 'Reexamining the Relationships among Dementia, Stigma, and Aging in Immigrant Chinese and Vietnamese Family Caregivers'. *Journal of Cross-cultural Gerontology* 23(3): 283–299.

Liu, Y., While, A. E., Norman, I. J., and Ye, W. (2012). 'Health Professionals' Attitudes toward Older People and Older Patients: A Systematic Review'. *Journal of Interprofessional Care* 26(5): 397–409.

Low, L. F., Anstey, K. J., Lackersteen, S. M., Camit, M., Harrison, F., et al. (2011). 'Recognition, Attitudes and Causal Beliefs Regarding Dementia in Italian, Greek and Chinese Australians'. *Dementia and Geriatric Cognitive Disorders*, Special Issue: *Dementia: The Asia-Pacific Perspectives* 30: 499–508.

Luoma, J. B., Hayes, C. S., and Walser, R. D. (2007). '*Learning ACT: An Acceptance and Commitment Therapy Skills-training Manual for Therapists*'. Oakland, CA: New Harbinger.

Luszcz, M., Giles, L., Eckermann, S., Edwards, P., Browne-Yung, K., et al. (2007). *The Australian Longitudinal Study of Aging: 15 years of Aging in South Australia*: Adelaide: South Australian Department of Families and Communities.

McLaughlin, D., Adams, J., Almeida, O., Brown, W., Byles, J., et al. (2011). 'Are the National Guidelines for Health Behaviour Appropriate for Older Australians? Evidence from the Men, Women and Aging Project' (invited paper). *Australasian Journal on Aging* 30(S2): 13–16.

McLaughlin, D., Vagenas, D., Pachana, N. A., Begum, N., and Dobson, A. (2010). 'Gender Differences in Social Network Size and Satisfaction in Adults in their 70s'. *Journal of Health Psychology* 15(5): 671–679.

Martiny, C., Cardoso de Oliveira, A., Nardi, A. E., and Pachana, N. A. (2011). 'Translation and Cross-cultural Adaptation of the Brazilian Version of the Geriatric Anxiety Inventory (GAI)'. *Revista de Psiquiatria Clínica* 38(1): 8–12.

Pachana, N. A., Byrne, G. J., Siddle, H., Koloski, N., Harley. E., et al. (2007). 'Development and Validation of the Geriatric Anxiety Inventory'. *International Psychogeriatrics* 19: 103–114.

Pachana, N. A., Emery, E., Konnert, C. A., Woodhead, E., and Edelstein, B. (2010). 'Geropsychology Content in Clinical Training Programs: A Comparison of Australian, Canadian and U.S. Data'. *International Psychogeriatrics* 22(6): 909–918.

Pachana, N. A. and Byrne, G. J. A. (2012). 'The Geriatric Anxiety Inventory: International Use and Future Directions'. *Australian Psychologist* 47(1): 33–38.

Pachana, N. A., Helmes, E., and Koder, D. (2006). 'Guidelines for the Provision of Psychological Services for Older Adults'. *Australian Psychologist* 41: 15–22.

Peterson, C. B. and Prasad, N. R. (2012). 'Assessing Assistive Technology Outcomes with Dementia'. *Gerontotechnology* 11(2): 259. doi:http://dx.doi.org/10.4017/gt.2012.11.02.414.00.

Pinquart, M. (2007). 'Main Trends in Geropsychology in Europe: Research, Training and Practice'. In R. Fernández-Ballesteros (ed.), *GeroPsychology: European Perspectives for an Aging World* (pp. 15–30). Göttingen, Germany: Hogrefe and Huber.

Poon, L., Jazwinski, M., Green, R. C., Woodard, J. L., Martin, P., et al. (2007). 'Methodological Considerations in Studying Centenarians: Lessons Learned from the Georgia Centenarian Studies'. *Annual Review of Gerontology and Geriatrics* 27(1): 231–264.

Prince, M., Bryce, R., Albanese, E., Wimo, A., Ribeiro, W., et al. C. P. (2013). 'The Global Prevalence of Dementia: A Systematic Review and Meta-analysis'. *Alzheimer's Dementia* 9(1): 63–72.

Quammen, D. (2012). '*Spillover: Animal Infections and the Next Human Pandemic*'. New York: W. W. Norton.

Schaie, K. W. (1993). 'The Seattle Longitudinal Studies of Adult Intelligence'. *Current Directions in Psychological Science* 2(6): 171–175. doi:10.1111/1467-8721.ep10769721.

Sousa, V. D. and Rojjanasrirat, W. (2011). 'Translation, Adaptation, and Validation of Instruments or Scales for Use in Cross-cultural Health Care Research: A Clear and User-friendly Guideline'. *Journal of Evaluation in Clinical Practice* 17(2): 268–274.

Stanley, M. A., Diefenbach, G. J., and Hopko, D. R., Novy, D., Kunik, M. E., et al. (2003). 'The Nature of Generalized Anxiety in Older Primary Care Patients: Preliminary Findings'. *Journal of Psychopathology and Behavioral Assessment* 25: 273–280.

Steverink, N., Lindenberg, S., and Ormel, J. (1998). 'Towards Understanding Successful Aging: Patterned Change in Resources and Goals'. *Aging & Society* 18: 441–467.

Steverink, N., Lindenberg, S., and Slaets, J. P. J. (2005). 'How to Understand and Improve Older People's Self-management of Wellbeing'. *European Journal of Aging* 2: 235–244.

Steverink, N. and Lindenberg, S. (2006). 'Which Social Needs are Important for Subjective Wellbeing? What Happens to them with Aging?' *Psychology and Aging* 21: 281–290.

Sun, F., Ong, R., and Burnette, D. (2012). 'The Influence of Ethnicity and Culture on Dementia Caregiving: A Review of Empirical Studies on Chinese Americans'. *American Journal of Alzheimer's Disease and Other Dementias* 27: 13–22.

Van de Vijver, F. J. R. and Hambleton, R. K. (1996). 'Translating Tests: Some Practical Guidelines'. *European Psychologist* 1(2): 89–99.

Verhaak, P. F. M., Bensing, J. M., and Brink-Muinen, A. (2007). 'GP Mental Health Care in 10 European Countries: Patients' Demands and GPs' Responses'. *The European Journal of Psychiatry* 21(1): 7–16.

Wetherell, J. L., Afari, N., Ayers, C. R., Stoddard, J. A., Ruberg, J., et al. (2011). 'Acceptance and Commitment Therapy for Generalized Anxiety Disorder in Older Adults: A Preliminary Report'. *Behavior Therapy* 42(1): 127–134.

Willis, S. L. and Marsiske, M. (1993). *Manual for the Everyday Problems Test.* University Park, PA: The Pennsylvania State University.

Woodhead, E. L., Emery, E. E., Pachana, N. A., Scott, T. L., Konnert, C. A., et al. (2013). 'Graduate Students' Geropsychology Training Opportunities and Perceived Competence in Working with Older Adults'. *Professional Psychology: Research and Practice* 44: 355–362.

World Health Organization (WHO). (2007). *Global Age-friendly Cities: A Guide.* Geneva, Switzerland: World Health Organization.

Yeo, G. and Gallagher-Thompson, D. (2006). *Ethnicity and the Dementias* (2nd edn). New York: Routledge.

Index